SURGERY

Official Publication SOCIETY OF UNIVERSITY SURGEONS

SOCIETY FOR VASCULAR SURGERY

Volume 67
January—June, 1970

St. Louis
The C. V. Mosby Company

VOLUME 67

Printed in the United States of America

1040

Volume 67 *Number* 1

SURGERY

CONTENTS, JANUARY, 1970

SOCIETY FOR VASCULAR SURGERY

page 1 **Presidential address: Standards in vascular surgery.** C. Rollins Hanlon, Chicago, Ill.

5 **An aortoiliac endarterectomy case series followed 10 years or more.** David B. Pilcher, M.D., Wiley F. Barker, M.D., and Jack A. Cannon, M.D., Los Angeles, Calif.

18 **Arterial autografts.** Ronald J. Stoney, M.D., and Edwin J. Wylie, M.D., San Francisco, Calif.

26 **Femorofemoral and axillofemoral grafts—compromise or preference.** Victor Parsonnet, M.D., Joseph Alpert, M.D., and Donald K. Brief, M.D., Newark, N. J.

34 **Aneurysmectomy in the aged?** Caldwell B. Esselstyn, Jr., M.D., Alfred W. Humphries, M.D., Jess R. Young, M.D., Edward G. Beven, M.D., and Victor G. deWolfe, M.D., Cleveland, Ohio

40 **Arteriovenous fistula: Results of management of congenital and acquired forms, blood flow measurements, and observations on proximal arterial degeneration.** Yoshio Sako, M.D., and Richard L. Varco, M.D., Minneapolis, Minn.

continued on page 9

Vol. 67, No. 1, January, 1970. The Journal of Surgery is published monthly by The C. V. Mosby Company, 3207 Washington Blvd., St. Louis, Mo. 63103. *Annual subscription rates*—United States and its possessions: institutional (multiple-reader) subscriptions,* $24.00; personal (regular) subscriptions,† $19.00; student, intern, and resident physician subscriptions,† $11.40. Canada and Mexico: institutional (multiple-reader) subscriptions, $26.50; personal (regular) subscriptions, $21.50; student, intern, and resident physician subscriptions, $13.90. Other countries: institutional (multiple-reader) subscriptions, $27.50; personal (regular) subscriptions, $22.50; student, intern, and resident physician subscriptions, $14.90. Single copies, $3.50 postpaid.

*Institutional (multiple-reader) subscriptions are available to both public and private libraries, schools, hospitals, and clinics; city, county, state, province, and national government bureaus and departments; and all commercial and private institutions and organizations.

†Personal (regular) subscriptions and all student-rate subscriptions must be in the names of, and billed to, individuals.

Second class postage paid at St. Louis, Mo. Printed in the U. S. A.

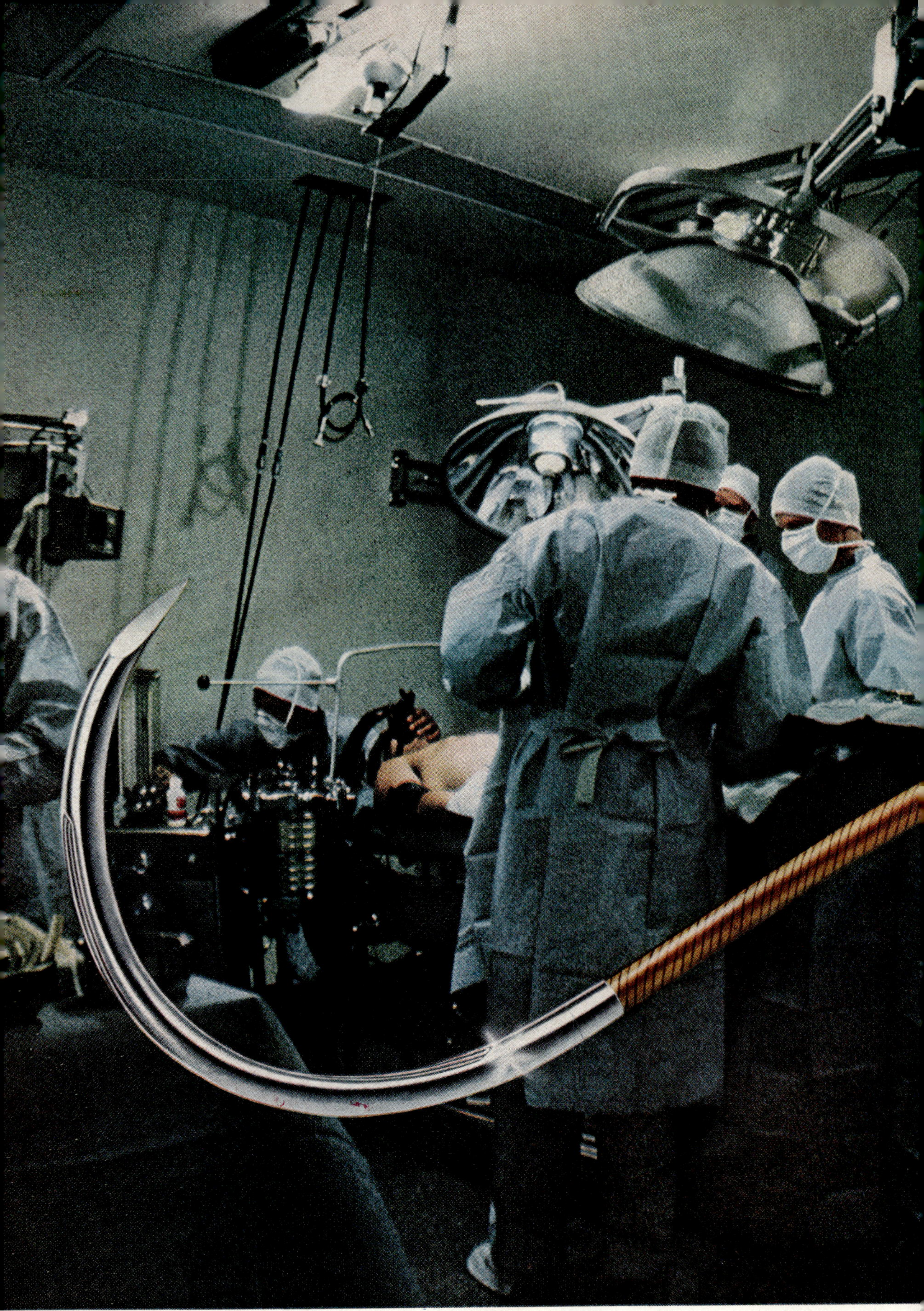

page 62 **Management of ischemia of the hand and fingers.** W. Andrew Dale, M.D., and Malcolm R. Lewis, M.D., Nashville, Tenn.

80 **Natural history of carotid bifurcation atheroma.** Hushang Javid, M.D., Ph.D., William E. Ostermiller, Jr., M.D., John W. Hengesh, M.D., William S. Dye, M.D., James A. Hunter, M.D., Hassan Najafi, M.D., and Ormand C. Julian, M.D., Ph.D., Chicago, Ill.

87 **Effect of CO_2 and systemic hypertension on downstream cerebral arterial pressure during carotid endarterectomy.** W. K. Ehrenfeld, M.D., F. N. Hamilton, M.D., C. P. Larson, Jr., M.D., R. F. Hickey, M.D., and J. W. Severinghaus, M.D., San Francisco, Calif.

97 **Conclusions from a controlled trial of the prophylactic portacaval shunt.** Allan D. Callow, M.D., Robert H. Resnik, M.D., Thomas C. Chalmers, M.D., Albert M. Ishihara, M.D., Arthur J. Garceau, M.D., and Edward T. O'Hara, M.D., Boston, Mass.

104 **Selective portal decompression.** Richard C. Britton, M.D., Arthur B. Voorhees, Jr., M.D., and John B. Price, Jr., M.D., New York, N. Y.

114 **Directional flow detection for localizing venous valvular incompetency.** Roland Folse, M.D., and Raymond H. Alexander, M.D., Seattle, Wash.

122 **Human heart transplantation for cardiomyopathy.** Donald R. Kahn, M.D., Ernest W. Reynolds, Jr., M.D., Joseph A. Walton, Jr., M.D., Marvin M. Kirsh, M.D., Sathaporn Vathayanon, M.D., and Herbert Sloan, M.D., Ann Arbor, Mich.

129 **Operation for cardiac complications following myocardial infarction.** George Schimert, M.D., Thomas Z. Lajos, M.D., Ivan L. Bunnell, M.D., David G. Greene, M.D., Herman L. Falsetti, M.D., Andrew A. Gage, M.D., David C. Dean, M.D., and Michael Bernstein, Buffalo, N. Y.

141 **Late results of heart valve replacement.** J. Richard Rees, M.D., Brian G. Miscall, M.D., George R. Holswade, M.D., Aldo Castaneda, M.D., and C. Walton Lillehei, Ph.D., M.D., New York, N. Y., and Minneapolis, Minn.

continued on page 13

page 151 **Aortic ball valve design based upon healing and hydraulic considerations.** Lester R. Sauvage, M.D., Robert F. Viggers, M.S., Knute Berger, M.D., Stephen J. Wood, M.D., Alloju M. Rao, M.D., Mark Dedomenico, M.D., Michael A. Ross, M.D., and Stephen B. Robel, M.S., Seattle, Wash.

168 **Direct coronary arterial revascularization for segmental occlusive disease.** E. D. Mundth, M.D., J. W. Harthorne, M.D., M. J. Buckley, M.D., R. E. Dinsmore, M.D., and W. G. Austen, M.D., Boston, Mass.

182 **Reappraisal of adjuncts to avoid ischemia in the treatment of thoracic aortic aneurysms.** E. Stanley Crawford, M.D., James M. Fenstermacher M.D., William Richardson, M.D., and Frank Sandiford, M.D., Houston, Texas

197 **The case for early closure of a patent ductus arteriosus.** James W. Kilman, M.D., Howard D. Sirak, M.D., H. William Clatworthy, Jr., M.D., Josepha Craenen, M.D., and Don M. Hosier, M.D., Columbus, Ohio

204 **Cardiovascular effects of glucagon following cardiac surgery.** Cecil C. Vaughn, M.D., Homer R. Warner, M.D., Ph.D., and Russell M. Nelson, M.D., Ph.D., Salt Lake City, Utah

212 **Arterial embolectomy: A 20 year experience with 163 cases.** Jesse E. Thompson, M.D., Luis Sigler, M.D., P. S. Raut, M.D., Dale J. Austin, M.D., and R. Don Patman, M.D., Dallas, Texas

221 **Microneurosurgical arterial reconstruction.** M. Gazi Yasargil, M.D., Hugo A. Krayenbuhl, M.D., and Julius H. Jacobson, II, M.D., New York, N. Y.

234 **Modification in the technique for femoropopliteal saphenous vein bypass autografts.** Robert R. Linton, M.D., and W. Laurence Wilde, M.D., Boston, Mass.

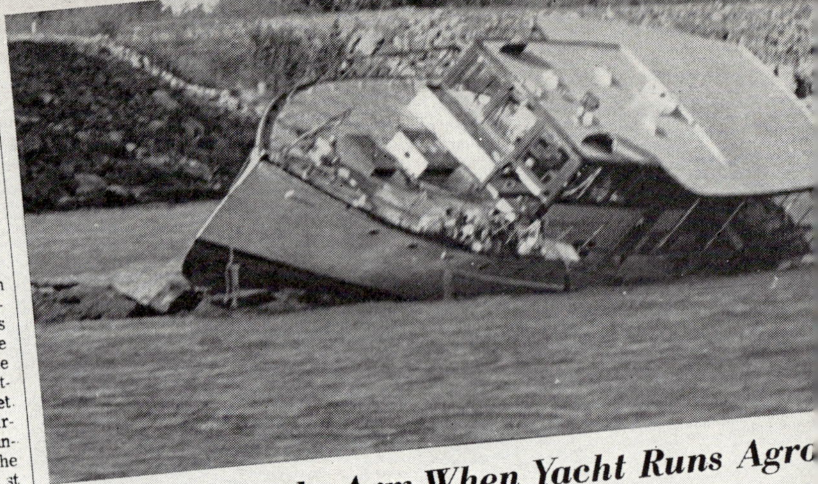

Owner Breaks Arm When Yacht Runs Agro

Schuyler, Oct. 31. Harry Waters of Covesville incurred a fractured arm ... large rock ... tially capsized. The fire d... had to rescue Waters by ... Damage to the yacht is es...

Hasn't the skipper had enough excitement for one day?

For the patient who has been through an accident, the worry and anxiety following the mishap may actually heighten the perception of pain. This is why there's a classic ¼ grain *sedative* dose of phenobarbital in Phenaphen with Codeine—to take the nervous "edge" off, so the rest of the formula can control the pain more effectively.

A. H. Robins Company, Richmond, Va. 23220 A-H-ROBINS

Phenaphen® with Codein

Phenaphen with Codeine Nos. 2, 3, or 4 contains: Phenobarbital (¼ gr.), mg. (warning: may be habit forming); Aspirin (2½ gr.), 162.0 mg.; Phena (3 gr.), 194.0 mg.; Hyoscyamine sulfate, 0.031 mg.; Codeine Phosphat gr. (No. 2), ½ gr. (No. 3), or 1 gr. (No. 4) (warning: may be habit form

The compound analgesic that calms instead of caffeina

Indications: Phenaphen with Codeine provides relief in severer grad pain, on low codeine dosage, with minimal possibility of side effects. Its frequently makes unnecessary the use of addicting narcotics. **Contrain tions:** Hypersensitivity to any of the components. **Precautions:** As wit phenacetin-containing products excessive or prolonged use shoul avoided. **Side effects:** Side effects are uncommon, although nausea, stipation and drowsiness may occur. **Dosage:** Phenaphen No. 2 and No 1 or 2 capsules every 3 to 4 hours as needed; Phenaphen No. 4—1 ca every 3 to 4 hours as needed. For further details see product literature

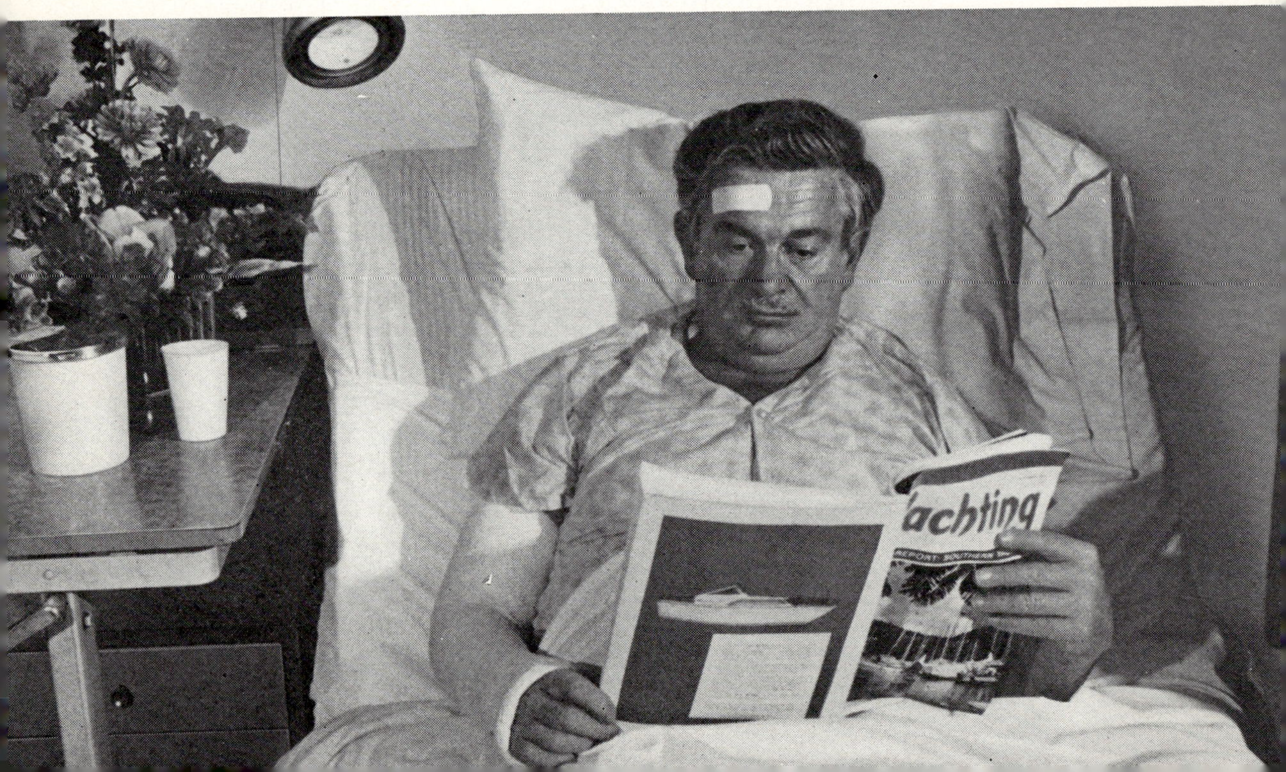

Volume 67 *Number* 2

SURGERY

CONTENTS, FEBRUARY 1970

CLINICAL SURGERY

page 249 **Use of diuretic agents during oliguria after renal transplantation.** Carl F. Anderson, M.D., Hugh O. O'Kane, M.B., F.R.C.S., Roy G. Shorter, M.D., William J. Johnson, M.D., and George A. Hallenbeck, M.D., Rochester, Minn.

255 **Biliary manometry: Its role in clinical surgery.** Clarence J. Schein, M. D., and Thomas C. Beneventano, M.D., New York, N. Y.

261 **Accelerated rejection of skin grafts in recipients sensitized with extracted human histocompatibility antigens.** H. F. Seigler, N. F. Mendes, and R. S. Metzgar, Durham, N. C.

267 **The influence of thermal burns on gastric acid secretion.** James A. O'Neill, Jr., M.D., Fort Sam Houston, Texas, and Columbus, Ohio

272 **Long-term sequelae of common femoral vein ligation in the treatment of thromboembolic disease.** Robert A. Nabatoff, M.D., Lester Blum, M.D., and Arthur S. W. Touroff, M.D., New York, N. Y.

277 **The duplicated saphenous vein in femoropopliteal bypass grafting.** H. Gaylis, Ch.M., F.R.C.S.(Eng.), Johannesburg, South Africa

279 **Venous presure monitor.** Bernard Vidne, M.D., Shaul Levinson, Eng., and Morris J. Levy, M.D., Tel Aviv, Israel

281 **Carcinoma of thyroglossal duct cyst: Case reports and review of the literature.** Belur S. Bhagavan, M.B., B.S., D. R. Govinda Rao, M.B., B.S., and Tobias Weinberg, M.D., Baltimore, Md.

continued on page 9

Vol. 67, No. 2, February, 1970. The Journal of Surgery is published monthly by The C. V. Mosby Company, 3207 Washington Blvd., St. Louis, Mo. 63103. *Annual subscription rates*—United States and its possessions: institutional (multiple-reader) subscriptions,* $24.00; personal (regular) subscriptions,† $19.00; student, intern, and resident physician subscriptions,† $11.40. Canada and Mexico: institutional (multiple-reader) subscriptions, $26.50; personal (regular) subscriptions, $21.50; student, intern, and resident physician subscriptions, $13.90. Other countries: institutional (multiple-reader) subscriptions, $27.50; personal (regular) subscriptions, $22.50; student, intern, and resident physician subscriptions, $14.90. Single copies, $3.50 postpaid.

*Institutional (multiple-reader) subscriptions are available to both public and private libraries, schools, hospitals, and clinics; city, county, state, province, and national government bureaus and departments; and all commercial and private institutions and organizations.

†Personal (regular) subscriptions and all student-rate subscriptions must be in the names of, and billed to, individuals.

Second class postage paid at St. Louis, Mo. Printed in the U. S. A.

CONTENTS *continued*

page 293 **Management of malignant esophagobronchial fistula.** G. B. Ong and K. H. Kwong, Hong Kong

302 **Elevation of serum creatine kinase following amputation of the leg.** Raymond Penneys, M.D., and J. Henry Wilkinson, D.Sc., Ph.D., Philadelphia, Pa.

INVESTIGATIVE SURGERY

306 **A technique for prolonged splenic perfusion.** Robert Atkins, M.B., M.R.A.C.P., Cleve Trimble, M.D., and Ben Eiseman, M.D., Denver, Colo.

313 **Arteriography as an adjunct to the diagnosis of splenic injury.** Stanton G. Polin, Commander, MC, USNR, William D. Walklett, Commander, MC, USN, and Osbey L. Sayler, Lieutenant Commander, MC, USN, Portsmouth, Va.

319 **The effect of liver disease on the need for venous decompression during the anhepatic phase of canine orthotopic liver transplantation.** Reginaldo S. Picache, M.D., Brij M. Kapur, F.R.C.S., and Thomas E. Starzl, Ph.D., M.D., Denver, Colo.

322 **Effects of phytohemagglutinin on humoral antibody response, delayed hypersensitivity and homograft rejection.** Keiji Ono, M.D., Herve Blanchard, M.D., Noboru Kashiwagi, M.D., Roderick, N. M. MacSween, M.B., Henry N. Claman, M.D., and Thomas E. Starzl, M.D., Denver, Colo.

328 **Demonstration of humoral immunity against aortic leaflet heterografts.** George E. Pierce, M.D., Ingegerd E. Hellström, M.D., Hitoshi Mohri, M.D., D.M.Sc., Dennis D. Reichenbach, M.D., and K. Alvin Merendino, M.D., Ph.D., Seattle, Wash.

332 **Autoradiographic studies on the incorporation of foreign DNA and RNA into kidney allografts.** Gottfried Lemperle, Wolf Michaelis, and Ulf Wieczorek, Freiburg, Germany.

338 **The role of vasoconstriction in the suppression of hemorrhage from arteries. I. The completely severed artery.** Stephen L. Wangensteen, M.D., Stephen F. Kiechel, B. A., Robert M. Ludewig, M.D., and James J. Madden, Jr., M.D., Charlottesville, Va.

342 **Blood viscosity in the normal man.** Martin S. Litwin, M.D., Kenneth Chapman, B.S., and J. Bruce Stoliar, M.D., New Orleans, La.

346 **Cholesterol excretion following chronic ileal bypass.** Marshall Z. Schwartz, B.S., Richard B. Moore, M.D., and Henry Buchwald, M.D., Ph.D., Minneapolis, Minn.

continued on page 13

CONTENTS *continued*

page 350 **Potassium vasoactivity—a biphasic effect.** Scott J. Boley, M.D., Neil Kamil, B.S., Bernard S. Levowitz, M.D., William F. Treiber, Jr., B.S., Girhar P. Agrawal, M.D., and Frank J. Veith, M.D., New York, N. Y.

PEDIATRIC SURGERY

355 **A new type subcutaneous arteriovenous fistula for chronic hemodialysis in children.** Juan J. Pérez Alvarez, M.D., F.A.C.C., Rubén Vargas-Rosendo, M.D., Ramón Gutiérrez-Bosque, M.D., Manuel Matos Díaz-Ordaz, M.D., and David Santos-Atherton, Mexico City, Mexico.

360 **Gastric secretion in the canine fetus following maternal stimulation: Experimental studies on placental transfer of insulin, histamine, and gastrin.** Walter L. Bruckner, M.D., Harold D. Snow, D.V.M., and Eric W. Fonkalsrud, M.D., Los Angeles, Calif.

364 **Jejunoileocolic intubation and plication for intestinal obstruction caused by massive adhesions in infancy.** Thomas C. Moore, M.D., Arnold M. Salzberg, M.D., and E. Armistead Talman, M.D., Richmond, Va., and Los Angeles, Calif.

RECENT ADVANCES IN SURGERY

369 **Infections: Prophylaxis and management—a symposium.** William A. Altemeier, M.D., Benjamin A. Barnes, M.D., Edwin J. Pulaski, M.D., William R. Sandusky, M.D., John F. Burke, M.D., and George H. A. Clowes, Jr., M.D., Cincinnati, Ohio

383 **Amniocentesis: A new approach to some old problems in obstetrics.** Henry A. Thiede, M.D., Jackson, Miss.

SURGICAL TECHNIQUES

389 **Ligation, stripping, and excision of varicose veins.** W. Andrew Dale, M.D., Nashville, Tenn.

394 **A method of salvaging the bifurcated saphenous vein for use in femoral-to-popliteal bypass grafts.** W. Jason McDaniel, M.D., and George Johnson, Jr., M.D., Chapel Hill, N. C.

EDITORIAL

396 **Cancer immunology and the surgeon.** Donald L. Morton, M.D., Bethesda, Md.

399 **The crisis in surgical training.** Basil R. Meyerowitz, M.B., B.Ch., M.D., F.R.C.S., San Mateo County and Palo Alto, Calif.

401 **Letters to the Editors**

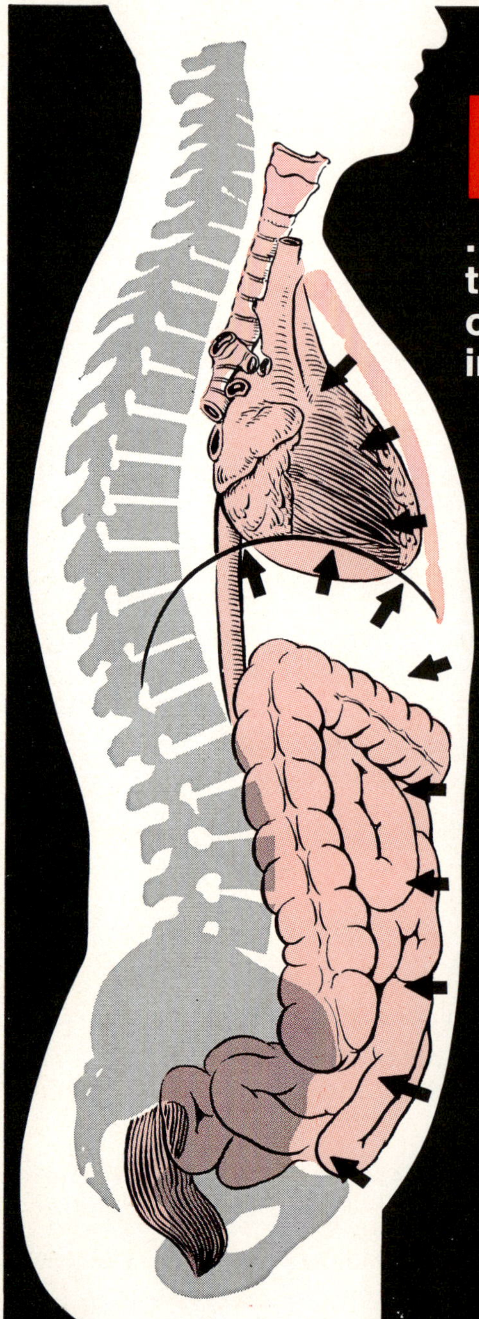

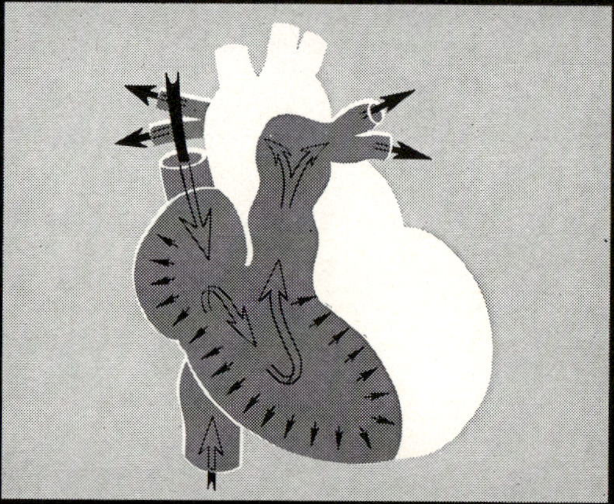

Volume 67 *Number* 3

SURGERY

CONTENTS, MARCH 1970

CLINICAL SURGERY

page 403 **A study of the danger of antibiotic preparation of the bowel for surgery.** E. Thurston Thieme, M.D., and George Fink, M.D., Ann Arbor, Mich.

409 **Transabdominal ligation-resection of the esophagus in cases of bleeding esophageal varices.** I. Boerema, M.D., F.A.C.S.(Hon.), P. J. Klopper, M.D., and A. A. Holscher, M.D., Amsterdam, The Netherlands

414 **An intensive care bed for the initial diagnosis and treatment of severely ill patients.** J. Donald Hill, M.D., and Elmer E. Johnson, San Francisco, Calif.

418 **Primary malignant tumors of the gallbladder: Report of 43 cases.** Manikchand Rukmanappa Tanga, M.B., B.S., M.S., and J. Burke Ewing, M.D., C.M., F.R.C.S.(C), F.R.C.S.(E), F.A.C.S., F.I.C.S., Ottawa, Ontario, Canada

427 **Polyarteritis nodosa of the gallbladder.** Paterno Remigio, M.D., and Edward Zaino, M.D., New York, N. Y.

432 **The clinical use of intraperitoneal cephalothin.** Martin H. McMullan, M.D., and William O. Barnett, M.D., Jackson, Miss.

continued on page 9

Vol. 67, No. 3, March, 1970. The Journal of Surgery is published monthly by The C. V. Mosby Company, 3207 Washington Blvd., St. Louis, Mo. 63103. *Annual subscription rates*—United States and its possessions: institutional (multiple-reader) subscriptions,* $24.00; personal (regular) subscriptions,† $19.00; student, intern, and resident physician subscriptions,† $11.40. Canada and Mexico: institutional (multiple-reader) subscriptions, $26.50; personal (regular) subscriptions, $21.50; student, intern, and resident physician subscriptions, $13.90. Other countries: institutional (multiple-reader) subscriptions, $27.50; personal (regular) subscriptions, $22.50; student, intern, and resident physician subscriptions, $14.90. Single copies, $3.50 postpaid.

*Institutional (multiple-reader) subscriptions are available to both public and private libraries, schools, hospitals, and clinics; city, county, state, province, and national government bureaus and departments; and all commercial and private institutions and organizations.

†Personal (regular) subscriptions and all student-rate subscriptions must be in the names of, and billed to, individuals.

Second class postage paid at St. Louis, Mo. Printed in the U. S. A.

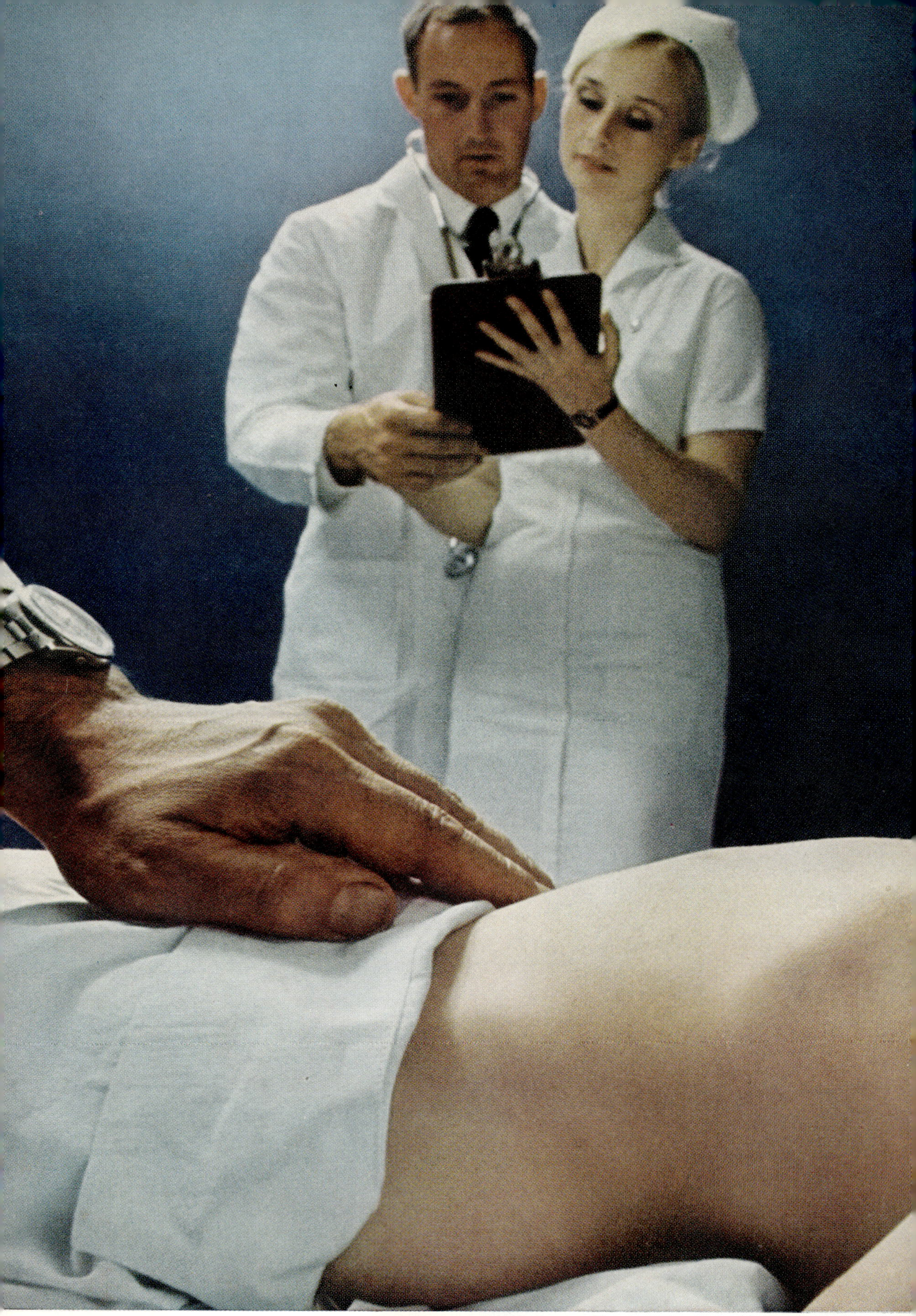

CONTENTS *continued*

page 437 **Mortality factors in major limb amputations for vascular disease: A study of 176 procedures.** Norman Rosenberg, M.D., Edgardo Adiarte, M.D., Leslie J. Bujdoso, M.D., and Klaus D. Backwinkel, New Brunswick, N. J.

442 **Contralateral arterial grafts.** León Bialostozky, M.D., Raúl Legaspi, M.D., Lorenzo Rish F., M.D., and Federico Morales M., M.D., Mexico City, Mexico

452 **Arteriovenous vein graft for chronic hemodialysis: A preliminary report.** Mark Mozes, M.D., F.A.C.S., Baruch J. Hurwich, M.D., Raphael Adar, M.D., Heskel E. Eliahou, B.A., M.D., and Harry Bogokowsky, M.D., Tel Aviv, Israel

455 **Long-term arterial catheterization for repeated blood sampling.** Roger V. Moseley, M.D., and Donald B. Doty, M.D., Washington, D. C.

457 **Catheter embolism.** Emil Blair, M.D., Robert Hunziker, M.D., and Martin E. Flanagan, M.D., Burlington, Vt.

INVESTIGATIVE SURGERY

462 **Studies on the effect of 2-phenyl-2-(2-pyridyl)-thioacetamide (antigastrin) on canine gastric acid secretion.** Jaime Isaza, M.D., Kyoji Sugawara, M.D., Richard Tiongco, M.D., and M. Michael Eisenberg, M.D., Gainsville, Fla., and Minneapolis, Minn.

468 **Esophageal mucosal regeneration following experimental prosthetic replacement of the esophagus.** Bernard J. Leininger, M.D., Howard Peacock, and William E. Neville, M.D., Hines, Ill.

474 **Cholesterol absorption following reversal of the upper and lower halves of the small intestine.** Roger L. Gebhard, M.D., and Henry Buchwald, M.D., Ph.D., Minneapolis, Minn.

478 **Intestinal strangulation in rats monocontaminated with *Sphaerophorus necrophorus*.** C. E. Yale, M.D., D.Sc., and V. R. Dowell, Jr., Ph.D., Cincinnati, Ohio

484 **Lymphatic absorption of intraperitoneal endotoxin in the dog.** Ronald Daniele, M.D., Hira Singh, M.D., Hubert E. Appert, Ph.D., Frederick W. Pairent, Ph.D., and John M. Howard, M.D., Philadelphia, Pa.

488 **Studies on the functional and biochemical changes during kidney preservation.** Paul A. Lotke, M.D., and Sorell L. Schwartz, Ph.D., Bethesda, Md.

continued on page 13

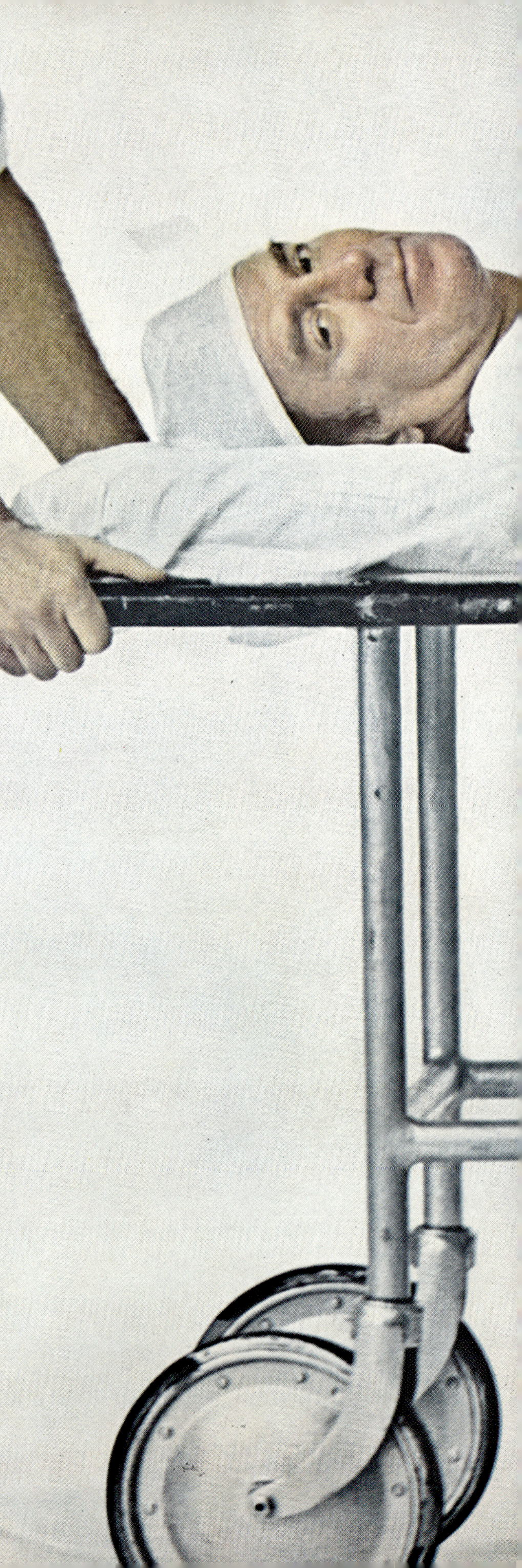

Before prescribing, please consult complete product information, a summary of which follows:

Indications: Tension and anxiety states; somatic complaints which are concomitants of emotional factors; psychoneurotic states manifested by tension, anxiety, apprehension, fatigue, depressive symptoms or agitation; acute agitation, tremor, delirium tremens and hallucinosis due to acute alcohol withdrawal; adjunctively in: skeletal muscle spasm due to reflex spasm to local pathology; spasticity caused by upper motor neuron disorders; athetosis; stiff-man syndrome. Injectable form may also be used adjunctively in status epilepticus and severe recurrent seizures; anxiety prior to gastroscopy, esophagoscopy, and surgical procedures; cardioversion (I.V.); tetanus.

Contraindications: Use of Injectable in infants and tablets in children under 6 months of age; known hypersensitivity to drug; acute narrow angle glaucoma; may be used in patients with open angle glaucoma who are receiving appropriate therapy.

Warnings: *Tablets:* Not of value in treatment of psychotic patients, and should not be employed in lieu of appropriate treatment. As with most CNS-acting drugs, caution patients against hazardous occupations requiring complete mental alertness (*e.g.*, operating machinery, driving). When using Oral adjunctively in convulsive disorders, possibility of increase in frequency and/or severity of grand mal seizures may require increase in dosage of standard anticonvulsant medication; abrupt withdrawal in such cases may also be associated with temporary increase in frequency and/or severity of seizures. Advise patients against simultaneous ingestion of alcohol and other CNS depressants. Withdrawal symptoms (similar to those with barbiturates and alcohol) have occurred following abrupt discontinuance. Keep addiction-prone individuals (such as drug addicts or alcoholics) under careful surveillance because of their predisposition to habituation and dependence. Use of any drug in pregnancy, lactation or in women of childbearing age requires that potential benefit be weighed against possible hazard. *Injectable:* I.V. should be injected slowly, directly into vein, taking at least one minute for each 5 mg (1 cc) given; do not mix or dilute with other solutions or drugs; do not add to I.V. fluids; not recommended as the sole treatment for psychotic or severely depressed patients; should not be administered to patients in shock, coma, or in acute alcoholic intoxication with depression of vital signs.

Precautions: If combined with other psychotropics or anticonvulsants, carefully consider individual pharmacologic effects—particularly with known compounds which may potentiate action of Valium (diazepam) such as phenothiazines, narcotics, barbiturates, MAO inhibitors and other antidepressants. Employ usual precautions in the severely depressed or in those with latent depression; suicidal tendencies may be present and protective measures necessary. Observe usual precautions in impaired renal or hepatic function. Limit oral dosage to smallest effective amount in elderly and debilitated to preclude ataxia or oversedation (initially 2 to 2½ mg once or twice daily, increasing gradually as needed or tolerated). *Injectable:* Not recommended for bronchoscopy, laryngoscopy, obstetrical use, or in diagnostic procedures other than gastroscopy and esophagoscopy; laryngospasm is a possible reaction during gastroscopy and necessary countermeasures should be available; drug has produced hypotension, respiratory depression or muscular weakness particularly when used with narcotics, barbiturates or alcohol; since effect with narcotics may be additive, appropriate reduction in narcotic dosage is possible; use lower doses (2 to 5 mg) for elderly and debilitated; safety and efficacy in children under 12 not established.

Adverse Reactions: Side effects most commonly reported: drowsiness, fatigue and ataxia. Infrequently encountered: confusion, constipation, depression, diplopia, dysarthria, headache, hypotension, incontinence, jaundice, changes in libido, nausea, changes in salivation, skin rash, slurred speech, tremor, urinary retention, vertigo and blurred vision; with Injectable, hiccups, hypoactivity, phlebitis at injection site, syncope and urticaria. Paradoxical reactions such as acute hyperexcited states, anxiety, hallucinations, increased muscle spasticity, insomnia, rage, sleep disturbances and stimulation have been reported; should these occur, use of the drug should be discontinued. Because of isolated reports of neutropenia and jaundice, periodic blood counts and liver function tests are advisable during long-term therapy. Minor changes in EEG patterns (low-voltage fast activity) observed during and after therapy and are of no known significance.

ROCHE
Roche
LABORATORIES
Division of Hoffmann-La Roche Inc.
Nutley, New Jersey 07110

CONTENTS *continued*

page 493 **Use of saphenous vein homografts for arterial reconstruction: A preliminary report.** David A. Tice, M.D., and Ernesto Santoni, M.D., New York, N. Y.

499 **The progressive nature of pulmonary contusion.** Robert L. Fulton, M.D., and Edward T. Peter, M.D., Ph.D., Albuquerque, N. Mex.

507 **Responses of skeletal muscle pH to injury: A new technique for determination of tissue viability.** Irwin R. Berman, M.D., Michael D. Lemieux, M.D., and Gene V. Aaby, Lieutenant Colonel, MC, USA, Washington, D. C., and New York, N. Y.

PEDIATRIC SURGERY

513 **Massive megacolon and megaileum in childhood due to tuberculous stenosis of the ascending colon.** James J. Patton, M.D., and Thomas C. Moore, M.D., Torrance and Los Angeles, Calif.

519 **Intrauterine midgut strangulation in a gastroschisis defect.** Jay L. Grosfeld, M.D., and H. William Clatworthy, Jr., M.D., Columbus, Ohio

522 **Improved operative technique for gastric duplication.** John J. White, M.D., C.M., and W. W. Morgan, M.D., Baltimore, Md.

527 **Surgery for duodenal and gastric ulcer in infancy and childhood.** J. E. Strode, M.D., and John F. Balfour, M.D., Honolulu, Hawaii

536 **Repair of intracardiac defects after previous constriction (banding) of the pulmonary artery.** Jaroslav Stark, M.U.Dr., C.Sc., Michael Tynan, M.B., B.S., Eoin Aberdeen, F.R.C.S., D.C.H., David J. Waterston, M.B.E., F.R.C.S., Richard E. Bonham-Carter, M.A., F.R.C.P., Gerald R. Graham, B.A., M.D., and Jane Somerville, M.R.C.P., London, England

RECENT ADVANCES IN SURGERY

548 **Localization of gastrointestinal hemorrhage by selective angiography.** Charles F. Frey, M.D., Stewart R. Reuter, M.D., and Joseph J. Bookstein, M.D., Ann Arbor, Mich.

SURGICAL TECHNIQUES

556 **Hemostasis during liver resections.** William R. Clark, Jr., M.D., and Robert P. Leather, M.D., Albany, N. Y.

EDITORIAL

558 **A Pacific-wide view of surgery.** Sir Douglas Robb, Auckland, New Zealand

Made

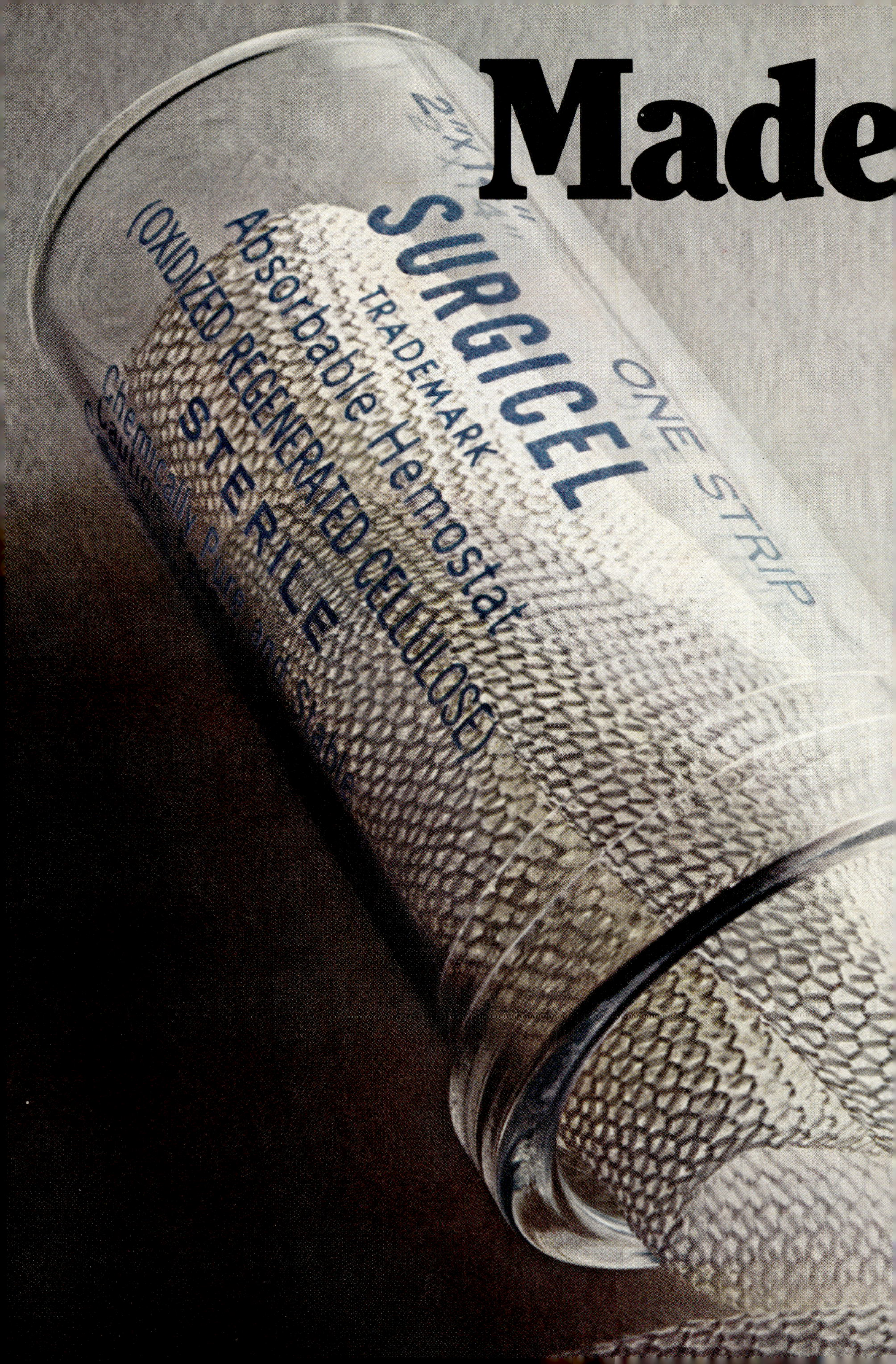

SURGICEL
TRADEMARK
ONE STRIP
Absorbable Hemostat
(OXIDIZED REGENERATED CELLULOSE)
STERILE
Chemically Pure and Stable

Volume 67 *Number* 4

SURGERY

CONTENTS, APRIL 1970

CLINICAL SURGERY

page 561 **"Fiberduodenoscopy"—early diagnosis of cancer of the papilla of Vater.** Itaru Oi, M.D., Tadayoshi Takemoto, M.D., and Komei Nakayama, M.D., Tokyo, Japan

566 **Removal of residual biliary tract calculi without reoperation.** R. Mazzariello, M.D., Buenos Aires, Argentina

574 **Local gastric hypothermia in gastroduodenal hemorrhage.** Boris A. Petrov and Nicolay N. Korenev, Moscow, Union of Soviet Socialist Republics

577 **Hemodynamic alterations and results of treatment in patients with gram-negative septic shock.** George J. Motsay, M.D., Ronald H. Dietzman, M.D., Robert A. Ersek, M.D., and Richard C. Lillehei, M.D., Ph.D., Minneapolis, Minn.

584 **Use of heparinized priming blood after whole-body perfusion.** Sait Tarhan, M.D., Emerson A. Moffitt, M.D., Richard O. Lundborg, M.D., and Robert B. Wallace, M.D., Rochester, Minn.

590 **Intensive care unit flow sheet.** Scott G. Kramer, Captain, MC, USN, and Charles S. Lipson, Commander, MC, USNR, Chelsea, Mass.

593 **Improved surgical technique for arteriovenous shunt implantation: Experiences with an all-Silastic shunt.** Luis A. Aravena, Leo Kaplan, M.D., Arthur Golding, M.D., Arthur Gordon, M.D., and Morton H. Maxwell, M.D., Los Angeles, Calif.

continued on page 9

Vol. 67, No. 4, April, 1970. The Journal of Surgery is published monthly by The C. V. Mosby Company, 3207 Washington Blvd., St. Louis, Mo. 63103. *Annual subscription rates*—United States and its possessions: institutional (multiple-reader) subscriptions,* $24.00; personal (regular) subscriptions,† $19.00; student, intern, and resident physician subscriptions,† $11.40. Canada and Mexico: institutional (multiple-reader) subscriptions, $26.50; personal (regular) subscriptions, $21.50; student, intern, and resident physician subscriptions, $13.90. Other countries: institutional (multiple-reader) subscriptions, $27.50; personal (regular) subscriptions, $22.50; student, intern, and resident physician subscriptions, $14.90. Single copies, $3.50 postpaid.

*Institutional (multiple-reader) subscriptions are available to both public and private libraries, schools, hospitals, and clinics; city, county, state, province, and national government bureaus and departments; and all commercial and private institutions and organizations.

†Personal (regular) subscriptions and all student-rate subscriptions must be in the names of, and billed to, individuals.

Second class postage paid at St. Louis, Mo. Printed in the U. S. A.

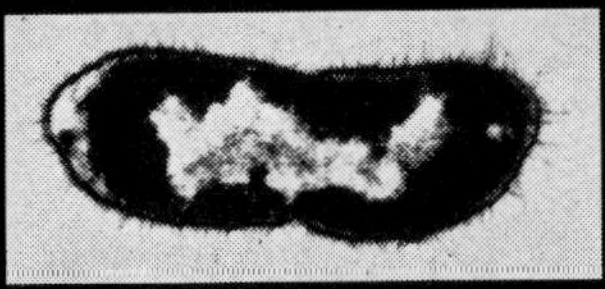

CONTENTS *continued*

page 601 **Scapulectomy: Indications and technique.** Tapas K. Das Gupta, M.D., Ph.D., Chicago, Ill.

607 **Spontaneous rupture of the esophagus.** Saul F. Salinas Izaguirre, M.D., James T. Haggerty, M.D., and Gerald Eckert, M.D., Rochester, N. Y.

614 **Thymoma arising from undescended cervical thymus.** C. E. Ridenhour, M.D., J. H. Henzel, M.D., M. S. DeWeese, M.D., and S. Earl Kerr, M.D., Columbia, Mo.

620 **A new operation for varicocele: Use of microvascular anastomosis.** Koichi Ishigami, M.D., Yoshiyuki Yoshida, M.D., Masao Hirooka, M.D., and Kikuo Mohri, M.D., Kyoto, Japan

624 **High systemic origin of the sole artery to the basal segments of the left lung: Findings, surgical treatment, and embryologic interpretation.** Eugene A. Hessel, II, M.D., Edward A. Boyden, Ph.D., Stanley J. Stamm, M.D., and Lester R. Sauvage, M.D., Seattle, Wash.

633 **Pulmonary resection for massive hemoptysis.** Antonio A. Garzon, M.D., Marcial Cerruti, M.D., Anatole Gourin, M.D., and Karl E. Karlson, M.D., Brooklyn, N. Y.

INVESTIGATIVE SURGERY

639 **Recurrent pulmonary emboli following inferior vena caval plication.** G. A. E. Coupland, M.B., F.R.A.C.S., and T. S. Reeve, M.B., F.A.C.S., F.R.A.C.S., Sydney, Australia

644 **Silver sulfadiazine and Sulfamylon Cream in the burned rat model: A comparative evaluation.** Donald P. Dressler, M.D., and William A. Skornik, M.S., Cambridge, Mass.

650 **Vasodepressor factor in declamp shock production.** Bolek Brant, M.D., Richard P. Armstrong, M.D., and R. Mark Vetto, M.D., D.Sc., Portland, Ore.

654 **The permanence of adequate incomplete vagotomy: A preliminary study in dogs.** Guy Legros, M.D., and Charles A. Griffith, M.D., Seattle, Wash.

658 **Circulating lymphocyte depletion: Effect on lymphoid tissue.** Jay C. Fish, M.D., Gerald Beathard, M.D., Harry E. Sarles, M.D., August R. Remmers, Jr., M.D., and Stephan E. Ritzmann, M.D., Galveston, Texas

667 **The immunologic response to intravascular skin allografts.** William J. Donawick, D.V.M., and Arthur E. Baue, M.D., Kennett Square and Philadelphia, Pa.

continued on page 13

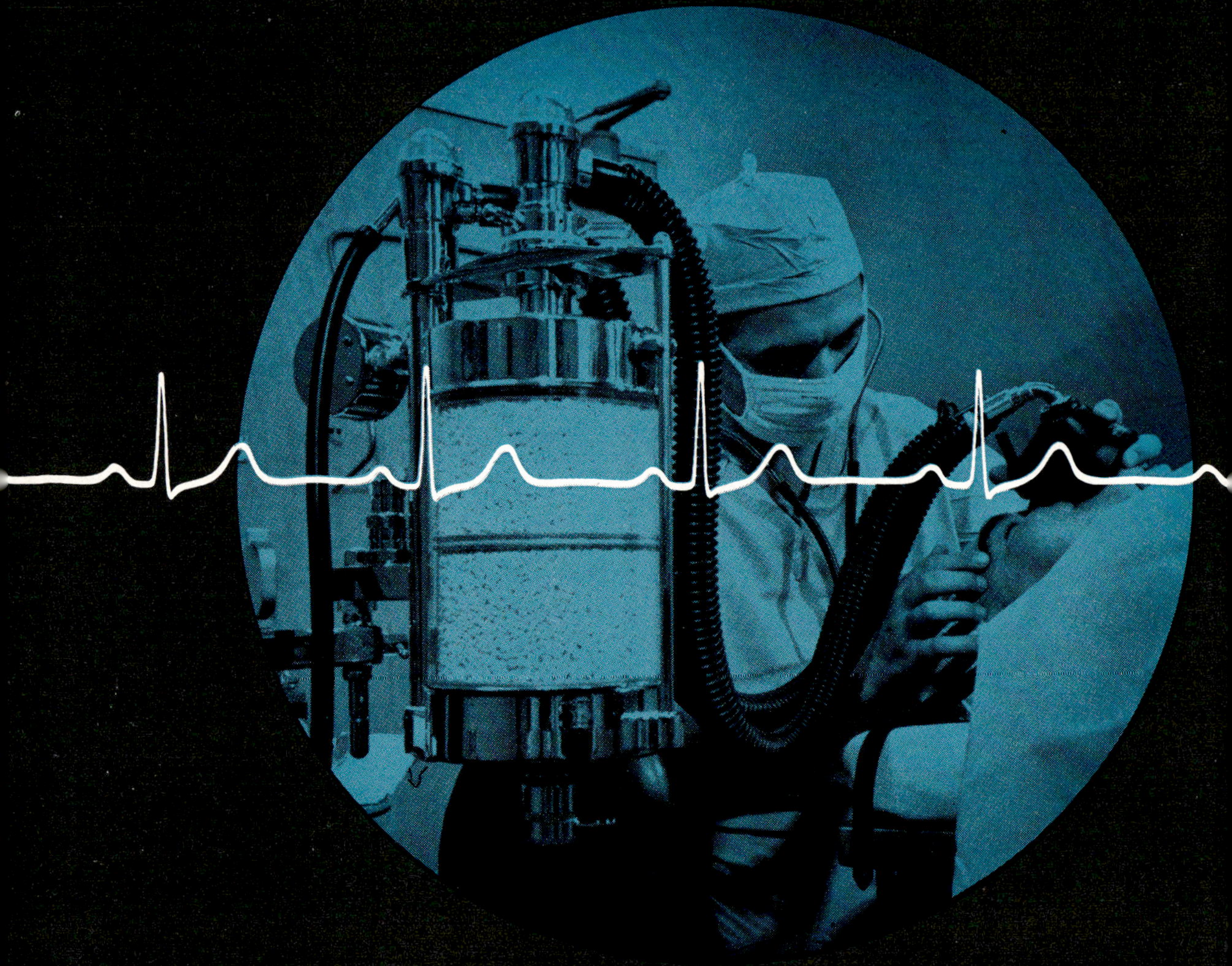

CONTENTS *continued*

page 672 **Experimental studies on the effect of dimethyl sulfoxide on pedicle flaps.** H. E. Koehnlein, M.D., and G. Lemperle, M.D., Freiburg, Germany

678 **Auxiliary homotransplantation of the porcine liver into the retroperitoneal space.** V. Novak, L. Hill, R. Rothwell-Jackson, A. Velasquez, R. Wright, B. Eiseman, Denver, Colo.

687 **Adaptation of functioning and bypassed segments of ileum during compensatory hypertrophy of the gut.** M. David Tilson, M.D., and Hastings K. Wright, M.D., New Haven, Conn.

694 **Vena cava catheter for asanguineous liver resection.** Federico Chávez-Peón, M.D., Eduardo Gonzalez, M.D., and Ronald A. Malt, M.D., Boston, Mass.

PEDIATRIC SURGERY

697 **Emergency separation of thoracopagus (twins conjoined at thorax) in the newborn period: Importance of careful preoperative cardiac evaluation.** James S. Simpson, M.D., W. T. Mustard, M.D., C. A. F. Moes, M.D., and T. Izukawa, M.D., Toronto, Ontario, Canada

703 **Torsion of the testis in the newborn infant.** Melvyn J. Michaelian, M.D., G. H. Mahour, M.D., M.S. (Surgery), and Paul W. Johnston, M.D., Los Angeles, Calif.

706 **Complete transposition of the great vessels: Surgical results of emergency Blalock-Hanlon operation in infants.** Rolando Zamora, M.D., James H. Moller, M.D., Russell V. Lucas, Jr., M.D., and Aldo R. Castaneda, M.D., Minneapolis, Minn.

RECENT ADVANCES IN SURGERY

711 **The current status of immunosuppressive therapy.** John A. Mannick, Boston, Mass.

SURGICAL TECHNIQUES

720 **Control of the hepatic parenchyma by direct compression: A new instrument.** Donald B. Doty, M.D., Heinz W. Kugler, and Roger V. Moseley, M.D., Washington, D. C.

EDITORIAL

725 **Experiments in delivery of surgical care.** B. Eiseman, M.D., M. Pomerantz, M.D., F. Merkel, M.D., and D. Cowen, M.D., Denver, Colo.

IN THE SURGICAL SETTING:

To help you cope with hospital bacterial infections...before they become life-threatening

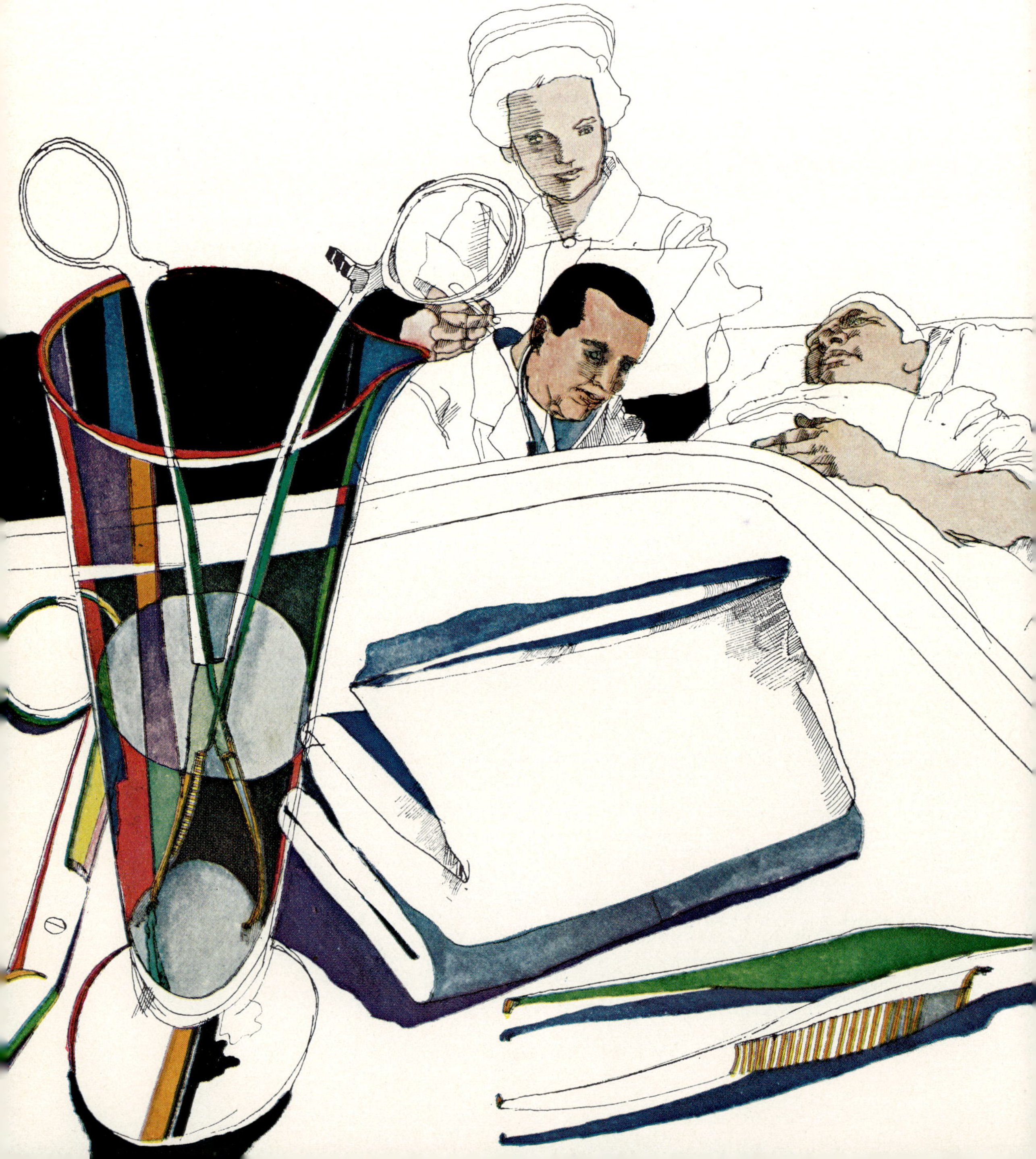

Volume 67 *Number* 5

SURGERY

CONTENTS, MAY 1970

CLINICAL SURGERY

page 727 **Perforated duodenal ulcer: Long-term follow-up.** George J. Nemanich, M.D., and Demetre M. Nicoloff, M.D., Ph.D., Minneapolis, Minn.

735 **Studies of the "gastroesophageal sphincter mechanism": The role of the phrenoesophageal membrane.** Cedric G. Bremner, M.Ch., F.R.C.S., Jerry F. Schlegel, B.S., and F. Henry Ellis, Jr., M.D., Ph.D., Rochester, Minn.

741 **The value of pneumoperitoneum in the diagnosis of hernia in the inguinal region.** Ored Arner, M.D., and Ingmar Fernström, M.D., Stockholm, Sweden

748 **Role of mammography with palpable breast lesions.** Ezri S. Sokol, M.D., Barry Walker, M.D., Jose J. Terz, M.D., and Walter Lawrence, Jr., M.D., Richmond, Va.

754 **Hemodynamic alterations in acute cardiac tamponade after penetrating injuries of the heart.** W. C. Shoemaker, M.D., J. S. Carey, M.D., S. T. Yao, M.D., P. A. Mohr, M.D., J. J. Amato, M.D., K. J. Printen, M.D., R. D. Corley, M.D., D. O. Monson, M.D., S. Youssef, M.D., and N. J. Shoemaker, R.N., New York, N. Y., and Chicago, Ill.

765 **Hypoxemia during the first twelve hours after battle injury.** Roger V. Moseley, M.D., and Donald B. Doty, M.D., Washington, D. C.

continued on page 9

Vol. 67, No. 5, May, 1970. The Journal of Surgery is published monthly by The C. V. Mosby Company, 3207 Washington Blvd., St. Louis, Mo. 63103. *Annual subscription rates*—United States and its possessions: institutional (multiple-reader) subscriptions,* $24.00; personal (regular) subscriptions,† $19.00; student, intern, and resident physician subscriptions,† $11.40. Canada and Mexico: institutional (multiple-reader) subscriptions, $26.50; personal (regular) subscriptions, $21.50; student, intern, and resident physician subscriptions, $13.90. Other countries: institutional (multiple-reader) subscriptions, $27.50; personal (regular) subscriptions, $22.50; student, intern, and resident physician subscriptions, $14.90. Single copies, $3.50 postpaid.

*Institutional (multiple-reader) subscriptions are available to both public and private libraries, schools, hospitals, and clinics; city, county, state, province, and national government bureaus and departments; and all commercial and private institutions and organizations.

†Personal (regular) subscriptions and all student-rate subscriptions must be in the names of, and billed to, individuals.

Second class postage paid at St. Louis, Mo. Printed in the U. S. A.

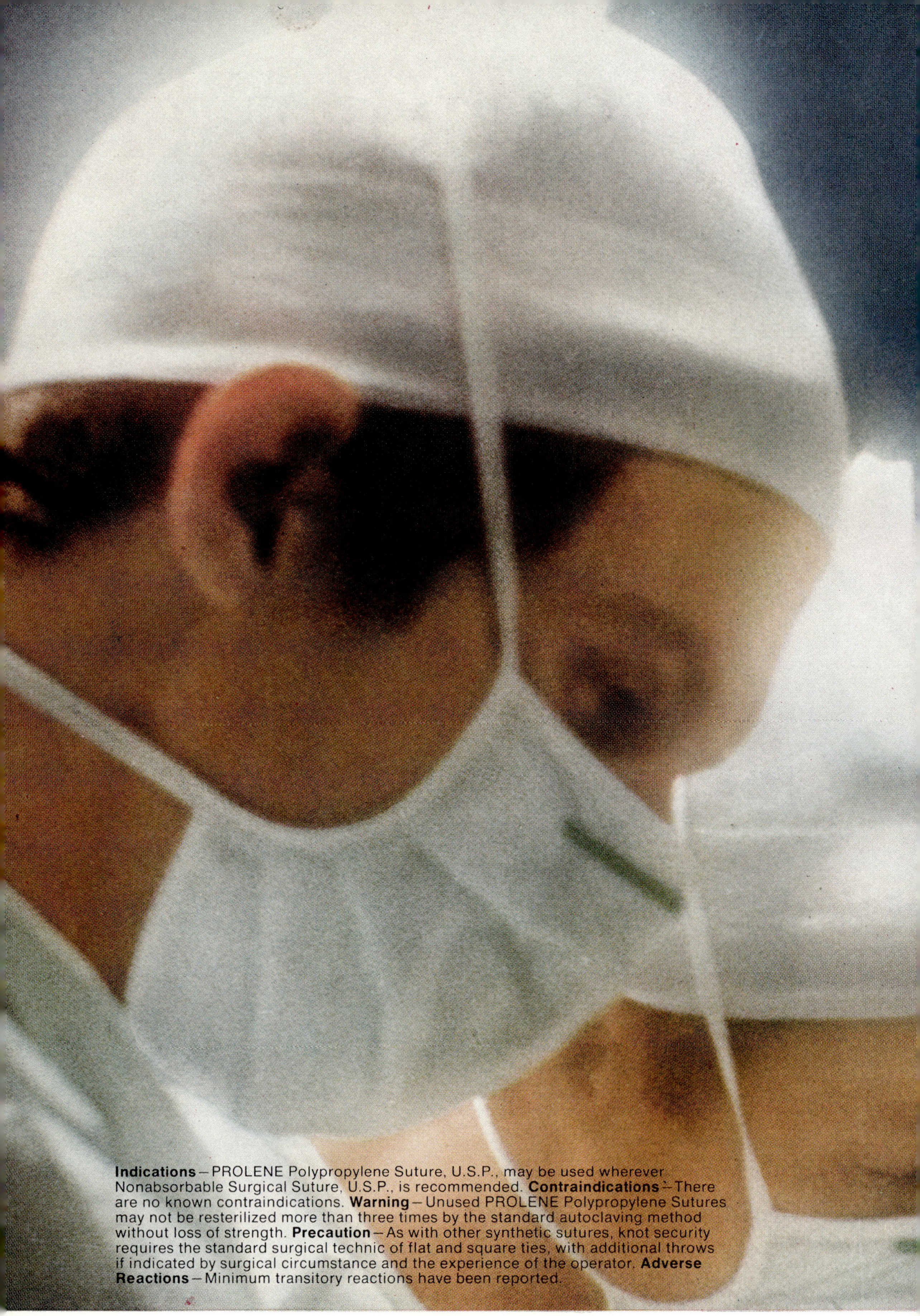

CONTENTS *continued*

page 773 **A simple and accurate manometer for monitoring central venous pressure.** Gerald Moss, Ph.D., M.D., Troy and Albany, N. Y.

775 **Extra-abdominal management of late aortofemoral graft thrombosis.** Lawrence H. Cohn, M.D., Wesley S. Moore, M.D., and Albert D. Hall, M.D., San Francisco, Calif.

780 **Metabolic changes in surgical delirium tremens.** E. Truman Mays, M.D., Herbert T. Ransdell, M.D., and Bob M. DeWeese, M.D., Louisville, Ky.

INVESTIGATIVE SURGERY

789 **Antibody localization in horse, rabbit, and goat antilymphocyte sera.** Noboru Kashiwagi, M.D., David Scherer, M.D., Courtney M. Townsend, M.D., Roberta Jacobs, M.A., Keiji Ono, M.D., Brij Kapur, M.D., and Thomas E. Starzl, M.D., Ph.D., Denver, Colo.

799 **Hemodynamics and blood gas exchange in allografted canine lungs. I. Immediate effects.** Kazuo Momma, M.D., Leonard M. Linde, M.D., Eric W. Fonkalsrud, M.D., Gary H. Stevens, M.D., Decio M. Rangel, M.D., and Yozo Yakeishi, M.D., Los Angeles, Calif.

807 **The value of dextrans in the treatment of experimental pancreatitis.** Philip W. Wright and Bernard Goodhead, Torrance and Los Angeles, Calif.

816 **Dissociation of the hyperglycemic and vascular effects of glucagon.** Sten Tibblin, M.D., Nils G. Kock, M.D., and Worthington G. Schenk, Jr., M.D., Buffalo, N. Y.

826 **Synthetic thromboresistant surfaces from sulfonated polyelectrolyte complexes.** Lita Nelsen, Robert A. Cross, Mary Ann Vogel, Vincent L. Gott, and A. Moniem Fadali, Lexington, Mass., and Baltimore, Md.

831 **The effect of epicardiectomy on the function and diastolic compliance of the normal canine left ventricle.** Hamner Hannah, III, M.D., Lee P. Enright, M.D., and Robert L. Reis, M.D., Bethesda, Md.

836 **Local irrigation with an antibiotic solution in the prevention of infection in vascular prostheses.** John W. D. DiGiglia, M.D., George L. Leonard, M.D., and John L. Ochsner, M.D., New Orleans, La.

continued on page 13

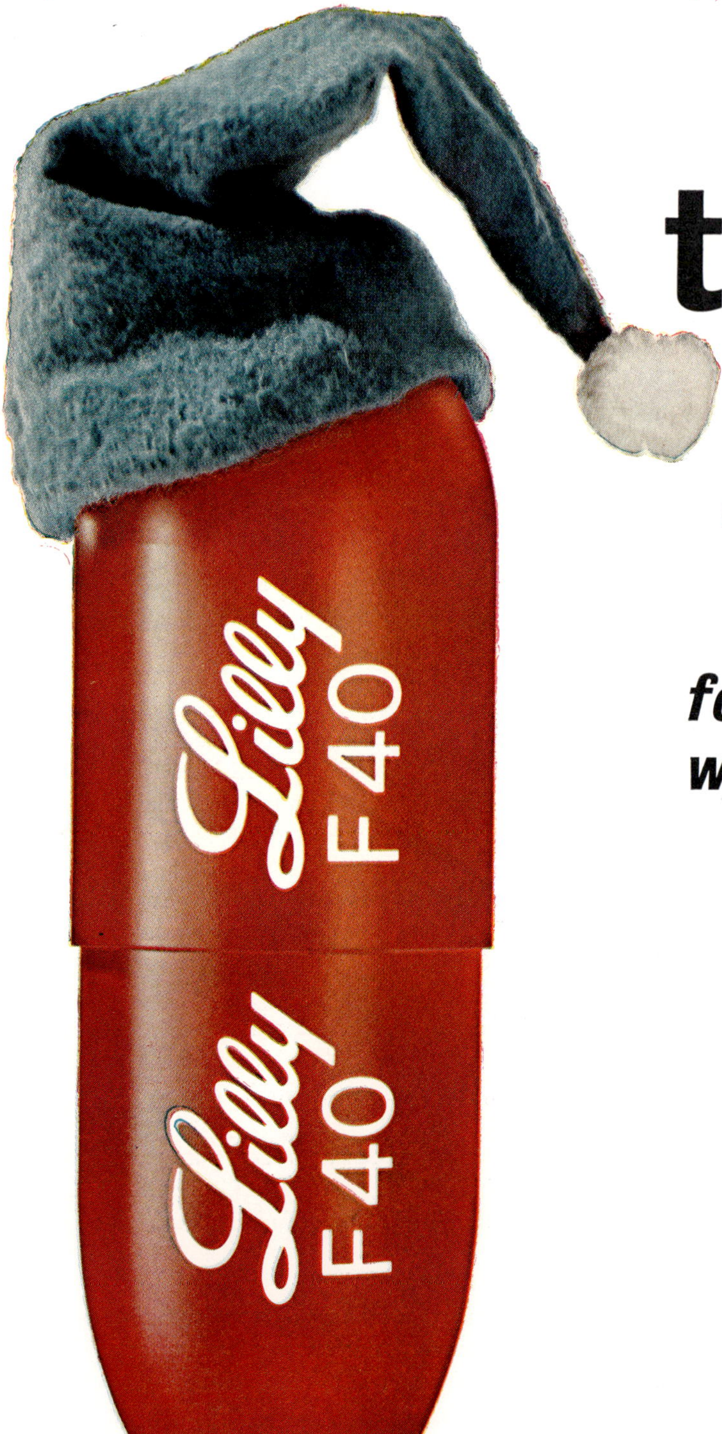

the night "cap"

for patients with insomnia

CONTENTS *continued*

PEDIATRIC SURGERY

page 841 **Appendicitis in the newborn infant.** John M. Parsons, M.D., Brian G. Miscall, M.D., and Charles K. McSherry, M.D., New York, N. Y.

844 **Traumatic pseudodiverticulum of the esophagus in the newborn infant.** Raymond G. Armstrong, Lieutenant Colonel, USAF (MC), Evan F. Lindberg, Lieutenant Colonel, USAF (MC), William Stanford, Lieutenant Colonel, USAF (MC), Robert M. Takamoto, Major, USAF (MC), Richard D. Wolfe, Lieutenant Colonel, USAF (MC), and James W. Dietz, Major, USAF (MC), Lackland Air Force Base, Texas

847 **Idiopathic edema of scrotum in young boys.** J. L. Nicholas, F.R.C.S., A. Morgan, F.R.C.S., and R. B. Zachary, F.R.C.S., Sheffield, England

851 **Total prosthetic transplantation of the inferior vena cava, with venous drainage restoration of the one remaining kidney on the graft, successfully performed on a child with Wilms' tumor.** Lorenzo Sarti, M.D., Milan, Italy

856 **Vascular obstruction of the superior renal infundibulum in children.** Peter J. Deckers, M.D., Elwin E. Fraley, M.D., David F. Paulson, M.D., and John C. Harbert, M.D., Bethesda, Md.

863 **External iliac artery occlusion in a newborn infant.** Felix Salerno, M.D., O. Dale Collins, M.D., and Daniel C. Redmond, M.D., Fort Hood, Texas

RECENT ADVANCES IN SURGERY

867 **Prevention of prosthetic cardiac valve detachment.** Noel H. Fishman, M.D., John C. Hutchinson, M.D., and Benson B. Roe, M.D., San Francisco, Calif.

SURGICAL TECHNIQUES

874 **Diagnostic peritoneal irrigation—a simple and reliable technique.** Joseph M. Civetta, Major, USAF (MC), M. J. Williams, Colonel, USAF (MC), and Robert E. Richie, Lieutenant Colonel, USAF (MC), Keesler Air Force Base, Miss.

EDITORIAL

878 **A fork in the road: The geographic full-time system.** Richard H. Egdahl, M.D., Boston, Mass.

881 **The retrievable error.** John R. Derrick, M.D., Galveston, Texas

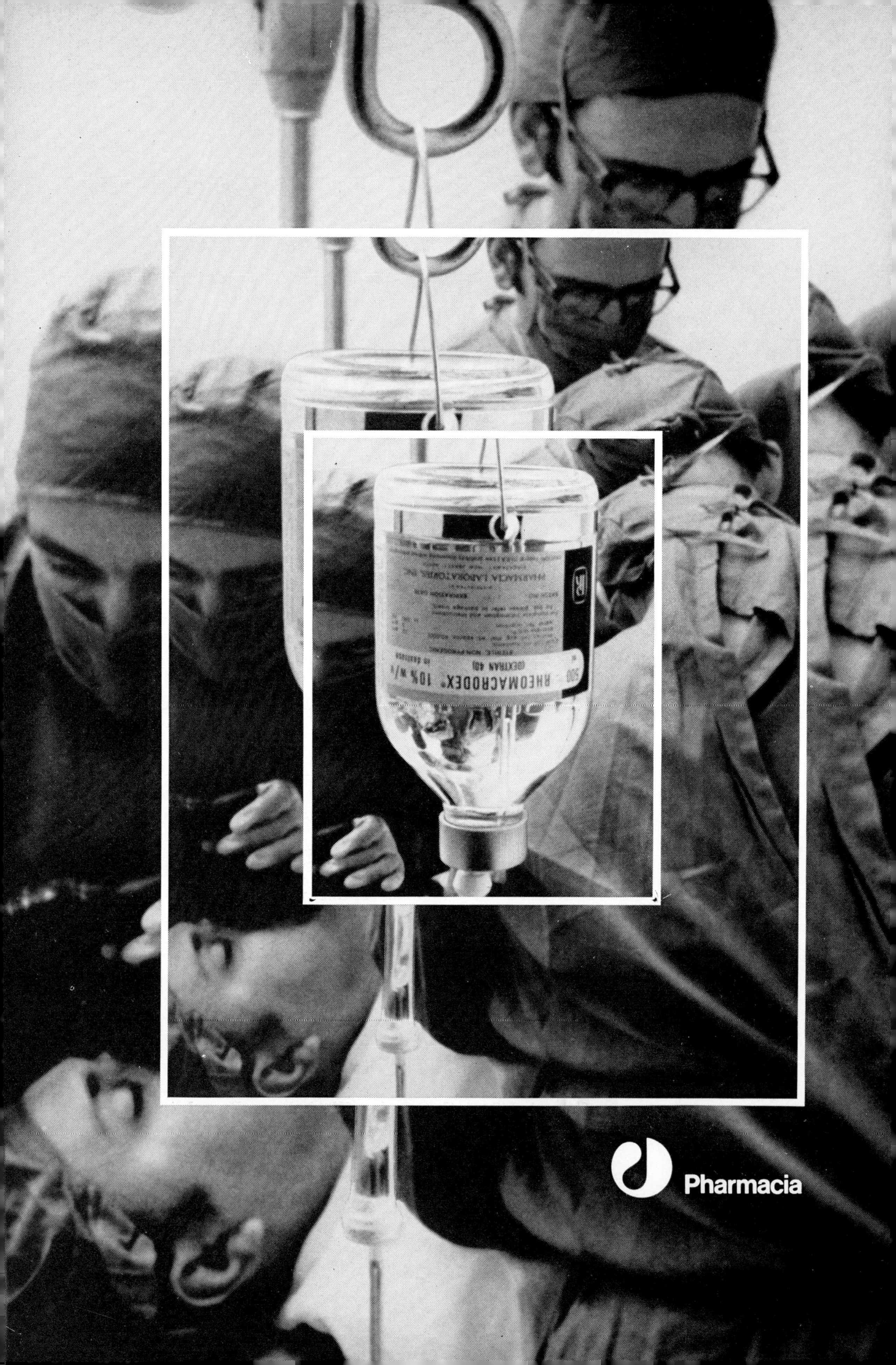
RHEOMACRODEX® 10% w/v
(DEXTRAN 40)
Pharmacia

Volume 67 *Number* 6

SURGERY

CONTENTS, JUNE 1970

CLINICAL SURGERY

page 883 **Arterialization of the liver with portacaval shunt in the treatment of portal hypertension due to intrahepatic block.** Jean-Noël Maillard, M.D., Jean-Pierre Benhamou, M.D., and Bernard Rueff, M.D., Clichy, France

891 **Cystic degeneration of the popliteal artery.** S. J. A. Powis, D. M. Morrissey, and E. L. Jones, Edgbaston, Birmingham, England

895 **Renal artery thrombosis following blunt trauma: Report of four cases.** Oscar M. Grablowsky, M.D., Rudolph F. Weichert, III, M.D., Jacob B. Goff, M.D., and Jorgen U. Schlegel, M.D., New Orleans, La.

901 **Scoliosis and acute vascular compression of the duodenum.** Wilton Bunch, M.D., and John Delaney, M.D., Minneapolis, Minn.

907 **Clinical and experimental use of thoracic impedance plethysmography in quantifying myocardial contractility.** John H. Siegel, M.D., Miklos Fabian, Charles Lankau, M.D., Michael Levine, M.D., Andrew Cole, M.D., and Michel Nahmad, M.D., Bronx, N. Y.

continued on page 9

Vol. 67, No. 6, June, 1970. The Journal of Surgery is published monthly by The C. V. Mosby Company, 3207 Washington Blvd., St. Louis, Mo. 63103. *Annual subscription rates*—United States and its possessions: institutional (multiple-reader) subscriptions,* $24.00; personal (regular) subscriptions,† $19.00; student, intern, and resident physician subscriptions,† $11.40. Canada and Mexico: institutional (multiple-reader) subscriptions, $26.50; personal (regular) subscriptions, $21.50; student, intern, and resident physician subscriptions, $13.90. Other countries: institutional (multiple-reader) subscriptions, $27.50; personal (regular) subscriptions, $22.50; student, intern, and resident physician subscriptions, $14.90. Single copies, $3.50 postpaid.

*Institutional (multiple-reader) subscriptions are available to both public and private libraries, schools, hospitals, and clinics; city, county, state, province, and national government bureaus and departments; and all commercial and private institutions and organizations.

†Personal (regular) subscriptions and all student-rate subscriptions must be in the names of, and billed to, individuals.

Second class postage paid at St. Louis, Mo. Printed in the U. S. A.

To help you cope with susceptible hospital bacterial infections... before they become life-threatening

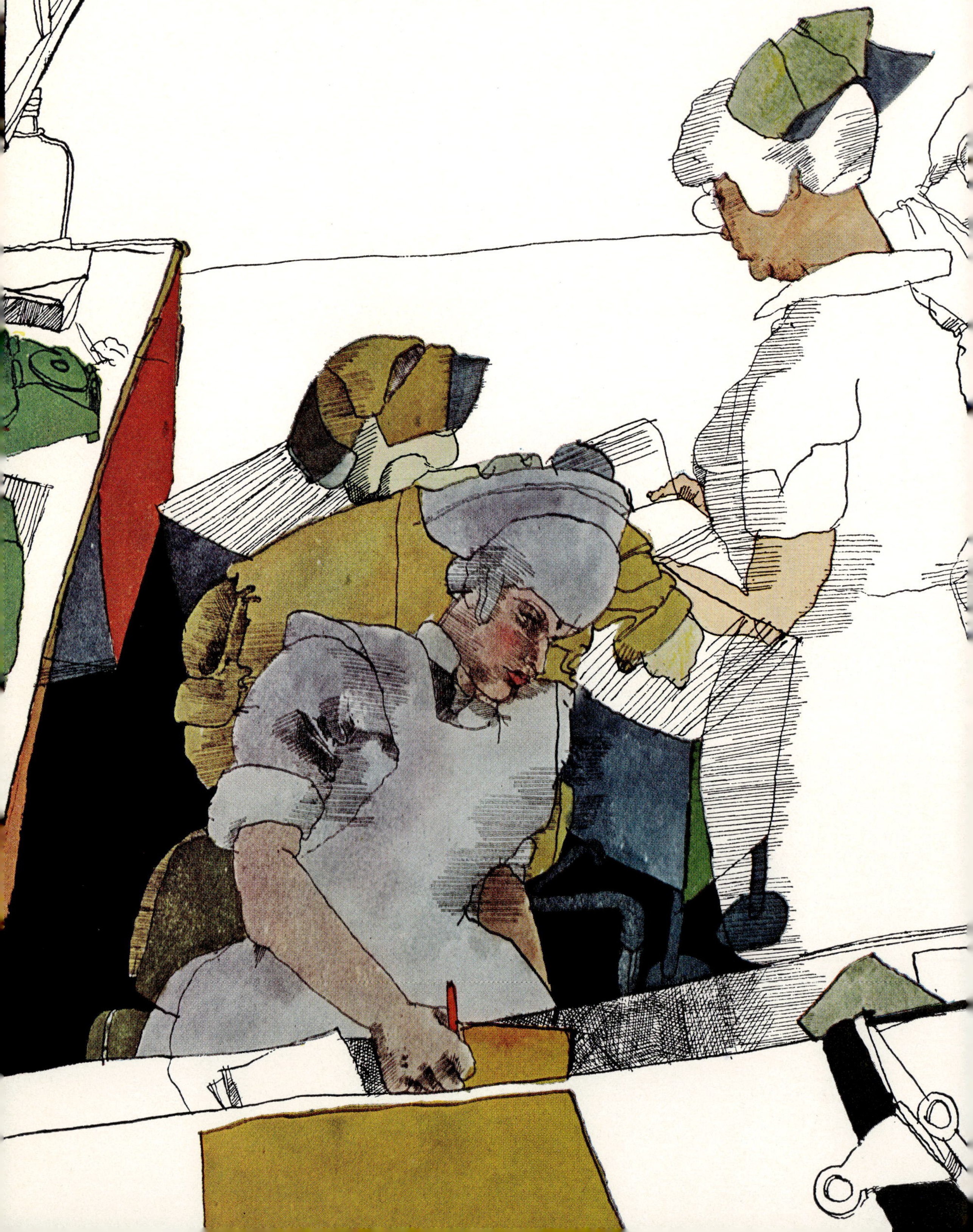

CONTENTS *continued*

page 918 **Decompression of the colon with complete diversion of the fecal stream by an in situ colonic catheter: A pilot study.** Norman H. Schulman, Lieutenant Commander (MC) USNR, Howard G. Pritham, Lieutenant (MC) USN, and Stanton G. Polin, Commander (MC) USNR, Portsmouth, Va.

922 **Diverticulosis of the appendix.** Alfredo R. Esparza, M.D., and Charles M. Pan, M.D., Providence, R. I.

929 **Anterior mediastinitis as a complication of median sternotomy incisions: Diagnostic and surgical considerations.** Manuel Jiménez-Martínez, Rubén Argüero-Sánchez, Juan José Pérez-Alvarez, Pedro Mina-Castañeda, Mexico City, Mexico

INVESTIGATIVE SURGERY

935 **Influence of hemodialysis on a myocardial depressant factor in hemorrhagic shock.** Stephen L. Wangensteen, M.D., J. David deHoll, B.S., Stephen F. Kiechel, A.B., Julian Martin, B.A., and Allan M. Lefer, Ph.D., Charlottesville, Va.

944 **Successful 24 hour renal perfusion-preservation with monitoring by surface electrometry during the storage interval.** J. L. Alexander, M.D., J. R. Dmochowski, M.D., J. E. Murray, M.D., and N. P. Couch, M.D., with the technical assistance of A. M. Macey, B.S., and N. A. Prentiss, B.S., Boston, Mass.

951 **Collagen arterial graft of bovine origin: Seven-year observations in the dog.** Norman Rosenberg, M.D., Geoffrey H. Lord, D.V.M., Ph.D., John Henderson, M.D., James W. Bothwell, Ph.D., and Eugene R. L. Gaughran, Ph.D., New Brunswick, N. J.

957 **Prolonged left ventricular bypass by transvalvular aortic catheterization. I. Physiologic effects and rationale of surgical concept.** R. E. Schuhmann, L. A. Geddes, and H. E. Hoff, Houston, Texas

969 **Circulating lymphocyte depletion: Effect on renal allograft survival in calves.** Jay C. Fish, M.D., Kenneth R. T. Tyson, M.D., Gerald A. Beathard, M. D., Harry E. Sarles, M.D., August R. Remmers, Jr., M.D., and Stephan E. Ritzmann, M.D., Galveston, Texas

976 **Reduction of postoperative thrombocytosis.** Paul Atkins, M.S., F.R.C.S., and Robert E. Lempke, M.D., Indianapolis, Ind.

981 **Body temperature monitoring via the tympanic membrane.** William Thomas Dickey, E. Warner Ahlgren, M.D., and C. R. Stephen, M. D., Dallas, Texas

continued on page 13

the night "cap"

for patients with insomnia

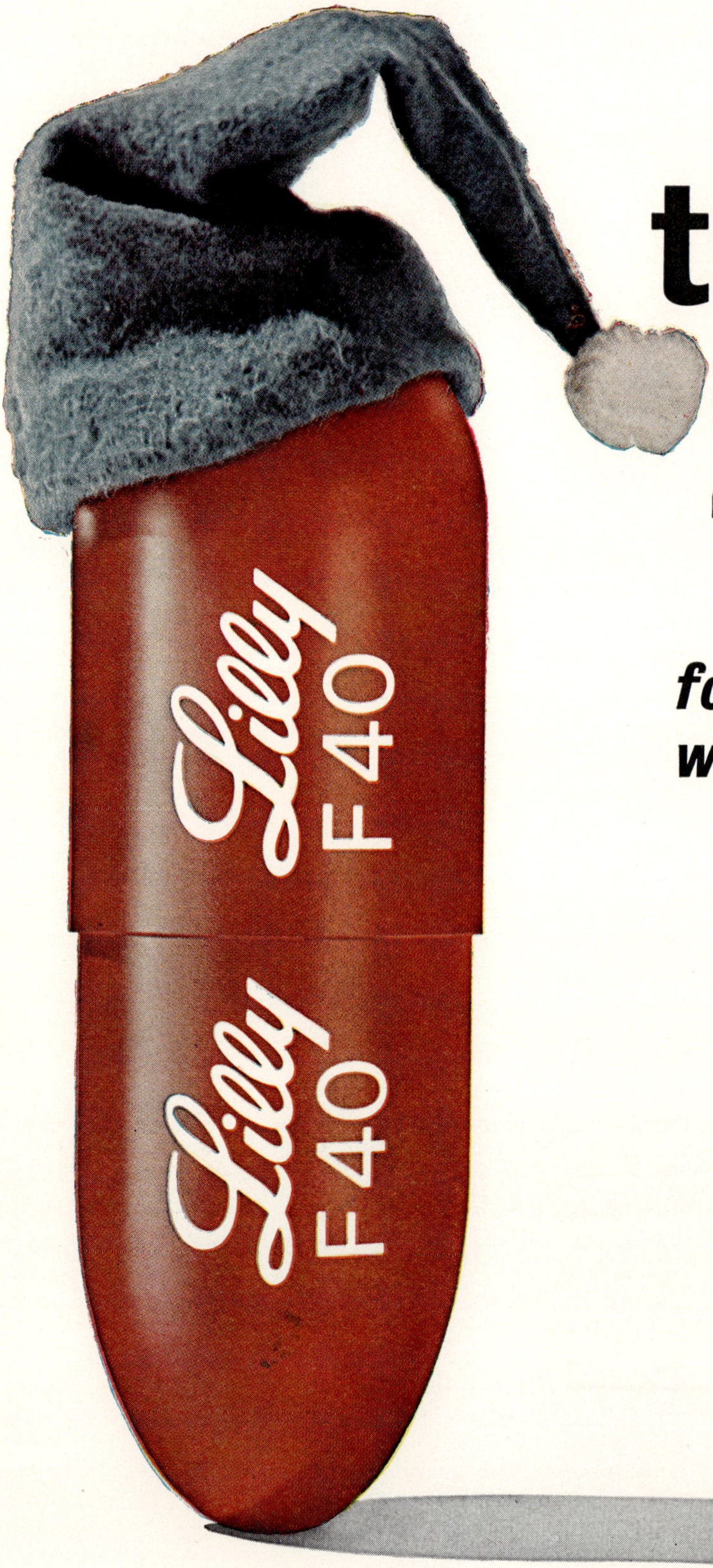

CONTENTS *continued*

PEDIATRIC SURGERY

page 985 **Coronary artery-right ventricular fistula with congestive heart failure: Surgical correction in the neonatal period.** Thomas M. Daniel, M.D., Thomas P. Graham, M.D., and David C. Sabiston, Jr., M.D., Durham, N. C.

995 **Studies of carbohydrate metabolism and serum electrolytes during surface-induced deep hypothermia with prolonged circulatory occlusion.** Edward A. Rittenhouse, M.D., Hitoshi Mohri, M.D., Dr.Med.Sci., and K. Alvin Merendino, M.D., Ph.D., Seattle, Wash.

1006 **Repair of aortic arch interruption in the neonate.** Kenneth R. T. Tyson, M.D., Leonard C. Harris, M.D., and Quang X. Nghiem, M.D., Galveston, Texas

1011 **Aortic arch atresia with transposition of the great vessels: Physiologic considerations and surgical management.** J. B. Norton, Jr., M.D., Danel J. Ullyot, M.D., Edward T. Stewart, M.D., A. M. Rudolph, M.D., and L. Henry Edmunds, Jr., M.D., San Francisco, Calif.

RECENT ADVANCES IN SURGERY

1017 **The surgical treatment of peptic ulcer: A critical analysis of results from subtotal gastrectomy and from vagotomy plus partial gastrectomy.** Alton Ochsner, M.D., Paul R. Zehnder, M.D., and Shirley W. Trammell, B.A., New Orleans, La.

SURGICAL TECHNIQUES

1029 **Technique of gastric mobilization for esophageal replacement.** E. P. Simkin, M.Chir., F.R.C.S., and P. M. Stell, M.B., F.R.C.S., Liverpool, England

1031 **An electromagnetic probe for the quantitation of intracardiac flows.** Byrn T. Williams, M.D., Robert K. Worman, M.D., Rae R. Jacobs, M.D., and Worthington G. Schenk, Jr., M.D., Buffalo, N. Y.

EDITORIAL

1035 **Considerations regarding the coming of National Health Insurance.** C. Barber Mueller, M.D., Hamilton, Ontario, Canada

INDEX

1041 **Index**

If the pH of the gastric contents is raised, the irritant effects of aspirin are diminished.[1]

1. Woodbury, D. M.: *In* The Pharmacological Basis of Therapeutics, 3d ed., 1965, L. S. Goodman and A. Gilman, eds., Macmillan, New York, p. 319.

Volume 67 Number 1

SURGERY

JANUARY, 1970

Society for Vascular Surgery

Presidential address: Standards in vascular surgery

C. ROLLINS HANLON*
CHICAGO, ILL.

The Society for Vascular Surgery was founded more than two decades ago. Having passed its legal majority and with its twenty-fifth year clearly in view, it may properly be considered as mature—as is the field of vascular surgery.

One of the signs of maturity is the setting of goals and the assessment of progress toward their achievement. In a free society, when one sets a well-defined goal, there are no formal taskmasters as there were in the shameful building of the Egyptian pyramids; rather we must be our own taskmasters, measuring our achievement by the standards originally set out in our Constitution.

At the end of this twenty-third meeting of the Society, let us examine briefly our standards and our progress.

The purposes of the Society for Vascular Surgery are directed, obviously enough, at the field of vascular diseases—the promotion of their study, the definition of the role of surgery in their therapy, the *standardization* of their study and management, the *standardization* of the nomenclature of vascular diseases, and the encouragement of adequate teaching and training programs for individuals and for institutions.

More than half of the seven stated objectives in Article II of the Constitution are explicitly or implicitly concerned with *standardization*.

Reading further in the Constitution of the Society, beyond the objectives of the organization to the qualifications for membership, we see that this membership privilege is limited to physicians in good standing in their state or provincial medical societies. Moreover, these physicians are to be certified by one of the American boards, by one of the Royal Colleges, or they should show evidence of measuring up to the equivalent of these formal standards.

This is not the occasion for a discussion of certifying boards, but since we have already mentioned standards more than half a dozen times we should pause to consider the significance of the word.

Most commonly we think of standards in the rather dull sense defined in scientific and technical encyclopedias, for example, "standard: an accepted reference sample used for establishing a unit for the measurement of physical quantities." This is precise but deadly dull. Or again, in a shorter but desiccated phrase, "standard: a physical

Presented at the Twenty-third Annual Meeting of the Society for Vascular Surgery, New York, N. Y., July 12-13, 1968.

*Reprint requests: 55 Erie St., Chicago, Ill. 60611.

quantity specified by a numerical factor and a unit." There is nothing wrong with these definitions in 1969, as long as we recognize the derivation of their current sense from a different original meaning more than eight hundred years ago. At that time "standard" was specifically or by implication "the King's standard," that is, the military ensign planted at the point where the commands originated and where the army reunited around its commander in the midst of battle. Indeed, the first known use of the word was in reference to the "Battle of the Standard" in 1138. So in earlier days, a standard was a rallying point because it marked the site of command and direction, and it was a source of inspiration before it became merely a unit of reference. It was to the king and leader that the soldiers returned, not merely to his ensign high on its staff.

Isaac Watts at the turn of the seventeenth century captured this meaning in his book on "False Greatness" when he wrote:

"Were I so tall to reach the pole
Or grasp the ocean with my span
I must be measured by my soul.
The mind's the standard of the man."

There is no time today to dilate on the minds of the great men in vascular surgery, much less on the phraseology in which they presented their contributions.

Many of them, in addition to their surgical achievements, were masters of a clear and elegantly stylish prose. There is far too little of this today, partly from lack of interest, deficiency of effort, or hesitancy to depart from the clichés which dominate the scientific journalese of so many surgical contributions. Who, in 1969, would venture to refer to ligation of a major vessel in the words used by Halsted,[7] ". . . the moment of tying the ligature is indeed a dramatic one. The monstrous, booming tumor is stilled by a tiny thread, the tempest silenced by the magic wand."

If modern, published surgical contributions display a striking literary poverty, what may we expect of the abstracts for a program such as this? One concedes the ephemeral nature of such abstracts and recognizes that they are often constructed in haste between operations or committee meetings and dispatched on the deadline date after a telephone call to the secretary of the Society. Such circumstances are scarcely conducive to elegance in language; unfortunately there are numerous instances where not even the basic essential of clarity in expression is achieved. This bespeaks carelessness, lack of application, or both.

Some have maintained that we shall not see again the vascular surgical giants of old, born in an era of less intense competition and restricted development of the field, when major achievements seemed more readily accessible because so few were present to seek them. Others maintain that the men entering the field today are of intrinsically poorer capacity than those of old. I deny this as a valid premise, much as Alan Gregg did in his delightful anecdote of the old convict who explained the outrageous behavior of his fellow inmates to the state governor after a prison riot, with the statement, "Governor, they're not getting the class of men in here that they used to!"

Our vascular surgeons today are carrying out new operations under circumstances quite different from those of past centuries. But the underlying principles are the same. So too are the standards, as one may easily see by analysis of our 1969 program in an historical frame of reference. The first paper yesterday[8] on a series of patients followed for more than 10 years after endarterectomy is a demonstration of patient and critical study for a long time so that no one could level the charge of hasty and premature reporting. This is laudable, exemplary, and impressive but we must match it against the standards of Rudolph Matas who reported a patient with an abdominal aortic operation with follow-up observations of half a century.

The fourth paper on aneurysmectomy in the aged[5] concludes that it is safer to do the operation than it is to withhold it under the misapprehension that inaction is safer than a potentially dangerous operation. We are reminded of Astley Cooper, who in another century ligated the aorta in a bold and temporarily successful procedure, embarked upon only after imminence of fatal hemorrhage was clearly demonstrated.[2]

In the eighth paper on ipsilateral cerebral perfusion pressure during carotid endarterectomy[4] we find a record of careful analytical testing in the operating room in order to provide a rational basis for the clinical technique used. And again—we recall Astley Cooper's successful ligation of the carotid artery in 1808[2] and the detailed and thorough experiments he carried out on ligation of the carotid and vertebral arteries in experimental animals.

In the paper of Britton and others[1] we see preliminary observations suggesting that better understanding of mechanisms in portacaval shunts for a complex disease could lead to more rational and effective therapy. But the preceding paper[3] shows that rational hopes may turn to disappointment in the face of long-range observations on the inefficacy of prophylactic portacaval shunts. This cooperative, interhospital study is a fine example of the constitutional objective to ". . . pool the experience and knowledge of the membership."

In a scientific discipline, the published reports of a given individual or group become standards or marks for others to equal or surpass. As specialists we are characteristically striving for individual excellence in our specialty, which implies rigid standards for entry to the profession, stern demands on training programs, and rejection of individuals who fall below the norms during or after the course of their training. It is disturbing to many that new and complex socioeconomic factors have been introduced into the equation. We can cite the problems of inadequate manpower, of disadvantaged groups understandably eager for entry to a given field despite their deficiencies, and finally a more intense and aggressive public scrutiny of professional behavior by citizens and their government. We cannot escape the social and political realities of our time; neither can we relax into what John Gardner[6] styled an "amiable mediocrity" just because the effort for excellence is so much more difficult in our present society.

In his well-known book on "Excellence" Gardner[6] has gone beyond the problem of excellence as it confronts the specialist striving for the highest reaches of performance in his particular field. Gardner is concerned with excellence in an entire society, and he identifies a difficulty among the general public in thinking about and talking about excellence in their daily round of life.

To the credit of our profession, it may be said that our problem is the reverse, for we think regularly of excellence as a standard, with little care and sympathy for deviation, despite the humbling possibility of mediocrity and failure that may haunt our individual performance.

Thus we approach the end of our brief excursion into semantics and superficial analysis of the meaning of standards in our profession and in our current society. We have come aside in this twenty-third scientific session, as in all of our annual meetings, to reconsider more or less explicitly our objectives, to define them more precisely, to understand them more clearly, to assess our progress and our failings so that we might return with fresh insight and a renewed sense of high purpose to the tasks to which these objectives of the Society commit us.

As Thornton Wilder[9] said in *The bridge of San Luis Rey,* "We come from a world where we have known incredible standards of excellence, and we dimly remember beauties which we have not seized again."

Let us give the lie to Wilder's gentle indictment as we pause today to seize again the dimly remembered beauties of past performances in vascular surgery, to freshen the memory of William Halsted, Rudolph Matas, Astley Cooper, and a host of illustrious forbears, whose example should challenge us to strive toward their incredible standards of excellence.

REFERENCES

1. Britton, R. C., Voorhees, A. B., Jr., and Price, J. B., Jr.: Selective portal decompression, SURGERY **67:** 104, 1969.
2. Brock, R. C.: The life and work of Astley

Cooper, Edinburgh, 1952, E. & S. Livingstone, Ltd.

3. Callow, A. D., Resnick, R., Chalmers, T., Ishihara, Albert M., Garceau, J., and O'Hara, Edward T.: Conclusions from a controlled study of prophylactic portacaval shunt, SURGERY **67:** 97, 1969.
4. Ehrenfeld, W. K., Hamilton, F. N., Larson, C. P., Jr., Hickey, R. F., and Severinghaus, J. W.: Effect of CO_2 and systemic hypertension on downstream cerebral arterial pressure during carotid endarterectomy, SURGERY **67:** 87, 1969.
5. Esselstyn, C. B., Jr., Humphries, A. W., Young, J. R., Bevan, E. G., and deWolfe, V. G.: Aneurysmectomy in the aged? SURGERY **67:** 80, 1969.
6. Gardner, J. W.: Excellence, New York, 1961, Harper & Row, Publishers.
7. Halsted, W. S.: Ligations of the left subclavian artery, The Johns Hopkins Hospital Report, Vol. XXI, Baltimore, 1920.
8. Pilcher, D. B., Barker, W. F., and Cannon, J. A.: An aortoiliac endarterectomy case series followed 10 years or more, SURGERY **67:** 5, 1969.
9. Wilder, T.: The bridge of San Luis Rey, New York, 1927, A. and C. Boni.

An aortoiliac endarterectomy case series followed 10 years or more

DAVID B. PILCHER, M.D.*
WILEY F. BARKER, M.D.**
JACK A. CANNON, M.D.
LOS ANGELES, CALIF.
From the Department of Surgery, University of California, School of Medicine

Since the reports of Wylie and associates[12] in 1951 and Barker and Cannon[2] in 1953, aortoiliac endarterectomy has gained an accepted place in the procedures of reconstructive vascular surgery. Synthetic grafts have been in use only since 1957 when they largely replaced homografts.

Several reports of aortoiliac endarterectomy have shown the durability of this technique in follow-up studies extending to 9 years,[1, 8, 9] but in all of these reports the cases followed over 5 years have been few. The 5 year patency rate of aortoiliac endarterectomy from these reports varies from 51 to 76 percent, with the poorest results in those with distal occlusive disease or severe ischemia. Cannon and co-workers[5] and Darling and Linton[6] reported 95 to 97 percent good-to-excellent relief of symptoms in series followed up to 5 years.

Aortoiliac endarterectomy remains our procedure of choice for aortoiliac obstructive disease. It is the purpose of this paper to review a series of patients followed for 10 years or more to evaluate the durability of endarterectomy and the long-term results.

CLINICAL MATERIAL

Included in this study are the cases of all patients undergoing aortoiliac endarterectomy from 1954 through the first half of 1959 performed by J. A. C. or W. F. B. or by the resident staff at UCLA.

The 69 aortoiliac endarterectomies performed in this period can be considered as 134 limbs for follow-up purposes, as pointed out by Humphries and associates.[8]

Only three patients were operated upon for severe ischemia and one for a probable embolic occlusion. The remainder were operated upon for relief of claudication. The average age of these patients was 52 years and 63 percent were male.

Of the 69 patients, 37 were followed for more than 10 years and 16 died before 10 years elapsed. Follow-up with a detailed questionnaire answered by the patient with an examination by a physician known to us was accepted in seven of the long-term follow-ups, but all other living patients were examined by one of us after the 10 year interval. One patient could not be traced after hospital discharge. The remaining patients were lost to follow-up at varying intervals prior to 10 years.

The cumulative patency curves include all of the patients but the early failures. This is in accord with the method proposed by Stokes, Sugg, and Butcher[10] and compensates for those lost to follow-up from death or other reasons.

RESULTS

Early failures. There were four early failures (with early failures defined as those occurring prior to discharge from the hospital), a rate of 6 percent. One of these patients died of acute renal failure 3 days

Presented at the Twenty-third Annual Meeting of the Society for Vascular Surgery, New York, N. Y., July 12-13, 1969.

*Present address: Department of Surgery, University of Vermont, College of Medicine, Burlington, Vt. 05401.

**Reprint requests: University of California, Los Angeles, Calif.

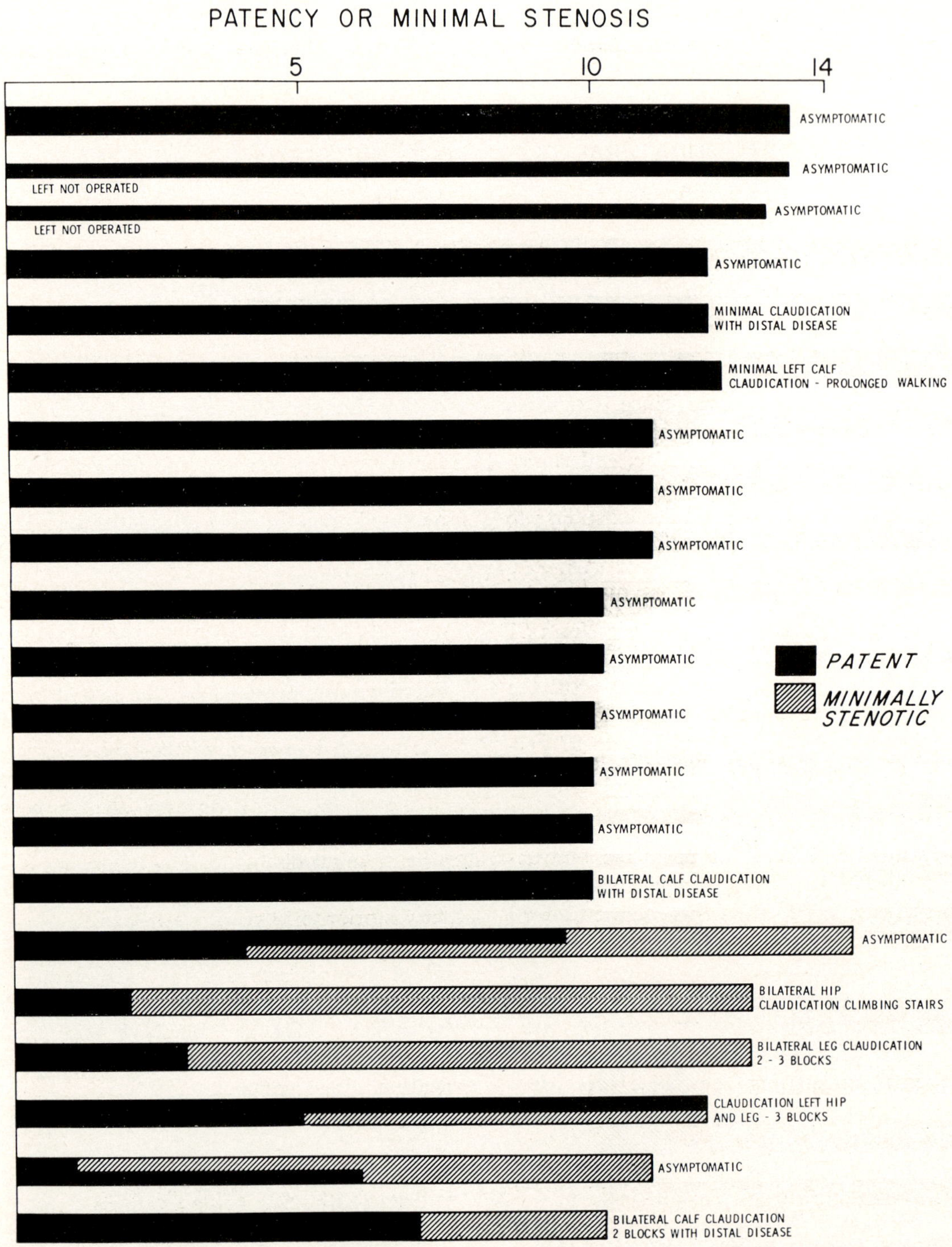

A

Fig. 1. *A* and *B,* Graphic representation of all cases of aortoiliac endarterectomy followed for more than 10 years.

postoperatively. One patient who was operated on for acute ischemia had a postoperative occlusion because of severe distal disease and required above-the-knee amputation. One patient died 3 years after his early occlusion, and the last patient was salvaged by an aortofemoral graft to survive for 4 years. These cases most likely represent technical failures, the cause of which has been reviewed by Buckberg and co-workers.[3]

Deaths. There was one death in the post-

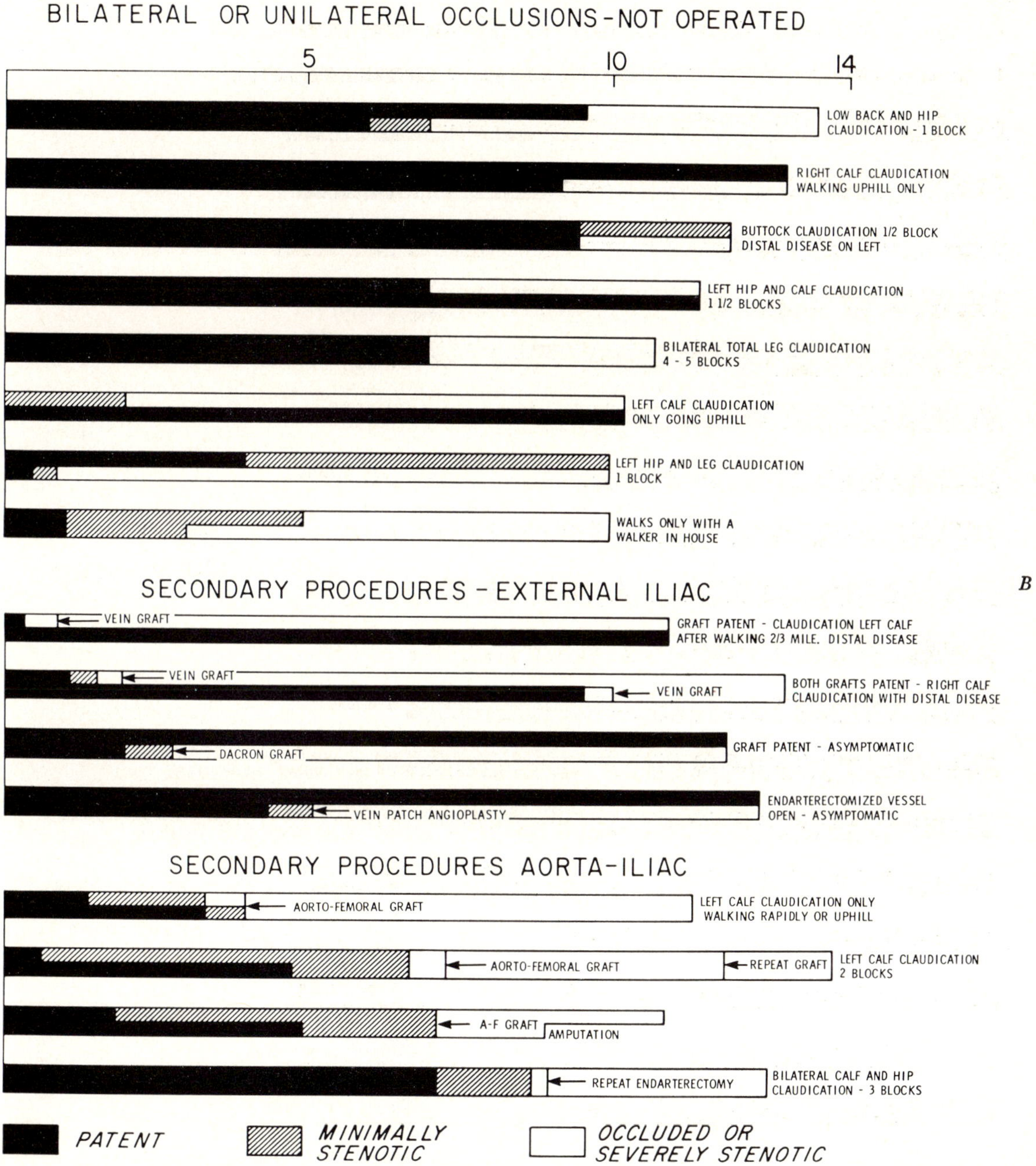

Fig. 1—Cont'd. *For legend see opposite page.*

Table I. *Deaths in endarterectomy series*

Time of death after endarterectomy	*Status of endarterectomy*	*Cause of death*
3 days	Occluded	Acute renal failure
2 months	Patent	Pulmonary embolus
4 months	Patent	Coronary thrombosis
10 months	Patent	Cerebrovascular accident
1 year	Patent	Cancer of cervix and postirradiation necrosis of bowel
2½ years	Patent	Cancer of floor of mouth
3 years	Patent	Unknown
3 years	Occluded left, stenotic right	Myocardial infarction
4 years	Unknown	Cerebrovascular accident with pneumonia
6 years	Occluded right in hospital, left not operated	Unknown
6 years	Patent	Cerebral and pulmonary emboli 3 days postoperatively mitral commissurotomy
8 years	Patent	"Arteriosclerotic cardiovascular disease"
8 years	Unknown	Leukemia
8 years	Patent	Heart attack
8 years	Stenotic (since 6 years)	Heart failure
9½ years	Stenotic (since 1 year)	Unknown
11 years	Unknown (patent at 2 years)	Unknown
11 years	Patent	Myocardial infarction
12 years	Unknown (patent at 3 years)	Heart disease
12 years	Patent left, stenotic right (since 8½ years)	Heart failure and lymphosarcoma of stomach
13 years	Unknown (patent at 7 years)	Myocardial infarction

operative period and one death 2 months postoperatively from a pulmonary embolus. No other death can be attributed to operation or its sequelae.

There were 16 deaths in the 10 year period after operation and five more in the period after 10 years. Eight deaths are known to have been due to arteriosclerotic heart disease and three more to cerebrovascular accidents. The causes of death and status of endarterectomy at time of death are presented in Table I.

Long-term patency. Thirty-seven patients (72 limbs) were followed 10 years or more (Fig. 1). Forty-eight of these iliac endarterectomies were still patent at 10 years.

Although angiographic proof of patency would be desirable in all cases, we have not felt ethically justified nor have we been financially equipped to make such a study. Arteriography has been performed only when indicated for symptoms of arterial insufficiency or for some other problem. Clinical evaluation of femoral pulses, oscillometrics, and symptoms generally give an adequate basis for a diagnosis of patency of the aortoiliac segment.

Thirty-five of the limbs considered above were widely patent at 10 years with no evidence of stenosis. A typical aortogram is shown in Fig. 2.

Thirteen of the limbs considered patent at 10 years showed some evidence of stenosis manifested by minimally decreased femoral pulses with bruits and oscillometric decrease from normal or angiographic evidence of stenosis. Many of these patients have some

Table II. *Number of limbs at risk for the intervals compared in the cumulative patency curves (Fig. 6)*

	0-1 yr.	*4-5 yr.*	*9-10 yr.*
UCLA	122	78	52
Kouchoukos and associates[9]	256	110	—
Humphries and associates[8]			
Claudication	186*	20*	—
Ischemia	75*	8*	—

*Number of limbs estimated from graphs.

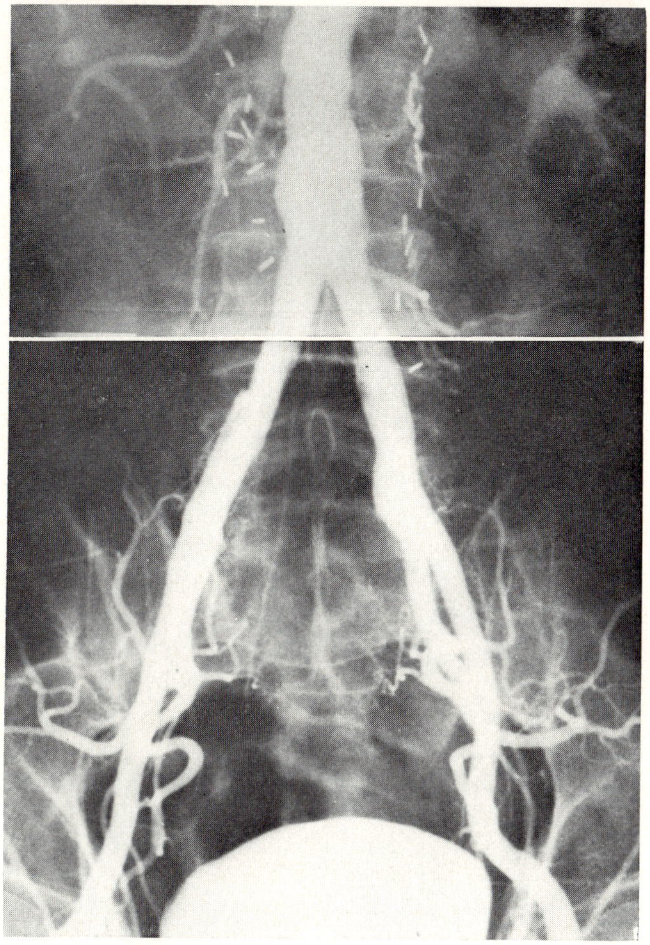

Fig. 2. Aortogram 6 years after aortoiliac endarterectomy, showing normal patency of the endarterectomized segments.

symptoms. Fig. 3 is an aortogram of a patient categorized as occluded on one side and stenotic on the other.

Weak femoral pulses without bruits and absent femoral pulses are considered as adequate evidence of occlusion in those patients in whom occlusion cannot be documented angiographically. Patients who have grafts for either stenosis or occlusion are considered to have been occluded, regardless of their present status. An aortogram of one patient treated with aortofemoropopliteal bypass graft for relief of symptoms mostly on the basis of distal disease shows stenosis, not occlusion of the aortoiliac segment (Fig. 4), but is tabulated as occlusion. Similarly all four of the illiofemoral grafts performed 1 to 10 years after the original endarterectomy and the vein patch angioplasty presented an identical picture of external iliac occlusion with the endarterectomy remaining patent as far as the hypogastric artery (Fig. 5). In all of these cases the endarterectomy was initially terminated at the origin of the external iliac artery.

The cumulative patency curves are presented in Fig. 6 and Table II, showing the rates for those widely patent without any stenosis. A second curve includes those in whom minimal stenosis is considered patent. The curves presented by Humphries and associates[8] and Kouchoukos and co-workers[9]

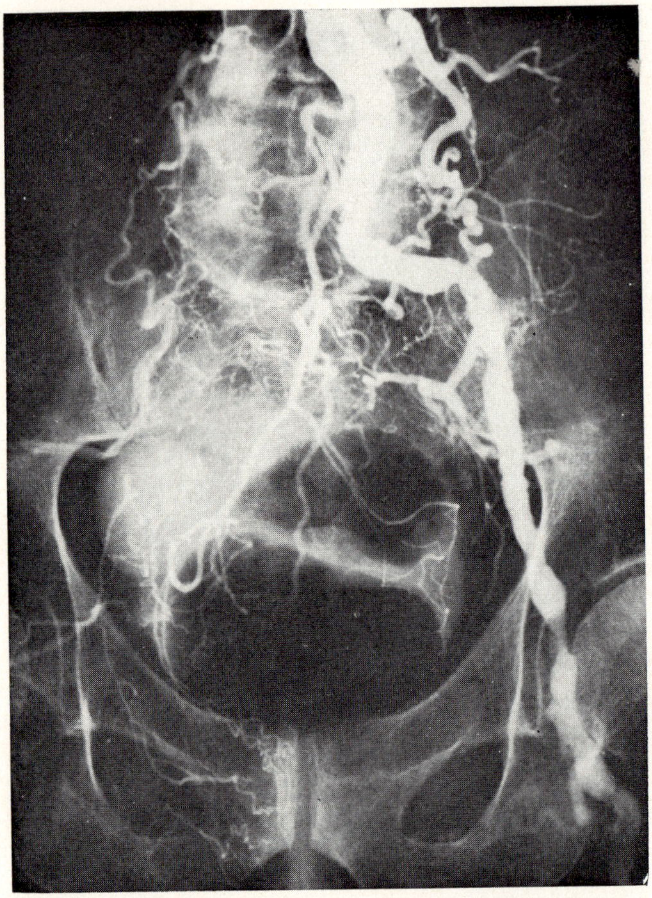

Fig. 3. Aortogram 12 years after aortoiliac endarterectomy, demonstrating occlusion of the right side and stenosis of the left common and external iliac arteries.

Table III. *Status of aortoiliac endarterectomies followed 10 years*

Condition	*No. of limbs*
Widely patent	35
Minimal stenosis	13
Occluded	11
External iliac grafts	5
Aortofemoral grafts	8
Total	72

are included for comparison. The cumulative patency rate at 10 years is 50 percent for widely patent limbs, and 69 percent if minimal stenosis is considered to be patent. The status of these endarterectomies followed 10 years is summarized in Table III.

Relation of symptoms to patency. Many of the patients with stenosis and some with complete occlusion were not having severe symptoms of arterial insufficiency in the legs. Several of the patients with stenoses have no symptoms referable to the legs, but these patients do not exercise vigorously. Several more have symptoms of claudication only when walking uphill. Others claudicate at a normal rate of walking after two to five blocks.

All of the patients with occlusions have some symptoms of claudication. In several, symptoms are present only on climbing stairs or walking uphill.

Three of the patients with patent endarterectomies have calf claudication from femoropopliteal occlusive disease. The individual cases presented in Fig. 1 are summarized as to symptoms of claudication

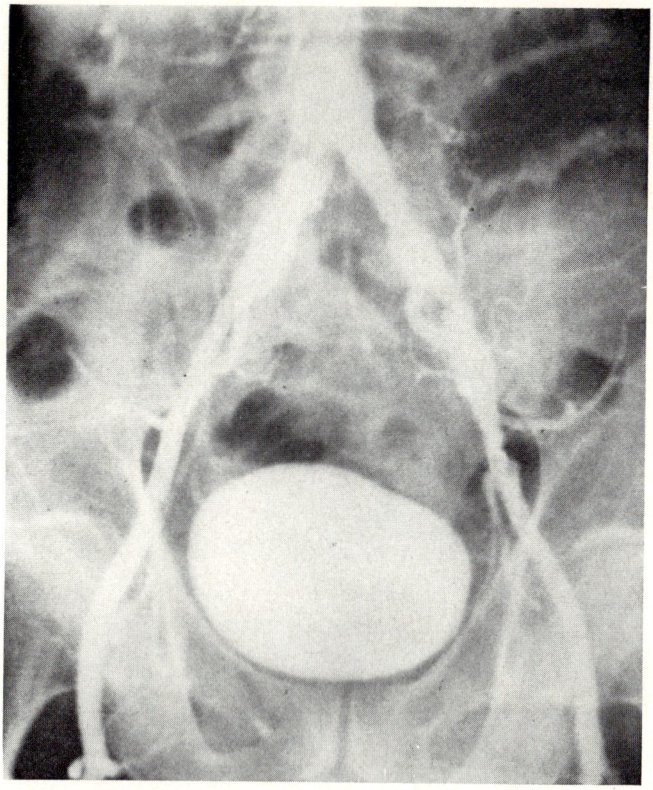

Fig. 4. Aortogram 7 years after aortoiliac endarterectomy, demonstrating severe segmental stenosis at the origin of the right common iliac artery. The minimal dilation of the terminal aorta does not behave as an aneurysm.

in Table IV showing 62 percent good-to-excellent results at 10 years.

Sympathectomy. Nineteen of the 27 patients followed 10 years had lumbar sympathectomy at the time of endarterectomy, but there is no discernible difference in patency rates of the aortoiliac segment between them and those not having sympathectomy. Definite progression of distal occlusive disease had occurred in 75 percent of those without sympathectomy and only 40 percent of those with sympathectomy.

Effect of diet. All patients followed a low saturated fat, low cholesterol diet with varying faithfulness. Emphasis was given to decreasing weight and avoiding obesity. Weight loss or gain appeared to have no correlation to outcome of endarterectomy in the survivors.

Three patients maintained a weight of at least 20 pounds less than their preoperative weights. Two of these patients had widely patent endarterectomies at 10 and 11 years. The third experienced an occlusion at 9½ years.

Three patients gained more than 20 pounds. Two of these had stenoses at 1 and 7 years postoperatively. The other patient in this group with no further problems gained

Table IV. *Results of aortoiliac endarterectomy followed 10 years in terms of clinical symptoms*

Condition	*No. of patients*	
Asymptomatic	17	62%
Minimal symptoms (uphill or prolonged walking)	9	
Claudication 2 to 5 blocks	6	
Claudication > 2 blocks	4	
Amputation	1	
Total	37	

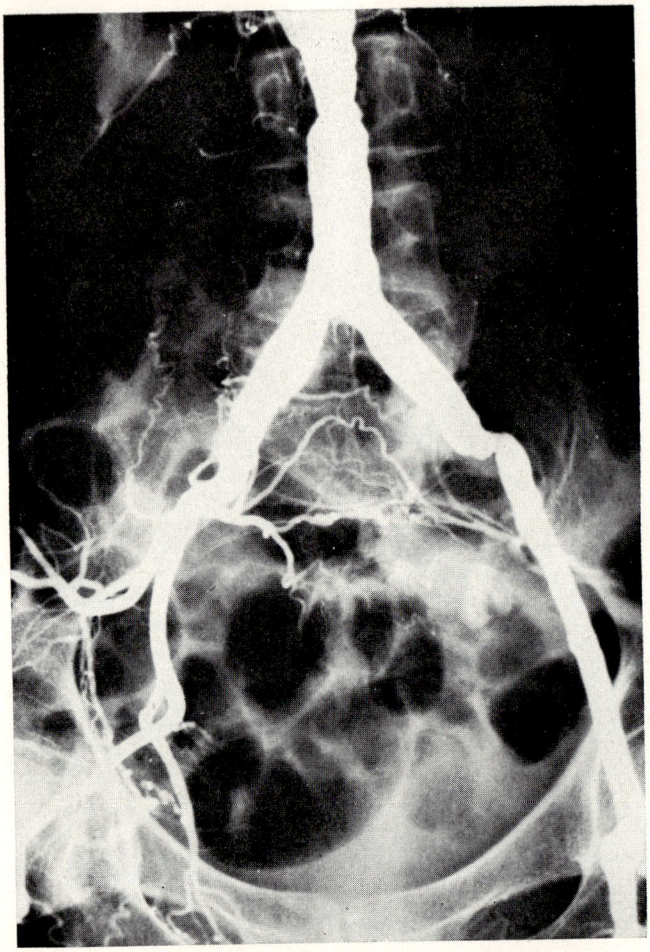

Fig. 5. Aortogram 10 years after aortic and common iliac endarterectomy. Patent vein graft on the left placed for external iliac occlusion 2 years after original endarterectomy. External iliac occlusion now present on the right.

weight (25 pounds) only when he stopped smoking 5 years after endarterectomy.

The serum cholesterol levels of most patients fell within the normal range, but the progressive decreases in serum cholesterol in patients who had serial determinations suggest some effect of adherence to diet (Fig. 7). Normal values are reported to increase with age, especially in female patients.[7]

Smoking. All but one of the patients in this 10 year follow-up study smoked prior to operation. Despite advice to stop smoking, only seven patients of the 37 who were followed 10 years stopped smoking. Correlation of smoking history with results of endarterectomy does not show a definite relationship.

COMPLICATIONS

Aneurysm. We are aware of only two cases of aneurysm formation in our total experience with aortoiliac endarterectomy and these were both false aneurysms. One of these is a part of this series. In this case a pulsatile mass became evident 1 month postoperatively following a septic arthritis of the knee. This aneurysm was removed 7 years later at the time of aortofemoral bypass graft and was found to be a false aneurysm of the terminal aorta.

Vessels which have been endarterectom-

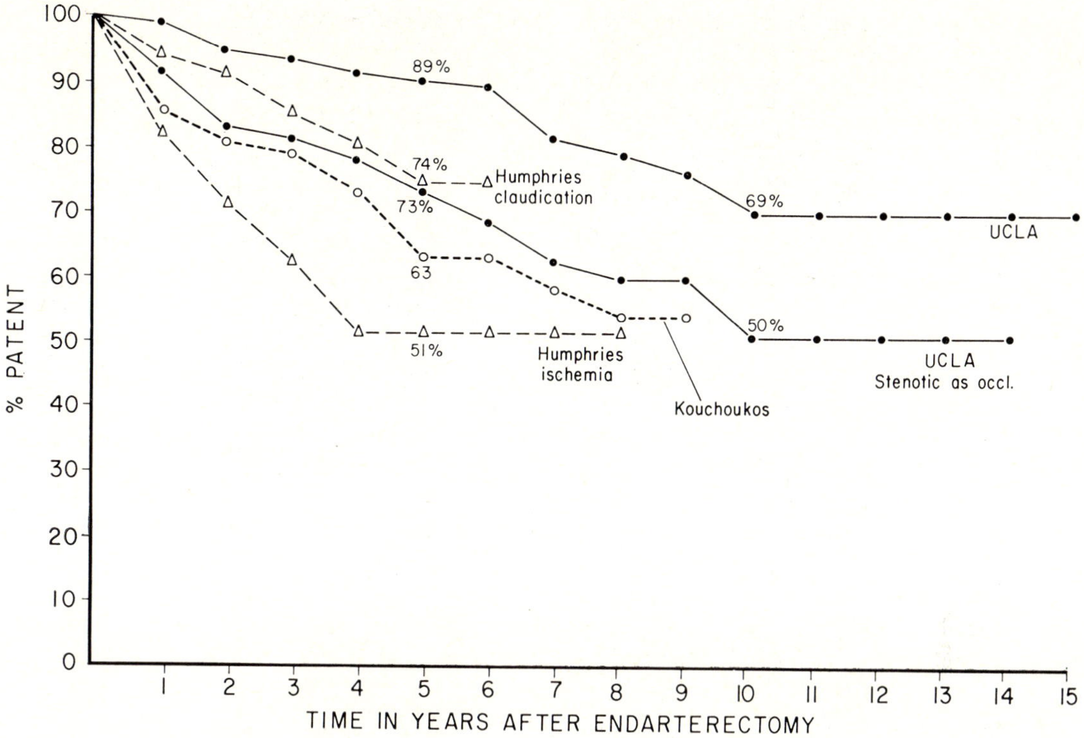

Fig. 6. Accumulative patency curves of aortoiliac endarterectomies performed more than 10 years ago. The curves of Kouchoukos and associates[9] and Humphries and co-workers[8] are included for comparison. (Early failures are excluded.)

ized are frequently larger than normal, but progressive dilation does not occur. One patient was operated upon at another hospital with a diagnosis of aneurysm of the abdominal aorta. We do not interpret the preoperative aortogram on which this diagnosis was based as demonstrating aneurysm (Fig. 4).

Infection. There were no major wound infections and only one superficial infection in this series. There was no proved instance of early or late infection of the arterial repair or its vicinity, although the above case of false aneurysm is suspect of infection. One bypass graft performed 7 years after endarterectomy subsequently became infected.

Amputations. There was one above-the-knee amputation 1 month postoperatively in a patient with severe distal disease. Failure of a bypass graft 9 years after endarterectomy (on the patient whose arterio-

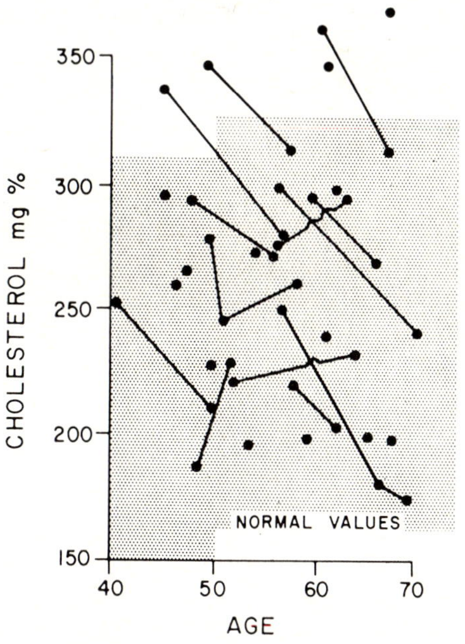

Fig. 7. Serum cholesterol in relation to age of endarterectomies followed 10 years.

gram is shown in Fig. 4) led to infection which necessitated the amputation.

One transmetatarsal amputation healed successfully following aortoiliac endarterectomy for severe ischemia and gangrene of the toes.

DISCUSSION

The technique of aortoiliac endarterectomy currently used at UCLA is well described by Buckberg, Henney, and Cannon.[3, 4] There are a few points in which the technique used in this early series of patients was different from that currently employed. Bilateral lumbar sympathectomy is now done as the first step of the operation in virtually all patients. In the series under discussion sympathectomy was done at the time of operation in 56 percent of the patients. The known increase of flow in the immediate postoperative period after endarterectomy should aid in maintaining early patency, and we believe that sympathectomy offers some long-term protection against the progression of the basic disease. The decrease incidence of progression of distal disease in the patients in this series who had sympathectomy supports this view.

Intravenous heparin, 25 to 50 mg., is administered immediately prior to clamping the aorta and a dilute solution of heparin in normal saline is used to irrigate the legs intermittently via red rubber catheters which remain in place while distal arteriotomies are sutured (Fig. 8).

We are no longer hesitant to incise the groin and start the endarterectomy in the femoral artery when significant disease extends that far. It appears now that endarterectomy should be carried to the femoral artery in more cases than the 8 percent in which it was. It was started in the groin in 62 percent of the last 150 cases of aortoiliac endarterectomy performed at UCLA.[3] The several cases of external iliac occlusions requiring grafts that followed an endarterec-

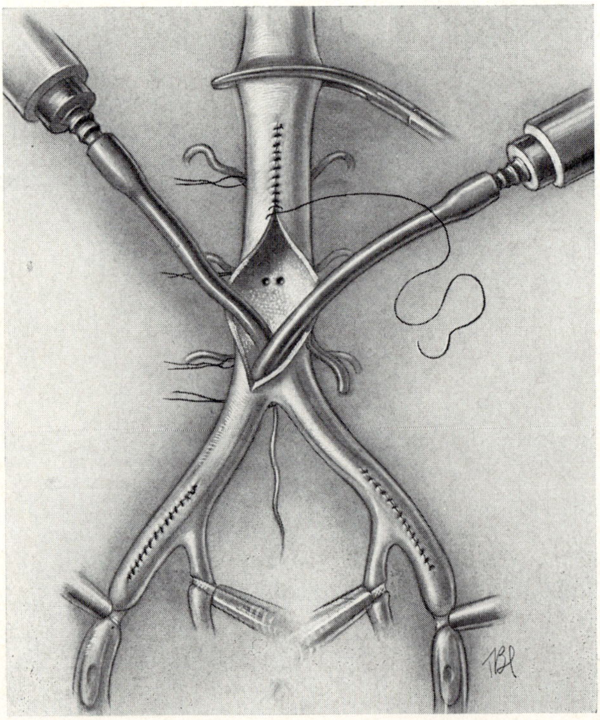

Fig. 8. Longitudinal arteriotomies are sutured over catheters which are used to irrigate distal vessels intermittently. (Reprinted from Arch. Surg. 82: 813, 1961.)

tomy of only the common iliac artery lend support to this hypothesis. We believe these cases do not represent failure of the endarterectomized vessel, but incompleteness of the endarterectomy.

We continue to use longitudinal arteriotomies closed with fine sutures over stents and feel that a vein patch is rarely indicated. Postoperative arteriograms do not show narrowing from this closure (Fig. 9).

Stenosis of the endarterectomized segment does not uniformly progress to occlusion, as Szilagyi[11] suggested with his observation that four of nine stenoses occluded within 2 years of their first appearance. A number of patients have had stenosis which has not changed with further follow-up. In those cases in which arteriography has been performed, the clinical judgment of stenosis rather than occlusion has been confirmed. In view of the lack of symptoms and lack of progression of disease in these cases, the higher rate of patency achieved by including these cases as patent seems valid. There would actually be some argument for including as patent those endarterectomies palliated by distal grafts by passing the external iliac arteries, which would further improve the late patency rate.

We believe that restoration of flow into inferior mesenteric, lumbar, and hypogastric arteries is often possible with aortoiliac endarterectomy and may offer real protection when more distal progression of main vessel

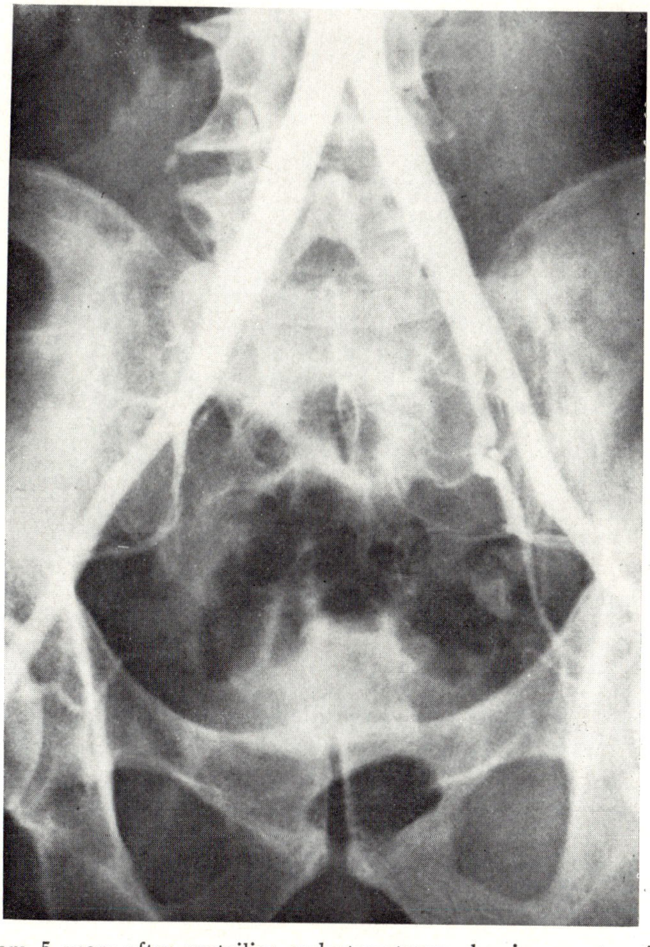

Fig. 9. Aortogram 5 years after aortoiliac endarterectomy, showing no stenosis from vertical incision and closure.

disease occurs. Bypass grafting does not offer this advantage.

Although false aneurysm may appear, as in the one case reported here, it is extremely rare after endarterectomy, and progressive aneurysmal dilation of the endarterectomized vessels has not been shown to occur.

CONCLUSIONS

Aortoiliac endarterectomy has now proved its durability with a low incidence of early failures followed by a late patency that encourages its continued use. Although a significant number of stenoses develop between the 5 and 10 year periods, the 5 year cumulative patency rate of 89 percent drops only to 69 percent at 10 years.

Many of the patients with stenoses and some with occlusions have mild symptoms not demanding further surgery. The opening of collaterals at the time of endarterectomy may be beneficial.

The external iliac artery is the site of frequent problems after endarterectomy, and we should not hesitate to start the endarterectomy in the groin when the disease extends that far.

One case of false aneurysm occurring in the immediate postoperative period is presented and no proved cases of infection involving the arterial repair. We believe that both of these complications are more frequent with bypass grafting than with endarterectomy.

Aortoiliac endarterectomy is a durable and effective reconstructive procedure, but the real challenge remains in the control of the underlying disease process.

REFERENCES

1. Barker, W. F.: Peripheral arterial disease, Philadelphia, 1966, W. B. Saunders Company, pp. 188-189.
2. Barker, W. F., and Cannon, J. A.: An evaluation of endarterectomy, Arch. Surg. **64:** 488, 1953.
3. Buckberg, G. D., Henney, R. P., and Cannon, J. A.: Postoperative complications of aortoiliac endarterectomy: Incidence, cause, and prevention, Surgery **63:** 121, 1968.
4. Cannon, J. A.: A current technique of aorto-iliac and femoro-popliteal endarterectomy for obliterative atherosclerosis, Springfield, Ill., 1965, Charles C Thomas, Publisher.
5. Cannon, J. A., Kawakami, I. G., and Barker, W. F.: The present status of aorto-iliac endarterectomy for obliterative atherosclerosis, Arch. Surg. **82:** 813, 1961.
6. Darling, R. C., and Linton, R. R.: Aortoilio-femoral endarterectomy for atherosclerotic occlusive disease, Surgery **55:** 184, 1964.
7. Henry, R. J.: Clinical chemistry, principles and techniques, New York, 1965, Paul B. Hoeber, Inc., Medical Book Division of Harper & Row, Publishers, p. 862.
8. Humphries, A. W., Young, J. R., and McCormack, L. J.: Experiences with aortoiliac and femoropopliteal endarterectomy, Surgery **65:** 48, 1969.
9. Kouchoukos, N. T., Levy, J. F., Balfour, J. F., and Butcher, H. R.: Operative therapy for aortoiliac arterial occlusive disease: A comparison of therapeutic methods, Arch. Surg. **96:** 628, 1968.
10. Stokes, J. M., Sugg, W. L., and Butcher, H. R., Jr.: Standard method of assessing relative effectiveness of therapies for arterial occlusive diseases, Ann. Surg. **157:** 343, 1963.
11. Szilagyi, D. E., Smith, R. F., and Whitney, D. G.: The durability of aorto-iliac endarterectomy: A roentgenologic and pathologic study of late recurrence, Arch. Surg. **89:** 827, 1964.
12. Wylie, E. J., Kerr, E., and Davies, O.: Experimental and clinical experiences with the use of fascia lata as a graft about major arteries after thromboendarterectomy and aneurysmorrhaphy, Surg. Gynec. Obstet. **93:** 257, 1951.

DISCUSSION

Dr. Weisman (Hanover, N. H.). I appreciated very much hearing this excellently documented report on the long-range outcome of successful endarterectomy on the aortoiliac segment.

I wish to report a single case of a 15 year follow-up on aortoiliac endarterectomy done in 1954 after the technique originally described by Jack Wylie.

This patient died approximately 14½ years after his original operation of a chronic suppurative pancreatitis, and at autopsy he had a 5 to 6 cm. aneurysm at the end of the operated segment.

This was, I believe, associated with atheromatous destruction or degeneration of the remaining media which was left behind. I could not find any cases in the literature which describe this kind of outcome.

I, too, used endarterectomy for several years but gave it up in recent years because of the incidence of stenotic segments that appear in the distal common iliac and external iliac areas which have necessitated reoperation.

Dr. Barker (closing). This is a progressive disease and it is not strictly located in the aortoiliac bifurcation. One cannot under play the fact that 16 of these 69 patients have died in 10 years.

I think that Dr. Weisman has put his finger on one of the problems, that is, the stenoses that occur at the end of the endarterectomized segment.

Dr. Jack Connolly has criticized the endarterectomies as usually failing to clear the external iliac artery. I think that this is one weak spot which we should treat more completely. I'm sure in some of this series we did leave residual disease at the start of the proximal external iliac which has caused us some of this trouble. One could see that from some of the arteriograms Dr. Pilcher showed. I think you also saw that we sometimes failed to get all of the atheroma out in the infrarenal aorta, but this, I don't believe, has caused any trouble. It gives a terrible-looking arteriogram, but it doesn't give us any trouble.

I want to thank Dr. Weisman for his comments, and I want to thank the Society for the privilege of presenting this material.

Arterial autografts

RONALD J. STONEY, M.D.
EDWIN J. WYLIE, M.D.
SAN FRANCISCO, CALIF.
From the Department of Surgery, University of California School of Medicine

Our preliminary experience with arterial autografts in 23 patients to overcome special problems in arterial replacement was presented in 1965.[2] The high rate of success prompted an expansion of this technique into other situations in which alternate methods have not been wholly satisfactory. The present report describes the immediate and long-term results of 101 arterial autografts in 95 patients.

The donor arteries were the hypogastric (36), the external iliac (38), the combined common and external iliac (15), and the superficial femoral (12). Although the hypogastric arteries were removed without bridging the resulting defect, only one patient described mild gluteal claudication postoperatively. The external iliac donor segments were usually obtained through a lower quadrant retroperitoneal approach. Except for one patient in whom redundancy of the iliac arteries permitted primary repair, the common and external iliac defects were bridged by Dacron prostheses. All but one of these prostheses have functioned normally. The one failure resulted from atherosclerotic occlusion of the common femoral artery and retrograde thrombotic occlusion of the graft 6 months postoperatively. Common femoral endarterectomy and graft thrombectomy restored a normal arterial lumen and patency which has persisted for the past 4 years.

Atherosclerotic occlusion or stenosis in 12 of the donor iliac segments was corrected by eversion endarterectomy of the resected segment before implantation. A similar technique was used for the superficial femoral donor segments, all of which were occluded by atherosclerosis.

Presented at the Twenty-third Annual Meeting of the Society for Vascular Surgery, New York, N. Y., July 12-13, 1969.

INDICATIONS

In six patients autografts were used because of sepsis at the site of intended repair or replacement. The local arterial lesions

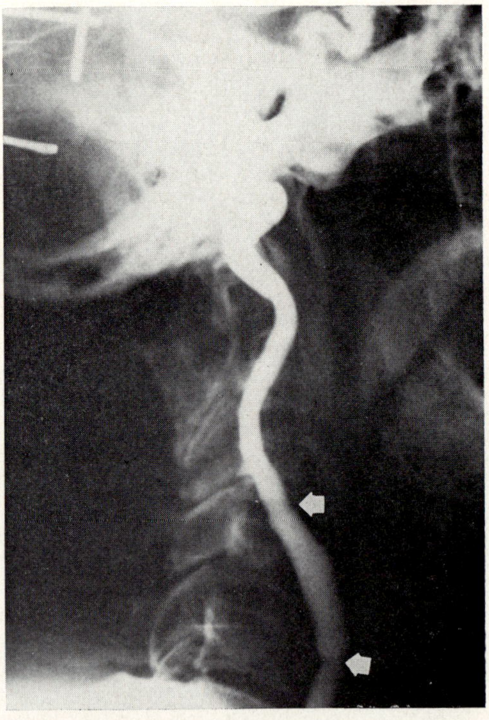

Fig. 1. Carotid arteriograms 4½ years following autograft replacement (arrows) of the distal common carotid artery for the management of an infected false aneurysm. The graft was anastomosed distally to the internal carotid artery.

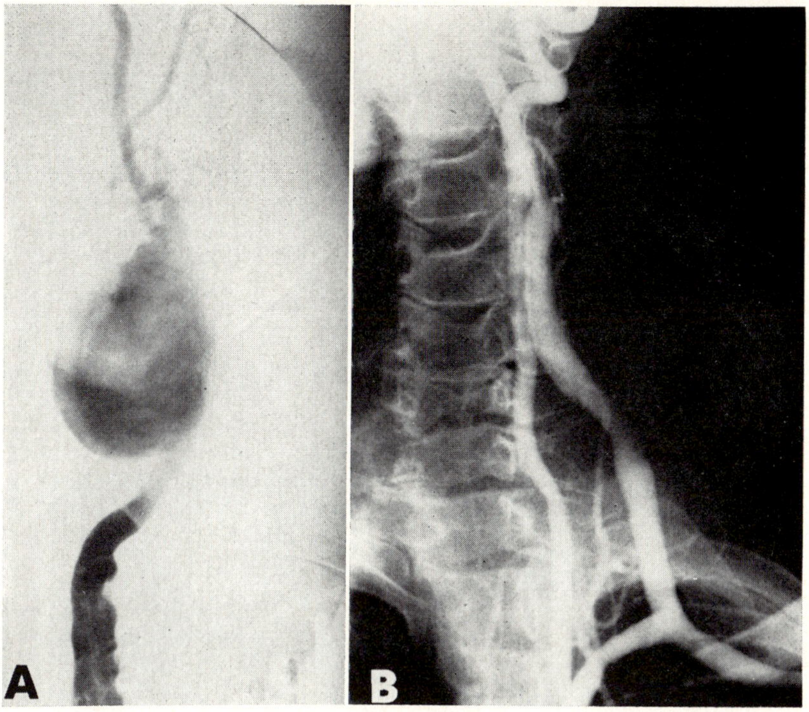

Fig. 2. Preoperative and postoperative arteriogram in a patient with ruptured and infected primary aneurysm of the left common carotid artery *(A)*. An arterial autograft was anastomosed from the left subclavian artery to the internal carotid artery *(B)*.

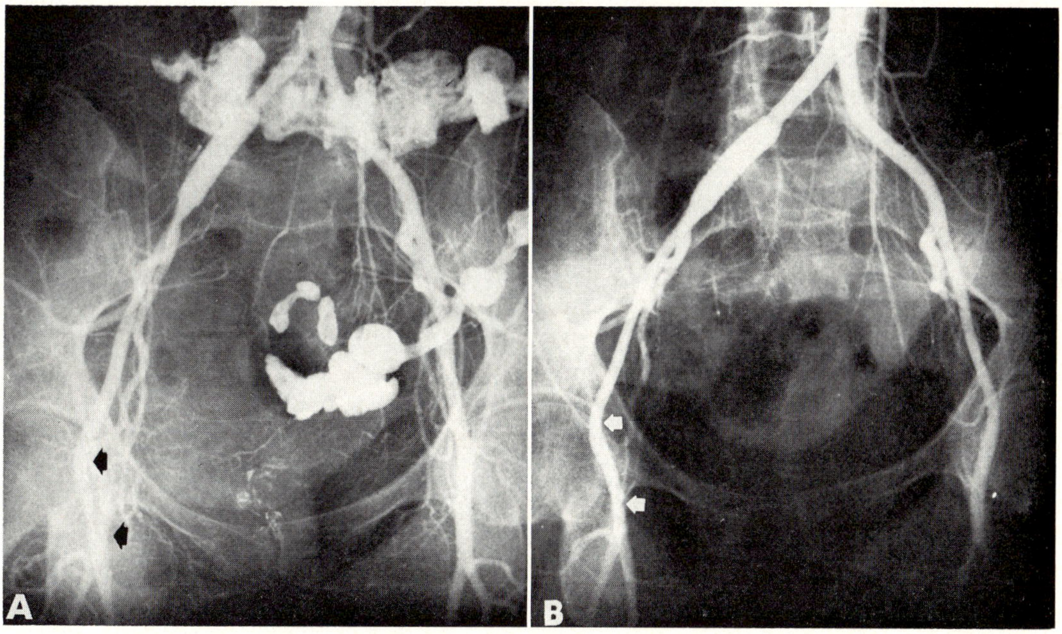

Fig. 3. Aortograms at 1 year *(A)* and 7 years *(B)* following replacement of the right common femoral artery with a right common iliac autograft (arrows). Previous irradiation to the right groin for the treatment of malignancy had caused sloughing of the skin and necrosis of the artery, leading to hemorrhage. Two weeks after arterial grafting, the wound was covered with a split-thickness skin graft.

were aneurysms of the carotid artery in two patients (Figs. 1 and 2), disruption of a Dacron graft anastomosis in the groin in two patients, bleeding from irradiation necrosis of the common femoral artery in an open wound (Fig. 3), and an abscess surrounding the full length of an aortobilateral common femoral Dacron bypass graft (Fig. 4). Normal arterial function was restored in all six. The patient with the abdominal abscess died of uremia secondary to inoperable bilateral renal artery stenosis 2 weeks after operation.

The need to replace or bypass a major artery in an area adjacent to an active joint prompted the use of an arterial autograft in 41 patients. The primary lesions were malignant invasion or primary aneurysm of the common carotid artery in seven patients, occlusion or aneurysm in the subclavian-axillary arteries in five patients (Fig. 5), occlusion, false aneurysm, or hemorrhage of the common femoral and profunda femoris arteries in 26 patients, and true or false aneurysm of the popliteal artery in eight patients. Seventeen patients needed a common femo-

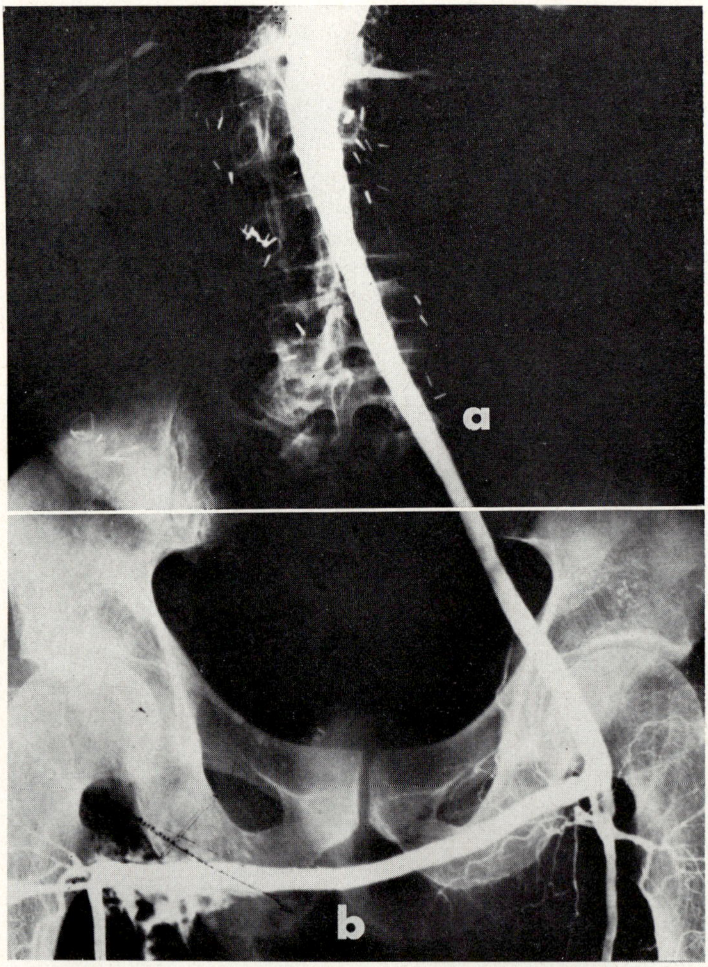

Fig. 4. Postmortem aortogram in a patient whose infected aortofemoral Dacron graft was replaced by an autograft. The previously occluded superficial femoral arteries were removed and opened by endarterectomy. One artery was grafted from the aorta to the left common femoral artery *(A)* The other graft was used for a femoral-femoral bypass *(B)*. The patient recovered from the infection but died from uremia 15 days postoperatively. Autopsy showed bilateral advanced nephrosclerosis.

ral arterial graft, and one patient needed a popliteal arterial graft because of anastomotic disruption or thrombosis of an earlier Dacron prosthesis. In each case technical factors and potential postoperative infection favored an arterial graft in preference to another Dacron prosthesis. In the patients with popliteal aneurysms the diameter of the popliteal artery distal to the aneurysm was more than double the diameter of the saphenous vein. The comparable diameters of the autograft and the distal popliteal artery favored the use of the larger vessel (Fig. 6). Whenever a vessel longer than the donor artery was needed, a composite graft of a synthetic and autogenous artery was fashioned. The autograft segment was applied at the mobile end and the synthetic graft was used for the portion in the midthigh or abdomen.

The most recent indication for arterial autografts has been the need for replacement of a stenosed or occluded visceral or renal artery. The donor artery was usually the hypogastric artery.

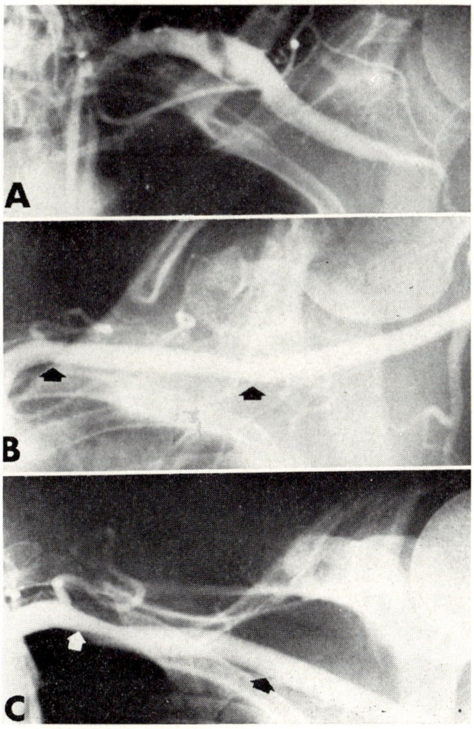

Fig. 5. Subclavian arteriogram preoperatively *(A)* and at 1 year *(B)* and 8 years *(C)* after autograft replacement of a subclavian aneurysm.

Compression of the celiac axis by the median arcuate ligament of the diaphragm is often complicated by secondary intimal hyperplasia or fibrosis.[1] In 14 of 20 patients operated upon for celiac axis compression, division of the arcuate ligament failed to restore a normal arterial lumen. Of the various techniques for management of residual stenosis of the celiac axis, autograft replacement of the celiac artery is the easiest to perform and was used in six patients (Fig. 7). The graft is anastomosed to the anterior surface of the aorta proximal to the celiac axis and to the divided end of the celiac axis beyond the level of stenosis.

Arterial autografts have been used most often in patients with renovascular hypertension secondary to fibromuscular hyperplasia of the main renal arteries.[3] The grafts were unilateral in 33 patients and bilateral in two. The ease of anastomosis to the fragile thin-walled renal artery distal to the level of stenosis is in marked contrast to the relative awkwardness which occurs when synthetic grafts are used. Because we can always obtain a hypogastric artery of suitable size through the original abdominal incision, we prefer to use this vessel rather than a segment of the saphenous vein. The graft is customarily anastomosed to the side of the aorta proximal to the origin of the inferior mesenteric artery and to the divided end of the distal renal artery (Fig. 8).

RESULTS

Early postoperative arteriograms were obtained in all patients. The autograft thrombosed in the early postoperative period in three patients. In one of these cases the graft had been used for renal artery replacement in a patient with residual minor stenotic lesions at the renal artery bifurcation beyond the distal anastomosis. In two patients occlusion of an endarterectomized external iliac donor artery used for common femoral artery replacement developed in the second postoperative week. Both operations were

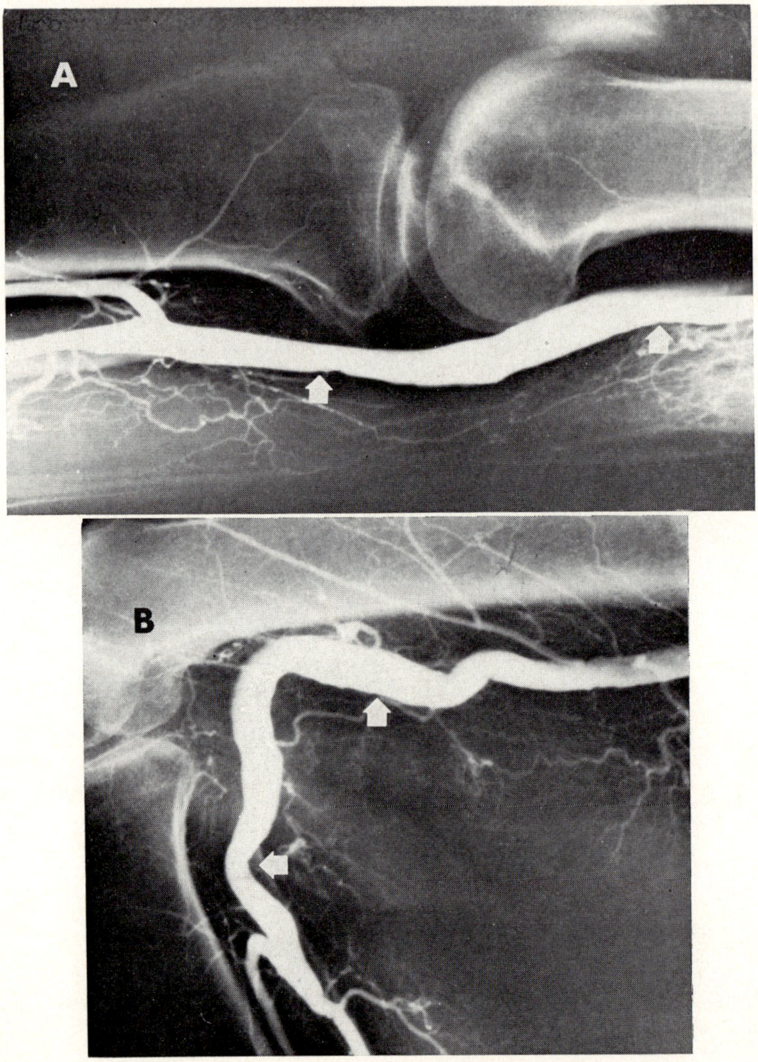

Fig. 6. *A* and *B,* Arteriograms at 1 year following replacement of a popliteal aneurysm by an external iliac autograft (arrows).

performed to overcome recurrent occlusions of aortofemoral synthetic bypass grafts in patients with previous occlusion of the superficial femoral arteries. Technical difficulties in developing an adequate profunda femoris lumen distal to the graft probably caused autograft thrombosis. One patient had postoperative hemorrhage from loss of the ligature on a branch of the autograft.

Ninety-one of 94 patients surviving operation were discharged from the hospital with 95 patent autografts. Late graft occlusion has developed in seven patients during a follow-up period of 2 months to 8½ years (average 4 years). Four of the late occlusions occurring 1 to 5 years postoperatively were in grafts anastomosed to the distal common femoral or profunda femoris arteries in patients with occlusion of the superficial femoral arteries. Progression of distal atherosclerotic lesions was considered to be the cause of graft occlusion. A composite Dacron autograft to the popliteal artery occluded at 7 months in a patient with obstructive outflow lesions. A celiac graft with an anastomotic defect demonstrated postoperatively

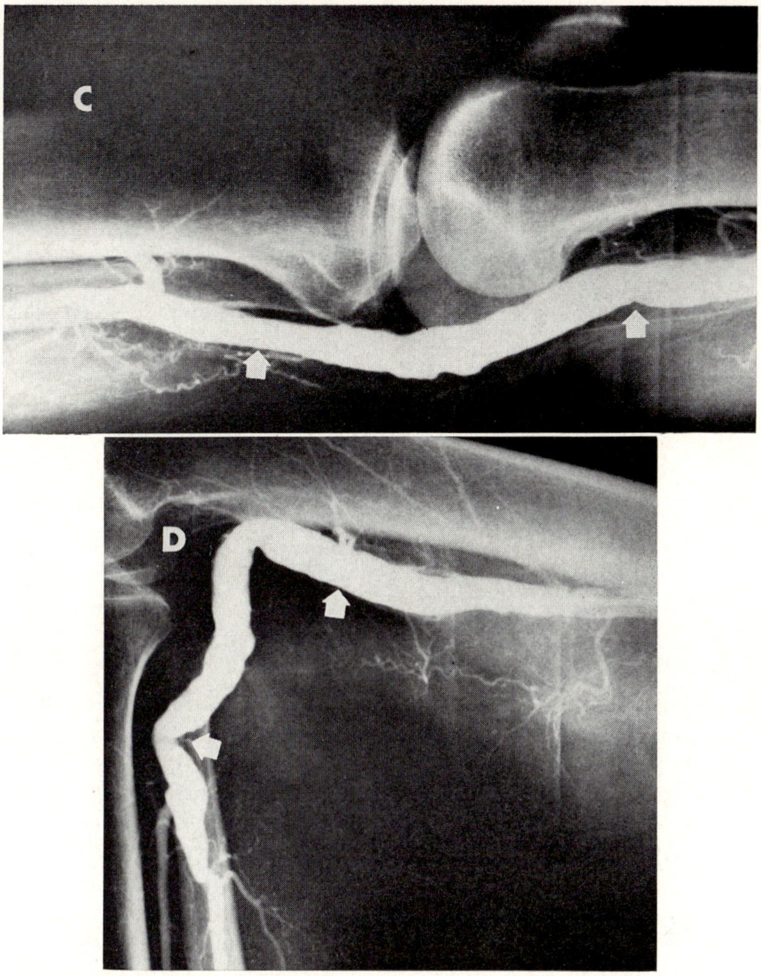

Fig. 6. *C* and *D*, Arteriograms at 8 years following replacement of a popliteal aneurysm by an external iliac autograft (arrows).

was shown to be occluded on a second postoperative arteriogram taken 3 years later. One occlusion was in an endarterectomized iliac autograft used to replace an aneurysm of the subclavian artery which preoperatively had been the source of recurrent emboli to the arm.

Eleven patients have died from causes unrelated to the grafting operations. The grafts were patent to the time of death during an average follow-up period of 3½ years. Seventy-four autografts in 72 living patients are still clinically patent in follow-up periods of 3 months to 8½ years. Recent arteriograms were obtained in 13 of the longest functioning autografts in each of the sites of application. The lumen of the grafts showed no change from that seen postoperatively in 11 patients. In one patient an external iliac graft used to replace a popliteal aneurysm showed slight irregular dilatation after 8 years (Fig. 6, *C* and *D*). This may represent progression of diffuse arterial ectasia which was seen in all of the major arteries on preoperative aortograms. In another patient, moderate narrowing of the full length of a femoral popliteal bypass autograft was evident after 3 years. Seven years after operation, this graft is still open, without further narrowing.

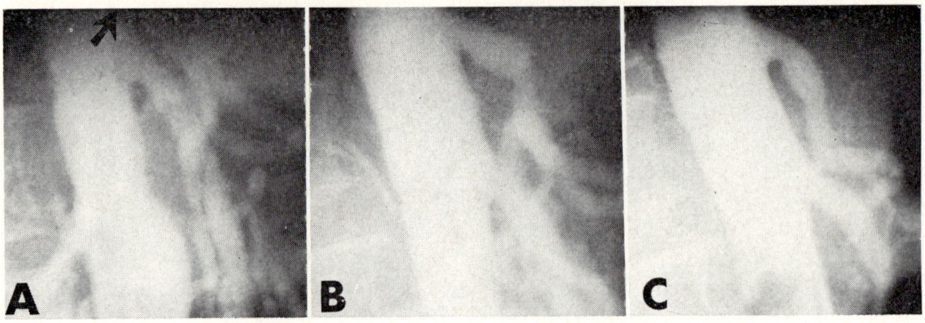

Fig. 7. Aortograms preoperatively *(A)* and at 1 month *(B)* and 3½ years *(C)* following replacement of the celiac artery with a hypogastric autograft. Stenosis of the celiac artery (arrow) persisted following division of the median arcuate ligament of the diaphragm.

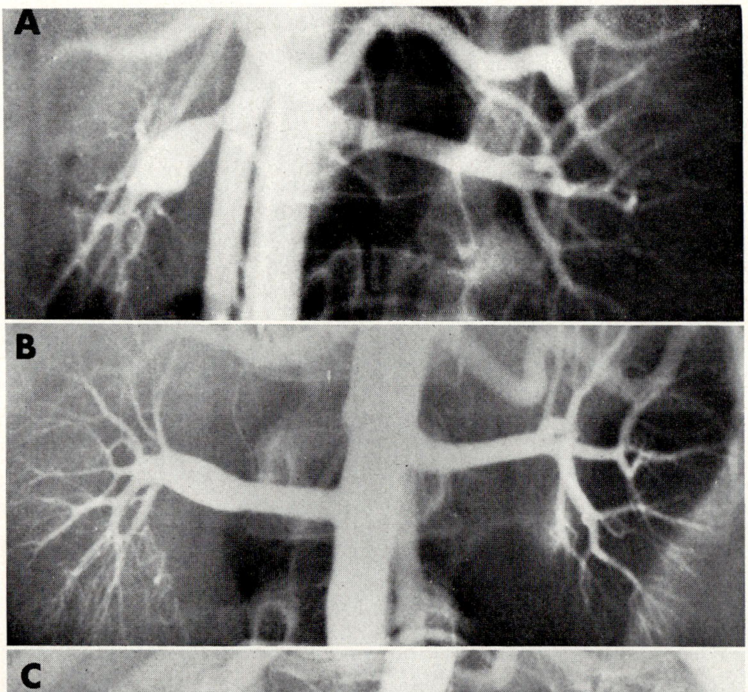

Fig. 8. Aortograms preoperatively *(A)* and at 1 month *(B)* and 5 years *(C)* following replacement of the right renal artery. The original stenosis was caused by fibromuscular hyperplasia.

SUMMARY

A total of 101 arterial autografts in 95 patients have been followed for periods extending to 8 years. The donor arteries were either segments of the iliac arterial system, or occluded superficial femoral arteries reopened by endarterectomy. Technical errors in three operations and progression of the original arterial disease in seven patients caused autograft occlusion. Normal function has persisted in 91 grafts. Arterial autografts appear particularly suited in clinical situations where graft mobility, resistance to infection, and ease of anastomosis are critical.

REFERENCES

1. Lord, R. S. A., Stoney, R. J., and Wylie, E. J.: Coeliac-axis compression, Lancet **2:** 795, 1968.
2. Wylie, E. J.: Vascular replacement with arterial autografts, SURGERY **57:** 14, 1965.
3. Wylie, E. J., Perloff, D. L., and Stoney, R. J.: Autogenous tissue revascularization techniques in surgery for renovascular hypertension, Ann. Surg. In press.

DISCUSSION

Dr. Jere W. Lord, Jr. (New York, N. Y.). This is a beautifully presented paper by Drs. Stoney and Wylie and prompts me to rise for two reasons.

First, I'm not sure that many in the audience realize that in Dr. Wylie's early career 25 years ago, he also had a distinguished career as a softball player when he was a resident at the New York Hospital. On one of these occasions in Central Park, he was warming up—he was selected as first baseman because, as you know, he's tall and lean. A ball was thrown to him and, subsequently, it was necessary to repair his mallet finger. Despite this he has gone on to do many distinguished surgical procedures.

Second, and the thing that really is important is that he has been a pioneer in the concept of using autogenous tissue in the repair of vessels, particularly in endarterectomies and more recently in arterial grafts.

It surprised me, in looking up the literature recently, that there was only one reference in the literature to the use of the autogenous saphenous vein to bypass from the common iliac or external iliac artery to the common, superficial, and profunda femoral arteries. Several angiograms in their paper showed the autogenous artery crossing the inguinal ligament.

It would appear obvious to all of us that autogenous tissue is better than a prosthesis when placed deep to the inguinal ligament into an artery in the thigh.

We have used the saphenous vein in a small number of cases, seven to be precise, with success in all, to bypass from the common and proximal external iliac arteries to the femoral vessels. One of them goes back 14 years.

I think the concept of using an endarterectomized autogenous artery is an exceedingly good one.

Our observation in operations for aneurysmal disease and also occlusive disease of the aortoiliac arteries is that the hypogastric arteries usually have far-advanced atherosclerotic changes.

Thank you very much for the privilege of discussing this excellent paper.

Dr. Stoney (closing). I would like to thank Dr. Lord for his comments.

We used an endarterectomized artery which had been previously occluded for an arterial autograft in 24 cases. The occluded vessel is excised and following thromboendarterectomy a satisfactory vessel is available for grafting. This type of autograft compared favorably to previously patent arterial segments removed and utilized as arterial autografts.

The hypogastric artery is usually removed and used as free graft for repairing renal or visceral artery stenosis. Patients who have fibromuscular hyperplasia of the renal artery or compression of the celiac axis have very little other arterial disease. The hypogastric artery is therefore normal and is available for these clinical instances.

I would like to thank the Society for the privilege of presenting this paper.

Femorofemoral and axillofemoral grafts—compromise or preference

VICTOR PARSONNET, M.D.
JOSEPH ALPERT, M.D.
DONALD K. BRIEF, M.D.
NEWARK, N. J.
From the Department of Surgery, Newark Beth Israel Medical Center

Axillofemoral[2] and femorofemoral[13] grafts originally were devised to salvage ischemic legs when aortoiliac reconstruction was not feasible. Some grafts have functioned so well, however, that one might consider the operation the procedure of choice in certain types of occlusive arterial disease.[11]

Various "donor" and "recipient" arteries have been interconnected, such as femorofemoral,[14, 18-20] iliofemoral,[13] femoropopliteal,[5] axillofemoral,[3, 6, 7-9, 10, 15, 16, 20] carotid-subclavian, and carotid-carotid grafts.[20] All of these operations are extraperitoneal and extrathoracic, and because the grafts are essentially subcutaneous only light general or local anesthesia is required. They are, therefore, particularly suitable for elderly and poor risk patients.

Our experience with 59 crossover grafts at the Newark Beth Israel Medical Center includes 10 carotid-subclavian, 11 axillofemoral, and 38 femorofemoral grafts. This report deals with the 49 operations performed for occlusive disease of the aorto-iliac segment.

METHOD

Both axillofemoral and femorofemoral grafts were performed in accordance with earlier descriptions of others.[1, 2, 18] The donor vessel for the axillofemoral graft was the second or third portion of the axillary artery. When the second portion was used it was necessary to divide the pectoralis minor tendon; this maneuver often simplified the anastomosis and permitted the graft to come off the artery at an oblique angle (Fig. 1). In a femorofemoral graft, in order to attach the graft to the external iliac or the proximal anastomosis, it was necessary it attach the graft to the external iliac or high on the common femoral artery. Most proximal anastomoses, however, were made at right angles to the common femoral artery (Fig. 2).

Twenty grafts were made of knitted and 28 of woven Dacron of 8 to 10 mm. diameter. One femorofemoral graft was done with a segment of reversed autogenous saphenous vein (Fig. 3).

Clinical case material. There were 49 complete operations in 47 patients (exclusive of early postoperative revisions); 33 of the patients were men and 14 women; the average age was 67 in the axillofemoral group and 62 in the femorofemoral group. The average follow-up was 9 months and 14 months, respectively (Table I).

Patients were selected for operation for impending or frank gangrene of the extremity in 31 cases, and for incapacitating claudication or rest pain in the remaining 18. With the exception of a few of the most recent patients in whom surgical indications were somewhat relaxed, all patients were unsuitable candidates for aortofemoral reconstruction because of old age, cardiopulmonary disease, or cancer. Twenty-one patients were diabetic.

Presented at the Twenty-third Annual Meeting of the Society for Vascular Surgery, New York, N. Y., July 12-13, 1969.

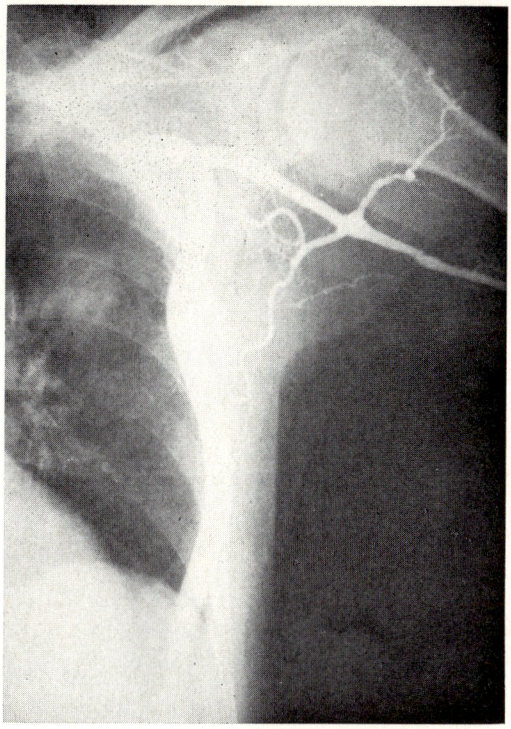

Fig. 1. Upper anastomosis of axillofemoral bypass to second portion of axillary artery. The graft leaves the artery at an oblique angle.

The site of inflow obstruction in the axillofemoral group was in the aorta or common iliac arteries; in the femorofemoral group most of the obstructions were in the common iliac artery, but one third were due to various combinations of external iliac and common femoral artery obstruction.

The outflow vessels were often severely diseased so that in 33 of the 47 patients thromboendarterectomy of the recipient artery was necessary before adequate runoff was obtained. An ultrasonic flowmeter, used in six patients, proved important in one, when despite an adequate pulse in the profunda femoris artery the flow was only 15 c.c. per minute. After endarterectomy of the profunda femoris artery 2 cm. from its orifice, the flow was over 200 c.c. per minute and the graft has remained patent. In 21 cases the only runoff vessel was the profunda femoris artery.

Axillofemoral grafts were indicated when the aorta or both iliac artery segments were obstructed. If obstruction was confined to one iliac artery, a femorofemoral graft was

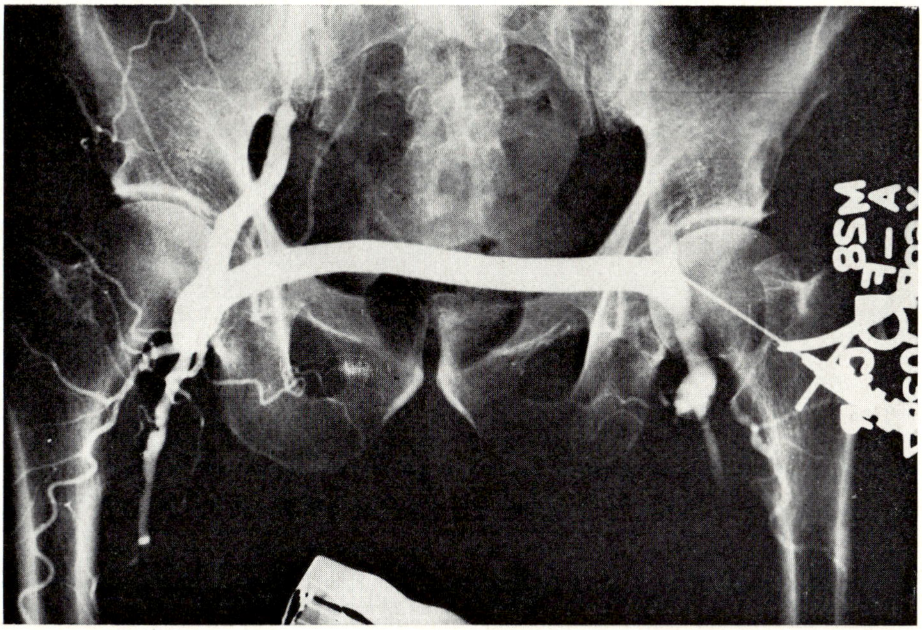

Fig. 2. Femorofemoral graft of woven Dacron. (Flow is from right to left.) The proximal anastomosis from the donor artery (to the reader's right) makes an angle of more than 90 degrees (see text).

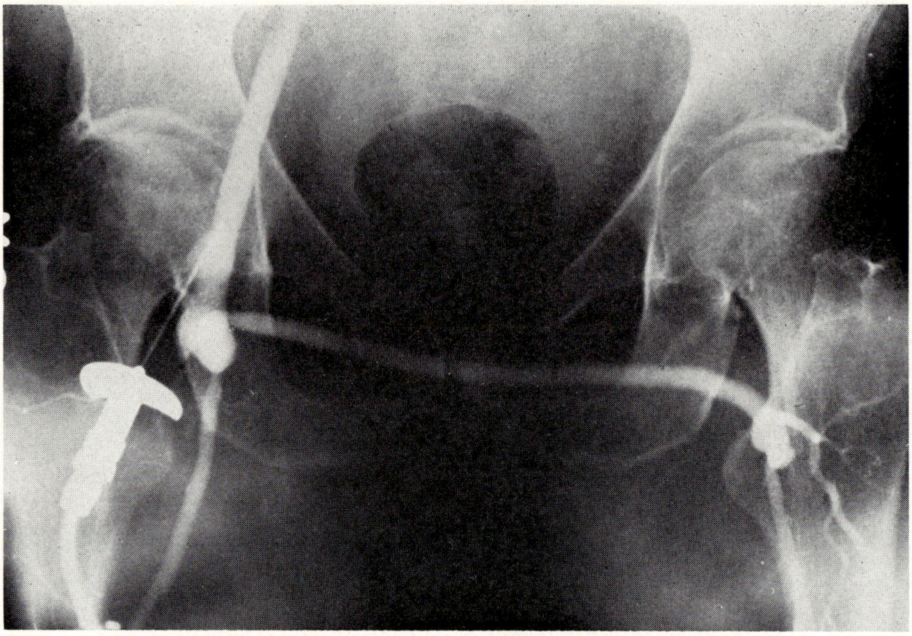

Fig. 3. Femorofemoral graft of reversed autogenous saphenous vein. (Flow is from left to right.) The distal anastomosis has been made to two separate branches of the profunda femoris artery; the superficial femoral artery is obstructed on both sides.

Table I. *Age, sex, and follow-up period of 47 patients with axillofemoral and femorofemoral grafts*

	No. of cases	*Sex*		*Ages*	*Follow-up*
		M	*F*		
Axillofemoral	9	6	3	58 to 88 (average 67)	1 to 18 (average 9)
Femorofemoral	38	27	11	45 to 85 (average 62)	1 to 27 (average 14)

performed. In four cases in which the inflow of the donor femoral artery was questionable, intra-arterial femoral artery pressures were compared to the pressure in the brachial artery. If the mean pressure differential was more than 5 mm. Hg, a femorofemoral graft was not done.

Of the nine patients with axillofemoral grafts, five were on the right and four on the left. In the femorofemoral group, however, 28 of the 38 obstructions were on the left.

Operative results. In the nine patients with axillofemoral grafts there were three early failures. One of these was completely revised and remained patent; the other two patients required leg amputations. There were three late obstructions, one of which was successfully revised, one was revised but failed and the limb remains ischemic, and the third was converted to a femorofemoral graft, because the axillary artery was thrombosed (Table II).

In the 38 femorofemoral grafts there were four early failures, one at the operating table that could not be revised, one in the immediate postoperative period that was not revised because the original obstruction in

Table II. *Early and late graft closures and long-term patency of axillofemoral and femorofemoral grafts*

	Axillofemoral	*Femoro-femoral*
No. of patients	9*	38
Early thrombosis	3	4
Results	1 revised 2 major amputations	2 revised 1 removed
Late thrombosis	3	—
Results	1 reoperation, patent 1 reoperation, failed 1 converted to femorofemoral	—
Long-term patency	4/8 (50%)	36 (95%)

*One early postoperative death (graft patent).

Table III. *Immediate and long-term limb salvage in patients with axillofemoral and femorofemoral grafts and impending gangrene*

	No. of patients	*Immediate*	*Long-term*
Axillofemoral	9	7	4*
Femorofemoral	22	20 (2 limbs lost despite patent grafts)	20

*One late failure (infection).

the external iliac artery had been removed and the functioning bypass was not necessary, and two that were revised and remained patent. There have been no late failures in this group, and no deaths.

There was one hospital death in the axillofemoral group. In seven there was immediate limb salvage, and long-term salvage in four of these. One patient lost his leg after 9 months when the graft was removed for infection that involved the entire length of the graft.

Of the 22 patients with impending or frank gangrene in the femorofemoral group, there was immediate and long-term limb salvage in 20. Two patients lost their limbs although their grafts remained patent, one from secondary venous gangrene that was due to phlegmasia cerulea dolens, and one for progressive small vessel disease in the distal leg (Table III).

Important postoperative problems were frequent in the axillofemoral group, half the operations being complicated by early thrombosis, hemorrhage, false aneurysm, or infection. In two cases there was late thrombosis of the axillary artery, one following the second repair of a false aneurysm due to sepsis and one occurring spontaneously. In neither case was the arm severely compromised and function has remained near normal. By contrast, there were only six (16 percent) complications in the femorofemoral group, and the patients' progress tended to remain relatively uneventful.

DISCUSSION

So far, crossover grafts have not been used in preference to aortofemoral grafts in relatively good risk patients. It has been suggested that the recipient artery will "steal" blood from the "donor" limb, especially if the graft produces a "borrowing-lending" phenomenon such as has been reported following sympathectomy.[12, 20] Common sense should tell us, however, that this will not occur. For example, exercise of the right arm does not steal blood from the brain, even though there is a common "donor" innominate artery. It has also been believed that flow through the donor artery may be inadequate for both legs. But consider, for example, that during cardiopulmonary bypass, the entire cardiac output of an adult can pass through a tube with a diameter of ⅜ inch. Further study has shown that the flow through an artery is in general not affected by the diameter, but by the peripheral vascular resistance. Ehrenfeld and associates[4] demonstrated that the flow can increase as much as 10 times normal in the donor artery. In experimental femorofemoral

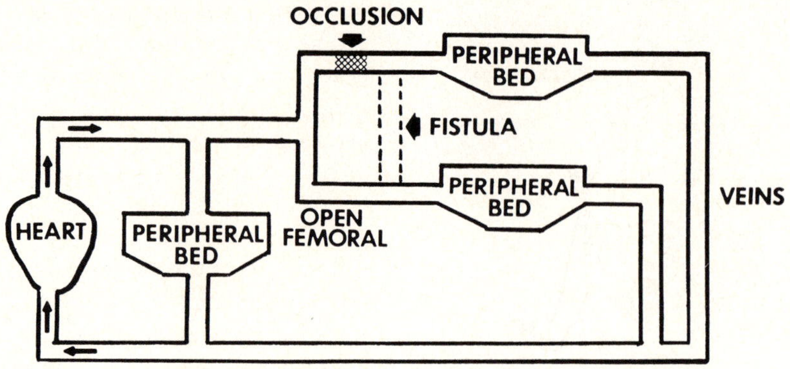

Fig. 4. Diagram of circulation to lower extremities. Note that the resistance beds of the legs are in parallel.

grafts, the flow of the donor artery doubled, and in the distal donor artery it remained the same after the graft was allowed to flow.

These flow patterns are shown diagrammatically in Fig. 4. One notes that the resistances of the limbs are in parallel. It has been stated that vascular resistances *in parallel* roughly obey electrical analogies.[21]

If the total resistance in parallel can be calculated by

$$\frac{1}{R} = \frac{1}{r_1} + \frac{1}{r_2 \;.\;.\; r_n}.$$

Then $$R = \frac{r_1 \quad r_2}{r_1 + \quad r_2}$$

or, substituting in Ohm's law, where $I = \dfrac{E}{R}$

$$I = \frac{E}{\dfrac{r_1 \quad r_2}{r_1 + r_2}}.$$

Therefore, if the new limb perfused by the donor artery has the same resistance as the donor limb, the total resistance would be half and the flow of the donor artery would double.

We have studied flow in three patients with crossover femoral grafts with the graft clamped and opened. (Typical findings are seen in Fig. 5.) When the graft was opened there was a transient drop in pressure in the donor artery; this rapidly returned to normal and was followed by an increase in flow to about double the original volume. In the distal donor artery (beyond the graft origin), both pressure and flow dropped for a few moments but quickly returned to their original levels.

Clinical observation has revealed no subsequent problems with the donor limb. This fact, plus the observed intraoperative findings, indicates that there are no deleterious rheologic effects of femorofemoral grafts on the donor artery or limb.

Atherosclerosis, although a generalized process, tends to be symmetrical. Therefore, in performing femorofemoral grafts for unilateral iliac artery occlusion we have been concerned that progression of the disease process in the *donor* iliac artery would eventually lead to its occlusion. Follow-up in our series has not been sufficiently long to assure us that this will not happen, but others have also observed continued patency of the donor vessel.[19] This lack of progression suggests that the increase in flow may have a protective effect, perhaps by a decrease in the lateral pressure associated with the increase in flow.

The sites of iliac artery occlusion in the femorofemoral group revealed one unusual feature in that 76 percent of the occlusions were on the left. This would occur by chance

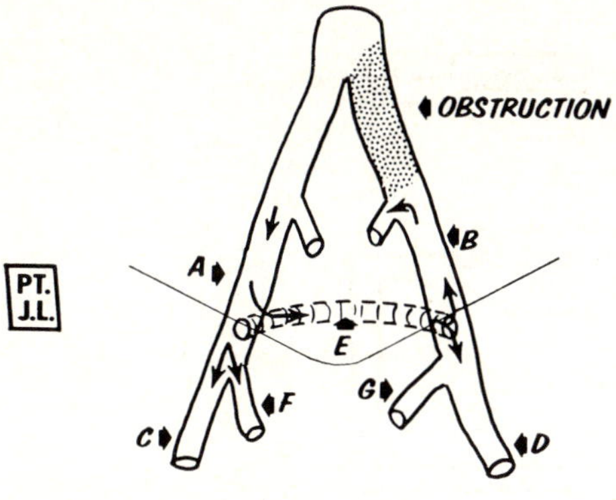

GRAFT	A	B	C	D	E	F	G
CLAMPED	300	260	100	200	0	?	?
OPEN	611	268*	100**	200	462	?	?

FLOWS - cc/minute

* DIRECTION OF FLOW REVERSED?
**POPLITEAL OCCLUSION DISTALLY

Fig. 5. Diagram of intraoperative flow studies with the femorofemoral graft clamped and opened. Probes were not applied to the profunda femoris artery (*F* and *G*), and therefore the precise distribution of the runoff is not known. Also, there was a peripheral block of the right superficial femoral artery *(C)* which explains the low flow rate in that vessel. Despite a flow of 462 c.c. per minute through the graft, there was no change in flow in the femoral artery below the proximal anastomosis *(C)*, and the flow in the proximal donor artery *(a)* doubled.

19 times in 10,000 cases—the odds against it are 500 to 1. The reasons for this difference are obscure but may have to do with the effects of flow patterns on atherogenesis at the aortic bifurcation, or perhaps with subtle difference in patient selection.

The possibility that there will be damage to the host artery from technical mishaps cannot be ruled out. With femorofemoral grafts this has not been reported so far, but in axillofemoral grafts arm claudication has been seen.[10, 16] There were two cases of thrombosis of the axillary artery in our series, one secondary to massive thrombosis of the graft caused by poor runoff, and the other caused by infection, false aneurysm, and repeated surgical intervention at the proximal anastomosis. In neither case was there any permanent damage to the arm.

The configuration of the anastomosis between the proximal femoral artery and the graft is not the best one for optimum flow, because the graft comes off at an angle greater than 90 degrees (see Fig. 2). It has been shown that an angle of about 15 degrees provides the best flow pattern,[16] and the least transition from laminar to turbulent flow.[22] Although a bruit, presumably from turbulence, can often be heard over the anastomosis, there have been no late failures in the femorofemoral group, and there has been no pressure differential between the graft and host artery in the two patients in whom such measurements were made.

We believe that the good immediate and long-term results in femorofemoral grafts can be explained by the fact that the grafts are short (approximately 17 cm.). In contrast, axillofemoral grafts are approximately 45 cm. long, and are, therefore, more prone to a closure from torsion, kinks, external pressure, or spontaneous thrombosis on the long graft surface not covered with neointima.

Despite advanced atherosclerosis in the recipient artery, all but two femorofemoral grafts were carried out successfully; in 21 cases the only runoff vessel was the profunda femoris artery.[19] Often this artery had also been occluded, and was opened by removing the atheromatous plug from its orifice. In two patients pedal pulses returned despite continued obstruction of the superficial femoral artery.

Major complication rate and immediate and late graft thrombosis were all more common in the axillofemoral than the femorofemoral grafts. Thirty-six of the 38 femorofemoral grafts remained patent over an average follow-up period of 14 months; but only four of the eight surviving patients in the axillofemoral group have patent grafts after 9 months.

CONCLUSION

Axillofemoral grafts are useful for the treatment of impending gangrene caused by occlusion of the aorta or both iliac arteries. The high complication rate and high incidence of late failure, however, suggest that they should not be used as a preferential procedure in patients who are able to tolerate standard aortofemoral bypass procedures.

Femorofemoral grafts are indicated in patients with unilateral iliac artery occlusion. Despite a wide angle at the proximal anastomosis and even when runoff is limited to the profunda femoris artery, these grafts tend to remain patent. Although originally intended for desperate situations, they may, in our opinion, be used in any patient with unilateral iliofemoral artery occlusion.

The curious preponderance of left-sided occlusions (76 percent) in this group was noteworthy.

REFERENCES

1. Alpert, J., Brief, D. K., and Parsonnet, V.: Vascular restoration for aortoiliac occlusion —an alternate approach to the poor risk patient, J. Newark Beth Israel Hosp. **18:** 4, 1967.
2. Blaisdell, F. W., and Hall, A. D.: Axillary-femoral artery bypass for lower extremity ischemia, Surgery **54:** 563, 1963.
3. DeAvila, R., Doyle, J., and Heaney, J. P.: Axillary-femoral bypass, Arch. Surg. **92:** 118, 1966.
4. Ehrenfeld, W. K., Harris, J. D., and Wylie, E. J.: Vascular "steal" phenomenon. An experimental study, Amer. J. Surg. **116:** 192, 1968.
5. Goetz, R. H., and Lord, J. W., Jr.: Cross-over femoropopliteal shunt, Surgery **64:** 681, 1968.
6. Gorman, J. E., and Douglas, F. M.: Axillary-femoral artery bypass, Arch. Surg. **91:** 509, 1965.
7. Jackson, B. B., and Ward, W. W.: Contralateral axillofemoral bypass graft, Amer. J. Surg. **110:** 926, 1965.
8. Kupic, E. A., and Mackenzie, J. R.: Angiographic demonstration of cross pelvic collateral circulation following bilateral axillary femoral bypass, Amer. J. Roentgen. **102:** 418, 1968.
9. Lewis, C. D.: A subclavian artery as a means of blood supply to the lower half of the body, Brit. J. Surg. **48:** 574, 1961.
10. Louw, J. H.: The treatment of combined aortoiliac and femoropopliteal occlusive disease by splenofemoral and axillofemoral bypass grafts, Surgery **55:** 387, 1964.
11. Mannick, J. A., and Nabseth, D. C.: Axillofemoral bypass graft. A safe alternative to aortoiliac reconstruction, New Eng. J. Med. **278:** 461, 1968.
12. May, A. G., De Weese, J. A., and Rob, C. G.: Effect of sympathectomy on blood flow in arterial stenosis, Ann. Surg. **158:** 182, 1963.
13. McCaughan, J. J., Jr., and Kahn, S. F.: Cross-over graft for unilateral occlusive disease of the iliofemoral arteries, Ann. Surg. **151:** 26, 1960.
14. Papadopoulos, C. D.: Cross-over femorofemoral bypass, Amer. J. Surg. **111:** 216, 1966.
15. Pierangeli, A., and Guernelli, N.: The axillofemoral bypass as a treatment of the obstruction of the aortoiliac junctions in the poor risk patients, J. Cardiov. Surg. **8:** 353, 1967.
16. Sauvage, L. R., and Wood, S. J.: Unilateral axillary bilateral femoral bifurcation graft: A procedure for the poor risk patient with aortoiliac disease, Surgery **60:** 573, 1966.
17. Szilagyi, D. E., Whitcomb, J. G., Schenker, W., and Waibel, P.: The laws of fluid flow and arterial grafting, Surgery **47:** 55, 1960.
18. Vetto, R. M.: The treatment of unilateral iliac artery obstruction with a transabdominal, subcutaneous, femorofemoral graft, Surgery **52:** 342, 1962.
19. Vetto, R. M.: The femorofemoral shunt. An appraisal, Amer. J. Surg. **112:** 162, 1966.
20. Warren, W. D., and Fomon, J. J.: Rerouting arterial flow to relieve ischemia: Femorofemoral, axillary-femoral, and carotid-carotid artery bypasses, Ann. Surg. **163:** 131, 1963.
21. Weale, F. E.: The values of series and parallel resistances in steady blood flow, Brit. J. Surg. **51:** 623, 1964.
22. Wesolowski, S. A., Sauvage, L. R., Pinc, R. S., and Fries, C. C.: Dynamics of blood flow in graft disproportions and in normal blood vessels, Surg. Forum **6:** 227, 1955.

DISCUSSION

Dr. Albert D. Hall (San Francisco, Calif.). I rise to compliment Dr. Parsonnet on his fine presentation.

His series interests us because 7 years ago when Bill Blaisdell and I first performed the axillary-femoral operation, we had the opportunity to utilize the procedure in several cases within a short period of time. All the patients operated upon were being treated for desperate conditions such as retroperitoneal sepsis, thrombosis of the aorta, and recent myocardial infarction. Many of these operations were performed under local anesthesia, and the grafts functioned very adequately in perfusing the lower extremities.

As a result of our initial experience we investigated the axillary-femoral bypass as an alternative procedure to conventional aortoiliac reconstruction in patients who were poor operative risks for laparotomy. In the years 1963 through 1966, we compiled an experience of 40 axillary-femoral operations and now have a combined series between the Veterans Administration Hospital and the San Francisco General Hospital of 55 axillary-femoral operations.

The 2 year patency rate has been 50 percent in these axillary-femoral operations and because of that, our current indications for doing the procedure are reserved for patients who have threatened loss of limb or are otherwise inoperable intra-abdominally because of sepsis or other contraindications to major operation. It has proved to be a lifesaving procedure in these instances.

With regard to cross leg grafts, we have a number of the axillary-femoral series in whom cross leg grafts have also been performed. The cross leg component of some of these patients has remained patent even though the axillary-femoral graft may have thrombosed. Our experience is similar to that of Dr. Parsonnet with a very high patency rate in the cross leg grafts.

Concerning complications, we have not seen false aneurysm formation. There are two technical factors on which I might comment. We place the proximal anastomosis at the first portion of the axillary artery adjacent to the first rib, so that there is virtually no motion of that anastomosis with abduction of the arm. At the distal anastomosis, we try to avoid anastomosing to an end-arterectomized common femoral or profundus femoral vessel, but have elected to use a patched open type end-to-side anastomosis with Dacron suture.

I appreciated the opportunity to discuss this paper.

Dr. John Keshishian (Washington, D. C.). I thought some of you might be interested in hearing of a desperate situation we had recently at the Andrews Air Force Base Hospital in Washington. A young woman who had metastatic carcinoma involving the glands in her groin was being treated with irradiation. She subsequently developed radiation necrosis and suddenly hemorrhaged from the right groin. This was stopped immediately, but the area became septic. Something had to be done to preserve the limb, even though she was dying of advanced carcinoma. Arteriograms showed that there was a distal runoff in the femoral artery.

So, we elected to join three segments of bovine heterografts kindly supplied by Dr. Henderson of Johnson & Johnson and performed an axillary-popliteal anastomosis without much difficulty. This saved the limb. We avoided the septic area, and she died of her carcinoma.

We've had a little experience with these heterografts now and have learned that they can be used with impunity above, under, and below the inguinal ligament in vascular reconstructive surgery.

Dr. Parsonnet (closing). I'd like to thank the discussants.

False aneurysm, in my experience, is usually due to complications of infection or hemorrhage at the site of the anastomosis. This is precisely the way it occurred in our case. Hemorrhage occurred and we had to take the graft out and replace it; it subsequently became infected which, eventually, led to the catastrophe.

It's also interesting that the patient had thrombosis of the graft in the early period, so we anastomosed the graft from the axillary to the femoral artery and with a branch down to the popliteal to take care of his runoff.

This graft stayed open and subsequently he got pedal pulses. But he eventually developed infection and we had to clamp his graft. There was no other way out of it. We couldn't bring it through the obturator foramen, or through the abdomen because he had had peritoneal sepsis. We eventually had to remove the functioning graft and he lost his limb. But, the axilla will supply the popliteal as attested now by two of us.

I appreciate the privilege of presenting this paper.

Aneurysmectomy in the aged?

CALDWELL B. ESSELSTYN, JR., M.D.
ALFRED W. HUMPHRIES, M.D.
JESS R. YOUNG, M.D.
EDWARD G. BEVEN, M.D.
VICTOR G. DEWOLFE, M.D.
CLEVELAND, OHIO
From the Departments of General Surgery, of Vascular Surgery, and of Peripheral Vascular Disease, The Cleveland Clinic Foundation

In general, surgical risk increases with chronologic age, because of a decrease in homeostatic reserve and an increase in frequency of associated disease. Therefore, a point may be reached when the surgical risk exceeds the danger of the primary disease.

Although it is generally conceded that aneurysmectomy and replacement with a graft is the indicated procedure in most patients with abdominal aortic aneurysm, the justification of this method of treatment in the aged has been questioned.[1] To help resolve this controversy, we are reviewing our experience with patients who were 75 years of age or older when first seen at the Cleveland Clinic with a diagnosis of abdominal aortic aneurysm.

CLINICAL MATERIAL

Between the years 1954 and 1968, we examined 152 patients with abdominal aneurysm who were 75 years of age or older at the time of diagnosis. The age range was 75 to 88 years; the average age was 78 years.

Eighty-two patients (54 percent) underwent resection and graft replacement of the aneurysm. Sixteen of these patients were operated on for ruptured aneurysm, 29 for symptomatic aneurysm, and 37 for asymptomatic aneurysm.

Seventy patients (46 percent)did not undergo operation. In 47 patients the risk of surgery was considered prohibitive because of the severity of associated diseases. Seven patients were found to be in good health, but operation was not performed because of the small size (5 cm. or less) of the aneurysm. Seven patients were seen in

Table I. *Cause of death (82 operative patients)*

Cause of death	No. of deaths: In-hospital	No. of deaths: Late
Myocardial infarct	7	5
Renal failure	3	3
Pneumonia	2	3
Peritonitis	2	2
Heart failure	2	1
Stroke	0	3
Ruptured thoracic aneurysm	0	3
Pulmonary embolus	1	2
Pulmonary failure	2	0
Aortoenteric fistula	1	1
Cancer	0	2
Hemorrhagic diathesis	1	0
Septicemia	1	0
Hepatitis	0	1
Shock	1	0
Hemorrhage	1	0
Not known	0	7
Subtotals	24	33
Total	57	

Presented at the Twenty-third Annual Meeting of the Society for Vascular Surgery, New York, N. Y., July 12-13, 1969.

other departments at the clinic and were not considered for surgery on the basis of age alone. Surgery was advised but was refused by eight patients.

As expected, the incidence of associated disease was high in these patients: 77 percent had arteriosclerotic heart disease, and 67 percent had significant hypertension.

We have been able to follow the progress of all patients in the operated group and all but one in the group who were not surgically treated.

RESULTS

Operated group. Of the 16 patients who were operated on for ruptured aneurysm ten (63 percent) died in the hospital; of the 29 patients operated on for symptomatic aneurysm, 12 (41 percent) died; of the 37 patients operated on for asymptomatic aneurysm, 5 (14 percent) died. The cause of these deaths as well as the cause of late deaths are listed in Table I.

The accumulative survival rates are shown in tabular and in graphic form in Tables II and III and Fig. 1, respectively.

Nonoperated group. Of the 69 nonoperated patients, 46 (67 percent) have died. The causes of death are listed in Table IV. It should be noted that 17 (37 percent) died of rupture of their aneurysm. The

Table II. *Accumulative survival rate in patients operated upon electively*

Months at risk	*No. of patients at risk*	*Died during interval*	*Interval survival rate (%)*	*Accumulative survival rate (%)*	*Patient's follow-up terminated in interval*
In-hospital period	37	5	86	86	0
2- 6	32	2	94	81	3
7- 12	27	0	100	81	2
13- 24	25	1	96	78	3
25- 36	21	3	86	67	4
37- 48	14	2	86	58	1
49- 60	11	2	82	48	2
61- 72	7	1	86	41	0
73- 84	6	3	50	21	0
85- 96	3	2	33	10	0
97-108	1	0	100	10	0
109-120	1	0	100	10	0

Table III. *Accumulative survival rate in patients operated upon for ruptured or symptomatic aneurysm*

Months at risk	*No. of patients at risk*	*Died during interval*	*Interval survival rate (%)*	*Accumulative survival rate (%)*	*Patient's follow-up terminated in interval*
In-hospital period	45	22	51	51	0
2- 6	23	2	91	46	1
7-12	20	1	95	44	0
13-24	19	1	95	42	5
25-36	13	2	85	36	0
37-48	11	1	91	33	1
49-60	9	4	56	18	0
61-72	5	0	100	18	0
73-84	5	2	60	11	1
85-96	2	1	50	6	1

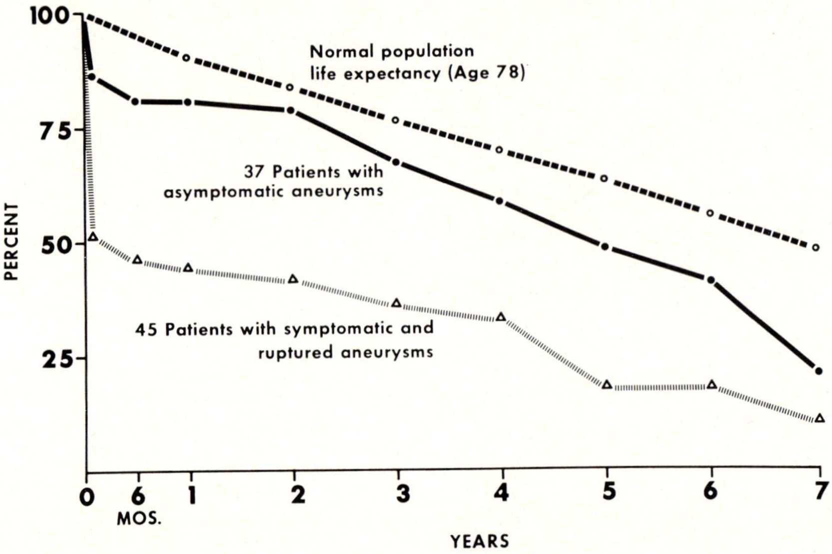

Fig. 1. Accumulative survival rates of 37 patients operated on for asymptomatic aneurysm, of 45 patients operated on for ruptured or symptomatic aneurysm, and the survival rate of the normal population, adjusted to age 78 years.

Table IV. *Causes of death (69 nonoperative patients)*

Causes	*Deaths*	*%*
Ruptured aneurysm	17	37
Myocardial infarction	9	19
Cerebrovascular accident	5	11
Other cardiovascular diseases	5	11
Pulmonary	4	9
Other	6	13
Total	46	100

Table V. *Time of death after diagnosis (69 nonoperative patients)*

	Cause of death	
Years	*Ruptured aneurysm*	*Associated diseases*
1	11	13
2	2	8
3	1	3
4	2	1
5	0	2
6	0	1
7	1	0
8	0	0
9	0	1
Subtotals	17	29
Total deaths	46	

survival time after diagnosis is listed in Table V.

The accumulative survival rate is shown in tabular and in graphic form in Table VI and Fig. 2, respectively.

DISCUSSION

In our experience, advanced age only slightly added to the risk of surgery. The in-hospital mortality rate of 14 percent among those patients operated on for asymptomatic aneurysm in the older age group compares favorably with our in-hospital mortality rate of 9 percent for asymptomatic aneurysm in patients of all ages. The in-hospital mortality rate of 49 percent among elderly patients operated on for symptomatic or ruptured aneurysms is identical to our in-hospital mortality rate for symptomatic and ruptured aneurysms in all age groups.

Once a patient has been successfully operated on, his life expectancy then parallels that of the general population in his age group (Fig. 1).

The danger of death by rupture of an abdominal aneurysm is real, regardless of

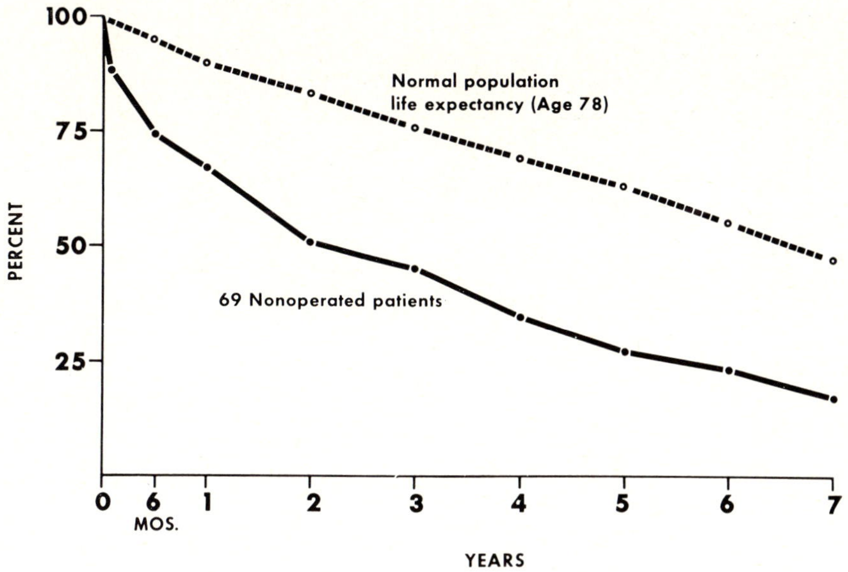

Fig. 2. Accumulative survival rate among 69 nonoperated patients.

Table VI. *Accumulative survival rate in nonoperative patients*

Months at risk	*No. of patients at risk*	*Died during interval*	*Interval survival rate (%)*	*Accumulative survival rate (%)*	*Patient's follow-up terminated in interval*
1	69	8	88	88	0
2- 6	61	10	84	74	0
7- 12	51	5	90	67	1
13- 24	45	11	76	51	6
25- 36	28	3	89	45	8
37- 48	17	4	76	34	4
49- 60	9	2	78	27	0
61- 72	7	1	86	23	2
73- 84	4	1	75	17	1
85- 96	2	0	100	17	1
97-108	1	0	100	17	0
109-120	1	1	0	0	0

the age of the patient. Of those patients in our series who were not operated on, rupture of the aneurysm was the cause of death of 37 percent. This percentage becomes highly significant when it is realized that of this group of 69 patients 54 were not operated on either because their aneurysm was small and believed to be unlikely to rupture, or their associated disease was expected to be the cause of death.

It is not possible to be dogmatic about the contraindications for surgery in patients with associated diseases. A decision for or against operation for aortic aneurysm must be based on such factors as the size of the aneurysm, the chronologic age of the patient, his estimated "physiologic age," and an estimation of his current ability to withstand major surgery. Imminently fatal diseases such as metastatic cancer, severe renal failure, severe emphysema, or incapacitating heart disease are obviously contraindications to elective surgery. In diseases of less severity, the risk of surgery must be weighed against the possible risk of rupture of the aneurysm. Since large aneurysms are more likely to rupture than small ones,[2] patients with mild angina or emphysema might not be considered candidates for surgery if their aneurysm is small, whereas patients with severe angina or mild renal failure might be operated on if the aneurysm is large. Patients with symptomatic or ruptured aneurysms undergo emergency operation regardless of the presence of associated disease.

SUMMARY AND CONCLUSION

We have reviewed our experience with 152 patients, 75 years of age or older, who had abdominal aortic aneurysms.

Of 69 nonoperated patients, 37 percent died of a ruptured aneurysm.

The in-hospital mortality rate for this older age group of 14 percent of 37 patients operated on for asymptomatic aneurysm compares favorably with our in-hospital mortality rate of 9 percent in patients of all ages operated on for asymptomatic aneurysms. The in-hospital mortality rate of 49 percent of 45 patients operated on for ruptured or symptomatic aneurysm is identical to our mortality rate for patients of all ages who were operated on for these types of aneurysms.

Once a patient has been operated on successfully, his life expectancy tends to parallel that of the normal population for his age group.

On the basis of these findings, we believe that age per se is not a contraindication to abdominal aneurysmectomy.

The authors herewith express their appreciation to their colleague, John R. Shainoff, Ph.D., for his help in making the statistical analyses.

REFERENCES

1. Bernstein, E. F., Fisher, J. C., and Varco, R. L.: Is excision the optimum treatment for all abdominal aortic aneurysms? SURGERY **61:** 83, 1969.
2. Szilagyi, E. D., Smith, R. F., DeRusso, F. J., Elliot, J. P., and Sherrin, F. W.: Contribution of abdominal aortic aneurysmectomy to prolongation of life, Ann. Surg. **164:** 678, 1966.

DISCUSSION

Dr. Wilfred Tam (Charlotte, N. C.). Thank you for the opportunity to present a few remarks on our experience in North Carolina.

We have made similar comparisons of aneurysmectomy in the aged and we have divided our patients in the past 10 years into two groups, ruptured and nonruptured.

The most important factor determining the operative risk of aortic aneurysm is whether or not the aorta is already ruptured. The age, general condition, and associated diseases the patient may be suffering bear only a secondary importance.

The different types of aneurysms of the abdominal aorta listed in order of increasing surgical mortality rates are as follows: asymptomatic (4.3 percent), symptomatic, nonruptured (12.5 percent), retroperitoneal rupture (50 percent), and intraperitoneal rupture (60 percent).

With good preparation and careful surgical technique, an excellent chance for survival and recovery is found in patients with nonreuptured aneurysms regardless of advanced age, associated heart disease, or disseminated arteriosclerosis.

The mortality rate of aortic resections for ruptured aneurysms is high, and the association of unfavorable factors such as advanced age, heart disease, or disseminated arteriosclerosis creates a rather hopeless situation.

On the basis of the data in the pertinent literature and our own experience, we recommend that all aneurysms of the abdominal aorta should be treated by resection and graft replacement soon after the diagnosis has been established unless the patient is extremely debilitated, has incurable malignancy, advanced renal insufficiency, or recent myocardial infarction.

Dr. James D. Hardy (Jackson, Miss.). I have certainly enjoyed this fine paper. The authors are to be congratulated on such a perceptive presentation of an important clinical problem.

We have resected abdominal aortic aneurysms in 26 patients who were 75 years of age or older. We do not distinguish so rigidly between patients who have symptoms and those who do not. However, we do distinguish between those patients whose aneurysm had ruptured and those whose aneurysm lesion had not ruptured. The patient with a ruptured aneurysm has blood volume deficit problems, he may have to be operated upon under extreme emergency conditions, and shock often occurs during anesthesia induction if it has not been present already. Suffice it to say that the patient with a ruptured aneurysm is taken immediately to the operating room, unmatched type O negative blood is secured while crossmatching is being carried out, and prompt operation is performed.

The aneurysm had ruptured in six of our patients, 75 years or older, and four died (66 percent)—as against our over-all mortality rate for ruptured aneurysms of about 40 percent.

Twenty patients were operated upon electively and three died, for a mortality rate of 15 percent. Most of these aneurysms were large, since small aneurysms are usually managed conservatively in the very elderly. The major contraindications to resection of a significant aneurysm are a recent myocardial infarction, marked debility, incipient uremia, and severe respiratory insufficiency. However, if resection of the aneurysm is indicated, and if the patient is active and in a reasonably fair general physiological state, a brisk operation is usually well tolerated.

It is important, we feel, to avoid excesses in the elderly patient. First, overtransfusion should be avoided and hypoxia and hypercarbia minimized, by an alert anesthetist. Second, the operation should be expeditiously performed. We quickly eviscerate the small bowel into a plastic Lakey bag, place a clamp across the aorta above the aneurysm, inject 20 mg. of heparin into the lesion to decrease the risk of clotting in the more distal arteries during aortic occlusion, then place a Crafoord clamp straight down across each common iliac artery without dissection, then incise the aneurysm anteriorly, oversew the few patent lumbar arteries, manage the inferior mesenteric artery, and then place the fabric prosthesis inside the aneurysm with synthetic suture material. With this technique, the size of the aneurysm makes little difference, just so long as it arises below the renal arteries. Performed in this way, the entire operation should take less than 2 hours, and alteration of the metabolic state of the very elderly patient is kept to a minimum.

Therefore, we agree with the authors that almost any patient in a generally stable psysiological condition can and should undergo resection of a threatening abdominal aortic aneurysm.

Dr. Jere W. Lord, Jr. (New York, N. Y.). Dr. Hanlon, I apologize for coming up so soon again. I'd like to ask Dr. Esselstyn a question.

In the slides, there was one group of eight patients all of whom apparently refused to have the operation. I thought it would be interesting to know what happened to these eight in comparison to the ones who did accept the operation because they certainly serve as a good control group.

Our experience has been like Dr. Hardy. We operated upon 19 patients, 75 years and older. Six were emergency operations and 13 were elective. There was one death in the emergency group and three deaths in the elective group.

The important thing, I think, is that we have learned in the last 2 years to do the procedure as Dr. Hardy described it and that two of the patients operated upon electively and who died would not have died if operated on by current techniques.

This would reduce the mortality rate to 11 percent, which is 4 percent above our mortality rate for all ages.

I agree with the conclusion of Drs. Esselstyn and Humphries that all of these patients with an abdominal aneurysm, 75 and over, who are reasonable operative risks should be offered the operation and not wait until a catastrophe develops.

President Hanlon. Would Dr. Esselstyn care to comment on the nature of those patients who served as unoperated "controls"? Some of them, I gather, were turned down because of poor general condition, and hence might constitute a peculiarly unfavorable group to contrast with the survival curve of the operative cases. I presume this is commented on in his manuscript.

Dr. Esselstyn (closing). I would like to thank the discussants for their comments.

Dr. Tam's experience with elderly patients who undergo aneurysmectomy appears to be in agreement with ours.

We agree with Dr. Hardy that elderly patients should be operated on under optimal conditions.

In reply to Dr. Lord's question regarding the fate of the eight patients who declined operation, two died of rupture of the aneurysm.

We would certainly agree with Dr. Hanlon's comment that the nonoperated group is not truly a control group, and we have not considered it as such, as most of those patients were too sick for surgical treatment. The only truly comparable group would be nonoperated patients who are followed a significant length of time before the era of aneurysmectomy and graft replacement.

I would like to thank the members of the Society for the opportunity to present our material.

Arteriovenous fistula: Results of management of congenital and acquired forms, blood flow measurements, and observations on proximal arterial degeneration

YOSHIO SAKO, M.D.
RICHARD L. VARCO, M.D.
MINNEAPOLIS, MINN.
From the Department of Surgery, University of Minnesota Hospitals and the Veterans Administration Hospital

Arteriovenous fistulas, both congenital and acquired, are abnormal connections between the artery and vein without the intervening capillary bed, but the similarity between the two groups, for the most part, ends there. Congenital fistulas result from abnormal maturation in one or more of the embryologic stages in the development of the vasculature. The lesions, thus, can range from capillary to macroscopic sizes and vary in appearance, number, extent, and behavior. Physicians and surgeons alike tend to look upon congenital arteriovenous fistulas with some sense of despair and futility. This is understandable because so many of these abnormalities are incurable and some are eventually lethal. Nevertheless, within the spectrum of these lesions, there are those in which prolonged palliation and even cures are possible by selection and timing of the surgical procedures.

An acquired arteriovenous fistula usually is single and occurs through external influence in a setting of a previously normal circulatory system. If the location, size, and duration of the fistula, all of which are fairly readily determinable, are known, the effect on the host and the treatment indicated are now fairly well understood. A fistula of long standing, however, may cause irreversible changes in the vessels and make attempts at surgical care hazardous.

This report is a review of our experience with a total of 57 patients with congenital and acquired arteriovenous fistulas of the extremities, abdomen, and chest wall during a 20 year period (1949-1969). Some of the patients in the congenital fistula group were reported on by Delaney[3] in 1960. An estimate of the frequency of arteriovenous fistulas as an over-all problem may be gained from the information that during the same period of our study, 23 patients with vertebral and carotid arteriovenous fistulas, six with pulmonary arteriovenous fistulas, and four with coronary arteriovenous fistulas were also seen and cared for.

CONGENITAL ARTERIOVENOUS FISTULA

There were 32 patients with congenital arteriovenous fistula, 15 male and 17 female, ranging in age from 3 to 79 years. Most of the older patients had had the lesion for many years prior to being seen, generally before puberty. Area of involvement, main

Presented at the Twenty-third Annual Meeting of the Society for Vascular Surgery, New York, N. Y., July 12-13, 1969.

The experimental aspects were supported by a grant-in-aid from the American Heart Association.

Reprint address: Surgical Service, 54th Street and 48th Avenue South, Minneapolis, Minn. 55417.

symptoms, features, angiographic findings, treatment, and results are listed in Table I. The diagnosis for the most part was made on the basis of the clinical features. Two thirds of the patients had birthmarks ranging from telangiectasia to lobular hemangiomas. Almost all of the patients have had prominent veins. Thirteen had thrill and 17 had bruit in the affected area. Nine had overgrowth of the involved member. Three had significant enlargement of the heart (Patient Nos. 2, 21, and 32). Two of these had congestive failure.

During the earlier period of the series, venous oxygen saturation was measured, an elevated level indicating direct arterial communications. Angiography was the most valuable of all diagnostic procedures that have been used (27 of 32). Visualization of the fistula itself (Fig. 1) or rapid venous opacification was indicative of abnormal shunts (Fig. 2).

Improvement in radiographic technique has made angiography even more valuable. In the earlier part of the series, rapid cassette changers, selective, and cineangiography were unavailable. Figs. 3 and 4 show the value of selective angiography in localization of the fistula.

There were six patients who had involvement of the arm and/or shoulder girdle who were operated upon and two who had no operation. There were 15 patients who had involvement of the lower extremities and/or pelvic girdle who were operated upon and seven who had no operation. Of the last two in the group, one had a splenic arteriovenous fistula and one had extensive involvement of the diaphragm and chest wall.

CASE REPORT I

Patient No. 22 is described in greater detail because of several unusual aspects about him. G. B., a 73-year-old man and veteran of World Wars I and II, was seen in March, 1966, with a history of progressive dyspnea for the previous 6 to 7 years. He was managed at home for congestive failure with diuretics, digitalis, and salt restriction until he became refractory to treatment.

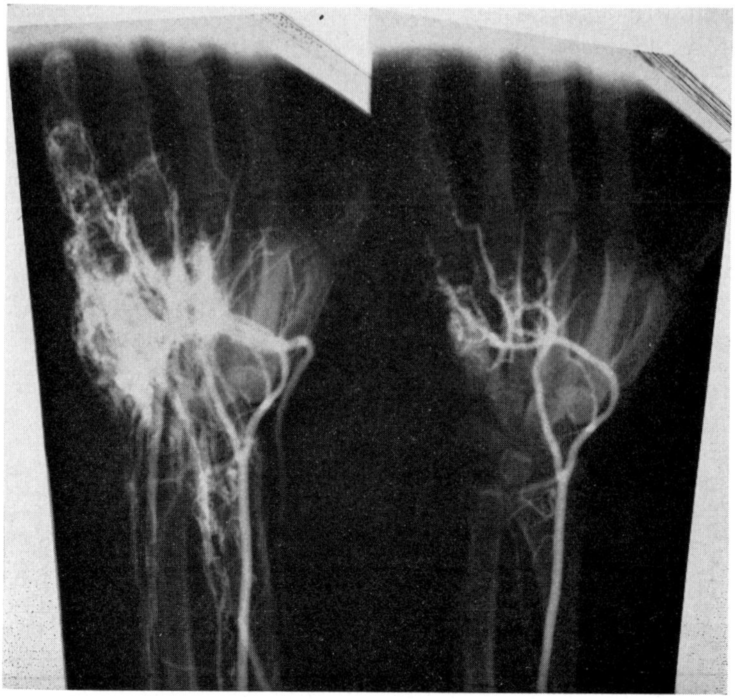

Fig. 1. Brachial artery arteriogram showing multiple A-V shunts in the medial half of the palm and the little finger (Patient No. 4).

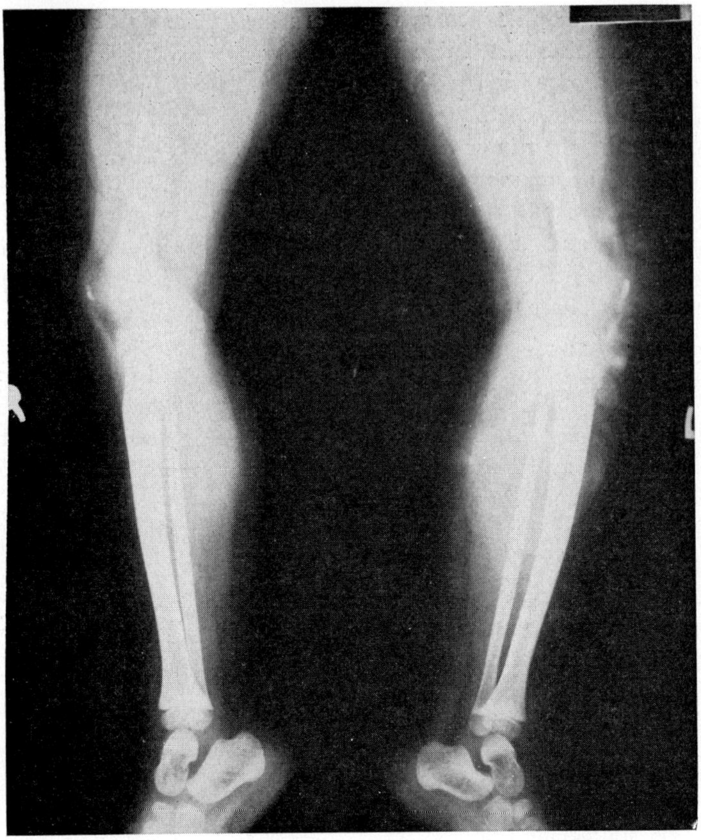

Fig. 2. Left femoral arteriogram showing only rapid venous filling (Patient No. 24). This shows limitation of the single film technique.

Examination showed that he had atrial fibrillation, cardiomegaly, murmurs of mitral and aortic valve insufficiency, blood pressure of 150/30 mm. Hg, pulse 120 per minute. There was an 8 by 10 cm. pulsating mass in the left lower abdomen, a thrill over the left common femoral artery, and a continuous bruit in the groin and left lower abdomen. Data from right and transeptal left heart catheterization showed biventricular failure, a large left-to-right shunt at the first portion of the inferior vena cava. Cardiac output was 11.3 L. per minute. The aortogram showed a left iliac artery aneurysm with immediate opacification of the inferior vena cava indicating an arteriovenous fistula.

In April, 1966, under the presumptive diagnosis of an arteriovenous fistula secondary to rupture of an arteriosclerotic aneurysm, he was operated upon and laparotomy revealed what is shown in Fig. 5. A tortuous left iliac artery and hypogastric artery aneurysm was excised and the distal end of the hypogastric artery was oversewn with multiple deep sutures. The point of communication with the iliac vein was not apparent. The maneuver obliterated the strong thrill for the most part, but it was not until the right hypogastric artery was also ligated that the thrill completely disappeared. The divided left iliac artery was reconstructed with a segment of Dacron graft. Blood flow measurements during the procedure showed 1,440 ml. per minute peak flow and 660 ml. per minute mean flow in the common iliac artery and after excision of the fistula 780 ml. per minute peak flow and 180 ml. per minute mean flow. Postoperatively, there was a rapid reduction in heart size and the symptoms of congestive failure disappeared. Dye-dilution curve showed no evidence of a left-to-right shunt.

Out-of-state hospital records were reviewed and they showed that the patient had been seen in 1946, at which time the presence of the abdominal aneurysm was noted but nothing was done because aneurysm operations were as yet unsatisfactory. In 1948, he had been seen again because of recurrent episodes of shortness of breath. At that time, slight enlargement of the heart, tachycardia, and a

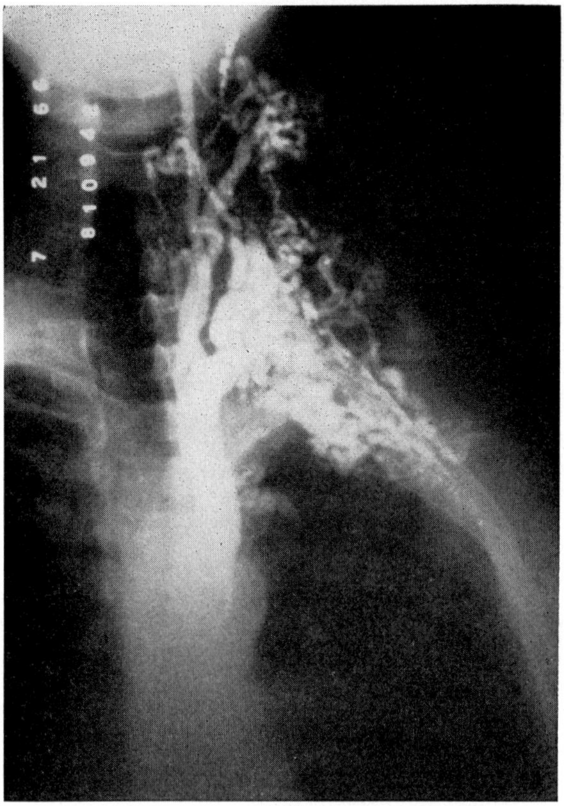

Fig. 3. Left subclavian arteriogram (Patient No. 2) showing extensive A-V fistula in the apex of chest. He already has had shoulder and arm amputation.

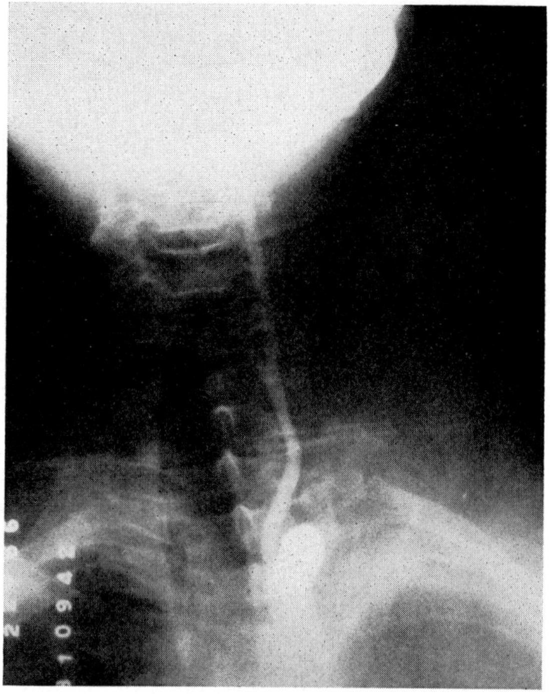

Fig. 4. Left subclavian arteriogram (Patient No. 2, Fig. 3) with the distal artery occluded with a balloon. The vertebral artery is selectively filled and appears not to be involved with the fistula.

continuous bruit over the left groin was noted. The working diagnosis was arteriosclerotic heart disease and abdominal aneurysm, and he was discharged from the hospital and did not seek medical attention again until the 1966 admission.

The patient was discharged from the current hospital admission following a rapid recovery and abatement of symptoms of cardiac failure. Discharge diagnosis was high output failure as a result of a left iliac artery arteriovenous fistula. The cause of the fistula was presumed to be a rupture of the iliac artery aneurysm. He was recalled for evaluation in June, 1969. In the interim between the discharge and recall, he had been cared for in his own state. He was asymptomatic, active for age 76, and in general good health, but his heart was again enlarged and a loud bruit could be heard in the lower abdomen. An aortogram showed a huge pelvic arteriovenous communication (Fig. 6). Cardiac output was 9.7 L. per minute and brachial artery pressure 140/42 mm. Hg. These findings indicated that the patient had always had a congenital arteriovenous fistula, proximal arterial degeneration, high cardiac output, marked relief for 3 years by ligation and excision of the hypogastric artery on the left and ligation of the hypogastric artery on the right. He was now 76 years old and still relatively free of symptoms but probably destined for more trouble because of progressive enlargement of arteriovenous channels in the pelvis. At this time, his heart is still smaller than before his operation 3 years ago and cardiac output is lower than before the operation (9.7 L. versus 11.3 L.).

COMMENTS

The clinical course of this patient is unusual in that the congenital arteriovenous fistula lay dormant for many years then progressed until high output failure provoked heart failure. He also benefited from the operation though it was not curative.

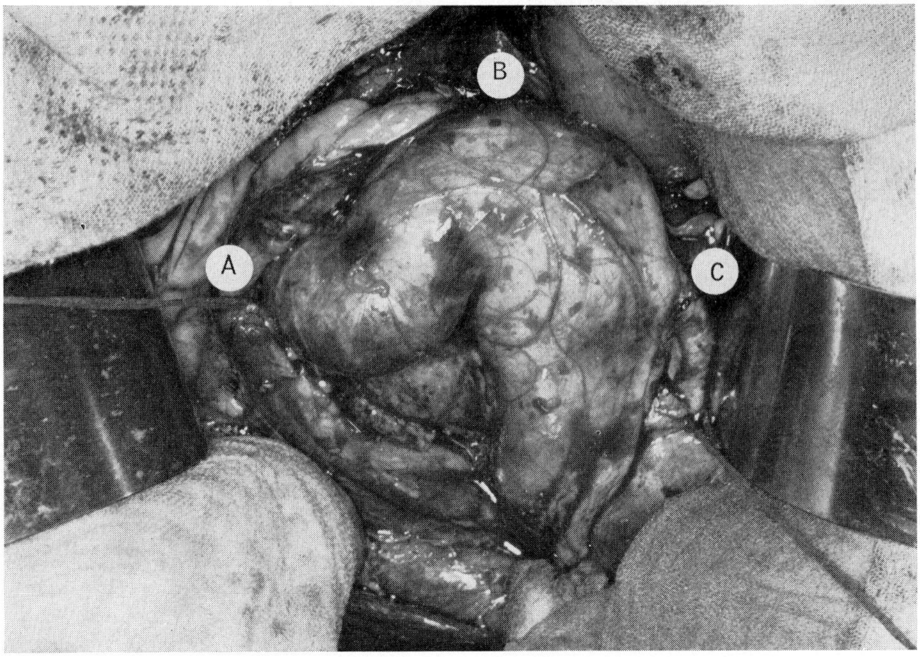

Fig. 5. Case Report I (Patient No. 21). Aneurysmal dilatation of the left common iliac (*A*) and hypogastric arteries (*B*). The external iliac artery (*C*) is normal in size.

RESULTS OF TREATMENT

The results were graded as *worse, unchanged, improved,* and *cured.* Those who were unchanged who also required amputation of any portion of the extremity were grouped as *worse.* On this basis, of six patients with upper limb and shoulder girdle involvement who were operated upon (Nos. 1 to 6, Table I), three were *worse,* one *unchanged,* and two were *cured.* In the two who had no operation, both were *unchanged* (Nos. 7 and 8, Table I).

In the lower extremity and pelvic girdle involvement, of 15 who were operated upon (Nos. 9 to 23), three were *worse,* one *unchanged,* eight *improved,* and three were *cured.* In the seven who had no operation (Nos. 24-30), two were *worse* and 5 were *unchanged.* In the last two patients (Nos. 31 and 32) the patient with the splenic arteriovenous fistula was *cured.* At operation, the splenic artery mean flow was 420 ml. per minute and after fistula closure it was 80 ml. per minute. The patient with the fistula involving the chest wall, back, and diaphragm died during operation from massive bleeding. Preoperative measurements showed 65 percent of the cardiac output going through the fistula. The surgical procedures, thus, in the 23 of the 32 patients resulted in six *cured,* eight *improved,* two *unchanged,* six *worse,* and one *death.* In the nine patients who had no operation, two were *worse* and seven were *unchanged.*

ACQUIRED ARTERIOVENOUS FISTULA

There were 25 patients operated upon for acquired arteriovenous fistula and two who required operations because of late complications related to their fistula which was removed years before. Ages ranged from 9 to 79 years and there were 5 female and 22 male patients.

The locations of the fistulas were as follows: lower extremities in 13 (seven femoral, 4 popliteal, two tibial), three in the iliac artery, and one each involving the gluteal, innominate, subclavian, radial, digital, internal mammary, left gastric, renal, and supraorbital arteries and veins.

The causes were as follows: small arms

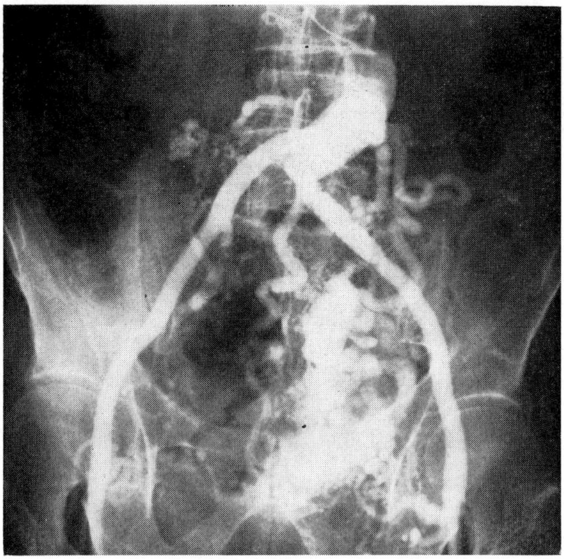

Fig. 6. Case Report I (Patient No. 22). Aortogram taken 3 years after operation showing extensive A-V shunts in the pelvis.

fire in nine, penetrating wound with knife or glass in six, war injuries with shell fragment or land mine explosion in three, multiple puncture for cardiac catheterization in two, and one each in blunt injury of the hand, pelvic fracture, renal needle biopsy, rupture of an arteriosclerotic iliac aneurysm, and one following gastrectomy which caused a left gastric artery arteriovenous fistula.

History of injury was readily obtained: diagnosis was easily established because of the characteristic local findings. Slowing of the pulse with fistula compression (Branham's sign) was present in nine, five had cardiac enlargement one had overt cardiac failure, and one had early failure. Twelve of these patients had had the fistula over 1 year before diagnosis and treatment. The intervals were 15 months in 2, 3 years in three, and one each at 6, 9, 10, 17, 20, and 43 years. Some of these patients will be discussed later.

Corrective procedures in the 25 patients with fistulas were quadruple ligation in six, excision of the fistula and artery and vein repair in 16, multiple ligation in two, and one patient with the ruptured iliac aneurysm had excision of an aortic and iliac artery aneurysm and replacement with a bifurcated Dacron graft. The two patients treated for late artery complications had had quadruple ligation previously. In arterial repair, primary anastomosis was used in 13, one had a homograft to an iliac artery, and three had autologous vein graft to the femoral artery.

CASE REPORT II

The following is a case report of unusual interest because the fistula went undetected for so long despite severe cardiac symptoms caused by the fistula: The patient was a Vietnam War veteran, aged 22, who sustained multiple wounds from a land mine explosion in September, 1967. The right leg was amputated below the knee because of extensive injuries to the soft tissue and bones. He required a long hospitalization for stump revision, skin grafting, and rehabilitation and was finally discharged from the hospital in June, 1968. Three months later he was seen at his local Veterans Administration Hospital because of bouts of tachycardia. Examination showed that his heart was slightly enlarged, cardiogram was normal, pulse 72, blood pressure 132/66 mm. Hg, and a Grade 1 systolic murmur was heard over the aortic and mitral valve areas. His symptoms progressed and by December, 1968, the heart was enlarged further (Fig. 7), and the physical signs of cardiomegaly and valve insufficiency became more prominent. Blood pressure was 130/0 mm. Hg. Differential diagnosis was ruptured aortic valve leaflet or Marfan's syndrome with aortic valve insufficiency, and he was referred to the Minneapolis Veterans Administration Hospital in January, 1969.

Examination confirmed the findings of cardiomegaly, tachycardia, and murmurs of aortic and mitral valve insufficiency; blood pressure was 160/55 mm. Hg. In addition, there was a strong thrill and bruit over the right femoral artery, most prominent in the midthigh with transmission of bruit to the knee. Compression of the right common femoral artery produced an abrupt fall of the heart rate from 100 to 65 beats per minute, and an elevation of the systolic and diastolic pressure. Femoral angiograms revealed a large arteriovenous fistula (Fig. 8). At operation, the femoral arteriovenous fistula measured 20 by 16 mm. externally and the fistulous opening was 12 by 8 mm. Proximal artery compression caused the blood pressure to rise from 120/68 to 160/100 mm. Hg, and heart rate to slow (Fig. 9). Blood flow measurements indicated proximal mean blood flow of 1,200 ml. per minute and 200 ml. per minute mean flow distal to the fistula (Fig. 10). Common femoral vein pressure was 30 mm. Hg with the fistula open and 10 mm. Hg with the fistula closed.

The fistula was corrected by resection of the

Table I

No.	*Sex*	*Age*	*Involvement*	*Main findings*
Shoulder girdle and arm—operative group				
1	F	30	Right thenar area	4 by 6 cm. mass, bruit, hand larger
2	M	30	Left arm and shoulder	Thrill, bruit, multiple hemangioma
3	M	15	Right hand, thenar area	Thrill, bruit, thumb and hand larger
4	F	14	Right hypothenar area	Thrill, bruit, finger overgrowth
5	F	18	Left arm	Thrill, bruit, 6 by 10 cm. mass
6	M	79	Left forearm	Thrill, bruit, progressive past 15 years
Shoulder girdle and arm—no operation				
7	M	5	Right shoulder, axilla	Thrill, bruit, many birthmarks
8	M	9	Right elbow	Thrill, bruit, 4 by 4 cm. mass
Pelvic girdle and leg—operative group				
9	F	32	Left leg	Prominent veins since 12 years
10	M	32	Right leg	Prominent veins since 18 years
11	M	5	Right leg	Thrill, bruit, birthmarks, leg 5 cm. longer
12	M	36	Right leg	Birthmarks, varices, entire leg bigger
13	F	14	Left leg	Bruit, 4 by 4 by 3 cm. mass dorsum of foot
14	F	13	Left leg	Varices leg, thigh, labia, birthmarks
15	M	52	Both legs	Prominent veins
16	F	16	Left leg	Thrill, bruit, 11 by 6 cm. pretibial hemangioma
17	M	31	Right thigh	Bruit in irregular 6 cm. mass
18	F	24	Right leg	Varices, right leg 1 inch longer
19	M	19	Both legs	Varicosities and stasis ulcers bilaterally
20	M	38	Left leg	Prominent veins since 14 years
21	M	73	Left iliac	Thrill, bruit, iliac aneurysm, intractable cardiac failure

*A-V = arteriovenous.

Angiography	*Treatment*	*Years followed*	*Results*
Not done	Radial and ulnar artery ligation	22	Bruit persists, index finger later amputated—*worse*
Extensive A-V* fistula in chest wall and arm	Ligation, eventual shoulder amputation	19	Extensive A-V fistula in chest and neck—*worse*
Multiple radial A-V fistulas	Ligation	13	Bruit persists, functional hand—*unchanged*
Multiple A-V fistulas	Ligation, excision, finger amputations	8	Occasional bleeding, index finger and thumb remain—*worse*
Multiple A-V fistulas	Mass and 10 A-V fistulas excised	5	Arm warmer than right, but no residual fistula—*cured*
[illegible] radial A-V fistulas	Ligation	4	No recurrence—*cured*
None	None	8	*Unchanged,* right arm 2 cm. longer
None	None	5	*Unchanged*
Multiple A-V fistulas knee, ankle	Fistula ligation and vein stripping	16	More surgery, edema, ulceration—*worse*
Rapid vein filling via genicular arteries	Ligation of 5 fistulas, vein stripping, supportive hose	15	Right leg bigger than left, not disabling—*improved*
Rapid vein filling via profunda femoris artery	Ligation right profunda femoris and hypogastric	14	No improvement, later leg amputation, intrapelvic A-V fistula multiple—*worse*
Multiple A-V fistulas right thigh	Ligation A-V fistula and excision subcutaneous 480 Gm. mass	12	Controlled with elastic support—*improved*
Multiple A-V fistulas foot and ankle	Staged ligation and excision 6 operations, 1958-1966	11	No bruit after last operation—*cured*
Rapid venous opacification	Excision mass, vein stripping	10	Chronic edema, minor vein surgery twice in 10 yr.—*improved*
Multiple small A-V fistulas	Vein stripping	10	Died of esophageal varices, bleeding, leg symptoms minimal—*improved*
Multiple A-V fistulas	Ligation, excision	9	Recurrent isolated anterior and posterior tibial A-V fistula, after 8 yr. ligated—*cured*
A-V fistulas outlined	Excision of subcutaneous mass and ligation	7	No recurrence—*cured*
Multiple A-V fistulas right thigh	Vein stripping and osteotomy	7	*Improved*
Multiple small A-V fistulas	Bilateral vein stripping, supportive hose	6	Episodic leg edema, but *improved*
apid venous opacification	Multiple vein operations and leg support	4	*Improved*
arge A-V fistula	Excision, multiple ligation	3	Gradual recurrence details in case history—*improved*

Continued on following page.

Table I—*Cont'd*

No.	*Sex*	*Age*	*Involvement*	*Main findings*
22	F	26	Right foot	5 by 7 cm. chronic ulcer, foot overgrowth
23	F	8	Left leg	Thrill, bruit, 1 cm. overgrowth, bulky spongy mass
Pelvic girdle and leg—nonoperative				
24	F	3	Left leg	Port wine–colored boggy mass below knee
25	F	17	Left leg	Ulcer left ankle
26	F	9	Both legs	Prominent leg veins since age 4
27	M	45	Left leg	Brawny leg, multiple purplish elevated skin lesion
28	F	26	Both legs	Prominent varices
29	F	69	Left thigh	Thrill, bruit, 7 by 7 cm. mass
30	M	6	Right foot	Prominent veins, foot overgrowth, multiple birthmarks
Other types—operative				
31	F	30	Splenic artery	Bruit
32	F	44	Diaphragm, chest wall	Thrill, bruit, cardiomegaly ascites, congestive failure

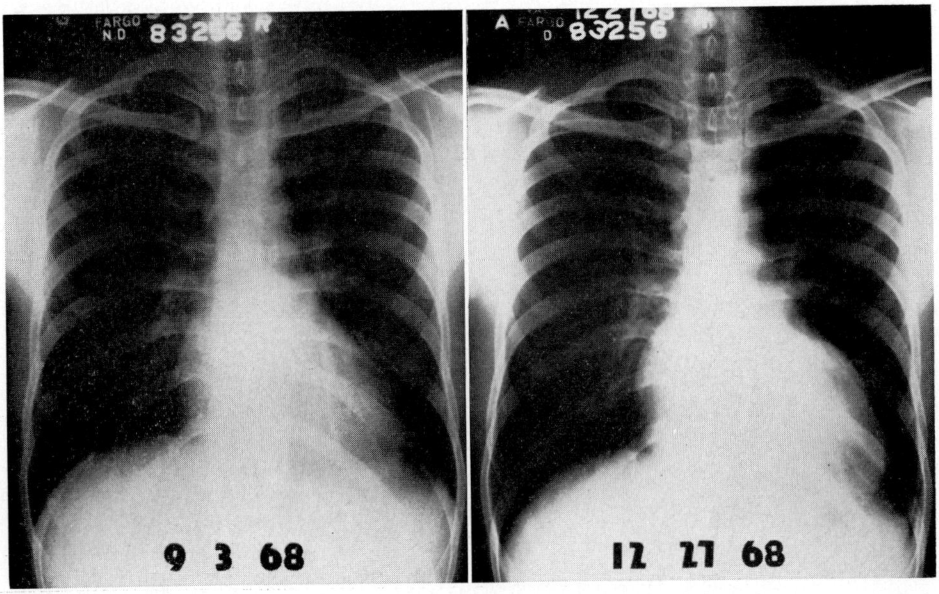

Fig. 7. Case Report II. Chest x-rays of patient depicting cardiac enlargement over a 3 month period.

Angiography	*Treatment*	*Years followed*	*Results*
Multiple A-V fistulas in foot and ankle	Excision and graft	1	Recurred 6 mo. later, below knee amputation
Multiple A-V fistulas	Ligation, vein stripping	½	Recent surgery, known residuals—*unchanged*
Rapid venous opacification, high venous O_2	Elastic support	22	Chronic induration left leg below distal thigh, needs crutches—*worse*
Multiple fistulas	Previous toe removal and leg support	10	Episodic ulceration in foot—*unchanged*
Multiple A-V fistulas	Elastic support	10	No disability, recurrent convulsions chief problem—*unchanged*
Thorotrast injection failed, extravasated	None	25	Invalid till death of urologic problems related to thorotrast—*worse*
Multiple fistulas, below and above the knee	Elastic support	23	Episodic foot and leg ulceration—*unchanged*
Tortuous calcified vessels on plain film	None	8	Asymptomatic—*unchanged*
Rapid venous opacification	Left heel elevation	6	Minimal disability—*unchanged*
A-V fistula	Division–ligation	4	No recurrence—*cured*
Multiple huge A-V fistulas	Multiple ligation	—	Operative death—hemorrhage during procedure, cardiac arrest

artery, oversewing of the fistulous tract flush with the vein, and bridging the arterial defect with a 4 cm. segment of autogenous vein graft. After reconstruction the mean blood flow was 700 ml. per minute in the superficial femoral artery which is about three times greater than normal, thus, another fistula was suspected and found by angiography to be between the anterior tibial artery and vein. The artery and fistulous tract were ligated just posterior to the interosseous membrane and the blood flow patterns in the popliteal artery before and after the ligation are shown in Fig. 11. Postoperatively, the patient's cardiac findings rapidly abated, but on the fifth day, a bruit was heard anterior to the tibia. An angiogram showed communication between the anterior tibial and peroneal artery and vein at a point distal to where the anterior tibial artery had been ligated previously (Fig. 12). Through an anterior incision, these were ligated and the bruit disappeared. Chest x-ray at time of discharge showed marked reduction in heart size (Fig. 13). Five months postoperatively, the cardiac murmurs were very faint, there was no bruit in the leg stump, and he was asymptomatic and able to wear his prosthesis without claudication.

COMMENT

No matter how the situation is analyzed, it seems incredible that the arteriovenous fistula was overlooked. The patient states that the buzzing sensation which he detected was described to his doctors soon after his convalescence from the traumatic amputation.

CASE REPORT III

The following is a brief summary on the patient who had a very unusual form of arteriovenous fistula: The patient was a 22-year-old man who, because of hematuria and history of nephritis at age 13, had a needle biopsy attempted in July, 1967, while in the army. Subsequently, he was discharged from the service with a diagnosis of chronic glomerulonephritis. In April, 1968, hypertension was discovered during an insurance ex-

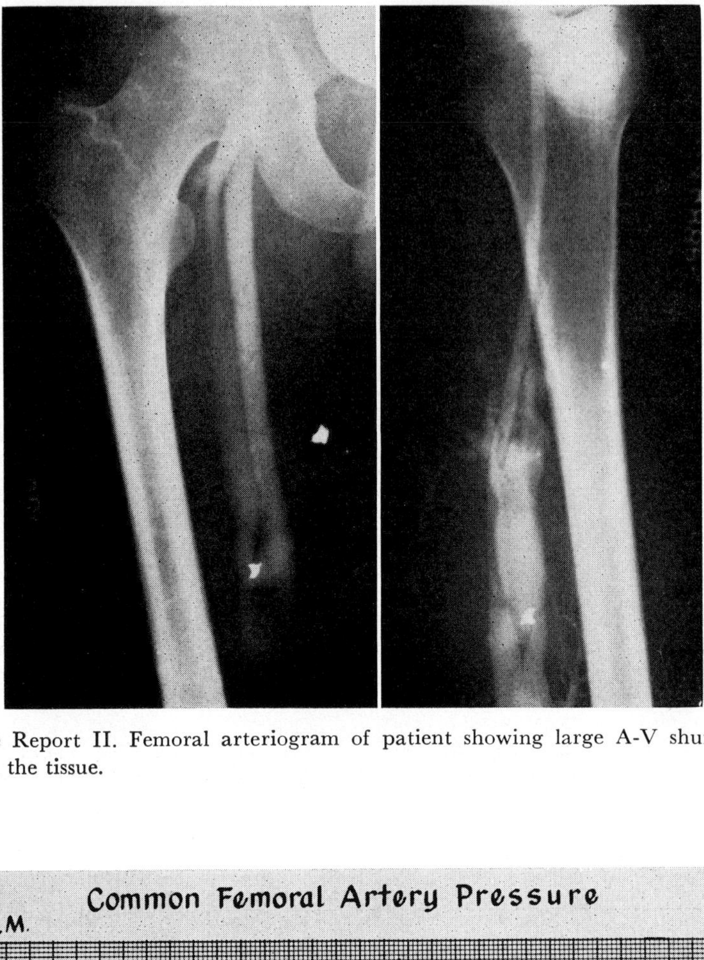

Fig. 8. Case Report II. Femoral arteriogram of patient showing large A-V shunt and metal fragments in the tissue.

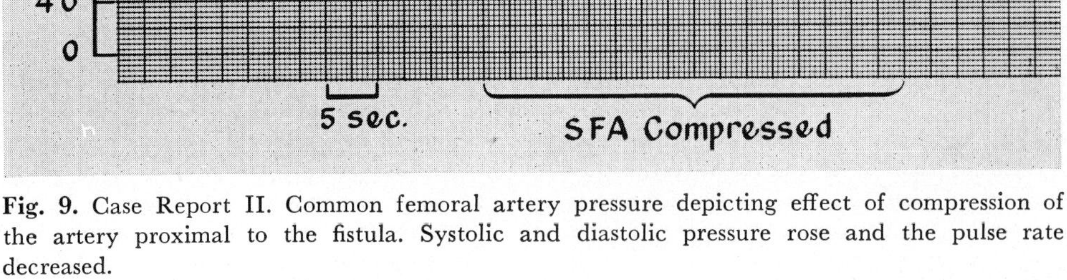

Fig. 9. Case Report II. Common femoral artery pressure depicting effect of compression of the artery proximal to the fistula. Systolic and diastolic pressure rose and the pulse rate decreased.

amination. He was admitted to the hospital in December, 1968, because of backache, abdominal pain, and easy fatigability. Blood pressure was 180/120 mm. Hg and a continuous bruit was heard over the left kidney area. Aortogram showed two left renal arteries and a renal arteriovenous fistula of the upper artery (Fig. 14). At operation in December, 1968, the arteriovenous fistula which was extraparenchymal was corrected by transvenous repair of the fistula. Blood flow measurements in the upper renal artery were 380 c.c. mean flow per minute before and 100 c.c. after closure

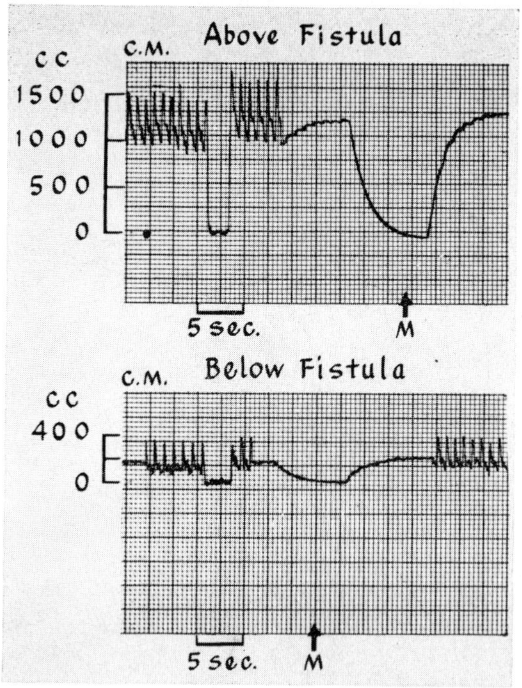

Fig. 10. Case Report II. Femoral artery blood flow above and below the fistula. The pattern of flow below the fistula shows no reverse flow in diastole which is indicative of low peripheral resistance. In this instance, the low resistance was caused by another fistula below the knee.

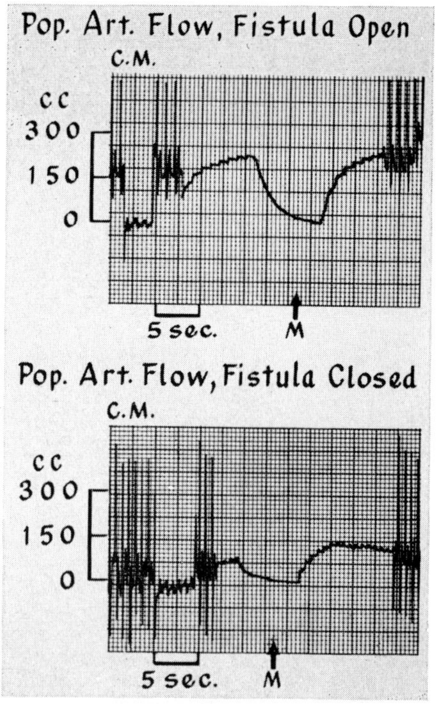

Fig. 11. Case Report II. Popliteal artery blood flow before and after closure of the anterior tibial A-V fistula. Following the fistula closure, normal reverse flow during diastole is evident.

of the fistula. Postoperatively, his hypertension promptly subsided and on the clinic visit, in July, 1969, blood pressure was 136/86 mm. Hg.

COMMENT

Renal arteriovenous fistulas have been found to occur following mass ligation of the renal pedicle during nephrectomy and other forms of trauma such as knife stab, bullet wounds, and as in this case, after needle biopsy. Renal ischemia provokes hypertension showing quite dramatically that tissues distal to an arteriovenous fistula have diminution in circulation.

DEGENERATION OF THE ARTERY PROXIMAL TO THE FISTULA

The most serious complication of an arteriovenous fistula of long standing is the proximal arterial degeneration that occurs because unlike cardiac enlargement which appears to be readily reversible upon closure of the fistula, the proximal arterial involvement not only fails to regress but also may become progressively worse. The following four case reports are examples of progression of disease in the artery proximal to the fistula even though the fistula was cured by operation.

CASE REPORTS IV TO VII

The first patient, Case IV, was a 49-year-old veteran who had had an anterior right tibial arteriovenous fistula that resulted from a 22 caliber bullet wound when he was 14 years old. The fistula was closed by quadruple ligation 21 years later while he was in the military service in World War II. He was seen 14 years after the fistula closure at the age of 49 because of multiple aneurysms of the femoral-popliteal segment (Fig. 15). This was excised and replaced with a segment of Dacron graft. The common femoral artery was 12 mm. in diameter; the profunda femoris artery was not involved. In the subsequent 6 years, there was progression of aneurysmal dilatation of the iliofemoral segment (Fig. 16), thus, this was

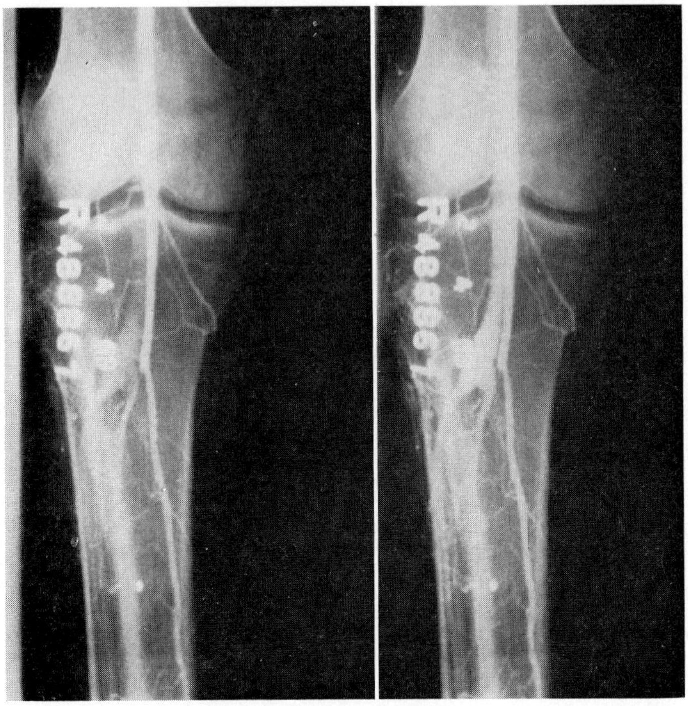

Fig. 12. Case Report II. Femoral arteriogram showing that there is retrograde flow from peroneal and anterior tibial artery into the vein.

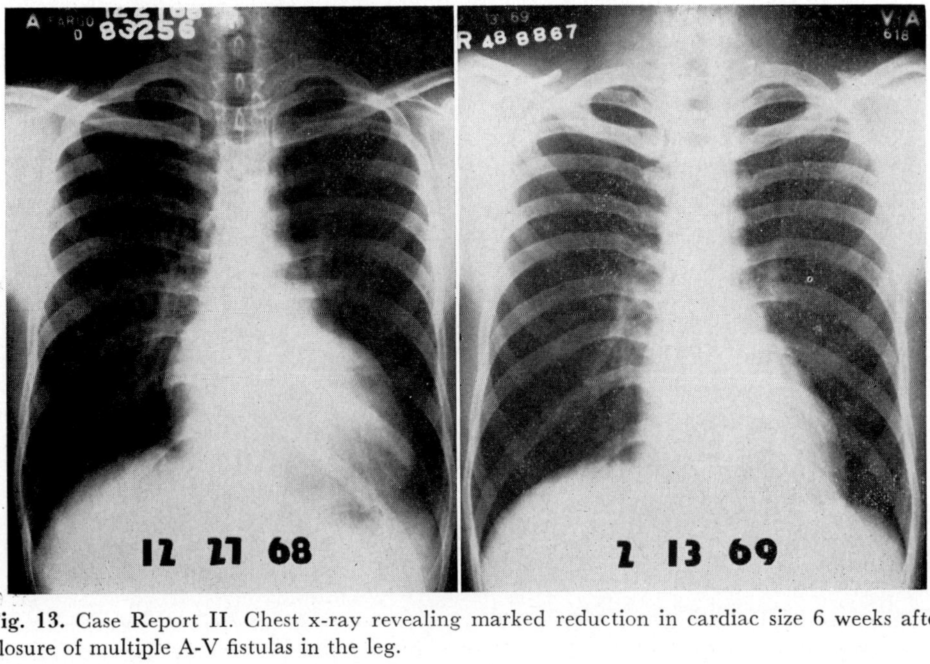

Fig. 13. Case Report II. Chest x-ray revealing marked reduction in cardiac size 6 weeks after closure of multiple A-V fistulas in the leg.

also replaced with a segment of Dacron graft. The aorta and left iliac and femoral artery were of normal size.

Case V was a 36-year-old man who at the age of 17 had had a gunshot wound of the left thigh which had produced a femoral arteriovenous fistula. This was removed by quadruple ligation 8 years later. Nine years later, after fistula closure, he was seen because of aneurysmal dilatation of the entire iliofemoral artery on the left. At operation, a tortuous iliofemoral artery 22 mm. in diameter was removed and replaced with a Dacron graft. The aorta and right iliac arteries were normal.

The third patient, Case VI, had had World War I injury to the right popliteal artery. He had been treated for recurrent phlebitis and leg edema for many years, but the presence of an arteriovenous fistula was not diagnosed until 43 years after injury. At operation, the popliteal artery proximal to the fistula was found to be 8 mm. in diameter and tortuous. Seven years later, after fistula closure and artery reconstruction, the popliteal artery had increased in size, the patient was now 73 years old and quite symptom free except for chronic varices.

The last patient in this group, Case VII, was a 51-year-old man who had had a right common femoral arteriovenous fistula from a 22 caliber

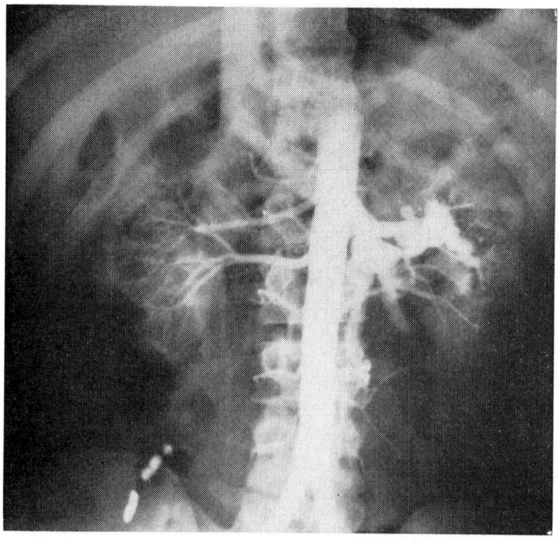

Fig. 14. Case Report III. Aortogram showing left renal A-V fistula occurring as a complication of renal needle biopsy.

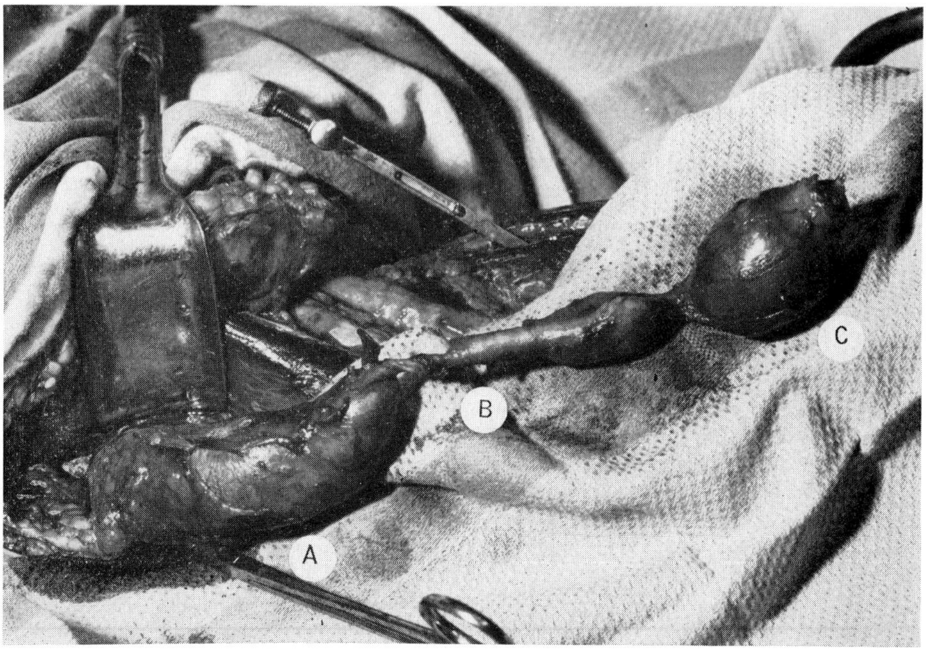

Fig. 15. Case Report IV. Aneurysmal dilatation of superficial femoral artery (*A*), narrow segment (*B*) where artery transversed Hunter's canal and popliteal artery aneurysm (*C*).

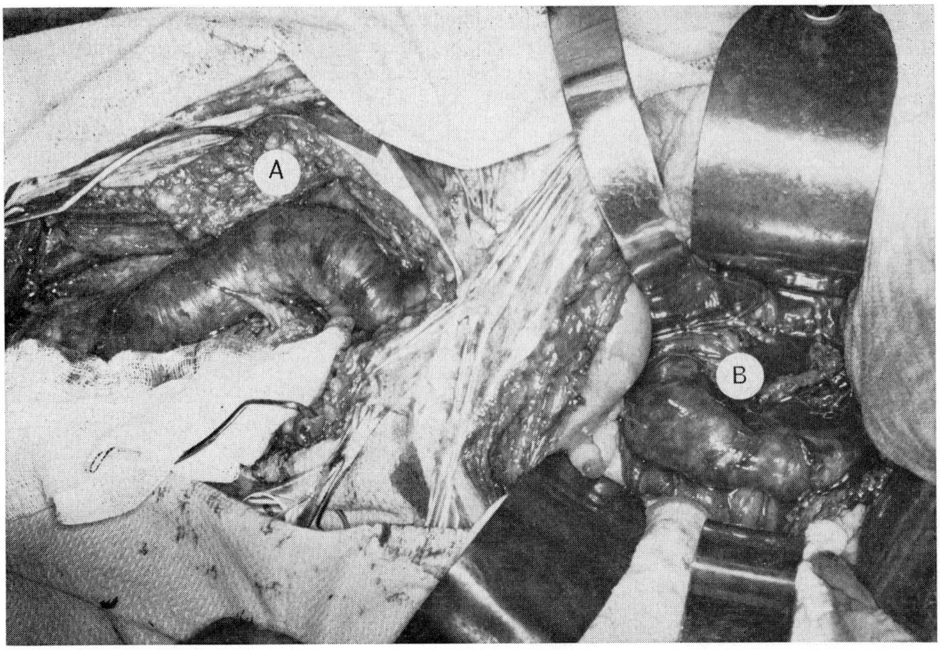

Fig. 16. Case Report IV. Aneurysmal dilatation of common iliac artery (*A*) and of common femoral artery (*B*).

bullet wound when he was 26 years old. The fistula was closed and artery and vein repaired 19 years later. At that operation, the common femoral artery was 8 mm. in diameter. Fifteen years after fistula closure, the patient was found to have a pulsatile right lower quadrant abdominal mass indicating that he had an aneurysm of the iliofemoral artery. The aneurysm was not discovered until the patient was recalled for a long-term evaluation of the operation for arteriovenous fistula.

RESULTS OF TREATMENT

The acquired fistulas were all cured without a death by the surgical procedures described. Long-term follow-up shows 14 of the 25 patients to be cured for 5 to 16 years, seven have been followed for over 2 years, and all are cured. One patient in this group had had a portion of the anterior tibial artery repaired after excision of the fistula, but the artery was occluded within the first year. Two were lost to follow-up after the first year, and one had had a quadruple ligation of the subclavian arteriovenous fistula. When last seen, he had symptoms indicating some ischemia of the arm. The other patient lost to follow-up had had a quadruple ligation of a gluteal artery arteriovenous fistula. The remaining two patients of this group were operated upon within the year. The two patients who had had aneurysmal dilatation in the proximal artery excised and replaced with a prosthetic graft were well 8 and 11 years after the operation. The other two patients with aneurysmal dilatation of the artery proximal to the fistula have not as yet had these corrected (Case Reports VI and VII). One patient who had had a portion of the iliac artery replaced with a 5 cm. segment of homograft was well 13 years since the procedure with no evidence of dilatation of the homograft.

DISCUSSION

The pathogenesis of congenital arteriovenous fistulas has been described by many, beginning over 40 years ago. The descriptions by Reid,[11] who has contributed much to our understanding of congenital and acquired arteriovenous fistulas, leave little to be improved upon. Subsequent additional case reports and reviews by Veal,[15] de Takats,[4] and Coursley and co-workers[1] have con-

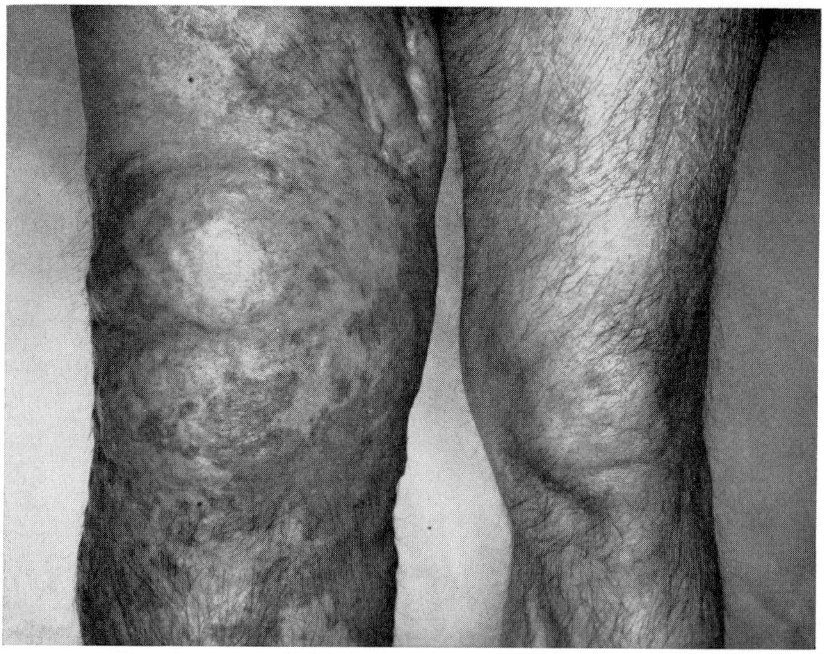

Fig. 17. Patient No. 12 (congenital A-V fistula). Present appearance of leg. The entire leg from ankle to groin is chronically edematous and enlarged. There are multiple hemangiomas and varicosities.

tributed further to our knowledge of the problems in management of patients with congenital lesions. More recently, Szilagyi and his associates[14] have described a clinical classification based on the angiographic features of the congenital lesions.

Difficulties in obtaining a cure except in those with an isolated or localized fistula are stressed by all. Multiple small arteriovenous fistulas in the lower extremities may be manageable for many years with elastic supports and vein stripping when large incompetent ones develop. In some by multiple operations, all the larger fistulas may be eliminated (Patient Nos. 6, 13, 16). Arteriovenous fistulas involving the hands are particularly difficult to manage (Patient Nos. 1 and 4, Fig. 1). If the greater portion of the fistula-bearing area is removed and limited amputations done, a functional hand may be the end result. Cross and associates[2] described two cases in which one patient ultimately required a hand amputation but another had an acceptable end result though multiple operations were needed.

Perhaps in only few other conditions is there a need for a close patient-doctor or parent-doctor relationship as when managing patients with extensive congenital fistulas because in the majority of patients, goals fall far short, both cosmetically and functionally, from what is usually understood as surgical success or cure. Generally, the situation is more a matter of degree of palliation. The present status of Patient No. 12, 9 years after operation, is shown in Fig. 17. The entire right leg from the ankle to the groin is involved, yet by wearing external support, the patient is able to work full-time. He is rated as improved, but the same situation in a woman might be rated as same or worse depending upon to what extent the patient expected the operation to correct the cosmetic aspects of the problem. In practically every group of patients with these lesions, there are a few who dissatisfied with the treatment seek assistance elsewhere and consent to a well-meaning but ill-advised operation. The end result may be a premature need for an amputation because of a painful limb provoked by proximal artery ligation.

The management for acquired arteriove-

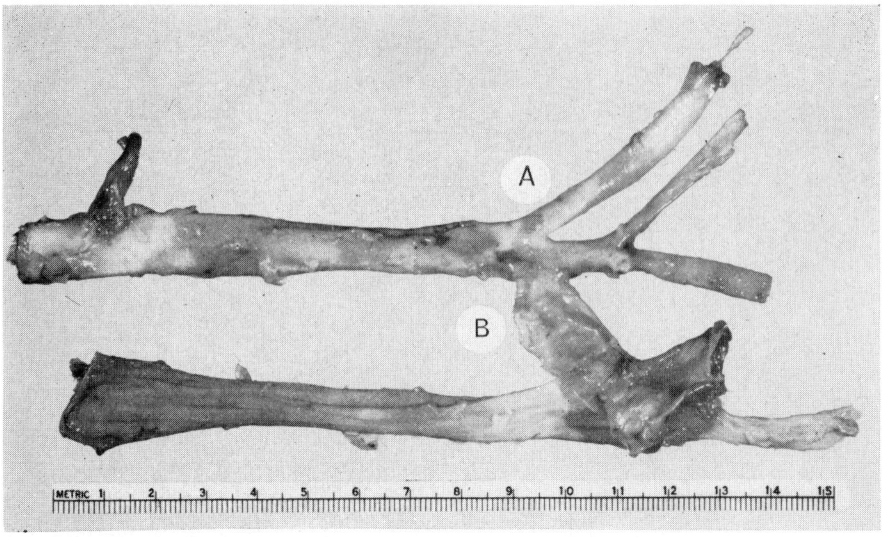

Fig. 18. Experimental iliac A-V fistula of 8 years' duration in a dog. (*A*) left iliac artery, (*B*) right iliac artery leading to fistula. The right iliac artery is dilated and thin.

nous fistula has largely been solved by current vascular surgical techniques. Much of what we know of acquired arteriovenous fistula was well established over 30 years ago because of the clinical and pathologic studies of Lewis and Drury,[9] Reid,[11] Rienhoff,[12] and Holman.[7] Holman,[7] in particular, is generally recognized as having clarified much of our understanding of the local and systemic effects of arteriovenous fistula through his sustained interest and investigation in patients and in the experimental laboratory.

Since trauma involving the artery and veins is the commonest cause of acquired fistulas, the largest series of such fistulas in any given period are such as those reported in battle casualties by Makins,[10] Elkins,[5] Shumacker,[13] Hughes and Jahnke.[8] Many of the principles of management were established from the experiences gained in treating these patients. With current techniques in vessel surgery, there is little need for quadruple ligation for treatment of arteriovenous fistula of the major arteries. Whether immediate repair is preferable even though there is no jeopardy to life or viability of the limb has not been completely settled, but Hewitt and Collins[6] report that such repairs are being done in battle casualties.

In our patients with acquired fistulas, delay in diagnosis for over 1 year occurred in one half of the group. Two patients, both children, were referred to the hospital for investigation of underdevelopment of one leg when in reality the problem was that of an acquired arteriovenous fistula in the opposite leg. Clearly there is greater need for awareness of the possibility of an arteriovenous fistula occurring in what may appear to be an innocuous or minor injury.

The occurrence of dilatation of the artery proximal to the fistula has long been known.[7] The mechanism underlying this is not completely clear, but it is thought to be due to stress, high blood flow, and interference with the function of the vasa vasorum. Microscopic sections of the arterial wall show fragmentation of the elastic tissue, atrophy of the muscles, increased fibrosis, intimal thickening, and calcification in some areas. The over-all appearance of the artery is similar to that of an arteriosclerotic aneurysm. The arterial dilatation noted in acquired arteriovenous fistulas may also occur in the congenital form (Fig. 5).

Degeneration of the artery proximal to the fistula can be demonstrated well experimentally. Figs. 18 and 19 show an example of an

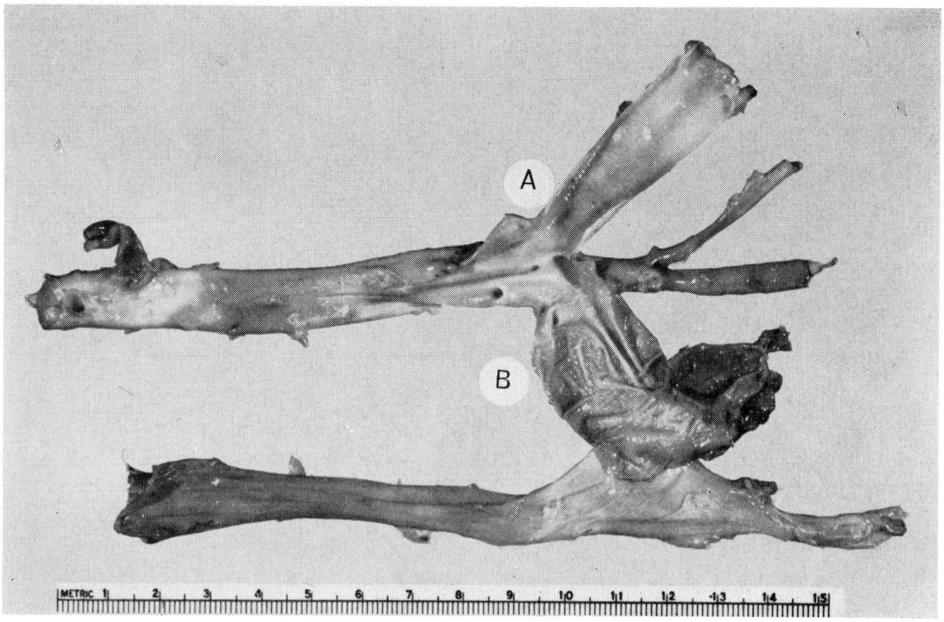

Fig. 19. Same specimen as in Fig. 18 with arteries opened. The right iliac artery (*B*) is dilated but the endothelial lining is smooth.

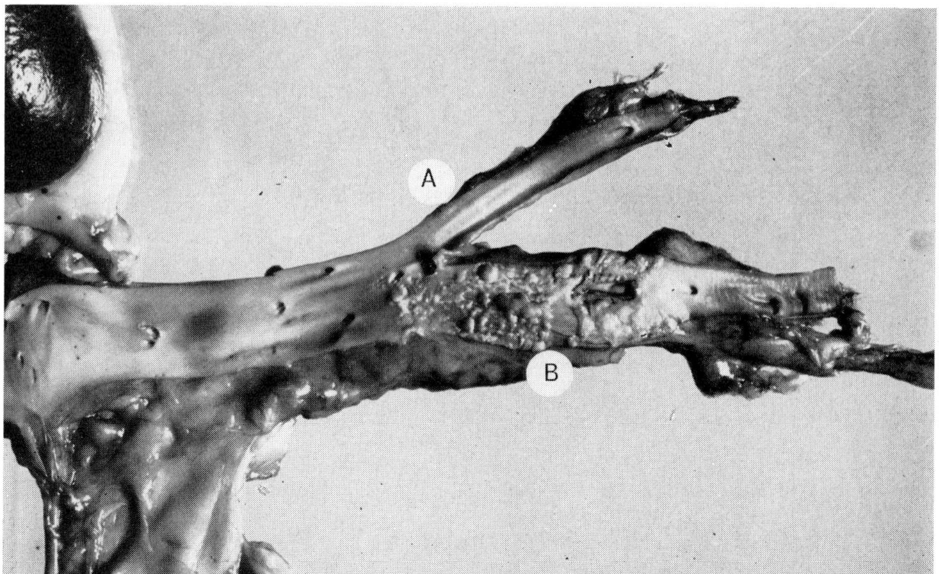

Fig. 20. Experimental A-V fistula comparable in size to the one shown in Figs. 18 and 19, but only of 6 months' duration and with cholesterol level maintained at 880 mg. percent. The left iliac artery is normal (*A*). There is atherosclerosis of the artery proximal to the fistula (*B*).

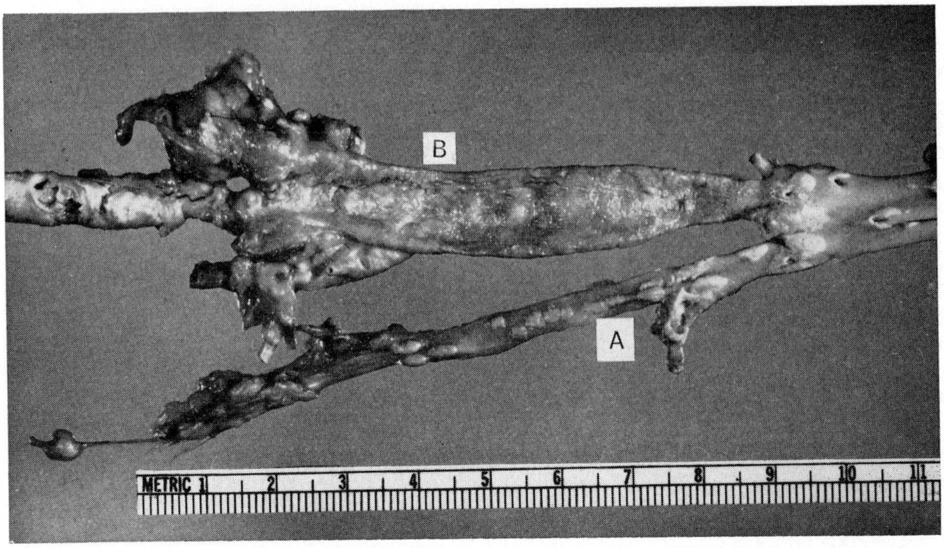

Fig. 21. Experimental A-V fistula and hypercholesterolemia of 1,080 mg. percent of 14 months' duration. There is some atheroma on the nonfistula side (*A*). There is marked dilatation of the artery and of atherosclerosis on the side of the fistula (*B*).

iliac arteriovenous fistula of 8 years' duration in a dog. The blood flow through the common iliac artery proximal to the fistula was 1,100 ml. per minute mean flow which is about five times normal flow. The proximal artery was twice the diameter of the opposite side and the vessel wall was markedly thinned but smooth. Fig. 20 shows another arteriovenous fistula of comparable size of only 6 months' duration, but the cholesterol level in the dog was maintained at 880 mg. percent by thyroidectomy and cholesterol feeding. The proximal segment was dilated and there was atherosclerosis of the proximal segment. Fig. 21 shows a specimen from another hypercholesterolemic dog with a fistula of 14 months' duration. It also shows marked dilatation of the artery and advanced atherosclerosis. These experiments show that the turbulent flow provokes arterial degeneration which in turn is aggravated by high cholesterol levels in the blood.

SUMMARY

The results of management of 32 patients with congenital arteriovenous fistulas of the extremities, abdomen, and the chest wall have been reviewed. The congenital fistulas may vary from diffuse to multiple but discrete lesions, thus, the evaluation of treatment of the group as a whole is extremely difficult.

Six patients, five of whom had extremity lesions, were cured by operation and eight were improved. Six patients who were operated upon were worse and two were unchanged.

In sharp contrast to the results attained in congenital fistulas, all 25 who had acquired lesions were cured. A significant problem encountered in patients with long-standing arteriovenous fistulas is that related to proximal arterial degeneration which may progress even after the fistula is removed. It is recommended that the possibilitiy of this occurrence be considered in every patient who has had a fistula of long duration.

REFERENCES

1. Coursley, G., Ivins, J. C., and Barker, N. W.: Congenital arteriovenous fistulas in extremities, Angiology **7:** 201, 1956.
2. Cross, F. S., Glover, D. M., Simeone, F. A., and Oldenburg, F. A.: Congenital arteriovenous aneurysms, Ann. Surg. **148:** 649, 1958.
3. Delaney, J. P.: Congenital arteriovenous fistulas of the extremities, Minn. Med. **44:** 160, 1961.

4. de Takats, G.: Aneurysms: General considerations, Angiology **5:** 173, 1954.
5. Elkins, D. C.: Vascular injuries of warfare, Ann. Surg. **120:** 284, 1944.
6. Hewitt, R. L., and Collins, D. J.: Acute arteriovenous fistulas in war wounds, Ann. Surg. **169:** 447, 1969.
7. Holman, E. H.: Clinical and experimental observations on arteriovenous fistulae, Ann. Surg. **112:** 840, 1940.
8. Hughes, C. W., and Jahnke, E. J., Jr.: The surgery of traumatic arteriovenous fistulas and aneurysms, Ann. Surg. **148:** 790, 1958.
9. Lewis, T., and Drury, A. N.: Observations relating to arteriovenous aneurysm, Heart **10:** 301, 1923.
10. Makins, G. H.: The Bradshaw lecture on gunshot injuries of the arteries, Lancet **2:** 1743, 1913.
11. Reid, M. R.: Studies on abnormal arteriovenous communications, acquired and congenital. I. Report of a series of cases, Arch. Surg. **10:** 601, 1925.
12. Rienhoff, W. F.: Congenital arteriovenous fistulae in children: An embryological study with report of a case, Bull. Johns Hopkins Hosp. **35:** 271, 1924.
13. Shumacker, H. B., Jr.: The problem of maintaining the continuity of the artery and vein in surgery of aneurysms and arteriovenous fistulae, Ann. Surg. **127:** 207, 1948.
14. Szilagyi, D. E., Elliott, J. P., DeRusso, F. J., and Smith, R. F.: Peripheral congenital arteriovenous fistulas, SURGERY **57:** 61, 1965.
15. Veal, J. R.: Congenital abnormal arteriovenous anastomoses of the extremities, Arch. Surg. **33:** 848, 1936.

DISCUSSION

Dr. Makis Tsapogas (Albany, N. Y.). I have very much enjoyed the paper by Drs. Varco and Sako; Dr. Cotton and I have also been interested in this difficult subject. I would like to bring up a few points on the diagnosis and management of the very diffuse congenital arteriovenous fistulas in the lower limb. In our series murmurs could be heard only sometimes over the affected vessels.

Significantly elevated venous pressures were recorded in the affected limb, and the oxygen saturation was usually considerably raised. Arteriographically the shunts could not be visualized in most instances. However, the whole arterial tree was enlarged, there were more tributaries than normal, and venous filling was very rapid.

The operative method we adopted aims in reducing substantially the arterial blood supply in the diseased limb. We ligate and divide the branches of the major arteries in the affected areas extensively, leaving the main trunk intact.

In selecting the arteries to be denuded of their branches, we found that arteriography and skin temperature contour maps offer valuable help. A most extensive ligation of branches of many arterial trunks, from the iliac down to the tibial vessels, may be found necessary. This is carried out in one or multiple procedures depending on the magnitude of the problem.

By this technique, clinical improvement over a long follow-up was achieved in the majority of cases.

I am grateful to the Society for the privilege of the floor.

Dr. John R. Derrick (Galveston, Texas). I would like to discuss just the acquired type of fistula to point out perhaps a technical problem that may be of help.

The high pressure in the venous system is usually the technical problem that most of us encounter in attempting to repair the acute or chronic fistula. We've had experience in the last 6 months with four fistulas; two of them were in the vertebral artery, one in the femoral, and one in the brachial artery.

By using a Fogarty catheter and passing it up until the bruit disappears, we are able to decompress the venous system. This makes the dissection simple and safe.

Another point of interest: Dr. Fred Volmer and I recently had an experience with a pelvic A-V fistula. This patient had recurring hemolysis, apparently from the jet effect that many of us have observed in the aortic valve leaks.

Thank you for the privilege of the floor.

Dr. Alfred W. Humphries (Cleveland, Ohio). I don't know what the conclusions of this paper are to be. If they are that the treatment recommended is either multiple ligations or observation of the disease, I must decry it.

I'm convinced that the treatment of this disease should be aggressively surgical. I've never seen one get smaller but many of them have enlarged, sometimes to the point where they are no longer amenable to surgical treatment.

Ligation, which we did do years ago, was notoriously unsuccessful—frequently within days. Other vessels picked up the blood supply and the fistula remained as large as before.

I think proper treatment is to excise everything involved other than nerve, primary artery, and essential muscle for function.

This is occasionally curative, but most often there's a bit left in some odd corner that can be corrected by a small procedure at a later time.

I think this should be treated surgically, aggressively and early.

Dr. James A. Key (Toronto, Ontario, Canada). I enjoyed Dr. Sako's paper and I would like to ask him if he has any observations to make on the appearance of fresh fistulas following either surgical procedures in an attempt to obliterate the fistula, or possible amputation.

We've had two patients in whom, despite radical surgery ending up in amputation, new fistulas have appeared proximal to the previous lesion which were previously unrecognized either clinically or by angiography.

Dr. Safuh Attar (Baltimore, Md.). I would like to address my remarks with regard to acquired arteriovenous fistulas which have not been discussed today.

In reviewing the literature, we found that there is very little written about acquired pulmonary arteriovenous fistulas of traumatic origin. Most of the reports concern congenital arteriovenous fistulas and we have the experience of a patient who presented at the accident room 3 years ago with eight gunshot wounds, one of them involving his chest, the others involving his abdomen and extremities.

The bullet was to the right of the midline and 4 L. of blood was evacuated. Immediate operation was performed repairing a 2 cm. laceration of the posterior aspect of the right lower lobe.

The patient was followed for 6 weeks and then was lost to follow-up, until 3 years later, when he presented again with clubbing cyanosis and shortness of breath. X-ray of the chest showed a coin lesion in the right lower lobe which on angiography proved to be an arteriovenous fistula.

The patient was catheterized and the pulmonary artery pressures and the right heart catheterization were within normal limits.

However, the oxygen tension was 34 mm. Hg (68 percent saturated) and the systemic arterial O_2 tension was only 46 mm. Hg (82 percent saturated). The cardiac output was normal. The 5-hydroxyindolylacetic acid in the urine was normal.

The patient was operated upon and immediately upon ligation of the inferior pulmonary artery, the arterial oxygen tension rose to 170 mm. Hg on 50 percent oxygen.

The point I want to make is twofold: First, the effects of the pulmonary arteriovenous fistula on the cardiac system are minimal. These patients do not present with heart failure. This patient did not have any evidence of cardiac insufficiency.

Second, whereas in congenital arteriovenous fistulas local excision has been advocated, we feel from our experience with this case that this could not have been possible since the fistula originated immediately after the takeoff of the inferior pulmonary artery.

Dr. Alton Ochsner (New Orleans, La.). Thank you, Dr. Hanlon. I rise only as a representative of that fast disappearing group—possibly not fast enough—the older surgeons Dr. Sako referred to!

We saw a good many of these congenital arteriovenous aneurysms long before we had the advantage of angiography. I can't help but agree with Dr. Humphries in believing that these cases must be treated most energetically. Because many of them will go on to ulceration of lower extremities, one should go in even without the benefit of angiography and remove or ligate most of the vessels involved without interfering with the vascularity of the area with the idea that later one will have to go back.

I know one lady upon whom I operated many years ago who required 12 operations. She had involvement of the lower part of her trunk and her left lower extremity. But, after 12 operations, we were able to control this well and she is still living today.

I'd like to make one note and I hope you won't think I'm too much of a purist—I notice that everyone today spoke of the word "bruit." I don't know why, but for some reason or another, we, being Anglo-Saxons, speak of a "murmur" in the heart but when it's anywhere else it is a "bruit"! Now, why should a "murmur" in the extremity be French and not Anglo-Saxon, when we are Anglo-Saxons?

Dr. Edward A. Edwards (Boston, Mass.). In examining patients with multiple fistulas, there are two helpful thoughts with regard to locating the fistulas.

The first is that although the murmur may be heard all the way, let us say, from the fingertips to the axilla, or toes to the groin, it is often the most distal fistula that gives rise to the proximal murmur. So one must not assume that there is necessarily a series of fistulas all the way up to the root of the limb. One should start by compressing the most distal part of the limb and find the proximal point at which all murmurs will disappear.

Second, because the fistulas arise in the embryo at a time when the entire vascular system is developing, the abnormal vessels often lie in the course of usually evanescent arteries.

In the upper extremity, for example, the fistulas may involve the median or anterior interosseous artery. In the lower extremity, the inferior gluteal or the saphenous artery territories may be involved in the formation of the fistulas.

This concept is helpful in planning the operative procedure.

Dr. Harwell Wilson (Memphis, Tenn.). I wish to briefly comment upon the management of acquired arteriovenous fistulas. Dr. Sako mentioned that the essential principles necessary for the cure of acquired fistula were established years ago and relatively little has changed in this regard. In general this is certainly true. The recognition of the site of the fistula, proximal and distal control of the vessels involved, followed by complete excision of the fistula result in a cure. Drs. Matas, Ochsner, Holman, de Takats, and many of our senior members made significant contributions to the problem.

In recent years, however, certain definite advances have been made in the surgical treatment of the acquired arteriovenous fistula.

The balloon catheter, as mentioned already today, can be very helpful in temporarily obliterating the fistula at the time of operation and may simplify the problem of proximal and distal control.

Dr. Joseph McCaughan, Jr., of our department reported the value of this method a few years ago in a group of patients at our Veterans Hospital, where he is now Director of Surgery.

Second, I think that where we were all taught that complete excision of the fistula, along with proximal and distal ligation of artery and vein, was very frequently necessary, the more usual procedure now would be to restore normal arterial continuity.

Dr. Sako (closing). Thank you very much. I'm a bit bewildered by the number of discussions, since I didn't have enough time to complete my presentation.

In the 32 patients with congenital fistula, six were cured. In five of these the fistulas were in the extremities. Two of these required multiple operations.

Our policy has been to recommend operation in most of the patients but realizing full well that occasionally this may result in the need for an amputation prematurely especially if one is forced to ligate the major artery for technical reasons. The fallacy of ligating major arteries for the treatment of congenital lesions is well known.

In response to the one question about recurrence of fistulas in new locations—yes, we have observed new ones appearing in muscle and under skin grafts which have been used to cover areas where blocks of tissue had been excised. These have been removed at reoperation 3 to 4 years later.

Management of ischemia of the hand and fingers

W. ANDREW DALE, M.D.
MALCOLM R. LEWIS, M.D.
NASHVILLE, TENN.
From the Vanderbilt University Medical Center, the St. Thomas Hospital, and the Mid-State Baptist Hospital

While occlusive arterial lesions of the upper extremities occur much less commonly than in the legs, diagnostic alertness permits helpful management of patients who develop coldness, pain, and necrosis in the fingers and hands because of these lesions (Fig. 1). The relative infrequency of patients with these problems, confusion between the several causes of their symptoms, and lack of a recognized program of management have been sources of difficulty in diagnosis and treatment. The 36 cases discussed below represent a variety of organic lesions which caused ischemia of the hands and fingers. Particular attention is focused upon distal arterial occlusions occurring in the vessels of the wrist, hand, and fingers. Patients with nonocclusive vasospastic disease are excluded from this report.

ETIOLOGY

Aside from *trauma,* the most common cause of arterial insufficiency of the hand and fingers is the presence of a clot within one or more arteries (Table I). *Arterial embolism* is to be immediately suspected when the onset is acute and there is found to be a recent or still present cardiac arrhythmia or myocardial infarction. Embolism from sources other than cardiac arrhythmia and infarction is uncommon.

Arterial thrombosis may also occur quite suddenly and mimic embolism. Absence of a primary embolic site as well as differences in the angiographic appearance aid the differential diagnosis between acute embolism and acute thrombosis. While many instances of thromboses of the hand and finger vessels caused by repeated occupational trauma are recorded,[4] we have not encountered such.

Phlegmasia cerulea dolens is an unusual cause of tissue ischemia in any event and its occurrence in the upper extremity is certainly rare. Our single case was secondary to acute venous thrombosis caused by pressure of the anterior scalene muscle upon the subclavian vein in a patient riding in an automobile for some hours with the left arm elevated on the opened window. Heparinization was ineffective in reversing the process and when the swelling and cyanosis increased to the point at which the radial and ulnar pulses ceased this anticoagulant therapy was stopped and venous thrombectomy was carried out with a Fogerty catheter placed through the brachial artery. Phlebograms later localized the site of compression (Fig. 2), and scalenectomy was performed electively to prevent recurrence.

Thoracic outlet syndrome as a cause of venous thrombosis is unusual but its effects upon the subclavian vein in terms of venous hypertension and arm edema have been described well by Adams and associates.[1]

Small arteries of the wrist and fingers may be occluded organically by lesions whose origins are difficult to determine specifically. These lesions usually occur as multiple sites of obstruction (probably because a single

Presented at the Twenty-third Annual Meeting of the Society for Vascular Surgery, New York, N. Y., July 12-13, 1969.

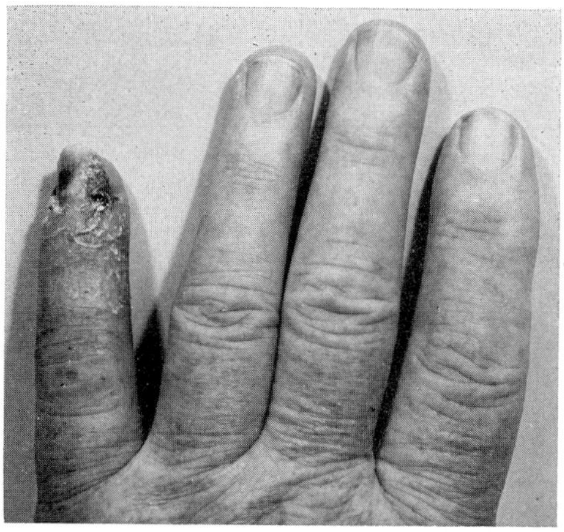

Fig. 1. L. B. Skin necrosis with severe pain as a result of digital arterial occlusions finally resulted in spontaneous amputation. Sympathectomy was contraindicated by severe coronary insufficiency.

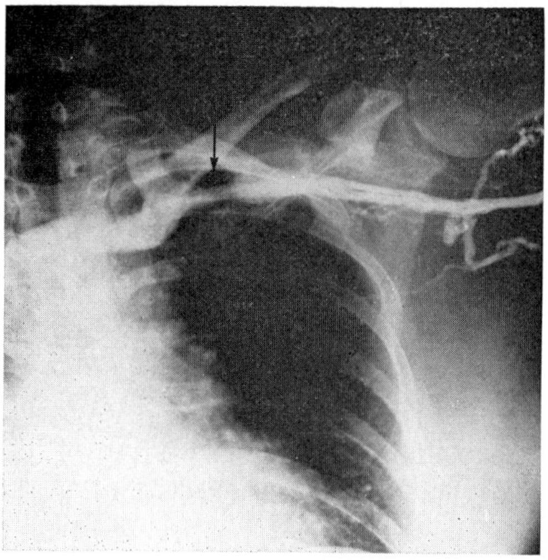

Fig. 2. V. G. Postoperative phlebogram shows patent venous system with compression by anterior scalene muscle and with irregular recanalized axillary and brachial vein following previous venous thrombectomy for phlegmasia cerulea dolens. Elective scalenotomy was done following this demonstration.

one would not produce symptoms) in the ulnar and radial arteries, the palmar arches, and digital vessels. We have treated 21 such patients (Table II).

The actual pathologic lesion has been determined in only one case (Fig. 3) where Buerger's thromboangiitis obliterans was

Table I. *Causes of ischemia of the hand and fingers*

1.	Trauma
2.	Arterial embolism:
	Cardiac arrhythmia or infarction
	Thoracic outlet syndrome
3.	Arterial thrombosis: acute or chronic
	Arteriosclerosis
	Thromboangiitis obliterans
	Repeated trauma
	Polycythemia
	Frostbite
	Collagen disease
4.	Phlegmasia cerulea dolens
5.	Vasospastic and miscellaneous conditions:
	Raynaud's disease
	Arteritis

found. Whether the other patients' occlusions were due to *arteriosclerosis* or to *Buerger's disease* has not been proved. The angiographic appearance leads us to suspect that they are arteriosclerotic in origin, but, in the absence of biopsy evidence in most, all have been herein classified simply as small artery occlusive disease.

Increasing use of angiography in the study of ischemia of the hand and fingers has raised doubt as to whether primary *Raynaud's disease* leads to ischemia of sufficient severity to result in fingertip necrosis or gangrene. Perhaps tissue necrosis is invariably preceded by arterial occlusion. It appears that our entire understanding (or confusion) in differential diagnosis may be greatly altered by the accumulating results of angiographic studies. Localization of the site and extent of the occlusive process, the results of arterial collateralization and differentiation from purely vasospastic disease by angiography allows new insight into these hand and finger problems.

CLINICAL SYNDROME

While claudication usually follows arterial occlusion of arteries of the leg, it is not common in the upper extremity because of less frequent prolonged use of the muscles, and because many of the lesions involve the arterial system at the wrist and hand distal to the large muscle mass. Changes in temper-

Table II. *Summary of 36 cases of ischemia of the hands and fingers*

Patient	*Age/ Sex*	*Duration of symptoms*	*Site of obstruction*	*Treatment*	*Comment*
I. Arterial embolism					
E. A.	76/M	7 hours	Brachial	Embolectomy	Good result
G. F.	54/F	30 days	Brachial	Bypass vein graft	Good 2 months, then graft thrombosed
T. G.	77/M	24 hours	Brachial bifurcation	Embolectomy, venous patch graft	Good result
L. L.	75/F	Few hours	Subclavian	Transbrachial embolectomy	Good result
L. H.	59/F	Few hours	Subclavian	Transbrachial embolectomy	Good result
I. W.	76/F	5 hours	Forearm vessel	Intravenous heparin	Salvage, slow improvement
S. T.	84/F	2½ hours	Brachial (first time)	Embolectomy	Good result
S. T.	85/F	5 hours	Brachial (second time)	Embolectomy	Good result
M. N.	70/F	Few hours	Brachial	Embolectomy	Good result
L. C.	68/F	Few hours	Radial	None	Good result
S. L.	76/F	3 hours	Axillary	Embolectomy	Good result
II. Phlegmasia cerulea dolens					
V. G.	46/F	24 hours	Axillary and brachial	Transbrachial thrombectomy	Good, later scalenotomy
III. Arterial thrombosis					
1. Large proximal artery					
C. H.	70/F	12 hours	Subclavian	Intravenous fibrinolysin	Arm improved, cerebrovascular accident, death
P. E.	68/F	Few hours	Brachial, radial, and ulnar	Brachial and radial thrombectomy	Loss of arm, death
N. A.	70/M	Few weeks	Subclavian	Vasodilators	Minor symptoms
2. Small distal arteries					
G. G.	49/M	3 months	Multiple in digital and palmar arch	Sympathectomy	Negative biopsy, finger healed
J. G.	53/F	6 months	First, second digitals	Sympathectomy	Simultaneous carpal tunnel release
G. R.	48/M	4 months	Ulnar artery, palmar arch, and digitals	Sympathectomy	Good
L. B.	69/F	5 months	Palmar arch and digital	Vasodilators	Spontaneous amputation one finger distally
L. S.	62/F	9 months	No arteriogram yet	None	No relief
G. J.	54/M	2 weeks	Ulnar and digital	Sympathectomy	Postthoracotomy neuritis, fingers good
H. C.	44/M	Few weeks	Radial and digital	Vasodilators	Negative biopsy
W. T.	39/M	5 years	Radial and ulnar	Sympathectomy	Good

Table II—*Cont'd*

Patient	*Age/ Sex*	*Duration of symptoms*	*Site of obstruction*	*Treatment*	*Comment*
T. T.	30/M	Several years	Radial and ulnar	Sympathectomy	Amputation finger tips, healed
A. D.	40/F	3 weeks	Radial and ulnar	Sympathectomy	Good
C. L.	58/M	3 weeks	Palmar arch, ulnar, digital	Sympathectomy	Good
J. A.	61/M	16 years	Indeterminate angiogram	Sympathectomy	Later multiple finger amputations
B. B.	46/M	4 weeks	Digital	Vasodilators cessation smoking	Improvement
W. M.	40/M	2 years	Ulnar and radial	Sympathectomy	Good
M. E.	29/F	2 months	Digital	Sympathectomy	Good
A. C.	58/M	Several years	Ulnar and digitals	Vasodilators	Still painful
H. Y.	58/F	Several years	Indeterminate	Vasodilators	No relief
J. J.	56/M	Several years	Digitals	Vasodilators	No relief
E. M.	48/M	7 months	No arteriogram	Vasodilators	No relief
A. S.	62/M	Several months	Ulnar and digital	Sympathectomy	Good, Horner's syndrome
S. P.	24/F	Several months	Radial and ulnar	Vasodilators	Undetermined

ature with symptomatic coldness are commonly acknowledged, and color changes associated with this often leads to the group of signs known as Raynaud's phenomenon.

A clear distinction between primary Raynaud's disease showing Raynaud's phenomenon and the same phenomenon secondary to other processes is important (Table III). Primary Raynaud's disease is uncommon, is usually seen in women, and is most often bilateral. The experience of others with large numbers of these cases has led to the recommendation that cases not be classified as primary until all studies have been accomplished and a considerable period (approximately 2 years) of careful follow-up has passed.[2] De Takats[6] points out that as careful follow-up continues over a period of time, more and more of such patients are found to have another primary cause which allows differentiation from primary Raynaud's disease.

The reason night pain in the fingers is less common than in lesions of the lower extremity is not clear, but this has proved to be typical. Some of the differential diagnostic characteristics of diseases causing pain in the hand and fingers are summarized in Table IV.

Table III. *Causes of Raynaud's phenomenon*

A. Primary Raynaud's disease
B. Raynaud's phenomenon due to:
  1. Arterial occlusion (arteriosclerosis, embolism, thromboangiitis obliterans, injury)
  2. Nerve lesions (thoracic outlet syndrome, causalgia)
  3. Intoxication (ergot, heavy metals)
  4. Miscellaneous (scleroderma, disseminated lupus, rheumatoid arthritis, dermatomyositis, leukemia, myeloma)

The pain which occurs in the arm and hand of patients with thoracic outlet syndrome is often supposed to represent arterial ischemia, whereas it actually is usually the result of nerve pressure. Actual ischemia is rare and the only instance in 60-odd patients seen by us is the one included in Table IV, G.

B. in whom embolism apparently originated in the subclavian artery and dropped down and lodged at the brachial arterial bifurcation in the upper arm (Fig. 6).

Finally, should be recognized the common occurrence of small areas of skin gangrene and the failure of minor wounds to heal. This has often led to incorrect management under the mistaken diagnosis of a retained foreign body or of osteomyelitis of the underlying bone without recognition of the vascular insufficiency which is the actual cause of necrosis and failure of healing.

PLAN OF MANAGEMENT

The diagnosis is often clear-cut from the history and examination, especially in trauma and acute arterial embolism secondary to heart disease. Appropriate therapy may be carried out on this basis. Angiography clarifies the situation so much that its use is almost mandatory.

Angiography. Radiographic visualization can be carried out easily with local anesthesia. A catheter may be passed retrograde through the femoral artery and the radiopaque material released into the subclavian

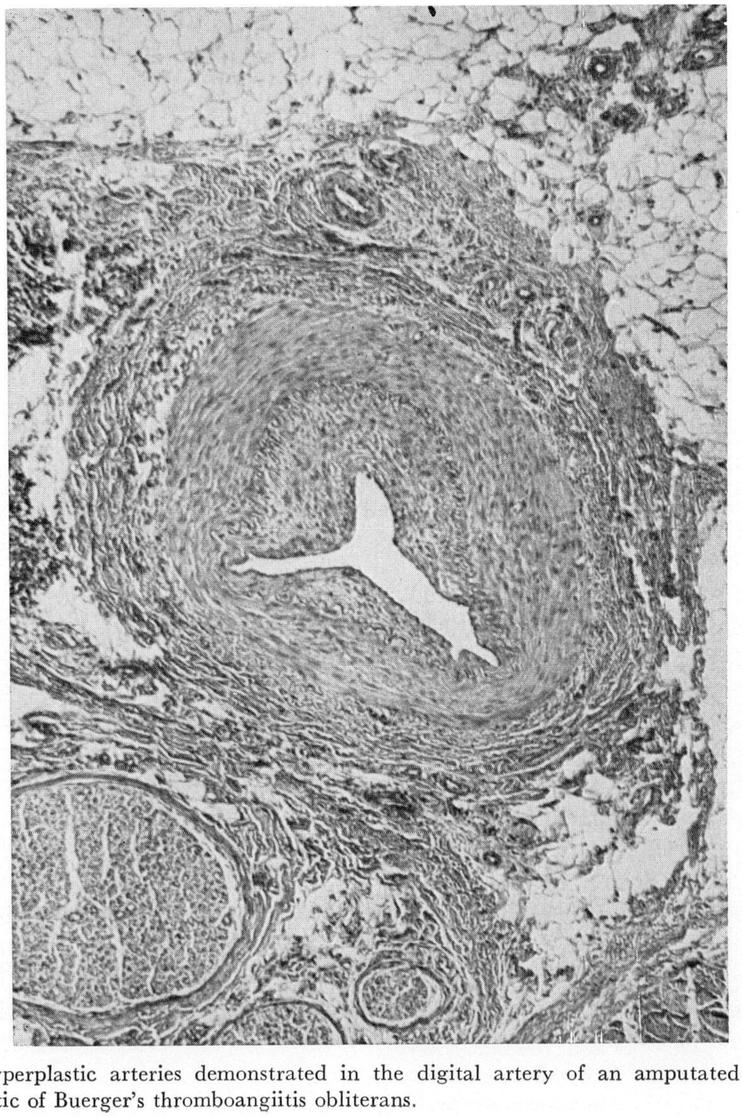

Fig. 3. Hyperplastic arteries demonstrated in the digital artery of an amputated finger tip characteristic of Buerger's thromboangiitis obliterans.

Table IV. *Differential diagnosis of hand and finger symptoms*

Arterial embolism: acute onset, recent cardiac arrhythmia or myocardial infarction, uniform tissue ischemia	
Arterial thrombosis: slow onset, minimal cyanosis, irregular distal distribution of tissue necrosis or gangrene with local pain	
Raynaud's "disease": usually female, episodic, bilateral, minimal tissue necrosis, absence of primary cause, long duration, triggered by cold and emotion	
Acrocyanosis: painless cyanosis of tips of appendages	
Reflex sympathetic dystrophy (causalgia): posttraumatic, decreased motion of joints, skin atrophy, pain prominent	
Thoracic outlet syndrome: pain due to nerve compression, arterial signs unusual, no tissue necrosis	

artery in the apex of the chest, or a needle may be passed into the brachial artery at the elbow for study of the wrist and hand. This latter is preferable because it allows more definitive vascular visualization than does the subclavian injection.

An 18 Cournand needle is passed through a bleb of local anesthesia in the skin directly into the brachial artery as it lies just proximal to the antecubital fossa. As soon as blood is obtained through the lumen of the indwelling needle, this is withdrawn leaving the blunt outer portion which is then advanced into the artery while a steady pulsatile stream of blood flows through it. The head of the needle is taped to the forearm and a connecting tube placed between the needle and a stopcock with syringe attached. Conray-60, 20 c.c., is injected through the needle (pointing in a cephalad direction). Blood flow from this point near the elbow to the distal fingers is slower than is usually anticipated and the multiple cassette changer

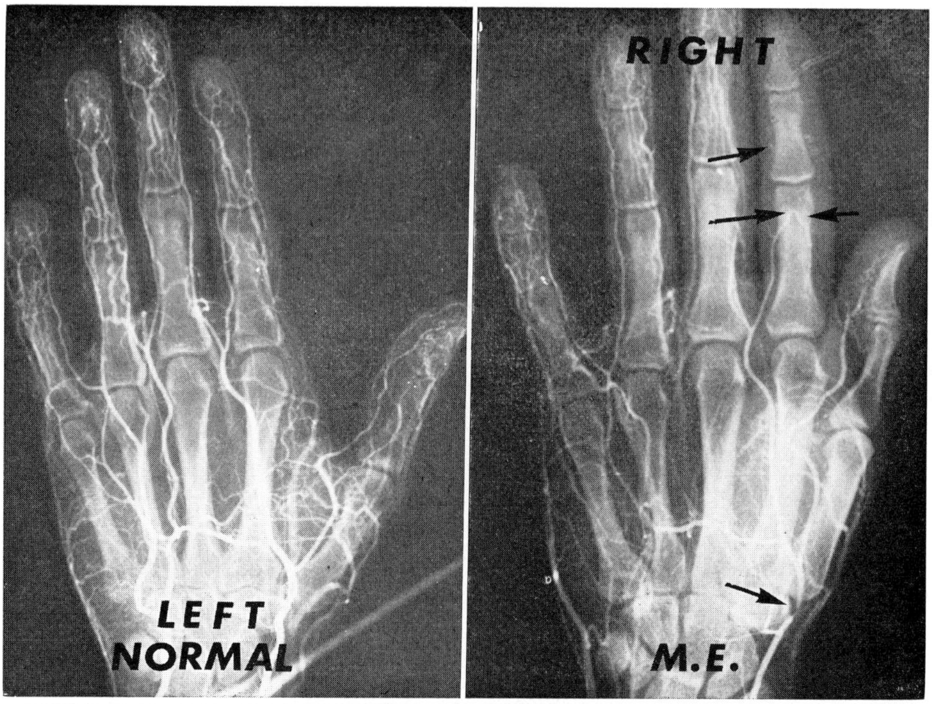

Fig. 4. M. E. Normal angiographic pattern of hand and fingers contrasted to distal radial arterial occlusion and multiple first finger digital arterial occlusion in a 29-year-old female. Healing occurred and pain ceased after thoracic sympathectomy.

should be set to expose 12 films at 2 second intervals in order to visualize all the vessels. In the event that there is difficulty with visualization of the distal hand and finger arteries, improvement may at times be obtained by intra-arterial injection of Priscoline just prior to repetition of the radiopaque injection.

The angiograms shown in Fig. 4 show normal arteries well opacified as well as a typical example of multiple blocks of the arteries of the wrist, hand, and fingers in the other hand of the same patient. Since a single film rarely delineates the entire arterial system, it is important to place all the films on a large viewing box so that each artery may in turn be traced to ascertain whether or not there is continuity or occlusion.

The distal brachial artery is occasionally difficult to cannulate with a needle and another alternative approach is the axillary artery. This is easily palpable with the arm extended above the head and lying on the same plane as on the back. Placement of the needle from above downward toward the wrist is not difficult.

Stellate block. Prediction of the effects of thoracic sympathectomy may to some extent be obtained by blocking the upper thoracic ganglionated chain with a local anesthetic solution. This can be easily accomplished in the patient's room in a few minutes and is not a technically difficult procedure.

The patient lies supine with a small pillow

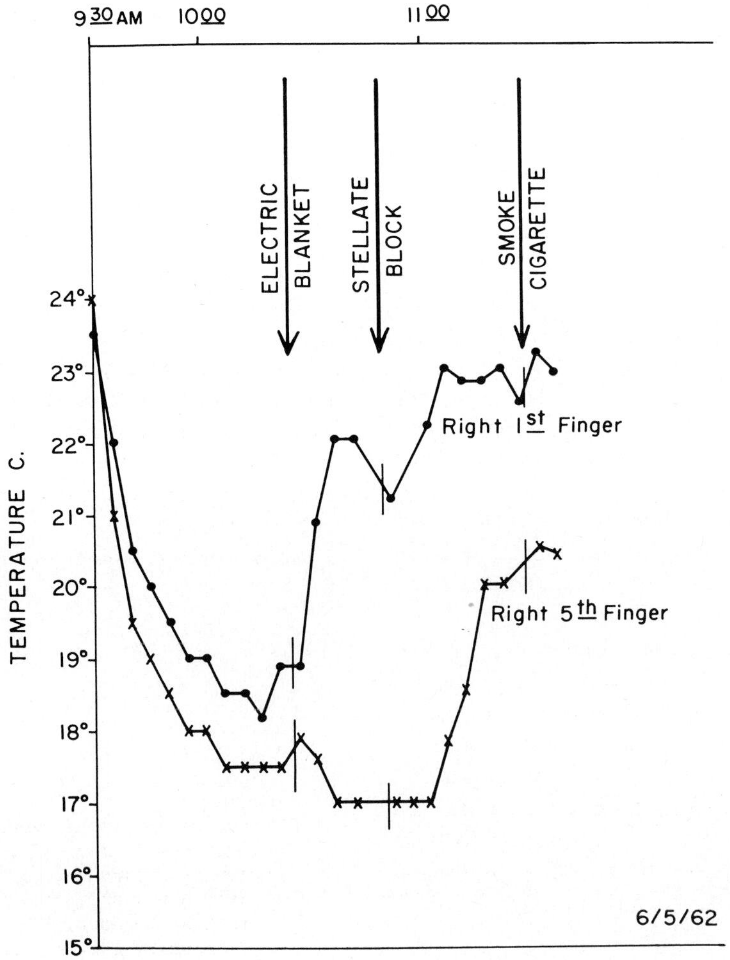

Fig. 5. Skin temperature studies show that general body warming did not completely release vasoconstriction as did the stellate nerve block. Thoracic sympathectomy relieved symptoms.

beneath the shoulders to force hyperextension of the cervical spine. The head of the bed may be elevated to 30 degrees to allow an easier position for the operator. A skin wheal is raised with 1 percent lidocaine just lateral to the trachea and a fingerbreadth cephalad to the clavicle, and through this is passed a long No. 22 needle directly posteriorly until it impinges upon the vertebral body or the disc. The needle then lies between the trachea medially and the carotid sheath laterally. After the needle impinges upon the bone or cartilage, aspiration assures that it does not lie within any large blood vessel. Five cubic centimeters of 1 percent lidocaine is placed as the needle is slightly withdrawn from the bony contact. Then another 5 c.c. is placed as the needle is slowly withdrawn another centimeter. This places a sufficient amount of lidocaine within the proper fascial space to insure prompt blockade of the lower cervical ganglia and the proximal thoracic ones since the anesthetic solution spreads widely following its deposition. The needle is immediately withdrawn and the patient observed for development of a Horner's syndrome within a few minutes. The anterior approach is very much easier than any other.

The patient is questioned after the block in regard to improvement of pain or feeling of warmth and objective measurements are made of the skin temperature of the fingers with a skin thermometer. Fig. 5 shows the results of such a study where general body warming released vasoconstriction to some extent but full vasodilatation was achieved only after stellate block was performed. The ensuing sympathectomy was highly successful.

Biopsy. Only a few biopsies have been done because of fear of failure of healing of the distal tissues as well as the knowledge that the biopsy often fails to aid diagnosis. The most rational approach for obtaining material for pathologic study is a lateral or medial incision over the proximal portion of the distal phalanx to find the neurovascular bundle and actually remove a small portion of this.

The hyperplastic arteritis with narrowing of the arteriolar lumen seen in Fig. 3 was obtained from an amputated digit tip and is believed to represent thromboangiitis obliterans. Most simple biopsies are not this determinative, since the lesions are irregular in distribution.

TREATMENT

While protection of ischemic fingers by gloves and use of vasodilators and cessation of smoking are important, the chief purpose of this presentation is to discuss surgical measures and, in particular, to recommend thoracic sympathectomy for hand and finger lesions.

Anticoagulation has been used in patients with acute thromboses of distal vessels where direct surgical intervention is not really practical. This is carried out by continuous administration of heparin intravenously. Table V summarizes an easy method of heparinization whereby a loading dose is followed by continuous intravenous administration of heparin in a dose designed to keep the Lee-White clotting time between 20 and 60 minutes continuously. The heparin dosage may be adjusted by increments of 25 mg. depending upon the reported clotting time. In doubtful situations a larger rather than a smaller dose should be used to ensure adequate anticoagulation. Since the clot is a dynamic continuing process, the period of 7 to 10 days is chosen to allow maximum resolution while preventing additional deposition of fibrin and platelets. This also carries the patient through the early period of arterial collateralization.

Embolectomy. Management of arterial em-

Table V. *Heparin anticoagulation regimen*

1. Immediate intravenous dose: 50 mg. aqueous heparin
2. Continuous intravenous drip: 500 c.c. D5W containing 125 mg. aqueous heparin each 8 hours
   a. Obtain Lee-White clotting time at 8 A.M. and 6 P.M. daily
   b. Modify heparin dosage ± 25 mg. dependent upon clotting time to maintain this at 20 to 60 minutes
   c. Continue program 7 to 10 days
   d. Reverse with protamine sulfate 50 mg. intravenously should bleeding occur

boli of the upper extremity has been similar to that of arterial emboli occurring elsewhere. Immediate anticoagulation therapy has been started by administration of 50 mg. of aqueous heparin intravenously. This has not resulted in troublesome bleeding at the time of operation in any instance and is used in an effort to prevent thrombosis in the arterial tree distal to the occluding embolus. Surgical embolectomy is done as soon as possible, and no effort is made to delay operation in order to allow conversion of rhythm, full digitalization, or other nonsurgical treatment.

Two patients had arterial occlusion of such a distal portion of the arterial tree that no operative intervention was necessary. Eight other patients had embolectomy via the medial upper arm approach to the brachial artery. This was usually done under local infiltration anesthesia. A Fogerty catheter was passed to remove the embolus from the subclavian artery or from the branchial artery itself. Adequacy of the cleanout was attested in each instance either by palpation of a pulse at the wrist or by postembolectomy angiography in the operating room.

One patient had two different brachial embolectomies from the same vessel 9 months apart. On the second occasion, this 85-year-old woman personally telephoned to state that since another clot had lodged in her

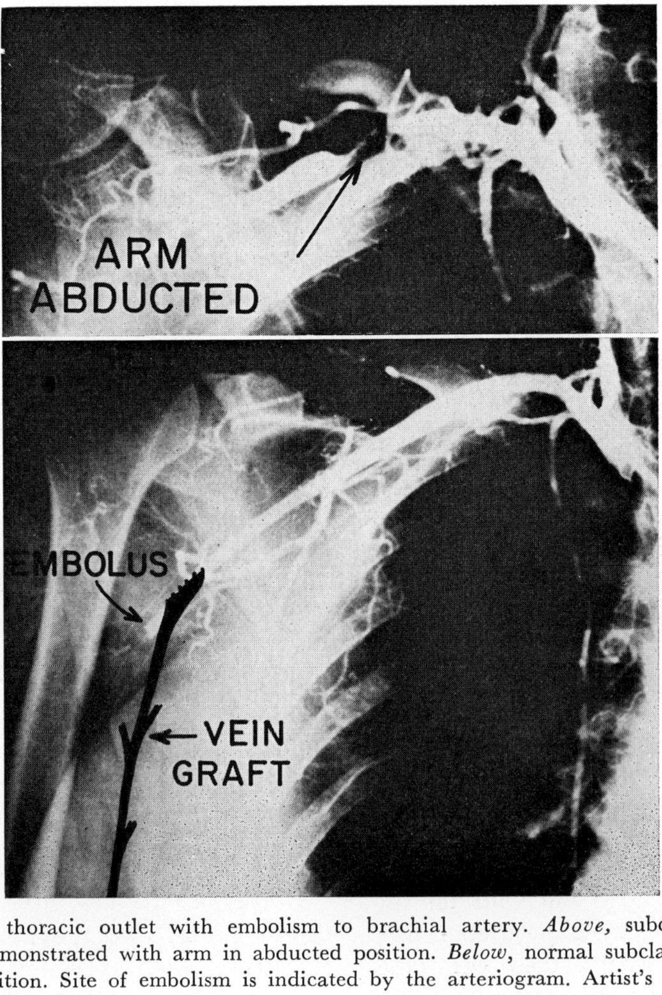

Fig. 6. G. B. thoracic outlet with embolism to brachial artery. *Above,* subclavian arterial occlusion is demonstrated with arm in abducted position. *Below,* normal subclavian with arm in neutral position. Site of embolism is indicated by the arteriogram. Artist's drawing shows proximal end of the bypassing vein graft.

arm she would again like to have it removed!

One embolus was operated upon 30 days after its occurrence. In this 54-year-old woman an apparently embolism occurred secondary to formation of a clot in the subclavian artery at the site of constriction by a cervical rib which had regenerated after its previous removal elsewhere. The first operation consisted of removal of the cervical rib and the underlying first rib to which it had fused. At the same time brachial embolectomy was carried out through through the usual midarm approach. The next day it was apparent that the hand and forearm not only were unimproved but were somewhat worse and since sensation was becoming impaired, a vein graft was removed from the contralateral forearm and used to bypass the rethrombosed site of embolectomy (Fig. 6). The result was excellent in terms of graft patency as well as of relief of the thoracic outlet syndrome and return of hand function for a period of 2 months when graft occlusion led to a recurrence of ischemia of the hand. No further procedure has yet been done.

This experience corroborates the general impression that embolectomy in the upper extremity is a perfectly easy procedure which should be carried out when needed[16] to avoid a functionally damaged extremity which may result after nonoperative management.

THORACIC SYMPATHECTOMY

The results of thoracic sympathectomy for ischemia of the fingers are good and, contrary to some earlier opinions of others,[8] impress us as better than those of lumbar sympathectomy for ischemia of the distal tissues of the lower extremity. It forms the basis of therapy for organic blocks of the small hand and finger vessels.

The sympathetic innervation of the upper extremity originates in preganglionic nerve cells whose bodies lie in the corresponding lateral horns of the gray matter of the spinal cord. The dendrites pass out with the anterior nerve roots into the paravertebral sympathetic chain and synapse there with postganglionic neurons. Dendrites from the latter pass through the rami into the peripheral nerves of the brachial plexus and then down the arm to supply the skin and vessels of the head, neck, and upper extremity.

There has been continuing difficulty in defining the proper nervous elements for ablation to denervate completely the vessels of the fingers and hand. Not only are there anatomic variations but also surgical failures have occurred because of inaccurate localization. While it was earlier believed that postganglionic sympathectomy caused hypersensitivity of the vessels to circulating epinephrine, it now appears that poor results after upper extremity denervation were the results of inadequate localization of the nerves or of incomplete operation.[5, 6] The preganglionic nerves enter the chain from the T_1 through T_{10} segments of the cord so the T_1 through T_5 resection should effectively sever the pathways. The occurrence of miosis, narrowing of the palpebral fissure, and enophthalmos (Horner's syndrome), if the sympathectomy disturbs the pupillociliary nerve pathway, limits the cephalad extent of resection of the chain. Sympathectomy of T_1 through T_5 fulfills the criteria of denervation without a high incidence of Horner's syndrome and is the preferred ablation.

The deep autonomic position of the nerves serving the upper extremity has resulted in a succession of favored surgical approaches. The earlier use of the transcervical route did not allow sufficiently low resection of the ganglionated chain for complete denervation and produced Horner's syndrome frequently by damaging the sympathetic pathways to the eye.

A more limited sympathectomy via a posterior thoracic approach was next popularized. After resecting a portion of the posterior third rib, a short length of the thoracic ganglionated chain (T_2 and T_3) could be disconnected from the spinal cord by severing the rami and cutting the chain below T_3. This resulted in a preganglionic form of sympathectomy since the postganglionic fibers were left intact in the disconnected but nonresected trunk. This retropleural approach was somewhat complicated, did not allow

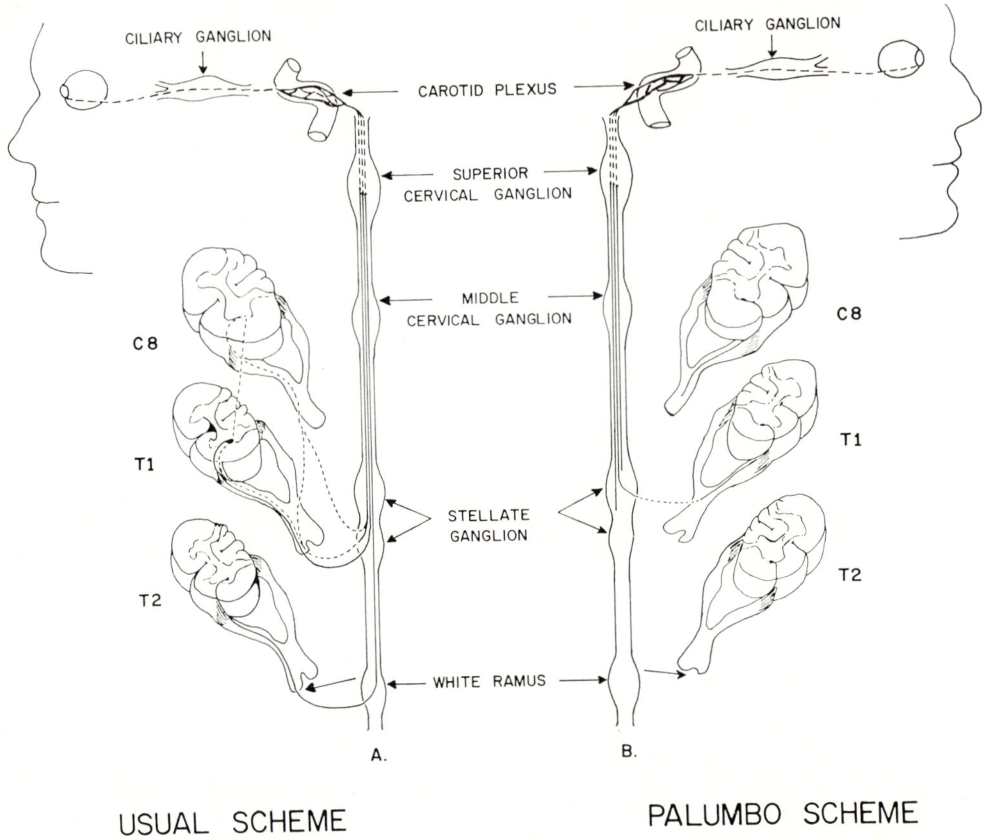

Fig. 7. Comparison of Palumbo's concept of sympathetic pathways to the eye with that thought to be usual. (From Palumbo, L. T.: A new concept of the sympathetic pathways to the eye, SURGERY **42:** 740, 1957, by permission.)

wide denervation of the upper extremity, and soon began to be changed by several variations to a wider transpleural approach.*

Louis T. Palumbo[12] in 1957 asserted that, previous authorities notwithstanding, the usual description of the anatomic pathway of the pupillociliary mechanism was incorrect and that it did not transverse the first ramus to the first thoracic ganglion but passed into the upper aspect of the stellate ganglion (Fig. 7). This allowed resection of the distal portion of the stellate ganglion (T_1) without production of Horner's syndrome in most patients. His and Lulu's[12, 13] experience was a significant contribution to proper denervation of the upper extremity.

*The interested reader is referred to the account of the development of variations of thoracic sympathectomy by Allen, Barker, and Hines.[2]

We have followed his technique in general but have now changed from the anterior approach to the axillary route (Fig. 8). This transaxillary approach does not cut muscles, allows better direct vision of the nerve chain, and heals with less pain and a more acceptable scar.

Technique. The patient is positioned laterally and the arm is supported on the anesthesia screen. The table may be rolled to either side to improve exposure later. An incision 4 to 5 inches long is made in the axilla in the line of the third intercostal space and carried through the fat. The medial pectoralis major and the lateral latissimus dorsi muscles are mobilized underneath to allow placement of retractors. The third interspace is entered and the intercostal incision is carried somewhat underneath the under-

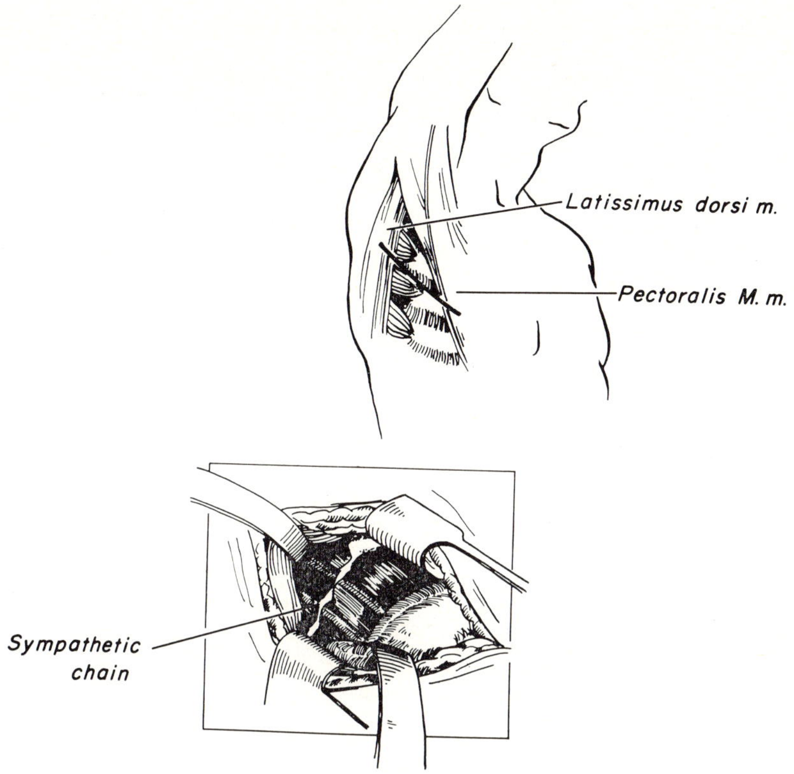

Fig. 8. Transaxillary approach through the third intercostal space allows downward retraction of the lung and easy visualization of the ganglionated chain as it lies on the rib ends beneath the posterior parietal pleura.

mined pectoralis major and latissimus dorsi muscles to allow better spreading of the ribs by the thoracic retractor.

Exposure is obtained by slowly opening the self-retaining retractor. The apex of the lung is held inferiorly by a malleable retractor placed over a gauze pad. The ganglionated chain is seen as it lies on the rib ends adjacent to the transverse processes of the thoracic vertebrae. The pleura is opened directly over the nerve chain to allow its dissection upward to the inferior border of the first rib where a clip is placed transversely and the chain is cut across. It is then elevated with a clamp and similarly dissected down to the lower border of the fifth rib where it is again clipped. No special attention need be made to clipping every attachment of the ganglionated chain, and the clips are primarily used for control of bleeding. The electrocautery is also useful for hemostasis. Particularly careful preservation of the azygos vein at the inferior aspect of the exposure is in order.

If the apical pleural space is obliterated by adhesions, these may require lysis. In this event it may be difficult to visualize the chain through the scarred parietal pleura, and this should simply be opened at the approximate location and search made for the nerve trunk in the extrapleural tissue.

At conclusion the lung is re-expanded, the ribs are closed with 2-0 chromic gut sutures placed pericostally, and the soft tissues are closed in layers.

While it may be unnecessary to provide tube drainage through a low lateral intercostal space, this has no particular disadvantage and it offers protection against the accumulation of fluid and a warning of intrapleural bleeding should that occur in the postoperative period.

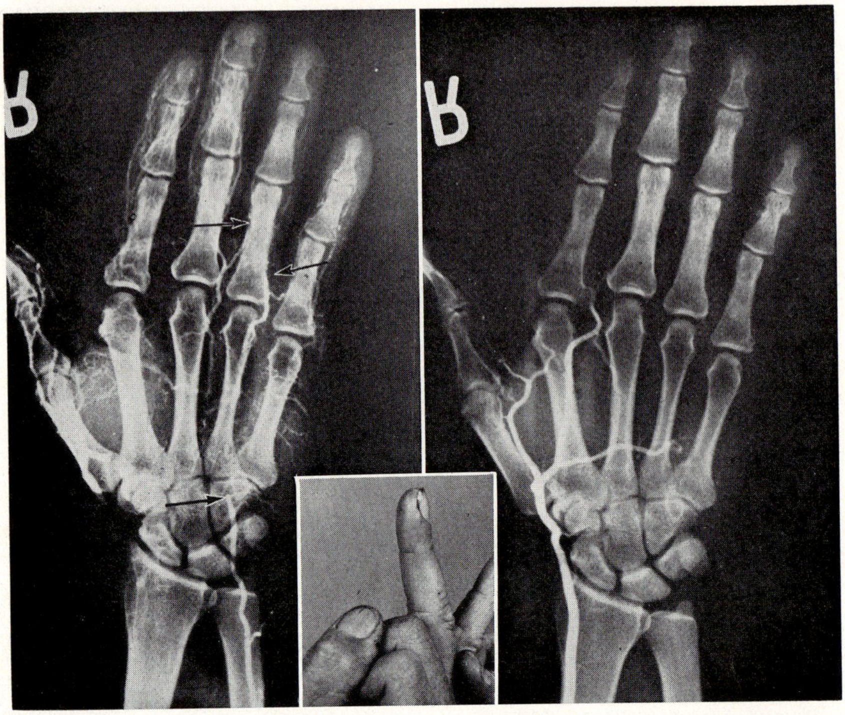

Fig. 9. A. D. painful finger with tip necrosis was caused by multiple small arterial blocks shown by arrows on left. Right is an earlier film which showed patent radial artery. Healing occurred after thoracic sympathectomy.

Postoperative care is similar to that for any thoracotomy. The tube may be removed at 24 to 48 hours depending on the amount of drainage. Wound dressings are removed at 48 hours and the patient is encouraged to move the shoulder and arm freely at once. Antibiotics are not necessary. Since many of these patients are relatively young and most are in excellent condition except for their hand problem, early discharge is often possible by the fifth to seventh hospital day.

Should there be a complicating thoracic outlet syndrome, the first rib can be easily resected through this basic approach after the technique described by Roos.[14] In the event that this is necessary the arm should not be fixed to the anesthesia screen because upward traction of this by an assistant greatly increases exposure of the subclavian vessels overlying the rib at the time of its dissection and removal. The arm is simply prepared and draped into the field with orthopedic stockinette rolled from the hand up to the shoulder.

Results. Twelve of the patients who had arterial blocks in the wrist, hand, or fingers had thoracic sympathectomy (Table II). There were no deaths. Results were excellent in terms of healing of skin lesions, relief of pain, improvement in nail nutrition, and increased fingertip temperature.

The patient (A. D.) whose painful cold ring finger is shown in Fig. 9 was a 40-year-old waitress. The distal ulnar arterial block and the digital arterial blocks are shown by arrows. Thoracic sympathectomy was done uneventfully and she soon returned to work. A warm, healed painless hand and fingers have persisted during the 9 year period which has elapsed since operation.

There were no deaths. Aside from the visible evidence of Horner's syndrome this did not cause particular difficulty to the 3 patients in whom it occurred. One patient was temporarily disabled by intercostal neuritis which persisted for several months (Fig. 10). Temporary relief by lidocaine block of the intercostal nerves was followed by later resolution of the pain.

The 9 patients with distal arterial blocks who have not yet had thoracic sympathectomy have done far less well. Despite vasodilators, a warm enviroment, and cessation of smoking (in some) the results have been poor and in direct contrast to the happy solution of the hand and finger problem in those similar patients who had sympathetic denervation.

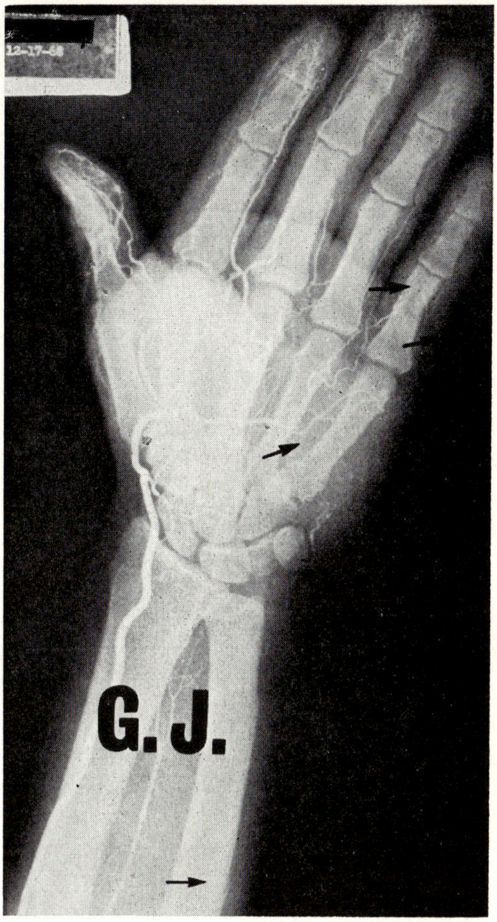

Fig. 10. G. J. Multiple blocks at arrows show occlusion of ulnar and digital arteries. Fifth finger promptly warmed and healed after thoracic sympathectomy. Convalescence was delayed by intercostal neuritis which persisted 3 months.

DISCUSSION

Far less interest, discussion, and systematization of diagnosis and treatment has occurred in ischemia of the upper than of the lower extremity. Indeed it is rather difficult to prepare a suitable bibliography because the reported experience is scattered under various titles. The common denominator of hand and finger ischemia has simply not been used to group patients.

Our interest in patients exhibiting hand and finger ischemia[5] has gradually led to formulation of the plan of management shown in Table VI which summarizes our current ideas regarding diagnosis and therapy. At least four points deserve further emphasis.

First, it is apparent that modern angiographic techniques aid diagnosis to such an extent that definitive arteriograms are always necessary. Experience with these patients as well as with patients having thoracic outlet syndrome, reflex sympathetic dystrophy, and other upper extremity lesions indicates the value of arteriography in differential diagnosis. There is now developing improved correlation between the clinical syndromes involved and the actual arterial lesions. A changing understanding of these problems is to be expected as experience increases.

Second, the importance of searching for distal arterial occlusions should be emphasized whenever hand symptoms suggest ischemia. For example, in the case of J. G. where the symptoms strongly suggested carpal tunnel syndrome the arteriograms showed digital vessel blocks in the index and long fingers and led to the performance of transaxillary thoracic sympathectomy as well as lysis of the volar carpal ligament at the same operation. In patient S. E. the apparent diagnosis of Raynaud's disease in a 29-year-old woman was changed to Raynaud's phenomenon secondary to distal digital arterial occlusions following angiography. The response to thoracic sympathectomy was dramatic.

Small vessel occlusions of the wrist, hand, and fingers are more common than have been supposed. Laws, El Sallab, and Scott[10]

Table VI. *Plan of management*

Diagnosis

1. History and examination often allows immediate recognition of cause and proper treatment
2. Test wrist arteries by occlusion and exercise
3. Angiography — to determine site and extent of occlusion
4. Stellate block — to determine effect of release of vasoconstriction upon finger temperature
5. Tissue biopsy

Treatment

1. Cessation of smoking
2. Vasodilators may be tried
3. Embolectomy for proximal acute lesions
4. Heparin anticoagulation (7-10 days) for acute distal occlusive lesions
5. Bypass graft for chronic proximal blocks
6. Thoracic sympathectomy for chronic distal occlusive lesions
7. Avoidance of sympathectomy for primary Raynaud's disease

studied the upper extremity by means of postmortem arteriograms on 94 random autopsies and concluded that complete arterial occlusion was rare prior to 50 years of age. The present group of patients, however, includes 11 (of a total of 21) patients with distal arterial occlusion prior to that age. Previously most of these people would very likely have been classed as examples of vasospastic disease but distal angiography has revealed the true organic nature of the lesions.

Some discussion of the differential diagnosis of arteriosclerosis versus Buerger's thromboangiitis is in order. After studying various reports it does not appear that this controversy is capable of scientific decision at present. To attempt etiologic classification on the basis of age, sex, angiograms, or therapeutic response appears useless. Rather than add another mere opinion to the multiplicity already recorded[2, 3, 13, 15] cases have been classified simply as "small arterial occlusion" without reference to specific etiology. The single exception has been discussed on the basis of the microscopic specimen.

Finally, it is suggested that current ideas of the role of thoracic sympathectomy require modification in the light of the newer surgical techniques as well as differences in diagnosis based on angiography and follow-up studies. Many physicians currently believe that lower extremity sympathetic ablation is more effective than is sympathectomy for the hand and fingers. Our experience leads us to believe that the reverse is probably true and that the bugaboo of recurrence of symptoms after upper extremity sympathectomy was based upon inadequate operation and poor case selection.

Currently there is also the opinion that patients with purely functional disease (such as primary Raynaud's) respond better to sympathectomy than do those with organic arterial occlusion. We submit that the reverse is true and that patients with organic obstruction of the small vessels of the hand and fingers may be expected to obtain considerably better results than the usual patient with primary Raynaud's disease without evidence of occlusion of the digital arteries. This statement cannot be fully documented yet and is certainly opposite to the opinion expressed by some others.[8] On the other hand there are experienced vascular surgeons who have previously come to the same conclusion. Gaza de Takats[6] 10 years ago stated that "lack of organic obstruction in the presence of clear-cut Raynaud's phenomenon is a warning signal of the the first order," and in 1967 Edwards[7] remarked that recurrence of symptoms was so common in primary Raynaud's disease that he found the operation inadvisable "except as a last-ditch effort."*

The present experience with thoracic sympathectomy outlined in Table II has evolved from cautious recommendation when the symptoms of small arterial occlusion were severe to enthusiastic expectation of postoperative benefit to the patient whose problem is small vessel organic disease rather than spasm. Operation is therefore regularly advised when disease of the small arteries of the wrist, hand, or fingers is found.

*Detailed discussion of the management of primary Raynaud's disease is not within the scope of this article. Our experience also indicates the results of sympathectomy to be poor and short-lived.

The improvement which occurs in terms of temperature increase, healing of finger ulcers, and cessation of pain appears to denote increase of blood flow due to prevention of vasoconstriction. In some instances the hand becomes warmer than the other at once while in others the full effect is noted only after a day or so. Continuation of a favorable course has been the rule and the progress of these sympathectomized patients has been strikingly better than the group who have not undergone operation.

SUMMARY

Experience in the management of 36 patients with arterial lesions of the upper extremity causing ischemia of the hand and fingers has led to formulation of a plan of diagnosis and treatment which affords relief for most. Only one extremity was lost.

The importance of angiography in localization of the lesion and in determination of cause is stressed. The role of stellate block is discussed.

Embolectomy is indicated for clots in the large arteries of the arm while intravenous heparin is useful for distal ones.

Thoracic sympathectomy (T_1 to T_5) via the axillary approach has resulted in good relief of ischemia due to multiple organic occlusions of the small wrist and hand arteries. Vasodilators and other nonoperative measures are far less satisfactory.

REFERENCES

1. Adams, J. T., DeWeese, J.A., Mahoney, E. B., and Rob, C. G.: Intermittent subclavian vein obstruction without trauma, SURGERY **63:** 147, 1968.
2. Allen, E. V., Barker, N. W., and Hines, E. A.: Peripheral vascular diseases, ed. 3, Philadelphia, 1962, W. B. Saunders Company.
3. Buerger, L.: The circulatory disturbances of the extremities, including gangrene, vasomotor and trophic disorders, Philadelphia, 1924, W. B. Saunders Company.
4. Butsch, J. T., and Jones, J. M.: Injuries of the superficial palmar arch, Trauma **3:** 505, 1963.
5. Dale, W. A.: Occlusive arterial lesions of wrist and hand, J. Tenn. Med. Ass. **57:** 402, 1964.
6. de Takats, G.: Vascular surgery, Philadelphia, 1959, W. B. Saunders Company.
7. Edwards, W. S.: Discussion of Kirtley, J. A., Riddell, D. H., Stoney, W. S., and Wright, J. K.: Ann. Surg. **165:** 878, 1967.
8. Kirtley, J. A., Riddell, D. H., Stoney, W. S., and Wright, J. K.: cervicothoracic sympathectomy in neurovascular abnormalities of the upper extremities, Ann. Surg. **165:** 869, 1967.
9. Kleinert, H. E., Cook, F. W., and Kutz, J. E.: Neurovascular disorders of the upper extremity, Arch. Surg. **90:** 612, 1965.
10. Laws, L. W., El Sallab, R. A., and Scott, J. T.: An arteriographic and histological study of digital arteries, Brit. J. Radiol. **40:** 740, 1967.
11. McKuseck, V. A., Harris, W. S., Ottesen, O. E., and Goodman, R. M.: The Buerger syndrome in the United States: Arteriographic observations, with special reference to involvement of the upper extremities and the differentiation from artherosclerosis and embolism, Bull Hopkins Hosp. **110:** 145, 1962.
12. Palumbo, L. T.: A new concept of the sympathetic pathways to the eye, SURGERY **42:** 740, 1957.
13. Palumbo, L. T., and Lulu, D. J.: Transthoracic upper dorsal sympathectomy, SURGERY **53:** 563, 1963.
14. Roos, D. B.: Transaxillary approach for first rib resection to relieve thoracic outlet syndrome, Ann. Surg. **163:** 354, 1966.
15. Theis, F. V.: Thromboangiitis obliterans: A thirty year study, J. Amer. Geriat. Soc. **6:** 106, 1958.
16. Trumbull, W. E., Urui, M., and Oberbrook, B. D.: Surgical therapy of acute upper extremity arterial occlusion, Amer. Surg. **149:** 388, 1959.

DISCUSSION

Dr. Geza de Takats (Skokie, Ill.) I had the privilege of reading Drs. Dale and Lewis's paper on a rather bumpy plane coming here from Chicago, and I must say there's a great deal more in their manuscript than Dr. Dale had time to discuss.

One of the first points that he brought up is the ill-repute of upper extremity sympathectomies which has prevailed for a long, long time, and he pointed out that we have not been removing enough segments, which is quite true. It is imperative to remove segments from T_1 to T_5 including the fifth in order to get a reliable sympathetic paralysis of the upper extremity.

In addition to an improved technique one's case selection must be carefully scrutinized.

Early in our vascular clinic at the University

of Illinois and later at Presbyterian–St. Luke's Hospital, we had operated on a large number of patients, well over 50, whom we diagnosed as having primary Raynaud's disease but who turned out to have collagen disease.

The old dictum that a Raynaud phenomenon remains a primary Raynaud's disease if no other disease shows up after 2 years is utterly erroneous.

We have seen patients develop typical scleroderma or lupus 15 or 20 years after the appearance of Raynaud's phenomenon.

Not only do you not influence the collagen disease by sympathectomy, but you can aggravate a quiescent lesion and we've seen acute fulminating lupus erythematosus after a dorsal sympathectomy.

Just as Dr. Dale has pointed out, we have come to prefer the transthoracic axillary approach.

We have gone, as you all have, through the anterior approach and the posterior approach. In 1954, Hedley Atkins, who's now Sir Hedley, in a very short but concise paper, described the trans-axillary approach and we started using it and have used it ever since. It is an excellent approach. To some of the young women who suffer also from diffuse hyperhidrosis, it's cosmetically highly acceptable.

There are two more points I would like to make.

One is in regard to the angiograms which Dr. Dale might want to say something about. These are exceedingly painful procedures, as many of you know. We have done them under brachial plexus block. We have done them after preliminary intra-arterial injection of papaverine and Novocain and the cases have to be individualized, but we have finally decided that a brachial angiogram, particularly when you're interested in small vessel disease and not when you're interested, of course, in subclavian occlusions done with preliminary intra-arterial injection of papaverine 15 to 30 mg., gives a very satisfactory picture.

Finally, I would like to say that with the routine use of punch biopsies done at the dorsal aspect of the proximal phalanx, which I think is safe—we have never seen an extension of any circulatory insufficiency from this procedure—has taught us a great deal and taught our pathologists a great deal.

I think one of the reasons why we're not getting any better diagnoses is because we do not give our pathologists enough material of this sort.

We have developed at Presbyterian–St. Luke's Hospital an awareness of vascular pathology to a point where we can really get a differential diagnosis of diabetic microangiopathy even before there's frank diabetes, of hypertensive arteriolar disease, of thromboangiitis obliterans, and of sensitization angiitis.

I'd like to again thank Dr. Dale and Dr. Lewis for this very timely and important discussion. I would like to say, also, in closing, that by being asked to discuss this paper I restrained myself from discussing congenital vascular anomalies which is one of my favorite subjects!

Dr. George Podgorny (Winston-Salem, N. C.). Mr. Chairman, if I may, I would like to make two remarks.

First, I would like to congratulate Dr. Dale and certainly agree with him. Some people indeed do feel that the thoracic sympathectomies have been in disrespect or disrepute.

Second, we have performed several thoracic sympathectomies which we feel have been very successful. I would like to point out the following: Despite the fact that we have a very active department of physiology, and this department has a constant temperature room and so forth, on a number of occasions patients have shown equivocal results on the temperature studies but have benefited from thoracic sympathectomy and also we have had one or two patients who showed very good result upon ingestion of alcohol but did not benefit from this operation.

At the time of sympathectomy, many people avoid getting the stellate ganglion because they are afraid Horner's syndrome may result.

What we do is we inject initially some lidocaine into the ganglion to ascertain if it is the stellate by production of a temporary stellate-to-ganglion block and Horner's syndrome. Later the lower part of this ganglion is injected; if no Horner's syndrome results it is excised being the first thoracic component (method of Dr. Jamel Kahn).

I want to add one more point to the etiology of the ischemia of the upper extremity, particularly the hands, and that is the deliberate iatrogenic problems that we occasionally encounter because of our orthopedic colleagues. They occasionally have the habit of resecting a portion of the brachial artery in cases of Volkmann's ischemia.

Briefly, a child was seen elsewhere who had fallen and had just a bruise on her forearm. This was thought not to be significant. She had some fever. The following day her forearm was swollen. She was seen by an orthopedist who x-rayed the arm and did not find any fractures. The next day the forearm was swollen even more and she had lost the pulses in the hand.

A fasciotomy was performed and it did not relieve the problem, so they proceeded to explore the forearm and found the brachial artery. It appeared to be normal and somewhat in spasm. They injected lidocaine without result and then resected a portion of it.

This apparently is recommended in Di Palma's Orthopedics. Even recently, there was an article in favor of this. Supposedly this maneuver relieves the spasm.

This child was then brought to our hospital

with impending loss of the hand. Interestingly enough, when we explained the situation to her mother, she refused to allow us to go into the leg to remove a vein for an autogenous graft and so we proceeded to put in a synthetic graft into the brachial artery to restore it which did save her hand. She required physiotherapy later on.

Since recently there have been articles in the literature to the effect of resection of brachial artery, I thought that this may be the proper time to discuss and condemn it.

Dr. Richard J. Sanders (Denver, Colo.). When patients with severe ischemic changes in their fingers respond to dorsal sympathectomy temporarily, only to have their symptoms recur, there is another procedure that can be performed when everything else has failed. Resection of the first rib has been performed in 2 patients by me, and in two patients by Dr. David Roos in exactly this situation. Each of these four patients had recurrent gangrene in the finger tips following temporary relief from dorsal sympathectomy. In three of the four patients, first rib resection resulted in fairly rapid healing of the finger tips. The longest follow-up is three years, and this patient is still improved, although not cured. In the fourth patient, the procedure was of no value, and she later was proved to have scleroderma.

The mechanism by which first rib resection relieves vasospastic symptoms in the hand is obscure. However, the answer may lie in the anatomic observations of Telford and Stopford (Brit. J. Surg. 18: 557, 1930-31) who demonstrated sympathetic fibers running in the lowest cord of the branchial plexus, the cord that runs closest to, and often in contact with the first rib.

Dr. Donald Silver (Durham, N. C.). I rise to compliment Drs. Dale and Lewis for their very fine presentation and to suggest another procedure that has not been mentioned.

I agree with Drs. Dale and de Takats that it's sometimes very difficult to identify the cause of ischemic lesions of fingers. I find that, as time goes on, more and more of these lesions are caused by the collagen disorders.

As has been pointed out by Dr. Dale and the other discussers, sympathectomy is not always the procedure of choice for these patients. However, one can perform a "medical sympathectomy" very easily, merely by injecting one milligram of reserpine intra-arterially. We have treated several patients with ischemic ulcers, like those presented by Dr. Dale, who have done very nicely with the injection of 1 mg. of reserpine at 3 to 6 month intervals.

I bring this procedure to your attention because it is a very nice way to treat these people until their diagnosis becomes obvious. This treatment will frequently control their symptoms for 1 or 2 years and let the underlying disease develop. If a collagen disorder does not appear, a surgical sympathectomy may be indicated.

Dr. Dale (closing). The fine applause for Dr. de Takats reflects his many contributions to this field and we appreciate his discussion.

Angiography is painful. Preparation with barbiturates and Demerol or with Valium makes it easier for the patient. One should delay between the injection of a vasodilator and the injection of the material for 3 to 5 minutes to obtain an optimal effect.

Dr. Podgorny has suggested that temperature studies are sometimes equivocal and we agree with this. Certainly one should not hesitate to do a sympathectomy simply because the temperature studies don't support it.

Horner's syndrome has occurred in about 15 percent of patients operated upon, as the paper shows. We warn all patients that this may occur. When it does, it looks a little odd as the lid droops down, but it has not been a functionally significant problem.

Dr. Sanders, we appreciate your suggestion of a first rib resection and recognize you as one of the authorities on that. Thank you.

Dr. Silver, we have no experience with the intra-arterial use of reserpine, but we shall certainly try it. Thank you for bringing it to our attention.

Natural history of carotid bifurcation atheroma

HUSHANG JAVID, M.D., Ph.D.*
WILLIAM E. OSTERMILLER, Jr., M.D.
JOHN W. HENGESH, M.D.
WILLIAM S. DYE, M.D.
JAMES A. HUNTER, M.D.
HASSAN NAJAFI, M.D.
ORMAND C. JULIAN, M.D., Ph.D.
CHICAGO, ILL.
From the Division of Surgery, Presbyterian–St. Luke's Hospital

The carotid sinus has a remarkable predilection for atheromatous changes. This special tendency has been reported on several occasions since 1900. Chiari[2] found atherosclerosis to be as frequent and as severe in the carotid sinus as in the aortic bifurcation. The frequency of carotid sinus atheroma was reported to be one in seven men beyond the age of 35.[6] Schwartz and Mitchell[6] also noted that if one carotid sinus is severely narrowed there is an 80 percent chance that the other side is also involved.

The relationship of carotid bifurcation atheroma and stroke has been recognized as early as 1914 when Hunt[4] recognized that atheromatous obstruction of the internal carotid artery in the neck can produce cerebral dysfunction. The effect of surgical removal of the obstructive atheroma in relieving transient ischemic attacks has been fully appreciated in the last decade.

Little has been written, however, regarding the natural course of the carotid sinus atheroma and its relation to the clinical course of the patient. A recent report on Cooperative Study[1] in 218 patients with unilateral internal carotid artery stenosis revealed that 42 months' survival in 111 patients after surgical removal of the atheroma was 81 percent when compared with 107 patients who were observed medically with a survival rate of 64 percent, suggesting that the progression of atheroma at the carotid bifurcation could have accounted for a 17 percent difference in survival rate. No arteriographic evidence was presented, however, to show the nature of these changes.

The present study was designed to evaluate the natural course of the carotid sinus atheroma and the speed of its progression.

MATERIAL

In a series of 1,040 patients studied for symptoms or physical findings of carotid bifurcation disease during the last 13 years, 140 patients were selected for this study. This group consisted of patients who had carotid sinus atheroma with varying degrees of internal carotid stenosis up to 60 percent of the lumen. All of these lesions were followed at least for a 12 month period, ranging from 1 year to 9 years for an average period of 3 years.

The object of the study was to evaluate the outcome of patients with carotid bifurcation disease and the speed of progression of carotid sinus atheroma.

Since the patients followed did not have

Supported in part by United States Public Health Service Training Grant No. I T 12 HE 5808.

Presented at the Twenty-third Annual Meeting of the Society for Vascular Surgery, New York, N. Y., July 12-13, 1969.

*Reprint requests: 1725 West Harrison Street, Chicago, Ill. 60612.

severe untreated lesions at the onset, the information obtained would not apply to patients with severely stenotic carotid bifurcation disease. Study consisted of a complete survey of patients' histories and physical findings during the original and subsequent admissions to the hospital. A critical evaluation of atheromatous plaque on posteroanterior and lateral view of carotid arteriograms was accomplished during each study. The percentile comparison of the degree of stenosis of the original and the last arteriogram was recorded. By dividing this figure into the number of years intervening between the two studies, the rate of change per year was obtained.

An attempt was made to determine the correlation between the rate of atheromatous change and age, symptoms of cerebral arterial insufficiency, hypertension, diabetes, extent of arteriosclerosis in other vessels, carotid bruit, and the degree of carotid bifurcation stenosis.

One hundred forty patients comprised the entire group. Twenty-five patients died during the study period. Twenty-two patients could not be restudied. Seven of these were octogenarian and disabled. Six patients refused repeated arteriograms, and we were unable to contact nine in this group. Ninety-three patients were studied by repeated arteriograms (Table I). A review of the records of patients who died revealed an age range of 57 to 76 years with a mean average of 66 years of age. Eighteen patients in this group were hypertensive. Four patients had complete occlusion of the internal carotid artery on one side. Eighteen patients had bilateral disease, and four patients had carotid endarterectomy on one side. Seven patients in this group were not operated upon because of acute and profound neurological deficit. Five of these patients died of stroke within 3 months after study.

Causes of death are shown in Table II. Chronic heart disease and myocardial infarction were responsible as causes of death in seven patients. Eleven patients died with profound neurological deficit. Two patients had severe intracranial pathologic conditions, and five patients never recovered from their original stroke. Fifty percent of patients who died from stroke had no symptoms referable to cerebral circulation prior to sudden development of neurological insult. Seven patients died of unrelated disease.

Repeated arteriograms in a group of 93 patients revealed no change or minimal change in the configuration of the carotid sinus atheroma in 35 patients. Moderate-to-severe changes were noted in at least one side of the neck in 51 patients. Seven patients had changes in the endarterectomized artery, recurrent stenosis was found in three and complete occlusion in four patients (Table III). Two of the latter group had stenotic lesions of the common carotid artery at the time of endarterectomy. Progression of the common carotid occlusion could explain the thrombosis of the entire carotid system.

Table I. *Natural course of carotid atheroma*

Material	*No. of patients*
Complete study	93
Died	25
Unable to contact	9
Octogenarian and disabled	7
Refused restudy	6
Total	140

Table II. *Causes of death*

Causes	*No. of deaths*
Cardiac	7
Cerebrovascular	11
Unrelated	7
Total	25

Table III. *Rate of atheromatous change*

Description	*No. of patients*
No change	35
Significant change	
Greater than 25% per year	32
Less than 25% per year	19
Recurrent stenosis or thrombosis	7
Total	93

Various factors which could conceivably influence the rate of atheromatous change were considered in studying three groups of patients. The first group consisted of 35 patients with an average age of 63 (48 to 83) in whom the repeated arteriogram did not reveal significant change in the appearance of the carotid atheroma during the interval studied. The second group consisted of 19 patients with an average age of 61 (50 to 86), whose arterial lesion changed at a rate less than 25 percent per year. The third group represents 32 patients with an average age of 62 (44 to 76) with a change in the degree of stenosis of more than 25 percent per year.

Age, sex, incidence of diabetes, presence of other vascular lesions did not appear to influence the rate of atheromatous changes in the carotid bifurcation. Hypertension, presence of symptoms, localized carotid bruit, and significant stenosis, however, appear to be prognostic factors in predicting the likelihood of rapid changes in the carotid sinus atheroma.

Fig. 1 shows that the mean average age for the three groups is about the same, and the rate of diabetes and other arteriosclerotic occlusive diseases does not vary greatly in the three categories. Patients with symptoms, however, had more likelihood of having a faster rate of atheromatous change.

Fig. 2 demonstrates the influence of hypertension on the rate of change. Seventy percent of patients whose carotid artery narrowing changed at a rate greater than 25 percent per year were hypertensive, compared to 37 percent in patients whose carotid lesion did not change significantly. One hundred thirty-five carotid bifurcations were observed in the series of 86 patients studied in the three categories. No changes were noted in 51 sides, less than 25 percent change was noted in 35 sides, and more than 25 percent change in 49 lesions. A correlation between these changes and the presence of carotid bruit and the extent of the lesion at the onset can also be seen in Fig. 2. Eighty percent of patients with rapid changes in the carotid bifurcation had a lesion greater than 25 percent, while only 36 percent of patients without atheromatous change had significant lesions at the onset.

The relationship of carotid bruit and the rate of change may relate to the extent of occlusive disease and the level of blood pres-

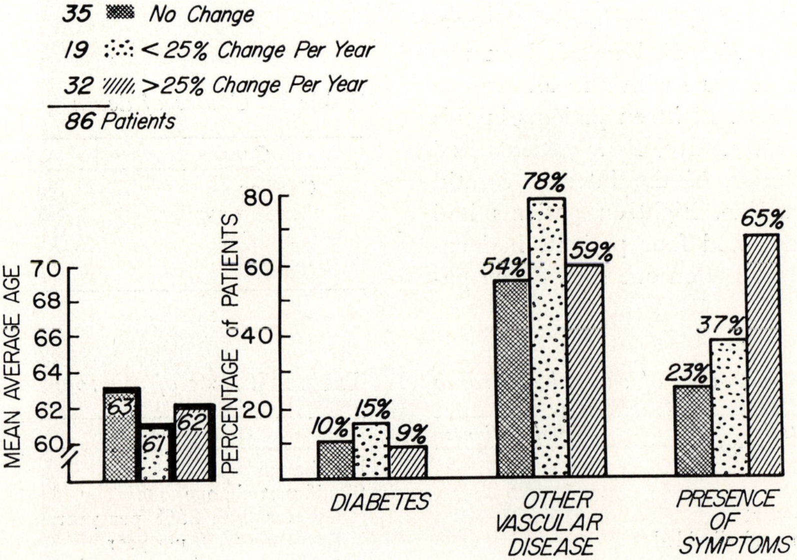

Fig. 1. The relationship of age, diabetes, other vascular disease, and symptoms on the rate of atheromatous change at the carotid bifurcation.

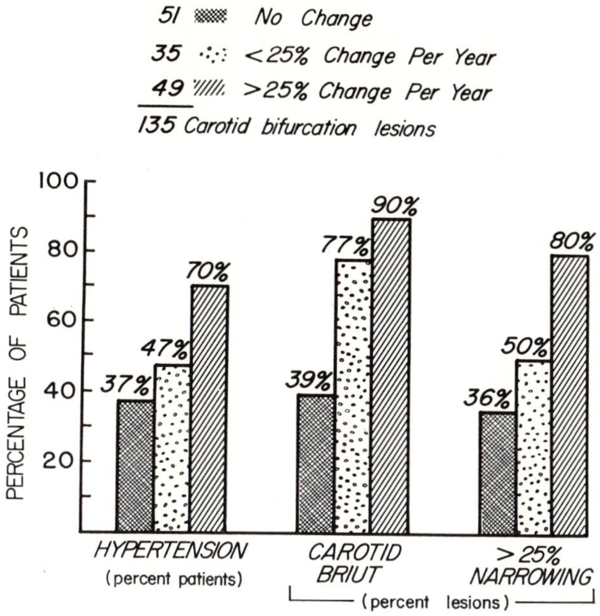

Fig. 2. The influence of hypertension on the speed of atheromatous change and the correlation between local factors such as presence of bruit or extent of disease and the rate of change.

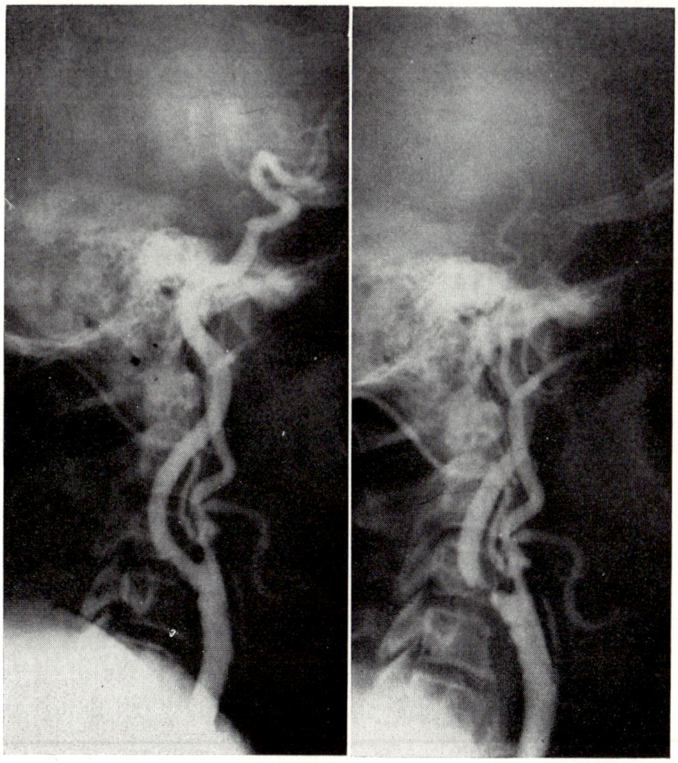

Fig. 3. Rapid changes in the degree of stenosis are demonstrated in a hypertensive individual over a 2 year period.

sure and only represents a positive correlation between the two.

From these observations it is realistic to assume that a hypertensive individual with persistent symptoms, a localized carotid bruit, and a carotid bifurcation stenosis of greater than 25 percent has a strong likelihood of developing rapid changes in the atheromatous plaque at the level of the carotid bifurcation.

Fig. 3 shows significant changes which were noted in a hypertensive individual within a 2 year period.

Recurrent stenosis and thrombosis were identified in seven patients coincidentally. Fig. 4 demonstrates a stenotic lesion at the distal end of the endarterectomized segment. A similar lesion was noted in the other two patients with recurrent stenosis. The location of the lesion and the appearance of the atheroma (Fig. 5) suggested the likelihood of inadequate removal of the tonguelike extension of the atheroma at previous operation. Removal of these recurrent atheromatous plaques which had developed during an interval of 3 to 6 years after endarterectomy was accomplished in the three patients.

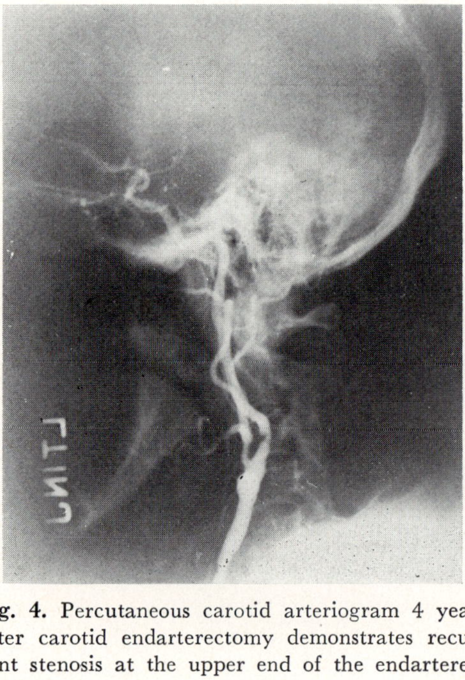

Fig. 4. Percutaneous carotid arteriogram 4 years after carotid endarterectomy demonstrates recurrent stenosis at the upper end of the endarterectomized segment.

DISCUSSION

Although no firm conclusions can be made on the basis of a small series, it appears, however, that the factors influencing the susceptibility of the carotid sinus to atherosclerotic changes and rapid rate of progression must be local rather than metabolic. The absence of atheromatous changes in the internal carotid between the carotid sinus and the base of the skull and the relative freedom of common carotid artery suggest the vulnerability of the carotid bifurcation. The direct relationship of the speed of atheromatous changes to hypertension, carotid bruit, and the degree of obstruction of the internal carotid artery suggests that increased stress caused by hypertension and turbulence could be important factors in progression of disease.

According to a number of studies[3, 5, 7] on human specimens, model hydraulic systems, and animal experiments, localization of the arteriosclerosis to the bifurcation can be explained on the basis of the laws of fluid mechanics.

The hydraulic effects responsible for the inception and progressive changes are diminished lateral wall pressure and increased velocity. Fig. 6 demonstrates the effect of a bifurcation and curved conduit on the velocity of flow and the lateral wall pressure.

Diminished lateral wall pressure produces a suction action of the tunica intima. The intima is thereby subjected to a lifting or pulling effect on the endothelial layer and superficial cells as the flowing blood tends to draw the wall inward toward the axial stream. The stiffness of the wall caused by atherosclerotic changes and turbulence of flow that are due to irregularity or thickening of the wall further cause bombardment of the atheroma and intimal proliferation extending along the direction of flow as a tonguelike projection. It is reasonable, therefore, to assume that once an atheromatous plaque reaches a critical level, the progressive changes may take place quite rapidly.

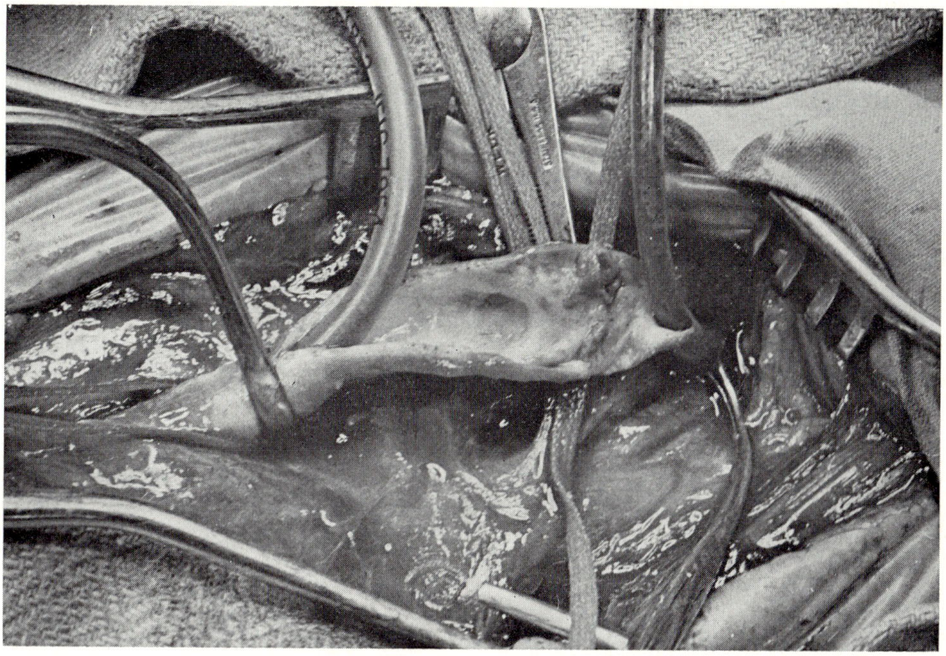

Fig. 5. An operative view of the recurrent atheromatous plaque in the internal carotid artery.

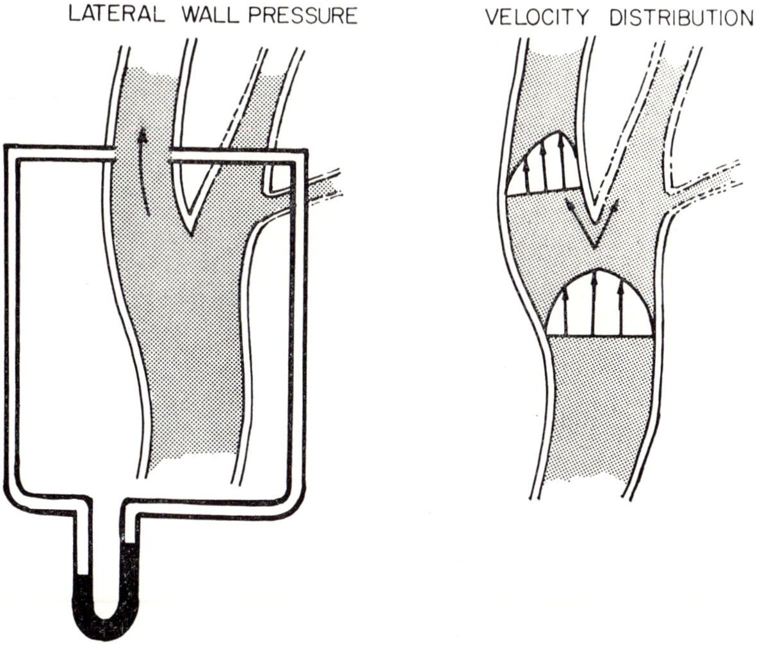

Fig. 6. The hydraulic effect of carotid bifurcation on lateral wall pressure and velocity of flow.

SUMMARY

In a series of 1,040 patients studied, 812 patients had severely stenotic lesions requiring carotid endarterectomy. A group of 140 patients with untreated stenotic lesions of the carotid bifurcation was selected and followed from 1 to 9 years. Eighty-six patients were available for repeated arteriograms and complete study. Thirty-five patients had no significant change in the appearance of the lesion, while 51 patients had increased severity of the degree of stenosis. Twenty-two patients in the latter group required carotid endarterectomy.

The rate of atheromatous change at the carotid bifurcation appears to be directly related to hypertension, presence of cerebral symptoms, localized carotid bruit, and the degree of stenosis.

REFERENCES

1. Bauer, R. B., Meyer, J. S., Fields, W. S., Remington, R., MacDonald, M. C., and Callen, P.: Joint study of extracranial arterial occlusion, J. A. M. A. **208:** 509, 1969.
2. Chiari, H.: Uber das Verhalten dis Teilungswinkels der Carotid Communis bei der Endarteritis chronica Deformans, Verh. Deutsch. Ges. Path. **9:** 326, 1905.
3. Fisher, C. M., Pritchard, J. E., and Mathews, W. H.: Arteriosclerosis of the carotid arteries, Circulation **6:** 457, 1952.
4. Hunt, J. R.: Role of carotid arteries in causation of vascular lesions of brain with remarks on certain special features of symptomatology, Amer. J. Med. Sci. **147:** 704, 1914.
5. Peterson, R. E., Livington, K. E., and Escohar, A.: Development and distribution of gross atherosclerotic lesions at cervical carotid bifurcation, Neurology **10:** 955, 1960.
6. Schwartz, C. J., and Mitchell, J. R. A.: Atheroma of the carotid and vertebral arterial systems, Brit. Med. J. **5259:** 1057, 1961.
7. Texon, M., Imparata, A. M., and Helpern, M.: The role of vascular dynamics in the development of atherosclerosis, J. A. M. A. **194:** 1968, 1965.

DISCUSSION

Dr. Jesse E. Thompson (Dallas, Texas). This is a very interesting and a very important study because of the practical aspects involved. I would like to comment on the asymptomatic carotid bruit as it relates to the natural history of the disease.

Over a 12 year period, my colleagues and I have done more than 700 endarterectomies on 550 patients. In our studies, we have found that a bruit appears at about 50 percent stenosis of the artery and that when a midcarotid bruit is heard, 90 percent of these arise from the internal carotid.

May I have that first slide, please.

The asymptomatic bruit is a troublesome and controversial problem. By liberalizing indications for arteriography in patients with asymptomatic bruits, we have learned a great deal about the natural history of carotid lesions and have now operated on more than 80 of these, as you see on the last line of the slide.

Now, the rationale is based on the following experience—next slide.

In a series of 30 patients with asymptomatic bruits followed but not operated upon, for various reasons, mostly because we didn't know what to do or what to expect, ten or one third of them have gone on to have frank strokes without an intervening episode of transient ischemia, usually from total thrombosis of the artery, at intervals ranging from 1 week to 3 years following detection of the bruit.

Two others had mild strokes, while six developed symptoms of transient ischemia. Thus 18, or 60 percent, of these patients developed symptoms of one sort or another.

So, we have been doing more operations for asymptomatic bruits in the last 5 years, especially when bilateral lesions are present in patients with known occlusions elsewhere in the peripheral vasculature and in those patients who are about to undergo major vascular operation of another sort.

With an internal shunt being used routinely in these patients, we have done 80 operations on 61 patients with no deaths and with one postoperative deficit.

Under these circumstances, I believe the operation is justified, especially after you have seen some relatively young, productive person permanently incapacitated from a stroke while you are following his asymptomatic bruit.

I enjoyed Dr. Javid's presentation very much indeed.

Dr. Javid (closing). I should like to thank Dr. Thompson for his many contributions in the field of carotid surgery and his informative slide showing the outcome of patients with carotid bruits.

We have seen many patients with carotid bifurcation bruit who had lesions involving the internal carotid artery of less than 50 percent stenosis. I fully agree with him, however that a carotid bruit in an asymptomatic patient cannot be considered innocent. As we have shown in our study, the atheroma will continue to progress and it may cause irreversible cerebral damage if the lesion is not removed surgically.

Effect of CO_2 and systemic hypertension on downstream cerebral arterial pressure during carotid endarterectomy

W. K. EHRENFELD, M.D.
F. N. HAMILTON, M.D.
C. P. LARSON, JR., M.D.
R. F. HICKEY, M.D.
J. W. SEVERINGHAUS, M.D.
SAN FRANCISCO, CALIF.
From the Departments of Surgery and Anesthesia, and the Cardiovascular Research Institute, University of California, San Francisco Medical Center

Regardless of the surgical precautions used during carotid endarterectomy, operative stroke from cerebral ischemia is an ever present possibility during clamp occlusion of the carotid artery. Anesthetic measures to increase the tolerance to cerebral ischemia during this critical period include general anesthesia, deliberate hypercarbia, and induced systemic hypertension.[11] The proposed mechanisms involved include: a decrease in cerebral oxygen consumption by general anesthesia, an increase in cerebral blood flow from hypercarbia, and an increase in cerebral perfusion pressure secondary to induced systemic hypertension. However, the beneficial effect of CO_2 in this circumstance has been questioned, since recent investigations in laboratory animals indicate that in the presence of cerebral ischemia hypercarbia may produce an intracerebral steal, that is, an increase in blood flow to normal brain and a decrease in flow to ischemic brain.[2, 12] The concept that cerebral perfusion pressure and hence cerebral blood flow (CBF) will be increased by inducing systemic hypertension during operation has also been questioned.[1, 10]

Supported in part by University of California School of Medicine Grant, Research 12, Clough Fund, and United States Public Health Service Grants H.E. 04850, 5T1 GM 00063, 1P01 GM 15571-01A1, and Research Career Award 5-K6-HE-19, 412.

Presented at the Twenty-third Annual Meeting of the Society for Vascular Surgery, New York, N. Y., July 12-13, 1969.

We reasoned that the arterial perfusion pressure available to the tissue beyond a surgically occluded internal carotid artery could be monitored by catheterizing the cephalad end of the occluded artery. As cerebral perfusion pressure decreases, autoregulation is ordinarily believed capable of maintaining adequate flow down to some critical level, below which flow will decrease with pressure, the resistance vessels being fully dilated. Regions of brain exposed to below-critical pressures may be thought of as ischemic, fully dilated, and thus incapable of further dilation with hypercapnia. We postulated that maneuvers such as induced hypertension, hypercapnia, or both should elevate the pressure monitored through the cephalad stump of the surgically occluded carotid artery. The following is a report of studies of the effect of CO_2 and induced systemic hypertension on this internal carotid stump pressure (P_{IC}) and on the oxygen saturation of jugular venous bulb blood on the same side.

METHODS

Ten studies were performed during carotid endarterectomy on nine patients ranging in age from 51 to 80 years. One patient had a staged bilateral procedure. Preoperative stenosis of the orifice of the internal carotid artery greater than 90 percent was present in all but one patient who had an ulcerated intimal plaque. Two patients had contralateral internal carotid occlusion, and three had severe contralateral carotid stenosis.

On the morning of operation, the patients were premedicated with atropine or scopolamine (0.3 to 0.4 mg.) alone or in combination with sodium pentobarbital (150 mg.) and morphine (8 to 10 mg.) or meperidine (100 mg.). Anesthesia was induced either with thiopental (100 to 375 mg.) given intravenously or by inhalation of halothane-oxygen, delivered by mask from a standard anesthesia circle system. Following orotracheal intubation, anesthesia was maintained with halothane-oxygen and d-tubocurarine (0.3 mg. per kilogram). Alveolar halothane concentration was determined at frequent intervals, with an infra-red halothane analyzer and sampling at end-expiration via a nylon catheter from the tracheal end of the orotracheal tube. The concentration ranged from 0.58 to 0.85 percent, but in any patient it was reasonably constant, varying by less than 0.1 percent during the

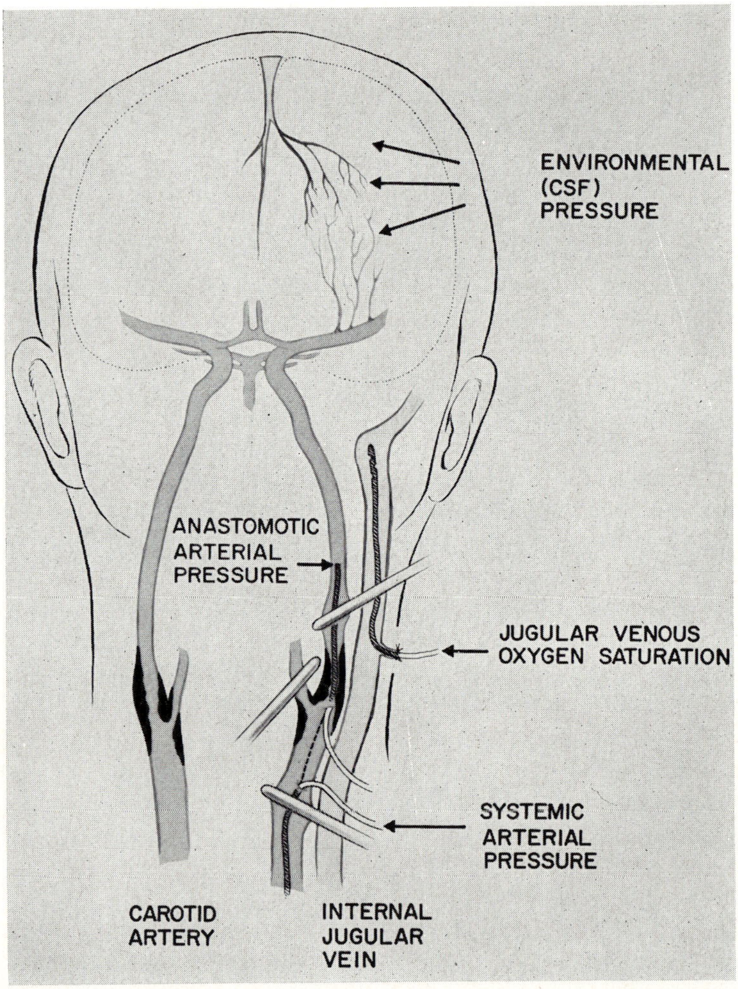

Fig. 1. Schematic diagram showing pertinent anatomic structures and placement of catheters for study of the effects of CO_2 and systemic hypertension on ipsilateral cerebral perfusion pressure during carotid endarterectomy. Catheters measured systemic carotid arterial pressure (P_{CC}), anastomotic or downstream cerebral arterial pressure (P_{IC}), and jugular venous oxygen saturation (S_vO_2) during carotid endarterectomy. Cerebral perfusion (environmental) pressure is the difference between P_{IC} and cerebral venous pressure.

period of study. Ventilation was controlled* at tidal volumes (8 to 13 ml. per kilogram) and respiratory frequencies (16 to 21 breaths per minute) required to decrease alveolar CO_2 tension ($PaCO_2$) to about 20 torr. $PaCO_2$ was monitored continuously with a microcatheter infra-red CO_2 analyzer, sampling from a 25 ml. extension tube interposed between the orotracheal tube and the Y-piece of the circle. CO_2 and halothane analyzers were calibrated with methods described previously.[8]

The common carotid artery and its branches and the ipsilateral common facial and jugular veins were isolated through a transverse cervical incision (Fig. 1). A polyethylene catheter† (dead space 0.4 ml.) was inserted into the transected end of the facial vein and threaded cephalad through the internal jugular vein to the region of the jugular bulb for sampling of cerebral venous blood. After heparin was given (2,500 to 3,500 I.U. intravenously), two rigid catheters‡ were inserted through a lateral arteriotomy at the carotid bifurcation and directed proximally and distally for measurement of common carotid (P_{CC}, i.e., systemic) and internal carotid (P_{IC}, i.e., stump or anastomotic) arterial pressures, respectively. Atraumatic Fogarty arterial clamps fixed the catheters in place. These pressures were transduced (Statham P-23d) and along with $PaCO_2$ were recorded continuously with a direct-writing polygraph.

A standard carotid bifurcation endarterectomy was then performed without an internal shunt. Average occlusion time was 33 minutes (range 23 to 40 minutes). During occlusion, two series of experiments were performed. First, while P_{CC} was kept constant, changes in P_{IC} were recorded while $PaCO_2$ was varied in a random manner from 20 to 60 torrs in about 20 torr increments by manual hyperventilation or by bypassing the soda lime and adding CO_2 to the inspired mixture. Allowing 5 minutes for equilibration, blood was drawn from the common carotid artery catheter for determination of pH, $PaCO_2$, and PaO_2. Simultaneously, blood was drawn from the venous catheter for determination of oxygen saturation (SvO_2) by reflection spectrophotometry and oxygen tension and pH. In seven studies, $PaCO_2$ was held constant at 46 torr and P_{CC} was varied randomly in 10 to 20 torr

*Air Shields Ventilation Ventimeter.

†K-33, Pharmaseal Laboratories, Glendale, Calif.

‡Teflon, No. 20 thin wall; Plastic Sales and Service, San Francisco, Calif.

Table I. *Values of internal carotid artery pressure distal to the site of surgical clamp (P_{IC}) and common carotid artery pressure proximal to the site of surgical clamp (P_{CC}) in torr at three levels of $PaCO_2$ in ten studies**

Study	*$PaCO_2$ (torr)*	*P_{IC} (torr)*	*P_{CC} (torr)*
1	25	38	127
	44	35	132
	65	41	143
2	32	61	138
	49	40	137
	68	41	137
3	29	85	103
	44	57	98
	59	67	103
4	29	22	72
	44	23	71
	62	26	76
5	21	54	100
	46	42	103
	51	48	112
6	22	95	110
	38	73	110
	65	76	93
7	19	85	122
	37	70	118
	59	64	119
8	25	40	86
	39	37	88
	55	42	90
9	23	84	107
	39	71	109
	61	75	108
10	27	65	115
	36	44	119
	54	40	122
Mean ± S.E.	25.2 ± 1.3	62.9 ± 9.7	108.0 ± 6.1
	41.6 ± 1.4	49.2 ± 5.5	108.5 ± 6.2
	59.9 ± 1.7	52.0 ± 5.4	110.3 ± 6.6

*Mean and one standard error (±S.E.) are included.

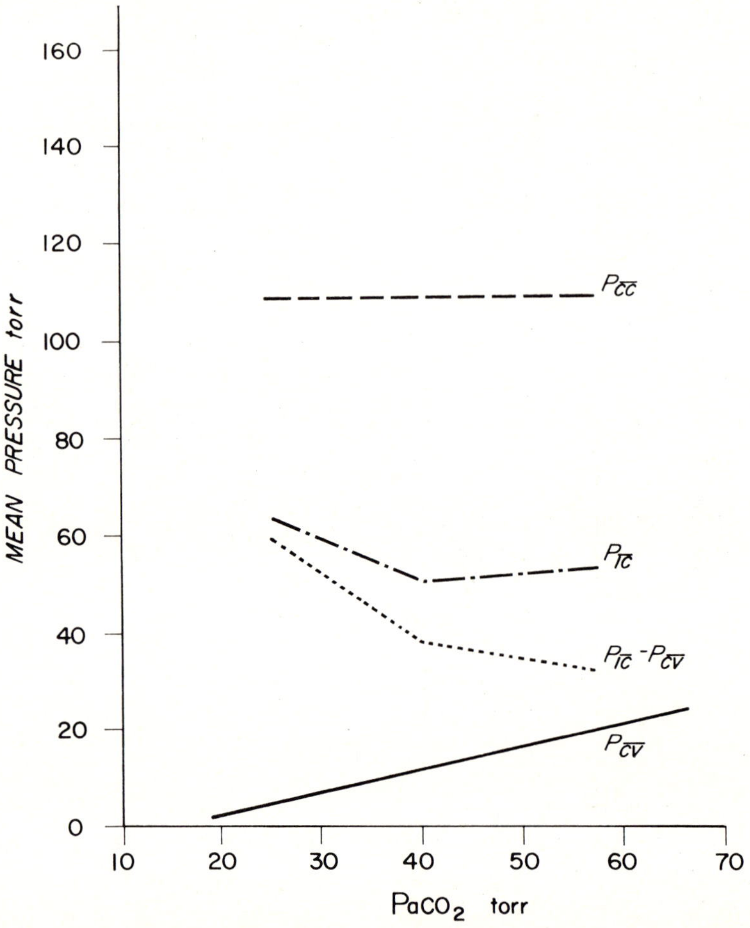

Fig. 2. Mean of ten slopes of common (P_{CC}) and internal (P_{IC}) carotid artery pressures below and above the site of clamp occlusion at three levels of $PACO_2$. $P_{\overline{CV}}$ is the mean change in sagittal sinus pressure observed by one of us (Severinghaus, unpublished data) in 12 dogs anesthetized with pentobarbital and exposed to varying concentrations of CO_2. $P_{\overline{IC}}$ minus $P_{\overline{CV}}$ is the theoretical reduction in cerebral perfusion pressure that might result by elevating $PACO_2$.

increments from a mean of 50 to 160 torr by infusion of norepinephrine intravenously. This was repeated in four studies at a mean $PaCO_2$ of 24 torr. Arterial and venous blood samples were drawn after 1 or 2 minutes at each new pressure increment. When the operative repair was completed, the catheters were removed and the wound was closed. Eight patients had an uneventful postoperative recovery. One patient had severe postoperative hypertension for 1 day which was treated with trimethaphan.

Arterial blood gases and pH were determined with the appropriate electrodes and were corrected to the patient's temperature. PaO_2 exceeded 300 torr throughout all studies. The correlation of measured (oximetry) and calculated (blood-gas) SvO_2 was similar to that published earlier.[6] Changes in pH were commensurate with changes in $PaCO_2$. Cerebral arteriovenous oxygen content difference was calculated and was used to determine the cerebral blood flow equivalent (milliliter of CBF per milliliter O_2 consumed). Paired analysis of data was made with Student's t test.

RESULTS

In eight of the ten studies, P_{IC} was highest at the lowest $PaCO_2$ (Table I, Fig. 2).

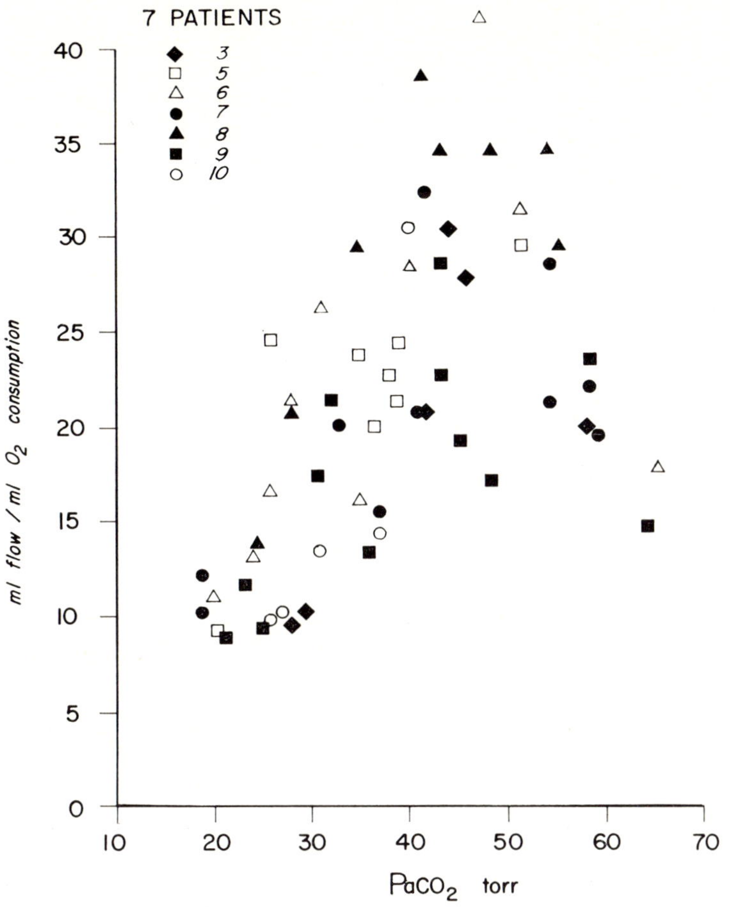

Fig. 3. Relation of total cerebral blood flow equivalent to P_ACO_2 in seven patients during carotid endarterectomy.

Comparison of P_{IC} values at the low (mean = 25.2 torr) and medium (mean = 41.6 torr) $PaCO_2$ levels indicates that P_{IC} decreased markedly in seven studies and remained unchanged in three as $PaCO_2$ was increased. This decrease in P_{IC} was highly significant ($p < 0.005$). Comparison of P_{IC} values at medium and high (mean = 59.9 torr) $PaCO_2$ levels indicates that P_{IC} increased in eight of ten studies as $PaCO_2$ was increased, but the P_{IC} changes were small and not statistically significant ($p < 0.2$). P_{CC} was maintained reasonably constant throughout this portion of the study at a mean pressure of 108 torr. With controlled ventilation, hypercarbia rarely resulted in any appreciable increase in P_{CC}.

As would be expected, CBF equivalent increased in all patients as $PaCO_2$ was increased (Fig. 3).

When arterial pressure was elevated at constant $PaCO_2$ (mean = 46 torr), P_{IC} increased proportionally with increase in P_{CC} in six of seven studies (Fig. 4). One patient showed no change in P_{IC} when mean P_{CC} was varied from 105 to 130 torr. Another patient showed an unusually marked and reproducible increase in P_{IC} when mean P_{CC} was increased from 145 to 153 torr. Decreasing $PaCO_2$ to a lower level (mean = 24 torr) displaced the curve relating P_{IC} to P_{CC} upward (to a higher P_{IC}) without any change in slope in three of four studies. One patient showed no displacement of P_{IC}–P_{CC} slope at $PaCO_2$ levels ranging from 26 to 54 torr. The initial P_{IC} and the P_{IC} re-

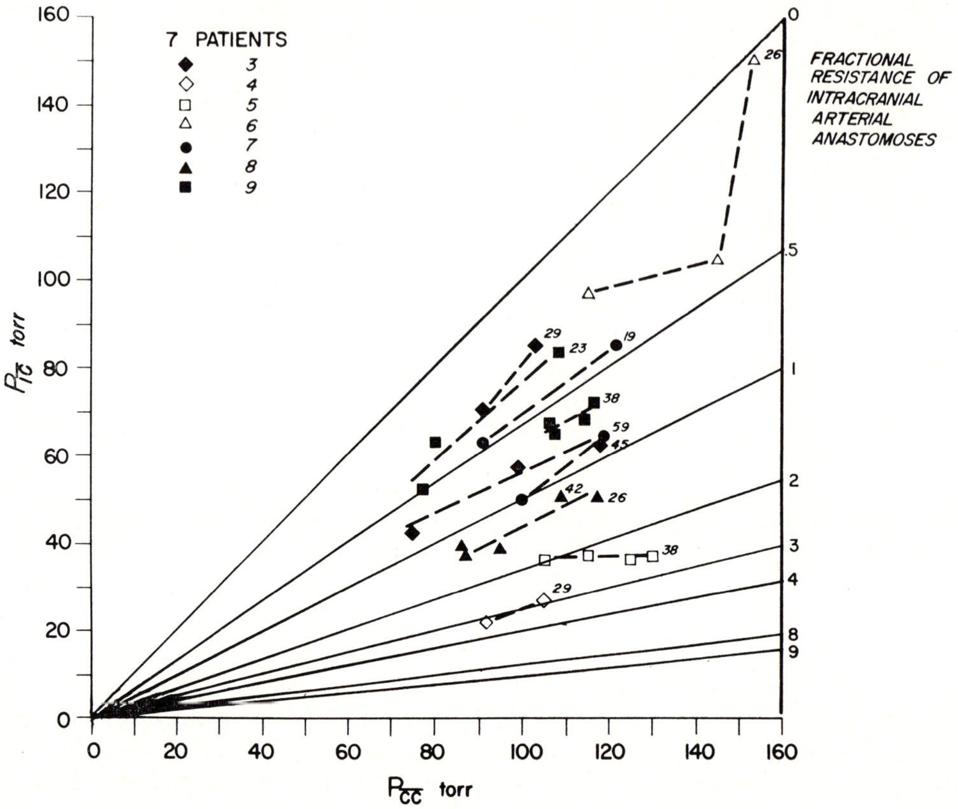

Fig. 4. Effect of changes in P_{CC} on P_{IC} at constant P_ACO_2. The P_ACO_2 values are indicated for the ten studies in seven patients. Isopleths are ratios of anastomotic resistance to downstream resistance assuming venous pressure equals zero. The data suggest that as systemic pressure was altered, this ratio remains constant at a mean of 2:1 irrespective of P_ACO_2.

sponses to changes in $PaCO_2$ or P_{CC} were unrelated to the presence or absence of contralateral carotid occlusive lesions.

DISCUSSION

The effect of changes in $PaCO_2$ or systemic blood pressure on cerebral perfusion to ischemic brain is currently the subject of considerable controversy. At issue is whether cerebral vessels made hypotensive or ischemic develop "vasomotor paralysis," that is, dilate maximally and lose the normal properties of autoregulation and responsiveness to CO_2. Presumably the mechanism is one of hypoxia and acute acidosis of brain tissue, which relaxes cerebral arterioles and renders them unresponsive to additional H^+ produced by CO_2 inhalation. Several lines of evidence support this concept. Cerebral vessels of dogs made severely hypotensive (mean pressure = 50 torr) show maximal vasodilatation and unresponsiveness to changes in $PaCO_2$.[3] Autoregulation is lost and cerebral blood flow is then entirely pressure dependent. Studies of regional cerebral blood flow suggest that similar changes occur in localized areas of cerebral ischemia.[4] However, in this circumstance, normal cerebral vasomotor responsiveness is maintained in the unaffected brain. As a result, increasing $PaCO_2$ has a paradoxical effect on regional cerebral blood flow, increasing blood flow to nonischemic brain and decreasing flow to ischemic brain. This intracerebral steal phenomenon has been observed in animals and in man with focal cerebral ischemic lesions during CO_2 inhalation.[2, 4, 12] As would be expected in this pressure-dependent system, an increase in systemic blood pressure by administration of a vasopressor increased blood flow to the ischemic area.

Additional evidence supporting the concept of vasomotor paralysis and altered responsiveness to CO_2 may be obtained from the report of Soloway and associates.[9] They found in dogs that hypocarbia ($PaCO_2$ = 25 torr) decreased markedly the magnitude of cerebral infarction resulting from occlusion of the internal and middle cerebral arteries over that observed at normocarbia ($PaCO_2$ = 38 torr). This finding suggests that hypocarbia increased blood flow to ischemic brain by increasing cerebrovascular resistance in nonischemic brain. Unfortunately, these investigators did not determine whether hypercarbia had the reverse effect, i.e., to enlarge the area of infarction. The phenomenon of increased regional blood flow provided by hypocapnia has been observed in man and has been named "the Robin Hood syndrome."[7]

In contrast to these findings, Kogure and associates[5] observed that middle cerebral artery ligation in dogs produced regional tissue ischemia but that this did not, in turn, result in maximal vasodilatation of the arteries visible in infra-red or fluorescein angiograms. In fact, the caliber of the cerebral arteries in the ischemic segment was much smaller than in normally perfused brain. Furthermore, autoregulation was retained in the ischemic zone and increasing $PaCO_2$ never decreased regional flow to the ischemic area. Support for this work is available from the studies of Waltz[10] in cats anesthetized with halothane. He found that blood flow to ischemic cerebral cortex was increased as mean systemic arterial pressure was increased from 35 to 120 torr but that further increases in systemic pressure did not produce a consistent increase in cortical blood flow.

In our experiments, the pressure monitored through the cephalad stump of the carotid artery (P_{IC}) may be regarded as controlled by the balance between two resistances: the anastomotic resistance delivering blood from open, normally perfused vessels to the occluded vessel's network, and the resistance of the tissue normally supplied by this occluded vessel. We found that stump pressure was raised by low $PaCO_2$. This could be due either to a higher pressure upstream of the anastomotic resistance due to vasoconstriction in normally perfused tissue, or to vasoconstriction in part of the distribution of the occluded vessel, raising runoff resistance. In either case, we assume that severely ischemic tissue would not respond to hypocarbia by vasoconstricting, but would be supplied with an increased perfusion pressure as a result of the vasoconstriction in more normal areas due to hypocarbia. Conversely, high $PaCO_2$ dilated only those vessels that were not already fully dilated, and hence not severely ischemic. During hypercarbia, the stump arterial pressure remained about constant, but for reasons discussed in the next paragraph, we believe the perfusion head of pressure, from artery to vein, decreased further.

Although not evaluated in this study, another mechanism whereby hypercarbia may decrease cerebral perfusion pressure during carotid occlusion is by its effect on cerebral venous pressure. Venous outflow from the skull is limited by the size of the bony orifices through which the major veins exit. As hypercarbia increases total cerebral blood flow, the fixed outflow resistance of the skull results in an increase in cerebral venous pressure and hence in brain tissue (environmental) and cerebrospinal fluid pressures (Fig. 1). One of us (J. W. S., unpublished observations) measured sagittal sinus pressure in 12 dogs anesthetized with pentobarbital, immobilized with gallamine, and artifically ventilated. As $PaCO_2$ was increased from 20 to 60 torr, mean sagittal sinus pressure increased from 2 to 20 torr. If hypercarbia produces a similar increase in cerebral venous pressure in man, cerebral perfusion pressure may decrease to a critically low value (Fig. 2).

The stump pressure (P_{IC}) generally remained below the critical pressure of 60 to 80 torr at which autoregulation is reported to begin. If, as P_{CC} was increased, autoregulation had held flow in the distribution of the stump constant, P_{IC} would have increased in parallel with P_{CC}. Instead, we observed a passive, proportionate change in stump pressure following induced alterations in systemic pressure. This indicates that the two resistances controlling stump pressure, the anastomotic and tissue resistances remained constant or changed proportionally.

SUMMARY

Pressure was measured distal to the surgical occlusion of the internal carotid artery during ten carotid endarterectomies, and the cerebral blood flow was estimated from jugular venous bulb blood oxygen saturation on the occluded side. Hyperventilation raised the distal "stump" pressure and lowered the flow, while hypercarbia increased flow with little effect on stump pressure, but may have decreased net perfusion pressure by elevating intracranial venous pressure. Systemic hypertension proportionally elevated stump pressure; the ratio between the two pressures averaged about 2:1. It is postulated that the distribution of the occluded carotid artery is partly well perfused, partly ischemic, and that the ischemic area is unresponsive to CO_2 changes. We conclude that procedures which increase the net arterial to venous perfusion pressure gradient should be chosen for maximum protection of brain during general anesthesia for carotid endarterectomy, and these appear to be systemic hypertension and hyperventilation with resultant hypocarbia.

REFERENCES

1. Bloodwell, R. D., Hallman, G. L., Keats, A. S., and Cooley, D. A.: Carotid endarterectomy without a shunt: Results using hypercarbic general anesthesia to prevent cerebral ischemia, Arch. Surg. **96:** 644, 1968.
2. Brawley, B. W., Strandness, D. E., and Kelly, W. A.: The physiologic response to therapy in experimental cerebral ischemia, Arch. Neurol. **17:** 180, 1967.
3. Harper, A. M., and Glass, H. I.: Effect of alterations in the arterial carbon dioxide tension on the blood flow through the cerebral cortex at normal and low arterial blood pressures, J. Neurol. Neurosurg. Psychiat. **28:** 449, 1965.
4. Høedt-Rasmussen, K., Skinhoj, E., Paulson, O., Ewald, J., Bjerrum, J. K., Fahrenkrug, A., and Lassen, N. A.: Regional cerebral blood flow in acute apoplexy: The "luxury perfusion syndrome" of brain tissue, Arch. Neurol. **17:** 271, 1967.
5. Kogure, K., Fujishima, M., Scheinberg, P., and Reinmuth, O. M.: Effects of changes in carbon dioxide pressure and arterial pressure on blood flow in ischemic regions of the brain in dogs, Circ. Res. **24:** 557, 1969.
6. Larson, C. P., Jr., Ehrenfeld, W. K., Wade, J. G., and Wylie, E. J.: Jugular venous oxygen saturation as an index of adequacy of cerebral oxygenation, SURGERY **62:** 31, 1967.
7. Lassen, N. A., and Pálvölgyi, R.: Cerebral steal during hypercapnia and the inverse reaction during hypocapnia observed by the ^{133}xenon technique in man, Scand. J. Clin. Lab. Invest. Suppl. 102, **13:** D, 1968.
8. Munson, E. S., Saidman, L. J., and Eger, E. I., II: Solubility of fluroxene in blood and tissue homogenates, Anesthesiology **25:** 638, 1965.
9. Soloway, M., Nadel, W., Albin, M. S., and White, R. J.: The effect of hyperventilation on subsequent cerebral infarction, Anesthesiology **29:** 975, 1968.
10. Waltz, A. G.: Effect of blood pressure on blood flow in ischemic and in nonischemic cerebral cortex: The phenomena of autoregulation and luxury perfusion, Neurology **18:** 613, 1968.
11. Wells, B. A., Keats, A. S., and Cooley, D. A.: Increased tolerance to cerebral ischemia produced by general anesthesia during temporary carotid occlusion, SURGERY **54:** 216, 1963.
12. Youmans, J. R., and Kindt, G. W.: Efficacy of carbon dioxide in the treatment of cerebral ischemia, Surg. Forum **19:** 425, 1968.

DISCUSSION

Dr. John E. Connolly (Irvine, Calif.). I rise because this recommendation made by Dr. Ehrenfeld, although attractive in theory, is diametrically opposite the procedure that we have adopted based on work done in our laboratory, principally by Dr. Stemmer.

I think that the authors' conclusions must be carefully considered because of the great hazards inherent in using systemic blood pressure as an index of regional blood flow for tissue perfusion in patients who are receiving vasopressors. This hazard is widely recognized in the treatment of hypovolemic shock and may also exist in normovolemic patients with regional ischemia.

Experimentally, we found that the commonly used vasopressors such as levarterenol, isoproterenol, phenylphrine, or ephedrine decreased carotid arterial blood flow even in the presence of systemic hypertension when hypercarbia was not employed. When hypercarbia was utilized, those agents which increased cardiac output such as levarterenol or isoproterenol did indeed increase cerebral blood flow. Even with hypercarbia, however, the administration of phenylephrine or ephedrine still caused a sharp decrease in carotid blood flow.

Many investigators, just as the authors have stated today, have shown that if you raise the pCO_2 you will raise the total cerebral blood flow. Also many investigators—and these particular slides are taken from the work of the Department of Anesthesia at the University of Pennsylvania—have shown that there's an inverse relationship between the pCO_2 and the cerebral vascular resistance, so that as the CO_2 goes down the pressure in the carotid artery will go up because the cerebral vascular resistance is greater. Therefore, if you were measuring the carotid blood flow with a flowmeter, you would find that while carotid pressure goes up, the flow goes down and vice versa. Because hypercarbia does increase total cerebral blood flow, we prefer to use it at the moment until there's more evidence about this so-called "Robin Hood steal."

We monitor blood gases during operation because we discovered from our experiments that a pCO_2 above 90 mm. Hg would decrease total cerebral blood flow. Maximum increases in cerebral blood flow occur with pCO_2 in the 60 to 80 range. We think that Penthrane anesthesia is important because arrhythmias often occur with the use of hypercarbia and halothane.

We also continue to use the Javid internal shunt and I suppose since many of you are going to be quite confused now as to whether one should use hypo- or hypercarbia, there's a good reason why we should continue to use a shunt since the consequences of ischemia of the brain are so severe.

Isoproterenol or levarterenol combined with hypercarbia may be beneficial in that the hypertension induced by these agents will further augment the increased carotid blood flow produced by hypercarbia but we have found it very difficult to maintain a stable elevated blood pressure with these drugs.

As you know, there are many cardiovascular surgeons who are using hypercarbia alone and getting very good results. I think that while the hypocarbia theory is interesting, we at least, are going to continue to employ hypercarbia and a shunt until there is more evidence that hypocarbia without a shunt is effective in preventing cerebral damage during cerebrovascular reconstruction.

Dr. Angelo Riberi (Youngstown, Ohio). The problems which have been discussed here are extremely important and I merely rise to comment and agree 100 percent with Dr. Connolly. Until we know for sure whether a shunt is needed or not, I do not believe that we are justified in taking chances which may produce cerebral ischemia and lead to disastrous results.

In our series, we have used cyclopropane, hypercarbia, and slight hypertension, but we definitely feel that internal shunting must be continued at the present time until proved otherwise.

Dr. Samuel R. Powers, Jr. (Albany, N. Y.). I rise to question the advisability of altering arterial carbon dioxide under any circumstances, either up or down.

Two years ago, we presented before this Society some studies on rhesus monkeys in which we separately measured cerebral and brainstem blood flow in animals that had a surgically produced subclavian steal.

When CO_2 was given, the two parts of the brain behaved in opposite directions. The brainstem blood flow went up and the cerebral blood flow went down.

I think there's an important principle concerning the use of pharmacologic agents to maintain cerebral blood flow. The brain is not homogenous. It consists of at least two parts, the cerebrum and medulla, which may be under separate control mechanisms. Increases in the arterial pCO_2 will probably dilate the vessels which don't need it and actually cut down on flow in those which you would like to have increased.

So, I would make a plea that agents which produce hypertension or that are presumed to dilate cerebral vessels should not be used until we understand a little more about the physiology of the intracerebral shunting of blood.

Dr. F. William Blaisdell (San Francisco, Calif.). Those of us who are part of the University of California have always followed the leadership of our senior vascular service but we must admit we are now a bit confused. This present paper advocates the use of hypocarbia in order to produce an elevation in intracranial arterial pressure. Prior to this, the authors advocated hypercarbia to increase cerebral blood flow during carotid artery surgery.

One wonders whether we couldn't combine hypocarbia with hypercarbia. Cerebral blood flow which is decreased by hypocarbia would be restored to normal and the hypotension produced in the cerebral arteries by the hypercarbia would be combatted by the hypertensive effects of the hypocarbia. Then, all one has to do is use an internal shunt and one can operate safely.

Dr. Julius Jacobson, II (New York, N. Y.). I rise to add still another approach to making carotid artery surgery safer. It has been our feeling that hypercarbia can be detrimental and we have abandoned it completely.

We have now done almost 100 cases of carotid endarterectomy under hyperbaric oxygenation at 3 atmospheres absolute. About 20 percent of these have been in patients with two, three, or four vessel involvement. Shunts have not been used simply because there has been no need for them.

Typically, if one measures the partial pressure of the blood going to and returning from the brain, it will be approximately 100 mm. Hg in the artery and about 45 mm. Hg in the veins. At 3 atmospheres absolute, with the patient breathing 99 percent oxygen and 1 percent Fluothane, the arterial pO_2 will be in the range of 1,600 to 1,800, while that in the veins will be 600 to 800. After 15 minutes of carotid occlusion, the jugular venous blood (facial veins having been ligated) is bright red and the measured oxygen tensions are in the range of 150 to 200.

We have not had a single case in this series of a patient waking up with a stroke. We certainly enjoyed Dr. Ehrenfeld's paper and the spirited discussion which has followed it.

Dr. Edwin J. Wylie (San Francisco, Calif.). Dr. Ehrenfeld's observations seem to be based on solid experimental data. They are particularly applicable to those vascular surgeons who have found that carotid endarterectomy is more effectively performed without the interference of an inlying shunt. A review of our own experience has indicated that it is necessary to augment collateral blood to the brain in approximately 9 percent of patients if endarterectomy is performed without a shunt. Of 357 patients operated upon under local anesthesia 32 patients were unable to tolerate test clamping or developed a stroke immediately following operation. Under general anesthesia alone the stroke rate dropped to 5 percent. In the last 161 carotid endarterectomies general anesthesia was supplemented by hypercarbia and induced hypertension. Although three patients developed temporary neurologic deficits in the postoperative period, only one was related to cerebral ischemia from carotid clamping. It is important to note, however, that whenever hypercarbia failed to elevate blood pressure, vasoconstrictors were added and carotid clamping was deferred until the blood pressure rose to at least 20 mm. Hg systolic over the patient's normal blood pressure. Dr. Ehrenfeld's data indicate that hypercarbia, if not accompanied by a rise in blood pressure, will actually decrease effective regional blood flow to the hemisphere normally supplied by the clamping carotid artery. Further studies to measure distal carotid pressures when hyper- and hypocarbia are combined with hypertension should give important additional information.

Dr. Ehrenfeld (closing). I would like to thank all of the discussants for their comments.

The observations that Drs. Connolly and Stemmer have made that vasopressors decrease cerebral blood flow are unique. There is a large body of evidence that vasopressors have no direct effect on cerebral vessels and hence do not alter cerebrovascular resistance or decrease cerebral blood flow by any direct mechanism. We certainly agree that CO_2 will increase cerebral blood flow; however. I would like to emphasize that we are concerned less with total cerebral blood flow and flow to "good" brain than with flow to ischemic or "bad" brain. If autoregulation in this area is lost, then flow to this area will be entirely pressure dependent, and we believe that techniques that prevent a reduction in perfusion pressure are beneficial.

With regard to Drs. Blaisdell and Riberi's remarks concerning the use of internal shunts, it has been the policy on our service to perform carotid endarterectomies without a shunt and I think this is true of many other centers. We have found that a better technical result can be accomplished without a shunt. The anesthetic management of these patients remains very important whether or not a shunt is used. Furthermore, I think that some of these data may be relative to the management of stroke patients in general, that is, many of these patients are treated with CO_2 and this may prove to be improper management.

Dr. Power's comments were of interest. To repeat, I do think that induced hypertension is quite important. I believe that further studies are perhaps necessary to further elucidate the phenomena of which I spoke.

I was interested in Dr. Jacobson's remarks regarding hyperbaric oxygen and we will look forward to reports of his work.

With regard to Dr. Wylie's statements, I would just re-emphasize the fact that there has been considerable improvement in our morbidity and mortality rates since turning from local to general anesthesia for carotid endarterectomy.

Conclusions from a controlled trial of the prophylactic portacaval shunt

ALLAN D. CALLOW, M.D.
ROBERT H. RESNICK, M.D.
THOMAS C. CHALMERS, M.D.
ALBERT M. ISHIHARA, M.D.
ARTHUR J. GARCEAU, M.D.
EDWARD T. O'HARA, M.D.
BOSTON, MASS.
From the Departments of Medicine and Surgery, Tufts University School of Medicine, Boston University School of Medicine, and Harvard Medical School

Of 471 patients with esophageal varices and cirrhosis studied and treated by the Boston Inter-Hospital Liver Group over a 3 year period, 51 percent experienced upper gastrointestinal hemorrhage. In 34 percent hemorrhage was the major cause of death. Only 31 percent were alive 1 year after demonstration of varices.[6] The calculated survival curve for this group closely duplicates curves obtained by Ratnoff and Patek[15] in their analysis of patients with decompensated cirrhosis studied during the years 1916 to 1938. Numerous reports are available attesting to the effectiveness of a therapeutic portacaval shunt in prevention of recurrent hemorrhage from varices in patients who have previously bled. Prevention of bleeding is taken as evidence that the over-all survival rate in survivors of hemorrhage is thereby improved.[3, 12, 19] Reduction of the mortality rate, however, may be more apparent than real, inasmuch as surgical therapy can be available only to survivors of the hemorrhage group, those in whom it has been pointed out already enjoy a more favorable prognosis.[35]

In the light of these many questions and with the considerable health care burden created by an increasingly larger number of patients with cirrhosis, it is not surprising that portacaval shunt as a prophylactic procedure has been advocated for the cirrhotic patient with esophageal varices.[14, 17, 18]

METHODS

During the 10 years from 1959 through 1968, members of the Boston Inter-Hospital Liver Group from seven participating hospitals* selected 93 patients with moderate-to-advanced cirrhosis of the liver in each of whom esophageal varices were unequivocally demonstrated by barium swallow on at least two occasions at least 4 weeks apart. Over three fourths of the patients came from The Lemuel Shattuck Hospital and the Boston Veterans' Administration Hospital. Diagnosis was established by clinical and laboratory criteria commonly accepted and detailed in a previous publication of the Boston Inter-Hospital Liver Group.[6]

Most of these patients required 2 to 3 months of in-hospital treatment. Although

Supported in part by United States Public Health Service Grants AM-09128 and FR05598-04.

Presented at the Twenty-third Annual Meeting of the Society for Vascular Surgery, New York, N. Y., July 12-13, 1969.

The following additional members of the Boston Inter-Hospital Liver Group have contributed to the collection of data for this report: Drs. C. F. Davidson, R. M. Donaldson, Jr., G. F. Grady, P. F. Gryska, F. J. Inglefinger, K. J. Isselbacher, J. F. Patterson, T. A. Wharthin, N. Zamcheck, L. Zetzel, E. Schimmel, Hugo Muench.

*Lemuel Shattuck, Boston Veterans' Administration, Boston City, New England Center, Massachusetts General, West Roxbury Veterans' Administration, and Beth Israel Hospitals.

seriously ill, they possessed enough hepatic reserve to recover sufficiently to permit inclusion in the study. Clinical criteria, such as general appearance, ascites, size of the liver and the spleen, dietary protein tolerance, and laboratory determinations including hemoglobin, serum bilirubin, albumin concentration, plasma prothrombin time, and serum enzymes denoting possible hepatic degeneration, were recorded at multiple intervals and at least twice before patients were admitted to the study. Such observations were made immediately after admission and before randomization into medical and surgical groups. Following the patient's consent to surgery, random assignment was then made to one of the two groups. Because surgical therapy could have been denied to some patients who were assumed to carry a high operative risk, rigid and somewhat arbitrary criteria for establishing operability were not utilized.[10, 11]

Although laboratory and clinical criteria were used as guides, randomization in essence was achieved independently by the medical and surgical teams on the basis of their individual appraisal and experience. Forty-five patients underwent construction of an end-to-side shunt, and three patients were given side-to-side anastomoses. In these three patients ascites was particularly troublesome, and it was believed at that time that a side-to-side shunt was preferable. Both groups of patients received careful in-hospital medical care and were observed after discharge in the same follow-up clinics. Particular attention was paid with respect to evidence of hepatic decompensation. Radiologic examinations for esophageal varices were performed annually. Because of the possibility of hemorrhage from varices in the nonshunted group, it was agreed that medical patients could be removed from the study for emergency surgical treatment as required.

RESULTS

Clinical condition at admission. Criteria utilized for determining severity of hepatic disease included clinical evaluation of jaundice, ascites, and encephalopathy. Patients were considered to have satisfactory hepatic function if none of these three complications was noted at the time of admission or in the history. A more serious degree of hepatic insufficiency was present if one or more of these three complications were present by history but had cleared with therapy in a hospital. Patients were considered to have advanced cirrhosis if any of these three conditions persisted despite therapy. Ascites was present at the time of admission or noted in the history in 83 percent of the patients. Encephalopathy was similarly noted in 48 percent. By the time of randomization, the mean duration of which for both medical and surgical groups was 10 weeks, ascites had diminished so that it was present in slightly less than two fifths of the patients. In no patient was symptomatic hepatic encephalopathy present. Moderate cirrhosis was judged to be present if the serum bilirubin was more than 1 but less than 2 mg. percent, the serum albumin between 2.5 and 3 mg. percent, and the prothrombin content below 100 but over 50 percent of normal. Advanced cirrhosis was considered to be present if the serum bilirubin was persistently greater than 2 mg. percent, the serum albumin less than 2.5 Gm. percent, and the prothrombin content under 50 percent of normal.

Clinical condition at selection. By the time of randomization and after optimal in-

Table I. *Classification at randomization*

Data	*Surgical*	*Medical*
No. of patients	48	45
Males	36	35
Females	12	10
Duration of cirrhosis in months (average)	22	27
Duration of hospitalization preceding selection in weeks (average)	10	10
History of:		
Jaundice	79%	87%
Ascites	83%	83%
Encephalopathy	41%	54%
Hepatomegaly	88%	87%
Splenomegaly	62%	62%

hospital therapy nearly 85 percent of patients in both groups demonstrated a serum bilirubin below 2 mg. percent, a prothrombin concentration above 40 percent, and a serum albumin concentration above 3 Gm. percent. In all but one patient in both groups excessive alcohol intake was considered to have played a major role in the development of cirrhosis. The 48 surgical and 45 medical patients at randomization were deemed to be comparable in all the variables studied (Table I).

MORTALITY RATE

The postoperative death rate was 2 percent at 30 days from operation and 10 percent if operative death is extended to include patients hospitalized for up to 90 days from operation. One patient died at 18 days and the remaining four patients between 47 and 69 days. Of these five operative deaths three patients demonstrated classic findings of the hepatorenal syndrome. Two of them at autopsy were found to have suffered thrombosis of the shunts. Five (10 percent) of the control patients ultimately developed variceal bleeding and died as contrasted to one surgical patient (2 percent). Seven of the surgical patients had shown occult blood loss before randomization. This was assumed to be most likely on the basis of bleeding from varices, since with additional studies no other diagnosis was possible. None of these patients, however, required transfusion for treatment of anemia prior to entry to the study and they were considered minor bleeders. Five of these so considered surgical patients died during the period of observation. In the medical group, six had shown occult bleeding insufficient to require transfusion and were considered minor bleeders similar to those in the surgical group. Four of these medical bleeders died during the period of observation. For the minor bleeders, therefore, the combined surgical and medical mortality rate is 75 percent and for the nonbleeders 46 percent ($p > 0.10$). The causes of death are summarized in Table II.

Table II. *Causes of death*

Cause	*Medical*	*Surgical*
Hepatic failure*	8	8
Combined hepatic and renal failure†	1	4
Variceal hemorrhage	5	1
Peptic ulcer	1	1
Trauma	0	2
Infection	0	1
Other	4	5
Total	19	22

*One postoperative death.
†Three postoperative deaths.

The survival experience of these two groups of patients is nearly identical and is represented graphically in Fig. 1. Two subjects in both the medical and the surgical groups have been lost to follow-up and do not influence this survival experience.

PERSISTENCE OF VARICES

Despite failure of the prophylactic portacaval shunt to alter survival experience of the two groups of patients, there was little doubt that the shunt exerted a beneficial effect upon the size of the varices, the reduction of portal pressure, and the prevention of hemorrhage. Among 26 surgical survivors and 26 medical survivors considered to be at risk, varices persisted by x-ray examination in three* surgical patients as contrasted to 15 of the medical patients. Varices were considered definitely smaller in six of the surgical survivors as contrasted to four of the medical patients and absent in 12 of the surgical patients as contrasted to four of the medical patients. No recent examination was available for meaningful interpretation in five of the surgical patients and in three of the medical patients. In the medical group therefore, varices were considerably more common ($p < 0.01$).

ESOPHAGEAL HEMORRHAGE

Among the surgical group bleeding from esophageal varices occurred in only one patient after construction of a shunt. This patient died from blood loss 33 months af-

*No decrease in size of the previously diagnosed varices was noted in 15 of 23 medical patients (74 percent), whereas only 3 of 21 (14 percent) surgical patients failed to show decrease in size.

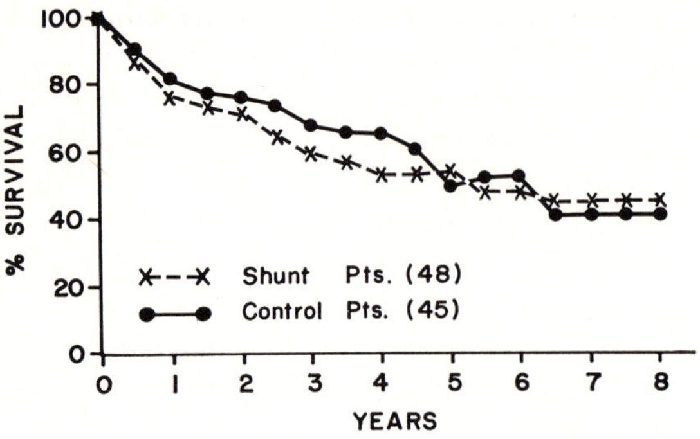

Fig. 1. Comparison of medically treated patients and patients with prophylactic shunts. A prophylactic portacaval shunt did not improve survival experience.

ter his operation as a consequence of repeated vomiting in association with excessive ingestion of alcohol. Twelve patients in the medical group experienced bleeding from esophageal varices. Five of these patients died as a consequence of hemorrhage, two of them despite the creation of a shunt as an urgent procedure. Both postoperative deaths were due to hepatic decompensation. Two patients died after 3 months of progressive liver failure which began after a bout of bleeding, and four patients died several months after shunting. Only one of the 12 bleeders in the medical group continues to survive. The effectiveness of the prophylactic shunt, therefore, in preventing hemorrhage from esophageal varices seems well established by a significant difference in frequency of hemorrhage ($p < 0.01$).

ENCEPHALOPATHY

The significant difference in the incidence of hepatic encephalopathy ($p < 0.05$) is apparent between the groups of patients. This is particularly true if one excludes the four medical patients who required an emergency portacaval shunt because of bleeding and in whom encephalopathy developed only after creation of the shunt. Of the 46 surgical patients, six developed mild encephalopathy, eight moderate, and ten severe, for a total of 24 or an incidence of 52 percent. Contrasted to this is the experience of 43 medical patients in whom four developed mild, ten moderate, and only two severe encephalopathy for a total of 16 or 37 percent. Severity of encephalopathy was based upon the length of time the complication existed since randomization together with the size of the dose of antibiotic required by the patient for its control. Encephalopathy was considered to be mild if it existed less than 1 month since the time of selection and the total dose of neomycin was not over 30 Gm. Moderate encephalopathy indicated duration not in excess of 6 months, and the total neomycin dosage was between 30 to 200 Gm. Encephalopathy was considered severe if it had been present for more than 6 months since selection and the requirement of neomycin was 200 Gm. or more. Encephalopathy occurred in the medical group largely as a consequence of severe liver failure, whereas in the surgical group it occurred in twice as many patients after randomization as in the medical group. Remissions were seen in 33 percent (14 of 43) of medical patients after selection as contrasted to only 20 percent (9 of 46) of the surgical patients.

ASCITES

Between the medical and surgical groups the frequency and severity of ascites were not significantly different. The remission rate after operation was 59 percent (27 of 46 patients) among the surgical patients as opposed to 43 percent (19 of 43) in the control group. After operation there were no new cases of ascites, whereas three new cases (8 percent) occurred among the medical patients. Reduction of portal pressure would seem to favor a lesser incidence of ascites and a less degree of severity when it occurs but these figures do not establish a significant difference ($p > 0.05$).

PEPTIC ULCER

Among the surgical patients six new cases of peptic ulcer (12 percent) occurred as contrasted to four new cases (9 percent) in the medical group. When one includes the ulcer hemorrhage occurring after therapeutic portacaval shunt in one of the control patients, ulcers occurred in seven of 48 surgical patients and three of 41 of the controls. The rate of ulcer formation after creation of a portacaval shunt, however, was not significantly increased ($p > 0.05$).

ALCOHOL

Contrary to a widely accepted belief, there was no difference observed in the surviving patients of both groups as to the incidence or the amount of consumption of alcohol ($p > 0.05$). Alcoholism was not significantly greater in either group who died of liver disease when compared to their respective surviving members. Nearly one half of the patients in both groups continued drinking after selection.

RISK OF HEMORRHAGE

Evidence has been put forth which suggests that the risk of hemorrhage from varices is considerably lessened in the patient whose varices have existed for at least 1 year.[1] In the present analysis 12 patients experienced variceal hemorrhage. Thirty-one patients in the medical group did not. Clinical features of these two groups of patients were compared in an attempt to determine if the potential bleeder demonstrated any factors of predictive significance. The duration of varices, dated from the time of discovery either by x-ray or by esophagoscopy, averaged 4.3 months for the medical patients who subsequently bled as compared to 9.4 months for those who did not. The duration of cirrhosis, dated from the appearance of its first objective evidence, was 19.9 months for those patients who bled as compared to 27.3 months for those who did not. Preselection hospitalization averaged 3 months. There were no significant differences in the values for serum bilirubin, serum albumin, or the prothrombin time. Encephalopathy was present in 41 percent of those patients who subsequently bled as compared to 58 percent of those who did not. A history of ascites was present in 75 percent of the subsequent variceal bleeders compared to 87 percent in the nonbleeders. It is seen, therefore, that the variables at the time of selection of the patient are not sufficiently precise to enable one to predict later variceal bleeding. The only exception was continued use of alcohol after selection. Nine of the 12 delayed variceal bleeders continued to drink after selection as compared to only 10 of the remaining 29 nonbleeders who resumed drinking after discharge ($p < 0.05$). In summary the patients who did develop variceal hemorrhage had a somewhat shorter duration of varices and cirrhosis. But this difference was not statistically significant ($p > 0.05$).

DISCUSSION

Justification for randomization of patients was based on the question of whether prevention of the initial variceal hemorrhage would result in a better survival rate than is available from the conventional practice of recommending operation as a therapeutic procedure among those individuals who survive their first and sometimes repeated hemorrhages. It was assumed among some investigators of the group that prophylactic portacaval shunt would indeed prolong life and ultimately would take precedence over the therapeutic shunt. Very few investigators[4, 13, 16] have questioned the efficacy and the propriety of therapeutic portacaval shunts. Most reports give enthusiastic endorsement to the operation. To have randomized patients for a therapeutic shunt would have been quite a different situation than randomizing patients for a prophylactic shunt. In the present state of the art such a proposal could be criticized on the grounds that it deprived patients of a form of therapy the benefits of which were widely accepted. The effect of the prophylactic shunt, however, was not known. The point has been made previously that unless a controlled study of this type is performed in the developing phase of a new form of therapy it may be impossible to do so subsequently. If clinical evaluation deems the treatment successful, one may not then deprive the patient of it.[2]

Application of these findings to all patients with all forms of cirrhosis with esophageal varices and without regard to distinguishing features such as the patient's socioeconomic status, the degree of risk, and the caliber of therapy must be avoided. The majority of patients in this study were treated in hospitals for the chronically ill. They came from a metropolitan setting and from a low socioeconomic level. Alcoholism was the major pathogenetic factor. Most of the patients were advanced cirrhotics with a high incidence of encephalopathy, ascites, jaundice, and malnutrition. The average hospital stay required to obtain clinical improvement sufficient to enter the study was 3 months. Lest these features be given undue importance, several additional factors are worthy of emphasis. The low surgical mortality rate of 2 percent in the 30 day period following operation indicates that these patients were not dead-end cirrhotics at the time of selection. The long in-hospital period of preoperative preparation permitting this unusually low surgical mortality rate indicated that substantial hepatic reserve was present. The patients selected for this study, whether in the surgical or medical group, demonstrated over a 10 year span a significantly better survival rate than that experienced among several hundred unselected patients with cirrhosis and varices hospitalized in the same institutions and without a history of bleeding.[7] The patients in the randomized study group, therefore, carried less risk than the other hospitalized patients with cirrhosis who had to be rejected because they were considered too ill to undergo a surgical procedure. Finally, it should be remembered that portal hypertension in the patient with early cirrhosis may diminish and even disappear on medical therapy. Conversely medical therapy may fail in the individual with advanced cirrhosis complicated by a persistent elevation of portal pressure.[9]

Similarly, these results should not be extrapolated in an effort to evaluate the usefulness of the therapeutic portacaval shunt. No objective justification for such judgment exists within the present study. It is tempting to conclude that if the prophylactic shunt does not improve survival, the therapeutic portacaval shunt will not do so. In the prophylactic shunt study operation is performed in an attempt to protect an indeterminate but probably small number of patients for whom variceal hemorrhage is inevitable. This is a distinctly different situation from that which exists among patients with cirrhosis who have already demonstrated their inability to tolerate portal hypertension without hemorrhage. Indeed, Hallenbeck and his associates[8] have pointed out that the patient who has experienced variceal hemorrhage and in whom a shunt is performed has already been selected by virtue of this surgical treatment as the patient who is most likely to live longer regardless of the type of treatment. With increasing skepticism expressed concerning the efficacy of the therapeutic shunt, it would no longer seem to be therapeutic heresy to evaluate the therapeutic shunt by means of a similar controlled trial. Indeed, early results from the Boston Inter-Hospital Liver Group suggests that patients in whom a portacaval shunt is created after hemorrhage enjoy a better survival experience than patients treated by medical means alone.

It is apparent from the present controlled study that creation of a prophylactic portacaval shunt did indeed reduce portal hypertension as manifested by disappearance or reduction in the size of varices and by a lesser incidence of variceal hemorrhage. Negating this benefit, however, was a higher mortality rate among the surgically treated patients. Insofar as survival is concerned, this study does not demonstrate any advantage to the prophylactic portacaval shunt. Further negating the presumed beneficial effect of reduction of portal hypertension by the shunt is the greater risk to which the shunt patient is subjected with regard to hepatic encephalopathy. One cannot, therefore, recommend prophylactic portacaval shunt in patients with alcoholic cirrhosis and with comparable social, economic, and nutritional characteristics.

CONCLUSIONS

1. Of 93 patients with cirrhosis and esophageal varices which had not bled, 48 under-

went a prophylactic shunt and 45 were given medical therapy. Choice of therapy was by random selection.

2. For the surgical group operative mortality rate was 2 percent at 30 days and 10 percent for all deaths occurring within 90 days of operation in the continuously hospitalized patient.

3. Ten percent of the medically treated patients died of variceal hemorrhage as contrasted to only one of the surgical patients.

4. The shunted patients demonstrated a greater prevalence of hepatocellular failure and a significantly increased incidence of hepatic encephalopathy.

5. Although surgical therapy greatly reduced the incidence of esophageal bleeding, it failed to improve longevity.

6. Abstinence from alcohol did not significantly improve survival among the unshunted patients although it appeared to exert a beneficial effect in a lower incidence of bleeding and less ascites.

7. Efforts to identify clinical factors at selection which might predispose to variceal hemorrhage were unsuccessful by retrospective analysis.

8. In this type of patient from the lower socioeconomic group with poor nutritional habits, prophylactic portacaval shunt does not exert a beneficial effect upon survival.

Invaluable assistance was provided by Dr. Hugo Muench, Mrs. Resna Veverbrants, Mrs. Carol Greene, and Mrs. Eva Borda.

REFERENCES

1. Baker, A. L., Smith, C., and Lieberman, G.: Natural history of esophageal varices; study of 115 cirrhotic patients in whom varices were diagnosed before bleeding, Amer. J. Med. **26:** 228, 1959.
2. Chalmers, T. C.: The management of hepatic coma. A continuing problem, Med. Clin. N. Amer. **52:** 1475, 1968.
3. Childs, C. G., III: Shattuck lecture: Portal circulation, New Eng. J. Med. **252:** 837, 1955.
4. Cohn, R.: A skeptical evaluation of portacaval anastomosis for gastro-intestinal hemorrhage of cirrhosis of the liver, Stanford Med. Bull. **9:** 231, 1951.
5. Cohn, R., and Blaisdell, F. W.: Natural history of patients with cirrhosis of liver with esophageal varices following first massive hemorrhage, Surg. Gynec. Obstet. **106:** 699, 1958.
6. Garceau, A. J., Chalmers, T. C., and the Boston Inter-Hospital Liver Group: The natural history of cirrhosis. Survival with esophageal varices, New Eng. J. Med. **268:** 469, 1963.
7. Garceau, A. J., Donaldson, R. M., Jr., O'Hara, E. T., Callow, A. D., Muench, H., Chalmers, T. C., and the Boston Inter-Hospital Liver Group: A controlled trial of prophylactic portacaval shunt surgery, New Eng. J. Med. **270:** 496, 1964.
8. Hallenbeck, G. A., Comess, M. S., Wollaeger, E. E., and Gage, R. P.: Bleeding varices due to cirrhosis. Survival after (1) nonsurgical treatment, (2) splenectomy with or without omentopexy, and (3) portacaval or splenorenal shunt, Arch. Surg. **78:** 774, 1959.
9. Leevy, C. M., Zinke, M., Baber, J., and Chey, W. Y.: Observations on influence of medical therapy on portal hypertension in hepatic cirrhosis, Ann. Intern. Med. **49:** 837, 1958.
10. Mackby, M. J.: Treatment of bleeding esophageal varices, J. A. M. A. **171:** 1916, 1959.
11. McDermott, W. V.: Amer. J. Med. **264:** 419, 1961.
12. McDermott, W. V., Jr., Palazzi, H., Nardi, G. L., and Mondet, A.: Elective portal systemic shunt. An analysis of 237 cases, New Eng. J. Med. **264:** 419, 1961.
13. Nachlas, M. M.: A critical evaluation of venous shunts for the treatment of cirrhotic patients with esophageal varices, Ann. Surg. **148:** 169, 1958.
14. Palmer, E. D., Brick, I. B., and Jahnke, E. J.: Esophageal varices without hemorrhage in cirrhosis: Proper indication for shunting procedures, New Eng. J. Med. **250:** 863, 1954.
15. Ratnoff, O. D., and Patek, A. J., Jr.: Natural history of Laennec's cirrhosis of liver: Analysis of 386 cases, Medicine **21:**207, 1942.
16. Strauch, G. O.: Second thoughts on cirrhosis and portosystemic shunts, Surgery **58:** 773, 1965.
17. Sullivan, P. H., Jr., Cohen, A., and Palmer, E. D.: Prophylactic portacaval shunts, Gastroenterology **39:** 414, 1960.
18. Welch, C. S., Kiley, J. E., Reeve, T. S., Goodrich, E. O., and Welch, H. F.: Treatment of bleeding from portal hypertension in patients with cirrhosis of the liver, New Eng. J. Med. **254:** 493, 1956.
19. Welch, C. S., and Ramos, A. G.: Results of portacaval shunts in treatment of portal hypertension, Surgery **41:** 756, 1957.

Selective portal decompression

RICHARD C. BRITTON, M.D.
ARTHUR B. VOORHEES, Jr., M.D.
JOHN B. PRICE, Jr., M.D.
NEW YORK, N. Y.
From the Departments of Surgery of the Brooklyn-Cumberland Medical Center and the College of Physicians and Surgeons, Columbia University

The absence of recurrent bleeding from esophagogastric varices in patients whose portacaval shunts were performed 5 to 20 years earlier has made it clear that adequate portal decompression is the most dependable method currently available for controlling the major complication of chronic portal hypertension. However, hepatic encephalopathy following these operations has proved to be a progressive complication which appears in 15 to 25 percent of patients within a year of operation and increases in incidence with prolonged follow-up. Among the many complications attributed to the diversion of portal blood around the liver, encephalopathy is the most common and the most disabling. It has seriously diminished the value of operation in the minds of many clinicians and has provoked a new examination of surgical goals and methods.

The technical goal of surgery has been the creation of large venovenous anastomoses to ensure continued patency and adequate portal decompression. In achieving this goal, the now standard portacaval and mesocaval shunts completely divert both intestinal and splenic venous drainage into the vena cava and abolish even the normal portal-systemic pressure gradient. A doubling of splanchnic flow through the stoma usually occurs,[6] and rate of intestinal absorption may be increased to greater than normal.[7] Doubling of hepatic arterial flow usually occurs also, but the total final hepatic blood flow is usually halved.[6] Together, these changes favor the development of encephalopathy by decreasing the efficiency of the liver in detoxifying cerebrotoxic substances present in blood of intestinal origin and by diverting such blood directly into the systemic circulation. In addition, reports of serious encephalopathy in patients with congenital or naturally acquired portacaval shunts without intrinsic liver disease indicate that a critical requirement for the development of encephalopathy is the hepatic bypass of blood of intestinal origin.[8]

Several investigators have recognized the deficiencies of standard shunt procedures and have begun to explore other methods for utilizing the tried principle of reducing pressure in the varices without the diversion of intestinal splanchnic blood into the systemic veins. In 1967, Warren and associates[10] reported an operation designed to drain only the splenic circuit and varices with preservation of superior mesenteric venous flow to the liver. This was accomplished technically by devascularization of the medial aspects of the abdominal esophagus and stomach, ligation of the splenic artery, division of the splenic vein in its midportion with ligation of the mesenteric end, and end-to-side anastomosis of the splenic end of the splenic vein

Presented at the Twenty-third Annual Meeting of the Society of Vascular Surgery, New York, N. Y., July 12-13, 1969.

to the side of the left renal vein. In a second report in 1969 with added cases, these authors recorded absence of variceal bleeding and encephalopathy in five survivors in a group of eleven patients treated in this manner.[9]

A similar study was begun in 1965 at the Presbyterian Hospital after recognition of a progressively unacceptable incidence of encephalopathy following standard shunt procedures, the necessity for avoiding the hepatic bypass of blood of intestinal origin, and the low incidence of encephalopathy following conventional splenorenal shunts. It was reasoned that a side-to-side anastomosis between the larger central portion of the splenic vein and the left renal vein would be less likely to become occluded than the end-to-side anastomosis, that it would selectively drain the splenic circuit and varices, and that it would permit continued mesenteric venous flow to the liver. Variations of the technical procedure have been reported by Clatworthy and Boles[3] in 1959, by Cooley[4] in 1963, and by Mason[5] in 1966. The goals of the study were to determine whether such anastomosis would significantly reduce variceal pressure, whether it would alter total hepatic blood flow and sinusoidal pressure, whether mesenteric flow would in fact continue to the liver, and whether encephalopathy would develop.

METHODS AND MATERIALS

Side-to-side central splenorenal venous anastomosis with preservation of the spleen was attempted in 19 patients and was successfully performed in 17 patients of whom one had schistosomiasis, two had extrahepatic portal obstruction without liver disease, two had Laennec's cirrhosis, and ten had posthepatitic cirrhosis. All patients had bled from varices. A clinical grading system included Grade I patients who demonstrated no evidence of hepatic decompensation prior to operation. Grade II patients may have had a history of reversible decompensation or developed symptoms after a recent hemorrhage but had stable jaundice or controlled ascites at the time of operation. Grade III patients had increasing jaundice, ascites, or both at the time of operation (Table I).

Table I. *Clinical data of 17 patients having central splenorenal shunt*

Case No.	Age	Sex	Disease	Clinical grade	Ascites	Ascites controlled	Prior surgery	Date of operation	Comment
1	61	M	EHB*	I	–	–	–	6/16/65	Splenectomy
2	62	F	PN	I	–	–	–	4/22/66	–
3	26	F	Sch.	I	–	–	–	6/16/67	–
4	59	M	PN	I	–	–	–	8/22/67†	–
5	44	M	PN	I	–	–	–	12/15/67	–
6	6	M	EHB	I	–	–	–‡	5/24/68	–
7	47	F	PN	II	+	+	–	12/ 3/66	–
8	6	M	PN	II	+	0	–§	6/ 9/67	–
9	52	F	PN*	II	+	+	–	4/30/68	–
10	64	M	PN	II	+	+	–	6/27/68	–
11	51	F	PN	II	+	+	–	9/10/68	–
12	42	F	L	III	+	+	–	4/18/67†	Splenectomy
13	47	F	PN	III	+	+	–	6/28/67	–
14	70	F	Bil.	III	+	0	–	8/17/67†	–
15	12	M	PN	III	+	+	–	10/23/67	–
16	63	M	L	III	+	+	–	5/10/68	–
17	51	M	L*	III	+	+	–	5/26/68	–

EHB = Extrahepatic block; PN = Postnecrotic cirrhosis; Sch. = Schistosomiasis; L = Laennec's cirrhosis; Bil. = Biliary cirrhosis.

*Diabetic.

†Emergency operation.

‡Mesocaval shunt, 1963.

§Mesocaval shunt, 1966.

Three patients had emergency operations for bleeding which did not respond to conservative measures.

It was considered essential at the outset that a suitable anatomic relationship and patency of the splenic and renal veins be established by preoperative splenoportography and retrograde renal vein catheterization and phlebography. This was not possible in all cases. In certain patients preoperative and postoperative catheterization studies were performed. These included estimation of hepatic blood flow by the indirect Fick method with indocyanine green.[2] Blood volume was estimated from the hematocrit and the 10 minute dilution of radioactive iodinated albumin. Pressures were measured by strain gauge and recorded with an electronic recorder. In postoperative patients, splenic vein pressures were recorded by passing a cardiac catheter through the shunt into the splenic vein at the hilum. Cardiac output estimations were obtained by averaging three dye-dilution curves.

The operation was usually performed through a midline incision. The transverse colon was retracted cephalad out of the wound to expose the ligament of Treitz which was taken down to permit retraction of the duodenum cephalad. This maneuver exposed the left renal vein which was mobilized from its junction with vena cava to its junction with the left adrenal vein. The duodenum was then retracted cephalad to expose the posterior aspect of the pancreas and the splenic vein coursing along its inferior border covered by peritoneum. The splenic vein was exposed a distance of approximately 2 inches, and in half the cases this was sufficient to permit the application of an exclusion clamp. In the other cases ligation of several venous branches between the vein and the posterior pancreas was necessary to give enough mobility for approximation of the two veins. Ellipses approximately 3.0 by 1.5 cm. were excised from each vessel and the side-to-side anastomosis completed. In several patients the inferior mesenteric vein joined the splenic vein near the midline and required ligation and division for adequate mobilization of the splenic vein.

RESULTS

Fifteen patients survived the operation, left the hospital, and have been followed from 4 to 48 months. Two patients died in the hospital. Patient No. 15, a 15-year-old boy with advanced posthepatitic cirrhosis, developed massive ascites postoperatively and required several paracenteses. He developed metabolic encephalopathy during intensive diuretic therapy and died with terminal coma 1 month after operation. Autopsy examination indicated a patent shunt and severe cirrhosis with extensive hepatic necrosis. Patient No. 17 developed congestive heart failure with pulmonary edema and ascites, and he required dialysis for renal insufficiency. He died 1 month after operation, and autopsy examination revealed pancreatitis and thrombosis of the portal and superior mesenteric veins but patency of the shunt. Three patients died after leaving the hospital. Patient No. 12, a 42-year-old woman with alcoholic cirrhosis, bled from the spleen after splenoportography. Emergency splenectomy and central splenorenal shunt were performed. Her postoperative course was complicated by fluid retention, but she finally recovered and was discharged from the hospital. She did well initially but resumed heavy alcohol ingestion and died from hepatic failure 1 year postoperatively. Patient No. 14 had multiple variceal hemorrhages in the hospital and had an emergency operation in the presence of hepatic decompensation. Early postoperatively she developed congestive heart failure, ascites, edema, urinary tract infection with systemic sepsis, and transient encephalopathy during diuretic therapy. She recovered sufficiently to leave the hospital but deteriorated steadily and died 4 months later. Patient No. 16 developed congestive heart failure during the first postoperative week and responded to cardiotonic and diuretic therapy with a 15 pound weight loss and coma. He improved and did reasonably well until death 6 months later following a stroke (Table II).

Table II. *Early and late postoperative courses of 17 patients having central splenorenal shunts*

Case No.	*Hospital death*	*Cause of death*	*Ascites*	*Heart failure*	*Encephalopathy*	*Follow-up (months)*	*Varix bleeding*	*Encephalopathy*	*Death*	*Cause of death*
1	–	–	–	–	0	48	0	0	–	–
2	–	–	–	–	0	38	0	0	–	–
3	–	–	–	+	0	24	0	0	–	–
4	–	–	–	+	0	22	0	0	–	–
5	–	–	–	–	0	18	0	+	–	–
6	–	–	–	–	0	13	0	0	–	–
7	–	–	–	–	0	30	0	0	–	–
8	–	–	+	–	0	24	0	0	–	–
9	–	–	–	–	0	14	0	0	–	–
10	–	–	–	–	0	12	0	0	–	–
11	–	–	–	–	0	9	0	+	–	–
12	–	–	+	?	+	12	0	0	+	Hepatic failure
13	–	–	–	–	0	24	0	0	–	–
14	–	–	+	+	+	4	0	0	+	Hepatic failure
15	+	Hepatic failure	+	–	0	1	–	–	–	–
16	–	–	+	+	+	6	0	0	+	Stroke
17	+	Renal failure	+	+	+	1	–	–	–	–

Preoperative portography was not performed in two patients who were subjected to needlessly long and difficult dissection before the operation was abandoned. In both patients anomalous splenic veins coursed along the superior border of the pancreas too far away from the renal vein for easy approximation. In one of these patients the left renal vein was divided at its junction with the adrenal vein and the caval end anastomosed to the side of the splenic vein. The anastomosis clotted and the patient's condition prohibited extending the operation. In one clinical Grade I patient being considered for operation, the portagram demonstrated thrombosis of the splenic vein. A side-to-side portacaval shunt was therefore performed, and she has been readmitted in the sixth, ninth, and twelfth postoperative months with encephalopathy without laboratory or clinical evidence of hepatic deterioration. In two patients splenectomy was performed at the time of the shunt operation. An attempt to perform a conventional splenorenal anastomosis after splenectomy in Patient No. 1 failed because of the poor quality and small diameter of the splenic vein at the hilum. The central anastomosis was carried out without difficulty and the proximal (splenic) end of the splenic vein was ligated. Patient No. 12 bled from splenic puncture for portography, and an emergency splenectomy was performed. Technical problems led to a decision to perform a central anastomosis. The remaining 15 patients had a central side-to-side anastomosis with preservation of the spleen.

The 13 surviving patients have been followed from 10 months to 4 years, and none has had recurrent bleeding from varices. Two patients who developed congestive heart failure in the early postoperative period had transient encephalopathy during intensive diuretic therapy. Both patients died within 6 months of operation with stroke and hepatic failure, respectively. Two patients have developed mild encephalopathy on an unrestricted diet. Patient No. 5 had several bouts of mild mental confusion beginning 11 months after operation, but these have not recurred following dietary protein restriction. Patient No. 11 had a bout of precoma 4 months after operation but has been asymptomatic with dietary protein restriction for the ensuing 5 months.

Ascites was present preoperatively in 11 patients of whom nine had the ascites controlled before operation. Postoperatively, three patients developed ascites in association with congestive heart failure, with pancreatitis and thrombosis of the portal vein and superior mesenteric vein, and with subacute hepatic failure, respectively. Late ascites has not appeared in any of the survivors to date. Congestive heart failure occurred in the early postoperative period in five patients in the absence of hypertension, myocardial infarction, or clinical heart disease. It responded to conventional cardiotonic and diuretic therapy but in three patients who were not simultaneously given supplemental potassium transient encephalopathy developed.

Preoperative and postoperative studies demonstrated lower final splenic vein pressures than those recorded at operation (Table III). The mean operative pressure after completion of the anastomosis was 19.9 mm. Hg while the postoperative catheterization pressure averaged 11.6 mm. Hg in the same six patients (Table IV). An average reduction in absolute portal pressure in the splenic circuit of 10.0 mm. Hg, with a range of 6.0 to 14.0 mm. Hg, resulted from operation. The residual measured splenic vein pressures ranged from 15.4 to 22.0 mm. Hg with a mean of 18.6 mm. Hg. The absolute splenic vein pressures, represented by the measured value minus the abdominal caval pressure, averaged 11.6 mm. Hg with a range of from 5.2 to 17.0 mm. Hg. In the six patients studied both before and after operation, total hepatic blood flow was reduced an average of 50 percent with a range of 10 to 69 percent. There were corresponding reductions in hepatic vein wedge pres-

Table III. *Operative portal pressure changes*

Case No.	Portal pressure*: Before shunt (mm. Hg)	Portal pressure*: After shunt (mm. Hg)	Change (mm. Hg)
1	29.2	20.0	- 9.2
2	18.5	12.3	- 6.2
3	—	—	—
4	28.4	20.8	- 7.6
5	22.3	16.8	- 5.5
6	37.0	21.5	-15.5
7	30.8	24.6	- 6.2
8	23.2	13.8	- 8.4
9	29.2	23.0	- 6.2
10	30.8	16.8	-14.0
11	29.2	24.5	- 4.7
12	25.0	17.3	- 7.7
13	27.8	20.0	- 7.8
14	26.1	15.4	-10.7
15	28.4	20.8	- 7.6
16	26.5	15.5	- 9.0
17	37.0	21.6	-15.4
Mean	28.0	19.0	- 9.0

*Portal pressures are expressed as portal pressure minus the abdominal vena cava pressure.

Table IV. *Data of preoperative and postoperative catheterization studies*

Case No.	Preoperative: Estimated hepatic blood flow (ml./min.)	Preoperative: Hepatic vein* wedge pressure (mm./Hg)	Preoperative: Cardiac output (L./min.)	Postoperative: Time after operation (weeks)	Postoperative: Estimated hepatic blood flow (ml./min.)	Postoperative: Hepatic vein wedge pressure (mm. Hg)	Postoperative: Splenic vein pressure (mm. Hg)	Postoperative: Cardiac output (L./min.)
1	1,940	13.0	4.00	8	600	2.9	—	4.77
2	1,123	15.6	—	3	756	4.2	11.2	13.45
7	713	19.4	6.32	2	645	7.9	9.4	8.20
9	—	—	—	4	—	8.0	14.0	—
11	650	28.2	5.58	4	400	9.0	17.0	4.81
12	1,345	15.6	7.01	—	—	—	—	—
13	1,300	14.2	4.28	2	507	—	12.5	8.35
16	976	16.5	6.67	4	490	13.0	5.2	12.30
Mean of paired studies	1,117	18.5	5.47		566	9.2	11.6	7.68

*Pressures are expressed in millimeters of mercury as pressure minus abdominal vena cava pressure.

sure which averaged 9.3 mm. Hg with a range of 3.5 to 19.2 mm. Hg. In six of the seven patients who had postoperative catheterization studies, hepatic vein wedge phlebography was performed. With cardiac catheter firmly wedged into a right lobe hepatic vein, contrast medium was injected by hand during filming on 35 mm. film with a frame speed of 48 frames per second. In all six patients contrast medium could be forced retrograde through the sinusoids into portal branches. With maximum hand injection pressure, it could be forced into the main portal trunk but could not be forced retrograde into the splenic vein except in one patient (Patient No. 11). In this patient retrograde flow into the splenic vein and the shunt from the portal trunk was possible only during maximum hand injection pressure and during deep inspiration. It was concluded that there was prograde flow to the liver of superior mesenteric vein blood. In three patients, estimation of splenic vein flow rate was obtained by repeatedly injecting small volumes of contrast medium through the catheter with its tip through the shunt and lodged at the splenic hilum during filming at 48 frames per second. By a method previously described,[2] a gross estimate of flow rate was calculated. In Patient No. 13 the rate was 1,850 c.c. per minute. In Patient No. 9 the rate was 1,650 c.c. per minute. In Patient No. 16 the rate was 4,800 c.c. per minute. The velocity of flow in all three patients exceeded 10 cm. per second. No flow of contrast medium into the distal splenic vein to the right of the shunt stoma was observed. The velocity of flow through the shunt was noted to increase during inspiration.

DISCUSSION

The side-to-side central splenorenal shunt appears to be effective in preventing recurrent bleeding from varices despite the fact that it incompletely decompresses the splenic circuit. Unlike the standard portacaval and mesocaval shunts which abolish any pressure gradient between the portal bed and the vena cava, this shunt leaves a low grade hypertension in the splenic vein and, presumably, the esophagogastric varices. Nevertheless, disappearance of varices by barium study of the esophagus has resulted in all seven of the patients studied by this method. Reduction in splenic size has also occurred, but no significant changes in blood platelet count or leukocyte count have been observed.

The control of ascites, including two patients whose ascites was not controlled by usual means before operation, was associated with significant reductions in sinusoidal pressure as indicated by hepatic vein wedge pressure. This is of interest since in those patients who were studied postoperatively there was persistent superior mesenteric flow to the liver. If sinusoidal hypertension is considered a major cause of ascites formation, the relief of ascites in these patients may be explained by alterations in the relationship where *resistance equals pressure divided by flow.* A reduction in the denominator, i.e., flow, must result in a reduction in the numerator, i.e., pressure, if resistance is constant. In cirrhosis the resistance is predominantly anatomic and functionally constant although it may steadily increase in time with progression of obliterative changes in the hepatic veins.[1] Thus, diversion of the splenic circuit inflow alone should affect the pressure-flow relationship with reduction in sinusoidal pressure. From the data obtained in the studied patients, it would appear that the splenic circuit contribution was nearly 50 percent of total hepatic blood flow before operation.

The appearance of encephalopathy in two patients would suggest that hepatic resistance has increased and that increasing amounts of mesenteric blood are being diverted retrograde into the splenic vein and the shunt. If this explanation is correct, it would be expected that eventually most patients with cirrhosis and with a central shunt would develop encephalopathy if they survive long enough. It would seem logical to consider ligating the distal (mesenteric) end of the splenic vein after completion of the anastomosis to prevent reflux of mesenteric blood into the splenic vein and the shunt. In effect, this is accomplished by the operation described by Warren and associates.[10] The potential hazard of inducing acute ascites may result, as it did in one of their patients. This might be avoided if the occluded portal hepatic pressure were measured as a guide to the severity of hepatic vascular resistance. If the pressure were significantly less than free portal pressure, the splenic vein could probably be ligated with impunity. However, if it were approximately the same as the free portal pressure, it would be safer to leave the splenic vein open and accept the possibility that reflux and encephalopathy may develop.

The significant increases in cardiac output observed in three of the patients raises the question of the importance of this change in relation to the high incidence of congestive heart failure early in the postoperative period. Studies in patients having standard portacaval shunts have indicated that the cardiac output usually increases in direct proportion to the amount of flow through the shunt. A higher than expected incidence of early congestive heart failure in the absence of demonstrable cardiac disease has also been observed in these patients. Ligation of the splenic artery would affect associated hypersplenism favorably and should reduce the volume of shunt flow and the likelihood of high output congestive heart failure.

CONCLUSIONS

The central splenorenal shunt appears to function for an indeterminate period of time in some patients as a selective shunt which drains only the splenic circuit and preserves superior mesenteric blood flow to the liver. Although it reduces splenic circuit pressure, it does not abolish the portal-systemic venous pressure gradient. The pressure reduction obtained has been sufficient to prevent further bleeding from varices during prolonged follow-up periods. It reduces total hepatic blood flow and sinusoidal pressure to the same degree as conventional portacaval shunts and is effective in controlling ascites. Although it is effective in selective decompression of varices, it retains a pathway through which blood of intestinal origin may reflux into the shunt and contribute to the development of encephalopathy. Progressive changes in the venous outflow tract of the liver in association with cirrhosis may be expected to increase hepatic vascular resistance with the passage of time and increase the amount of reflux. The concept of selective portal decompression has merit and deserves further study.

REFERENCES

1. Britton, R. C.: The hepatic outflow tract and ascites, Amer. J. Gastroent. **44:** 443, 1965.
2. Britton, R. C., Voorhees, A. B., Jr., and Price, J. B., Jr.: Perfusion of the liver following side-to-side portacaval shunt, SURGERY **62:** 181, 1967.
3. Clatworthy, H. W., and Boles, E. T., Jr.: Extrahepatic portal bed block in children: Pathogenesis and treatment, Ann. Surg. **150:** 371, 1959.
4. Cooley, D. A.: Side to side splenorenal anastomosis with splenic preservation for portal hypertension, Surg. Gynec. Obstet. **116:** 626, 1963.
5. Mason, E. E.: Splenectomy and side-to-side splenorenal shunt for portal hypertension, SURGERY **60:** 536, 1966.
6. Price, J. B., Jr., Britton, R. C., and Voorhees, A. B., Jr.: The significance and limitations of operative hemodynamics in portal hypertension, Arch. Surg. **95:** 843, 1967.
7. Price, J. B., Jr., McCullough, W., Petersen, L., Britton, R. C., and Voorhees, A. B., Jr.: Effect of portal-systemic shunting on intestinal absorption in the dog and man, Surg. Gynec. Obstet. **125:** 305, 1967.
8. Raskin, N. H., and Price, J. B., Jr.: Portal-systemic encephalopathy due to intrahepatic shunts, New Eng. J. Med. **270:** 225, 1964.
9. Warren, W. D., Fomon, J. J., and Zeppa, R.: Further evaluation of selective decompression of varices by distal splenorenal shunt, Ann. Surg. **169:** 652, 1969.
10. Warren, W. D., Zeppa, R., and Fomon, J. J.: Selective trans-splenic decompression of gastroesophageal varices by distal splenorenal shunt, Ann. Surg. **166:** 437, 1967.

DISCUSSION*

Dr. George Johnson, Jr. (Chapel Hill, N. C.). The data presented by Dr. Callow is important additional information in evaluating surgery to control portal hypertension.

I would like to present some additional thoughts

*This discussion also applies to the previous paper by Callow and associates on the control of portal hypertension that I believe will be appropriate.

We have recently reported and published our long-term experience with 55 patients subjected to an ablative procedure.

Our results demonstrated no deterioration of liver function with time, no encephalopathy, and a long-time survival paralleling that reported for portacaval shunt. The incidence of recurrent gastrointestinal bleeding was higher than that following a shunting procedure.

It has been well documented that cirrhosis of the liver has a profound effect on the systemic cardiovascular system.

A portacaval shunt may control portal hypertension, may alter the portal system hemodynamics, yet cause a severe and devastating alteration of liver and systemic hemodynamics leading eventually to the death of the patient.

Since both the ablative and shunt procedures have their merits and demerits, we need to improve our methods of selecting the operation for these patients. Although we are currently evaluating systemic hemodynamics, local hemodynamics, angiography, liver and splenic blood flow, as yet, none of these correlates with our results.

Perhaps studies such as Dr. Britton has presented will give us some insights into this problem.

I would like to ask Dr. Callow if they have been able to correlate any of the local or systemic hemodynamics with their long-term results.

Dr. W. Dean Warren (Miami, Fla.). First, I would like to compliment Dr. Callow and his co-authors on this excellent paper. I believe that this is one of the important studies in the field of portal hypertension in the last decade and has been an enormous contribution. I tend to agree with their conclusion, and this is one of the reasons that made us search for a new type of operative procedure.

Regarding the therapeutic group, in which the results have not been clearly established, I think one can safely say that there will still be certain people for whom a portacaval shunt is harmful. One of the great needs in this field is the development of information and techniques to allow proper selection of candidates for any type of operative procedure.

However, I rise primarily to discuss Dr. Britton's paper. As some of you know, we have devoted several years in an unsuccessful attempt to "educate" the group at the Columbia Presbyterian Medical Center. I think that our failure may have been due in large part to their being unduly concerned about the fact that they could not reproduce our experimental results, and this has led them to look askance at some of the concepts and procedures which we have developed! In a serious vein, however, I must say that I fail to see how continued perfusion of the liver will generally follow an open side-to-side splenorenal anastomosis. In some instances this has been shown to decompress the portal venous system completely and, physiologically, is similar to a side-to-side portacaval shunt except perhaps in the degree of decompression related to the size of the anastomosis.

Could I have the first slide, please?

We have recently advocated a new procedure in which we attempt to shunt only the blood draining the spleen and the stomach into the left renal vein. All communications between the intestinal portal system and the gastrosplenic portal system are divided insofar as possible. Despite this deliberate attempt, we have found in two cases that we have not been able to perfuse the liver in the postoperative period. This first slide shows a wedged hepatic venogram preoperatively which demonstrates a very sluggish hepatopetal portal flow. In other words, there is perfusion of the liver preoperatively and this was confirmed by splenoportography. However, following this selective decompression of the splenic system, there was a reversal of flow in the portal vein as demonstrated by this slide. Whereas preoperatively the portal flow was into the liver, it is now out of the liver (and this was confirmed by superior mesenteric angiography). Note that down at the bottom of the slide the dye flowing out of the liver becomes so diluted that one cannot follow it past the junction wtih the major collaterals of the portal vein. I think this is the reason that Dr. Britton has not been able to see the dye pass out through his splenorenal shunt. Although he did not point this out on both of the wedged hepatic venograms which he demonstrated in postoperative patients, the major portal veins were filled throughout their length that could be seen on the slide. Today he has used a devilishly clever method of showing the slide upside down so as to throw everybody off, but we managed to identify this point anyway.

In fact there is a very simple way to show whether or not you are perfusing the liver, and this is demonstrated on the next slide. This is superior mesenteric angiography, and on the venous phase you can see clearly that the portal vein is filled, its intrahepatic branches are filled, and there is a good liver blush indicating good perfusion of the liver. As you can see, the surgeon who did this particular operation (and he shall remain nameless) failed to ligate the coronary vein, one of the cardinal points in this operation; he intended to cut down the amount of communication between the two systems and to help prevent losing blood from the liver perfusate.

The last slide simply shows the splenorenal shunt which we have demonstrated in every survivor. This has been demonstrated either by direct splenoportography or by splenic angiography studying the venous phase.

When I recently reported the results of this procedure at the Southern Surgical Association we had only five survivors out of 11 patients in whom the operation was completed. We now have accomplished the operation in 17 patients and have ten survivors. There has been only one death in our last six cases and this was in a patient who had an undiagnosed but extensively infiltrating hepatoma and chronic active hepatitis.

I am most impressed by the excellent achievement of a very low mortality rate with a difficult group of patients and a difficult operation. They have had three late deaths and some encephalopathy. In our ten survivors we have had no late deaths, no encephalopathy, and no gastrointestinal bleeding.

Dr. Robert R. Linton (Brookline, Mass.). I feel I must get up and defend myself and also those who have advocated the end-to-side splenorenal shunt. I still don't understand why surgeons find it so difficult to do an end-to-side splenorenal shunt, and then they find it so easy to do a side-to-side splenorenal shunt or a Warren splenorenal shunt. It seems to me that these are much more difficult to carry out than the end-to-side.

The end-to-side splenorenal shunt, in our hands, has stood up now for approximately 23 years. The 10 year follow-up, that is, on patients who were operated upon 10 years ago or more, gives a survival rate for splenorenal shunts of 33 percent and for direct portacaval for 14 percent so that there isn't any question in my mind that the splenorenal shunt is superior to the portacaval shunt. It is my opinion that the portacaval shunt should be done only in rare instances as when you have a small splenic vein which usually can be determined preoperatively by angiography, or if the patient has had a splenectomy, or a splenorenal shunt that has failed.

One of the criticisms that I would have of the Boston Inter-Hospital Liver Group study in Boston is that the prophylactic procedures were direct portacaval shunts.

I still am in hearty agreement with Dr. Callow and his associates, however, in that there is no place for prophylactic shunts in the treatment of esophageal varices and cirrhosis of the liver.

In closing, I would like to thank the essayists for two very interesting papers and I enjoyed them very much.

Dr. Allan D. Callow (closing). I wish to thank the audience for their attention and the discussants for their comments.

When one begins a study such as this which was begun some 10 years ago, one always runs the risk of being put out of business by the introduction of new shunts before the study is completed.

The shunts that Drs. Britton and Warren have described have much to offer and should be very helpful in alleviating the problem of postshunt encephalopathy which is seen with such troublesome frequency with a standard portacaval shunt.

In relation to the pressure studies discussed by Dr. Johnson, we do not have sufficient data to permit a valid opinion at this time.

Dr. Linton, the answer to your question is very simple: There are very few people in this world of portacaval shunts who can do the shunts as well as you can! I think that's the reason most surgeons have preferred the easier portacaval anastomosis.

Thank you for the privilege of the floor.

Dr. R. C. Britton (closing). Dr. Warren has put great faith in his interpretation of what is seen on wedged hepatic phlebography. In the cirrhotic liver there are such large numbers of portal vein-hepatic vein intrahepatic shunts that these may invalidate his isotopic method for determining total hepatic blood flow and lead to erroneous interpretation of retrograde phlebography. It takes very little pressure in most cirrhotic livers to force dye, even preoperatively, back into the portal trunk.

The slides, which were apparently shown upside down, are clips from cine films. The cineangiograms shot at high camera speed showed that portal blood did not go back into the shunts in six patients at that time. In the two patients who subsequently have developed encephalopathy, some portal diversion must have begun to occur, and this represents a flaw in the basic concept of the operation.

Because of an enormous cardiac output measured later in one of the patients, a celiac arteriogram was attempted to determine whether large arteriovenous shunts existed in the spleen. The catheter slipped, resulting in both splenic and mesenteric injections and demonstrating mesenteric perfusion of the liver.

I would echo what Dr. Callow said to Dr. Linton and add that there are individual technical problems, particularly in the postsplenectomy patient. Bill Clatworthy pointed out years ago that the central portion of the splenic vein may be twice as large as the hilar portion. This permitted us to do central shunts in three patients in whom we could not have done the conventional shunt.

This is a relatively easy operation in which we have used a midline incision, lifted up the colon, dissected the left renal vein, and then dissected the anterior aspect of the splenic vein posterior to the pancreas on its inferior border. One advantage is that there are no vascularized adhesions such as occur in the upper quadrants following cholecystectomy and those which occur naturally between the spleen and diaphragm.

A third group not represented today is the emergency shunt group which depends for its efficacy upon the use of one of the standard shunts. I think where Dean Warren and I agree is that it is medically wrong and perhaps morally wrong today to impose a shunt which will cause disabling encephalopathy in a large proportion of patients. Of 490 adult cirrhotics followed at the Presbyterian Hospital up to 25 years, 30 percent have developed encephalopathy of mild-to-moderate degree within 5 years of operation and 60 percent after 5 years. This does not represent a clinical gain.

Directional flow detection for localizing venous valvular incompetency

ROLAND FOLSE, M.D.
RAYMOND H. ALEXANDER, M.D.
SEATTLE, WASH.
From the Department of Surgery of the University of Washington, School of Medicine, and the Second University Surgical Service of the Harborview Medical Center

Successful treatment of the complications of venous insufficiency in the lower leg depends upon accurate localization and ligation of perforating veins. When stasis dermatitis and edema are present, precise localization of perforators by clinical means is difficult. Because of this difficulty in identifying individual incompetent perforators, subfascial approaches to the perforating veins through a long medial incision have been used most often. Although these methods give very satisfactory results, the risk of wound necrosis is significant in wide flaps fashioned in areas of brawny edema, fibrosis, or ulceration.

The complications of large incisions can be avoided by localizing the perforators individually preoperatively and ligating each one through a separate small incision just as it perforates the fascia. Since removal of all veins which communicate with the deep system is important, a means of accurately locating each perforator is necessary. Recently, a directional ultrasonic flow detector has become available which allows a simple transcutaneous assessment of venous dynamics and also can be used to accurately identify incompetent perforating veins. This report describes the application of the ultrasonic flow detector in the identification of incompetent perforating veins and their treatment by local interruption through multiple small incisions.

Supported in part by a grant from the Washington State Heart Association.

Presented at the Twenty-third Annual Meeting of the Society for Vascular Surgery, New York, N. Y., July 12-13, 1969.

METHODS

The directional ultrasonic flow detector utilizes the principle that transmitted ultrasonic waves shift in frequency as they are reflected from moving blood particles. The frequency shift is proportional to the velocity of the moving particles. The ultrasonic flow detector consists of a small probe with transmitting and receiving crystals connected with the appropriate electronic circuitry to convert the reflected waves into an audible signal or a written record of instantaneous velocity changes. Changes in the intensity and frequency of the audible signal reflects alteration in the velocity of blood flow.

Venous flow in the leg can easily be monitored by placing the probe over a distal superficial vein. In patients with normal veins which contain competent valves, compressing the calf results in flow of blood toward the heart. The probe placed over a vein distal to the compression point will detect no flow, as competent valves prevent retrograde flow of blood. Upon release of pressure, flow is detected as blood rushes past the probe into the compressed space.

With incompetent veins, a different set of events occurs. Calf compression initiates forward flow toward the heart but also causes reverse flow through incompetent valves. When compression is released, flow resumes as in the normal case. Therefore, when detecting flow from a point distal to the compression site, the presence of both reverse and forward flow indicates incompetent intervening valves (Fig. 1).

In order to distinguish between an incompetent superficial vein and an incompetent perforator, a tourniquet is placed between the compression point and the probe (Fig. 2). With compression the retrograde flow of blood through superficial veins is prevented. Venous flow detected at this time would necessarily be due to incompetent perforating veins.

When the ultrasonic probe is passed over various levels of the leg in a systematic fashion, localized areas of reverse flow can be identified which represent the precise sites of incompetent perforating veins.

This method of identifying incompetent perforators has been used in the evaluation of patients with chronic venous insufficiency. All patients had edema and many had overt ulceration. All were examined with the ultrasonic flow detector, and the sites of their perforating veins were mapped and photographed (Fig. 3). Persons who refused operative treatment or whose disease did not warrant operation were followed at intervals. Those who were candidates for surgical intervention were operated upon either in the outpatient minor surgery clinic or as inpatients. In all but two cases, the operation performed consisted of local ligation of the perforators which had been previously marked. Small incisions, 1 to 2 cm. in length were used to isolate the veins. In all cases, the perforating veins were dissected and followed as far down toward the fascia as possible before ligation. The superficial veins from which the perforating vein arose were then ligated or stripped proximally and distally. This procedure was combined with greater saphenous ligation and stripping in patients with incompetent superficial systems who had not received this procedure as a part of prior treatment. In the remaining two patients, subfascial ligations through long vertical incisions were performed.

In general, those patients with severe ulceration were admitted to the hospital. After the acute inflammation and edema had subsided, the ulcer was excised and covered with a split skin graft either immediately or after a few days' delay. As soon as healing occurred, the perforating veins were identified and ligated.

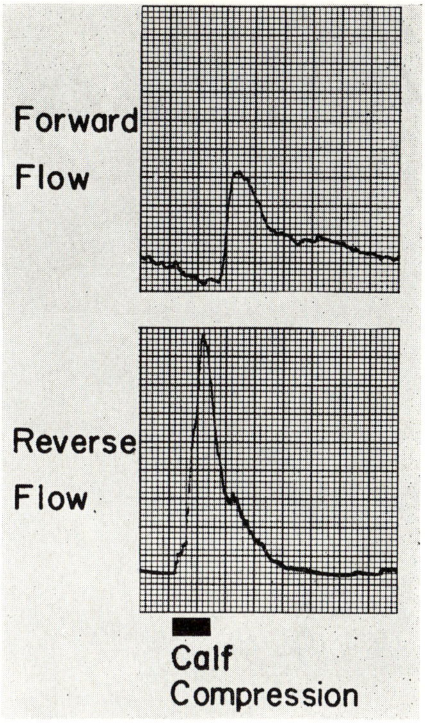

Fig. 1. Bidirectional flow in an incompetent perforating vein with calf compression.

RESULTS

Of 31 patients studied, 28 underwent operations. Five patients had very localized disease and were operated upon as outpatients. The remaining 23 were hospitalized. Thirteen of the series had interruption of perforators in conjunction with high ligation and stripping of the greater saphenous vein. Another 13 had interruption of perforators only, as the saphenous system was competent or a saphenous stripping had been performed previously. Two had subfascial ligations through long incisions.

The number of perforators found at operation ranged from one to as many as 18; the average number interrupted was seven. No good correlation was apparent between

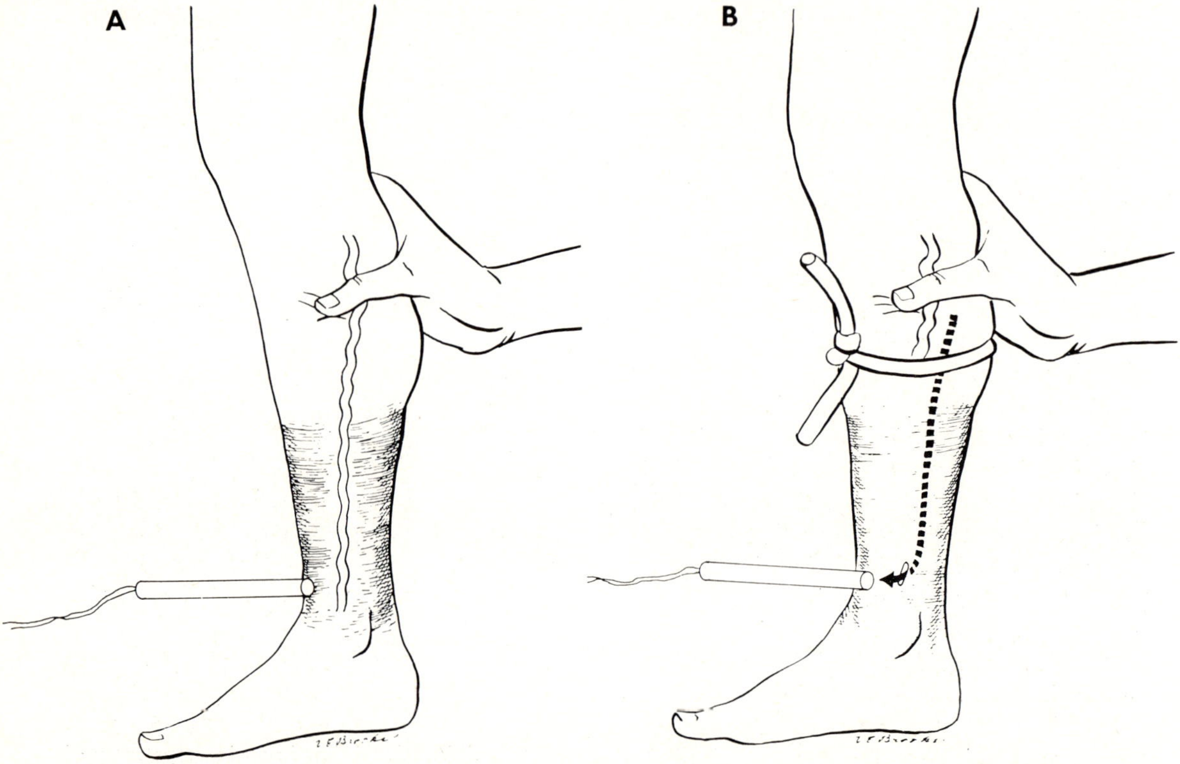

Fig. 2. *A,* An incompetent superficial vein detected with calf compression. *B,* Obliteration of reverse flow in the superficial vein by use of a tourniquet allowing detection of only perforating vein.

the number of perforators present and the clinical severity of the disease.

In almost every case an incompetent vein was found at operation beneath the previously marked area. In a few cases an incompetent connecting superficial vein was found rather than a vein which could be found to penetrate the deep fascia. All perforating veins were interrupted at the fascial level, and radiating superficial tributaries were removed.

In two cases more extensive subfascial ligation procedures were performed to test the accuracy of the method for localizing perforators. In the first case, nine perforators were marked. Two marks lay over superficial communicating veins which did not directly perforate the fascia, and two unmarked perforators were found. The remainder of the perforators had been accurately localized by the ultrasonic flow detector. In the second subfascial operation, 18 perforators were marked. Two marks lay over superficial veins but no perforating veins were found. No unmarked perforators were found. In this case, dissection was carried beyond the usual limits of the procedure to ligate perforators which would have been entirely missed except for prior knowledge of their presence.

Three major complications occurred. One patient developed thrombophlebitis after his operative procedure, and clinically exhibited evidence of pulmonary embolus. He was treated with heparin and left the hospital asymptomatic. A second patient had wound infections involving two of the local incisions. A third complication occurred in a woman who had a subfascial ligation. The edges of her wound became necrotic postoperatively requiring extended hospital therapy for complete healing.

The advantages of the local interruption

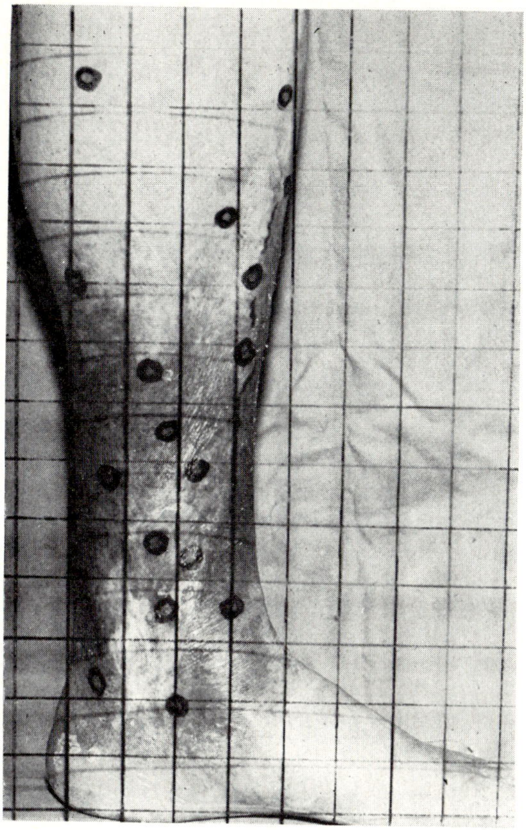

Fig. 3. Method of recording the exact position of perforating veins. The grid photograph can be used for comparison at a later time.

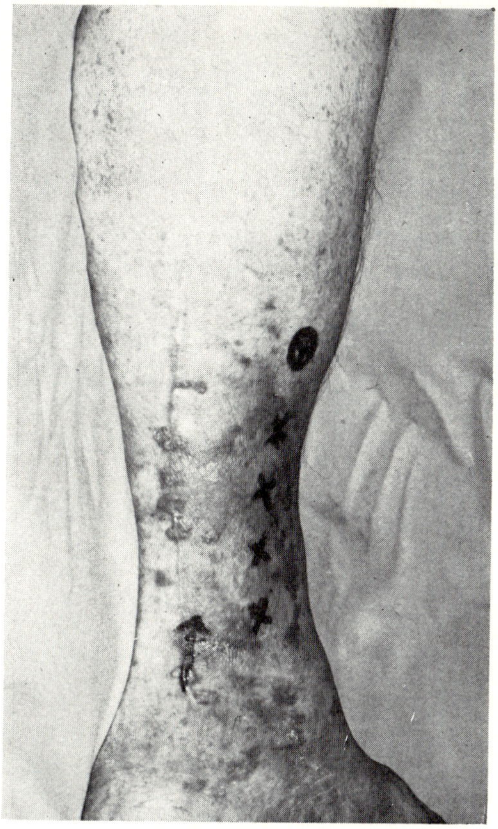

Fig. 4. Preoperative photograph of an 80-year-old man who had a subfascial ligation. A single perforator and its superficial connection are shown.

of perforating veins are best demonstrated by several examples. Fig. 4 is the preoperative photograph of an 80-year-old patient who 8 years previously had subfascial ligation for incompetent perforators. Local edema and skin fragility prompted examination of his leg with the ultrasonic flow detector. A solitary perforator feeding a short segment of superficial vein was found. The communicating vein was ligated and the superficial one stripped under local anesthesia in the minor surgery clinic. Prompt resolution of the skin changes followed.

Fig. 5 is the photograph of a 61-year-old man who had stasis ulcers for 8 years prior to his admission. The severity of the disease had resulted in his not being able to work. His ulcers were excised, grafted, and followed by a saphenous ligation and stripping combined with local interruption of 12 perforating veins. He is now working and his ulcers have not recurred.

Fig. 6 is the photograph of a 51-year-old man who had a circumferential leg ulcer for which amputation had been advised. He was admitted to the hospital and the ulcer was excised and covered with a split-thickness skin graft. He was then mapped with the ultrasonic flow detector, and a significant number of the perforating veins were under the old ulcer bed. These veins were ligated and a saphenous stripping was performed. Thus far, the patient has shown no recurrence of the communicating veins or skin breakdown.

Fig. 7 shows the leg of a 31-year-old woman who presented with a history of "tiredness" and slight swelling in her right

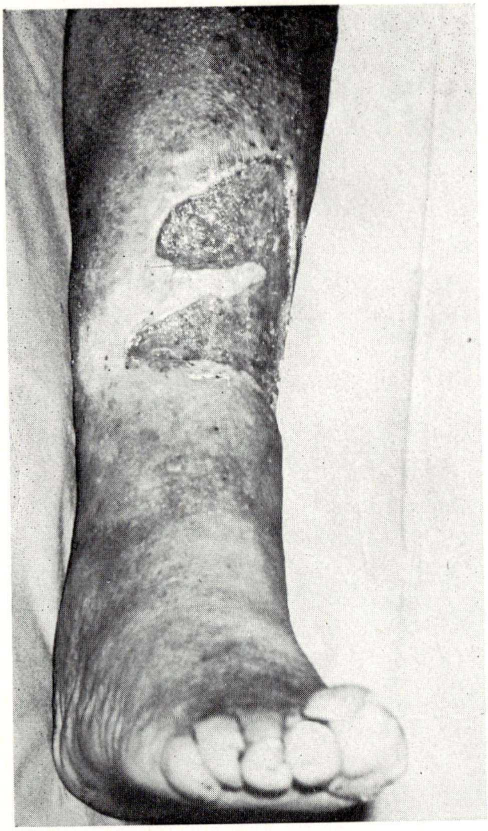

Fig. 5. Preoperative photograph of a 61-year-old man with severe stasis ulceration. After grafting, the incompetent perforating veins were ligated.

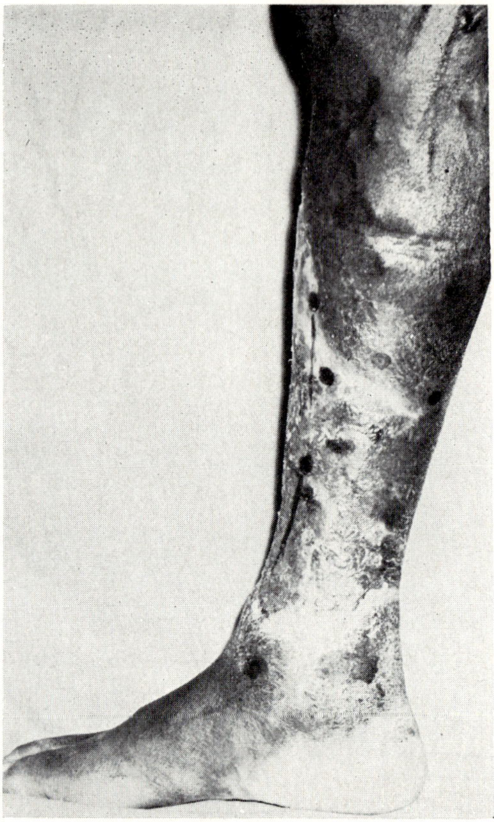

Fig. 6. Appearance after skin grafting in a patient with a severe circumferential stasis ulcer. Note the number of perforating channels which overlie the old ulcer bed.

leg. Examination with the flow detector revealed venous insufficiency and a significant number of incompetent perforating veins which were not apparent by clinical means. She, too, underwent local ligation of perforators and saphenous stripping with marked relief of her symptoms.

This group of patients represents a spectrum of venous pathology: postoperative recurrent disease, severe stasis dermatitis with ulceration, and perforator incompetency associated with varicose veins. All were treated by local procedures and complications were minimized. Perforating veins were located easily despite fibrosis, discoloration, and thickened skin.

In only one of the operative cases has skin complication recurred during the follow-up period, and this was due to patient neglect rather than the development of recurrent perforators.

Preoperative venograms were performed in 15 patients. Although helpful in some cases, they were found to be misleading and confusing in other cases. Orientation without multiple views or markers made localization of the exact sites of fascial perforation difficult. In some cases, perforating veins which were obvious by directional flow detector examination and at operation were not visible on venogram. Conversely, apparent incompetent veins appeared on the venogram which could not be confirmed by clinical or ultrasonic flowmeter examination. The ultrasonic flow detector proved to be a more reliable and simpler means of localizing perforating veins with less discomfort and potential risk to the patient.

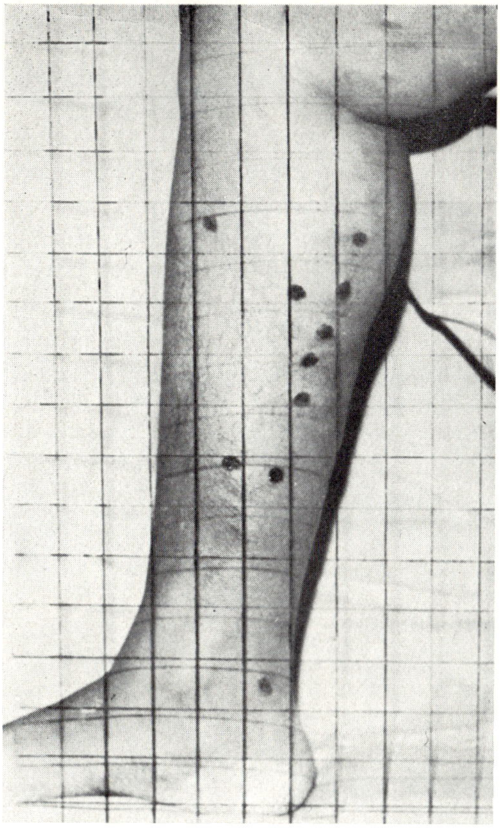

Fig. 7. A 31-year-old woman with minimal physical signs of venous insufficiency. A significant number of perforating veins were found on examination with the transcutaneous flow detector.

DISCUSSION

The work of Linton,[3] Cockett and Jones,[1] Sargeant,[4] and others has demonstrated that the complications of venous insufficiency can be controlled by preventing retrograde flow from the deep venous system of the leg to the superficial veins.

Two alternatives exist for surgical treatment of venous insufficiency. The subfascial ligation of perforating veins is presently the most popular of these. This procedure may produce dramatic reversal of brawny edema and ulceration. The operation requires a long incision, usually from the level of the tibial tubercle distal to a point just below the medial malleolus. Medial and lateral subfascial dissection is then carried out, creating two large flaps. Areas complicated by edema, dermatitis, or scar may be slow to heal. Of 11 subfascial ligations performed on patients with severe skin changes prior to the use of the local method, five developed significant wound complications requiring prolonged hospitalizations.

An alternative method of interrupting incompetent perforating veins is to ligate each separately through a small incision. This method has had limited usefulness because of inadequate methods of identifying the perforating channels. The use of the directional ultrasonic flow detector in the identification of perforators has proved accurate and reliable. The device can be used in areas of thickened skin and ulceration without discomfort of the patient.

The directional ultrasonic flow detector provides a means for a dynamic assessment of the entire venous system of the leg, as well as precise localization of the sites of perforators. The diagnosis of deep venous insufficiency is often inaccurate when made purely on clinical grounds. All too often edema, pigmentation, dermatitis, or ulceration due to other causes are improperly credited to incompetent venous valves. Such errors in diagnosis were noted by Haeger,[2] who warned against acceptance of clinical criteria alone as rationale for operation. If deep venous insufficiency cannot be detected by the ultrasonic flow detector, then other causes for the skin complication must be sought.

In many cases the clinical distinction between congenital superficial varicose veins and deep venous insufficiency is difficult. However, when skin complications develop, incompetent perforating vein valves are inevitable. In postphlebitic or postraumatic venous insufficiency the saphenous system may be entirely competent and removal unnecessary. Therefore, complete assessment of the entire deep and superficial venous system for valvular incompetency is an essential part of the preoperative assessment and with precise localization removal of only the incompetent veins is advised.

The technique of mapping perforators is simple and requires little experience for speed and accuracy. The examination can be performed in a physician's office or in the hospital with little equipment other than a tourniquet and the light, portable, battery-powered flow detector. A physician or trained technician can completely examine a severely affected leg in 20 to 30 minutes.

The operative procedure consists of multiple small 1 to 2 cm. incisions over the perforating veins. In cases where few perforators are present, operation can be carried out in an outpatient clinic under local anesthesia. The patient experiences little discomfort and is immediately ambulatory after the procedure. Patients with numerous perforators are operated upon under general or regional anesthesia. When perforating channels communicate with an incompetent saphenous system, a high ligation and stripping should be performed. The identification and ligation of perforating veins are quite simple at the operating table as the perforators are branches of a superficial vein lying just under the skin. It should be noted, however, that the perforators may not dive directly down to the fascia but often take oblique or parallel courses to superficial veins before penetrating the deeper tissues. Both the superficial veins and perforators should be ligated. After the skin incisions are closed, a snug elastic bandage is used to wrap the leg.

The patient is ambulated the first postoperative day and may be discharged from the hospital by the third postoperative day. The small incisions heal readily, even in areas of fibrotic, edematous skin. There is little tendency to infection when pre-existing stasis ulcers are grafted and healed before the venous ligation.

Close follow-up of the patient is necessary even after the immediate postoperative period. Continuous compressive bandages or elastic stockings are strongly advocated. Recurrences of symptoms in patients with chronic venous insufficiency are common, including those with perforator ligations. Edema and ulceration which follow a period in which the patients are asymptomatic are suggestive of new incompetent perforators. Often a single incompetent channel is the cause of symptoms.

SUMMARY

The ultrasonic flow detector offers a precise, simple way of examining the venous system in patients suspected of having venous insufficiency. Incompetent perforators can be accurately located in lower extremities with ulceration, discoloration, and brawny edema. With precise localization the individual ligation of perforating veins through separate incisions is possible. Postoperatively, patients are able to ambulate quickly and hospital stay is shortened. Subfascial ligation, a successful but much more extensive operation, is avoided. In addition, the technique allows for simple follow-up reevaluation, and recurrent perforators can be treated on an outpatient basis.

REFERENCES

1. Cockett, F. B., and Jones, D. E. E.: The ankle blow-out syndrome, Lancet **1:** 17, 1953.
2. Haeger, K.: Venous incompetence and concomitant diseases of the leg, J. Cardiov. Surg. **6:** 482, 1965.
3. Linton, R. R.: The post-thrombotic ulceration of the lower extremity: Its etiology and surgical treatment, Ann. Surg. **138:** 415, 1953.
4. Sargeant, T. R.: Surgical anatomy in the treatment of venous stasis, Surg. Clin. N. Amer. **44:** 1383, 1964.

DISCUSSION

Dr. Norman Rosenberg (Highland Park, N. J.). I would like to compliment Dr. Folse on his unique approach to an admittedly difficult problem.

For the past 6 or 7 years, we, too, have been involved in trying to attack these perforators through small incisions and have used a somewhat different method of localization consisting of the use of thermographic techniques and a hand-held infra-red radiometer.

We put the patient in a cold room, made so just by using a simple air-conditioner or opening the windows in wintertime. The patient stands in the erect position, and the veins are marked in preparation for operation.

Careful palpation for fascial defects are carried out. Our previous experience showed that only one out of every six so-called fascial defects turned out to be an incompetent perforator at the time of operation.

We found that a 2° F. rise in temperature compared to the temperature of the surrounding skin areas was indicative of blood refluxing from the deeper tissues out to the surface, usually through incompetent perforators. By the use of this technique, we have improved our ability to localize perforator veins approximately twofold when compared with simple palpation for fascial defects.

We still feel, however, that it is imperative to explore every defect that one encounters with the examining finger.

Other observations that we have made at operation to help distinguish a normal, competent perforator vein from an incompetent perforator are (1) the increased size of the vessel as it emerges through the fascia, (2) the increased thickness of its wall, and (3) whether retrograde bleeding can be induced from the cut end of the vein when the table is placed in a foot-down position.

This is an admittedly incomplete approach to the complicated problem of stasis syndrome, but I'd like to add these diagnostic suggestions because of their simplicity.

Dr. Geza de Takats (Skokie, Ill.). I have long been an admirer of the work of Dr. Strandness and his group, and have used it in pulmonary embolism, in venous occlusions, and in peripheral arterial disease.

I'd like to ask Dr. Folse about an almost intractable and inoperable group of patients, where the valvular incompetence is in the iliofemoral segment.

I don't know whether he can apply ultrasound at this level, but we know that no matter what you do, unless you transplant a valve-bearing segment, postural hypertension will open up more and more previously competent perforators.

If the method is applicable at this level, then it will really solve a difficult diagnostic problem because in this group of patients no matter what we have done in the periphery, we have always gotten a recurrence.

Dr. D. E. Strandness (Seattle, Wash.). I would like to emphasize that surgeons should be grateful to our engineering colleagues who have developed the directional flow detector.

I hope the audience realizes the significance of the fact that we can now detect the direction of blood flow by a transcutaneous method. While Dr. Folse didn't have time to consider this in some detail, future studies of arterial and venous disease are going to bring out some new and interesting concepts on the pathophysiology of these problems. I have followed Dr. Folse's work with a great deal of interest and feel it represents an important contribution to our understanding of deep venous disease.

Dr. Folse (closing). I'd like to thank Dr. Rosenberg for his comments. I have been familiar with his method of localizing perforators. Although we have not used it, we, too, have found that the clinical assessment of perforators is extremely inadequate and very difficult.

In answer to Dr. de Takats' question concerning iliofemoral incompetency, yes, it's very easy to detect iliofemoral incompetency. We've done a considerable amount of work in this area and I hope it will be the subject of some future presentation.

I think the dynamic assessment of all valves, both superficial and deep, is necessary in making a decision. I think we cannot lump together varicose veins, venous insufficiency of the lower leg, and iliofemoral venous incompetency. We have to make a distinction, and we now have the techniques for making distinctions and thus providing the proper operation at the proper site.

Human heart transplantation for cardiomyopathy

DONALD R. KAHN, M.D.
ERNEST W. REYNOLDS, Jr., M.D.
JOSEPH A. WALTON, Jr., M.D.
MARVIN M. KIRSH, M.D.
SATHAPORN VATHAYANON, M.D.
HERBERT SLOAN, M.D.
ANN ARBOR, MICH.
From the Departments of Surgery and Medicine, the University of Michigan Medical Center

At the University of Michigan Medical Center the first heart transplant operation was carried out in September, 1968. Two more patients have since been operated upon, one in December, 1968, and the other in March, 1969. The patients were men, aged 50, 39, and 43, respectively, and at present all are alive and well.

The three patients differed from most of those reported elsewhere in that all represented idiopathic myocardial disease rather than disease involving the coronary circulation. This was not a matter of selection, however; it was only by chance that such similar candidates for heart transplantation appeared within a relatively short period. Otherwise, the indications for operation were much the same as in other centers: In all patients the disease was in the end stages, no longer responding to medical management, and no other cardiac surgical procedure was possible. All patients were so ill that they could not safely be discharged from the hospital even for 2 or 3 month periods.

Cardiac catheterization in all three patients confirmed the clinical evidence of severe congestive heart failure, with significantly increased pressures in all the heart chambers. Left ventricular cineangiocardiograms showed a generalized poorly contracting left ventricle. Physical limitations in all three patients were such that they could not walk more than a few steps. The first patient experienced four or five episodes of cardiac shock during his period of waiting until the operation became possible.

Supported by United States Public Health Service Grant No. 5 RO 1-HE-09385 and Michigan Heart Association Grant No. 34760.

Presented at the Twenty-third Annual Meeting of the Society for Vascular Surgery, New York, N. Y., July 12-13, 1969.

MATERIALS AND METHODS

Histocompatibility. Histocompatibility studies were performed by Dr. Paul I. Terasaki.[4] Tests were performed for ABO red cell compatibility, lymphocyte cross-matching for preformed antibodies and lymphocyte antigen matching, with the use of the Terasaki microdroplet lymphocyte cytotoxicity testing technique and grading scale. In all three patients the tissue was classified as type C; each patient showed one major incompatibility at the HLA_2 (human lymphocyte antigen) locus in the first case, HLA_8 in the second, and HLA_5 in the third. The blood type was A in the first and third patients, both of whom received hearts from type O donors; in the second patient the blood type was B for both patient and donor.

Surgical procedure. In each instance, the clinical evidence of the donor's death was confirmed by two isoelectric encephalograms, the second being recorded after an interval of 24 hours during which respiration and blood pressure were artificially maintained in the donor's body. Only after this proof had been obtained were the recipient and donor taken to the operating room. The donors also had dilated fixed pupils and absent reflexes before the first electroencephalograms were obtained.

At operation the first step was to institute cardiopulmonary bypass for the recipient. The donor heart was then removed and immediately connected to the pump oxygenator for perfusion through a Bardick tube placed in the aorta, where a temperature of 32° C. and pressures of 70 to 80 mm. Hg were obtained. The recipient heart was excised, leaving an atrial cuff but removing the atrial appendages. Installation of the donor heart began with left atrial anastomosis, followed by the interatrial septum and the right atrium. In keeping with Barnard's[1] modification of the Lower-Shumway[2] technique the superior vena cava was tied off, the right atrium was split open toward the atrial appendage, and the left and right atrial walls of the donor heart were sutured to the interatrial septum of the recipient. Thus the sinoatrial node was not injured and no sutures were placed in the interatrial septum of the donor heart. The pulmonary artery was anastomosed after the atrial anastomoses were complete. The donor heart was then disconnected from the pump oxygenator and aortic anastomosis in the transplanted heart was completed.

The establishment of normal sinus rhythm posed no difficulty. In the first patient a normal sinus rhythm developed spontaneously, in the second patient defibrillation occurred with the first electric shock, and in the third a normal rhythm was maintained throughout the entire operative procedure.

As a possible aid in the management of immune responses, the operation included removal of the thymus in every case. The blood pressure, pulse, and cardiac output were normal in all three patients at the end of the operation.

Postoperative problems. Our experience with laboratory animals, both dogs and calves, indicated that isoproterenol was needed after cardiac transplantation, and it appears that the drug should be given prophylactically in any case of human heart transplantation. This was not done in our first patient, and it became necessary to reopen the incision when sinus arrest was followed by a brief period of inadequate cardiac output 2 hours after the operation. This patient showed an excellent cardiac output just after the cardiopulmonary bypass was removed; oxygenation was adequate, blood volume was normal, and no arrhythmia was apparent. After 2 hours, however, the patient's blood pressure dropped to about 20 mm. Hg, and the emergency administration of isoproterenol was necessary to restore heartbeat and cardiac output. In the subsequent patients, the drug was given prophylactically for 48 hours, and these patients did not experience similar postoperative difficulty.

The severe preoperative congestive heart failure and hypervolemia in all three patients were found to have considerable bearing on calculations of blood loss and blood replacement immediately after the operation. It was noted that the pump oxygenator contained a large amount of the patient's blood following the bypass procedure. Since this large volume was no longer needed when myocardial function was restored, the postoperative volume was lower by a considerable amount—2,000 ml. in the first patient, 3,500 in the second, and 5,000 in the third. The third patient was particularly dramatic. Before the operation this patient's liver had been noted to extend below the right iliac crest; afterward it was at the right costal margin even before the patient was moved to the recovery room. Apparently such patients have a great deal of excess blood pooled in their hepatic system, and any attempt to restore the preoperative blood volume after adequate cardiac function has been achieved may create a typical picture of hypervolemic heart failure.

Our single instance of major postoperative infection occurred after the chest was reopened under nonsterile conditions in the first patient in order to correct sinus arrest. As a result, a Pseudomonas infection developed in the right pleura, mediastinum, and lower lobe of the right lung. Treatment involved tube drainage of the chest and the administration of colistin, on the basis of sensitivity studies, as well as Pseudomonas-immune globulin. Immunosuppressive therapy was not interrupted, and the infection cleared during the patient's 3 month period of convalescence in the hospital. The other two patients had uncomplicated postoperative courses and were discharged about 6 weeks after operation.

Immunosuppression. Thymectomy was carried out at the time of cardiac transplantation. Our experience with animal studies, as well as that reported by other workers,[3] had shown that survival time was greatly increased in adult animals when thymectomy was added to other types of immunosuppressive therapy.

Treatment with azathioprine and prednisone was started 12 hours before the operation at a daily level of 200 and 150 mg., respectively, and continued for 3 weeks after the operation. The prednisone dosage was then lowered to 75 mg. per day between the third and fourth week and gradually decreased during the next 3 months to a maintenance level of 30 mg. per day. Azathioprine was decreased to 150 to 175 mg. per day after 2 months and maintained at that level.

Although there is as yet little information regarding the possible value of anticoagulant therapy following heart transplantation, there is some evidence that it may decrease the incidence of small-vessel involvement and help to maintain a more normal coronary blood flow. Accordingly, heparin administration was started on the fourth postoperative day and continued for 6 weeks. At that time Coumadin replaced heparin for maintenance therapy. In two patients studied with radioactive cesium^{131} immediately after operation and again 2 to 8 month after operation, coronary blood flows have been shown to be relatively unchanged from the immediate postoperative values.

Rejection episodes. The early detection of rejection phenomena has been based on examination of lactic acid dehydrogenase (LDH), with isozyme 1, platelet counts, as well as electrocardiograms, chest x-rays to reveal heart size, changes in the leukocyte count, and the general condition of the patient from the clinical viewpoint. The first two patients have shown no abnormality that would suggest an acute rejection episode. The LDH value, initially high after the operation, returned to normal and has remained so. Heart size has not changed, and the patients have remained clinically well. The platelet counts have always remained above 150,000.

The third patient developed a rejection episode 3 months after transplant. He gained weight and had pulsations in his neck veins although his general condition remained good. His electrocardiographic voltage dropped, and his platelet count acutely decreased to 80,000. He was treated with 1 Gm. per day of antilymphocytic globulin and intravenous heparin for 4 days. His platelet count returned to above 150,000, his electrocardiographic voltage rose, and he lost weight, and the venous pulsations disappeared. He has been maintained on subcutaneous heparin.

Electrocardiogram. There have been some variations in the electrocardiograms, the significance of which we are uncertain. The only arrhythmia occurred in the first patient who developed atrial flutter in the donor heart on the thirty-eighth postoperative day. He had a mediastinal infection at the time. He returned to sinus rhythm 20 days later on digitalis therapy.

The sum of the QRS voltage in Leads I, II, and III dropped markedly in the first patient on the third postoperative day and even more on the ninth postoperative day. It did not increase appreciably until the thirty-ninth postoperative day. He was not treated for rejection. The second patient's voltage has remained relatively constant since the time of his transplantation. The third patient showed a progressive decline in voltage starting after the second month until his rejection episode at 3 months.

All three patients developed marked terminal inversion of the T waves in V_4 to V_6 between the third and thirteenth postoperative day. T wave inversion occurred somewhat later in the limb leads. These changes fluctuated, but they had largely disappeared by the fiftieth postoperative day in two of the three patients.

Effect on lymphocytes. Immediately before the operation, all three patients showed a normal leukocyte count with a normal proportion of lymphocytes—25 to 30 percent. During the first month after the operation, the leukocyte count in all patients rose to 15,000 to 20,000, which was judged to represent the effect of the large doses of prednisone. Subsequently the leukocyte count dropped to the range of 6,000 to 8,000 and remained at that level. Meanwhile the percentage of lymphocytes in the total leukocyte volume dropped precipitously, so that during the first month after the operation the level varied between 0 and 5 percent. After the prednisone dosage was reduced at the end of the first month, the lymphocyte content rose to about 10 percent and has remained at about this level.

Pathologic features. The first patient clearly had a family history suggesting a familial type of cardiomyopathy. His father and his father's brother died of a similar type of heart disease before their fiftieth birthday. The patient has no brothers; he

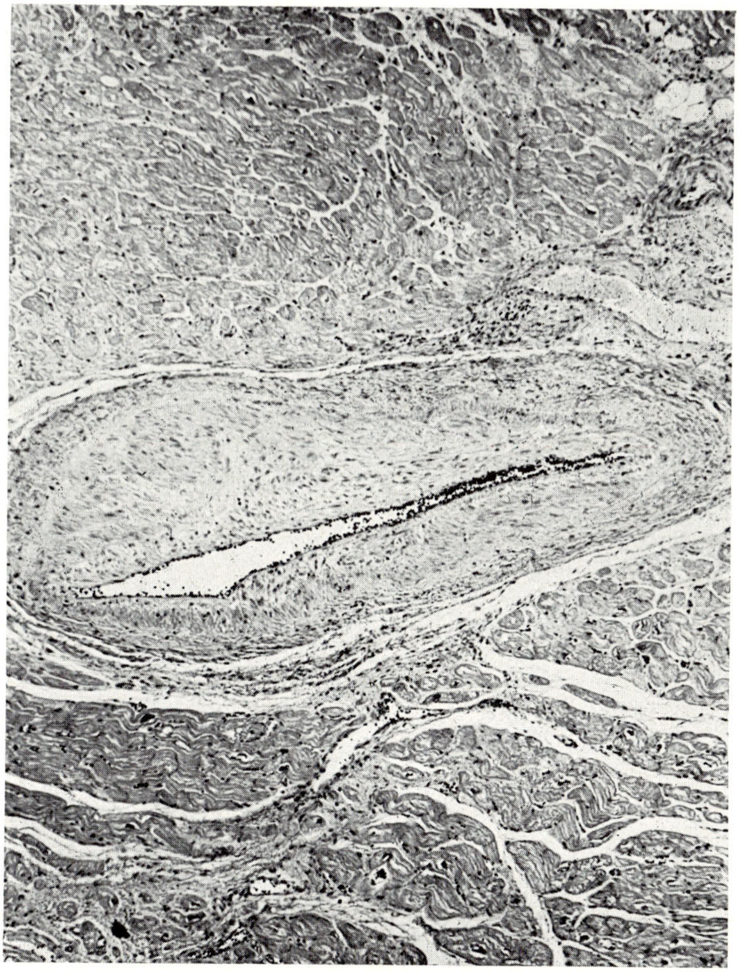

Fig. 1. Microscopic picture of the myocardium of the first patient. Hypertrophy of the muscle fibers and marked muscular hypertrophy of the small arteries are seen.

does have younger sisters who have not shown any cardiac disorder so far. Our other two patients had no familial history, and their personal histories disclosed no etiologic factor such as alcoholism or myocarditis.

The heart ventricles were greatly enlarged in all three patients, the hearts weighed 533, 476, and 522 grams, respectively. Microscopic findings in the first and third patients were similar, showing extreme hypertrophy of the muscle fibers and some focal vacuolar changes in the myocardial fibers. There was endocardial scarring secondary to the chronic heart failure. The large coronary arteries showed mild atherosclerosis, but no artery was narrowed more than 50 percent. In the small arteries, however, the hearts in these two patients showed marked muscular hypertrophy which had resulted in narrowing of these vessels (Fig. 1). There was no significant myocardial fibrosis. In the second patient there was not only muscle hypertrophy but also diffuse microinfarction throughout the heart (Fig. 2). The small arterioles, however, were normal, in contrast to those in the other two patients. There was some coronary arteriosclerosis in this patient, also, with narrowing to 30 percent of the lumen of the right coronary artery, but this was not considered a significant degree of obstruction to explain his diffuse myocardial fibrosis.

Hemodynamic features. Cardiac output in all three patients, which had amounted to

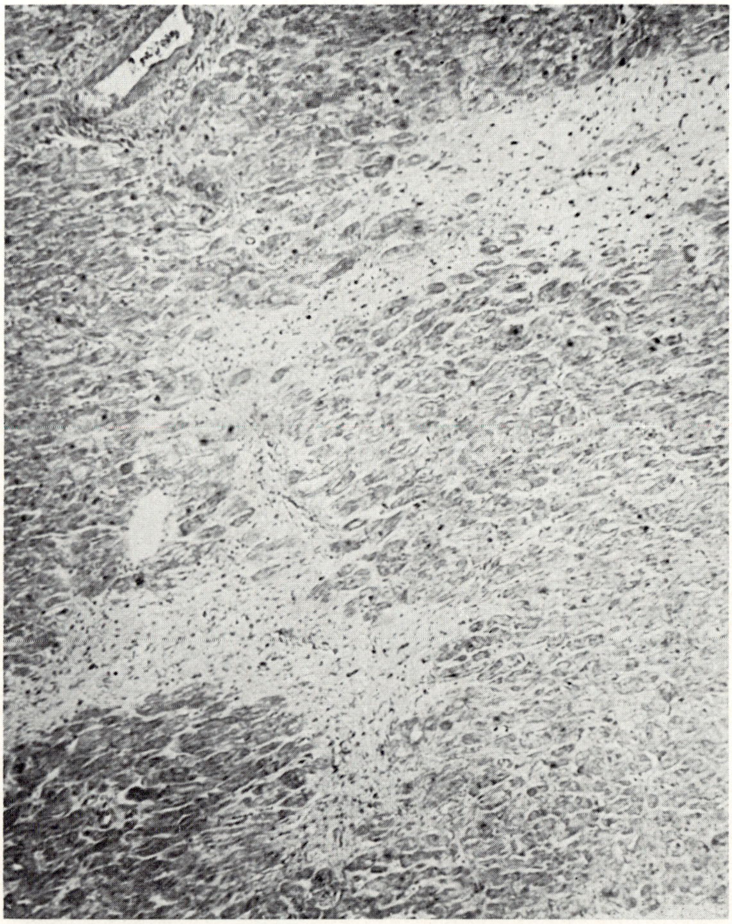

Fig. 2. Microscopic picture of the myocardium of the second patient. Muscle hypertrophy and diffuse microinfarction are seen throughout the heart.

less than a liter before the operation, increased afterward to 5 or 6 L. per minute. One patient has been studied by graded exercise tests at 3 and 6 months after the operation. On both occasions his cardiac output was over 6 L. per minute at rest, with a heart rate of 100, and with exercise, output rose to over 9 L. and the heart rate to 130. His heart rate did not change with carotid sinus pressure or 0.6 Gm. atropine indicating that the heart has not, as yet, become reinervated. The other two patients have not yet undergone exercise tests; their cardiac outputs at rest range from 5 to 6 L.

SUMMARY

Three patients with end-stage myocardial disease have undergone heart transplantation with excellent results in terms of hemodynamic improvement, general physiologic well-being, and only one rejection episode. Immunosuppression was achieved by thymectomy and chemotherapy involving azathioprine, prednisone, and anticoagulant agents. With this program the number of circulating lymphocytes was lowered to under 5 percent for the first month and under 10 percent for 8 months. In one patient a major infection by Pseudomonas organisms, introduced during an emergency operation, was successfully treated without interruption of the immunosuppressive treatment. The third patient had an acute rejection episode 3 months after transplant that was reversed by antilymphocytic globulin and intravenous heparin.

All three patients differed at one HLA locus from their donor, making them a type C tissue match. Hemodynamic studies show that these patients have a normal resting cardiac output postoperatively and that the cardiac output in one patient increased with exercise with both an increase in heart rate and an increase in stroke volume.

REFERENCES

1. Barnard, C. N.: Human cardiac transplantation: An evaluation of the first two operations performed at the Groote Schuur Hospital, Cape Town, Amer. J. Cardiol. **22:** 584, 1968.
2. Lower, R. R., and Shumway, N. E.: Studies on orthotopic homotransplantation of the canine heart, Surg. Forum **11:** 18, 1960.
3. Monaco, A. P., Wood, M. L., and Russell, P. S.: Adult thymectomy: Effect on recovery from immunologic depression in mice, Science **149:** 432, 1965.
4. Terasaki, P. I., Marchioro, T. L., and Starzl, T. E.: Sero-typing of human lymphocyte antigens: Preliminary trials on long-term kidney homograft survivors, *in* Russell, P. S., Winn, H., and Amos, D. B., editors: Histocompatibility testing, Washington, D. C., 1965, National Academy of Sciences Publication 1229.

DISCUSSION

Dr. Denton A. Cooley (Houston, Texas). We have performed 20 cardiac allografts in 19 patients in our hospital since May, 2, 1968. Of these patients, 15 had coronary occlusive disease, one infant had an arteriovenous canal defect with severe pulmonary hypertension, a 5-year-old child had endocardial fibroelastosis plus myocardiopathy, and an adult had idiopathic myocardiopathy. Both of the patients with myocardiopathy had fatal rejection on the seventh or eighth day after an initially uncomplicated course.

Our method of immunosuppression had varied from Dr. Kahn's in that we have not used anticoagulants routinely until the rejection crisis appears. We have used intensive therapy with antihuman-lymphocyte globulin (ALG) throughout. Perhaps Dr. Kahn's program is superior and we will consider the regimen which reserves ALG to combat impending rejection.

A summary slide will show our experience with cardiac transplants. Beginning May 2, 1968, we performed our first cardiac transplantation on a 47-year-old patient who had multivalvular rheumatic disease complicated by coronary insufficiency.

This is the only patient in our series who had a second transplant, some 7 months later. He lived only 72 hours following his second transplantation.

A 47-year-old man, operated upon April 4, 1969, had two-staged cardiac replacement with an orthotopic cardiac prosthesis being used for the first 64 hours, and a cardiac allograft for the next 36 hours, which terminated in his death caused by Pseudomonas pneumonia and septicemia.

To summarize the survival in our patients, 12 of the 19 recipients survived 1 month, 10 survived 2 months, 8 survived 3 months, 7 survived 4 months, 6 survived 5 months, 3 survived 6 months, and 2 patients continued to live more than 9 months.

So you can see our attrition rate has been not particularly enviable. Most of our patients have had tissue-matching grades, according to Terasaki, of C and D: two thirds in the C category and one third in the D category. We have had no B matches. In fact, we have had only one classified as C+, and that man lived 9 months.

Again, I compliment Dr. Kahn on his splendid results and I hope that this will encourage others to continue with cardiac transplantation. This is not the time to abandon this technique; this is the time to accumulate more experience. I am convinced that in properly selected patients there is ample justification for using cardiac transplantation as a palliative therapeutic procedure.

President Hanlon. Thank you, Dr. Cooley. Are there additional comments? I suppose there are none because we have heard from Dr. Kahn a report of three operative cases, all surviving, and these results cannot be improved on; from Dr. Cooley we have heard of the world's largest individual series, so I can understand why there is hesitancy about further comments.

In regard to the practice by the Ann Arbor group of maintaining their patients on catecholamines for 2 days because of catecholamine depletion, I might mention that Drs. Willman and Cooper and others in our laboratories demonstrated some time ago in autotransplants that the depletion is not instantaneous but occurs over a couple of days. Whether this sequence is precisely duplicated in clinical allotransplants is of some practical significance in deciding on the need for supplemental catecholamines during the early period after operation.

Operation for cardiac complications following myocardial infarction

GEORGE SCHIMERT, M.D.
THOMAS Z. LAJOS, M.D.
IVAN L. BUNNELL, M.D.
DAVID G. GREENE, M.D.
HERMAN L. FALSETTI, M.D.
ANDREW A. GAGE, M.D.
DAVID C. DEAN, M.D.
MICHAEL BERNSTEIN
BUFFALO, N. Y.
From the Departments of Surgery and Medicine, State University of New York at Buffalo, the Buffalo General Hospital and the Veterans Administration Hospital

Myocardial infarction impairs left ventricular function by a primary insult and by secondary changes subsequently affecting the noninfarcted muscle fibers. Power failure may range from cardiogenic shock noted after acute infarction to chronic congestive heart failure seen in patients with ventricular akinesis or aneurysm. Because damage to the ventricular wall, papillary muscles, or septum is usually a reflection of local coronary artery lesions, we believe that the factors causing cardiac failure are often more discrete than was previously thought.

The effects of the primary insult upon the noninfarcted muscle fibers are even more important than the dead muscle itself. According to Herman and associates,[11] when a noncontracting segment approaches 20 to 25 percent of the left ventricular surface area, the extent of fiber shortening required of the remaining heart begins to exceed physiologic limits, and ventricular dilatation may ensue. Similar changes will occur after precipitous development of mitral regurgitation or intracardiac shunt. Therefore, protection of noninvolved myocardium and cardiac reserve is essential for recovery.

Ellis and associates[4] have reported heart failure in 17 to 45 percent of patients with coronary artery disease, bearing a rough relationship to the severity and extent of the associated vessel lesions. Wiggers,[20] Tennant and Wiggers,[19] and later Harrison[9] showed that localized disorders of ventricular systole can cause cardiac failure; this was carefully analyzed and documented by Gorlin and his group.[5, 12] Surgical efforts to correct specific postinfarction abnormalities, both in the acute and chronic stages, have been recently reported by Heimbecker and associates,[10] Daicoff and Rhodes,[3] Austen and co-workers,[1] and the authors.[13, 16, 17]

Surgical procedures to salvage patients suffering from severe congestive heart failure or status anginosus are relatively hazardous and rarely alter the basic nature and progressive course of coronary artery disease. Therefore, to understand the indications for surgery and selection of these patients, we present our experience in the surgical treatment of postinfarction heart failure. Patients with classical ventricular aneurysms have been excluded from this study.

This investigation was supported in part by research grants from the Heart Association of Western New York, New York State Heart Assembly, and Research Grant HE-07539-06 from the National Heart Institute.

Presented in part at the Twenty-third Annual Meeting of the Society for Vascular Surgery, New York, N. Y., July 12-13, 1969.

Table I. *Clinical and cardiac catheterization data in 24 patients*

Patient	*Age*	*Infarct location*	*Mo.*	*Shock*	*V.F.**	*Mitr. insuff.**
Group I: Excision of localized akinesis						
1. N. M.	53	Anteroapical	8			
2. M. W.	44	Anterolateral	8			2+
3. A. F.	48	Anterior	16			1+
		Posterior	8			
4. W. B.	44	Anterolateral	12			2+
5. M. L.	65	Anteroapical	3	+	+	
6. J. P.	68	Anterior	24			4+
7. L. D.	54	Anterolateral	12			1+
		Septal	18			
8. J. B.	41	Anteroseptal	8	+		
9. F. H.	63	Anteroseptal	13	+		1+
10. M. S.	57F	Apical	7			
11. L. F.	64	Anteroseptal	8	+	+	
12. E. B.	49	Posterolateral	11			
Group II: Excision of localized akinesis and mitral valve replacement						
13. S. Z.	50	Anterior	12	+		4+
		Posterior	8			
14. A. H.	63F	Posterior	18		+	4+
15. F. H.	65	Anterolateral	8			4+
16. J. L.	64	Anteroseptal	2			
		Posterior	12			
17. R. T.	53	Anterolateral	4	+		4+
18. M. P.	53F	Anterolateral	2			
		Posterior	2			
19. D. C.	54	Anterolateral	7			2+
Group III: Excision of acute infarct and closure of ruptured ventricular septum						
20. H. G.	46	Anterior	5	+		
		Septal	3 wk.	+		
21. J. G.	59	Anteroseptal	2 wk.	+		
Group IV: Mitral valve replacement for ruptured papillary muscle						
22. L. S.†	41	Posterior	3 da.	+		
23. H. G.	68	Posterior	4 da.	+		
Group V: Coronary thrombectomy						
24. V. D'A.	37	Status anginosus	3 da.	+	+	

*Abbreviations: V.F. = ventricular fibrillation; Mitr. insuff. = mitral insufficiency; LVEDP = left ventricular end diastolic

LVEDP* (mm. Hg)		ESV* (ml.)		EDV* (ml.)		R.F.*		
Pre-operative	Post-operative	Pre-operative	Post-operative	Pre-operative	Post-operative	Pre-operative	Post-operative	Result
27		305		350		0.87		Home
18	10	270	220	415	350	0.65	0.63	Unlimited activity
25		246		332		0.74		Home
27		215		275		0.78		Unlimited activity
21	30	370	315	440	385	0.84	0.82	Home
25		275		345		0.80		Home
40		223		260		0.86		Operative death
27		224		280		0.80		Died second post-operative day
35	25	300	260	375	325	0.80	0.80	Home
15	7	40	30	135	135	0.30	0.22	Unlimited activity
25	17	264	295	335	400	0.79	0.74	Home
15		135		200		0.68		Unlimited activity
34	10	375	360	470	450	0.80	0.73	Unlimited activity
17	10	190	55	310	135	0.61	0.41	Unlimited activity
20	2	75	35	205	125	0.37	0.28	Unlimited activity
18		335		405		0.83		Operative death
27	12	130	85	230	200	0.57	0.43	Unlimited activity
18		230		305		0.75		In hospital
23		170		270		0.63		In hospital
22	15	284	250	342	378	0.83	0.66	Unlimited activity
27	15	255	88	335	116	0.76	0.76	Home
Not catheterized, patient in shock, pulmonary edema, and anuria								Unlimited activity
22				235		0.49		Operative death

Preop. coronary arteriogram (4/10/66): 75% occlusion anterior descending coronary artery just beyond bifurcation
Postop. coronary arteriogram (5/5/68): venous patch patent with good distal runoff

pressure; ESV = end systolic volume; EDV = end diastolic volume; R.F. = residual fraction (ESV/EDV).

MATERIALS AND METHODS

In the past 3 years, we have operated upon 24 patients suffering from severe congestive heart failure as a result of coronary artery disease. The authors have divided the patients into five groups. Group I includes those patients with congestive heart failure that is due to localized akinesis of the ventricular muscle, requiring excision of the akinetic segment. Group II consists of those patients with localized akinesis of the ventricular wall in combination with papillary muscle dysfunction, requiring resection of the akinetic segment and mitral valve replacement. Patients in Group III had anteroseptal infarction, resulting in rupture of the ventricular septum; they underwent operation for excision of the acute infarct and closure of the ruptured septum. Patients in Group IV suffered from rupture of the posterior papillary muscle and required replacement of the mitral valve. One patient, tentatively identified as Group V, had early coronary occlusion with impending infarction and underwent acute coronary thrombectomy.

The clinical and cardiac catheterization data are summarized in Table I. The patients ranged in age from 37 to 68 years and included 4 women. They all had cardiac enlargement radiologically and electrocardiographic evidence of myocardial ischemia or infarction. Nineteen patients had chronic heart failure, in 17 of whom the symptoms and signs had reached the point of unresponsiveness, with fluid retention, peripheral edema, and severe limitation of exercise tolerance. Two patients (Cases 10 and 12) with angina, chronic fatigue, and self-imposed limitation of exercise, were maintained ambulatory on digitalis, diuretics, and coronary vasodilators. Four patients had acute congestive heart failure resulting from an acute myocardial infarction (Cases 20, 21, 22, and 23). All 4 of these patients suddenly developed a systolic murmur. Ventricular septal perforation occurred 12 and 17 days after the acute infarct (Cases 20 and 21). Papillary muscle rupture occurred 3 and 4 days after the acute infarct (Cases 22 and 23). These 4 patients were in shock and pulmonary edema, as were 3 others in the chronic group who had progressed and were in both acute and chronic failure (Cases 5, 13, and 19). One patient, Case 24, had status anginosus, and because of hypotension and repeated episodes of ventricular fibrillation had coronary thrombectomy 72 hours after admission. These 7 patients were operated on as emergencies, 1 without even preoperative catheterization.

As might be expected, most of the patients had episodes of previous ischemia or infarction. Twenty-three of the patients in this series had previously documented infarcts. Table I describes the approximate age and location of the infarcts as determined by history, enzyme studies, and electrocardiographic tracings. The anterior wall was involved in 19 patients, the posterior wall in 8, and the septum was involved in 6 patients. At least 8 patients had repeated episodes of infarction, often involving different areas. The salient features of the preoperative electrocardiographic findings in the 24 patients were reasonably consistent with the pathologic indications noted on the ventriculograms and observed during operation. These findings are presented in Table II. Severe arrhythmias varying from rapid atrial fibrillation to ventricular tachycardia were present in seven patients. One in the acute group (Case 24) and 3 in the chronic heart failure group (Cases 5, 11, and 14) had ventricular fibrillation requiring electrical defibrillation before operation. Cases 1, 2, and 3 form the basis of a previous preliminary report, and

Table II. *Summary of electrocardiographic findings in 24 patients*

	No. of patients
Anterior M.I.*	5
Anteroseptal M.I.	3
Anterolateral M.I.	6
Apical M.I.	2
Inferior M.I.	3
Inferolateral M.I.	1
L.B.B.B.	4
Total	24

*M.I. = Mitral insufficiency.

Case 21 has been accepted for publication as a single case report.

Twenty-three were studied by cardiac catheterization and angiographic techniques. In each patient the valvular, septal, or muscular pathology was demonstrated by the altered characteristics of each particular area. Left ventricular cineangiograms were made in both the right anterior oblique and left anterior oblique positions in all patients. A thorough appraisal of the state of the remaining heart muscle was made by end diastolic and end systolic volume measurements and estimation of forward flow. Coronary angiograms were performed frequently but were omitted in the acute patients or when the pathologic condition was sufficiently and clearly demonstrated by ventriculograms.

Table I summarizes preoperative and postoperative cardiac catheterization data. Preoperatively, end diastolic pressure was elevated in all patients; pressures were referred to a zero level 10 cm. above the tabletop. Left ventricular volumes were determined by a one-plane cineangiographic method previously described in man by Greene and associates[7] and confirmed in animals by Leshin and co-workers.[14] The end diastolic volume (normal is less than 200 ml.) was elevated in all patients. The residual fraction (end systolic volume divided by end diastolic volume) was abnormally large in all but three patients (Cases 10, 15, and 23). The measurement of left ventricular volume by the one-plane cineangiographic method must be applied with caution in these patients. It has not been validated in subjects such as these, whose noncontractile segments may alter the critical dimensions. We therefore present the figures only as a relative indication of cavity volume.

MANAGEMENT OF THE PATIENTS

In the 5 patients with cardiogenic shock refractory to medical management, assisted circulation under local anesthesia was instituted as soon as possible until corrective operation could be performed 1 to 2 hours later. In the less acute patients, preoperative preparation included breathing exercises, avoidance of smoking, and oral or intravenous administration of potassium chloride, as recommended by Sodi-Pallares and coworkers.[18] Twelve hours before operation, an infusion of 1,000 ml. of 5 percent dextrose in water with 60 mEq. KCl and 10 units of insulin was started in some patients and continued until completion of operation.

Halothane, methoxyfluorane, or continuous morphine infusion anesthesia was used in order to maintain optimal tissue oxygenation. The chest was opened by a sternum-splitting incision. In elective surgery, a high-flow normothermic perfusion combined with 20 percent hemodilution was maintained by the Mayo-Gibbon pump oxygenator. In emergency cases, if the patient needed assisted circulation, a Travenol oxygenator, primed with 1,500 ml. of 5 percent glucose in water, was used in the initial femoral vein to femoral artery bypass. Within minutes after the initiation of a 2,000 ml. bypass through the assister, peripheral tissue perfusion usually improved. After the chest was opened, the assisted circulation system was converted into total cardiopulmonary bypass by cannulating the superior vena cava. Particularly in patients with pulmonary edema, endotracheal intubation and positive-pressure ventilation with 100 percent oxygen were instituted early. Paralyzing agents were used to control the patient's respiratory efforts and to prevent voluntary muscle movements.

The surgical pathology is only partially revealed by inspection of the intact, beating heart. While effective contractions were usually seen near the atrioventricular groove, they became less forceful toward the apex, and the heart wall appeared to be distended and tense during the entire cardiac cycle. Opening the left ventricle through the apex provided good exposure of the interior of the chamber, with little damage to myocardium or coronary blood vessels. In an empty, beating left ventricle, noncontractile areas could most accurately be outlined by observing the contractions from both the endocardial and the epicardial surfaces. The quality of the contractions, or their absence, could also be

A

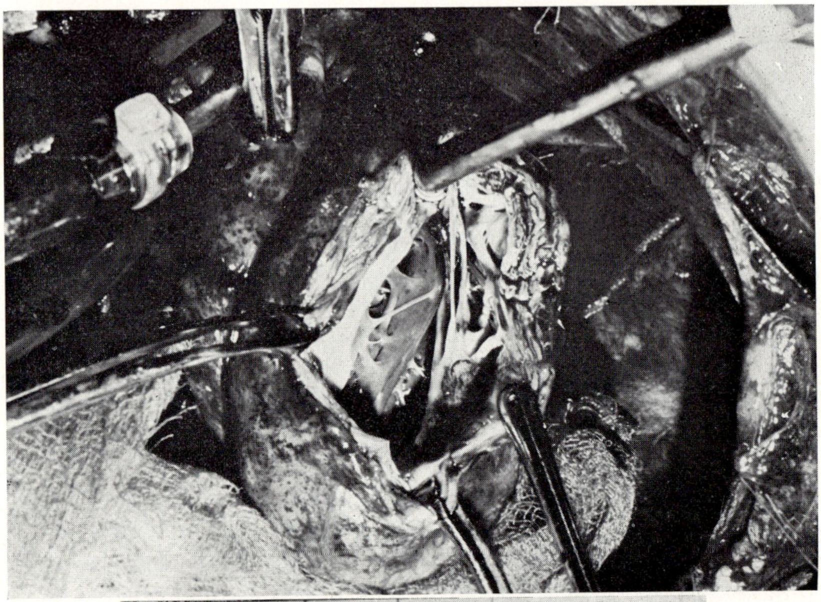

B

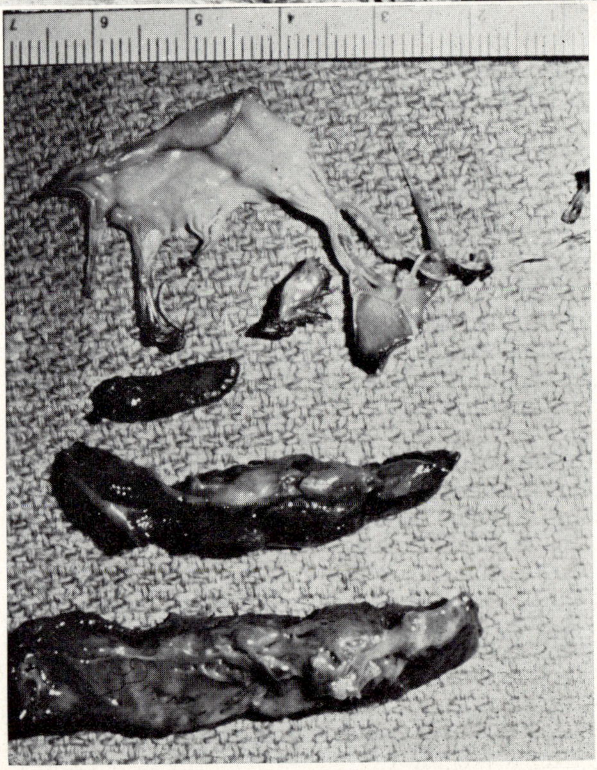

Fig. 1. *A,* Fibrosed papillary muscles in Case 18, as seen during operation. *B,* Excised mitral valve (Case 18) showing elongated chordae tendineae. Also shown are two fragments of the akinetic area.

evaluated by simple palpation, confirming the location of the area to be excised.

In planning the removal of the apparently noncontractile muscle, some consideration was given to the pattern of coronary artery distribution, so that functional vessels were injured as little as possible. After excision, the defect in the left ventricular wall was closed with interrupted sutures, using Teflon felt strips along the line of closure. The effect was to reduce substantially the size of the left ventricular cavity, since functioning myocardium was approximated by closure. The pericardium was left open to avoid impairment of cardiac function by compression. Wire electrodes were implanted into the atrium or ventricle to permit pacing in the postoperative period, if this were necessary.

In patients with associated massive mitral regurgitation due to rupture or dysfunction of the papillary muscle (Fig. 1, *A* and *B*), concomitant mitral valve replacement was carried out. In our patients, the mitral prosthesis was inserted through the ventriculotomy in a retrograde fashion. In fact, the excision of the mitral valve and subsequent insertion of the prosthesis was accomplished more easily through a ventriculotomy than through the conventional left atrial approach (Fig. 2).

Patients with acute ventricular septal defects merit careful consideration since the septum itself will seldom hold suture material firmly, hence the reluctance of Campion and associates[2] to operate at an early stage. Daicoff and Rhodes,[3] however, resected an early aneurysm and closed a ventricular septal defect at the same time. We approached the perforation from the left side, since we had to perform concomitant inferior apical infarctectomy in one patient (Case 21) and excision of an early aneurysm in a second patient (Case 20). The closure of the ventriculotomy incorporated the septal defect in the suture line, buttressing the remainder of the diseased septum by normal myocardium from the left as well as the right side. In the majority of cases this is possible since most of the acute ventricular septal defects are in the apical portion of the septum and are associated with left ventricular wall pathology.

In the postoperative period, the maintenance of adequate cardiac output was stressed. In order to ensure ventricular filling, pressure in the right atrium was kept be-

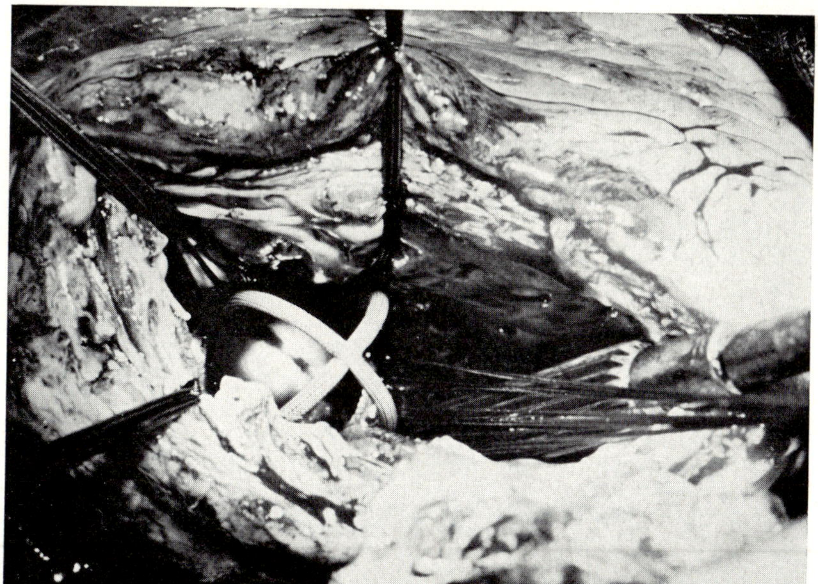

Fig. 2. Case 15: Mitral prosthesis being inserted in retrograde fashion through ventriculotomy.

tween 15 and 20 mm. Hg. Low output failure was treated with an intravenous solution of isoproterenol, and the increased heart rate achieved by fast pacing was beneficial in overcoming possible low output states. In order to insure normal saturation and maximal oxygen utilization, all patients were kept on volume-controlled respirators for at least 48 to 72 hours. Two patients required respiratory assistance for 10 to 14 days. Intravenous succinylcholine infusion was used when necessary to control voluntary respiratory movements.

Cardiac arrhythmias were avoided by careful attention to digitalis dosage and serum potassium levels, particularly since low serum potassium is apt to occur in the postperfusion period. Although most of the patients on diuretics were on potassium replacement therapy, additional intravenous administration of potassium chloride was begun immediately after termination of cardiopulmonary bypass, particularly in patients who had hemodilutional perfusion. In the immediate postoperative period, daily determination of serum electrolytes guided further potassium replacement and administration of digoxin.

PATHOLOGY

The excised heart wall was measured, weighed, and fixed in 10 percent formalin. The sections were stained with hematoxylin and eosin. The microscopic interpretation of the lesions was done by one pathologist. The ages of the infarcts were determined according to Mallory and associates.[15] Since the dating by histopathology is not clear-cut, the microscopic findings were correlated with available clinical data.

Several problems were encountered when interpreting the gross lesions. The measurements of the excised specimens do not exactly correspond with the surface areas occupied in the beating heart, since the intracavitary distending force is no longer being applied. Similarly, a fibrosed, thinned-out section of wall weighs less than a full thickness of muscle.

The microscopic examination of the 23 specimens showed a wide variety of tissue composition. The most interesting finding was normal-looking myocardium of full thickness, with only slight hypertrophy of myocardial fibers being found upon microscopic examination (Cases 2 and 5). Our studies, therefore, confirm the findings of Gorlin, Klein, and Sullivan[5] that normal-looking viable muscle can be identified within a localized akinetic segment.

In Cases 20 and 21, the diagnosis of acute, recent infarction was confirmed by sections prepared from excised necrotic or degener-

Table III. *Operative or hospital deaths*

Patient	*Age*	*Clinical condition*	*Infarction*	*Cause of death*
7. L. D.	54	Pulmonary emboli, left ventricular failure, right ventricular failure R.F.* = 0.85	Anteroseptal and posterior wall	No effective cardiac contractions after terminating cardiopulmonary bypass
8. J. B.	41	Mitral regurgitation, pulmonary emboli, tachyarrhythmia, left ventricular failure R.F. = 0.80	Anteroseptal infarction	Doing well for 48 hours—died of hypokalemia
16. J. L.	65	Severe mitral regurgitation, left ventricular failure R.F. = 0.85	Anteroseptal and posterior wall	No effective cardiac contractions after terminating cardiopulmonary bypass
23. H. G.	68	Shock, pulmonary edema, anuria R.F. = 0.49	Posteroinferior and rupture of posterior papillary muscle	Hemorrhage due to left atrial tear near the atrioventricular groove next to aortic root

*R.F. = residual fraction = end systolic volume/end diastolic volume.

ated septum and anterior wall; in Cases 22 and 23, this same diagnosis was confirmed by sections prepared from the ruptured papillary muscle which had been removed. A separate report on the histopathology of excised heart wall is now under preparation.

RESULTS

Three patients died during operation and a fourth died 48 hours after operation. Table III summarizes the causes of death in these 4 patients. In Case 23 the immediate cause of death was hemorrhage from a left atrial tear. In Cases 7 and 16, two thirds of the left ventricular myocardium was severely damaged, and the ventricle failed to contract effectively after termination of cardiopulmonary bypass. Both of these patients also had extensive septal involvement. In some clinics they might have had cardiac transplantation. One patient, Case 8, died from electrolyte imbalance, and particularly from low serum potassium. In this patient hemodilution was utilized in conducting cardiopulmonary bypass, and this may have further compounded his electrolyte imbalance. It is now our policy to use not more than 20 percent hemodilution in patients with coronary artery disease.

Of the 24 patients, 18 were improved when they were discharged from the hospital; two patients are still in the hospital. Four of the patients who had shown improvement in their symptoms died at 6 weeks, 7 weeks, 4 months, and 6 months after operation. The deaths in 3 of these patients appeared to be due to progression of their coronary artery disease (Cases 1, 3, and 5); Patient 6 died because of a massive stroke 6 weeks after operation. Patient 20, in Group III, had made an uneventful recovery after closure of a ruptured septum and excision of an early aneurysm involving the anterior wall and the apex of the left ventricle. He had returned to work as a mechanic, but died 15 months after operation because of hemorrhagic pancreatitis.

The surviving 16 patients have shown varying degrees of improvement. The patient with acute coronary thrombectomy (Case 24) had an uneventful recovery and still had, 2 years later, a patent left anterior descending coronary artery with good runoff. He is presently performing light work. Two patients (Cases 9 and 11), while vastly improved, still require digitalis and diuretic therapy. Thirteen patients are on unlimited exercise, and 11 have returned to work. Postoperative complications were uncommon. However, 1 patient bled from the ventricu-

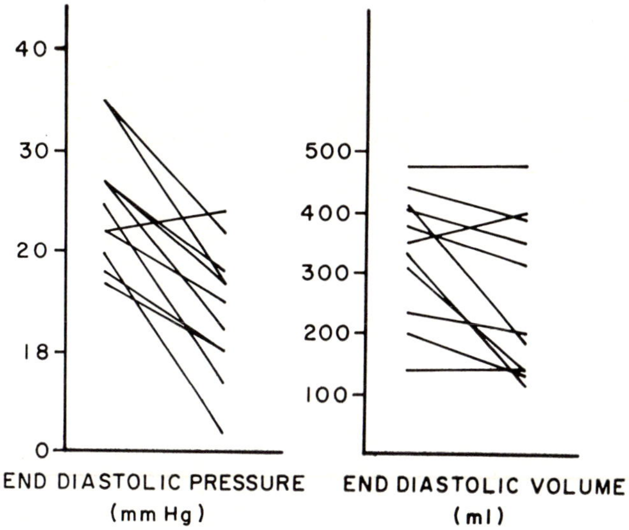

Fig. 3. Changes with operation in 11 patients.

lotomy the seventh day after operation; he was explored and the bleeding was arrested. One patient had to be explored three times for bleeding; he had polycythemia, and the bleeding was arrested by fresh blood transfusions. The 7 patients with mitral valve replacement were placed on anticoagulant therapy within 48 to 72 hours after operation, and continued on this regimen. No thromboembolic phenomena have been noted to date.

Eleven patients have been recatheterized 3 weeks to 9 months after operation (Fig. 3 and Table I). These results show an improvement in end diastolic pressure in all but one patient (Case 13). Similarly, there has been an improvement in end diastolic volume in all but 1 patient (Case 15). Of the 5 surviving patients not recatheterized (Cases 4, 12, 18, 19, and 22), all but 2 (Cases 18 and 19) have returned to work.

DISCUSSION

Acute or chronic intractable heart failure following myocardial infarction is difficult to manage because the hemodynamic overload cannot be compensated for by the damaged and poorly contracting ventricle. Surgical elimination of such an overload and re-establishment of left ventricular synergy, or both, appear to be theoretically attractive and surgically feasible. According to LaPlace's law, the ventricle will function more effectively as its radius is decreased. Reversal of intractable heart failure can therefore be accomplished by excising dead, fibrotic, or noncontractile heart wall. Such a procedure, by reducing the size of the left ventricle, decreases tension of the left ventricular wall and re-establishes synergy over the remaining contracting myocardium. Furthermore, a decrease in the tension required to generate pressure within the left ventricle should increase the rate of fiber shortening. According to Graham and associates,[6] this should result in a decrease in myocardial oxygen consumption. Postoperative ventriculograms have revealed, in the majority of patients restudied, a substantial reduction of left ventricular cavity volume. We have also noted that the over-all synergistic efforts were more favorable.

Acute coronary thrombectomy may improve blood flow to marginally surviving ischemic myocardium, as was seen in Case 24. The authors feel that many patients could be saved if an accurate and rapid diagnosis of coronary thrombosis could be made preop-

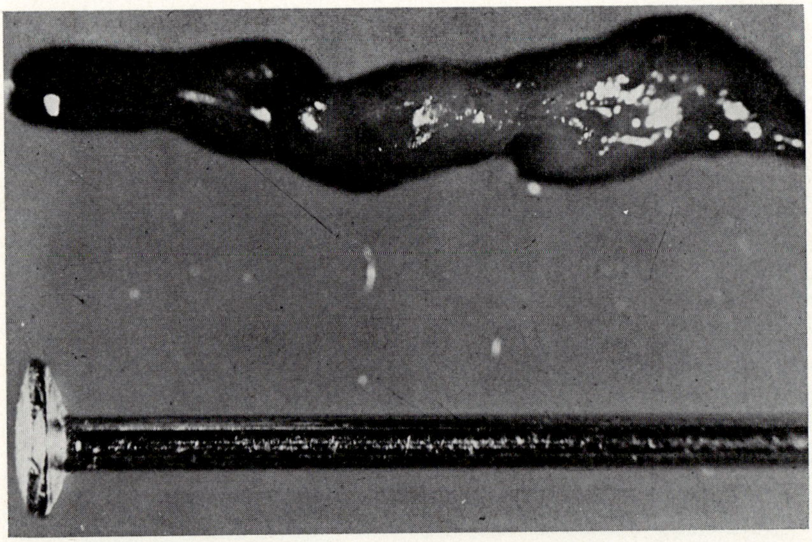

Fig. 4. Recent thrombus removed from a previously documented narrowing of the left anterior descending coronary artery, 72 hours after development of status anginosus.

eratively. In our case, the operation was performed on the assumption that the pathologic narrowing of the left anterior descending coronary artery, which had been diagnosed by coronary arteriography 1 month prior to operation, had become thrombosed (Fig. 4).

Although surgical correction of these defects is possible, there are many problems associated with this approach. The question arises as to how to delineate the damaged portions of the ventricular muscle, and how to assess the quality and contractility of the remaining myocardium. How much of the left ventricular wall can be removed without reducing the left ventricular cavity to such an extent that this in itself impedes ventricular function also must be determined.

In our experience, ventriculograms have been highly accurate in outlining the akinetic areas. These findings have corresponded with observations made during operation, at which time we tried to estimate the amount of left ventricular surface area involved. If only 20 to 30 percent of the left ventricular surface area is damaged, the patient will probably have an excellent clinical result. However, benefit from operation will decline with progressively increasing myocardial involvement. If more than 50 percent of the left ventricular wall is involved, and satisfactory contractions on ventriculograms are noted only near the atrioventricular groove, then it is likely that these patients either will not survive the operation or the clinical benefit derived from the resection will be minimal. It is striking that patients with significant mitral regurgitation who had mitral valve replacement have done exceptionally well.

In a highly selected group such as this, the mortality rate under medical management is difficult to predict. We estimate that the majority of these patients would have died in less than a year without operation, and 7 had operation as a desperate emergency measure. The worse the medical outlook for a given patient, the poorer surgical risk he is. However, any salvage from the worst group may represent improvement over nonoperative results. We have, therefore, not rejected any patient as too sick for surgery, but have excluded patients with generalized left ventricular muscle weakness as demonstrated angiographically. Some of the sickest patients overlap the group who may become suitable for transplantation. On the other hand, as experience accumulates, it may be justifiable to extend left ventricular reconstruction to better risk patients.

SUMMARY

Twenty-four patients with congestive heart failure had operations for the complications of coronary artery disease. In 21 patients, congestive heart failure was due to localized akinesis of the left ventricular wall, associated with mitral regurgitation in seven patients and with rupture of the ventricular septum in two patients. One patient with status anginosus, with previously documented left descending coronary artery narrowing, had acute coronary thrombectomy. Four had been defibrillated, and in two patients the only lesion found was rupture of the papillary muscle with mitral regurgitation. Seven patients were in shock and pulmonary edema and were operated upon as emergencies. There were four hospital deaths, four late deaths, and variable degrees of improvement in the other 16 patients, 11 of whom are now working or are fully active.

Selection of patients was based on a high index of suspicion and careful preoperative clinical evaluation, with identification of all lesions by angiocardiography. Operative success depended upon meticulous attention to preoperative preparation and postoperative management, as well as upon the surgical procedure. Postoperative physiologic studies confirmed the improvement seen clinically in 11 patients.

REFERENCES

1. Austen, W. G., Sokol, D. M., DeSanctis, R. W., and Sanders, C. A.: Surgical treatment of papillary muscle rupture complicating myocardial infarction, New Eng. J. Med. **278**: 1137, 1969.
2. Campion, B. C., Harrison, C. E., Giuliani, E. R., Ellis, F. H., Jr., and Schattenberg, T. T.: Ventricular septal defect after myo-

cardial infarction, Ann. Intern. Med. **68:** 1152, 1968.
3. Daicoff, G. R., and Rhodes, M. L.: Surgical repair of ventricular septal rupture and ventricular aneurysm, J. A. M. A. **203:** 457, 1968.
4. Ellis, L. B., Allison, R. B., Rodriguez, F. L., and Robbins, S. L.: Relation of the degree of coronary-artery disease and of myocardial infarctions to cardiac hypertrophy and chronic congestive heart failure, New Eng. J. Med. **266:** 525, 1962.
5. Gorlin, R., Klein, M. D., and Sullivan, J. M.: Prospective correlative study of ventricular aneurysm, Amer. J. Med. **42:** 512, 1967.
6. Graham, T. P., Cowell, J. W., Sonnenblick, E. H., Ross, J. R., and Braunwald, E.: Control of myocardial oxygen consumption: Relative influence of contractile state and tension development, J. Clin. Invest. **47:** 375, 1968.
7. Greene, D. G., Carlisle, R., Grant, C., and Bunnell, I. L.: Estimation of left ventricular volume by one-phase cineangiography, Circulation **35:** 61, 1967.
8. Harman, M. A., Baxley, W. A., Jones, W. B., Dodge, H. T., and Edwards, S.: Surgical intervention in chronic postinfarction cardiac failure, Circulation **39:** 1, 1969. (Suppl. 1.)
9. Harrison, T. R.: Some unanswered questions concerning enlargement and failure of the heart, Amer. Heart J. **69:** 100, 1965.
10. Heimbecker, R. O., Lemire, G., and Chan, C.: Surgery for massive myocardial infarction, Circulation **37:** 2, 1968. (Suppl.)
11. Herman, M. V., Heinle, R. A., Klein, M. D., and Gorlin, R.: Localized disorders in myocardial contraction, New Eng. J. Med. **277:** 222, 1967.
12. Klein, M. D., Herman, M. V., and Gorlin, R.: Hemodynamic study of left ventricular aneurysm, Circulation **36:** 614, 1967.
13. Lajos, T. Z., Greene, D. G., Falsetti, H. L., Bunnell, I. L., Federico, A. J., and Schimert, G.: Surgery for acute myocardial infarction, Ann. Thorac. Surg. In press.
14. Leshin, S. J., Pomposiello, J. C., Sharma, G. V. R. K., Snow, J. A., and Messer, J. V.: The influence of systole and diastole on the accuracy of ventricular volumes calculated from single plane cineventriculography, Fed. Proc. **27:** 378, 1968. (Abst.)
15. Mallory, K. G., White, P. D., and Salcedo-Salgar, J.: The speed of healing of myocardial infarction, Amer. Heart J. **18:** 647, 1939.
16. Schimert, G., Falsetti, H. L., Bunnell, I. L., Dean, D. C., Gage, A. A., Grant, C., and Greene, D. G.: Excision of akinetic left ventricular wall for intractable heart failure, Ann. Intern. Med. **70:** 437, 1969.
17. Schimert, G., Lajos, T. Z., Greene, D. G., Falsetti, H. L., Dean, D. C., and Bunnell, I. L.: Surgery for postinfarction complications, Circulation **38:** 4, 1968. (Suppl. 4.)
18. Sodi-Pallares, D., Bisteni, A., Medrano, G. A., Testelli, M. R., and DeMicheli, A.: The polarizing treatment of acute myocardial infarction, Dis. Chest **43:** 424, 1963.
19. Tennant, R., and Wiggers, C. J.: Effect of coronary occlusion on myocardial contraction, Amer. J. Physiol. **112:** 351, 1935.
20. Wiggers, C. J.: Physiology in health and disease, Philadelphia, 1934, Lea & Febiger, Publishers, p. 1156.

DISCUSSION

Dr. Russell M. Nelson (Salt Lake City, Utah). I'd like to emphasize a point to which Dr. Schimert made reference, and stress again the marked amount of mitral regurgitation the patient can have by just having infarcted papillary muscles which are not ruptured and whose chordae tendineae are intact.

Patients who have intact mechanisms but with infarcted muscle may have massive regurgitation, and I think an aggressive approach on these patients is very rewarding even relatively early after myocardial infarction. I've done a mitral valve replacement on such a patient 5 weeks after a myocardial infarction with very good results.

This concept of massive mitral regurgitation due to infarcted papillary muscles which have not ruptured and have intact chordae tendineae is one which many of our colleagues have not yet obtained.

I'd like to congratulate Dr. Schimert on an excellent presentation.

Late results of valve replacement

J. RICHARD REES, M.D.
BRIAN G. MISCALL, M.D.
GEORGE R. HOLSWADE, M.D.
ALDO CASTANEDA, M.D.
C. WALTON LILLEHEI, PH.D., M.D.
NEW YORK, N. Y., AND MINNEAPOLIS, MINN.
From The New York Hospital–Cornell University Medical Center and The University of Minnesota Medical Center

Replacement of damaged heart valves not amenable to plastic procedures is being employed with benefit in an ever-increasing number of patients. Because valve replacement has been in general use for only 8 years, few reports of the long-term follow-up results have appeared in the literature. This paper reports the late results in 389 patients from two university medical centers.

The case records of 213 patients from The University of Minnesota Medical Center and 175 patients from The New York Hospital were reviewed. All patients included in this study were those operated upon by the authors and were well at the time of discharge from the hospital. The patients from The University of Minnesota Medical Center all underwent operation prior to August, 1967; those from The New York Hospital underwent operation prior to July, 1968.

Only patients upon whom complete follow-up data were available were included; however, the late follow-up was 93 percent complete.* The length of the follow-up period was from 1 to 8 years. All deaths and complications have been included regardless of the cause of death and regardless of the interval following operation that each occurred provided the patient had been discharged from the hospital well.

Presented at the Twenty-third Annual Meeting of the Society for Vascular Surgery, New York, N. Y., July 12-13, 1969.

*Deaths clearly due to other causes, such as cancer, suicide, auto accidents, etc., were included in the mortality calculations.

No attempt was made to compare the patient's preoperative and postoperative cardiac status. All effort was directed toward evaluating the function and/or complications of the prosthesis. The incidence of complications directly attributable to the prosthesis, such as thromboembolic phenomena, infection, valve detachment, and ball variance, was tabulated. Factors necessitating reoperation were closely scrutinized.

Cerebral vascular accidents due to embolism, thrombosis, or hemorrhage were all considered to be thromboembolic complications as the authors found it impossible to separate these categories completely with the information available. Episodes in any way suggestive of thromboembolism were recorded as such, regardless of the presence or absence of residual damage.

OPERATIVE PROCEDURES

Mitral valve replacement. Long-term follow-up material was available on 207 patients who had undergone isolated mitral valve replacement. One-hundred forty-one had had Starr-Edwards prostheses inserted, of whom 5 received the Model 6300. Smeloff-Cutter prostheses had been implanted in 45 patients. Eleven had received Gott-Daggett valves. In an additional 10 patients, two Alvarez, five Kay-Shiley, and three Lillehei-Nakib valves had been used.

Aortic valve replacement. Information regarding the status of 157 patients who had received prosthetic aortic valves was studied. Magovern sutureless valves have been used in 68 patients. Starr-Edwards prostheses had been used in 89 patients of which 9 received Model 2300 valves.

Replacement of multiple valves. Twenty-five patients who had undergone replacement of two or more valves had complete follow-up material available in their records. Caged-ball valves were used in all instances.

Among the 25 patients, 17 had undergone aortic and mitral valve replacement, 4 mitral and tricuspid replacement, 2 aortic and tricuspid replacement, and one patient replacement of the aortic, tricuspid, and mitral valves. Sutureless prostheses were used in the aortic position in 6 patients and for both the aortic and mitral valves in one. Smeloff-Cutter prostheses were used in the mitral position in 5 patients and in the tricuspid position in 2. Starr-Edwards valves were used in all other instances.

RESULTS

Mitral valve replacement with Starr-Edwards prostheses. Among 141 patients with Starr-Edwards prostheses, 31 died during the follow-up period (Fig. 1). The causes of death and the intervals after operation at which they occurred are shown in Table I.

Fatal thrombosis of the valve cage occurred in 3 patients. Six had fatal cerebral vascular accidents. One patient sustained a fatal myocardial infarction secondary to an embolus from the prosthetic valve. Cerebral vascular accidents have occurred in 26 patients now living. In 8 the strokes have been multiple. Six patients have had transient episodes suggesting cerebral emboli though none exhibit residual damage. One patient sustained cerebral and renal artery emboli. Isolated retinal artery emboli occurred in 2 patients. One patient had a probable renal artery embolus, though this was not documented. Thus, the total incidence of thromboembolic complications ranging from fatal to mild and transient was 45 of 141 patients or 32.8 percent.

Infection of the prosthesis occurred 15 months postoperatively in one patient and resulted in valve detachment and death. Another suffered partial detachment and died 14 months postoperatively having refused any further operative procedures. Suc-

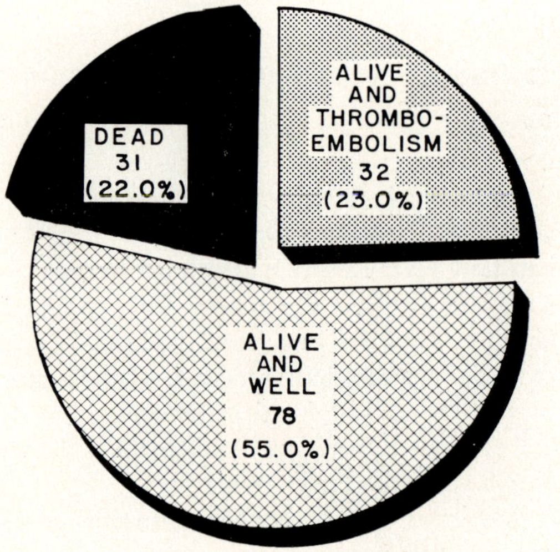

Fig. 1. Starr-Edwards mitral valve prostheses: 1 year or more follow-up of 141 patients.

Table I. *Starr-Edwards mitral valve prostheses: Late deaths (31 patients)*

	Follow-up year				
Causes of death	*1*	*2*	*3*	*4*	*5*
Sudden death, unknown cause	2			2	
Arrhythmia	1	1			
Thrombosis valve	2	1		1	
Coronary thrombosis				1	2
Cerebral vascular accident	2	1	1	1	1
Congestive heart failure	4	1*	1		
Bacterial endocarditis		1			
Unrelated disease†	2	2	1		

*Prosthesis partially detached.
†Four patients died of malignancy.

Table II. *Cutter-Smeloff mitral valve prostheses: Late deaths (3 patients)*

	Follow-up year		
Causes of death	*1*	*2*	*3*
Coronary thrombosis	1		
Cerebral vascular acident		1	1

cessful resuturing of a detached prosthesis was carried out in a third patient 4 months after the first procedure.

The longest survival since operation has been eight years. The distribution of the remaining survivors is found in Fig. 2. A finding of significant interest is the well-being and freedom from fatal complications in the 21 patients whose follow-up interval is now 5 to 8 years (Fig. 2).

Mitral valve replacement with Smeloff-Cutter prostheses. There were 3 late deaths among 45 patients with Smeloff-Cutter prostheses (Table II). Cerebral vascular accidents accounted for 2 of these deaths (Fig. 3). Among the living patients one has sus-

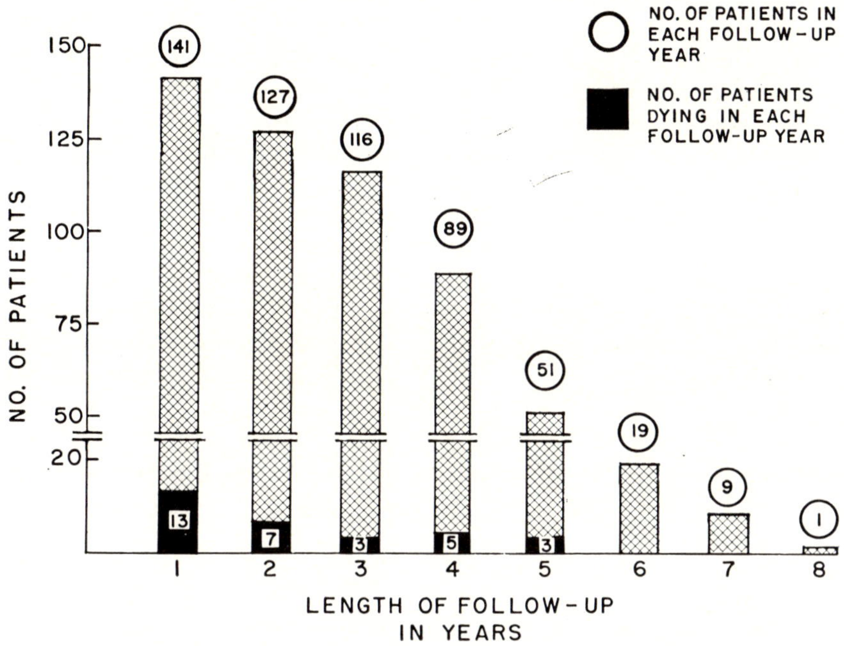

Fig. 2. Starr-Edwards mitral valve prostheses: results of follow-up of 1 to 8 years. Note the reduced mortality in the late follow-up after 5 years.

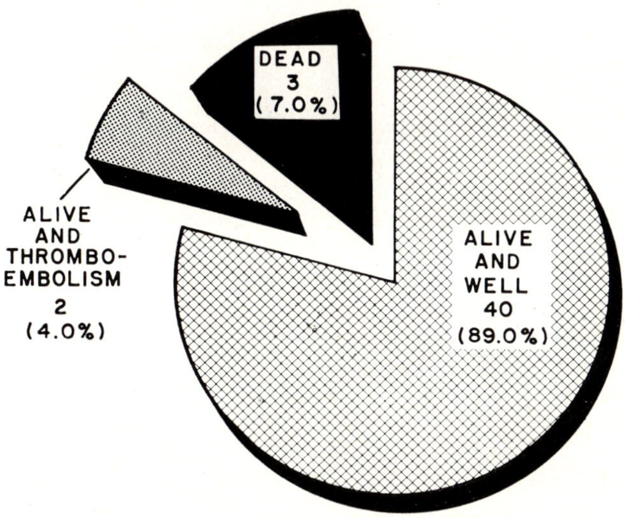

Fig. 3. Cutter-Smeloff mitral valve prostheses: 1 year or more follow-up of 45 patients.

tained a documented cerebral embolus and another a probable one. The remaining patients are all alive and well (Fig. 4).

Mitral replacement with Alvarez, Kay-Shiley, Gott-Daggett and Lillehei-Nakib prostheses. Among 11 patients with Gott-Daggett valves, 3 died during the first year after operation, two of thromboembolic complications and the other of pneumonia and sepsis. A fourth patient died 18 months after operation of an unknown cause. There have been 7 long-term survivors, of whom 3 have had cerebral emboli. One of the 3 underwent removal of the Gott-Daggett prosthesis and insertion of a Starr-Edwards valve because of recurrent cerebral emboli.

Two patients with Alvarez prostheses and two with Kay-Shiley valves are alive and well. One patient with a Kay-Shiley prosthesis sustained a cerebral embolus and

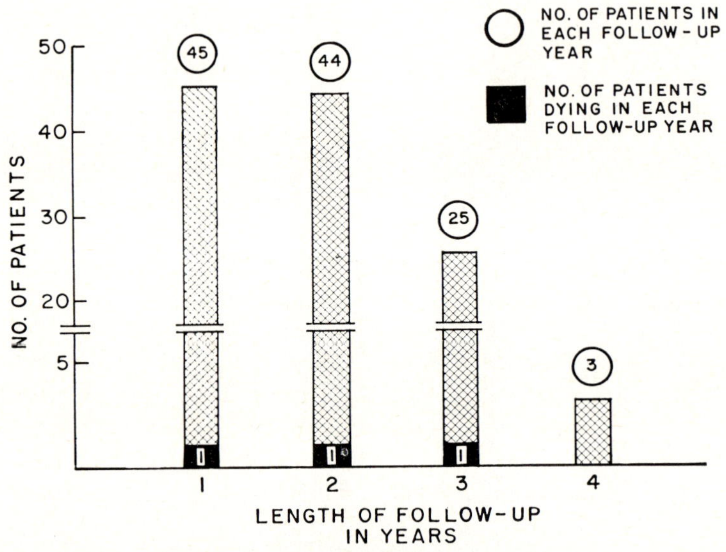

Fig. 4. Cutter-Smeloff mitral valve prostheses: results of follow-up of 1 to 4 years.

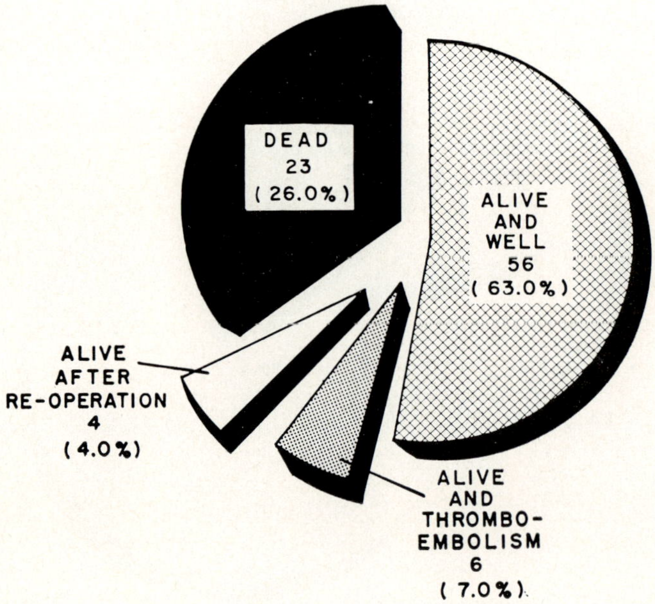

Fig. 5. Starr-Edwards aortic valve prostheses: 1 year or more follow-up of 89 patients.

another a retinal artery embolus. Valve detachment necessitated reoperation in a third patient with a Kay-Shiley valve. The patient died during the procedure.

Lillehei-Nakib toroidal prostheses have been used in 3 patients each followed for 1 year. All are alive and well.

The patients with Gott-Daggett prostheses have been followed from 3 to 5 years; the 2 patients with Alvarez valves have been followed for 2 years; the surviving 4 patients with Kay-Shiley prostheses one to 2 years.

Table III. *Starr-Edwards aortic valve prostheses: Late deaths (23 patients)*

Causes of death	*Follow-up year* 1	2	3	4
Sudden death, unknown cause	8		1	1
Arrhythmia		1		
Cerebral vascular accident	1	1	2	
Reoperation	3			
Congestive heart failure	3*			
Ball variance			1	
Unrelated disease	1			

*One patient developed leakage (no autopsy).

Starr-Edwards aortic prostheses. Late deaths occurred in 23 patients among 89 with Starr-Edwards aortic prostheses (Fig. 5). The causes of death and the postoperative year of occurrence of each are listed in Table III.

Cerebral vascular accidents resulted in death in four patients. One had a proved embolus and the other three subarachnoid hemorrhages. Another patient who died suddenly of an unknown cause sustained a peripheral embolus. Among 66 survivors four have had cerebral emboli, one a questionable cerebral embolus and another a peripheral embolus. Thus, the total incidence of thromboembolism in the group was 11 of 89 patients or 12.3 percent.

Infection of the prosthesis has occurred in 4 patients and all have been treated operatively. There was one survivor. This patient sustained an infection of the second prosthesis but is well after a third operation during which a homograft valve was substituted for the Starr-Edwards valve.

Known ball variance has occurred in 4

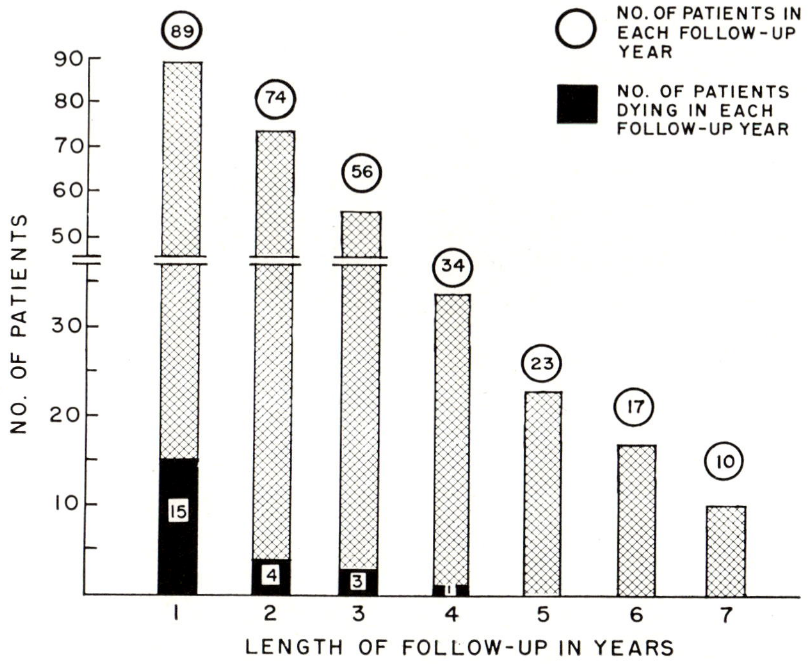

Fig. 6. Starr-Edwards aortic valve prostheses: results of follow-up of 1 to 7 years. Note again the reduced late mortality in the patients followed.

patients. Fracture of the ball occurred in one with multiple peripheral emboli and death. Three patients underwent reoperation successfully. In one of these the mitral valve was replaced at the time the aortic ball was changed. No instance of valve detachment in the absence of bacterial endocarditis was encountered.

Table IV. *Magovern aortic valve prostheses: Late deaths (29 patients)*

	Follow-up year				
Causes of death	1	2	3	4	5
Sudden death, unknown cause	4	2		1	
Arrhythmia	1	1			
Thrombosis valve	1		1	1	1
Coronary thrombosis	1	1		2*	
Cerebral vascular accident	1†		2		
Reoperation	1	1	1		2
Congestive heart failure	1				
Bacterial endocarditis with embolism		1			
Superior mesenteric artery embolism	1				
Pneumonia and sepsis			1		

*One patient with ball variance.
†Prosthesis partially detached.

Hemolytic anemias were noted in 8 patients. Six of the patients had either ball variance or aortic insufficiency. In 2 the cause of the anemia has not yet been explained.

Length of survival is found in Fig. 6. Noted here again is the freedom from complications in patients followed from 4 to 7 years.

Magovern aortic valves. The late mortality rate was highest among patients receiving Magovern aortic valves. Forty-two percent of 68 patients have died (Table IV, Fig. 7).

Thrombosis of the valve cage occurred in 4 patients with this prosthesis. Three patients died of cerebral vascular accidents. In 2 the cause was an embolus. One patient died after sustaining a superior mesenteric artery embolus. Three of the surviving patients have sustained cerebral and peripheral emboli, 3 cerebral emboli alone, and one a cerebral and retinal artery embolus. An additional 3 patients have had episodes suggesting cerebral embolization but do not have residual damage. The total incidence of thrombolic complications for the group was 19 of 68 patients or 22.9 percent.

Reoperation was required in 7 patients because of variance (2), variance and detachment (1), detachment alone (3), and superimposed mitral valve disease (1).

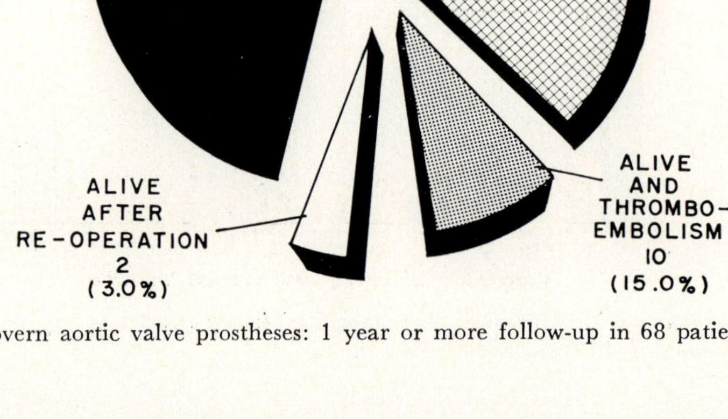

Fig. 7. Magovern aortic valve prostheses: 1 year or more follow-up in 68 patients.

A fatal yeast infection of the prosthesis occurred in one patient who sustained multiple septic emboli prior to death. Demonstrated paravalvular leaks with resultant aortic insufficiency are currently present in two patients. One patient with variance exhibited hemolytic anemia.

Thirty-two patients have been followed 4 years or longer. Fatal complications have continued to occur into the fifth postoperative year (Fig. 8).

Replacement of multiple valves. Follow-up material is available in 24 patients who underwent replacement of two valves and one patient who underwent replacement of three valves. Eight of the 25 patients are now dead (Table V, Fig. 9). The cause of death was sudden and unknown in 3, thrombosis of the cage in one, and cerebral vascular accidents in 2. A final patient died after a traumatic rupture of the spleen.

There have been no thromboembolic episodes among the survivors (Fig. 10). One patient developed a streptococcal endocarditis 18 months after operation that was successfully treated with high doses of intravenous penicillin. Another with a Starr-Edwards aortic prosthesis and a Smeloff-Cutter mitral prosthesis has a paravalvular leak in the aortic area.

DISCUSSION

That prosthetic heart valves may function well for long periods of time is evident in that 108 patients in our series followed from 3 to 8 years have had no late complications directly attributable to the presence of a prosthesis. However, thromboembolism, valve detachment, mechanical failure (variance), and infection continue to plague the sur-

Table V. *All types of multiple valve replacements: Late deaths (8 patients)*

	Follow-up year			
Causes of death	*1*	*2*	*3*	*4*
Sudden death, unknown causes	3			
Thrombosis valve		1		
Cerebral vascular accident			1	1
Ruptured spleen, spontaneous	1			
Arrhythmia	1			

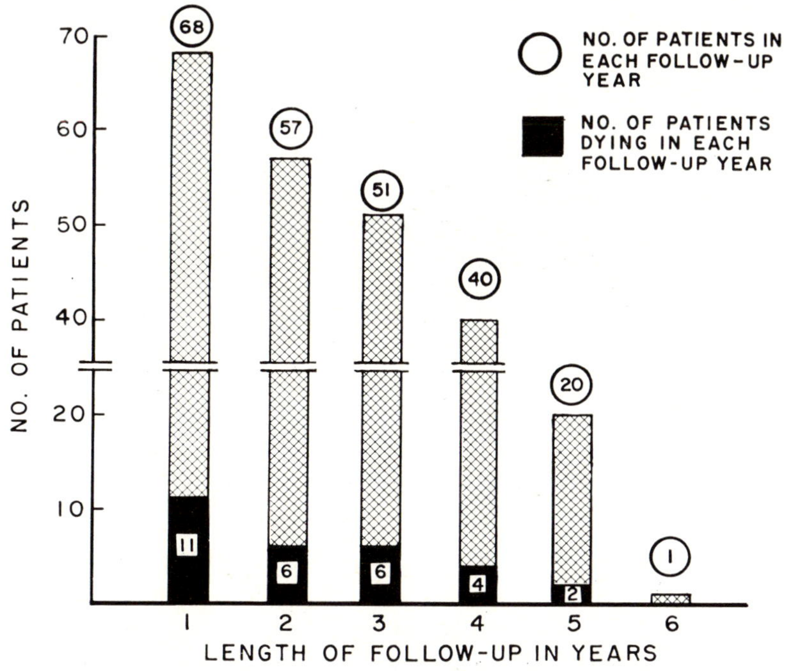

Fig. 8. Magovern aortic valve prostheses: results of follow-up of 1 to 6 years.

geon, physician, and patient after successful cardiac valve replacement surgery.

Thromboembolism was more common among our patients with mitral prostheses. Starr, Herr, and Wood[8] recently reported an incidence of 37 percent thromboembolic complications among 153 patients with Starr-Edwards mitral valves. This coincides closely with the incidence of 32.8 percent of 141 patients in our series.

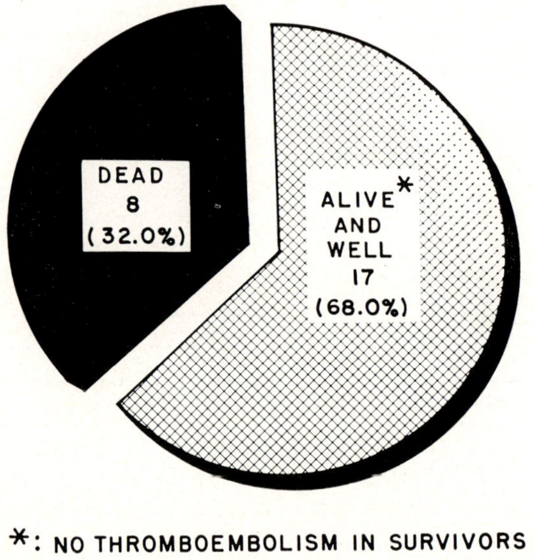

Fig. 9. All types of multiple valve replacements: 1 year or more follow-up of 25 patients.

A low-pressure system, persistent atrial arrhythmias, obstruction to flow at the atrioventricular level (most prosthetic valves tested have measurable diastolic flow gradients at rest) or ventricular outflow level (projection of the prosthesis into the outflow tract) and the presence of a foreign body in the bloodstream are contributing factors toward the formation of septic thrombi.

Control of the ventricular response to atrial arrhythmias, careful management of anticoagulation, and use of a prosthesis least obstructive to flow at both levels should reduce the incidence of thromboembolic complications. Currently we are of the opinion that the Smeloff-Cutter prosthesis is the one of choice for the mitral position especially in patients with a small left ventricular cavity.

Thromboembolism occurs after aortic valve replacement but is less common. Duvoisin, Wallace, Ellis, Anderson, and McGoon[1] recently reported a late incidence of

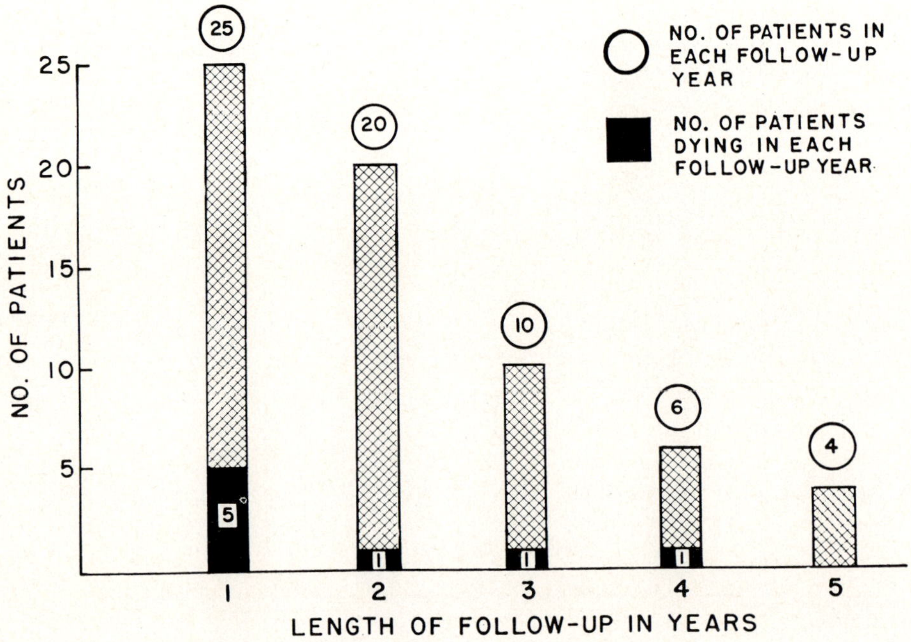

Fig. 10. All types of multiple valve replacements: results of follow-up of 1 to 5 years. The low incidence of late mortality in these far advanced disease patients is of particular interest.

thromboembolism of 8.4 percent among 452 patients with Starr-Edwards aortic valves. Starr[7] and Nelson, Jensen, and Jones[6] reported an incidence of 19 percent late thromboembolic complications among 216 and 105 survivors, respectively. In our study 22.9 percent of 68 patients with Magovern valves sustained thromboembolic complications. Among 89 patients with Starr-Edwards prosthetic aortic valves the incidence was 12.3 percent.

Many complications attributable to the prosthesis following aortic replacement are probably initiated by small tears in the aortic annulus or the sewing ring of the valve at the points of pin or suture fixation. These tears result from the battering the prosthesis receives in the high pressure left ventricular outflow tract and set the stage for detachment, infection, and paravalvular leak. Fixation of a well-aligned aortic prosthesis to the annulus using interrupted mattress sutures of 2-0 Tevdek backed with 6 mm. Teflon spaghetti minimizes damage to the annulus and sewing ring.[3] Though initially pleased with the results with the sutureless aortic prosthesis,[4] we now use it only under unusual circumstances because of the high incidence of late complications.

Infection of the prosthesis is more common with those in the aortic position for the reasons previously mentioned. Duvoisin and associates[1] reported an incidence of 7.1 percent for this complication among 452 patients with Starr-Edwards valves. Four of 89 patients with Starr-Edwards valves in our series and one with a Magovern developed infections. Reoperation was performed in 3 with only one survivor. We have had recent apparent success in medically treating 2 patients with infected aortic prostheses; however, we still favor removal of the valve when infection has become definitely established.

Ball variance has been treated successfully by replacement with aortic prostheses in 6 patients. We feel this complication is more common than is recognized and deserves immediate attention. Use of Model 2300 and 2310 series Starr-Edwards valves should eliminate this problem.

The occurrence of hemolytic anemia should arouse suspicion of valve dysfunction or paravalvular leak.[2] Among 9 of our patients who were markedly anemic after aortic valve replacement, 7 were eventually proved to have variance or paravalvular leaks (often due to partial detachment) and 4 required additional operations.

SUMMARY

The late results following replacement of one or more heart valves in 387 patients are reported. Transient or fatal thromboembolic complications were most common among patients with mitral prostheses. Late results were better among patients with Smeloff-Cutter valves.

Infection of the prosthesis, detachment, and ball variance were complications more commonly encountered among patients with prosthetic aortic valves. The sutureless aortic prosthesis incurred the greatest incidence of prosthesis-related complications and deaths.

Suggestions are made regarding lessening the incidence of complications as well as their treatment when they arise.

REFERENCES

1. Duvoisin, G. E., Wallace, R. E., Ellis, F. H., Jr., Anderson, M., and McGoon, D. C.: Late results of cardiac valve replacement, Circulation **38:** 75, 1968. (Suppl. II.)
2. Kastor, J. A., Akbarian, M., Buckley, M. J., Dinsmore, R. E., Sanders, C. S., Scannell, J. G., and Austen, W. G.: Paravalvular leaks and hemolytic anemia following insertion of Starr-Edwards aortic and mitral valves, J. Thorac. & Cardiov. Surg. **56:** 279, 1968.
3. Lillehei, C. W., Levy, M. J., Lillehei, R. C., Wang, Y., Cruz, A. B., Kaster, R. L., and Bonnabeau, R. L.: Mitral, aortic, and tricuspid valve replacement with the ball valve, SURGERY **54:** 184, 1965.
4. Lillehei, C. W., Lillehei, R. C., Castaneda, A. R., and Ferlic, R. M.: Aortic valve replacement utilizing the sutureless (Magovern) prosthesis, J. Thorac. & Cardiov. Surg. **54:** 333, 1967.
5. McGoon, D. C., Ellis, F. H., Jr., and Kirklin, J. W.: Late results of operation for acquired aortic valvular disease, Circulation **31:** 108, 1964. (Suppl. 1.)
6. Nelson, R. M., Jensen, C. B., and Jones, K. W.: Aortic valve replacement, Ann. Thorac. Surg. **6:** 343, 1968.

7. Starr, A.: Clinical and laboratory experience with ball valve prostheses, Presented at the Third Annual Postgraduate Seminar on Frontiers of Cardiovascular Surgery, Fortieth Annual Session, American Heart Association, San Francisco, Calif., Oct. 19, 1967.
8. Starr, A., Herr, R. H., and Wood, J. A.: Mitral replacement-review of six years experience, J. Thorac. & Cardiov. Surg. **54:** 333, 1967.
9. Kaster, R. L., Lillehei, C. W., Helgerud, R. J., Rassman, W. R., and Nakib, A.: The design features and the development of the toroidal heart valve, Trans. Amer. Soc. Artif. Intern. Organs **15:** 206, 1969.
10. Kaster, R. L., Bonnabeau, R. C., Tanaka, S., and Lillehei, C. W.: *In* Brewer, L. A., III, editor: A comparative analysis of the flow characteristics of seven different prosthetic heart valves in vitro, Proc. II National Conference on Prosthetic Heart Valves, Springfield, Ill., Charles C Thomas, Publisher, pp. 137-147, 278-284.

DISCUSSION

Dr. Denton A. Cooley (Houston, Texas). Dr. Rees' presentation has been most informative and raises some important questions.

Using the Cutter-Smeloff prosthesis in about 1,200 replacements, we had 4 patients who developed ball variance—3 mitral replacements and one aortic. The swelling that occurred in the Silastic ball caused it to stick in the metal ring. This prosthesis has such a tendency because the ball enters completely into the ring.

This complication, rare in our experience, should be almost eliminated by the current technique reported of curing the Silastic at a lower temperature. Ball variance in the future should be reduced for all poppets.

In the reported series the Cutter-Smeloff valve was not used in the aortic annulus, yet for the past several years it has been our favorite.

Dr. Rees reported a significant incidence of hemolytic anemia among his patients in the aortic group with the Starr-Edwards prostheses. Dr. Rees, was incidence in prostheses with cloth-covered cage and a metal ball?

We discontinued the use of a similar prosthesis made especially for us by the Surgitool Company because of a high incidence of hemolytic anemia.

Apparently the blood jetting past the cloth-covered aortic cage at high velocity results in excessive trauma and hemolysis. I believe in aortic replacements one should use a cage which does not have a cloth covering. On occasion one can remove these prostheses months later and the cloth covering will have an incomplete endothelial covering.

Our choice of a mitral prosthesis at present is the Wada-Cutter hingeless valve. This valve has been inserted without postoperative anticoagulation; and only two definite thromboembolic complications have occurred in a series of 110 cases.

Dr. Rees (closing). Yes, thank you, Dr. Hanlon.

As to the complications of hemolytic anemia, in 9 of our patients (all of these patients were operated on prior to July of 1968) we had inserted the Model 2300 valves and 4 hemolytic anemias have developed among these patients.

Maybe the incidence might be due to the fact that we have a hematologist interested in studying hemolytic anemia in patients who have aortic prostheses, but 2 of the patients have had significant perivalvular leaks and 4 had ball variance.

So, I think we only have 2 patients in whom we can't explain the problem.

As to the use of the cloth-covered prosthesis, we have discontinued the use of the Model 2300 valve because we had a significant number of patients with hemolytic anemia and thrombosis and very high gradients postoperatively.

As a matter of fact, a man came in yesterday who appears to have the same problem.

We've adopted the use of the Model 2310 valve, which we hope will help alleviate some of these problems. Recently we have been using the Cutter-Smeloff valve in the aortic position with good results. The latter is an excellent prosthesis and both hemodynamically in the pulse duplicator 10 and in the patient has proved in the mitral position to be superior to the Starr-Edwards prosthesis and this may prove to be true in the aortic position as well.

As to sticking of the ball, you'll notice in our series, as in any series, there are sudden deaths, cause undetermined. I'm sure in some of these cases, dysfunction of the prosthesis with sticking of the ball could have occurred and remained undetected and we haven't always had autopsies.

However, in 15 of our patients with sudden and unexpected deaths where we had autopsies we have no documented evidence that the ball became stuck.

Last, in the series of 200 patients in whom the toroidal valve[9] has been inserted in the mitral position during the past 18 months we have been very pleased with the low mortality and absence of early embolic episodes and this valve has become our prosthesis of choice for all mitral replacements.

Aortic ball valve design based upon healing and hydraulic considerations

LESTER R. SAUVAGE, M.D.
ROBERT F. VIGGERS, M.S.
KNUTE BERGER, M.D.
STEPHEN J. WOOD, M.D.
ALLOJU M. RAO, M.D.
MARK DEDOMENICO, M.D.
MICHAEL A. ROSS, M.D.
STEPHEN B. ROBEL, M.S.
SEATTLE, WASH.
From The Reconstructive Cardiovascular Research Laboratory, Providence Hospital, School of Engineering, Seattle University, and the Department of Surgery, University of Washington

Our criteria for an acceptable prosthetic aortic valve are: (1) The valve must not have a mean systolic gradient of more than 20 mm. Hg for pulsatile flow rates of 2,500 c.c. per minute per square centimeter of valve orifice. (2) The valve must not have regurgitation greater than 10 percent of the forward flow. (3) The fabric portion of the prosthesis should be healed within 6 months. (4) The destructive effect of the valve action upon the blood should be minimal. (5) The healed valve should be essentially free of thrombotic or embolic complications. (6) The attachment of the valve to the host must remain secure. (7) There must be no deterioration of the hydraulic efficiency of the valve, either as a result of complications of healing (thrombosis or dehiscence) or from failure of component parts (such as ball wear).

Our data relate primarily to the hydraulic function of prosthetic aortic valves and to the healing response of the host to their presence. In this paper we shall consider those results that appear important to the design of aortic ball valves.

HYDRAULIC CONSIDERATIONS

1. An implanted prosthetic aortic valve attached to the inner aspect of the annulus presents an obvious physical obstruction to the ejection of blood from the left ventricle, as the body and sewing ring of the valve require space and therefore encroach significantly upon the outlet channel of the left heart (Fig. 1). Unfortunately, it is difficult to design a valve with a minimum channel *diameter* larger than about 70 percent of the outside diameter of the valve, and thus the valve orifice *area* tends to be only 50 percent of that of the natural valve.

Assuming the same stroke volume and ventricular ejection rate, the velocity of blood flow through the restricted orifice of the prosthetic valve is therefore approximately twice that in the ventricular exit channel.* Of necessity, greater force is required by the ventricle to generate the higher blood velocity through the reduced cross sec-

Supported by The John A. Hartford Foundation, Inc., and United States Public Health Service Grant HE-11749-01.

Presented at the Twenty-third Annual Meeting of the Society for Vascular Surgery, New York, N. Y., July 12-13, 1969.

*The blood velocity at the exit of the natural valve leaflets is about one and one-half times that found in the ventricular exit, because the valve leaflets form a tapering tube whose final area is approximately two-thirds that of the ventricular exit channel.

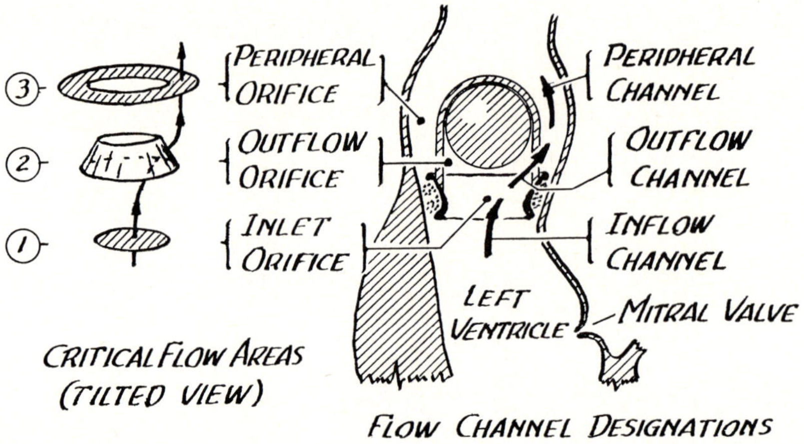

Fig. 1. Schematic diagram showing the blood flow channel through an aortic prosthesis divided into three parts: an inflow channel; outflow channel; and peripheral channel. The critical areas in these channels should be such as to gradually reduce blood velocity from a maximum in the inlet orifice to half the maximum or less in the peripheral channel orifice. Flow path is indicated by arrow. The guided-flow valve is designed with an exit orifice area 150 percent of the inlet orifice area and a nominal peripheral orifice of 300 percent of the inlet orifice. (Based upon relative size data taken by Sauvage and associates,[1] 300 percent is larger than desired, but necessary to insure an adequate channel with a contracted sinus area during times of low aortic pressure.)

tion represented by the prosthetic valve. At the valve inlet the ventricular energy (largely static pressure) now develops a substantial kinetic component which is reconvertible to static pressure energy if eddy currents can be prevented. The goal of our hydraulic approach is to return this kinetic energy to pressure energy as completely as possible.

The liability to eddy formation (turbulent flow) is increased by the following conditions: (1) abrupt change in channel cross section, (2) abrupt change in channel direction, and (3) abrupt change in fluid velocity (pulsatile flow). Obviously, we can work only on the first two conditions. Hence, after the designer has expended every effort to keep the valve passages large, he should, in addition (for a ball valve), shape the channel formed by the valve body (lateral) and the ball (medial) so as to minimize eddy formation. This is the essence of flow guidance.

2. Thus far, we have been able to achieve modest reduction (about 20 percent) in the loss of kinetic energy due to turbulence by extending the outflow bell of the prosthesis beyond the point of ball seating by 2 mm. at an angle of 30 degrees from the center line of the valve. The outflow extension of the valve body at this angle acts with the ball occluder to guide the blood flow and keep substantial eddy formation from occurring until the flow is in the vicinity of the valve outlet, at which point (assuming an adequate peripheral channel) the blood velocity has been reduced from that at the valve inlet (Fig. 1).

3. In a ball valve, the ball itself is not a functional site of obstruction if there is an adequate peripheral channel for flow between the aortic wall and the ball (Fig. 2). *Assuming an adequate peripheral channel, a central-flow prosthetic valve is not more efficient than a ball valve unless the open configuration of the central flow valve decreases turbulence,* as is so beautifully accomplished by the natural aortic leaflets.[2] Many valves that are termed "central-flow" are really not. Instead, they have a modified type of asymmetrical lateral flow, with greater turbulence

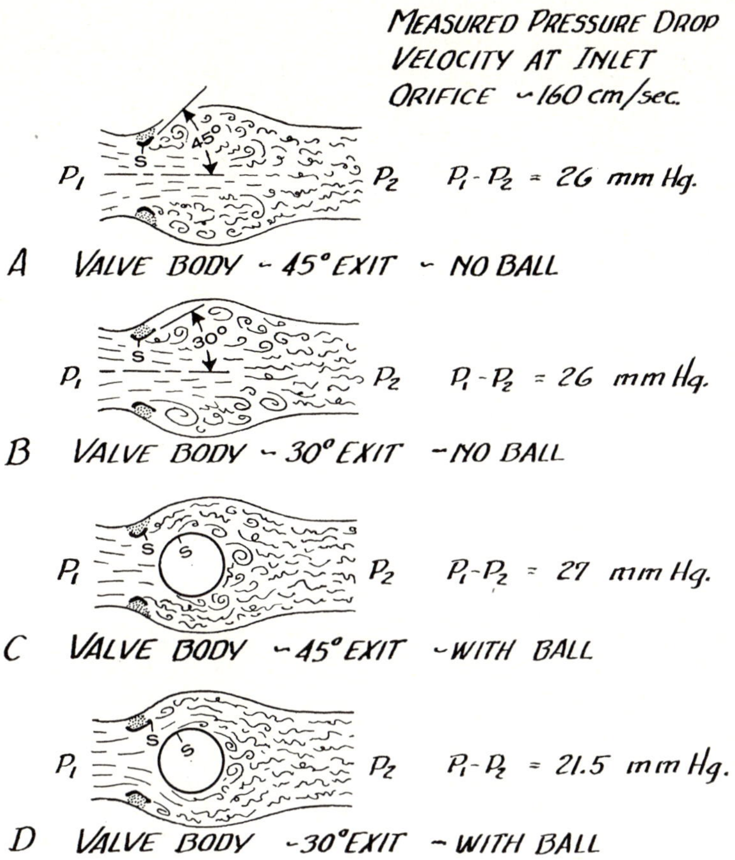

Fig. 2. Eddy-filled wake distal to the valve seating ring in the sinus area and beyond, with and without a ball occluder in place, for valve bodies with a 45 degree exit skirt and a 30 degree extended exit skirt. Pressure drop P_1-P_2 was measured in a pulsatile flow test at the time of maximum flow with a fluid velocity of 160 cm. per second in all 4 cases. Fluid was a mixture of 35 percent glycerin and water. *A* and *B:* Flow separation occurs at approximately the same place(s) in each of the two valve body contours. This has been inferred from the fact that the measured pressure drop, and therefore, energy content of each wake, was the same in both cases. *C* shows that the energy in the combined wakes trailing from valve body and ball is nearly the same as that in a single wake from the valve ring alone (with no occluder). We interpret this to mean that the presence of the ball has delayed flow separation for a short, but important distance along the valve body contour, and decreased the energy content of the wake off the valve ring. *D* shows that by changing the angle of the exit skirt on the valve ring the flow may be further guided, with the ball occluder in position, causing flow separation to be delayed to a point near the end of the skirt. Further energy reduction in the wake off the valve body is believed responsible for the reduction in pressure drop shown.

and, therefore, a higher pressure gradient than a ball valve. It is worthy of re-emphasis that the ball is part of a guidance channel, and the presence of the ball in conjunction with an appropriately contoured valve body can result in a reduction of turbulence (Fig. 2, *D*). It is very important to realize that the main cause of inefficiency of prosthetic valves is their failure to convert the kinetic energy of the high velocities of blood flowing through the narrowed orifices back to static pressure energy.

4. Regurgitation is an important cause of energy loss with an aortic ball valve, as the ball is closed by backward flow. In contrast to the normal, natural aortic valve, which

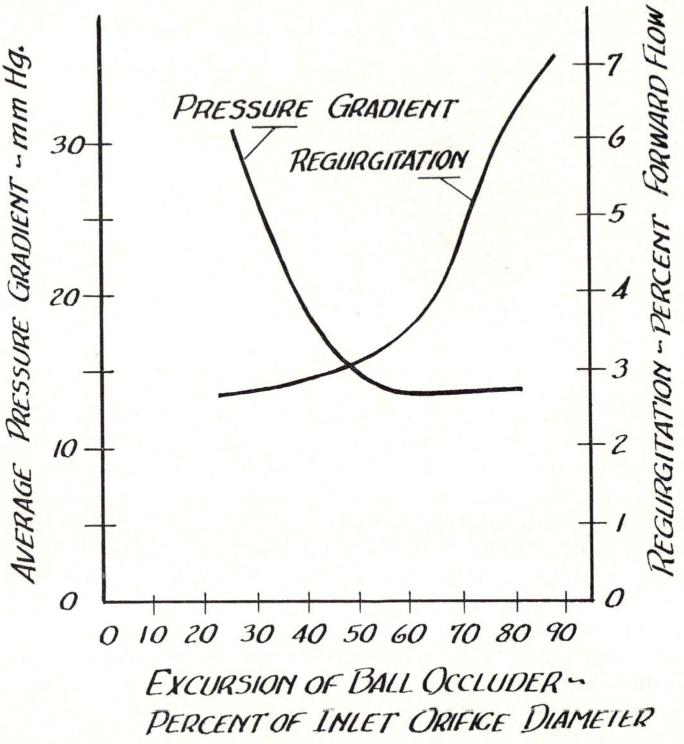

Fig. 3. Effect of cage length (ball excursion) upon pressure gradient and regurgitation for the guided-flow valve. The data show a "natural" excursion (near optimal) of about 50 percent of the valve orifice diameter.

Table I. *Incidence of significant thrombosis*: 79 aortic ball valves† in the calf without anticoagulants (1-504 days)*

Valve	*Total*	*Days*	*Average days*	*Significant thrombosis*	
				No.	*%*
Guided-flow, hidden sewing ring	27	5-318	105	3	11
Starr-Edwards 1000, small sewing ring	8	5-183	62	1	12
Starr-Edwards 1000	27	1-504	140	11	40
Starr-Edwards 1200	7	9-273	107	5	71
Starr-Edwards 2300 (cloth-covered)	10	1- 51	16	10	100
Total	79				

*"Significant thrombosis" as used here: more than 2 mm. thick, highly friable, and/or located along struts or projecting into ball path or inlet orifice.

†All valves constructed of Stellite-21.

has minimal regurgitation, an aortic ball valve has significant regurgitation (5 to 10 percent). The degree of regurgitation is influenced by the relationship of cage length to the diameter of the ball. It is obvious that if the cage is very short the gradient across the valve will be excessive, and that if the cage is very long, the degree of regurgitation will be high. There is an optimal ratio of cage length to ball diameter as expressed in the curves of Fig. 3. The forward flow across an aortic valve has to be increased by the amount of regurgitant flow to obtain a given net blood delivery and, as a result, blood velocities will be increased. The energy losses concomitant with these larger blood velocities

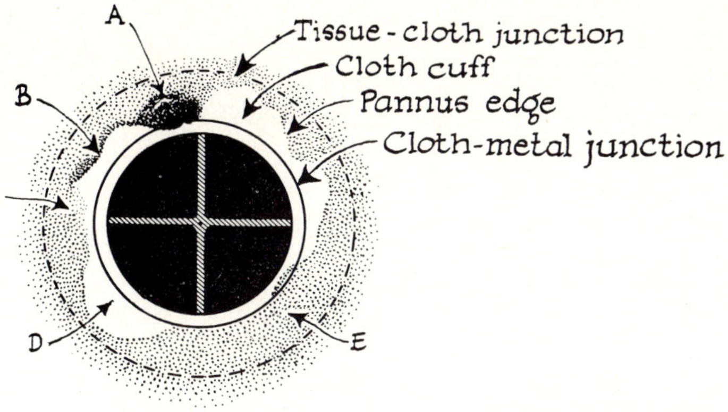

Fig. 4. Diagrammatic summary of gross and microscopically verifiable healing phenomena of valve sewing rings in man. Healing tends to be eccentric or erratic in terms of total tissue coverage. Stipple equals tissue. *A:* Pannus may merge into thrombus which may or may not lap onto metal. *B:* Pannus may halt rather abruptly, forming a little ledge with "bare" cloth beyond or *C:* pannus may fade gradually off to bare cloth, as at *D. E:* Pannus may extend and halt neatly at cloth-metal junction, or may overlap metal to various degrees. The healing (tissue coverage) has both benign and malignant components. Complete tissue coverage of cloth beyond about 5 mm. appears to be unreliable in adult man. Children may have greater potential in this regard. Evidence points increasingly to the probability that tissue coverage of exposed cloth is more feasible in the right heart than in the left. An A-V valve is used for this schematic because the sizable flat fabric surface enables the different phenomena to be shown clearly. However, these occur in all valve sites.

Table II. *Starr-Edwards aortic valves in man: maximum extent, tissue coverage of sewing ring*

Patient	Sex	Age (years)	Implant time (mos.)	Inflow aspect		Outflow aspect	
				Distance	To C-M junction*	Distance	To C-M junction*
1	M	45	1.3	Beginning	No	Beginning	No
2	F	46	3.5	Bare	No	5 mm.	Yes†
3	M	54	4	6 mm.	Yes	Thrombosis	No
4	M	27	8	5 mm.	No	7.5 mm.	Halfway
5	M	39	10	—	—	5 mm.	?
6	M	55	10.5	2 mm.	Yes†	5 mm.	Halfway
7	M	36	12	3 mm.	?	5 mm.	Halfway?
8	F	16	20	2 mm.	Yes†	7 mm.	Yes†
9	M	40	60	—	—	3 mm.	Yes

*Cloth-metal junction.
†Complete tissue coverage.

are of a size which may appreciably add to the work load of the ventricle. It is of interest to realize that with a regurgitant flow of 10 percent the increased velocity necessary to maintain a given flow will result in an energy loss about one third larger than if there were no regurgitation.*

*Calculations upon which these estimates are based have a rational basis, even though they cannot be considered exact because of the variability of hydraulic parameters from patient to patient.[1]

HEALING CONSIDERATIONS

Pertinent conclusions from our studies follow:

1. The incidence of significant thrombosis about an aortic ball valve in the calf is reduced markedly by decreasing the exposed fabric of the prosthesis to the minimum required for an effective sewing ring (Table I).

2. The calf has great ability to cover and to incorporate by tissue the exposed fabric in

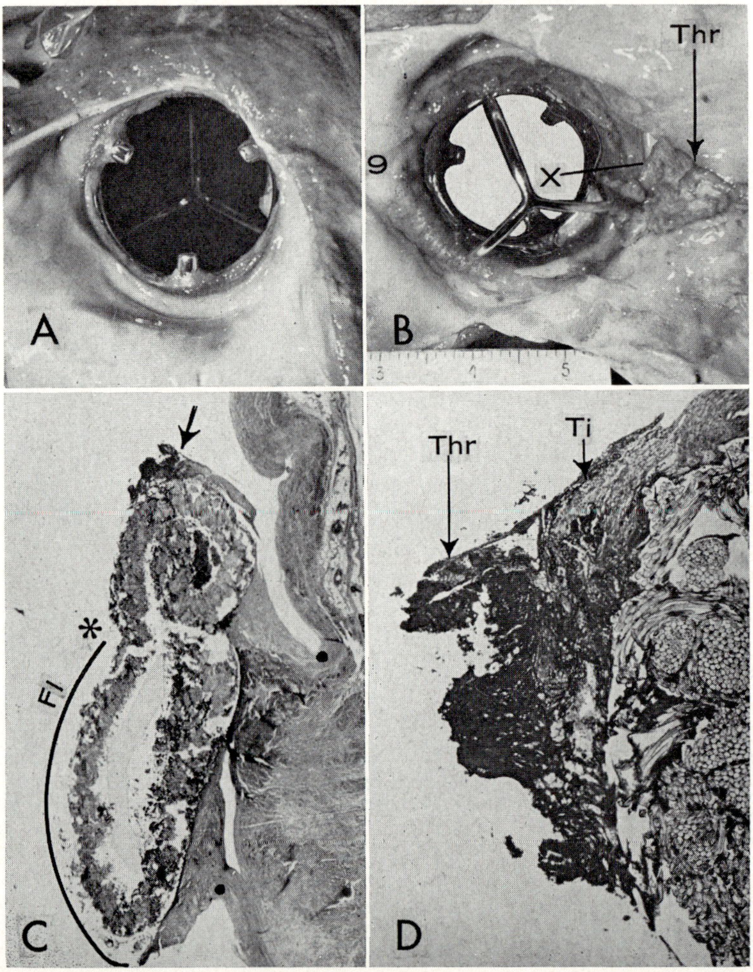

Fig. 5. Healing of 10A Starr-Edwards Model 1000 valve in 55-year-old nonanticoagulated patient 314 days after implant. *A:* Inflow aspect. Tissue reaches cloth-metal junction 3 mm. from annulus. Thin layer of fibrinous thrombus laps onto metal. *B:* Outflow aspect. Pedunculated thrombus (*Thr*) occludes left coronary orifice—the cause of death in this patient. Note the variable degree of tissue coverage of the fabric. Even where grossly it appears to be completely covered with tissue, such as at 9 o'clock (9), the tissue does not reach downward to the cloth-metal junction. The bare-looking area at 7 o'clock is devoid of tissue and only contains bits of fibrin in the crevices of the cuff. *C:* Low-power photomicrograph of section taken at *X* shows healing pattern characteristic of this specimen. Position of metal flange (*Fl*) is indicated. Superiorly, tissue merges with thrombus at summit of cuff (arrow). The distance from the dot at the bottom of the cul-de-sac to the arrow is 4 mm. To completely cover the cuff down to the cloth-metal junction (*), the tissue would have to go 7 to 8 mm. The distance for tissue coverage of the cloth of the inflow aspect is but 8 mm., which is within man's apparent limited ability to grow pannus. *D:* Detail showing tissue-thrombus junction in region of arrow in *C*. Organization of a tissue layer is not being assisted by transinterstice growth from inside the cuff. The cuff is densely constructed and there is no tissue observable inside it.

cardiac valve sites. For example, in the calf we have observed pannus to extend as far as 32 mm. over the surface of a cloth-covered aortic ball valve within 51 days. It is not surprising, then, that this animal tissue incorporates the small cuff of the guided-flow prosthesis within one month.[1]

3. In adult man, tissue coverage of sewing rings is limited and tends to be eccentric, irregular or erratic, especially in the aortic valve site. This variability is summarized in Fig. 4, and an example is shown in Fig. 5.

Our observations of the healing of Starr-Edwards aortic valves in man (Table II)* suggest that in an adult the maximum distance tissue can extend over the surface of an aortic valve cuff is about 5 to 7 mm. The extent of tissue coverage appears to be unpredictable. In these studies it was often difficult to measure, principally because some patients showed prosthetic valve complications at death. This is indicated by dashes and question marks in Table II. It is of interest to note that complete tissue coverage in this series was observed in a 16-year-old girl with a prosthesis implanted for 2 years.

4. Tissue that extends into the flow path of a prosthesis is undesirable, as it is prone to thrombotic complications (due to trauma and turbulence) and it decreases the orifice of the valve.[1]

5. A lateral cul-de-sac about the inlet and the outlet of the valve is not, per se, a nidus for thrombus formation.[1]

6. Residual valve tissue must not protrude over the inlet rim of the prosthesis into the flow tract, as this may be thrombogenic and lead to the secondary complications of obstruction, embolism, or infection.

DESIGN OF AN AORTIC BALL VALVE BASED UPON THE FOREGOING CONSIDERATIONS

As our studies of current prosthetic aortic valves have shown significant hydraulic and healing problems, we have designed a ball

*Of 23 specimens made available for study by Drs. Richard Varco and Jesse Edwards of the University of Minnesota (NHA Research Grant No. 5R01HE05694), 8 were suitable for analysis of tissue coverage of fabric.

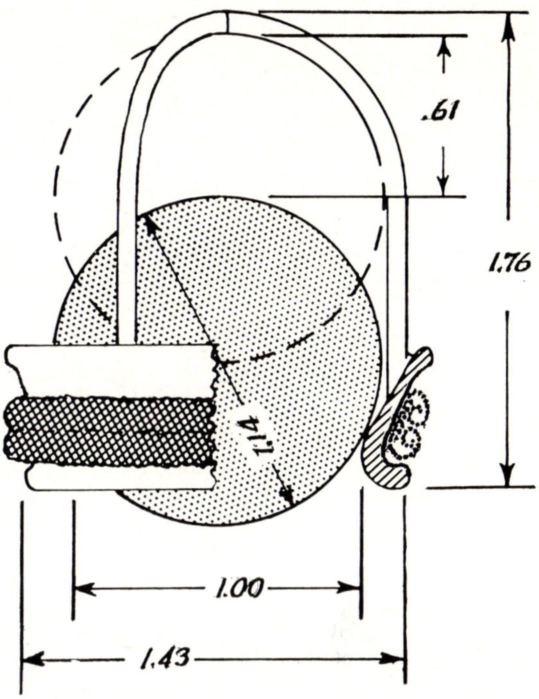

Fig. 6. Dimensions of the guided-flow, hidden sewing ring aortic valve in terms of its inlet orifice size.

valve which may aid in the solution of these problems. The important features of this prosthesis are: (1) maximum I.D. to O.D. ratio; (2) flow guidance; (3) minimum amount of exposed fabric; (4) "non"-thrombogenic metal body and cage; (5) valve body designed to prevent tissue access to flow tract; and (6) a small, strong, extensible (5 mm.), conformable, porous* fabric sewing ring that is shielded from the flow tract by the design of the valve body.

We have termed this new prosthesis a "guided-flow, hidden sewing ring aortic ball valve." It has been developed in consultation with Philip N. Sawyer and Sigmund A. Wesolowski. The important features of the prosthesis are shown in Figs. 6, 7, and 12.†

*Water porosity per square centimeter of flat fabric: 7,000 c.c. per minute at 120 mm. Hg.

†We are indebted to the following companies for working with us in the development of this valve: Austenal Division, Howmet Corporation, N. Y., Edwards Laboratories, Santa Ana, Calif., and Shiley Laboratories, Santa Ana, Calif. The prosthesis will be available through Shiley Laboratories.

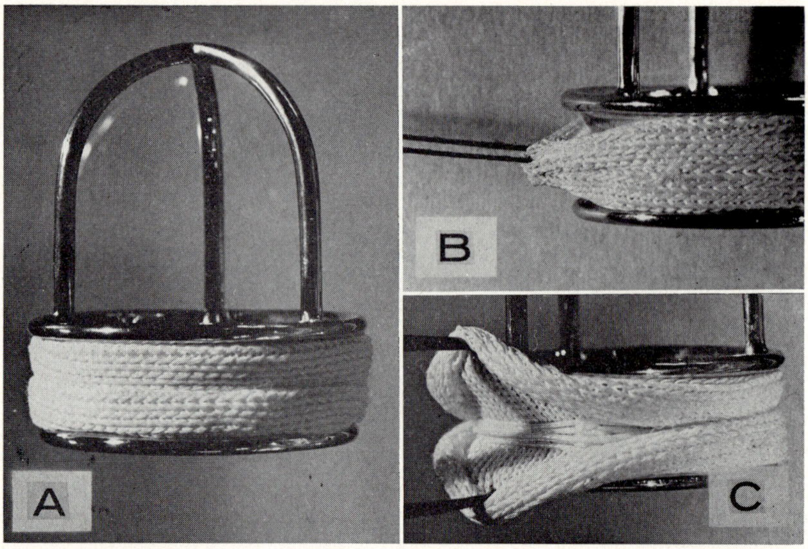

Fig. 7. Guided-flow, hidden sewing ring aortic valve. *A:* The rounded metal lips of the valve ring extend out a millimeter from the struts so as to decrease the likelihood of tissue overlapping into the ball path. *B:* Small sewing ring is yieldable when sutures are placed. Mattress sutures catch both rolls of fabric as shown in Fig. 8. *C:* Shows construction of cuff. There is no sewn seam. The fabric is highly porous, and this, coupled with the "open seam" renders it highly accessible to tissue ingrowth. (From Sauvage, L. R., Berger, K. E., Wood, S. J., Sameh, A. A., Dedomenico, M. P., and Viggers, R. F.: Amer. J. Surg. 116: 261, 1968.)

Recommended suture method for the guided-flow, hidden sewing ring aortic ball valve. A suture technique has evolved[3] which reduces the time of implantation, achieves secure fixation without distortion, and has proved effective for proper attachment of the open sewing ring to the annular tissues. We are in the process of testing other modifications of suture technique for this prosthesis.

The suture technique which we have used for the majority of our implants is as follows. All sutures are taken as horizontal mattresses. Those at the commissures are taken down so as to bring them more into line with those in the sinuses and reduce the vertical distance between the high and low points of the suture line. The stitches placed in the sinus portions of the annulus are taken upward so that they exit above the annulus. These mattress sutures are then brought up through the upper and lower rolls of the open sewing ring, thereby binding all portions of the cuff together. This method is illustrated in a porcine heart in Fig. 8. We have found temporary removal of the ball to be of assistance in assessing the proper positioning of the valve with respect to the annular tissues. It is very important that no tissue protrude into the inflow tract of the prosthesis.

RESULTS OBTAINED WITH THE GUIDED-FLOW, HIDDEN SEWING RING AORTIC BALL VALVE

We have both experimental and clinical data concerning the new valve. The experimental data pertain to in vitro hydraulic testing and biologic evaluation in the calf. The clinical data pertain to 15 implants, including 3 postoperative hemodynamic studies after significant intervals, and one autopsy examination 8 months after implantation.

Experimental data.

Hydraulic studies.

TEST METHOD. The hydraulic characteristics of a large number of aortic valve prosthesis geometries have been experimentally determined with the apparatus shown sche-

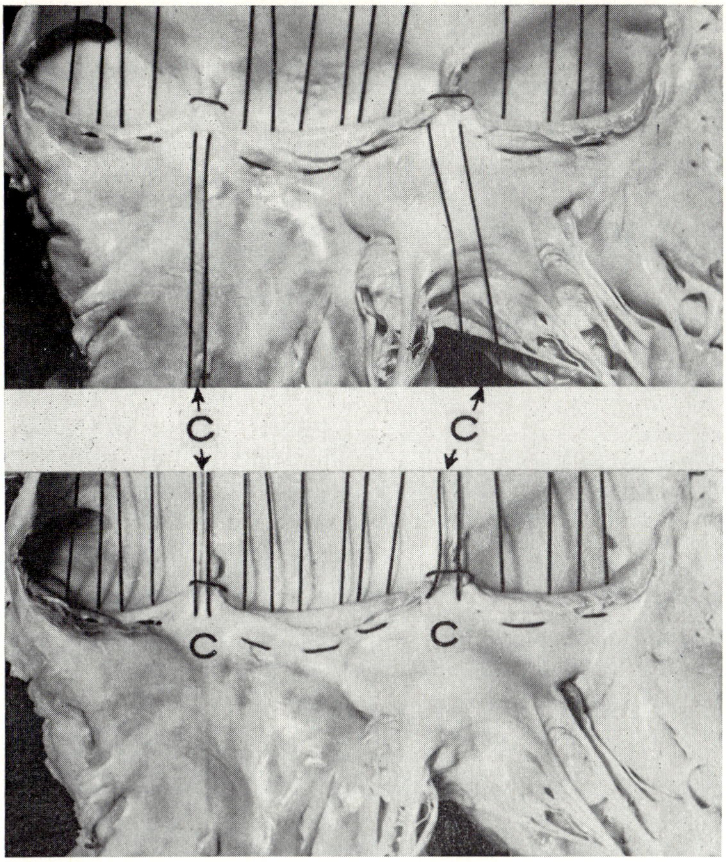

Fig. 8. Mattress suture placement along aortic valve annulus as viewed in the opened porcine heart. Leaflets have been excised. The mattress sutures are placed so as to emerge out the sinus side of the annulus. Those at the commissures (*C*) are placed so as to emerge downward and ventricularly (*top*). Thus, when all sutures are pulled up, their line of emergence is in an essentially single plane (*bottom*). (From Wood, S. J., and Sauvage, L. R.: J. Thorac. Cardiov. Surg. 54: 91, 1967.)

matically in Fig. 9. This apparatus creates a near-physiologic environment of pressure and pulsatile flow in the valve test chamber, which is appropriately sinus-shaped, allowing evaluation of any valve opening stickiness and valve closing regurgitation, as well as measurement of valve pressure gradient. In addition, the test chamber has been made transparent, which allows direct viewing of eddy formation as the valve operates.*

RESULTS. All experiments performed with this apparatus have conclusively shown the dissipative component of the pressure drop across the aortic valve to be due to eddy formation,[2] with pressure drop varying with the square of the instantaneous flow rate through the valve.

The pressure drop versus flow characteristic of several aortic valve prosthesis types is compared with that of the natural valve in Fig. 10. Data for the construction of the plot were obtained with the apparatus in Fig. 9, using a working fluid of 35 percent glycerin in water to simulate the viscosity and density of blood. The pressure gradient (dissipative component) of the natural valve has been estimated for this diagram, using the relative passage sizes as found by Sauvage and associ-

*A vanadium pentoxide sol transilluminated with polarized light is used for flow visualization.

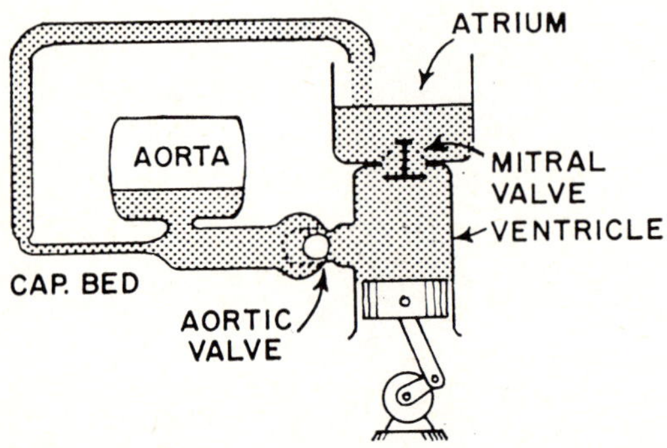

Fig. 9. Schematic of pulsatile flow valve testing apparatus. The hydraulic circuit is composed of a pump (ventricle), sinus-shaped test chamber for testing aortic valve prostheses, air chamber energy storage (simulation of aorta), a laminar flow resistance (capillary bed), and an open sump (atrium) communicating with a simulated mitral valve to the main pump chamber.

ates,[1] and the laws of conservation of energy and conservation of momentum.

The hydraulic improvement of the guided-flow, hidden sewing ring valve over others is due to two factors of essentially equal importance: (1) an improved channel profile, which guides the flow through its highest velocity region with less energy going to eddy formation, and (2) a larger orifice diameter (for the same outside or tissue diameter). The latter is possible because of the reduced bulk of the sewing ring.

Implantation studies. Results from 27 calves are compared with those from 52 implants of other types of ball valves in the calf (Table I). It is of interest to note that the incidence of significant thrombosis with the guided-flow, hidden sewing ring valve is practically the same as the incidence with the Model 1000 Starr-Edwards valve from

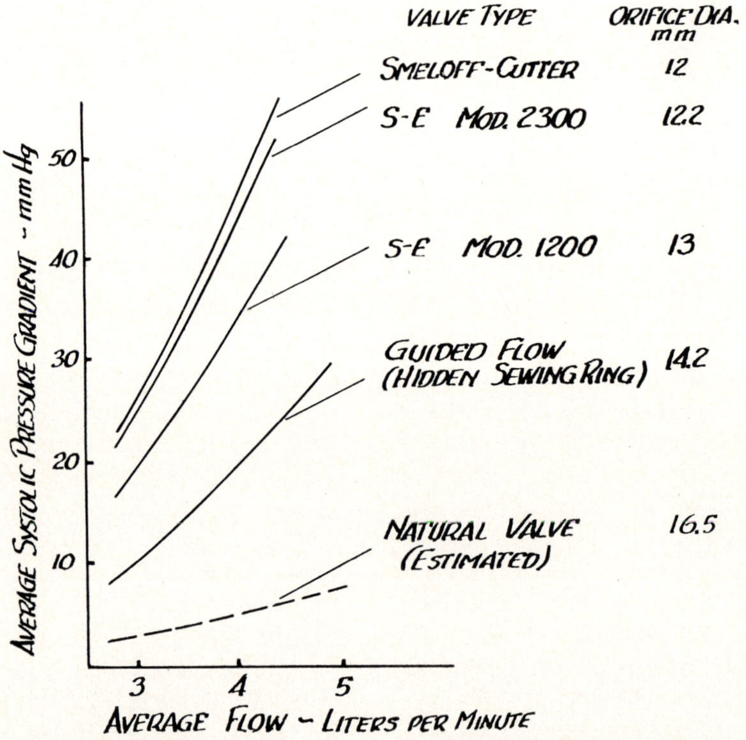

Fig. 10. Comparative pressure drop versus flow data from pulsatile in vitro tests for various prosthetic valve geometries all appropriately sized for the same implantation site. *All valve geometries were scaled to have the outside diameter of the inflexible portion of the sewing ring equal to 20 mm. (tissue diameter = 20 mm.).* The outflow tube formed by the natural leaflets tapers to a triangular area with an equivalent diameter of 16.5 mm.[1]

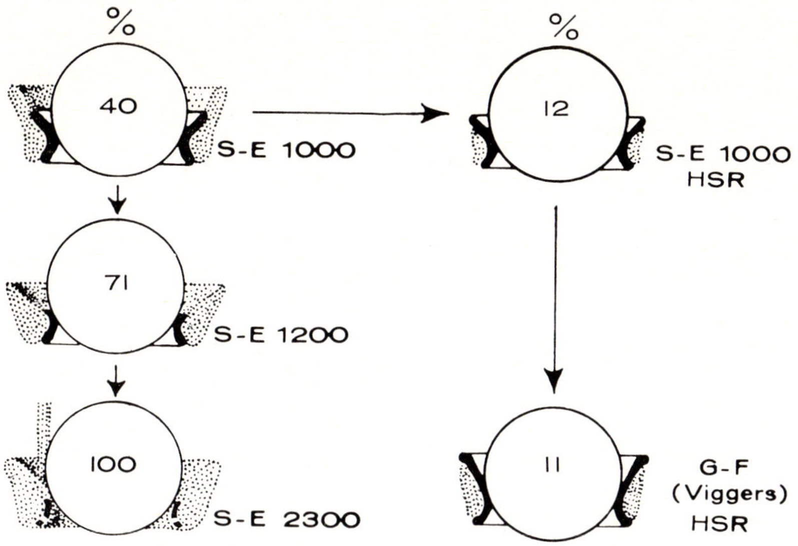

Fig. 11. Diagram showing relative extents of cloth and metal with percentages of significant thrombosis with various prostheses in the calf, as detailed in Table I.

Table III. *Fifteen patients with guided-flow, hidden sewing ring aortic ball valve*

Patient	*Operation date*	*Postoperative studies (mos.)*	*Alive (No. of days) as of 7/1/69*	*Died (days)*
L. G.	10/ 6/67	12	632	
F. K.	1/26/68	9.5	520	
L. W.	2/ 9/68		506	
L. S.	5/ 7/68	5	419	
J. B.	7/ 3/68		363	
P. A.	9/10/68			Night of surgery*
W. W.	9/13/68		290	
M. DeV.	10/11/68 (3 valves)			241†
S. D.	11/ 8/68 (3 valves)			Night of surgery‡
M. B.	11/26/68		216	
H. W.	12/ 6/68		206	
L. S.	1/31/69 (2 valves)		150	
A. H.	2/14/69 (2 valves)		136	
V. K.	3/28/69		94	
B. E.	5/29/69		32	

*Massive cerebral hemorrhage.
†Bacterial endocarditis (Pseudomonas).
‡Low cardiac output.

which the large sewing ring had been removed and replaced with a very small one. The high incidence of significant thrombosis with the Model 2300 valve in the calf probably reflects the tendency of this animal to layer an exposed fabric surface with thrombus. The relationship of the incidence of significant thrombosis to the amount of exposed fabric and the design of the outflow channel is shown in Fig. 11.

A representative specimen from the guided-flow valve series is shown in Fig. 12. It is to be noted that the design of the valve body has effectively prevented tissue from gaining access to the flow tract of the prosthesis. The microscopy shows that the small, porous sew-

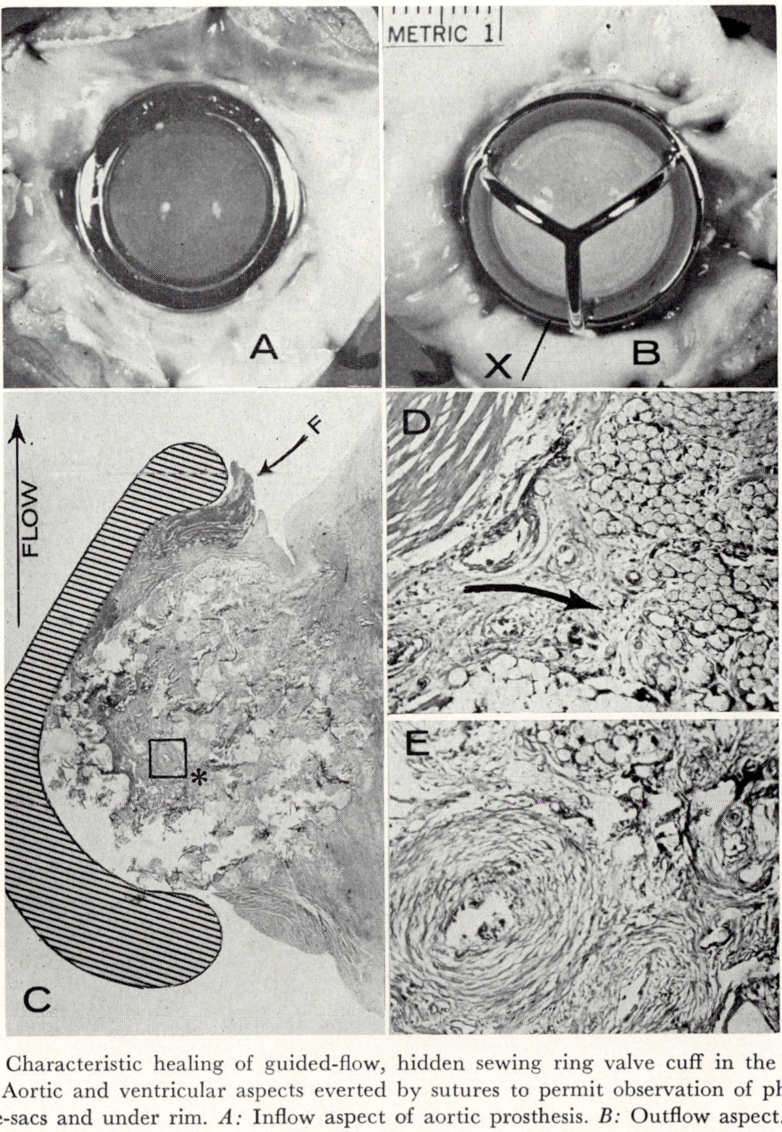

Fig. 12. Characteristic healing of guided-flow, hidden sewing ring valve cuff in the calf at 7 months. Aortic and ventricular aspects everted by sutures to permit observation of phenomena in cul-de-sacs and under rim. *A:* Inflow aspect of aortic prosthesis. *B:* Outflow aspect. "Clean" healing of valve remnants. No gross thrombus on either ventricular or aortic aspects. *C:* Section *X* as indicated in view *B*. Metal component indicated by hatched shape. Outflow is toward top. The small bulk of the cloth cuff is readily apparent. Arrow *F* indicates a small wedge of fibrin that remains to be organized under the upper lip of the metal. (Masson's trichrome. ×14.) *D:* View of annular zone where cloth abuts. Vascular collagenous connective tissue can be seen traversing fabric interstices in general direction of arrow. (Masson's trichrome. ×35.) *E:* Nature of tissue, well into hollow or "lumen" of cuff in region of square with asterisk in view *C*. The entire interior of the cuff has been colonized with mature vascularized collagenous connective tissue. (Masson's trichrome. ×135.)

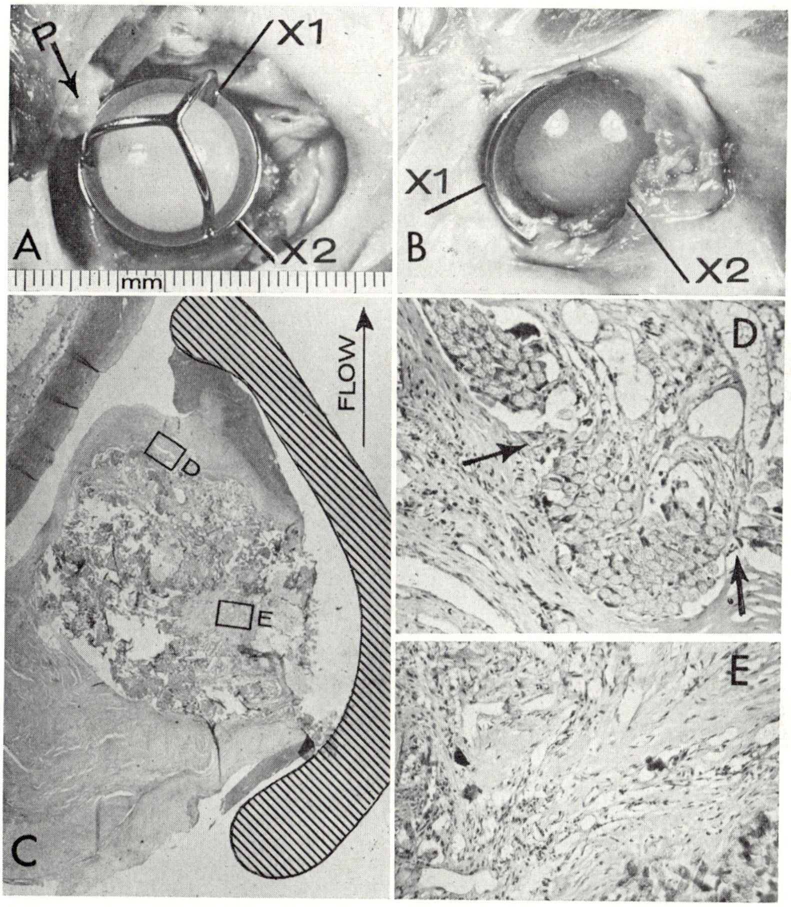

Fig. 13. Thirty-nine-year-old man with triple valve replacement expiring with Pseudomonas infection and cerebral embolus 8 months after operation. The infection arose from the ventricular aspect of the guided-flow, hidden sewing ring aortic prosthesis. *A:* Outflow side. Protrusion (*P*) is not thrombus, but a calcific remnant in the right coronary sinus 4 mm. above the valve rim. *B:* Inflow aspect, showing thrombus and degree of thrombotic occlusion of orifice. Tissue block taken at ×2 demonstrated bacteria-containing thrombus and nonunion of annular tissues to sewing cuff. Block taken at ×1 demonstrates salutary healing as depicted in the ensuing views. *C:* Low-power (×13) view of hidden sewing cuff with metal profile drawn in. Wedges of unorganized fibrin remain under the lips of the metal, but the cloth exposed in the sinus area is covered with mature fibrous tissue and the cuff hollow is filled with collagenous connective tissue that is highly vascularized. *D:* Detailed view shows tissue traversing cuff interstices indicated by arrows. (Hematoxylin and eosin. ×95.) *E:* Far out toward metal, cuff hollow is well filled with vascularized collagenous connective tissue. (Hematoxylin and eosin. ×95.) The capability of man to heal a small, open, and porous cuff is demonstrated. But in contrast to the calf, healing in man may be altered by the pathologic environment in which the prosthesis must be placed.

ing ring has been thoroughly infiltrated by host tissue to bind it securely to the annular tissues.

Clinical data. The guided-flow, hidden sewing ring prosthesis was first used clinically in October, 1967, and through May, 1969, this valve has been implanted in 15 patients. The results of the implants are shown in Table III. Three patients have died, two the night of surgery, one of cerebral hemorrhage and the other of low cardiac output associated with a triple valve replacement. The

Table IV. *Pre- and postoperative pressure gradients in 3 patients with guided-flow, hidden sewing ring aortic ball valve**

	L. S.		*F. K.*		*L. G.*	
Pressure gradient	*Pre-operative (mm. Hg)*	*Post-operative (mm. Hg)*	*Pre-operative (mm. Hg)*	*Post-operative (mm. Hg)*	*Pre-operative (mm. Hg)*	*Post-operative (mm. Hg)*
Average	64	16	88	13	45	26
Peak-to-peak	46	0	110	3	6	6
Maximum instantaneous	80	19	120	30	70	38

*Valve orifice area: 158 mm.².

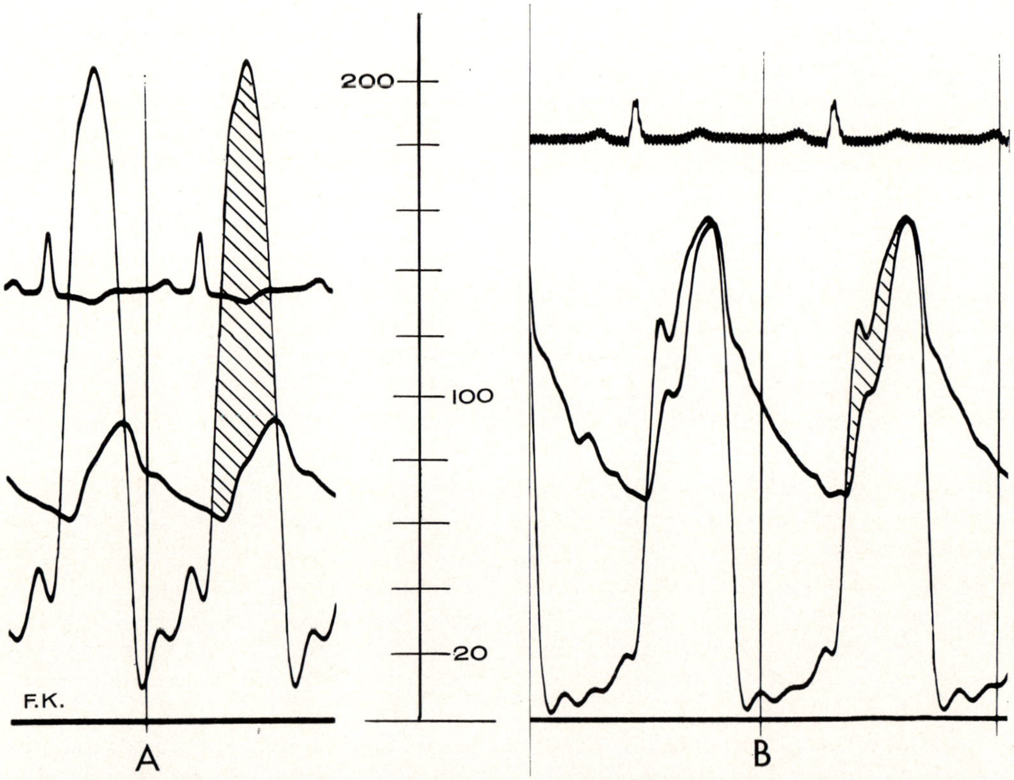

Fig. 14. Preoperative and 9½ month postoperative pressure versus time tracings for Patient F. K. having implantation of guided-flow, hidden sewing ring aortic ball valve. The shaded area, which equals the time integral of the systolic ventricular-aortic pressure difference, when divided by systolic time, gives the "average" pressure gradient. The preoperative pressure gradient (*A*) shows an *average* value of 88 mm. Hg and a *peak-to-peak* value of 110 mm. Hg; the postoperative (*B*) *average* pressure gradient is 13 mm. Hg and the *peak-to-peak* gradient is 3 mm. Hg. We feel that the average pressure gradient is the more meaningful figure.

third patient died 8 months after surgery from complications of Pseudomonas bacterial endocarditis affecting the under side of the aortic prosthesis, as shown in Fig. 13. One of the 12 surviving patients, a 76-year-old man not on anticoagulants, had a nonfatal cerebral embolus (probable) 3 months after operation. The other 11 patients, now an average of 297 days postoperative, are in excellent clinical condition and have shown no evidence of valve dysfunction, embolism, or infection. They are receiving moderate doses of Coumadin.

Hemodynamic studies. We have been able to carry out postoperative hemodynamic studies on 3 patients at intervals of 5, 9½, and 12 months after operation. Comparative pre- and postoperative pressure gradients are shown in Table IV, and the pressure tracings on one of the patients are shown in Fig. 14. We have measured the maximum instantaneous pressure drop, the average pressure drop and the terminal peak-to-peak pressure drop in each instance. The wide difference in these values is of interest, and emphasizes the importance of using the same method of measurement in comparing hemodynamic results from various laboratories. The average pressure drop appears to be the most meaningful figure, especially when the drop is small. Although only three patients have been studied comparatively, the results are impressive when compared with the much higher gradients reported for similarly sized totally cloth-covered ball valves. We believe that the high gradients observed in the totally cloth-covered prostheses result from diminution of the diameter of the inlet orifice of the valve.

Tissue studies. Despite the fact that the aortic valve of the patient who succumbed from a cerebral embolus at 8 months was partially involved with Pseudomonas infection, much of value can be obtained from study of the noninfected portions of this specimen. The embolus presumably arose from the site of infection on the inflow side of the prosthesis. The gross and the microscopic findings from a noninfected area are shown in Fig. 13. This human implant shows that a cul-de-sac about the upper side of the valve (view *C*) was not a nidus for thrombus formation. Invasion of the sewing ring by highly vascularized fibrous tissue, as seen in Fig. 13, *D* and *E*, is remarkably similar to the healing observed in the calf (Fig. 12). This small, highly porous hidden sewing ring requires only 3 to 5 mm. of tissue extension for complete incorporation.

DISCUSSION

The hydraulic efficiency of an implanted prosthetic valve is not going to improve with time, but one hopes that there will be no deterioration of its function after implantation. The reactions of the host to the valve, including tissue ingrowth, must not interfere with the hydraulic efficiency of the prosthesis if a suitable result is to be obtained. Hence, the goal of the surgeon is to replace the diseased valve with an efficient hydraulic appliance that will be healed permanently in stable position, and whose effectiveness will not be compromised by tissue or by reactions of the blood to its presence. Our observations suggest that the reactions of the host to the prosthesis are comparatively benign, provided that certain spatial relationships of the healable portions of the prosthesis to the healing sources are obtained. In essence, we believe that the smaller the amount of fabric, the better, and that it is important to keep the fabric and residual tissue fragments well shielded from the flow tract of the prosthesis by the design of the body of the valve. By so doing, we believe that the incidence of thrombosis and, hence, of embolism, can be reduced to a very low level.

In addition, if the 5 to 7 mm. maximum tissue extension which we have observed in the aortic site in man represents an accurate picture, the rationale for reduction in the amount of cloth exposed to the blood is clear. It is our hope that information from other centers will be forthcoming concerning the distance tissue can extend from the annulus out over fabric cuffs in the aortic valve location in man.

There are two factors that must be considered in the choice of a prosthesis for valve replacement for a given patient. First, what are the physiologic needs of the patient for flow? Second, what size prosthesis will the root of the aorta accept?

We believe that a mean gradient of more than 20 mm. Hg at rest is unacceptable for a prosthetic aortic valve. It is of interest to realize that with a mean valve pressure gradient of 20 mm. Hg at a regurgitant flow of 10 percent of the forward flow, the increase in ventricular work is 40 percent over that of the normal valve. Hence, it is apparent that prosthetic valves return the patient toward normal if the preoperative hemodynamic abnormality is large, but they do not attain the normal. Accordingly, it is desirable for the surgeon to plan to use a valve that will allow at least resting physiologic flows at a mean gradient of less than 20 mm. Hg. For example, a patient of 1.5 $M.^2$ body surface area should have a basal cardiac output at rest of 4,500 c.c. per minute. A valve size should be selected that will allow a pulsatile flow rate of this magnitude without a mean gradient greater than 20 mm. Hg.

The second point the surgeon must face is the size of the aortic root. Will the root accept a valve of the size that the patient needs? If the root is not of adequate size, it should be enlarged by a gusset to allow implantation of a large enough valve. However, most aortic roots will accept a valve that is adequate for the patient's minimum needs. With appreciable increase of cardiac output (exercise) all prosthetic valves present significant obstruction unless the root is very large, allowing an unusually large valve to be placed.

At present, aortic valve operation is indicated for symptomatic patients with major hemodynamic abnormalities and for asymptomatic patients if they show significant increase in heart size and decrease in contractility. Asymptomatic patients with major hemodynamic abnormalities, whose contractility is good and whose heart is not greatly enlarged, are not candidates for operation because the risk of an implanted prosthesis of any type is still appreciable, or at least unknown for the newer ones, and because the duration of the asymptomatic period in this type of patient cannot be predicted. This delay is not ideal, as the left ventricle is allowed to develop major structural changes before the patient is subjected to the risk of prosthetic replacement. Our goal must be to develop prostheses having such excellent attributes that their implantation will be indicated earlier in the course of aortic valve disease than is justified with current prostheses.

CONCLUSIONS

Our studies of aortic ball valves support the following: (1) The energy losses across an aortic ball valve are due, in the main, to orifice constriction, with resultant turbulence of the blood flowing through the valve passages. (2) The degree of turbulence can be reduced by flow guidance and the energy losses decreased moderately. (3) The ball is not a functional site of obstruction if there is an adequate peripheral channel for flow around the ball. (4) Even though the calf has great ability to cover the fabric surface of an aortic ball valve by fibrous tissue, the incidence of significant thrombosis in this species is reduced by decreasing the amount of exposed fabric. (5) Man has much less ability to cover the fabric surface of an aortic ball valve than does the calf.

The lasting value of any of the clinically used prostheses, including the one presented in this paper, will be determined by time. However, we believe that the prosthesis described embodies design features important to long-term success.

We wish to express our gratitude to the following for their contributions to our program: American Silk Sutures, Inc., Roslyn Heights, N. Y. (Dacron sutures); Ayerst Laboratories, New York, N. Y. (Fluothane); Cutter Laboratories, Berkeley, Calif. (intravenous fluids); Ethicon, Inc., Somerville, N. J. (Mersilene sutures); Eli Lilly & Company, Indianapolis, Ind. (Keflin).

For assistance in our experimental studies, we wish to thank Miller Packing Company, Renton, Wash.; Seattle Packing Company, Seattle, Wash.; and Smith Brothers Farms, Kent, Wash.

REFERENCES

1. Sauvage, L. R., Viggers, R. F., Berger, K. E., Wood, S. J., and Robel, S. B.: The aortic valve: Studies pertinent to prosthetic replacement, Springfield, Ill., Charles C Thomas, Publisher. In preparation.
2. Viggers, R. F., Robel, S. B., and Sauvage, L. R.: A hydraulic figure-of-merit for heart valve prostheses, J. Biomed. Mater. Res. **1:** 103, 1967.
3. Wood, S. J., and Sauvage, L. R.: Single plane fixation for prosthetic aortic valves, J. Thorac. Cardiov. Surg. **54:** 90, 1967.

DISCUSSION

Dr. William W. L. Glenn (New Haven, Conn.). Dr. Sauvage, do you have any concern about using the Silastic poppitt under these circumstances?

Dr. Sauvage (closing). I think that all of us who deal with materials that may break down have real concern for them and, Dr. Glenn, I think the poppitt is a weak point in the prosthesis.

The wear of the poppitt is related to the amount of oscillation. We hope that stabilization of flow through a prosthesis will decrease poppitt oscillation and wear.

Direct coronary arterial revascularization for segmental occlusive disease

E. D. MUNDTH, M.D.*
J. W. HARTHORNE, M.D.
M. J. BUCKLEY, M.D.
R. E. DINSMORE, M.D.
W. G. AUSTEN, M.D.
BOSTON, MASS.
From the Department of Surgery, Medicine and Radiology, Massachusetts General Hospital and Harvard Medical School

Because of the frequency of proximal segmental occlusive lesions in patients with symptomatic coronary artery disease, direct arterial reconstruction has gained increasing acceptance as a logical approach to myocardial revascularization. Early experience with direct arterial reconstruction of the coronary arteries, particularly the left coronary artery and its two major branches, was associated with a considerable operative mortality thereby limiting wide clinical application.[8] With increasing experience and improvement in the technical aspects of coronary artery reconstruction and careful patient selection, the operative risk has approached acceptable levels.[10]

A number of procedures for coronary artery reconstruction have been applied clinically, including endarterotomy with patch angioplasty,[9] endarterectomy,[6, 7, 18] segmental saphenous vein interposition,[10] internal mammary-coronary artery bypass,[13] and saphenous vein aortocoronary bypass.[14] Long-term evaluation and comparison of the advantages of each procedure related to the anatomic distribution of the occlusive disease and preoperative clinical manifestations are not yet complete. Careful selection for myocardial revascularization and choice of the appropriate procedure are of great importance for a successful surgical approach to coronary artery disease. The purpose of this study has been to review our recent experience with direct coronary arterial reconstructive procedures for the treatment of proximal segmental coronary artery occlusive disease with analysis of the criteria used for patient selection, type of procedure selected, and technical aspects of the surgical procedure.

CLINICAL MATERIAL

Between November, 1967, and May, 1969, 21 patients underwent direct coronary artery reconstructive procedures at the Massachusetts General Hospital. Sixteen were men and 5 were women. The average age was 51 years at the time of operation and ranged from 34 to 67 years. Routine preoperative evaluation was carried out followed by selective cine coronary angiography using the Sones' technique. This included complete right and left coronary artery studies before and after nitroglycerin. In several patients, metabolic studies, including coronary arteriovenous lactate differences, were determined before and after isoproterenol stimulation. Left ventricular angiocardiography was carried out in all patients in whom it was tolerated.

The indications for study are tabulated in Table I. Three main categories of patients with coronary artery occlusive disease have

Supported in part by the United States Public Health Service Grants HE-12489-01 and HE-0-6664.

*Fellow, Medical Foundation, Inc.

been accepted for evaluation and considered for operation: (1) progressive angina intractable to medical management, (2) one or more myocardial infarctions in the asymptomatic younger age patient, and (3) progressive and disabling congestive heart failure without angina on the basis of coronary artery disease. Of the 21 patients who were studied and operated upon, 15 had progressive and intractable angina, 3 were asymptomatic in the younger age group having had one or more myocardial infarctions, and 3 had progressive disabling congestive heart failure without angina. In the intractable angina group, 10 of the 15 patients had previous myocardial infarctions, 4 of them multiple, based upon a clinical diagnosis at the time of the infarct and persistent electrocardiographic changes consistent with a previous infarct. Additionally in the angina group there were 5 patients who had clinical evidence of intermittent cardiac failure. All 5 of these patients had a previous myocardial infarct and in all 5 a left ventricular aneurysm was present. In the third group of 3 patients with progressive congestive heart failure as a manifestation of coronary artery disease, 2 had a previous myocardial infarct.

In all 15 patients with intractable angina, careful medical management failed to control the symptoms. Medical treatment included short- and long-acting nitrites, diet and activity restriction, digitalis when cardiac failure was associated, and propanolol when tolerated. Propanolol frequently improved the condition when cardiac failure was not present, but in these selected cases the degree of disability remaining warranted consideration of operation.

The arteriographic findings of the 21 patients undergoing operation are summarized in Table II. The criteria for the extent and significance of coronary arterial disease was modified after the classification of Diethrich and associates.[5] Stenosis of greater than 75 percent or total occlusion of one of the four

Table I. *Clinical characteristics of 21 patients undergoing evaluation for coronary artery disease and subsequent direct coronary artery reconstructive surgery*

Category	*No. of patients*	*Average age*	*Previous myocardial infarction*	*Left ventricular aneurysm*	*Associated vascular disease*
Intractable angina	10	51	5	0	2
Intractable angina + cardiac failure	5	54	5	5	4
Previous myocardial infarct, asymptomatic	3	39	3	0	0
Cardiac failure without angina	3	52	2	0	2
Total	21	51	15	5	8

Table II. *Arteriographic findings of 21 patients undergoing evaluation for coronary artery disease and subsequent direct coronary artery reconstructive surgery*

	Extent of coronary artery disease				
Category	*No. of patients*	*1 Vessel*	*2 Vessel*	*3 Vessel*	*4 Vessel*
Intractable angina	10	3	4	3	0
Intractable angina + cardiac failure	5	0	2	2	1
Previous myocardial infarct, asymptomatic	3	0	3	0	0
Cardiac failure without angina	3	0	3	0	0

major coronary arteries, including the right coronary artery (RCA), the main left coronary artery (LCA), the anterior descending artery (ADA), and circumflex artery (CA), was considered significant. Frequently, diffuse distal disease involves one or more of the major coronary artery branches in combination with proximal segmental occlusive disease. When it could be estimated arteriographically that greater than 50 percent of the outflow of a given major coronary artery was obliterated either by diffuse distal disease alone or in combination with proximal stenosis it was considered to be hemodynamically significant.

In this series there were 3 patients with single vessel disease, one each involving the RCA, ADA, and CA. Two of the 3 patients had a previous myocardial infarction, perhaps indicating the severity of involvement of the single possibly dominant artery in each case. There were 12 patients with 2 vessel disease including 10 patients with RCA-ADA disease and 2 patients with RCA-CA disease. Five patients had 3 vessel disease, all involving the RCA-ADA and CA. There was one patient with 4 vessel disease who in addition had an apical left ventricular aneurysm.

OPERATIVE PROCEDURES

An attempt was made to pattern the operative procedure to each individual patient in terms of anatomic distribution of the disease, presence or absence of diffuse distal disease, presence or absence of a ventricular aneurysm or dyskinetic areas of the left ventricular wall, presence or absence of left ventricular failure, and the patient's over-all clinical status. Where proximal occlusive disease was involved, endarterectomy or a bypass graft procedure was used, usually in association with internal mammary artery implants. The latter have been implanted in areas of significant diffuse distal disease when direct arterial reconstruction was not feasible. The various operative procedures employed in these 21 patients are summarized in Table III. There were 14 direct arterial reconstruction procedures involving the RCA and 10 involving the LCA or its branches.

Direct arterial reconstruction of two major coronary arteries was carried out in 3 patients, all involving the RCA and ADA. In 2 instances this was accomplished by RCA endarterectomy and saphenous vein aorto-ADA bypass and in one instance by a saphenous vein aorto-RCA bypass and saphenous vein aorto-ADA bypass. In 4 patients a left ventricular aneurysm was resected in association with coronary arterial reconstruction. The aneurysmectomy was accompanied by an internal mammary-RCA shunt in one patient, and RCA endarterectomy in one, a saphenous vein aorto-RCA bypass in one, and in one patient with saphenous bypass grafts to both the RCA and ADA. Either anterolateral and/or posterior internal mammary artery implants were added to each procedure.

The technical aspects of coronary arterial reconstructive surgery are of considerable

Table III. *Coronary arterial reconstruction procedures in 21 patients*

Type of procedure	*RCA*	*LCA*	*ADA*	*CA*	*Total*	*Complementary internal mammary artery implants:* *Anterolateral and posterior double*	*Single anterolateral*	*Single posterior*
Endarterectomy	7*	1	0	0	8	4	0	1
Internal mammary—coronary artery bypass	3*	0	1	1	5	0	1	3
Staphenous vein aorto-coronary artery bypass	4*	0	7*	0	11	11	0	0
Total	14	1	8	1	24	15	1	4

*Left ventricular aneurysmectomy associated with direct coronary artery revascularization in 4 patients, one of whom had a double bypass.

importance. The prevention of even relative hypotension in these patients is extremely important during induction of anesthesia, intraoperatively, and postoperatively. Most positive inotropic drugs have a β-adrenergic action causing an increase in heart rate, myocardial contractility, and myocardial oxygen demand, all of which may cause significant myocardial ischemia due to the anatomically fixed limited capacity of coronary circulation. Thus, relatively pure α-adrenergic drugs as phenylephrine may be used effectively to support the blood pressure without markedly increasing myocardial oxygen and coronary blood flow requirements. Since coronary blood flow decreases in a linear fashion when coronary perfusion pressure falls to relative hypotension levels it is essential to maintain the mean central aortic blood pressure in a normal range for each patient in order to prevent myocardial ischemia and infarction.[20] Phenylephrine was used to maintain the mean aortic blood pressure in the range of 80 to 110 mm. Hg in all but 3 of the patients in this series. In certain patients with a very marginal cardiac reserve, particularly those with an elevated left ventricular end diastolic pressure at rest, exposure of the femoral vessels under local anesthesia may be advisable so that prompt cannulation and partial cardiopulmonary bypass may be instituted for circulatory assistance if refractory hypotension develops during induction of anesthesia or in the early operative phase. This

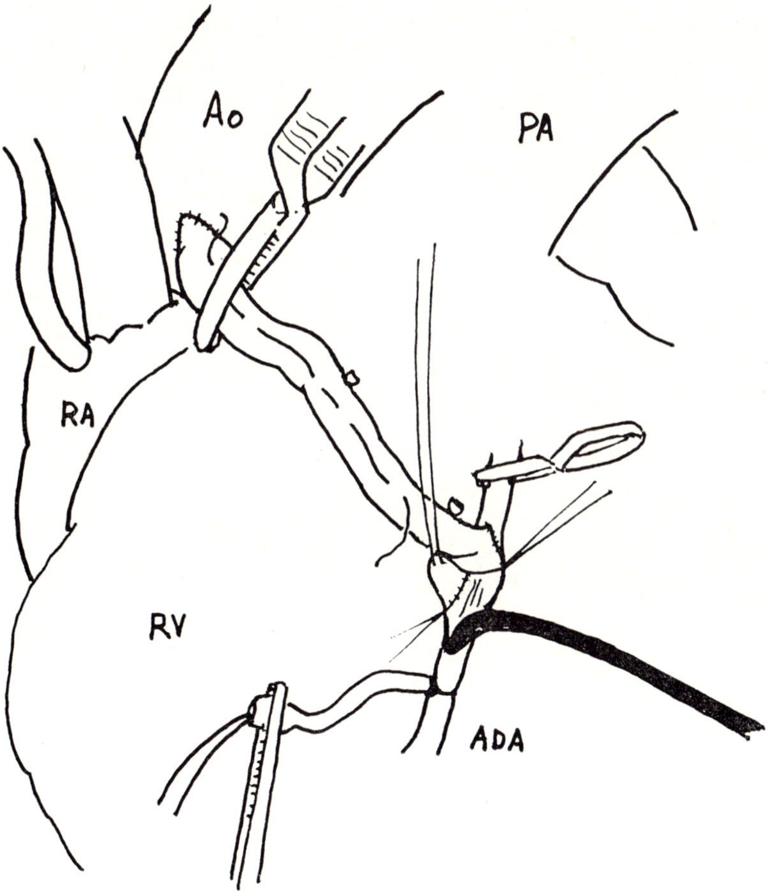

Fig. 1. Method of distal coronary artery perfusion during saphenous vein aortocoronary bypass graft to the anterior descending artery. Perfusion is achieved via the coronary perfusion line from the heart-lung machine.

technique was used in 4 patients in this series and in one patient early cannulation and cardiac assistance was required. The latter patient had severe 3 vessel disease, a large aneurysm involving the entire anterior left ventricular wall and a resting left ventricular end diastolic pressure of 30 mm. Hg.

We have found an anterior approach through a median sternotomy incision the most useful. This allows access to both internal mammary arteries, the right coronary, and anterior descending arteries but does not allow good exposure of the main left coronary or circumflex arteries. A left thoracotomy approach was used in the 2 patients where these 2 arteries required reconstruction. In the early phase of the procedure both internal mammary arteries are dissected out using a modified Sewell technique[19] in addition to a 8 to 12 inch length of proximal saphenous vein. The patient is heparinized and the internal mammary vessels prepared for implantation or coronary artery bypass. When one or more saphenous vein aortocoronary bypass grafts are contemplated, the reversed saphenous vein segments are anastomosed to the root of the aorta in an oblique end-to-side fashion, care being taken to direct the axis of the anastomosis toward the coronary artery being bypassed in order to avoid kinking. The right coronary artery may be dissected without using cardiopulmonary bypass. Prior to dissection of a major coronary artery branch, 1 percent lidocaine is carefully infiltrated around the artery proximally to avoid coronary arterial vasoconstriction. To dissect the anterior descending artery it is generally necessary to place the patient on cardiopulmonary bypass so that lifting the heart does not cause hypotension. Prior to occluding any of the major coronary arteries, the patient is placed on total cardiopulmonary bypass using systemic moderate hypothermia (28° C.) and left ventricular decompression. Left ventricular distention has been shown to have a persistent adverse effect on subsequent left ventricular function[22] and care is taken to prevent this throughout the procedure.

There is considerable controversy concerning the effect of coronary ischemia during cardiac surgery, but certainly in patients with severe coronary artery occlusive disease, coronary ischemia may be very deleterious to subsequent myocardial function and possibly result in myocardial infarction. Protection of the ischemic myocardium during reconstruction of the involved coronary artery requiring a period of coronary artery occlusion is accomplished by combining topical profound cardiac hypothermia (4°C.) and distal coronary perfusion by means of a small cannula attached to the coronary perfusion line (Fig. 1) or an internal shunt if the vessel is of adequate size and an endarterectomy being done (Fig. 2). Ventricular fibrillation occurs with profound cardiac hypothermia and provides a quiet field. Because of the small size of diseased coronary arteries, microsurgical vascular techniques are required using two power operating loupes. Bypass anastomoses or arteriotomy closures following endarterectomy must be done with extreme care gaining exact intima-to-intima apposition without kinking or distortion. We have used a running 7-0 suture for this. Bypass grafts are cut obliquely allowing a more capacious anastomosis.[15] It is important to measure the length of bypass graft needed so as to prevent

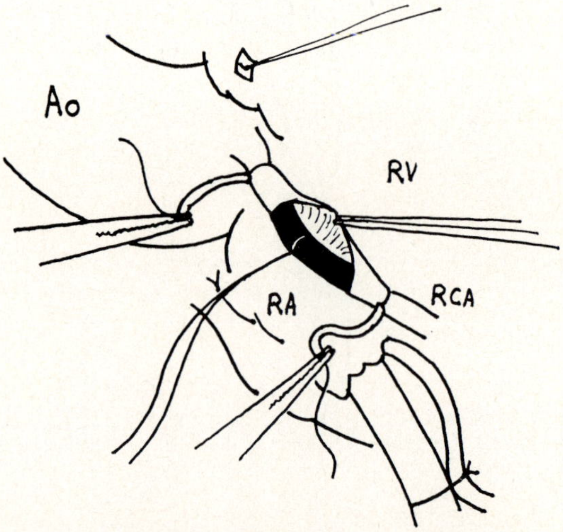

Fig. 2. Method of distal coronary artery perfusion by means of an internal shunt during right coronary endarterectomy.

redundancy, kinking, or excessive tension. A linear marking adventitial suture on the vein graft prevents twisting of the graft. Following completion of the direct reconstruction and during rewarming, the internal mammary implants are placed in intramyocardial tunnels anteriorly and posteriorly in the standard fashion.

Every effort is made to maintain the mean aortic pressure between 80 and 110 mm. Hg when cardiopulmonary bypass is discontinued and the patient resumes his own circulatory support. Phenylephrine has been used at this stage of the procedure in all patients except the first 3 in this series because of the tendency for peripheral vasodilation and relative hypotension. Six of the 21 patients required some form of inotropic support ranging from one to 4 days postoperatively. Following direct coronary arterial reconstruction coronary blood flow is increased with a resultant increase in tolerance and response to inotropic agents without producing ischemia on the basis of increased myocardial oxygen demand. Because of the propensity to postoperative arrhythmias, temporary epicardial atrial and ventricular electrodes are placed in most patients and have been effective in both diagnosing and treating arrhythmias.[17]

POSTOPERATIVE MORBIDITY AND EARLY RESULTS

There were 4 hospital deaths in the series of 21 patients, 3 occurring intraoperatively (Table IV). All 3 patients had terminal severe coronary artery disease, but since their prognosis was estimated to be hopeless, they elected to undergo operation. All 3 of these patients presented with progressive angina, chronic congestive heart failure, and left ventricular aneurysms. One of the patients represented our first attempt at a direct arterial reconstruction of a major branch of the left coronary artery. All had massive intraoperative myocardial infarctions. In 2, profound cardiac hypothermia was not used as a method of myocardial protection. There was one additional hospital death, 2 weeks following operation, associated with a myocardial infarction. This was the first patient undergoing direct coronary artery surgery and residual near total occlusion of the proximal right coronary artery adjacent to an incomplete endarterectomy was found at autopsy. Another patient in this group had crescendo coronary insufficiency pain 12 hours preceding operation, and although the electrocardiogram did not show infarction, serum enzymes taken at the time were subsequently reported as elevated, indicating the possibility of an acute myocardial infarction just prior to operation. There were 6 patients with documented intraoperative myocardial

Table IV. *Operative mortality of direct coronary arterial reconstruction in 21 patients*

Category	No. of patients	Hospital mortality
Intractable angina	10	1
Intractable angina, cardiac failure, left ventricular aneurysm	5	3
Previous myocardial infarct, asymptomatic	3	0
Cardiac failure without angina	3	0
Total	21	4

Table V. *Complications of operation in 21 patients undergoing coronary arterial reconstruction*

Complication		No.
Low cardiac output		6
Exploration for excessive bleeding		2
Arrhythmias		13
Atrial	6	
Nodal	4	
Ventricular	3	
Renal insufficiency		5
Mild, BUN < 100	3	
Severe, BUN > 100	2	
Dialysis	0	
Respiratory insufficiency		4
Minor	2	
Tracheostomy	1	
Tracheal stenosis	1	
ECG changes		6
MI	2	
Nonspecific ischemia	3	
LBBB	1	
Wound complications		5
Minor	2	
Major, debridement	3	
Thromboembolic (CVA)		1

infarcts, 4 of whom died as indicated above. The complications of surgery in this group of 21 patients are shown in Table V. Worthy of note is the number of renal complications. Two of the 5 patients had pre-existing renal disease and both of these patients became azotemic but did not require dialysis. The other 3 had very mild transient elevations of the BUN probably related to somewhat reduced cardiac output in the early postoperative phase. The number of major wound complications, 3 in 21 patients, probably reflects the lengthy duration of these procedures and perhaps may be related to devascularization of the midsternum by virtue of removing both internal mammary arteries.

The time of follow-up is too early and the series still rather small to draw any conclusions regarding early results of operation. Only 2 patients of the group of 21 have been followed one year or more. However, of 9 patients with intractable angina, 7 are improved, ranging in follow-up time from 1 month to 1 year, and 4 of these have had no angina. Of 2 patients with angina and cardiac failure surviving operation, one died 3 months postoperatively of a myocardial infarct and one is improved just one month postoperatively. Of 3 young asymptomatic patients with previous myocardial infarctions, all are alive and well ranging from 1 month to 1 year postoperatively. Of 3 patients with cardiac failure as a sole manifestation of coronary artery disease, all are alive with questionable improvement in two and definite improvement in one.

Postoperative angiogram study has been accomplished in 5 patients at 6 to 8 months postoperatively with patency of the arterial reconstruction demonstrated in 3, questionable in one, and occluded in one.

DISCUSSION

Unquestionably, the single most important contribution in the development of coronary artery surgery was the technique of coronary cine angiography pioneered by Sones.[21] Accurate determination of the localization, character and extent of coronary artery disease by this method has allowed the cardiovascular surgeon to apply direct vascular reconstructive techniques to coronary artery disease.

Although the coronary angiogram yields a graphic illustration of anatomic involvement, it does not, however, provide direct information as to the hemodynamic or physiologic significance of the observed occlusive disease. Gorlin and Taylor[12] have attempted to gain a more objective method of determining the physiologic significance of arteriographically demonstrated coronary artery disease by studying coronary arteriovenous lactate differences during cardiac catheterization. They have shown a correlation between excess myocardial lactate production and arteriographically demonstrated coronary disease. However, myocardial lactate production may be extremely variable even during the course of a catheterization study thereby decreasing the reliability of the method in case selection.

Anatomically and physiologically normal coronary arteries are essentially end arteries in the human heart without demonstrable intercoronary collateral coronary circulation.[2] The presence of intercoronary collaterals indicate ischemic myocardium and supports the probability of physiologically significant coronary artery disease. If distal retrograde filling of a major coronary artery occurs at the time of angiography when the contralateral coronary artery is injected it is an indication of hemodynamically significant disease proximally. Arteriographic evidence of hemodynamically significant occlusive disease may also be inferred when there is slow transit of contrast medium through a diseased vessel compared to the other vessels, and restricted outflow capacity may be inferred if there is prolonged retention of contrast medium within a major vessel. These observations require expert cine coronary angiography and interpretation but are extremely helpful in deciding the appropriate revascularization procedure.

If several vessels are involved as is frequently the case, it may be impossible to determine which vessel or areas of the myocardium are responsible for the patients' clinical manifestations. In this situation, if operation is to be effective, a combination of procedures may be necessary.

Frequently an aneurysm or akinetic area

of the ventricular wall is seen on cine ventriculography and it may be impossible to decide whether the poorly contracting area is due to ischemia of viable contractile myocardium or is due to fibrous scar. When cardiac failure alone is present, resection of the poorly contracting area of ventricular wall, if resectable, is the procedure of choice without associated revascularization. In the present series, there were three patients with progressive cardiac failure as their only clinical manisfestation of coronary disease, but in all 3 cine left ventricular angiography revealed a large dilated poorly contracting left ventricle without evidence of a discrete aneurysm or akinetic ventricular wall. Coronary arterial revascularization was carried out in the 3 patients in this series in the hope that myocardial ischemia contributed to the left ventricular failure. The patients' prognosis on the basis of the expected natural history of end stage coronary artery disease was virtually nil, perhaps justifying the operative risk.

When intractable angina is the predominant clinical manifestation in association with left ventricular failure and a left ventricular akinetic area or aneurysm, selection of the appropriate operative procedure may be difficult. Because of the presence of angina, myocardial revascularization in addition to resection of the aneurysm or akinetic area would seem advisable. In the present series there were 5 patients in this category all with severe occlusive disease involving 2, 3, or 4 major coronary arteries. All had markedly elevated left ventricular end diastolic pressures at rest and were totally incapacitated by their symptoms. The immediate operative mortality was considerable with 3 of the 5 patients unable to maintain their own circulatory support with cessation of cardiopulmonary bypass. Patients in this category and those with cardiac failure alone represent patients with end stage coronary artery disease; with increasing experience it may become clear that this group should not be considered for coronary arterial reconstructive surgery.

The selection of patients with inractable angina alone for myocardial revascularization is less uncertain. Encouraging results from both indirect revascularization procedures[11] and direct coronary arterial reconstruction[10] indicate that operative revascularization of the ischemic myocardium is effective in the treatment of disabling angina.

Little is known regarding what effect myocardial revascularization procedures will have upon the natural history of coronary artery occlusive disease in terms of the rate of progression of the disease and the incidence of further complications. Diethrich and associates[4] have found in a relatively controlled series that myocardial infarction occurred three times more frequently in patients not operated upon compared to operatively treated patients. Differences in over-all survival between operative and nonoperative patients were less impressive because of the operative mortality rate. These studies support the concept that operative myocardial revascularization may provide a significant degree of protection from subsequent myocardial infarction in the patient with symptomatic coronary artery disease. It seems reasonable to extend this concept to include patients who are not symptomatic from coronary artery disease but previously have had one or more myocardial infarctions. In the present series, 3 such patients in the younger age group underwent myocardial revascularization in the hope that this will afford them protection against the probability of further myocardial infarction. In this situation, the operative risk has to be weighed against (1) the risk of further occlusion of the involved vessels with the probability of myocardial infarction and (2) the effectiveness of myocardial revascularization in preventing myocardial infarction. The latter is unknown and the answer can come only from clinical experience.

Selection of an appropriate myocardial revascularization procedure for the individual patient depends upon a number of factors, including (1) the number of major coronary arteries involved with estimated hemodynamically significant disease, (2) the location and character of the occlusive disease in each vessel and its anatomic accessibility, (3) the estimated left ventricular functional capacity, (4) the presence or absence of a left ventricular aneurysm or akinetic area and (5) the presence or absence of intercoronary collaterals and their location.

Although indirect myocardial revascularization using internal mammary artery implantation, or a variant thereof, could be uniformly selected as applicable for all patients undergoing coronary artery surgery, it is questionable whether this procedure is the most effective. Experimental studies have indicated there is little or no effective forward flow through acutely implanted internal mammary arteries which could contribute to coronary blood flow at the time of operation.[3] Gaining an immediate increase in coronary blood flow undoubtedly may be very important in patients with severe coronary artery disease, particularly if they have had a previous myocardial infarct or have a reduced left ventricular functional capacity. Although chronic internal mammary implants provide an extra cardiac source of arterial blood to the coronary circulation via collaterals, the actual proportion of the coronary blood flow supported by the implant and its physiologic significance may be questionable.[1] Direct coronary arterial reconstruction has the advantage of immediately increasing coronary blood flow. Blood flow through coronary artery bypass grafts has been determined intraoperatively using electromagnetic flow probes with a finding of flow rates in the range of 40 to 150 ml. per minute.[16]

The decision regarding applicability of direct coronary arterial reconstruction for a given patient is derived primarily from the findings of coronary angiography. Two criteria must be satisfied: (1) the involved vessel must be anatomically accessible and (2) the vessel must be patent distally with acceptable runoff. The right coronary artery is accessible from its point of origin distally to the proximal 2 to 3 cm. portion of the posterior descending branch located inferiorly in the right atrioventricular groove. The anterior descending artery is accessible throughout its entire length on the anterior surface of the heart. The anatomic approach to these vessels is best gained through a median sternotomy although the anterior descending artery may also be approached from a left thoracotomy. The main left coronary artery can be approached satisfactorily only from a left thoracotomy. The circumflex artery is the most inaccessible but may be exposed in the left atrioventricular groove over its proximal 3 to 4 cm. from a left thoracotomy. It usually is necessary to ligate and divide the great cardiac vein which overlies it distally in the left atrioventricular groove.

Although scattered atherosclerotic disease involving the terminal branches of the major coronary arteries is nearly always evident on coronary arteriography of patients with symptomatic coronary artery disease, the majority of these patients have significant proximal segmental occlusive disease in one or more major vessels. If this disease is located within anatomically accessible areas of the major vessels and if the vessel is patent distally at an accessible point as determined angiographically, it will be amenable to a direct reconstructive procedure. Acceptable runoff of the involved vessel is difficult to define but precludes major occlusion or stenosis in the vessel distal to an anatomically accessible area. If intercoronary collaterals are present between the involved vessel distally and terminal branches of another major coronary artery, this is good evidence of adequate runoff. Prominent intercoronary collaterals which were judged to indicate adequate runoff of the involved vessel were noted in 16 of the 21 patients in the present series.

Endarterectomy was selected as the procedure of choice if the occlusive disease was focal (not extending over 1 cm. in length), easily accessible anatomically and if the vessel proximally and distally was minimally involved by disease and 5 mm. or greater in diameter. In this series, 8 endarterectomy procedures were done, 7 involving a relatively large right coronary artery in its midproximal portion. The one remaining endarterectomy was of the main left coronary artery requiring patch angioplasty. Patch angioplasty was required only twice for right coronary endarterectomy. In the other 5 patients, meticulous closure of the arteriotomy did not result in narrowing of the vessel. Focal obstructing lesions located at the origin of the right coronary artery were not considered amenable to endarterectomy because proximal control could not be obtained without cross-clamping the aorta.

Although 5 internal mammary–coronary artery bypass procedures were done early in this series, this technique has now been omitted in favor of the reversed saphenous vein aortocoronary bypass graft. The saphenous vein segment is larger, less friable and technically easier to handle. Larger anastomoses may be accomplished with the vein graft and because of the larger size and lack of vasoconstriction there is less resistance in the bypass graft. Size discrepancy has not been a problem, and with the vein graft, there is no restriction in length. Use of the saphenous vein aortocoronary bypass graft also allows implantation of both internal mammary arteries as a complementary procedure.

Acute intraoperative flow studies were accomplished in 8 of the 21 procedures. Graft blood flow through the internal mammary-coronary artery bypass grafts was an average of one-half to one-third the flow obtained with reversed saphenous vein aortocoronary bypass grafts in comparable situations.[16]

A reversed saphenous vein aortocoronary bypass graft was selected as the procedure of choice for revascularization of the right coronary artery when the occlusive disease was at the origin or in the midproximal portion and not limited to less than 1 cm. in length or if the artery was less than 5 mm. in diameter. The vein graft is now the procedure of choice in all cases of revascularization of the anterior descending or circumflex arteries.

Because of the high incidence of scattered disease involving major coronary artery branches other than those revascularized by a direct reconstructive procedure, complementary internal mammary artery implants were placed in intramyocardial tunnels in 20 of the 21 cases in this series. In 15, double implants have been used. The implants were placed whenever possible in areas where collaterals had been noted in the angiogram.

In each of 3 patients in this series, direct arterial reconstruction of two major coronary arteries was undertaken because of near total occlusion of both vessels by proximal segmental disease. In all 3 patients reconstruction involved the RCA and ADA.

The methods used to protect the myocardium against ischemia during the time of coronary arterial reconstruction appear to be very important. These consist of profound cardiac hypothermia and distal coronary artery perfusion. Even though distal coronary arterial perfusion can be achieved throughout most of the time of direct surgery on the involved coronary artery, there is an irreducible brief period of time when perfusion cannot be accomplished and profound cardiac hypothermia affords protection against this period of ischemia. Although brief, this period of time may be significant in a heart with marginal coronary blood flow. Both of these methods for myocardial protection were used in 16 patients of this series with only one operative death occurring in a patient with end stage coronary artery disease and left ventricular failure undergoing left ventricular aneurysmectomy and double saphenous vein bypass grafts to nearly occluded right coronary and anterior descending arteries. Intraoperative myocardial infarction occurred in all 5 patients early in this series where myocardial protection was not used and resulted in 3 deaths, although in 2 patients the operative risk was known to be inordinately high because of severe multivessel disease, left ventricular aneurysm, and left ventricular failure. In contrast there were only 3 intraoperative myocardial infarctions, one of which resulted in death, in the 16 patients protected by profound cardiac hypothermia and distal coronary artery perfusion.

SUMMARY AND CONCLUSIONS

1. Clinical experience with 21 patients undergoing direct coronary arterial revascularization for proximal segmental coronary artery occlusive disease over an 18 month

period has been reviewed. The operative mortality for the over-all group was 19 percent.

2. Criteria for patient selection for direct coronary artery reconstruction is based upon accurate coronary angiography, left ventricular angiography, and complete cardiac hemodynamic assessment by left and right heart catheterization. The clinical categories of patients with coronary artery disease which have been considered for direct myocardial revascularization included (1) intractable angina, (2) previous myocardial infarction in an asymptomatic patient in the younger age group, (3) intractable angina with cardiac failure, and (4) cardiac failure without angina.

3. Selection of an appropriate myocardial revascularization procedure for the individual patient depends upon (1) the number of major coronary arteries involved with estimated hemdynamically significant disease, (2) the location and character of the occlusive disease in each vessel and its anatomic accessibility, (3) the estimated left ventricular functional capacity, (4) the presence or absence of a left ventricular aneurysm or akinetic area, and (5) the presence or absence of intercoronary collaterals and their location.

4. Endarterectomy was selected as the procedure of choice for focal ($\leq$ 1 cm.) disease limited to the midproximal right coronary artery and if the vessel proximally and distally is minimally involved by disease and is 5 mm. or greater in diameter.

5. A reversed saphenous vein aortocoronary bypass graft was selected as the direct revascularization procedure of choice for proximal segmental occlusive disease of the anterior descending artery, the circumflex artery, and the right coronary artery if the occlusive disease was at the origin, in the midproximal portion but not focal, or if the vessel was less than 5 mm. in diameter.

6. Profound cardiac hypothermia and distal coronary artery perfusion as a method of myocardial protection during direct coronary arterial reconstruction has been shown to be important in decreasing the incidence of intraoperative myocardial infarction and mortality rate.

REFERENCES

1. Barner, H. B., Kaiser, G. C., Mudd, J. G., Jellinek, M., and Hanlon, C. R.: Internal mammary artery implantation. Effects upon coronary flow and ventricular function, J. Thorac. & Cardiov. Surg. **56:** 43, 1968.
2. Baroldi, G., Mantero, O., and Scomazzoni, G.: The collaterals of the coronary arteries in normal and pathologic hearts, Circ. Res. **4:** 223, 1956.
3. Carlson, R. G., Edlich, R. F., Landé, A. J., Bonnabeau, R. C., Gans, H., and Lillehei, C. W.: A new concept for the rational of the Vineberg operation for myocardial revascularization, Surgery **65:** 141, 1969.
4. Diethrich, E. B., Liddicoat, J. E., Kinard, S. E., and De Bakey, M. E.: An analysis of operated and non-operated patients with documental coronary arterial disease, J. Thorac. & Cardiov. Surg. **57:** 115, 1969.
5. Diethrich, E. B., Liddicoat, J. E., Kinard, S. A., Garrett, H. E., Lewis, J. M., and De Bakey, M. E.: Surgical significance of angiographic patterns in coronary arterial disease, Circulation **35:** 155, 1967. (Suppl. 1.)
6. Dilley, R. B., Cannon, J. A., Kattus, A. A., MacAlpin, R. N., and Longmire, W. P., Jr.: The treatment of coronary occlusive disease by endarterectomy, J. Thorac. & Cardiov. Surg. **50:** 511, 1965.
7. Effler, D. B., Groves, L. T., Sones, F. M., Jr., and Shirey, E. K.: Endarterectomy in the treatment of coronary artery disease, J. Thorac. & Cardiov. Surg. **47:** 98, 1964.
8. Effler, D. B., Groves, L. K., Suarez, E. L., and Favaloro, R. G.: Direct coronary artery surgery with endarterotomy and patch-graft reconstruction. Clinical application and technical considerations, J. Thorac. & Cardiov. Surg. **53:** 93, 1967.
9. Effler, D. B., Sones, F. M., Jr., Favaloro, R. G., and Groves, L. K.: Coronary endarterotomy with patch-graft reconstruction. Clinical experience with 34 cases, Ann. Surg. **162:** 590, 1965.
10. Favaloro, R. G.: Saphenous vein autograft replacement of severe segmental coronary artery occlusion, Ann. Thorac. Surg. **5:** 334, 1968.
11. Favaloro, R. G., Effler, D. B., Groves, L. K., Sones, F. M., Jr., and Ferguson, D. J. G.: Myocardial revascularization by internal mammary artery implant procedures, J. Thorac. & Cardiov. Surg. **54:** 359, 1967.
12. Gorlin, R., and Taylor, W. J.: Selective revascularization of the myocardium by in-

ternal mammary artery implant, New Eng. J. Med. **275:** 283, 1966.
13. Green, G. E., Stertzer, S. H., and Reppert, E. H.: Coronary arterial bypass grafts, Ann. Thorac. Surg. **5:** 443, 1968.
14. Kerth, W. J.: Aorto-coronary bypass grafts, J. Thorac. & Cardiov. Surg. **57:** 487, 1968.
15. Linton, R. R.: Some practical considerations in the surgery of blood vessel grafts, SURGERY **38:** 817, 1955.
16. Mundth, E. D.: Unpublished data.
17. Nathan, M., Mundth, E. D., Buckley, M. J., and Austen, W. G.: A new method for the placement of epicardial atrial pacing electrodes, J. Thorac. & Cardiov. Surg. In press.
18. Sawyer, P. N., Kaplitt, M., Sobel, S., Karlson, K. E., Studkey, J., Wechsler, B. M., Summers, D. N., and Dennis, C.: Experimental and clinical experiences with coronary gas endarterectomy, Arch. Surg. **95:** 737, 1967.
19. Sewell, W. H.: Results of 122 mammary pedicle implantations for angina pectoris, Ann. Thorac. Surg. **2:** 17, 1966.
20. Sokol, D. M., Mundth, E. D., and Austen, W. G.: Optimal levels of coronary perfusion pressure during cardiopulmonary bypass, Surg. Forum. In press.
21. Sones, F. M., Jr., and Shirey, E. K.: Cine coronary arteriography, Mod. Conc. Cardiov. Dis. **31:** 735, 1962.
22. Taylor, R. S.: The significance of left intraventricular pressure during early resuscitation after temporary total myocardial ischaemia. Presented at the joint meeting of The Society of University Surgeons, Surgical Research Society and the European Society for Experimental Surgery, London, July, 1969.

DISCUSSION

Dr. William Neville (Hines, Ill.). Dr. Hanlon, Members, and Guests: Our group at Hines agrees with the principles outlined by the Boston group, in so far as the reversed saphenous vein graft is concerned for revascularization of the heart. This procedure is certainly better if it can be performed rather than doing an internal mammary implant, since it permits immediate vascularization of the myocardium. In the beginning we tried to do the vein graft without initially placing the patient on cardiopulmonary bypass, believing that this should lessen the period of extracorporeal circulation. However, it's much easier when the pump oxygenator is used throughout the entire procedure in order to attain a relatively quiet operative field.

In the past nine months, we have had a modest series of 14 patients in whom it was possible to perform an aorta-coronary artery vein bypass. Thirteen individuals are living and well at the present time; one patient died in the immediate postoperative period. In this group, we did 12 right aorta-coronary vein grafts. In 2 patients, vein grafts were placed in the anterior descending branch of the left coronary artery. Of the 14 patients, 12 had internal mammary implants and three had a concomitant ventricular aneurysmectomy. We also believe that distal perfusion of the coronary artery is necessary and for this purpose an ordinary 14 or 15 gauge Intra-Cath is used with an extension to pressure and flow monitored coronary perfusion pump.

Unfortunately, in only about 50 percent of the patients can one perfuse the distal coronary artery because there is some element of obstruction beyond that area. If the pressure rises or flow cannot be obtained the coronary perfusion is discontinued but the Intra-Cath is left in the distal artery. This facilitates performing the distal anastomosis. Thus there is some advantage in placing a catheter in the tiny distal coronary artery even though the coronary artery cannot be perfused.

Dr. George Green (New York, N. Y.). I enjoyed the paper very much.

At New York University, we have been pursuing the same goal in a somewhat different way.

Dissections of arteriosclerotic coronary arteries in the morgue have convinced me that the segments of the coronary tree that usually remain normal are very small in diameter, about 1.5 mm., so we've gone directly to the use of the operating microscope.

I'd like to describe the patients we've seen.

Thirty-six patients have been referred for consideration for operation, had angiograms, and have been scheduled for surgery. Of those patients, 7 died between the time they were scheduled for operation and the time that operation would have taken place.

Most of these patients have had several previous infarctions and angina at rest and almost half of them have had clinical congestive heart failure as well.

Following operation, 4 patients died in the hospital. One patient died 5 months following operation.

The operation performed was direct coronary anastomosis to the anterior descending coronary artery in 29 patients. The anastomosis was done about 2 inches from the apex of the heart, using the operating microscope at 16 magnifications and 9-0 monofilament nylon sutures.

In 26 cases the internal mammary artery was used as a graft and in 3 instances vein grafts were interposed from the ascending aorta to the distal anterior descending. Twelve of these patients also had vein grafts to the distal right coronary.

In almost all of the patients, there was a complete proximal occlusion and distal perfusion has not been performed during the operation.

Our flow studies show that flow through the internal mammary artery and the vein grafts have been very similar. The mammary artery flow averaging about 50 ml. per minute and the vein grafts running about 70 ml. per minute.

We've had much better luck with the mammary artery anastomosis than with the vein graft. Going back about 18 months, in the 26 patients who have had mammary artery anastomoses, only one has had a recurrence of any angina.

This patient is also the only patient who had an intraoperative infarction. I'm not certain when it took place. He was having unusually severe angina the morning of operation, and it may not have been related to my manipulation of his coronary arteries.

Two of the 3 patients who had vein grafts to the anterior descending have had a recurrence of angina, one at 18 days and one at about 3 months.

They are still improved. They both also had anastomoses to the distal right coronary artery, so that may be what has maintained improvement.

Dr. W. Sterling Edwards (Birmingham, Ala.). I enjoyed very much Dr. Mundth's paper and I think we're heading in an exciting new direction.

I rise to support Dr. Green's approach to direct surgery of the left anterior descending coronary artery, using real operating microscopic technique and very small 9-0 nylon suture. He has convinced me that end-to-side anastomosis of the left internal mammary to the distal left anterior descending coronary near the apex of the heart can be done with the heart fibrillating without undue difficulty. The great advantages of this technique are: (1) Almost all patients with angina and a diffusely obstructed left anterior descending coronary still have a widely patent distal bed with good runoff. (2) Temporary occlusion of a 1 cm segment of the coronary at this level to perform the anastomosis causes little or no permanent myocardial damage without a shunt and with only mild hypothermia (28°). (3) End-to-side anastomosis allows perfusion both ways, both proximal and distal, so that distal anastomosis is the preferred and safest technique even in proximal obstructions.

I believe the mammary is a better conduit for the left anterior descending than a saphenous vein bypass. The mammary is larger than the coronary and there is even greater disproportion if a vein is used. Use of the vein requires two anastomoses whereas the mammary requires only one. Because the right coronary is much larger than the left, aorto-coronary vein bypass is probably preferable in right coronary obstruction.

Review of the coronary arteriograms in our patients who have undergone mammary implants for left coronary obstruction have convinced us that almost all would have been candidates for a distal mammary coronary shunt with the advantage of immediate revascularization rather than delayed and somewhat uncertain revascularization.

Six consecutive patients have successfully undergone this operation, 4 had aorto-right coronary vein bypass at the same time and all have done well.

Dr. Paul Field (Sudbury, Ont., Canada). I rise to congratulate the speakers and also to emphasize that this operation does have tremendous value in the patient who has been assessed as being a bad operative risk by currently accepted criteria.

We have operated on 22 cases in the last eight months and many of these have preoperatively shown a Grade 3 or 4 ventriculogram. We think that some of these patients have muscle that just cannot contract because it has no blood supply.

We think that some of these so-called akinetic areas are not actually areas of myocardial fibrosis, but portions of muscle that just have an inadequate blood supply and therefore cannot work.

May I have the first slide, please?

[Slide] This slide shows what we have been doing. The aorta is at the top. A reversed saphenous vein graft is crossing over the right atrium and going into the right coronary at the acute margin of the heart. The lower anastomosis is shown.

We have done all with cardiopulmonary bypass. We have used anoxic arrest for short periods, particularly for reconstruction of the left anterior descending coronary artery.

Next slide, please!

[Slide] This is a typical postoperative angiogram where you can see the upper anastomosis. Selective injection is made into the graft and here it is filling the dominant right coronary and passing down the posterior descending coronary artery to the apex of the heart.

We have had 2 deaths in the series of 22 patients. The most dramatic observation has been the tremendous improvement from this "instant revascularization." This has been seen in a few different ways: A patient may require support with a pump oxygenator while the chest is being opened. We have had 2 patients who required such support immediately following induction of anesthesia because of hypotension. In these 2 patients, we exposed the femoral artery and femoral vein before induction because the possibility of this hypotension was anticipated. Yet, these and all the other patients came right off bypass without any difficulty, and this we attribute to the improvement in the coronary blood flow.

We have found significant reduction in the values of the left ventricular and diastolic pressure. For example, one patient who had a pressure of 58 mm. Hg—the highest in the series—dropped to 30 mm. Hg postoperatively. Many people with a level of 30 mm. Hg dropped to a normal range.

The left ventriculogram has improved and we have found a decrease in heart size in patients with cardiac enlargement.

I would therefore try to contribute this one thing—that a patient having a poor left ventriculogram and other untoward criteria rendering him unsuitable for internal mammary implantation should not be rejected for this operation because he may well end up with a very good heart. This may be because muscle which could not contract before will now be able to work due to a better blood supply.

Dr. Mundth (closing). I would like to thank the various discussants for their comments. I certainly agree with Dr. Neville that cardiopulmonary bypass is necessary for myocardial protection during direct coronary arterial reconstructive procedures. About 50 percent of our patients had lesions of the left coronary artery which, in the past, has been associated with a considerable mortality. Improved methods for myocardial protection and for coronary arterial reconstruction have lessened the risk, however. Interestingly, Dr. Neville reported three aneurysmectomies associated with direct vascular reconstruction. We have had experience with 5 patients similarly treated. These patients had angina in addition to left ventricular failure which I think is an indication for direct revascularization in addition to aneurysmectomy. When left ventricular failure is the only manifestation of the ventricular aneurysm, we have preferred to limit the surgery to aneurysmectomy alone.

I was interested in Dr. Green's comments. In our study, intraoperative bypass graft flow studies were obtained in 8 patients, these being equally divided between internal mammary artery bypass and vein bypass grafts. In comparable situations, there was a mean blood flow of 50 ml. per minute for the internal mammary bypass grafts and 100 ml. per minute in vein grafts.

Because of the frequency of severe occlusive disease involving the major coronary artery branches proximally, we have found that bypass of the anterior descending artery frequently can be accomplished in the mid portion or even the mid proximal portion rather than distally. Unquestionably, the most important criteria for determining where the bypass graft should be anastamosed to the coronary artery is the presence or absence of disease in the coronary artery.

I would agree with Dr. Edwards that bypass grafts can be anastamosed to terminal branches of the anterior descending artery and consequently more patients may be selected for direct revascularization rather than an indirect procedure. The internal mammary artery would seem to be a reasonable selection for a bypass graft to these terminal branches of the coronary arteries. Certainly one can harvest the saphenous veins more distally in the leg and obtain a satisfactory sized vein for the purpose of bypass grafting without having problems as far as size discrepancy.

Dr. Field emphasized that many patients undergoing direct revascularization were seriously ill prior to operation. We had to use exposure to the femoral vessels under local anesthesia in 4 patients in the series reported and one patient required partial circulatory assistance at an early phase of the operative procedure.

Reappraisal of adjuncts to avoid ischemia in the treatment of thoracic aortic aneurysms

E. STANLEY CRAWFORD, M.D.
JAMES M. FENSTERMACHER, M.D.
WILLIAM RICHARDSON, M.D.
FRANK SANDIFORD, M.D.
HOUSTON, TEXAS
From the Cora and Webb Mading Department of Surgery, Baylor College of Medicine and the Surgical Service of the Methodist Hospital

Ischemic damage of the spinal cord was not uncommon in the early days of excisional therapy of thoracic aortic aneurysm. This led to development and application of various methods to prevent this complication, including hypothermia, simple external and internal shunts, and pump bypass shunts, including left atriofemoral artery and femoral vein to femoral artery, using a pump oxygenator. Consequent to the application of these techniques, the incidence of ischemic damage to the spinal cord and other organs beyond the region of operation is thought to have been reduced. The first sizable series of thoracic aortic aneurysms treated by excisional therapy employing these techniques was presented in 1958 by De Bakey and associates[3] and, using left atriofemoral artery bypass, 2 (5.5 percent) of 36 patients developed partial paraplegia after operation. Austen and associates[1] in 1967 reported no cases of paraplegia occurring in 23 patients with dissecting aortic aneurysm treated by excision of the origin of dissection employing the same technique. In the same year, Neville and associates[11] reported no incidence of distal organ damage following thoracic aortic operation in 18 patients using femoral vein to femoral artery bypass with pump oxygenator. Dillon, Young, and Sealy[4] reported in 1967 no distal organ damage in 31 patients in whom the thoracic aorta was cross clamped for elective excisional therapy; femoral vein to femoral artery pump oxygenator bypass was employed in 21, left atriofemoral artery bypass in one, and hypothermia in 9 patients. Kahn, Vathayanon, and Sloan[9] in 1968 reported a series of 13 patients using an external shunt and distal organ damage was avoided.

These reports are very encouraging indeed; however, Bloodwell, Hallman, and Cooley[2] in 1968 reported the development of partial paraplegia in 3 (17.6 percent) of 17 patients submitted to operation using the more recently developed idea of femoral vein to femoral artery bypass technique. A close scrutiny of these studies would indicate that the discrepancy lies primarily in the fact that Bloodwell, Hallman, and Cooley's series contained a higher percentage of more extensive aneurysms with more pressing indications for operation. Thus, it may be assumed that distal organ damage possibly varies with a number of factors, including the nature and extent of disease; type and extent of treatment, including methods to protect organs distal to operation; and duration of aortic clamping. The purpose of this report is to present the senior author's entire experience in the treatment of thoracic aortic aneurysms of all types and manifestations arising beyond the left subclavian artery, and to compare results in patients in whom various shunts

Supported in part by United States Public Health Service Grant HE-0-5435.

Presented at the Twenty-third Annual Meeting of the Society for Vascular Surgery, New York, N. Y., July 12-13, 1969.

were employed with those in whom no shunts or other protective methods were used.

CLINICAL MATERIAL

During the period between Dec. 12, 1956, and March 17, 1969, excisional therapy was employed in 58 patients with aneurysm of the thoracic aorta arising distal to the left subclavian artery. During the first 10 years of this experience, some type of bypass was employed to protect the organs, especially the spinal cord, distal to operation, and also to reduce left ventricular strain from proximal aortic occlusion (Table I). During the latter part of this period, temporary bypass occasionally was not employed; either because the method had to be abandoned for technical reasons at the time of aortic clamping or because operation was employed for rupture and time did not permit institution of bypass. The results in the latter cases appeared to be as good as in the former and the operation less complicated. For these reasons, operation has been routinely employed without bypass during the past 2 years. Thus, this series of cases is divided into two groups, an earlier one consisting of 38 cases in whom some type of bypass was used, except femoral vein to femoral artery bypass using pump oxygenator, and another or more recent group consisting of 20 patients in whom no bypass or other method of protection was employed (Table II).

The etiology of aneurysm in the two groups was similar except that there were no chronic dissecting aneurysms in the no-shunt group (Table III). The location and extent of operation again was similar, but with some differences (Fig. 1). Approximately half the patients in both groups had operation limited to the proximal one third of the descending thoracic aorta (Figs. 2-4). Most of the descending thoracic aorta was replaced in 25 percent of the no-shunt group and 34 percent in the shunt group (Figs. 5 and 6). Lower thoracic or thoracoabdominal aneurysms were replaced in 6 patients without shunts and in 5 patients with shunts. The entire descending thoracic and abdominal aorta was excised in 2 patients with chronic dissecting aortic aneurysms in the latter group, employing permanent bypass grafts to which the major visceral arteries were attached in both. In one case a button of posterior wall of uninvolved aorta, from which arose two large lumbar arteries at the level of the fourth lumbar vertebra, was also attached as suggested by Spencer and Zimmerman.[12]

Operation, regardless of aneurysm etiology,

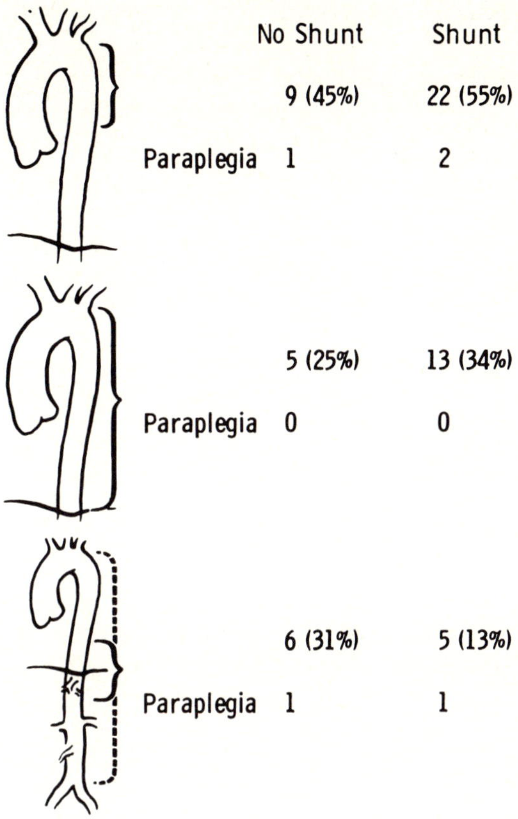

Fig. 1. Location of aneurysm and incidence of paraplegia in 58 cases.

Table I. *Descending thoracic aortic aneurysm results according to type of shunt (38 cases)*

Type of shunt	*No. of cases*	*Deaths*	*Paraplegia*
Left atriofemoral	28	4	2
Internal shunt	2	1	0
External shunt	8	3	1
Total	38	8	3

Table II. *Descending thoracic aortic aneurysm clinical data in patients treated without shunts (20*

Case No.	Sex	Age	Aneurysm: Type	Aneurysm: Extent	Operation: Indication	Operation: Type
1	M	63	Fusiform	Lower thoracic abdominal	Elective	Replacement
2	F	52	Traumatic	Upper thoracic	Elective	Replacement
3	M	54	Saccular	Upper thoracic	Elective	Resection
4	F	64	Fusiform	Descending	Elective	Replacement
5	M	62	Saccular	Upper thoracic	Elective	Replacement
6	F	36	Marfan	Descending thoracic Upper abdominal	Elective	Replacement
7	F	67	False	Lower thoracic	Hemorrhage	Repair
8	M	70	Fusiform	Descending	Pain	Replacement
9	M	63	Sacciform	Mid descending	Elective	Replacement
10	M	68	Dissecting	Descending	Elective	Replacement
11	M	58	Traumatic	Upper thoracic	Acute	Repair
12	M	65	Dissecting	Thoracoabdominal	Rupture	Replacement
13	M	68	Fusiform	Distal thoracic	Elective	Replacement
14	F	62	Fusiform	Descending	Elective	Replacement
15	M	77	Dissecting	Thoracoabdominal	Paraplegia major artery occlusion	Replacement thoracic and abdominal
16	M	66	Fusiform	Descending	Rupture	Replacement
17	M	58	Fusiform	Descending	Elective	Replacement
18	M	68	Saccular	Descending	Elective	Replacement
19	F	62	Fusiform	Lower thoracic Upper abdominal	Elective	Replacement
20	M	43	Fusiform	Lower thoracic Upper abdominal	Elective	Replacement

Table III. *Type of aneurysm and incidence of paraplegia (58 cases)*

Type	No shunt: Cases No.	No shunt: Cases %	No shunt: Paraplegia No.	No shunt: Paraplegia %	Shunt: Cases No.	Shunt: Cases %	Shunt: Paraplegia No.	Shunt: Paraplegia %
Dissecting	3	15	1	33*	14	37	3	21
Acute	3					9		2
Chronic						5		1†
Arteriosclerotic	13	65	1	7	21	55		
Trauma	2	10			3	8		
Syphilis	1	5						
Marfan's syndrome	1	5						
Total	20	100	2	10	38	100	3	8

*Paraplegia before operation.

†Entire aorta replaced from subclavian to iliac arteries.

cases)

Aortic occlusion time	Operative time	Transfusion	Complication	Results
13 min.	1 hr., 40 min.	5	None	Survived
24 min.	2 hr., 40 min.	18	Postoperative bleeding	Survived
12 min.	3 hr.	5	None	Survived
18 min.	2 hr., 15 min.	6	None	Survived
11 min.	1 hr., 45 min.	6	None	Survived
33 min.	3 hr., 30 min.	7	None	Survived
10 min.	2 hr.	10	None	Survived
19 min.	2 hr., 30 min.	4	None	Survived
12 min.	2 hr., 30 min.	4	None	Survived
34 min.	2 hr., 50 min.	4	None	Survived
6.5 min.	2 hr., 20 min.	4	None	Survived
64 min.	5 hr.	24	Cerebral insufficiency	Died p.o. 2
27 min.	2 hr., 50 min.	7	None	Survived
14 min.	2 hr., 5 min.	5	None	Survived
17 min.	2 hr., 15 min.	9	Paraplegia renal failure	Died p.o. 2
46 min.	3 hr.	13	Paraplegia pulmonary emboli	Died p.o. 9
20 min.	2 hr., 55 min.	4	None	Survived
10 min.	2 hr., 15 min.	4	None	Survived
33 min.	2 hr., 50 min.	5	None	Survived
34 min.	6 hr.	8	None	Survived

Table IV. *Results according to indications for operation (58 cases)*

Indication	Cases No.	Cases %	Deaths No.	Deaths %	Paraplegia (No.)
Emergency					
No shunt	5	25	3	60	2*
Shunt	8	21	4	50	2
Elective					
No shunt	15	75	0		0
Shunt	30	79	4	13	1
Total	58	100	11	19	5 (8.6)

*Paraplegia before operation in one case.

was considered elective if performed during the regular operative schedule after appropriate study and preparation. Operation was considered and performed as an emergency in the presence of progression of dissection, major vessel occlusion producing ischemic changes, airway compression, or signs of rupture. The indication for operation was virtually the same in the two groups of cases (Table IV). It is considered significant that 2 patients had paraplegia as a symptom at the onset of aortic dissection. This symptom

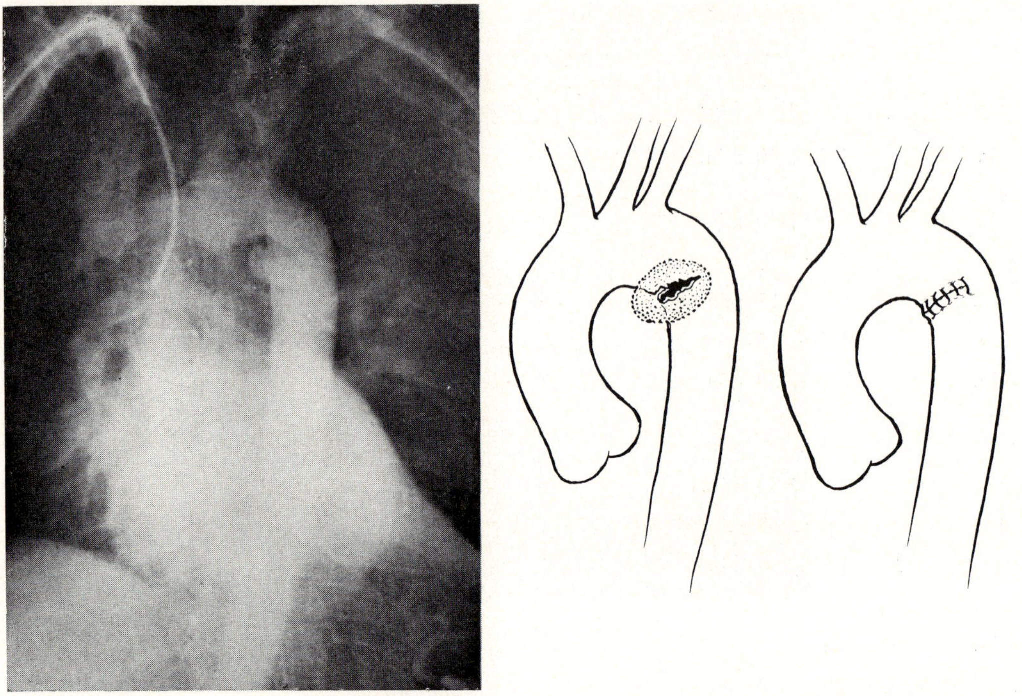

Fig. 2. Angiogram and diagrams showing excision and primary repair of acute laceration of aorta resulting from blunt trauma without shunt. Aortic occlusion time and operating time 6.5 minutes and 2 hours and 20 minutes, respectively. Patient doing well.

Table V. *Operating time (58 cases)*

Time (hr.)	*No shunt*			*Shunt*		
	Cases		*Paraplegia No.*	*Cases*		*Paraplegia (No.)*
	No.	*%*		*No.*	*%*	
1 - 2	3	15		1	3	
2 - 3	14	70	2	10	26	1
3 - 4	1	5		17	45	
4 - 5	1	5		4	11	
	1	5		3	8	1
6 - 7				3	8	1
Total	20	100	2 (10%)	38	100	3 (8%)

Table VI. *Aortic occlusion time (58 cases)*

Time (min.)	*No shunt*				*Shunts*			
	Cases		*Deaths (No.)*	*Paraplegia (No.)*	*Cases*		*Deaths (No.)*	*Paraplegia (No.)*
	No.	*%*			*No.*	*%*		
5 - 10	1	5	0	0	0			
10 - 15	6	30	0	0	0			
15 - 30	7	35	1	1*	13	34	2	
30 - 60	5	25	2	1	17	45	4	1
60 - 120	1	5			8	21	2	2
Total	20	100	3 (15%)	2 (10%)	38	100	8 (21%)	3 (8%)

*Paraplegia before operation.

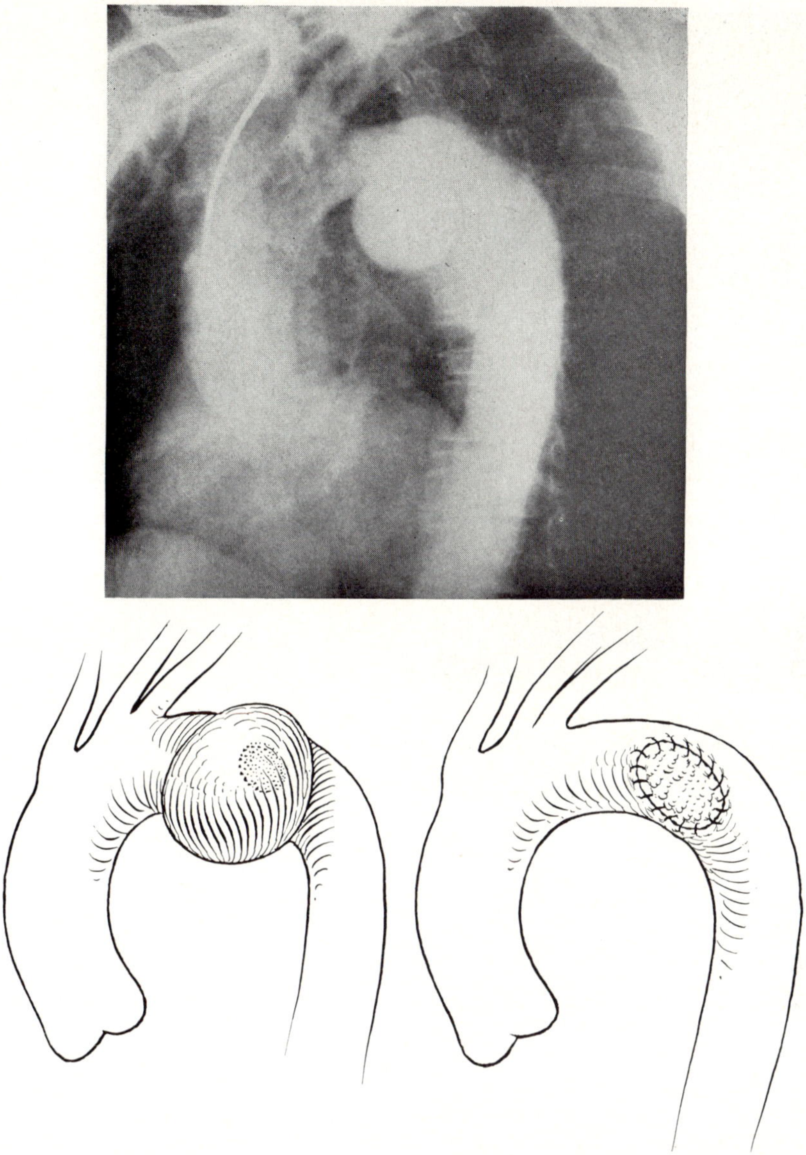

Fig. 3. Angiogram and diagrams showing excision and patch graft repair of saccular aneurysm of aorta without shunt. Aortic occlusion time and operating time 11 minutes and one hour and 45 minutes, respectively. Patient doing well.

cleared in one patient before operation, but not in another patient, submitted to operation without a shunt because of major artery obstruction.

TECHNIQUE OF OPERATION

The majority of patients in the shunt group had total excision of aortic circumference and graft replacement of the aneurysm, after ligation and division of the intercostal and lumbar arteries arising from the involved segment using shunts shown in Table I. More limited operation was performed in 3 patients; excision and patch graft replacement of saccular aneurysm in 2 and excision and end-to-end anastomosis in one patient. Similar limited procedures were performed in five of the no shunt group; saccular aneu-

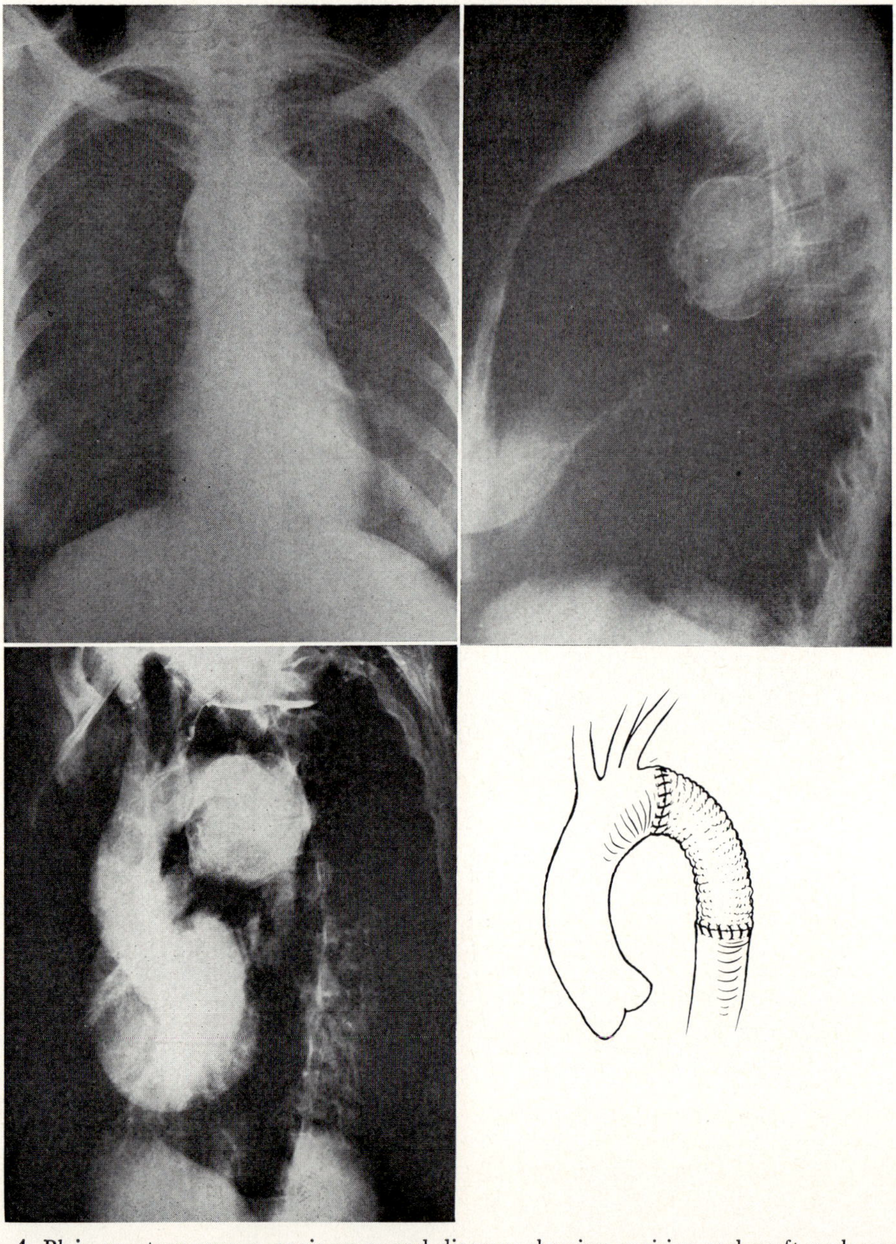

Fig. 4. Plain roentgenograms, angiogram, and diagram showing excision and graft replacement of traumatic aneurysm of thoracic aorta without shunt. Aortic occlusion time 24 minutes and total operating time 2 hours and 40 minutes. Patient doing well.

rysms were replaced with large patch grafts in three (Fig. 3), and end-to-end anastomosis was performed in two patients (Fig. 2). Total circumferential replacement was performed in the remainder of this group, including 5 (25 percent) patients in whom the entire descending thoracic artery was replaced (Fig. 4 through 6). There was, however, a major difference in the method of replacement in the majority of the no-shunt cases. Exposure of the involved aortic segment was facilitated in many cases by complete collapse of the left lung using a double-lumen Carlens endotracheal tube.

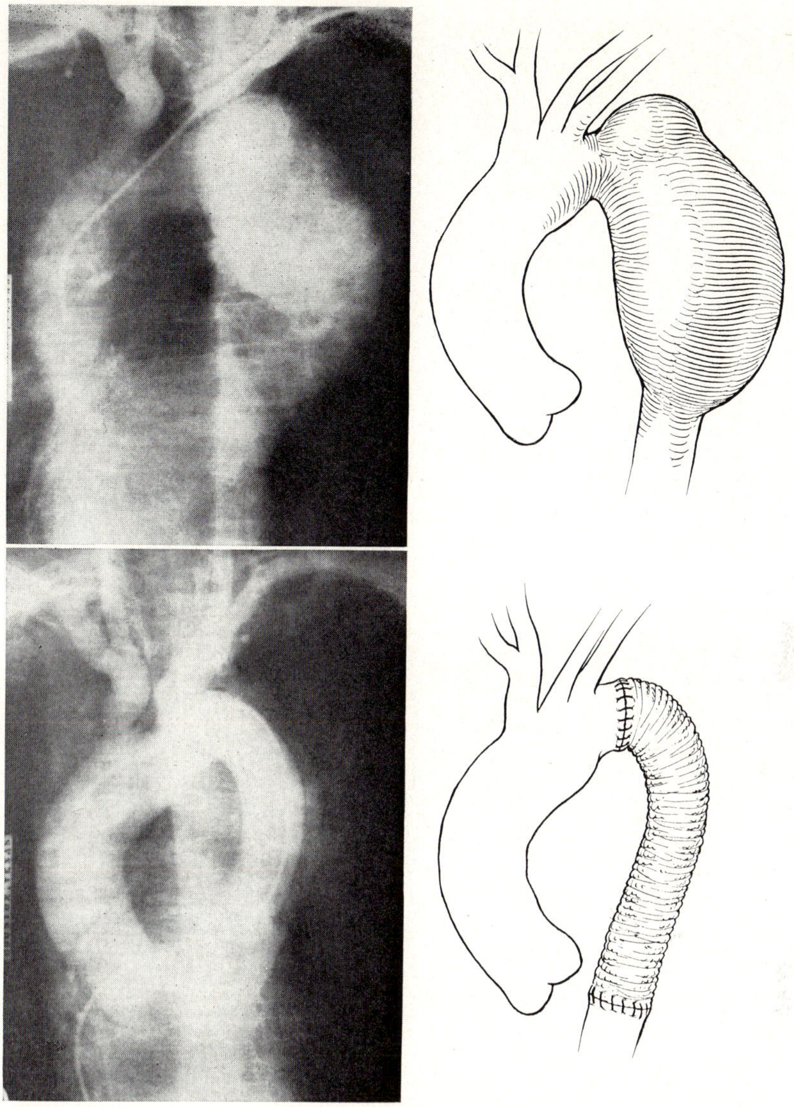

Fig. 5. Angiograms and diagrams made before and after operation showing excision and graft replacement of extensive aneurysm involving descending thoracic aorta without shunt. Aortic occlusion time 20 minutes and operating time 2 hours and 55 minutes. Patient doing well.

Most intercostal and lumbar arteries arising from the involved segment were ligated but not divided. The aorta was clamped proximal and distal to the aneurysm. The aneurysm was not excised but opened longitudinally, clot removed, and bleeding intercostal arteries suture ligated. The graft was then inserted by end-to-end anastomosis; the intima of aneurysm removed; and finally, the outer layer of aneurysm sutured around the graft. This technique saved time and reduced operative bleeding (Tables II and V).

Proximal blood pressure and pump flow were monitored in patients in whom atrio-femoral bypass was employed. The proximal blood pressure was maintained at normal levels by rates of flow varying from 1,200 to 3,000 c.c. per minute. This was not always possible in the emergency group because of reduced blood volume, due either to rupture

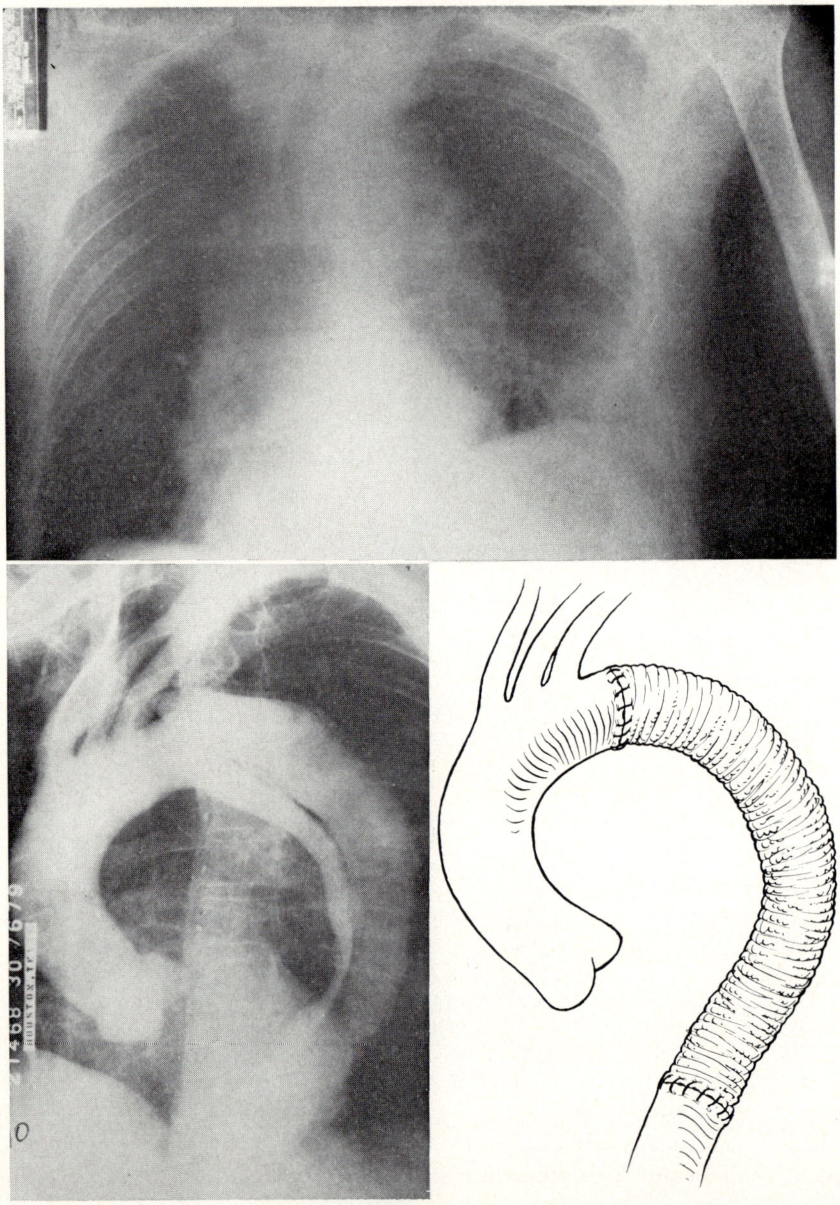

Fig. 6. Plain roentgenogram, angiogram, and diagram showing excision and graft replacement of extensive chronic dissecting aneurysm of descending thoracic aorta without shunt. Aortic occlusion time 34 minutes and operating time 2 hours and 50 minutes. Patient doing well.

or excessive hemorrhage during operation. Proximal blood pressure was monitored in the no-shunt group and hypertension controlled during aortic clamping with narcotics, halothane, and, when necessary, D-tubocurarine. Aortic occlusion time in the no-shunt patients varied from 7 to 64 minutes. Occlusion time was less than 30 minutes in 70 percent of the cases and less than 46 minutes in 18 (90 percent) patients (Table VI). Aortic occlusion time in the shunt group varied from 20 to 95 minutes, with only 34 percent being clamped less than 30 minutes. This difference was due more to technique of operation and

Table VII. *Blood transfusion (58 cases)*

Transfusions (500 c.c.)	*No shunt*		*Shunt*	
	No.	*%*	*No.*	*%*
1 - 5	10	50	2	5
5 - 10	6	30	21	55
10 - 15	2	10	9	24
15 - 20			6	16
20 - 25	2	10		
Total	20	100	38	100

Table VIII. *Cause of death after treatment (58 cases)*

Cause	*No shunt*	*Shunt*
Cerebral	1	
Renal failure	1	
Pulmonary embolus	1	1
Myocardial infarct		4
Hemorrhage		3
Total	3 (15%)	8 (21%)

operative experience at the time than extent of disease. Both due to the presence of a normal clotting mechanism (lack of heparin administration) and the shortened operation, 50 percent of patients in the no-shunt group received less than five transfusions, compared with only 5 percent in the shunt group (Table VII).

RESULTS

The results of treatment varied with a number of factors, including complications of the disease leading to operation, the type of aneurysm, and the method of operation. Of the 58 patients submitted to operation 47 (81 percent) patients survived. The survival rate was 85 percent for the no-shunt group and 79 percent for the series in which shunts were employed. The survival in patients submitted to emergency operation was 40 percent in the former and 50 percent in the latter. All 15 patients submitted to elective operation without the use of a shunt survived; and 87 percent of patients in whom shunts were employed for elective operation survived. The cause of death was myocardial infarction in 4, hemorrhage in 3, pulmonary embolus in 2, renal failure in one, and cerebral disturbances in one patient (Table VIII).

DISTAL ORGAN DAMAGE

Partial paraplegia was present in one patient before and after operation and in 4 other patients after operation; a total of 5 (8.6 percent) patients. The first-mentioned patient had acute dissection of the entire descending thoracic and abdominal aorta. Paraplegia in this case was considered due to his disease. Thus, the real incidence of spinal cord ischemia associated with operation in this series is considered to be 6.8 percent. Of the 4 patients developing this condition during operation, 3 were submitted to emergency operation, revealing diffuse dissecting aortic aneurysms in 2 cases and ruptured arteriosclerotic aneurysm of the descending thoracic aorta in one case. Partial paraplegia was present after elective operation in one of the 2 patients, in whom the entire descending thoracic and abdominal aorta was replaced for chronic dissection and dilatation. Death, resulting from factors other than neurological dysfunction, occurred in 3 of the 5 patients with paraplegia. The remaining 2 walk with crutches.

Paraplegia was present in 2 (10 percent) patients submitted to emergency operation without shunt. Since paraplegia was present in one patient before operation, the authors feel that paraplegia resulted from factors occurring during operation in only one (5 percent) case submitted to operation for rupture of arteriosclerotic descending thoracic aortic aneurysm. It is considered significant that none of the elective operations done without a shunt was associated with either death or paraplegia. Partial paraplegia occurred in 3 (8.6 percent) patients submitted to operation for dissecting aortic aneurysms using shunts; in 2 patients after emergency operation using atriofemoral bypass, and in one after extensive aortic removal without reattachment of either intercostal or lumbar arteries. Thus, paraplegia was either present or occurred in patients with acute extensive dissecting aortic aneurysms requiring extensive resection, in a hypotensive patient with rupture of lower thoracic aneurysm, and in a patient in whom the entire descending thoracic and abdominal aorta was removed.

Aortic occlusion time in patients developing paraplegia during operation was 46 minutes in the patient in whom no shunt was used and 55, 92, and 95 minutes, respectively, in 3 patients submitted to operation with a shunt. In the former group of patients aortic occlusion time was less than 46 minutes in all except one in whom the aorta was clamped for 64 minutes (Table II). Paraplegia did not occur in this case. Renal failure from bilateral renal artery obstruction occurred in one patient with acute dissecting aortic aneurysm which involved both renal arteries and was not corrected by operation. Detectable signs of transient or persistent distal organ ischemia, other than in the spinal cord, did not occur in any patient as a result of aortic clamping for operation in either group of patients.

DISCUSSION

Visceral organ damage did not occur as a result of operation in the series of 20 patients in whom shunts were not employed. Temporary periods of aortic clamping ranging from 6½ to 64 minutes were well tolerated. Thus, interruption of descending thoracic aortic blood flow for operation should, in itself, rarely if ever be a factor in distal organ ischemic damage except the spinal cord, provided that damage has not already occurred from the aneurysmal process and provided that branch occlusion is not produced by embolism. More likely causes for visceral organ damage during such operations are long periods of systemic hypotension and hemolysis resulting both from transfusion reactions and from trauma in the bypass apparatus.

The cause for spinal cord damage occurring during operation in these cases is not at all clear, but this series of cases suggests that the permanent removal of the blood supply to a segment of the spinal cord is considerably more of a factor than temporary aortic clamping. The blood supply of the lower spinal cord normally is derived from the intercostal and lumbar arteries. Occlusion of some of these vessels by the disease process is common and varies with the duration and extent of the process. Significant, in this regard, is the fact that approximately 10 percent of patients admitted for acute dissecting aortic aneurysms have a history of transient paraplegia. Of the 12 patients in this study, two had this history. Moreover, paraplegia—as reported by others—was persistent in one case.[7] Thus, it must be assumed that the blood supply to the lower spinal cord in patients with descending thoracic aortic aneurysms is abnormal and by collateral circulation arising from sites unknown, unpredictable, and undeterminable by the surgeon. Additional evidence of the possible limited blood supply to the lower cord is evident by the development of paraplegia by ligation of lumbar artery in the performance of sympathectomy, during replacement of abdominal aortic aneurysm, and in patients with thrombosis of the abdominal aorta.[6, 8] Thus, the more extensive the resection, the more acute the disease process, and the more limited the origins of collateral, the more likely operation may be associated with paraplegia as a result of permanent removal of the blood supply. It is considered significant that 4 of the 5 patients in this series had extensive resections for dissecting aortic aneurysm. In fact, as previously indicated, all of the aorta beyond the left subclavian artery was resected in 2 patients and this complication occurred in the patient in whom neither intercostal nor lumbar arteries were attached to the graft.

The systemic blood pressure has been shown in animals to be the most important factor controlling blood flow in the vessels of the spinal cord.[5] Paraplegia has been observed in man following periods of hypotension.[10] Thus, systemic hypotension may be a factor in the development of this complication in some patients submitted to lower thoracic aortic aneurysm operation. Of the 4 cases developing paraplegia during operation in this study, 3 patients were submitted to emergency operation (one without shunt and two with shunts) associated with periods of hypotension.

It is difficult to prove that temporary clamping alone of a segment of descending thoracic aorta involved by aneurysm will result in paraplegia and no attempt to deny it is made; however, this study appears to indicate that periods of occlusion up to 46 minutes are well tolerated. Moreover, with refinements in technique available today, aneurysmal removal and aortic repair can be accomplished with periods of aortic occlusion within this period of time. Considering the advantages of shortened operation, less blood loss, and the lack of need for special equipment, along with its special complications, the thoracic vascular surgeon may consider selection of cases for temporary bypass. It would seem more important to recommend operation electively, limit the extent of resection, preserving every possible intercostal and lumbar artery, and when extensive resections are performed, reattach either lumbar or intercostal artery to the graft.

Finally, since paraplegia occurred in this series of patients in whom shunts were employed after 46 minutes, namely, 55, 92, and 95 minutes, respectively, in the 3 patients developing this complication, it could be argued that the shunt technique increased the period during which the aorta could be safely clamped temporarily. The fallacy of this argument lies in an analysis of the 3 cases. All three patients had diffuse dissecting aneurysm of the lower thoracic aorta. The entire aorta beyond the left subclavian artery was removed in one, and extensive resections of the descending thoracic aorta was removed for rupture in the other 2 patients. Therefore, paraplegia more likely occurred from permanent deprivation of cord blood supply in these cases than from temporary aortic clamping.

SUMMARY

Distal organ ischemic damage has occurred with varying frequency during operations on the descending thoracic aorta despite the use of various methods of protection including hypothermia and temporary bypass techniques during the period of aortic clamping required for operation. A number of factors obviously contribute to these complications and the true value of the protective techniques are not known. This report is concerned with the author's entire experience in the treatment of descending thoracic aortic aneurysm to compare results in patients in whom various shunts were employed with those in whom no shunts or other protective methods were used.

During the period between Dec. 12, 1956, and March 17, 1969, excisional therapy was employed in 58 patients. Earlier, some type of bypass shunt was employed in 38 cases and, more recently, 20 patients were submitted to operation without shunt. The indications for operation, the type of aortic lesion, and the location and extent of operation was similar in the two groups, although the entire descending thoracic and abdominal aorta was replaced in 2 of the former and persistent paraplegia was present at operation in one of the latter cases of acute diffuse dissecting aortic aneurysm.

Graft replacement was the most common treatment employed. The lesion was circumferentially excised and replaced in the earlier cases using shunts. In the later cases in which shunts were not employed, the tube graft was inserted into the aneurysm by end-to-end anastomosis to proximal and distal normal segments through a longitudinal incision after removing clot. The outer layers of aneurysm were then sutured around the graft. Aortic occlusion time in the former varied from 20 to 95 minutes, with only 34 percent being clamped less than 30 minutes. Operation required over three hours in 69 percent of the cases and 95 percent of the cases required more than five blood transfusions. Aortic occlusion time in the latter cases was less than 30 minutes in 70 percent of the cases and operation completed in less than 3 hours in 85 percent of the cases using less than five blood transfusions in 50 percent of the patients.

Of the 58 patients submitted to operation

47 (81 percent) patients survived, 85 percent of the no-shunt group and 79 percent in the shunt group. All 15 patients submitted to elective operation without the use of a shunt survived and 87 percent of patients in whom shunts were used for elective operation survived.

Paraplegia developed during operation in 4 patients (6.8 percent); one in the no-shunt group, submitted to operation for rupture of descending thoracic aortic aneurysm, and 3 in the shunt group, submitted to extensive resection for complications of dissecting aortic aneurysm. Ischemic damage of other organs was not produced by operation in any case.

A critical study of these cases suggests that the most important factors producing paraplegia using present excisional techniques are the amount of aorta excised, the number of its branches ligated, and the nature and extent of disease rather than the period of cross clamping of the aorta required for operation. The dangers of paraplegia are much greater following extensive resection for dissecting aortic aneurysm because the disease process itself obliterates both intercostal and lumbar arteries. Excisional therapy of an extensive nature may include removal of collateral routes of cord circulation and produce ischemic damage. Extensive resections in such cases may benefit from reattachment of intercostal or lumbar arteries. The latter is mandatory in cases where the entire descending thoracic and abdominal aorta is excised.

REFERENCES

1. Austen, W. G., and De Sanctis, R. W.: Dissecting aneurysm, Surg. Clin. N. Amer. **46:** 573, 1966.
2. Bloodwell, R. D., Hallman, G. L., and Cooley, D. A.: Partial cardiopulmonary bypass for pericardiectomy and resection of descending thoracic aortic aneurysms, Ann. Thorac. Surg. **6:** 46, 1968.
3. De Bakey, M. E., Cooley, D. A., Crawford, E. S., and Morris, G. C., Jr.: Aneurysms of the thoracic aorta: analysis of 179 patients treated by resection, J. Thorac. Surg. **36:** 393, 1958.
4. Dillon, M. L., Young, W. G., and Sealy, W. C.: Aneurysms of the descending thoracic aorta, Ann. Thorac. Surg. **3:** 430, 1967.
5. Field, E. J., Graysen, J., and Roger, A. F.: Observations on the blood flow in the spinal cord of the rabbit, J. Physiol. (Lond.) **114:** 56, 1951.
6. Hara, M., and Lipin, R. J.: Spinal cord injury following resection of abdominal aortic aneurysm, Arch. Surg. **80:** 419, 1960.
7. Hill, C. S., and Vasquez, J. M.: Massive infarction of spinal cord and vertebrae bodies as a complication of dissecting aneurysm of the aorta, Circulation **25:** 997, 1962.
8. Hughes, J. T., and Macintyre, A. G.: Spinal cord infarction occurring during thoracolumbar sympathectomy, J. Neurol. & Neurosurg. Psychiat. **26:** 418, 1963.
9. Kahn, D. R., Vathayanon, S., and Sloan, H.: Resection of descending thoracic aneurysms without left heart bypass, Arch. Surg. **97:** 336, 1968.
10. Madow, L., and Alpers, B. J.: Involvement of the spinal cord in occlusion of the coronary vessels, Arch. Neurol. & Psychiat. **61:** 430, 1949.
11. Neville, W. E., Cox, W. D., Leininger, B., and Pifarre, R.: Resection of the descending thoracic aorta with femoral vein to femoral artery oxygenation perfusion, J. Thorac. & Cardiov. Surg. **56:** 39, 1968.
12. Spencer, F. C., and Zimmerman, J. M.: The influence of ligation of intercostal arteries on paraplegia in dogs, Surg. Forum **9:** 340, 1958.

DISCUSSION

Dr. J. Harold Harrison (Atlanta, Ga.) I certainly enjoyed this paper, and Dr. Crawford and his associates are to be congratulated on this worthwhile and timely presentation. We have operated on five aneurysms of the descending thoracic aorta utilizing this technique with similar results.

One patient having a recurring dissecting aneurysm died. An extensive endarterectomy was done extending from the subclavian to below the renal arteries. Death was due to cardiac complications not felt related to the period of occlusion. We have occluded the descending thoracic aorta in these patients for periods of 17 to 30 minutes without the development of spinal cord paralysis. Most of the spinal arteries occluded are in the area of involvement and will be ligated in the process of resecting the aneurysm. I doubt that this technique, providing the period of occlusion is kept below 45 minutes, will significantly increase this problem. The advantages of greater simplicity and avoiding the use of a bypass apply here as in any other area of surgery.

I cannot help but take this opportunity to say a few words regarding the numerous discussions yesterday on the merits of shunts for protection of the brain while operating on carotid arteries.

We have, during the past 11 years, operated upon over 2,500 cerebral arteries going through the varying stages that you have over the years heard reported at these meetings. We have gradually abandoned the use of shunts of any variety and now don't even have them in the operating room. It is my feeling that shunts in arterial surgery will ultimately become obsolete.

Dr. Max Gaspar (Long Beach, Calif.). Dr. Crawford mentioned that cord damage also occurs with operations on the abdominal aorta. We have had a little experience with this. We have had 5 cases of our own. There have been 8 others reported in the literature.

The anterior spinal artery is a long artery that is very tenuous throughout its course, becoming small particularly just before the major anterior radicular artery joins it. This usually comes in at about D_{12} but can be down as low as L_4.

The anterior spinal artery supplies most of the anterior portion of the cord sparing only a portion of the posterior portion.

When the anterior spinal artery is occluded the findings are paraplegia, incontinence, loss of deep tendon reflexes, loss of superficial sensation, and loss of superficial pain and light touch; but deep pain, vibratory sense, and position sense are preserved.

Of the 13 cases that have been reported, 8 have been ruptured abdominal aortic aneurysms, 3 in elective resection of aneurysms and 2 in occlusive aortic disease.

[Slide] This was a patient with occlusive disease. A bypass graft was used. We didn't recognize until later that there were huge lumbar arteries showing on the aortogram. These turned out to be the major supply to the spinal cord. They became occluded during the operation and the patient was paraplegic after operation.

We have concluded that if an aortogram has been done, it should be studied for large lumbar arteries. One of them might be the major anterior radicular artery because it can occur as low as L_4. All large lumbar arteries should be preserved if possible.

There has been a combination of suprarenal aortic clamping and hypotension in a large majority of these patients (most of them because they have ruptured aneurysms) and this combination should be avoided.

Dr. Rodman E. Taber (Detroit, Mich.). I'd like to compliment Dr. Crawford and his associates on this nice presentation and excellent illustrations.

We, too, have seen spinal cord paralysis in patients having left heart bypass, but we have preferred to ascribe this to operative sacrifice of intercostal vessels, rather than inadequate left heart bypass.

If I can show the first of three slides [Slide], I'd like to demonstrate some other reasons why we think left heart bypass shouldn't be given up completely. This data was gathered experimentally by one of our residents in the laboratory using left heart bypass in dogs.

If one is to provide something approximating a physiologic perfusion state when the descending aorta is clamped, it is necessary to bypass in the neighborhood of 70 percent of left heart output. Otherwise, left heart distention, left atrial hypertension, and pulmonary congestion, etc. will of course follow if the clamping is carried on sufficiently long.

The next slide shows that in this experimental data, bypass of even 60 c.c. per kilogram per minute in some animals with the aorta clamped may result in marked elevations in left atrial pressure.

Here is the original end diastolic pressure in the left ventricle before aortic clamping. Here, it's beginning to climb after clamping even with flow rates of 40 to 60 c.c. per kilogram per minute, and the only time when it didn't do this was when we failed to maintain normovolemia in the animal and therefore he had a reduced cardiac output.

The final slide shows a way that we prefer doing left heart bypass, which we've called arbitrarily a variable bypass flow rate. We monitor left atrial pressure and maintain the flow rate according to what is required to keep atrial pressure within normal limits. To maintain a normal left atrial pressure may require on occasions flow rates getting up to 80, 90, and even 100 c.c per kilogram per minute.

Granted that if the patient is hypovolemic, these pressure changes will not be present because output is low. However, we think that the variable bypass to maintain a normal atrial pressure is a little more of a physiologic situation.

Dr. W. G. Austen (Boston, Mass.). I would like to make just two brief comments.

We certainly agree with Dr. Crawford as to conserving as much thoracic aorta as possible. For example, in the treatment of dissecting thoracic aneurysms, we try very hard to remove only the area of origin of the dissection.

I would like to ask Dr. Crawford a question regarding renal problems. I wonder what his thoughts are specifically in the older age group who have marginal renal function. We worry particularly in these cases and try to maintain as normal a distal perfusion pressure to the kidneys as possible. Even very short periods of distal hypotension may cause acute tubular necrosis in patients with significant renal arteriosclerosis.

Dr. Donald R. Kahn (Ann Arbor, Mich.). I would like to congratulate Dr. Crawford on an excellent paper. Dr. Crawford's tremendous speed in resecting thoracic aneurysms must play an important part in preventing a higher incidence of spinal cord ischemia.

We should be cautious about giving up perfusion of the distal aorta during aortic cross clamping for thoracic aortic aneurysms. Experimental evidence shows that paralysis from spinal cord ischemia starts only after 20 to 30 minutes of aortic cross clamping and increases in incidence thereafter.

For the past 3 years we have operated upon 20 patients with thoracic aortic aneurysms and 6 patients with a traumatic rupture of the aorta with the use of a temporary bypass. The bypass consists of Tygon tubing connected with two metal cannulas. One of the cannulas is placed in the ascending aorta and another distal to the aneurysm. No heparinization is required as clotting does not occur as long as flow exists in the bypass shunt. Sufficient flow is maintained to prevent paraplegia as long as a 9 mm. cannula is used. In only one of the 26 patients did a paresis occur, and in this patient a 7.5 mm. cannula had been used.

Dr. Crawford (closing). I would like to thank the discussants for their kind remarks and additional knowledge which they have given to the subject and would like to recognize the fact that there are other very eminent individuals who could have contributed equally as well to the discussion had they not been so modest.

For example, in the paper on thoracic aneurysms published by De Bakey in 1958, he reported upon 4 patients submitted to operation without shunts. Dr. Neville had rather extensive experience using femorofemoral pump oxygenator bypass shunts with great success.

Dr. Kahn's method of bypass is intriguing both because it is simple and the fact that it does not require heparinization. The latter, of course, eliminates the bleeding problems in general and hemorrhagic lung problems in particular. If it is as simple as it sounds, this may be the ideal way to eliminate problems requiring temporary occlusion of the thoracic aorta.

I, like the other discussants, have found my greatest problems in the acute emergency cases and I am relieved to hear this to be their experience. My biggest problems, however, have been in the dissected aortic group, and I have been an admirer of the good results achieved by Dr. Gerald Austen. I have enjoyed all of his papers, and it is my suspicion that the key to his success is the fact that he has been conservative in aortic resection. I think it should be pointed out that he very meticulously identifies the origin of the dissection using angiographic technique, and he limits grafting placements to this area. Thus, he does a conservative resection and preserves the maximum number of intercostal arteries, which conforms to one of the principles recommended in this paper.

I cannot answer Dr. Austen's question regarding the patients with renal artery disease and impaired renal function because in general these will be in the high-risk category in many instances. In general, however, I think this study presented today would indicate that, with the exception of the spinal cord, no particular concern should be given to the circulation in the distal organ systems.

The case for the early closure of a patent ductus arteriosus

JAMES W. KILMAN, M.D.
HOWARD D. SIRAK, M.D.
H. WILLIAM CLATWORTHY, Jr., M.D.
JOSEPHA CRAENEN, M.D.
DON M. HOSIER, M.D.
COLUMBUS, OHIO
From the Division of Thoracic Surgery, Department of Surgery, and Division of Pediatric Cardiology, Department of Pediatrics, Ohio State University College of Medicine

The early closure of the patent ductus arteriosus has not become an established procedure, and certain standard textbooks in thoracic surgery and pediatric cardiology still suggest that the ideal time for operative intervention is between 6 years and 12 years of age. Clatworthy and McDonald,[5] in 1958, proposed that the patent ductus arteriosus should be closed before the age of 5 years in asymptomatic children and in children who are symptomatic the operation should be done as soon as the diagnosis is established. This policy has been used at the Children's Hospital, Columbus, Ohio, since that time. The concept was designed to reduce the morbidity and mortality in early infancy from the cardiorespiratory effects of patent ductus arteriosus and to eliminate the effects of this anomaly on growth patterns and to prevent complications from this lesion such as fixed pulmonary hypertension. This review was made to evaluate the influence of the early closure of the patent ductus arteriosus on growth patterns and to determine any effect that this concept has had on operative morbidity and mortality in the infant age group at our hospital.

Presented at the Twenty-third Annual Meeting of the Society for Vascular Surgery, New York, N. Y., July 12-13, 1969.

PATIENT MATERIAL

All of the patients admitted to the Children's Hospital, Columbus, Ohio, with the sole diagnosis of patent ductus arteriosus from 1950 to 1967 were included in the review. The diagnosis was proved by cardiac catheterization, autopsy, or at the time of operation in each case. All included cases had no other cardiac or pulmonary anomaly. There were 306 patients that fulfilled these criteria. Thirteen patients did not have surgery. Five of these had spontaneous closure of a ductus previously demonstrated by cardiac catheterization. Five infants died prior to operation. All of the infants that died were admitted to the hospital in a moribund state and prior to 1961. All 5 died of unrelenting congestive failure. Three patients were shown to have reversal of their shunt by cardiac catheterization. Closure of the ductus was not done in any of these patients with evidence of shunting right to left through the patent ductus arteriosus.

A rubella infection or exposure history in the mother was noted in 12 percent of the patients. Twenty percent of the patients were noted to be premature infants. There was a familial history of patent ductus arteriosus available in 3 percent of the patients. There was one family with 5 children, all

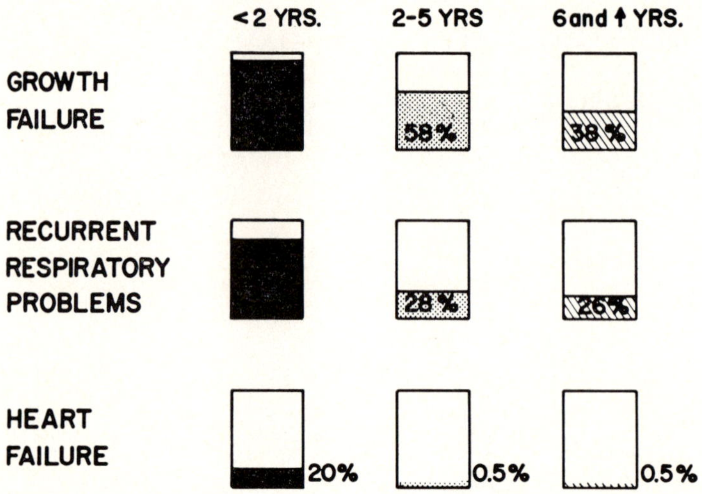

Fig. 1. Manifestations of growth failure, recurrent respiratory problems, and heart failure noted in infants and children with patent ductus arteriosus.

having patent ductus arteriosus. There was one set of identical twins with patent ductus arteriosus and one of brother and sister siblings with this anomaly. One patient's father had his patent ductus resected 18 years previously at three years of age and one patient's mother had her patent ductus arteriosus repaired following the repair of her son's anomaly.

Manifestations of growth failure, recurrent respiratory problems, and heart failure were most commonly noted in the group of patients below 2 years, but were also present in the older children (Fig. 1). These manifestations were quite incapacitating in the infant group below 2 years of age. Eleven newborn infants or neonates were admitted to the hospital in profound congestive failure and severe distress. All of these patients were refractory to medical therapy and were successfully managed by an emergency surgical procedure. One hundred and ten of the 306 patients were at or below the tenth percentile on an anthropometric chart for weight. Ninety-two percent of the infants below 2 years of age fell in this group. Twenty infants having closure of their ductus in infancy and 20 infants closed after 2 years of age had a comparison of percentile change in weight during a 5 year follow-up period. These data show a definite increase in percentile weight in the group having operation before 2 years of age as compared to the group having operation after 2 years of age (Fig. 2).

Cardiac enlargement by x-ray examination, pulmonary hypertension by catheterization and an abnormal ECG were the most common findings in these patients with isolated patent ductus arteriosus. Sixty-two of the children had cardiac catheterization to aid in diagnosis and increased pulmonary resistance was noted slightly more often in the older children (Fig. 3).

In the period of time from 1950 to 1956, 18 percent of the patients had their operation prior to 2 years of age. In the last 7 years, 50 percent of the patients had the closure of their ductus prior to 2 years of age. In this same period of time, 80 percent of these anomalies have been repaired prior to 5 years of age (Fig. 4). This earlier closure time has not changed the mortality and the immediate postoperative complication rate remains at about 14 percent, mainly consisting of atelectasis. The infants have a postoperative complication rate of less than 7 percent.

All of the patients were operated upon without a death or a serious postoperative complication. Transection of the patent ductus arteriosus was used in all patients except

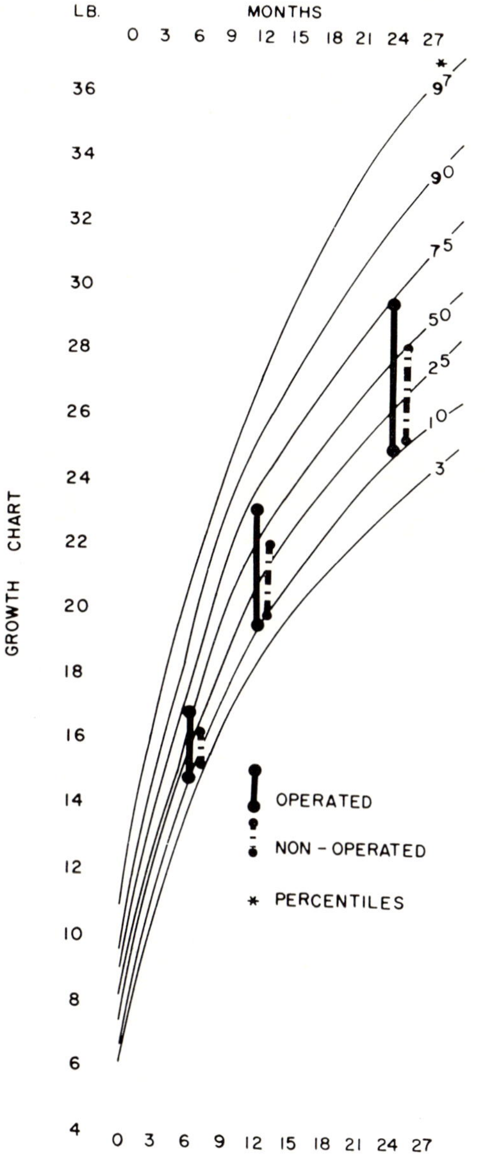

Fig. 2. An anthropometric chart for weight of children followed for 5 years (20 patients having their ductus closed prior to 2 years and 20 after 2 years of age). (Original mean percentile weights calculated at time of diagnosis in non-operative cases and at time of operation in the operative cases at 6 months, 12 months, or at 24 months.) Follow-up percentile weights at 5 years indicates that closing the patent ductus arteriosus prior to 2 years allows better growth.

2 who had ligation of their anomaly as an emergency. There was no instance in this series of a recurrent patent ductus arteriosus following the operative procedure.

DISCUSSION

Patent ductus arteriosus has been related to maternal rubella infections in the first trimester and this series supports this thesis with an incidence of 12 percent of the children having this history.[10] Lynch and associates[18] demonstrated that patent ductus arteriosus is probably a recessive familial anomaly. A familial history of patent ductus arteriosus was given by 3 percent of the patients reviewed. Prematurity has been associated with patent ductus arteriosus.[14] Twenty percent of this series had a history of prematurity. Powell[23] demonstrated that the incidence of patent ductus arteriosus in 400 cases reviewed was about the same in the prematures as in full-term infants. Danilowicz, Rudolph, and Hoffman[8] feel that delayed closure in premature infants may be associated with inadequate muscular development of the ductus of premature infants. Spontaneous closure of the ductus in the premature may be associated with high oxygen atmospheres in the Isolettes.[23] Spontaneous closure of the patent ductus arteriosus does occur as shown in the 5 cases in this series of patients. Mark and Young[20] have stated that in most cases if the ductus does not close within 2 months after birth, it will probably remain open.

The child with a patent ductus arteriosus may develop cardiac failure. The congestive failure seen with this lesion is most often seen in children under 2 years of age.[9] Five newborn infants with this anomaly died prior to operation due to unrelenting congestive failure. Newborn infants and neonates should be treated as surgical emergencies if the congestive failure cannot be controlled with medical management. Eleven infants under one month of age in unrelenting heart failure have had their patent ductus arteriosus divided with no mortality. Ziegler[30] has shown that the infant with the atypical ductus may be destroyed by this lesion. Those

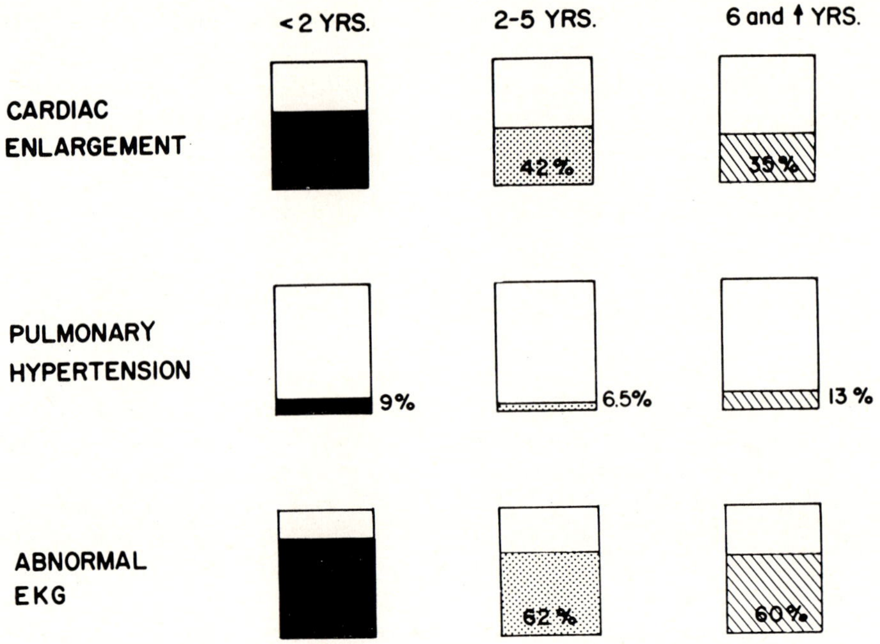

Fig. 3. The physical findings of infants and children with patent ductus arteriosus.

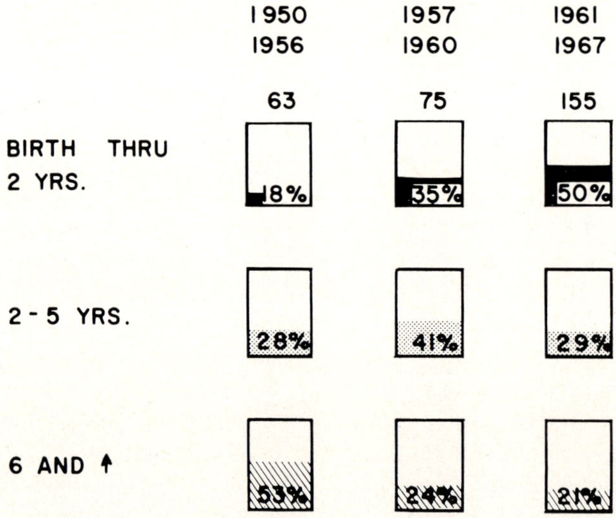

Fig. 4. The operative closure of the patent ductus arteriosus is done now at an earlier age with no increase in morbidity or mortality.

infants that are not destroyed have serious incapacity due to repeated cardiopulmonary problems and respiratory infections. Operative risk in the infant group is so low now that delaying operation until later childhood may subject the child to more hazard than the surgery in early infancy.

Adams and Forsyth[1] have shown that a patent ductus arteriosus diminished the rate of growth when the surgery was performed in late childhood. Growth failure is demonstrated in 92 percent of all of the patients below 2 years of age in this review and is present in a large percent of the older children with the diagnosis of patent ductus arteriosus. A review of 20 children repaired in early infancy and 20 repaired after 2 years of age demonstrates a greater increase in mean percentile weight attainment in the group repaired prior to 2 years of age with a 5 year follow-up in each of the groups (Fig. 2). This finding, with no increase in mortality due to early closure of the patent ductus arteriosus, should encourage the earlier closure of the anomaly by surgeons familiar with thoracic surgery in small infants (Fig. 4). It has been demonstrated by many authors[2, 3, 5, 9, 10, 12, 13, 16, 19, 28] that the patent ductus arteriosus can be closed in infants with the same mortality as in older children. This fact is more impressive when one realizes that infants have most of the symptoms that disable and are much more seriously ill than the older children. These infants actually have less postoperative morbidity than the older children especially if cared for by highly trained pediatric nurses in a special infant intensive care unit.

Cardiac enlargement by roentgenographic studies is present most commonly in the infants and seen frequently in the older children[6] (Fig. 3). Electrocardiograms are abnormal in a high percentage of the patients. This abnormality is usually left ventricular hypertrophy[26] (Fig. 3). Cardiac catheterization is not done as a routine in all patients, but in this series was done at times to aid in clinical diagnosis. No patient with evidence of a right-to-left shunt was taken to surgery. Several patients with balanced shunts or pulmonary hypertension were operated upon. The method of management in these patients was to clamp the ductus at the time of operation and if pressures in the pulmonary artery decreased slightly the ductus was closed. Sirak and Humphreys[25] have shown that the young individual with pulmonary hypertension tolerates closure of their ductus much better than the older child. Pulmonary hypertension in the majority of the patients below 2 years of age receded following operative closure of the patent ductus arteriosus, as shown by Dahl[6] and Tuuteri and Borkowska.[26] Only 3 children in this series demonstrated a reversal of their shunt contraindicating closure of the patent ductus arteriosus and in all cases this was found in patients well above 2 years of age. This late onset of fixed pulmonary hypertension again reflects the need for early closure of the patent ductus arteriosus.

The preferred method of closure of the patent ductus arteriosus in this series has been to transect it and oversew the ends. Two patients had ligation of the anomaly as an emergency. It has been stated that in all cases of patent ductus arteriosus the ductus should be divided and sutured. Others have championed simple multiple ligation as the safest approach. Wilcox and Peters[28] reported a large series of surgical closure of the patent ductus arteriosus in which both methods were used with no significant difference in mortality or morbidity related to the surgical procedure. Oldham and associates[21] reported a series of patients with giant patent ductus arteriosus in which there was an increased mortality in the patients who had ligation of the ductus. They also reported a higher incidence of aneurysm formation following ligation and a higher incidence of recurrence or recanalization of the ductus following ligation. There has been no mortality in this present series associated with the operative management. There has been no aneurysm formation or recurrence of the ductus noted in this group of patients.

Complications in the present group of operative patients have been minor. Pulmonary atelectasis and pneumonitis is frequent. Three patients were re-explored for bleeding with a good outcome. One chylothorax occurred that cleared with tube drainage. Earlier closure of the ductus has not increased the incidence of complications, in fact, the infants have a smoother postoperative course, seem to recuperate much more rapidly, and their frequency of pulmonary complications is less than in the older children in spite of the fact that the infants are more often in congestive failure and have a higher incidence of pulmonary hypertension when catheterized.

SUMMARY

The early surgical closure of the patent ductus arteriosus has been proposed and successfully used in a series of 306 patients. A method of management has been developed to surgically divide the patent ductus arteriosus of all patients with symptoms at the time of diagnosis and to close the patent ductus arteriosus of all asymptomatic patients prior to 2 years. Closure of the ductus in 115 infants in this series has resulted in no increased mortality, a slightly decreased morbidity and better growth and development of those children having closure of their ductus prior to two years of age. Early closure may be instrumental in preventing the development of fixed pulmonary hypertension which is more prevalent in the older child.

REFERENCES

1. Adams, F. H., and Forsyth, W. B.: Effect of surgery on growth of patients with patent ductus arteriosus, J. Pediat. **39:** 330, 1951.
2. Adams, P., Jr., Adams, F. H., Varco, R. L., Dammann, J. F., Jr., and Muller, W. H.: Diagnosis and treatment of patent ductus arteriosus in infancy, Pediatrics **12:** 664, 1953.
3. Anderson, R. C., Adams, P., Jr., and Varco, R. L.: Patent ductus arteriosus with reversal of flow: Clinical study of 10 children, Pediatrics **18:** 410, 1956.
4. Civin, H. W., and Edwards, J. E.: Postnatal structural changes in intrapulmonary arteries and arterioles, Arch. Path. **51:** 192, 1951.
5. Clatworthy, H. W., Jr., and McDonald, V. G., Jr.: Optimum age for surgical closure of patent ductus arteriosus, J. A. M. A. **167:** 444, 1958.
6. Dahl, G.: Ductus arteriosus with pulmonary hypertension: Physical findings in 20 children under the age of two years, Danish Med. Bull. **12:** 149, 1965.
7. Dammann, J. F., Jr., and Ferencz, C.: Vascular bed in congenital heart disease. III. Defects between ventricles or great vessels in which both increased pressure and blood flow may act upon lungs and in which there is common ejectile force, Amer. Heart J. **52:** 210, 1956.
8. Danilowicz, D., Rudolph, A. M., and Hoffman, J. I. E.: Delayed closure of the ductus arteriosus in premature infants, Pediatrics **37:** 74, 1966.
9. Gerbode, F., O'Brien, M. F., Kerth, W. J., and Robinson, S. J.: Surgical aspects of heart disease in infants under two years of age, Amer. J. Surg. **108:** 224, 1964.
10. Gross, R. E., and Longino, L. A.: Patent ductus arteriosus: Observations from 412 surgically treated cases, Circulation **3:** 125, 1951.
11. Gustafson, J. E., and Hill, L. F.: Patent ductus arteriosus in young infants, J. Iowa Med. Soc. **52:** 534, 1962.
12. Hara, M., Dungan, W. T., Lincoln, B. M., and McCutcheon, F. B.: Patent ductus arteriosus in early infancy, SURGERY **52:** 396, 1962.
13. Hardy, J. D., Webb, W. R., Timmis, H., Watson, D. G., and Blake, T. M.: Patent ductus arteriosus: Operative treatment of 100 consecutive patients with isolated lesions without mortality, Ann. Surg. **164:** 877, 1966.
14. Holman, E., Gerbode, F., and Purdy, A.: Patent ductus: Review of 75 cases with surgical treatment including aneurysm of ductus and one of pulmonary artery, J. Thorac. Surg. **25:** 111, 1953.
15. Hubbard, J. P., Emerson, P. W., and Green, H.: Indications for surgical ligation of patent ductus arteriosus, New Eng. J. Med. **221:** 481, 1939.
16. Krovetz, L. J., and Warden, H. E.: Patent ductus arteriosus: An analysis of 515 surgically proven cases, Dis. Chest **42:** 46, 1962.
17. Lindert, M. C. F., and Correll, H. L.: Rupture of pulmonary aneurysm accompanying patent ductus arteriosus: Occurrence in 67-year-old woman, J. A. M. A. **143:** 888, 1950.
18. Lynch, H. T., Grissom, R. L., Magnuson, C. R., and Krush, A.: Patent ductus arteriosus: Study of two families, J. A. M. A. **194:** 115, 1965.
19. Lyon, R. A., and Kaplan, S.: Patent ductus arteriosus in infancy, Pediatrics **13:** 357, 1954.
20. Mark, H., and Young, D.: Spontaneous closure of the ductus arteriosus in a young adult, New Eng. J. Med. **269:** 416, 1963.
21. Oldham, H. J., Jr., Collins, N. P., Pierce, G. E., Sabiston, D. C., and Blalock, A.: Giant patent ductus arteriosus, J. Thorac. & Cardiov. Surg. **47:** 331, 1964.
22. Payan, H., and Blaustein, A.: Aneurysm of the ductus arteriosus: Report of a case, Amer. J. Clin. Path. **44:** 449, 1965.
23. Powell, M. L.: Patent ductus arteriosus in premature infants, Med. J. Australia **2:** 58, 1963.
24. Ross, R. S., Feder, F. P., and Spencer, F. C.: Aneurysms of the previously ligated patent ductus arteriosus, Circulation **23:** 350, 1961.
25. Sirak, H. D., and Humphreys, G. H.: Atypical ductus: Physiologic and technical con-

siderations in its surgical therapy, SURGERY **41:** 112, 1957.
26. Tuuteri, L., and Borkowska, K.: Patent ductus arteriosus associated with pulmonary hypertension: Postoperative changes in the hemodynamics and in the electrocardiogram, Acta Paediat. **55:** 497, 1966.
27. Waterman, D. H., Samson, P. C., and Bailey, C. P.: Surgery of patent ductus arteriosus: Report of section on cardiovascular surgery, Dis. Chest **29:** 102, 1956.
28. Wilcox, B. R., and Peters, R. M.: The surgery of patent ductus arteriosus: A clinical report of 14 years' experience without an operative death, Ann. Thorac. Surg. **3:** 126, 1967.
29. Yauger, J. T.: Patent ductus arteriosus, J. Med. Ass. Georgia **52:** 337, 1963.
30. Ziegler, R. F.: Importance of patent ductus arteriosus in infants, Amer. Heart J. **43:** 553, 1952.

DISCUSSION

Dr. Arthur S. W. Touroff (New York, N. Y.). The paper which we have just heard concerning a large group of very young children suffering from patent ductus arteriosus, none of whom died following operation, is a fine achievement and reflects great credit on the surgeons involved. It also demonstrates how greatly the attitude of nonsurgeons has changed concerning the indication for operation over the years.

My interest in patent ductus arteriosus began early in 1940 but at that time few pediatricians and internists would turn over patients for operation until serious complications had already set in. Surgical treatment was considered to be a last resort rather than a means of protecting the patient against complications. The nonsurgeons, and even many well-informed surgeons, were of the opinion that once a complication had occurred when a young child was involved operation would invariably prove fatal.

Fortunately, it has now been demonstrated beyond question that young children and infants withstand major operation very well and often better than many of their elders.

As the authors have pointed out, failure of normal growth and development as well as cardiac failure are the two most common complications of patent ductus arteriosus. Both complications appear to be in direct proportion to the caliber of the ductus which in turn determines the volume of the left to right shunt. It should be stressed that interruption of blood flow within the ductus is a truly corrective procedure, for the surgeon accomplishes that which nature failed to do.

It is interesting to note that some adults who have a patent ductus arteriosus live out their normal life-span, are well developed, and do not suffer from cardiac failure. When a postmortem examination is performed upon such a person the ductus is found invariably to be of small caliber. Such a finding tends to support my personal opinion that the patient who has a patent ductus arteriosus of large caliber develops the well-known symptoms mentioned above very early in life.

A third complication and one which was not mentioned is the development of subacute bacterial endarteritis. A discussion of this complication of patent ductus arteriosus is not germane to the paper which we have just heard for the reason that foci of infection, usually close to the roots of the teeth, are not present in very young children and therefore such a complication is hardly to be expected. In passing it can be stated that all of the sulfonamides that were available in 1940 had absolutely no effect upon subacute bacterial endarteritis; today, however, antibiotics usually bring such infections under control promptly and the surgeon operates upon the patent ductus arteriosus when all evidence of sepsis has disappeared.

The lesson to be learned from the paper which the authors have presented so graphically today is that "the indication for operation in cases of patent ductus arteriosus is the very existence of a patent ductus arteriosus itself."

In an article in the July 15, 1949, issue of the *New York State Journal of Medicine* (pp. 1722-1726) I made the following statement: "The author is of the opinion that all children with patent ductus arteriosus, regardless of whether or not they present symptoms referrable to ductal patency, should be subjected to operation." At the time I was roundly criticized and met great resistance. I am grateful to the authors of the present paper for having vindicated me 20 years later, almost to the day.

Dr. Kilman (closing). I certainly appreciate Dr. Touroff's historical review and learned reflections on the subject and appreciate the opportunity to speak before this Society.

Cardiovascular effects of glucagon following cardiac surgery

CECIL C. VAUGHN, M.D.*
HOMER R. WARNER, M.D., PH.D.
RUSSELL M. NELSON, M.D., PH.D.
SALT LAKE CITY, UTAH
From the Surgical Research Laboratory, Latter-Day Saints Hospital, and the Department of Surgery, Latter-Day Saints Hospital, and the University of Utah

Glucagon, a polypeptide hormone produced by the alpha cells of the pancreas, has diverse physiologic actions. The hyperglycemic effect is well known. Other actions of glucagon include enhanced excretion of electrolytes and inhibition of gastrointestinal motility.[9] Recent work has demonstrated positive inotropic and chronotropic effects of glucagon on the heart.[3, 4, 5, 6, 13] Parmley, Glick, and Sonnenblick[8] and Linhart and associates[7] have studied the effects of glucagon in man at the time of cardiac catheterization, but the possible application of these hemodynamic effects following operation has not been reported. Therefore, this clinical study was undertaken to evaluate the cardiovascular effects of glucagon following cardiac surgical procedures.

METHODS

Glucagon† was administered on 25 occasions to 20 patients on the first postoperative day after various cardiac surgical procedures (Table I). Three patients received 3 mg., the others 10 mg. injected intravenously into a peripheral vein over a one minute period. Three patients received repeated injections of 10 mg. every 15 minutes up to one hour. Three studies were in patients with fixed rate cardiac pacing.

Following 6 base-line determinations at 5 minute intervals, glucagon was administered as described. The changes in stroke volume, heart rate, cardiac output, peripheral vascular resistance, and systolic and diastolic arterial pressures were monitored up to one hour by the computerized on-line pulse pressure wave analysis method of Warner and associates.[11, 12] Continuous electrocardiographic monitoring was utilized. Arterial blood gases, pH, and serum electrolyte changes were studied in 6 patients.

RESULTS

The stroke volume was increased in all but one patient. The maximal change of 16 ml. per stroke occurred without a rate increase in a patient with fixed rate cardiac pacing. The mean control level was 37 ml. per stroke, rising 19 percent to 44 ml. per stroke after glucagon. Diminished stroke volume after glucagon administration occurred in the patient who had excision of left ventricular aneurysm. The graph of peak responses for stroke volume following glucagon is shown in Fig. 1.

The heart rate was increased in 20 studies. The maximum rate increase was from 65 to 130 beats per minute. The mean base-line rate was 80 beats per minute with a mean rise of 24 percent to 99 beats per minute after glucagon. The rate was unchanged af-

Presented at the Twenty-third Annual Meeting of the Society for Vascular Surgery, New York, N. Y., July 12-13, 1969.

*Present address: 3411 North Fifth Avenue, Phoenix, Ariz. 85013.

†Eli Lilly and Company, Indianapolis, Ind.

Table I. *Cardiac procedures**

Aortic valve replacement
Mitral valve replacement
Open mitral repair
Double valve replacement
Clusure atrial septal defect
Resection left ventricular aneurysm
Resection dissecting thoracic aortic aneurysm (AVR)
Double mammary implant
Closed mitral commissurotomy

*Cardiac procedures included in the study involved extracorporeal circulation in all but the mammary artery implant and closed commissurotomy.

ter the ascending aortic resection and aortic valve replacement for a dissecting thoracic aortic aneurysm and in those patients with cardiac pacing. The graph of peak responses for heart rate is shown in Fig. 2.

Cardiac output following the administration of glucagon was increased in all cases. The maximum increase was from 1.7 to 4.1 L. per minute. The mean baseline value was 3.1 L. per minute with a rise of 25 percent to 3.8 L. per minute. The cardiac output following glucagon was increased only 400 c.c. per minute in the patient who had left ventricular aneurysm resection. Interestingly, with preoperative cardiac catheterization, the cardiac output decreased from 2.3 to 1.7 L. per minute with exercise. The graph of peak responses for cardiac output is shown in Fig. 3.

The graph expressing the mean percentage change of cardiac output in all 25 studies after glucagon is shown in Fig. 4.

The peripheral resistance calculations were decreased in 6, unchanged in 9, and increased in 10. These changes were variable at the dose level of 3 to 10 mg. and were not statistically significant. The variable responses were possibly related to the incidence of cutaneous flushing, nausea, and vomiting. The graph of peak responses for peripheral resistance is shown in Fig. 5.

The arterial systolic pressure was increased in 23 studies and unchanged in 2 (following left ventricular aneurysm resection and closure of atrial septal defect). The mean base-line value was 114 mm. Hg, rising 25 percent to a mean value of 148 mm. Hg, with a maximum rise of 64 mm. Hg. An increase of 50 mm. Hg resulted in one patient with fixed rate cardiac pacing. The graph for peak responses for arterial systolic blood pressure is shown in Fig. 6.

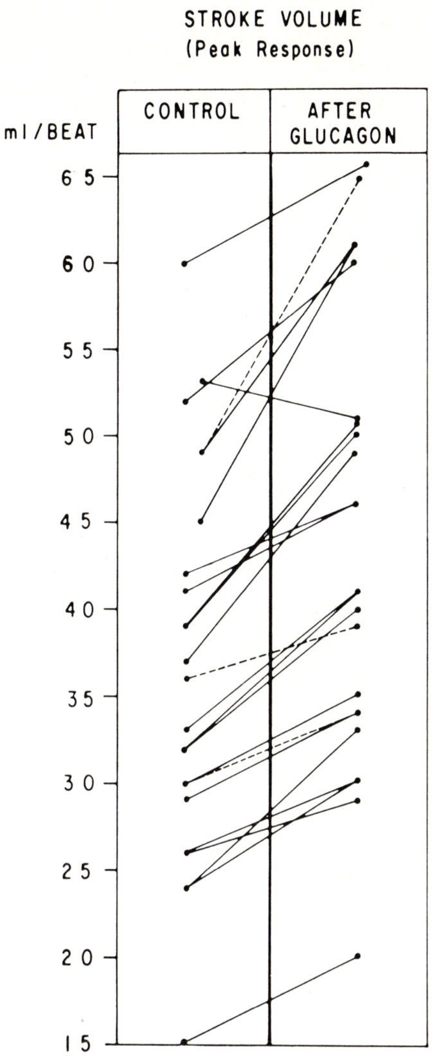

Fig. 1. Graph of peak responses for stroke volume after glucagon. Patients (in all graph slides) with fixed rate cardiac pacing are indicated by stippled lines.

The diastolic arterial pressure was increased in 20 studies, unchanged in 4, and decreased in one. The mean base-line value was 57 mm. Hg, rising 19 percent to a mean value of 80 mm. Hg. The graph of peak

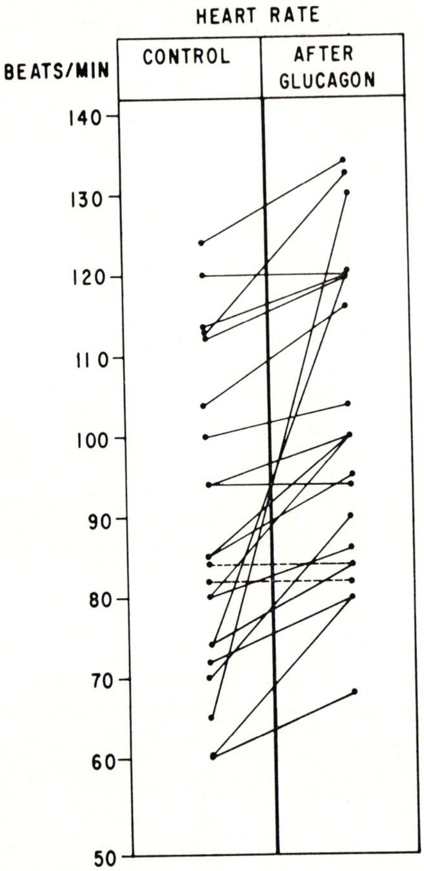

Fig. 2. Graph of peak responses for heart rate after glucagon. The maximum increase from 65 to 130 beats per minute occurred in a patient with low cardiac output syndrome following aortic valve replacement.

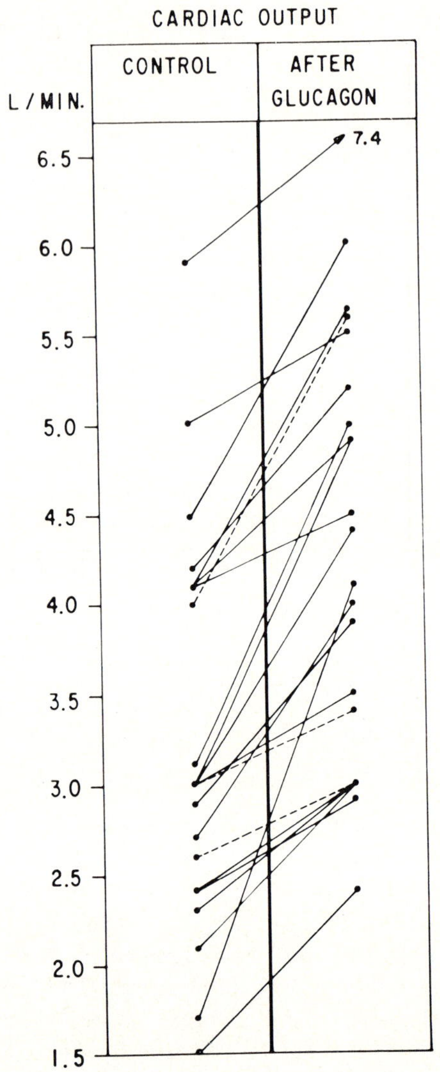

Fig. 3. Graph of peak responses for cardiac output after glucagon. Note the increase from 4.0 to 5.6 L. per minute in a patient with fixed rate pacing (stippled lines).

responses for diastolic arterial pressure is shown in Fig. 7.

Following the administration of glucagon in a peripheral vein the initial response was noted after 3 to 5 minutes, it became maximum at 7 to 10 minutes, and was apparently dissipated after 15 to 20 minutes. Repeated doses at 15 minute intervals were effective in eliminating the usual decay curve and sustained the inotropic and chronotropic effects up to one hour, which was the longest period tested. An example of the dosage response curve following repeated administration of glucagon is depicted in Fig. 8.

Observations noted in the three patients with cardiac pacing were of interest as the cardiac rate was constant. The stroke volume was minimally increased (2 and 4 ml. per stroke) in 2 patients. In the other, the stroke volume was increased 32 percent from the mean value of 49 to 65 ml. per stroke. Cardiac output was increased 13, 15, and 40 percent, respectively, in those patients with cardiac pacing. Systolic arterial pressure mean value was 115 mm. Hg, rising 24 percent to 143 mm. Hg.

There have been no disturbances of

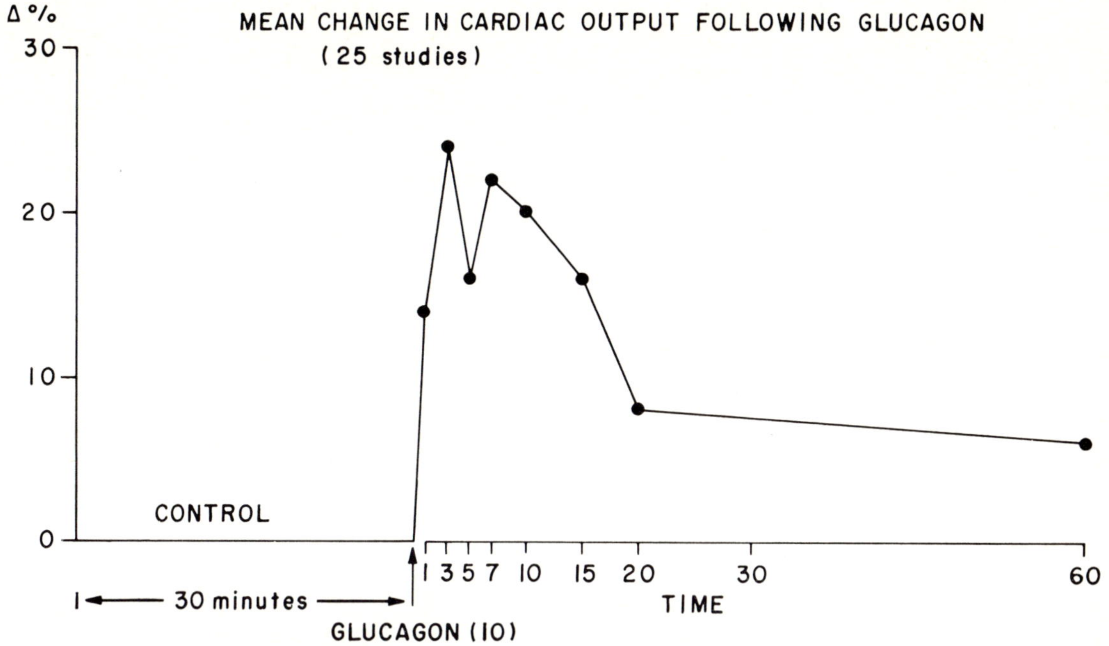

Fig. 4. Graph of mean change in cardiac output after glucagon. Six base-line control recordings at 5 minute intervals established the mean value for cardiac output. The maximum mean change of 25 percent occurred at 3 minutes. The characteristic decay curve is shown.

cardiac rhythm following the administration of glucagon.

Serum sodium, potassium, chloride, bicarbonate, arterial pH, and blood gas determinations were not significantly altered following glucagon administration. Moderate depression of the serum potassium level has been reported by others and this parameter should be monitored when glucagon is given.

Nausea and diaphoresis occurred in 8 patients following the administration of glucagon. One was profoundly nauseated and vomited on two occasions. The side effects were transient and abated without specific antiemetic therapy.

DISCUSSION

The metabolic effects of glucagon are only partially understood. The hyperglycemic effects are mediated through the liver by an increase in cyclic adenosine monophosphate (AMP) resulting in glycogenolysis through phorphorylase activation. The catecholamines activate the same enzyme system, but the inotropic action and the ability of the catecholamines to increase cyclic AMP levels are blocked by DL-propranolol.[10] The effects of glucagon are not altered by β-adrenergic blockade.[4, 6] However, the mechanism of the inotropic and chronotropic actions of glucagon on the human heart are being studied. Glick and associates[4] have noted that these responses are independent of digitalization, catecholamine depletion, or β-adrenergic blockade. The simultaneous administration of insulin has no effect on the inotropic response after glucagon.[4] The hemodynamic effects are of much shorter duration than the hyperglycemic effects and result possibly from a different mechanism. Braunwald, Ross, and Sonnenblick[1] have shown that glucagon increases myocardial contractility, cardiac index, and stroke work at a constant left ventricular end diastolic pressure.

The increased cardiac output following glucagon administration is not rate dependent. In animal experiments with fixed rate cardiac pacing, cardiac contractility is in-

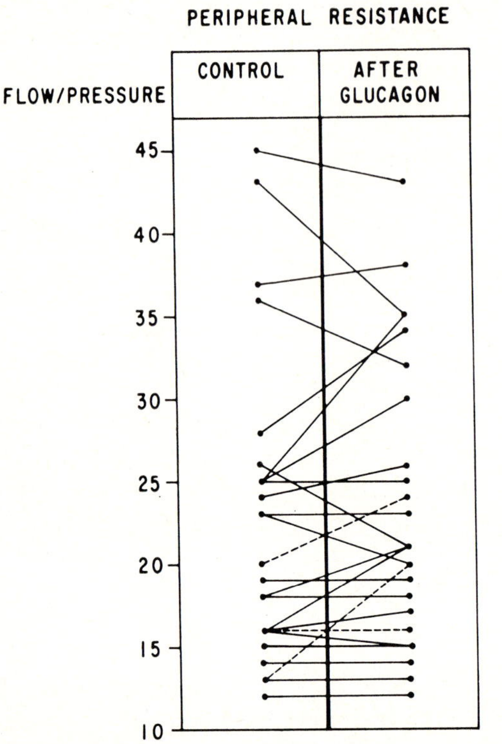

Fig. 5. Graph of peak responses for peripheral vascular resistance after glucagon. The variable responses are possibly related to the incidence of cutaneous flushing, nausea, and vomiting.

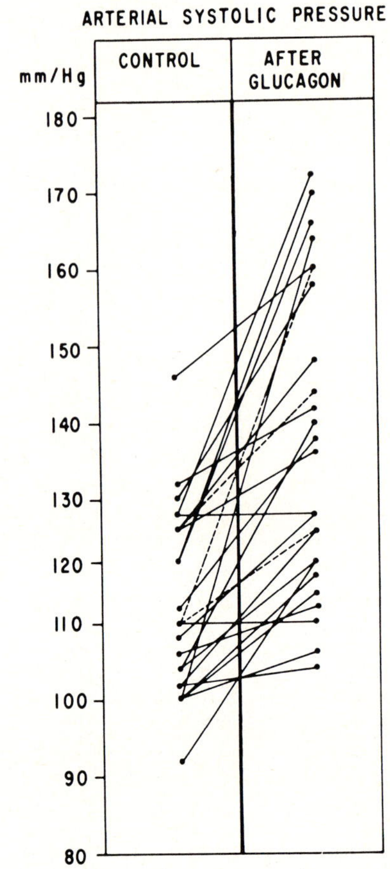

Fig. 6. Graph of peak responses of arterial systolic pressure after glucagon. An increase of 50 mm. Hg occurred in one patient with fixed rate cardiac pacing (stippled lines).

creased by glucagon according to Glick and associates.[4] In our studies, also the cardiac output was found to be increased up to 1.6 L. per minute (40 percent) following glucagon administration to patients whose rates were held constant by cardiac pacemakers.

Changes in peripheral vascular resistance following the administration of glucagon seem to be variable. Parmley, Glick, and Sonnenblick[8] reported a fall in peripheral resistance following the administration of 1 mg. of glucagon. Yet this was not noted consistently at dosage levels of 3 to 10 mg. in our study.

The possible role of glucagon in the management of the postoperative low cardiac output syndrome deserves consideration. Following open-heart surgery this is a many-faceted problem. Accurate repair of the cardiac defect, blood replacement, ventilatory management, acid-base balance, digitalization, cardiac pacing, and the judicious use of various cardiac agents are important. Glucagon, while not supplanting any existing treatment modality, may be added to the armamentarium of the physician in the management of the postoperative low cardiac output syndrome. In patients with increased myocardial irritability, glucagon may be safely used to augment cardiac output.

The utilization of glucagon in management of the low cardiac output syndrome is illustrated in the following case report. Aortic valve replacement was carried out in a 61-year-old white man with calcific aortic stenosis. He had taken digitalis for 5 years. His cardiac rhythm varied from normal sinus rhythm to atrial fibrillation. On

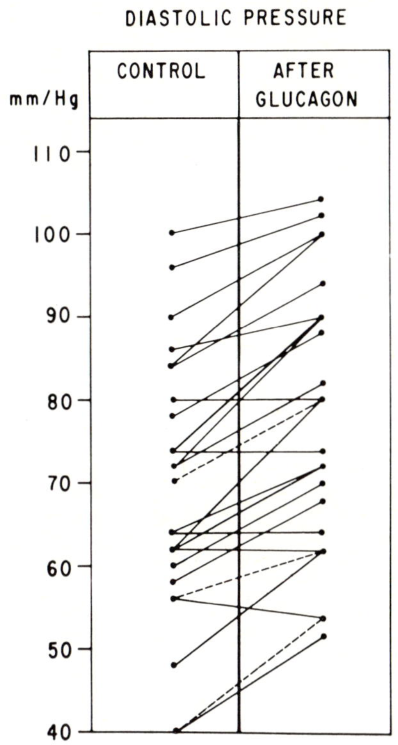

Fig. 7. Graph for peak responses of diastolic arterial pressure after glucagon.

the evening of operation, the patient was hypoxic, hypotensive, and he had convulsions. Emergency tracheostomy and management with a volume ventilator effectively restored respiratory cardiovascular dynamics. The following day, the patient had a bigeminal cardiac rhythm, and was oliguric, edematous, and hypotensive, with low cardiac output. The hematocrit, blood gases, and serum electrolytes were normal. Isoproterenol (Isuprel) was not given because of his increased ventricular irritability. The significant rise in cardiac output and arterial systolic pressure following the intravenous administration of 10 mg. of glucagon (two doses one hour apart) is recorded in Fig. 9. Electrocardiographic changes following glucagon administration in this patient are shown in Fig. 10.

SUMMARY

The cardiovascular effects of the intravenous administration of glucagon have been studied on 25 occasions in 20 patients on the first day following various cardiac surgical procedures. The positive inotropic and chronotropic effects of this pancreatic hormone were manifest by transient increases in cardiac rate, stroke volume, cardiac out-

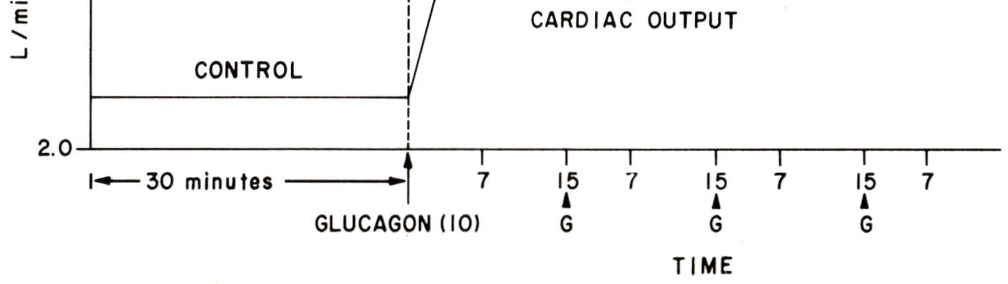

Fig. 8. Graph of cardiac output following repeated doses of glucagon. $G =$ repeated doses of 10 mg. glucagon at 15 minute intervals.

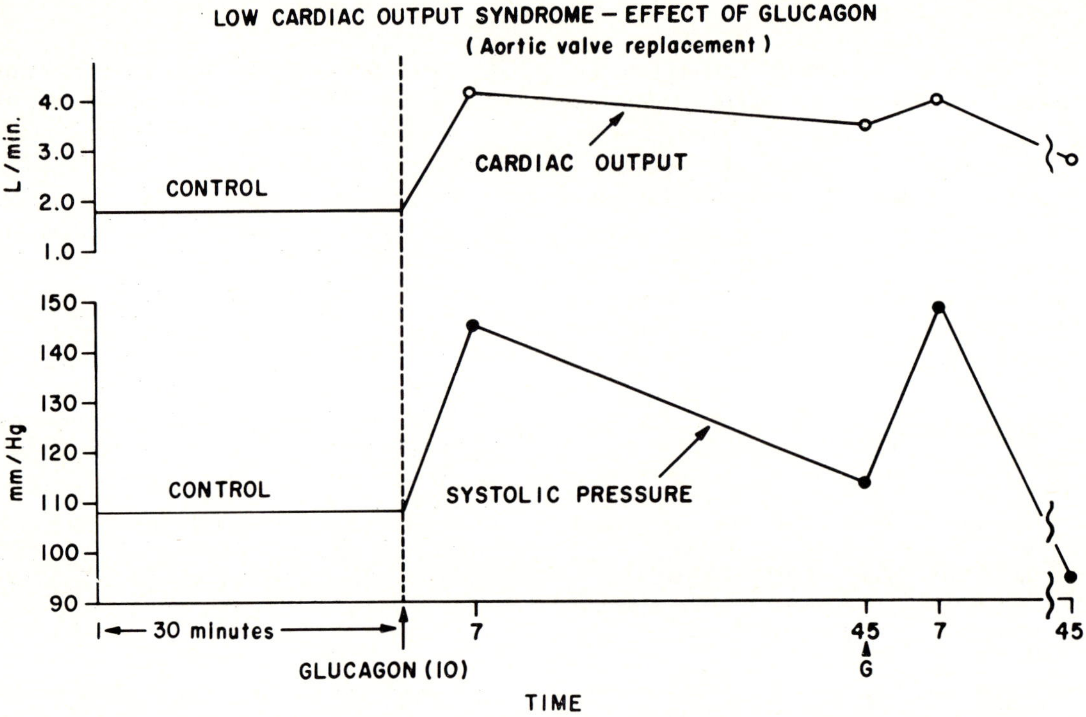

Fig. 9. Graph of arterial systolic pressure and cardiac output responses following repeated doses of 10 mg. of glucagon intravenously one hour apart in a patient with the low cardiac output syndrome following aortic valve replacement.

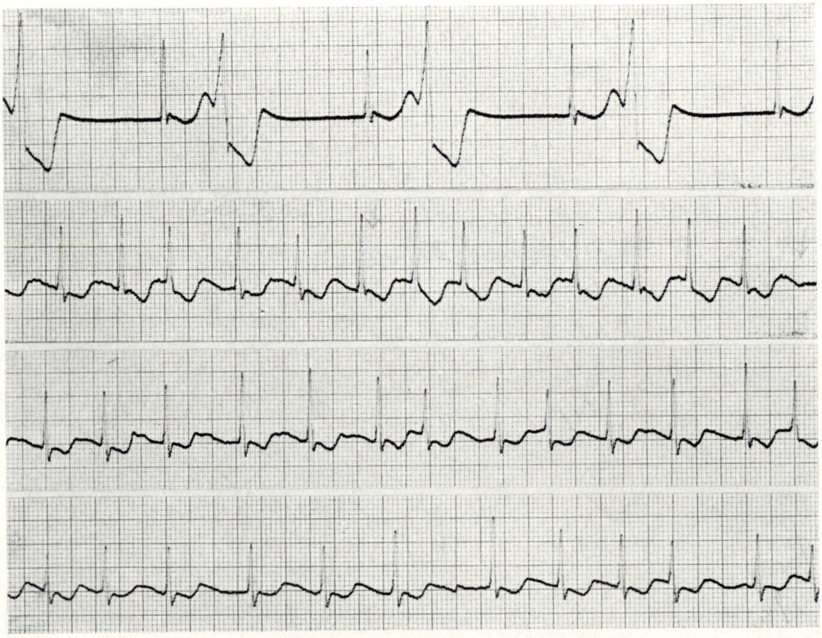

Fig. 10. Reproduction of electrocardiogram in a patient with low cardiac output syndrome. The upper panel depicts the bigeminal rhythm present which was associated with a low perfusion state. Three minutes following the administration of 10 mg. glucagon intravenously (second panel) rapid atrial fibrillation is evident. At 7 and 15 minutes (third and fourth panel, respectively) the atrial fibrillation was adequately controlled with intravenous digitalis preparation.

put, and arterial pressure. Changes in peripheral vascular resistance were variable and no significant alteration in electrocardiogram, arterial blood gases, pH, and electrolytes were evident. Side effects were minimal consisting of mild nausea and vomiting. Glucagon is a safe and moderately effective agent to augment cardiac function in selected situations of low cardiac output following cardiac surgery.

REFERENCES

1. Braunwald, E., Ross, J., Jr., and Sonnenblick, E. H.: Mechanisms of contraction of normal and failing heart, New Eng. J. Med. **277:** 794, 853, 910, 962, 1012, 1967.
2. Elrick, H., Huffman, E. R., Hlad, C. J., Whipple, N., and Staub, A.: Effects of glucagon on renal function in man, J. Clin. Endocr. **18:** 813, 1958.
3. Farah, A., and Tuttle, R.: Studies on pharmacology of glucagon, J. Pharmacol. Exp. Ther. **129:** 49, 1960.
4. Glick, G., Parmley, W. W., Weschler, A. S., and Sonnenblick, E. H.: Glucagon: Its enhancement of cardiac performance in cat and dog, persistence of its inotropic action despite beta receptor blockage with propranolol, Circ. Res. **22:** 789, 1968.
5. Glick, G., Parmley, W. W., Wechsler, A. S., and Sonnenblick, E. H.: Glucagon: Its positive inotropic and chronotropic properties as studied in a cat papillary muscle preparation, intact dog heart and conscious human subjects, Amer. J. Cardiol. **21:** 99, 1967. (Abst.)
6. LaRaia, P. J., Craig, R. J., and Reddy, W. J.: Glucagon: Biochemical mechanisms and contractility effects in heart, Amer. J. Cardiol. **21:** 107, 1968.
7. Linhart, J. W., Barold, S. S., Cohen, L. S., Hildner, F. J., and Samet, P.: Cardiovascular effects of glucagon in man, Amer. J. Cardiol. **22:** 706, 1968.
8. Parmley, W. W., Glick, G., and Sonnenblick, E. H.: Cardiovascular effects of glucagon in man, New Eng. J. Med. **279:** 12, 1968.
9. Sporn, J., and Necheles, H.: Effect of glucagon on gastrointestinal motility, Amer. J. Physiol. **187:** 634, 1956.
10. Sutherland, E. W., Robinson, G. A., and Butcher, R. W.: Some aspects of the biological role of adenosine 3′, 5′-monophosphate (cyclic AMP), Circulation **35:** 279, 1968.
11. Warner, H. R.: The role of computers in medical research, J. A. M. A. **196:** 944, 1966.
12. Warner, H. R., Gardner, R. E., and Toronto, A. F.: Computer based monitoring of cardiovascular function in postoperative patients, Circulation **37:** 68, 1968. (Suppl. II.)
13. Whitehouse, F. W., and James, T. N.: Chronotropic action of glucagon on sinus node, Proc. Soc. Exp. Biol. Med. **122:** 823, 1966.

Arterial embolectomy: A 20 year experience with 163 cases

JESSE E. THOMPSON, M.D.
LUIS SIGLER, M.D.
P. S. RAUT, M.D.
DALE J. AUSTIN, M.D.
R. DON PATMAN, M.D.
DALLAS, TEXAS
From the Surgical Service of Baylor University Medical Center

Peripheral arterial embolism continues to be a common clinical occurrence.[1, 6, 7, 13, 14, 19, 22] In fact the disease may be increasing somewhat in frequency because of the aging of our population, the improved care given cardiac patients, and the widespread use of prosthetic heart valves. It is now generally held that most accessible arterial emboli are best managed by surgical means. Despite innovations in therapeutic methods, mortality remains high because of the serious nature of the underlying cardiac disease, while amputation rates have progressively decreased. This report is based on a 20 year experience with 203 embolectomies performed on 163 private patients. A comparison is made of the older with the more recent results of treatment to point up improvements in therapy of the last decade.

DIAGNOSIS

In the usual case peripheral embolism is easily recognized by the sudden onset of pain in the extremity followed by coldness, pallor, numbness, and varying degrees of paralysis, with pulses absent distal to the site of lodgement, in patients with a history of cardiac disease, proximal aneurysms, or recent cardiovascular surgery. At times, however, the onset may be insidious, and differentiation from arterial thrombosis may be difficult without arteriography. Occasionally the early stage of acute deep thrombophlebitis is accompanied by such a degree of vasospasm and pain that the diagnosis of arterial embolism is entertained until further observation clarifies the situation.

Presented at the Twenty-third Annual Meeting of the Society for Vascular Surgery, New York, N. Y., July 12-13, 1969.

GENERAL PRINCIPLES OF MANAGEMENT

Once the diagnosis of peripheral embolism is made, the usual treatment is embolectomy without undue delay. Operation is contraindicated if the patient is moribund or if the extremity is gangrenous, when amputation may be the primary treatment of choice. Even in the presence of irreversible distal gangrene, however, it may be important in certain cases to attempt revascularization of the extremity in order to lower the level of amputation or insure its healing. Heparin in the appropriate dosage should be given immediately to prevent distal thrombosis.

A certain amount of delay occasionally may be necessary for treatment of arrhythmia, congestive heart failure, or shock, but delay should be kept at a minimum since best results from embolectomy are seen in patients with prompt restoration of peripheral blood flow. Arteriography, if necessary prior to embolectomy, may be done in the operating room.

Operative management. Since the usual patient with arterial embolism is a poor risk because of heart disease, local anesthesia for embolectomy is preferred to general anesthesia whenever possible. This is ordinarily feasible when incisions are made in the extremities. If laparotomy becomes necessary for aortic or iliac embolectomy, general anesthesia is used. With the advent of the Fogarty balloon catheters it is now possible in most instances to remove even aortic and iliac emboli through groin incisions, employing local anesthesia.

A transverse arteriotomy is made at the appropriate site. If over the embolus, this is gently removed with endarterectomy forceps. If the arteriotomy is distal to the site of lodgement, the Fogarty catheter is inserted proximalward for removal of emboli and thrombi. The balloon catheter should be passed routinely into the distal vasculature even when thrombosis is not apparent and backflow is satisfactory since small fragments of emboli and thrombi frequently will be found in the distal vessels. If the catheter will not traverse the entire length of the limb, one may be dealing with an atherosclerotic occlusion requiring arteriography on the operating table. Heparin is used liberally both proximal and distal to the occluding clamps. Papaverine or lido- the distal vasculature. Sympathetic blocks caine may be used to relieve vasospasm in are no longer used either pre- or postoperatively. Fasciotomy may be necessary in cases of extreme swelling.

All patients are routinely heparinized for a week or more following operation. At this time, depending upon the over-all clinical situation, they are usually started on Coumadin therapy. The appropriate cardiac management is carried out concomitantly.

CLINICAL MATERIAL

From October, 1948, through December 31, 1968, 203 arterial embolectomies were performed on 163 private patients of the authors. One hundred and forty-one patients had single embolic episodes, while 22 had multiple emboli. There were 82 males and 81 females. The ages ranged from 18 to 99 years, with an average of 62.5 years (Table I).

Table I. *Basic data on patients studied*

No. of patients	163
No. of embolectomy operations	203
Single embolic episodes (patients)	141
Multiple embolic episodes (patients)	22
No. of males	82
No. of females	81
Age range 18 to 99 years	
Average 62.5 years	

Table II. *Location of emboli*

Artery	*Patients*	*Episodes*	
		No.	*%*
Aorta	18	19	9.4
Iliac	34	38	18.7
Femoral	76	85	41.9
Popliteal	28	28	13.8
Posterior tibial	2	2	1.0
Anterior tibial	1	1	0.5
Subclavian	2	2	1.0
Axillary	13	13	6.4
Brachial	12	13	6.4
Carotid	2	2	1.0
		203	

Sites of embolization are given in Table II. As usual, femoral emboli were the most common (42 percent). No visceral emboli are included.

Table III shows the etiology of emboli in 163 patients. The heart was the predominant source (78 percent). The miscellaneous causes included lupus erythematosus, endocarditis, chest trauma, etc. The group of emboli with undetermined etiology is very interesting. A diligent search will at times reveal a proximal aneurysm or atherosclerotic plaque requiring definitive therapy. Occasionally, however, all efforts fail to uncover a specific source for the embolus.

RESULTS OF SURGICAL TREATMENT

Operative mortality. Twenty-four patients died following operation, giving a patient mortality of 14.7 percent and a procedure mortality of 11.8 percent (Table IV). The average time interval from operation to death was 7.3 days. The causes of death are given in Table V. Fifty-eight percent of the deaths were due to cardiac causes, either

Table III. *Etiology of emboli*

	No. of patients		*Total*
I. Cardiac causes			128
A. Myocardial infarction		53	
Recent	28		
Remote	25		
B. Auricular fibrillation		63	
Rheumatic	10		
Atherosclerotic	53		
C. Atherosclerotic without fibrillation or infarction		12	
II. Following cardiovascular surgery			11
III. Other known causes			7
IV. Undetermined etiology			17
Total			163

Table IV. *Mortality following embolectomy**

No. of patients		163
No. of operations		203
No. of deaths		24
Males	12	
Females	12	
Patient mortality		14.7%
Procedure mortality		11.8%

*Interval from operation to death: range – on operating table to 21 days; average interval – 7.3 days postoperation.

Table V. *Causes of 24 operative deaths*

Cardiac	14
Pulmonary embolism	5
Stroke	3
Mesenteric infarction	1
Hepatic coma	1
	24
Anesthesia used	
General	14
Spinal	1
Local	9

Table VI. *Operative mortality related to location of emboli*

Artery	*Deaths/ patients*	*Mortality (%)*
Aorta	4/18	22.2
Iliac	6/34	17.7
Femoral	7/76	9.2
Popliteal	2/28	7.1
Axillary-brachial	4/25	16.0
Carotid	1/2	50.0

cardiac arrest or congestive heart failure. This points up the seriousness of the heart disease in patients with embolism. The second most common cause of death was pulmonary embolism.

Table VI relates the deaths to the location of the emboli. It is obvious that aortic and carotid emboli carry the highest mortality. Among the four upper-extremity emboli deaths were two elderly patients, extremely ill with congestive heart failure, who were operated upon under local anesthesia in desperate attempts to relieve impending gangrene of the hand. A third patient died unexpectedly during cardioversion following successful axillary embolectomy.

Table VII relates the deaths to the underlying etiology of the emboli. Atherosclerotic heart disease, with or without myocardial infarction, carries the highest mortality.

Amputations. In the entire series there were 13 amputations necessary in 13 patients (Table VIII), a portion of one hand and 12 lower extremities. Nine of these were above-knee and 3 below-knee. The ages of these patients ranged from 37 to 85 years, with an average of 68.3 years. The over-all amputation rate among patients surviving embolectomy is 7.4 percent, or a limb salvage of 92.6 percent.

Table IX gives an analysis of the amputations based on location of emboli. Femoral emboli are responsible for the highest incidence of amputation as well as being the most common emboli. It is of interest to note that no patient with an aortic embolus lost an extremity. These patients either had good return of function or were so ill that they died following operation.

Table X relates the amputations to the time interval from embolic occlusion to operation. The amputation rate in patients operated upon within 24 hours of onset is 4.4 percent while for those operated upon after 24 hours is 19.4 percent. The highest

Table VII. *Operative mortality related to etiology of emboli*

Etiology	*Deaths/ patients*	*Mortality (%)*
Myocardial infarction-recent	6/28	21.4
Myocardial infarction-remote	4/25	16.0
Auricular fibrillation-atherosclerotic	7/53	13.2
Auricular fibrillation-rheumatic	1/10	10.0
Atherosclerotic heart disease without MI or AF	3/12	25.0
Other known causes	2/18	11.1
Undetermined etiology	1/17	5.9

Table VIII. *Amputations in surviving patients*

No. of embolectomies			176
No. of amputations			13
Amputation rate			7.4%
Limb salvage			92.6%
Total amputations			13
Lower extremities		12	
Above-knee	9		
Below-knee	3		
Upper extremity		1 hand	

Table IX. *Amputation related to location of emboli (survivors)*

Artery	*Amputation/ embolectomy*	*Amputation rate (%)*
Iliac	1/32	3.1
Femoral	10/75	13.3
Popliteal	1/25	4.0
Brachial	1/9	11.0

Table X. *Amputation related to time interval from embolism to embolectomy (survivors)*

Time interval embolism to operation (hr.)	*Amputation/ embolectomy*	*Amputation rate (%)*	
0- 6	2/64	3.1	4.4
7-12	3/50	6.0	
13-24	1/21	4.8	
25-48	4/11	36.4	19.4
>48	3/25	12.0	
Unknown	0/ 8	0	

Table XI. *Late embolectomy (> 48 hours)*

No. of embolectomies	25
No. of deaths	1
No. of amputations	3—12%
Era I—1/6 —17%	
Era II—2/10—20%	
Era III—0/8 — 0%	

incidence of amputation (36 percent) occurred in those patients operated upon between 24 and 48 hours after embolism occurred. Only one patient died after amputation, a 74-year-old woman who died 6 weeks postoperatively from cardiac causes secondary to massive gastrointestinal hemorrhage complicating heparin therapy for myocardial infarction.

Late embolectomy. Patients operated upon 48 hours or more after embolism occurred are designated delayed or late embolectomy cases. Table XI lists the data on these cases. The single death occurred unexpectedly during cardioversion three days following successful late axillary embolectomy. The 3 amputations all took place prior to the use of the balloon catheter. The time interval from embolism to operation ranged from 3 days to 10 months, with an average time of about 10 days. It is clear that successful embolectomy may be carried out from days to weeks after onset provided the extremity is viable or potentially viable.

Functional results. The immediate postoperative functional status of the extremities among survivors not requiring amputation was evaluated on the basis of distal pulses and symptoms. Eighty-four percent of these patients had an excellent or good result. An additional 13 percent had a satisfactory result, while 3 percent of the group had a poor result. Although not requiring amputation, the latter exhibited marked degrees of functional limitation requiring in some instances further vascular surgery for relief.

Miscellaneous data. Six patients required

subsequent vascular reconstructive surgery to relieve disabling symptoms of arterial insufficiency. Fifteen patients underwent lumbar sympathectomy either before, during, or after embolectomy. Twenty-two patients had arteriograms performed prior to operation, 5 during operation, and 8 following embolectomy. There were 2 wound infections and 4 wound hematomas requiring operative evacuation.

DISCUSSION

In the past two decades a number of therapeutic innovations have been introduced in the management of peripheral embolism. Perhaps the most significant one is the general acceptance of the thesis that early surgical removal of emboli is the primary treatment of choice in most cases rather than heroic or salvage therapy after failure of medical measures.

The administration of heparin as soon as embolism is recognized and its use during and after embolectomy have become routine. If there is delay in performing operation, heparin tends to prevent distal propagation of thrombi. However, the use of heparin has not been entirely successful in preventing embolization in patients with heart disease, especially after acute myocardial infarction. Twenty-four embolic episodes in our series occurred while patients were receiving anticoagulant therapy. In fact, Barker, Rosato, and Roberts[2] have pointed out that heparin may induce platelet agglutination on ulcerated endothelium and thus be responsible for embolization in certain cases. We have suspected this phenomenon on several occasions when patients on high doses of heparin had repeated embolic episodes. Nevertheless, heparin remains a very important adjunct.

Retrograde flush techniques were developed[5] to clear the distal vasculature of thrombi, the presence of which constitute the commonest cause of ischemia and gangrene even after removal of the embolus itself. These techniques have now been largely superseded by the balloon catheter.

Late embolectomy, or operation performed 48 hours or longer after the occurrence of embolism was described by several authors[16, 23] as a practical concept in cases where the extremity was still viable or potentially viable. Not only may an extremity be saved, but its functional result may be markedly improved by restoration of distal blood flow. It may also be employed to lower the level of amputation or insure the healing of an amputation stump.

The single most important advance in the management of embolism in the last decade has been the balloon catheter, which was developed and tested clinically by Fogarty and his associates.[4, 8, 9, 12] This single instrument has made the goal of embolectomy not simply preservation of life and limb, but rather restoration of distal blood flow in the limb with return of function to the pre-embolic state. This goal can now be achieved in a very high percentage of cases.

With the Fogarty balloon catheter one can apply a more aggressive surgical approach to patients suffering from embolism. Even in extremely ill patients one can successfully remove emboli from the aorta and iliac arteries through the femoral approach using local anesthesia.[18] Using the smaller caliber catheters it is also technically possible to remove emboli from the arteries in the arm and forearm[20] as well as from the arteries of the lower leg. Arteriography assumes a more important role also[26] since one can remove with the balloon catheter residual emboli and thrombi seen on the arteriogram but not suspected on clinical grounds.

Advances in cardiology, especially the management of arrhythmias and newer methods of cardiac resuscitation, have also contributed to the over-all results of management of patients with embolism.

To compare the effects of recent therapeutic innovations on mortality and amputation rates following embolectomy, we have divided our cases into three chronological eras (Table XII). Era I summarizes our first ten years' experience, previously reported.[25] Era II comprises the five years from January, 1959, through March 23, 1964. During this period we employed a

Table XII. *Mortality and amputation rates related to chronological eras*

Era	*No. of patients*	*No. of embolectomies*	*No. of deaths*	*No. of amputations (survivors)*	*Patient mortality (%)*	*Operative mortality (%)*	*Amputation rate (survivors, %)*
I October, 1948, through December, 1958	41	44	5	5	12.1	11.3	12.8
II January, 1959, through March 23, 1964	53	67	9	4	17.0	13.4	7.0
III March 24, 1964, through December, 1968 (Fogarty)	73	92	12	4	16.4	13.0	5.1

more aggressive surgical approach, used heparin more liberally, and attempted retrograde flush procedures. Era III encompasses the last five years since March 24, 1964, the date we first used a Fogarty catheter. In this period we have employed the catheter routinely and have operated more frequently upon popliteal and upper extremity emboli. We have also continued to perform late embolectomy. Analysis of the results shows that the operative mortality has increased a bit in the past decade, but this represents more liberal indication for operation on the seriously ill cardiac patients, especially those with acute myocardial infarction. During the first 10 years aortic and iliac embolectomies constituted 21 percent of our cases, while in the second decade they comprised 29 percent. This also reflects the severity of the heart disease in patients with embolism since only rarely do these patients die from complications of the operation itself. The amputation rate, on the other hand, has progressively declined with application of the innovations mentioned above, especially heparin and the Fogarty catheter. A limb salvage rate of 95 percent is now a practical goal in these patients. Not only have more limbs been saved during the past five years, but the functional results in these extremities have been markedly improved as a result of more complete removal of emboli and thrombi from the distal vasculature. The four amputations in Era III were a hand in a patient with lupus, previously mentioned, and three lower extremities in patients 80, 78, and 74 years of age, all with severe heart disease.

In Table XIII are listed some representative statistics on mortality and amputation rates following embolectomy taken from the recent literature.[2, 3, 4, 6, 9, 10, 11, 12, 15, 17, 21, 27] Haimovici's figures published in 1950 are included for comparison. In some instances comparative figures with and without the use of the Fogarty balloon catheter are available and are listed as such. Operative mortality is consistently high. Amputation rates have steadily declined with the advent of the balloon catheter. Our own figures compare favorably with those of Fogarty[9] and of Cranley and associates.[4]

Death following embolectomy is principally of cardiac origin, especially congestive heart failure. With continued refinements in cardiac management and with increasing use of local anesthesia made possible by the advent of the Fogarty catheter, it seems reasonable to hope for some further reduction in operative mortality without denying seriously ill patients the benefits of embolectomy.

A common cause of death reported in most series is pulmonary embolism. Stallone and associates[24] have recently examined this problem in detail and have concluded that both macro- and microemboli arising from the venous side of an extremity with arterial embolism may result in compromise of pulmonary function to a severe degree. In fact,

Table XIII. *Mortality and amputation following embolectomy*

*Author**		*Year*	*No. of cases*	*Operative mortality (%)*	*Amputation rate (%)*
Haimovici[10]		1950	29	51.8	48.3
Ouchi and Warren[17]		1962	80	38.6	14.0
Young and associates[27]		1963	74	36.0	14.0
Barker, Rosato, and Roberts[2]		1966	110	27.0	17.5
Krause and associates[12]	A	1966	133	34.0	9.0
	B		128	19.0	5.0
Fogarty[9]		1967	100	15.4	4.0
Billig, Hallman, and Cooley[3]		1967	76	18.4	18.0
Karageorgis[11]	A	1967	18	33.3	28.8
	B		8	25.0	12.5
Scheinin and Inberg[21]		1967	35	26.0	17.0
Darling, Austen, and Linton[6]		1967	224	19.2	8.9
McMahon and Sako[15]		1968	47	28.0	17.0
Cranley and associates[4]	A	1968	152	26.0	20.7
	B		128	12.0	7.0
Present series	A	1969	94	14.9	9.4
Thompson and associates	B		73	16.4	5.1

*A, without balloon catheter; B, with balloon catheter.

they recommend venous thrombectomy concomitant with arterial embolectomy in all severely ischemic limbs, together with vigorous ventilatory support, in an effort to reduce mortality and morbidity.

Recent experience indicates that no arbitrary limit need be set as to the time when embolectomy may be successfully performed after embolism occurs. Indeed operation may be done any time after occurrence provided the limb is viable or potentially viable. The fact that late embolectomy is frequently successful is indicative of adequate collateral circulation or a patent distal vasculature or both. However, it should be emphasized that the best results follow early embolectomy and that the commonest reason for amputation is delay in surgical treatment (Table X). Continued efforts should be made to educate the medical profession regarding the value of precise recognition of acute arterial embolism and the institution of prompt therapy. Operation should be carried out as soon as possible, while allowing for appropriate emergency evaluation and treatment of the underlying cardiac problem.

SUMMARY AND CONCLUSIONS

A series of 203 peripheral arterial embolectomies performed on 163 patients during a 20 year period has been presented. Patient mortality was 14.7 percent and procedure mortality 11.8 percent. Thirteen amputations were required, giving a limb salvage of 92.6 percent among survivors. The commonest cause of death was severe heart disease, while the chief reason for amputation was delay in the performance of embolectomy.

Recent innovations in therapy are discussed. These include the routine administration of heparin, late embolectomy, and especially the use of the Fogarty balloon catheter, which has facilitated embolectomy in all areas, has broadened the scope of embolectomy to include the upper extremity and the lower leg, and has simplified the removal of aortic and iliac emboli through the groins in seriously ill patients.

In the pre-Fogarty era our operative mortality was 14.9 percent and our amputation rate 9.4 percent; with the routine use of the Fogarty catheter during the past 5 years, the operative mortality has been 16 percent and the amputation rate 5.1 percent, in spite of a more aggressive surgical approach in extremely ill patients.

While no arbitrary time limit need be set for embolectomy, best results follow when diagnosis is made promptly and operation done without delay, especially within the first 24 hours after onset.

REFERENCES

1. Baird, R. J., and Lajos, T. Z.: Emboli to the arm, Ann. Surg. **160:** 905, 1964.
2. Barker, C. F., Rosato, F. E., and Roberts, B.: Peripheral arterial embolism, Surg. Gynec. Obstet. **123:** 22, 1966.
3. Billig, D. M., Hallman, G. L., and Cooley, D. A.: Arterial embolism, surgical treatment and results, Arch. Surg. **95:** 1, 1967.
4. Cranley, J. J., Krause, R. J., Strasser, E. S., Hafner, C. D., and Meese, E. H.: Unpublished data, 1968.
5. Crawford, E. S., and De Bakey, M. E.: Retrograde flush procedure in embolectomy and thrombectomy, SURGERY **40:** 737, 1956.
6. Darling, R. C., Austen, W. G., and Linton, R. R.: Arterial embolism, Surg. Gynec. Obstet. **124:** 106, 1967.
7. Flanc, C.: Saddle embolism of the aorta, Australia and New Zealand J. Surg. **37:** 384, 1968.
8. Fogarty, T. J., Cranley, J. J., Krause, R. J., Strasser, E. S., and Hafner, C. D.: A method for extraction of arterial emboli and thrombi, Surg. Gynec. & Obstet. **116:** 241, 1963.
9. Fogarty, T. J.: Catheter technic for arterial embolectomy, J. Cardiovas. Surg. **8:** 22, 1967.
10. Haimovici, H.: Peripheral arterial embolism: Study of 330 unselected cases of embolism of extremities, Angiology **1:** 20, 1950.
11. Karageorgis, B. P.: Experience with the catheter technique in arterial embolectomy, J. Cardiovas. Surg. **8:** 375, 1967.
12. Krause, R. J., Cranley, J. J., Strasser, E. S., Hafner, C. D., and Fogarty, T. J.: Further experience with a new embolectomy catheter, SURGERY **59:** 81, 1966.
13. Madoff, I. M., Thompson, J. E., and Streider, J.: Embolization in surgery of mitral stenosis, New Eng. J. Med. **251:** 730, 1954.
14. McCann, W. J.: The management of arterial emboli, Amer. J. Surg. **108:** 768, 1964.
15. McMahon, J. E., and Sako, Y.: Arterial embolism and embolectomy, Geriatrics **23:** 132, 1968.
16. Milliken, J. C.: Delayed arterial embolectomy, J. Irish Med. Ass. **61:** 390, 1968.
17. Ouchi, H., and Warren, R.: Arterial embolism. Modern concepts, Arch. Surg. **85:** 905, 1962.
18. Porter, J. M., Acinapura, A. J., and Silver, D.: Aortic saddle embolectomy, Arch. Surg. **93:** 360, 1966.
19. Rossi, N. P., Ehrenhaft, J. L., and Sensenig, D. M.: Acute brachial artery occlusion, Ann. Surg. **161:** 195, 1965.
20. Sachatello, C. R.: Technique for subclavian, axillary, and brachial artery embolectomy, Arch. Surg. **97:** 836, 1968.
21. Scheinin, T. M., and Inberg, M. V.: Management of peripheral arterial embolism, Acta Chir. Scand. **133:** 517, 1967.
22. Scheinin, T. M., Wegelius, U., and Inberg, M. V.: The role of embolectomy and angiography in arterial embolism of the arm, Vas. Surg. **2:** 12, 1968.
23. Spencer, F. C., and Eiseman, B.: Delayed arterial embolectomy, a new concept, SURGERY **55:** 64, 1964.
24. Stallone, R. J., Blaisdell, F. W., Cafferata, H. T., and Levin, S. M.: Analysis of morbidity and mortality from arterial embolectomy, SURGERY **65:** 207, 1969.
25. Thompson, J. E., Austin, D. J., and Lovett, V.: Peripheral arterial embolism, Texas State J. Med. **55:** 277, 1959.
26. Weston, T. S.: Arterial embolism of the lower limbs, Australian Radiol. **11:** 354, 1967.
27. Young, J. R., Humphries, A. W., DeWolfe, V. G., and LeFevre, F. A.: Peripheral arterial embolism, J. A. M. A. **185:** 621, 1963.

DISCUSSION

Dr. Henry Haimovici (New York, N. Y.). Our concepts of the management of arterial embolism have been changing in the past decade, as attested to by significant progress achieved, as indicated by Dr. Thompson in his presentation. In addition to the newer surgical techniques, a number of other facets have come to light in the diagnosis and understanding of arterial embolism. I wish to refer specifically to the biochemical changes secondary to ischemia of striated muscles due to arterial embolism. In the past few years, I have observed a few cases of an unusual complication consisting of severe ischemic myopathy associated with myoglobinuria (SURGERY 47: 734, 1960). I wonder whether Dr. Thompson has ever observed such a complication in his reported series. Personally, having scanned the literature and having found very little or nothing on this topic, I feel that it might be of interest to this Society that I mention briefly this unusual complication of arterial embolism.

Slide 1 indicates the clinical syndrome of arterial embolism and myoglobinuria which consists of excruciating pain, pronounced ischemia of the tissues, rigidity of the limb, and massive edema. Of these manifestations I have been particularly impressed by the rigidity of the limb, since neither passive nor active attempts at moving the joints are possible. Slide 2 summarizes the essential clinical data of 4 cases observed in the past few years. All these patients were seen within 6 to 10 hours after clinical onset and presented essentially the clinical manifestations as indicated in the previous slide. All displayed extensive gangrene of the extremity and two of these died of renal shutdown associated with "myoglobinuric nephrosis." Slide 3 is a cross section of a leg muscle which displays a mixture of necrotic areas with other less advanced ischemic changes of the muscular fibers. Slide 4 indicates the sequence of pathologic events which seem to take place in this syndrome: embolic occlusion, ischemic myopathy, and release of myoglobin (myoglobinemia) and myoglobinuria. Because of the acidity of the urine, the myoglobin has a tendency to precipitate in the tubules and thus leads to the nephrosis secondary to myoglobin. To overcome this often fatal complication, it is essential, as soon as the diagnosis is suspected or made, to alkalinize the patient in order to prevent precipitation of myoglobin in the renal tubules. Finally, slide 5 indicates the cross section of a kidney of one of these 4 patients who died from this condition in which one can see dilatation of the tubules containing a granular material which gave a positive chemical reaction for iron. The latter represents precipitated myoglobin in the tubules as mentioned above. It is hoped that these observations may stimulate the members of this Society in reporting similar observations in the future.

Dr. John J. Cranley (Cincinnati, Ohio). I enjoyed this excellent paper, which Dr. Thompson has presented so beautifully. I rise to make three points.

The first is that, since the most important determinant of the outcome of this disease when untreated is the degree of distal thrombosis, and since this can be modified by the fact that the patient may have been on long-term anticoagulants, that the first physician has given heparin (as he should), and for natural reasons, we can no longer set any arbitrary time limit on when a successful embolectomy can be performed.

As long as the limb is alive, there's a chance to revascularize it.

The only contraindication that we know of is advanced rigor. At times, you can operate successfully even on a limb that already has mild rigor.

The second point is this: Do not be fooled by a good backflow. Remember, there may be distal discontinuous clotting. It has been our repeated experience to remove a femoral artery embolus, have an excellent backflow, despite the fact that a great deal of soft clot can still be extracted from the artery from the level of the knee or lower with the Fogarty catheter.

I'll use that one slide to make the final point. It is now seven years since we had the first homemade Fogarty catheter and we too have divided our cases into two series, one before and one after its development.

We have never opened the abdomen for an aortic or iliac artery embolus since the first catheter became available. In Series I, there were 13 aortic emboli, of which 7 or 54 percent were removed successfully, and an over-all mortality of 62 percent. In the second group, using the catheter, there were 18 aortic emboli, all of which were successfully removed, and the over-all mortality dropped to 17 percent.

In Series I, 21 of 27 iliac artery emboli or 78 percent were removed successfully, with a 26 percent over-all mortality, while in Series II, 28 of 29 (96.5 percent) of the emboli were removed successfully, with an over-all mortality of 10 percent.

The use of the catheter, then, has permitted us to remove aortic and iliac emboli without laparotomy through a femoral arteriotomy under local anesthesia. We believe that it is the use of the local anesthesia that has largely been responsible for the improvement in the operative mortality.

Dr. Thompson (closing). I would like to thank the discussants.

In answer to Dr. Haimovici's question, I have not seen, or at least have not recognized, myoglobinuria. I suppose we simply haven't looked for it and I would think, as he said, that the use of heparinization and prompt operative therapy will do more than anything else to avoid this sort of thing.

I am in full agreement with what Dr. Cranley has said and, as we have learned also, one should not be fooled by a good backflow as soon as the embolus is removed because if you pass a Fogarty catheter down the entire extent of the limb at this point, frequently you will be rewarded by several small emboli or thrombi. This should be done routinely I think, even if one does operate very promptly and the backflow appears vigorous when the embolus is first removed.

We are all indebted to Dr. Cranley and his group and to Dr. Fogarty for the development of this simple instrument, which everyone in this Society wishes he had thought of 20 years ago!

Microneurosurgical arterial reconstruction

M. GAZI YASARGIL, M.D.
HUGO A. KRAYENBUHL, M.D.
JULIUS H. JACOBSON, II, M.D.*
NEW YORK, N. Y.
From the Department of Neurosurgery, University of Zurich, Zurich, Switzerland, and the Department of Surgery, Division of Vascular Surgery, The Mount Sinai School of Medicine, New York

Despite the widespread application of reconstructive vascular surgery in the extracranial segments of the carotid and vertebral arteries, intracranial arterial reconstruction has largely remained an unfulfilled but tantalizing goal. The development of microvascular surgical methods has made it practical, technically, to reconstruct intracranial arteries.[5, 6]

The purpose of this report is to briefly present our preliminary experience with intracranial arterial reconstruction. These operations on patients with occlusive intracranial vascular diseases have been approached with great apprehension and hesitation because the indication for operation in such cases has not been delineated. Clinical experience has shown that neither the extent nor the number of occlusions solely determine the symptoms and their evolution. In the individual case there is no precise method to determine whether spontaneous recovery or repeated attacks with progression of the disease will occur. In addition, the approach to the arteries at the base of the brain and in the Sylvian fissure is difficult. The arteries to be operated upon must be reached without damage to the neighboring cerebral structures; the cerebral circulation must not be interrupted for any prolonged periods during the surgical manipulation of the vessels.

Initially, microvascular operative techniques were applied to the intracerebral arteries of animals dealing with vessels varying in size from 0.5 to 0.8 mm. in diameter. The microinstruments and suture materials were further refined and intraluminal shunts for vessels of these sizes developed. The animal work included basilar artery segmental replacement, arteriotomy and patch grafting of cortical arteries, and extra cranial-to-intracranial shunts between the superficial temporal and the middle cerebral arteries. Details of this work and techniques used have been published in a symposium on microsurgery.[2]

CLINICAL EXPERIENCE

In view of the experience gained in animals, it seemed that identical methods could be applied in patients with greater ease in view of the larger size of human vessels.

Thus far, 20 patients have been operated on for the purpose of direct intracranial revascularization. In 9 patients an end-to-side anastomosis was performed between the end of the superficial temporal artery and the side of the temporal division of the middle cerebral artery. In 11 cases, a direct arteriotomy has been carried out in one or more segments of the middle cerebral artery

Presented at the Twenty-third Annual Meeting of the Society for Vascular Surgery, New York, N. Y., July 12-13, 1969.

*Reprint requests should be directed to J. H. Jacobson, II, M.D., 1176 Fifth Avenue, New York, N. Y.

Table I. *Superficial temporal-to-temporal cortical artery shunt*

Name age sex	*Date onset vascular accident and clinical description*	*Angiography*	*Operation and date*
N. K. 20 Male	Aug. 7, 1967 Hemiplegia, right aphasia	Occlusion of left middle cerebral artery; no collaterals	Oct. 30, 1967 Shunt
St. E. 61 Male	Oct. 22, 1967 (Case 1 in report) Syncope on turning head, hemiparesis, and homonymous hemianopia	Occlusion right and left internal carotid arteries and right vertebral artery	Nov. 7, 1967 Shunt
F. G. 51 Male	Dec. 5, 1967 Left hemiplegia and homonymous hemianopia	Occlusion of right internal carotid artery in siphon—no collateral	Jan. 4, 1968 Shunt
R. L. 66 Female	Jan. 29, 1968 Subarachnoid hemorrhage	Aneurysm of posterior communicating artery, right	Feb. 2, 1968 Shunt—clipping of aneurysm with narrowing of internal carotid artery
K. W. 39 Male	May 17, 1968 Severe hemiparesis, left homonymous hemianopia	Occlusion of right internal carotid artery in siphon. No collateral	June 17, 1968 Shunt
H. J. 19 Female	(Case 2 in report) Progressive weakness of left side—most marked in forearm and hand since 1964	Aneurysm of internal carotid bifurcation occlusion of right middle cerebral artery—poor collaterals	Dec. 18, 1968 Shunt
P. A. 56 Male	Vertigo and dysphagia for 2 years	Occlusion of left internal carotid in siphon	March 3, 1969 Shunt
W. R. 19 Male	(Case 3 in report) Progressive right hemiparesis and aphasia starting Nov. 8, 1968	Progressive stenosis of left internal carotid artery; no collaterals	March 17, 1969 Shunt
S. M. 42 Male	May 19, 1969 Left hemiplegia with homonymous hemianopia	Occlusion of left middle cerebral artery—segment too long (6 cm.) for embolectomy—poor collateral	June 10, 1969 Shunt

with either embolectomy or thrombectomy being performed. The two procedures are discussed individually in the following sections. A monograph will be published soon which provides detailed descriptions of the individual cases.[14]

Extracranial-to-intracranial shunting. The subcutaneously located superficial temporal artery is freed up just anterior to the tragus of the ear. A small bone flap is removed and the dura opened. Using the surgical microscope under low power, a superficial cortical artery lying on the temporal lobe in the immediate vicinity of the Sylvian fissure is chosen for the anastomosis. The arachnoid is opened adjacent to the artery and the artery dissected free for a distance of 10 to 12 mm. A rubber dam is laid under the artery in order to avoid touching or damaging the cerebral cortex.

The superficial temporal artery is then anastomosed end-to-side to the cortical artery with interrupted sutures of No. 10-0 monofilament nylon. Twenty-five times magnification is required for this. The occluding clamp on the proximal temporal artery is removed prior to those on the cortical arteries in order to wash out any air.

Five of the 9 patients undergoing the procedure showed marked improvement (Table I). In each of these, arteriography showed a patent anastomosis with the middle cerebral complex being filled by way of the superficial temporal artery. In the sixth patient who

Time elapsed from vascular accident	Follow-up clinical status	Follow-up angiography	Pulsation of superficial temporal artery
3 Months	Moderate improvement	Refused	Good
2 Months	Marked improvement in hemiparesis; can turn head freely	Bypass patent	Good
1 Month	Slight improvement	Poorly visualized ? Stenotic	Poor
3 Days	Left hemiparesis Moderately improved	Refused	Good
1 Month	Hemiparesis completely disappeared	Bypass patent	Good
4 Years	Hemiparesis completely disappeared	Bypass patent	Good
2 Years	Worse initially, slightly improved at present	Closed bypass—basilar artery stenosis not appreciated preoperatively	Absent
4 Months	Marked improvement	Bypass patent	Good
1 Month	Slight improvement	To be done	Good

was studied arteriographically and who showed moderate clinical improvement, the anastomosis was closed. The remaining three patients who showed no evidence of improvement have not, as yet, been studied.

CASE REPORTS

Case 1. This 62-year-old man had multiple episodes of transient hemiparesis, aphasia, and blurring of vision in the left eye during the 3 years prior to admission. Three weeks prior to admission he developed a permanent left hemiparesis and a left homonymous hemianopia. Angiography revealed occlusion of both internal carotid arteries and the right vertebral artery. The large left vertebral artery was the apparent source of bilateral filling of the infra- and supratentorial arteries. Pressure applied locally over the left vertebral artery origin induced syncope, as did turning the head to the extreme right.

Three weeks following the onset of the permanent hemiparesis, an end-to-side anastomosis was carried out between the superficial temporal artery and a temporal cortical artery. The operative and postoperative course was quite unremarkable. Gradual improvement occurred in the patient's neurological status. Eighteen months later he had only a slight distal paresis of the left arm and a quadrant visual field defect. Previous transient episodes which had been triggered by turning his head to the right could not be induced postoperatively.

A right carotid angiogram performed 12 weeks following the operation revealed patency of the anastomosis and filling of the cortical vessels with excellent delineation of the posterior temporal artery, the angular artery, and posterior parietal artery.

Comment. It is impossible to state whether the improvement would have occurred without the surgical intervention. However, the disappearance of syncope on head-turning and the cessation of transient ischemic episodes were clearly related in time to the performance of the surgery.

Case 2. This 19-year-old woman had a focal epileptic seizure followed by a pronounced left-sided hemiparesis. Right carotid angiography revealed partial thrombosis of a giant saccular aneurysm arising from the bifurcation of the right internal carotid artery (Fig. 1, *A* and *B*). Left carotid angiography showed filling of both anterior cerebral arteries, but no collaterals to the right middle cerebral artery (Fig. 2). The vertebral angiogram demonstrated a small posterior communicating artery on the right side with minimal filling of the right middle cerebral artery (Fig. 3).

At exploration through a frontotemporal craniotomy, the aneurysm was found to be totally thrombosed as was the right internal carotid artery. Therefore an end-to-side anastomosis was carried out between the superficial temporal artery and a cortical artery overlying the temporal lobe. The patient recovered without complications and showed rapid disappearance of the hemiparesis.

Arteriography 3 months later revealed the right internal carotid artery to be occluded with nonfilling of the aneurysm (Fig. 4). The branches of the right middle cerebral artery filled through the dilated superficial temporal artery via the surgically created end-to-side anastomosis.

Comment. While spontaneous improvement might well have occurred in this young woman, the filling of the middle cerebral complex via the shunt would seem to indicate that the filling pressure was higher from this source than in any collaterals that had also developed.

Case 3. This 19-year-old man developed a motor aphasia and a spastic right-sided hemiparesis following an epileptic seizure. The left carotid angiogram showed a stenosis of the internal carotid artery at the level of the upper siphon (Fig. 5). The aphasia and hemiparesis worsened during the 5 months following the original episode.

Another left carotid angiogram showed further obstruction of the internal carotid artery with only the anterior choroidal artery filling. The left middle cerebral artery was barely opacified and the left anterior cerebral artery was not filled at all. The vertebral angiogram showed a large posterior communicating artery but no filling of the middle cerebral artery even though the anterior cerebral was seen (Fig. 6).

A superficial temporal-to-temporal cortical artery shunt was performed. During an uneventful postoperative course, there was rapid lessening, but incomplete disappearance, of the hemiparesis and aphasia. An angiogram done 2 months postoperatively showed patency of the anastomosis and filling of the left middle cerebral artery and its branches (Fig. 7).

Comment. This is a particularly important case because time was allowed to elapse during which the neurological status worsened. The course of events was quite promptly reversed by the performance of the extra-to-intracranial shunt. The x-ray pathology in this patient suggests the possibility of the fibromuscular hyperplasia which, to our knowledge, has been unreported in the intracranial circulation.

MIDDLE CEREBRAL ARTERY

The middle cerebral artery has been opened eleven times with the clinical history and findings suggesting emboli in 5 and thrombi in 6 patients. The approach was through a frontotemporal bone flap. Thrombectomy or embolectomy was done in each case. In no instance was a true endarterectomy carried out as this term applies in peripheral vascular surgery. The middle cerebral artery in man is about 2 mm. in diameter and is more delicate, with a thinner wall, than that present in peripheral arteries of the same size.

Eight of the 11 patients showed improvement in their clinical status during their early postoperative period. In 4, the improvement was so rapid that the surgical intervention seemed clearly related. In 5 of the patients middle cerebral artery patency was demonstrated by angiography and in a sixth, at postmortem examination.

There were 2 deaths in the series directly attributable to the operation. The first was a 42-year-old man who had a thrombus removed 2 months following the stroke. He died suddenly on the third postoperative day of what was thought to be a pulmonary embolus. The second patient was operated

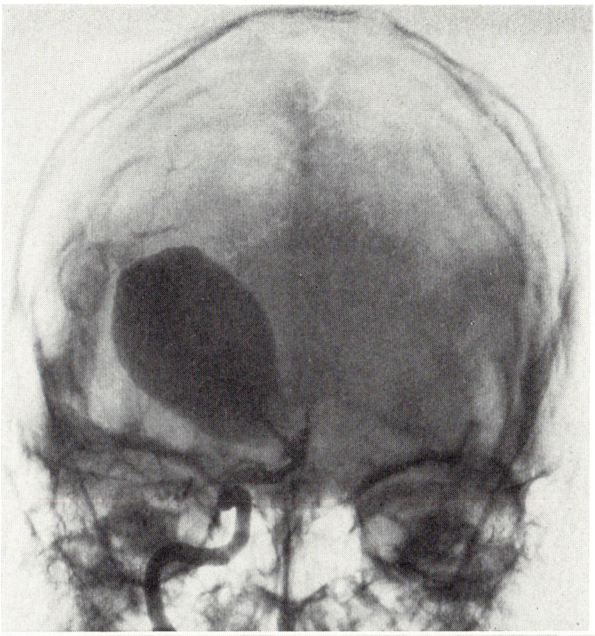

A

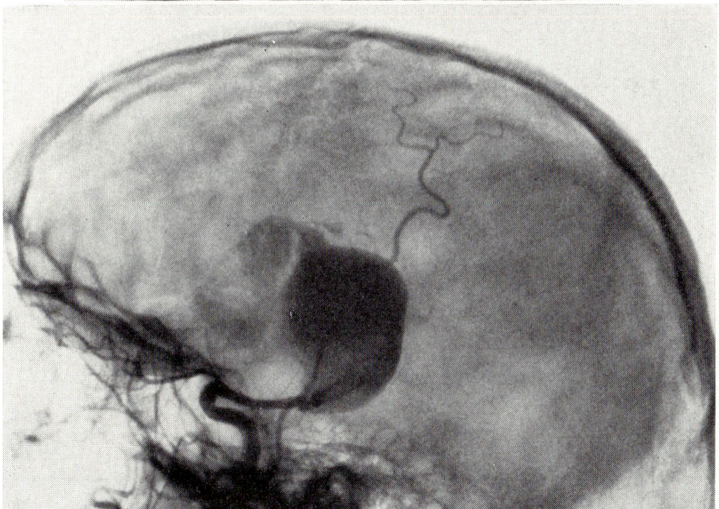

B

Fig. 1. Case 2. *A,* A right carotid angiogram showing a huge saccular aneurysm at the bifurcation of the internal carotid artery. *B,* Lateral view of the same angiogram showing a partial thrombosis of the aneurysm and stenosis of the internal carotid artery.

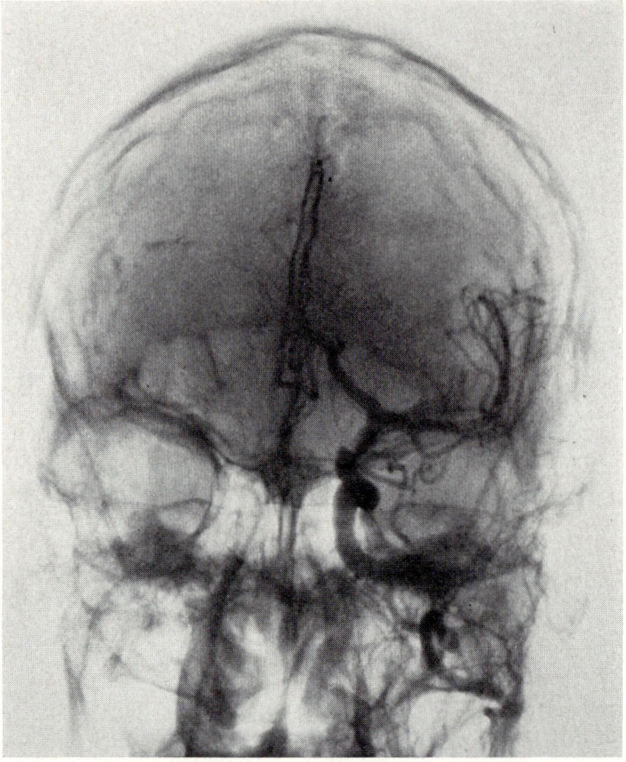

Fig. 2. Left AP carotid angiogram showing the absence of middle cerebral filling on the right, although both anterior cerebral arteries are clearly opacified.

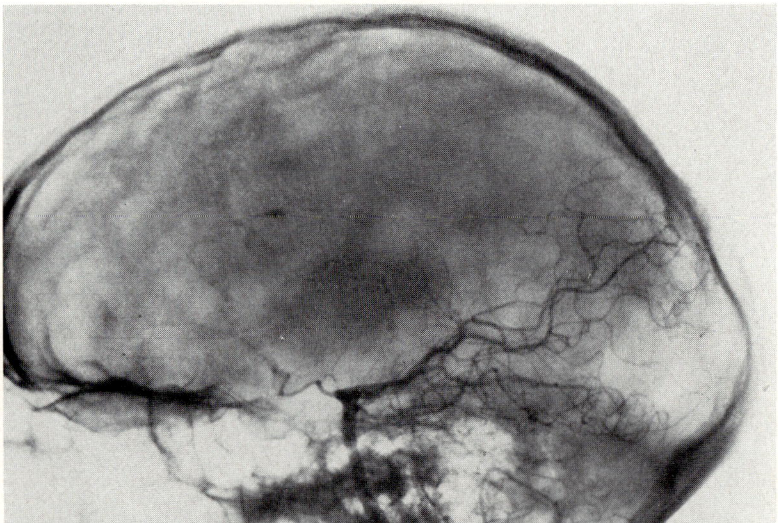

Fig. 3. Lateral vertebral angiogram demonstrating filling of the posterior communicating artery taken one month following the initial episode. Note that only a small twig communicates with the right cerebral artery.

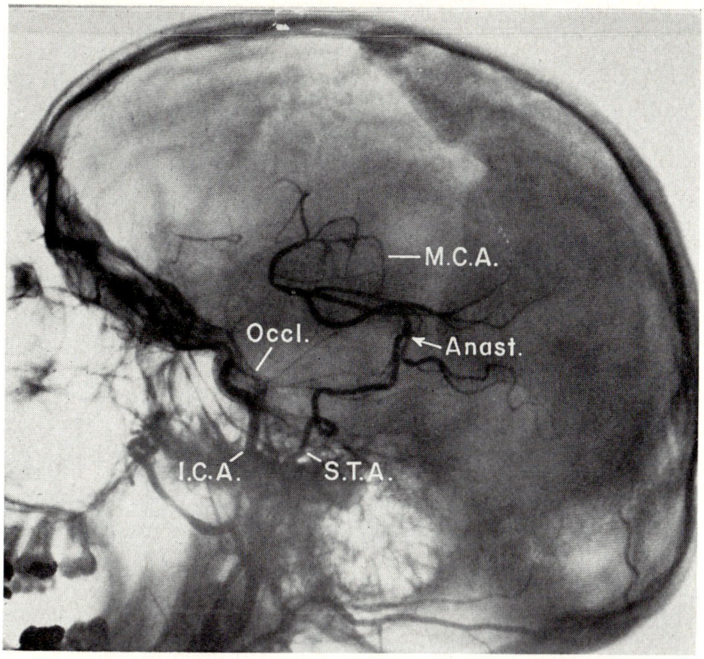

Fig. 4A. Right carotid angiography 3 months postoperatively showing occlusion of the right internal carotid artery at the siphon. The contrast media is filling middle cerebral branches through the patent enlarged superior temporal artery shunt which communicates with a temporal cortical artery. An arrow marks the anastomotic site. *I.C.A. Occl.,* Occluded internal carotid artery; *M.C.A.,* middle cerebral artery; *S.T.A.,* superficial temporal artery.

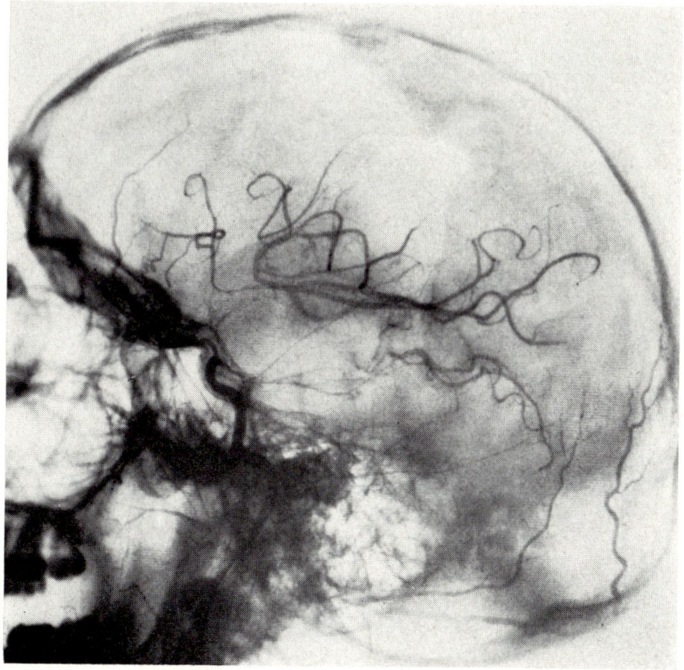

Fig. 4B. A later phase of the same angiogram showing further filling of the middle cerebral artery complex.

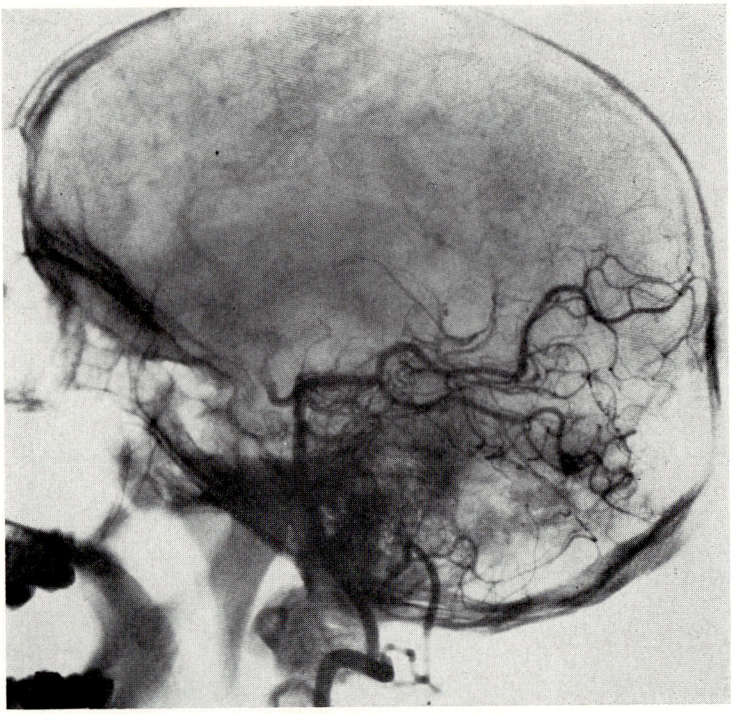

Fig. 5. Case 3. A left carotid angiogram showing stenosis of the internal carotid artery.

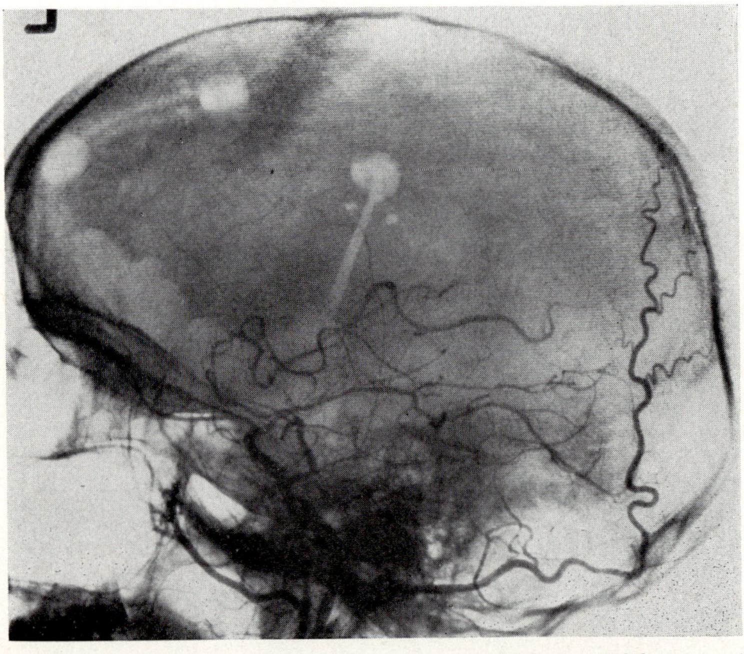

Fig. 6*A*. Left carotid angiogram 3 weeks after operation. The superficial temporal artery has been anastomosed to a temporal cortical artery which is in turn filling branches of the middle cerebral artery.

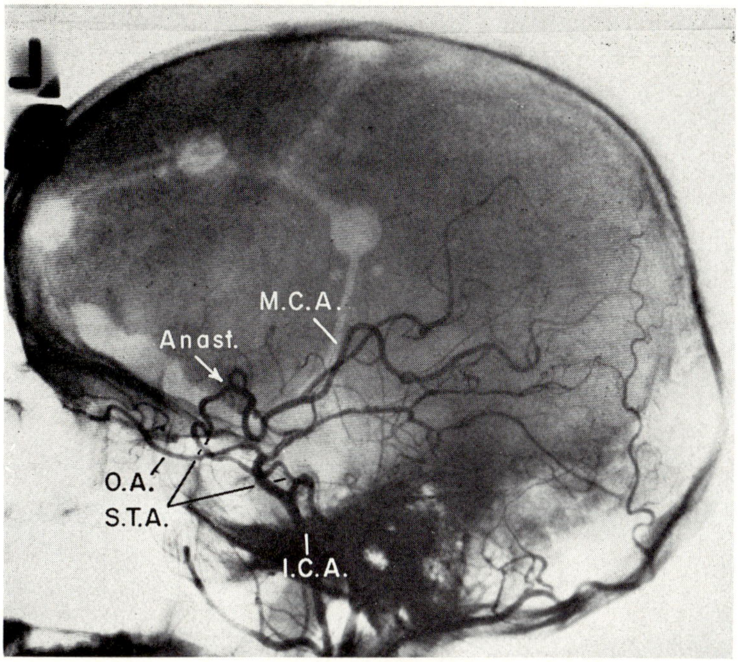

Fig. 6*B*. Two and a half months postoperatively, this left carotid angiogram shows marked enlargement of the superficial temporal artery and further improvement in the filling of the middle cerebral artery. *Anast.*, Superficial temporal-to-temporal cortical artery anastomosis; *M.C.A.*, middle cerebral artery; *S.T.A.*, superficial temporal artery; *I.C.A.*, internal carotid artery; *O.A.*, ophthalmic artery.

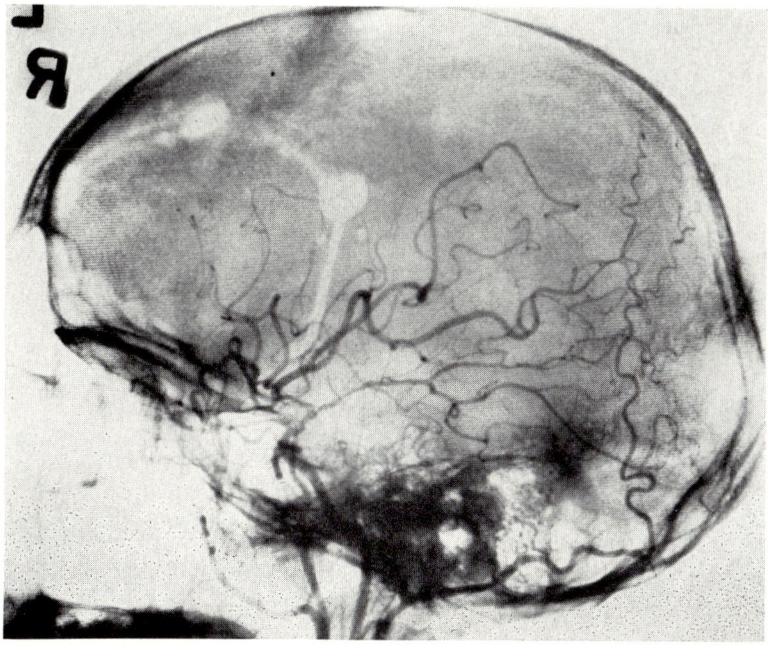

Fig. 6*C*. Later phase of the same study shown in Fig. 6*B*, demonstrating filling of the most distal branches of the middle cerebral artery.

Table II. *Direct middle cerebral artery reconstruction*

Name age sex	*Date of vascular accident and clinical description*	*Angiography*	*Date operation length of clot*
M. E. 48 Male	Aug. 7, 1966 Hemiparesis, aphasia, homonymous hemianopia	Occlusion left middle cerebral artery	Jan. 7, 1967 Thrombectomy 4 cm.
A. A. 31 Male	Aug. 12, 1967 Hemiparesis, aphasia, and homonymous hemianopia	Occlusion left middle cerebral artery	Aug. 14, 1967 Thrombectomy 1 cm.
R. H. 44 Male	Aug. 11, 1967 Myocardial infarct in 1960, hemiparesis and aphasia	Occlusion left middle cerebral artery	Aug. 27, 1967 Embolectomy 3 cm.
G. A. 29 Male	Jan. 19, 1967 Hemiplegia, left	Occlusion right middle cerebral artery	Jan. 27, 1967 Thrombectomy 2 cm.
W. E. 43 Male	Feb. 9, 1967 Hemiplegia and aphasia	Stenosis left internal carotid artery in neck Occlusion left middle cerebral artery	March 10, 1967 Carotid endarterectomy April 4, 1967 Embolectomy 3 cm.
M. A. 42 Male	Aug. 28, 1967 Hemiplegia	Occlusion right middle cerebral artery	Sept. 9, 1967 Thrombectomy 1 cm.
H. T. 44 Male	Starr-Edwards valve in 1965 Dec. 21 and 26, 1968 Hemiplegia worsening suddenly 5 days later	Occlusion right middle cerebral artery	Dec. 26, 1968 Embolectomy Two 0.5 cm. emboli
K. R. 43 Male	July 20, 1968, and Dec. 5, 1968 Hemiplegia and aphasia, homonymous hemianopia	Occlusion left middle cerebral artery	Dec. 12, 1968 Thrombectomy 1 cm.
M. R. 46 Male	March 28, 1969 Hemiparesis and aphasia	Occlusion left middle cerebral artery	April 4, 1969 Embolectomy 1 cm.
K. H. 44 Male	Feb. 13, 1969 Hemiparesis, right, and aphasia	Occlusion left middle cerebral artery	Feb. 21, 1969 Thrombectomy 1 cm.
P. L. 62 Male	April 21, 1969 Carotid—cavernous sinus fistula treated surgically by muscle embolization resulted in middle cerebral occlusion	Occlusion left middle cerebral artery	April 21, 1969 40 minutes after onset muscle embolus removed 0.5 cm.

on 18 hours following an embolus from a prosthetic aortic valve. He showed marked improvement during the early postoperative hours but at 10 hours required re-exploration for evacuation of a hematoma. A purulent meningtis subsequently developed. At postmortem examination 3 months postoperatively, the artery was found to be patent.

The reader is referred to Table II and the previously cited monograph[14] for further details of the cases.

DISCUSSION

Intracranial reconstructive vascular surgery has been performed in isolated cases without a microscope by Welch,[12] Shillito,[10] Driesen,[3] Scheibert,[9] Chou,[1] and Woringer and Kunlin.[13]

In 1960, Jacobson and Suarez demon-

Time elapsed from vascular accident	Easy follow-up clinical status	Angiography	Late follow-up status
5 Months	Marked improvement for 4 months	Not done	Died 6 months later of glioblastoma multiforme, left parietal
12 Days	Rapid improvement	Patent	No paresis Slight speech impairment
11 Days	Rapid improvement	Patent	No paresis No aphasia
2 Days	No improvement	Not done	Hemiplegia unchanged
1 Month	Moderate improvement	Patent	Moderate improvement Speech good
2 Months		Patent but stenosed	Hemiparesis remains
2 Months	No change for 3 days, then fatal pulmonary embolus	Not done	Died No postmortem
18 Hours	Improvement 10 hours, then coma due to intracranial hemorrhage—reoperation—infection	Not done	Died 3 months postoperatively of cerebral infection Postmortem showed patent artery
7 Days	Moderate improvement	Patent	Moderate improvement—walks alone but speech difficult
7 Days	Moderate improvement	Patent	Moderate improvement—walks alone, arm paresis persists, speech better but impaired
9 Days	Moderate improvement	Not done	Paresis improved—speech impairment
40 Minutes	Moderate improvement	Not done	Paresis better Speech impairment

strated the value of the surgical microscope in securing consistent patency in anastomosing arteries[5] and veins[7] and performing endarterectomy in vessels as small as 1 mm. in diameter. This work entailed the development of special instruments for microsurgery and ultrafine suture materials and needles. A small number of reconstructive procedures on intracranial arteries were then attempted, utilizing the microsurgical technique by Jacobson and Donaghy[6] in 1963 and Lougheed, Gunton, and Barnett[8] in 1965.

The presently reported experience can only be considered a very preliminary effort. The feasibility of surgically creating shunts from the extracranial to the intracranial arterial circulation has been demonstrated as has removal of blood clots directly from the middle cerebral artery. No mortality was encountered in the shunt group, while 2 of the 11 died in those undergoing direct middle cerebral artery reconstruction, one of a pulmonary embolus and the other of a purulent meningitis presumably secondary to re-exploration for postoperative bleeding.

Assessment of the improvement directly due to the surgical revascularization is obviously almost impossible in a small series of this nature; the speed and extent of spontaneous recovery in any individual case simply cannot be predicted. On the other hand, the demonstration of the anatomical revascularization demonstrated by angiography can certainly not be discounted as contributing to cerebral viability and function even by the most intransigent.

The debate which immediately arises, of course, centers around the viability of brain tissue exposed to various degrees of ischemia. Tissue which is dead cannot come back to life! Contrariwise, segments of brain tissue having marginal blood supplies may be nonfunctional and yet viable. To see the cogency of this viewpoint, one has only to think of the return of function of cerebral tissue, evidenced by the improvement in many patients having had acute strokes. Apparently an area of the brain damaged by ischemia is able to regain function, presumably concomitant with development of collateral circulation.

Furthermore, since the arterial circulation of the brain has relatively rich communications from one area to another, restoration of blood flow to one area might well have value in protecting against future vascular insults to another. It is not inconceivable that patients with organic mental syndromes may benefit from this type approach.

Better methods of assessing the viability of brain tissue are badly needed. Unfortunately, existing techniques of measuring brain blood flow do not help at all in assessment in a situation where a specific small region of the brain is in question. Hyperbaric oxygenation[11] may prove to be a useful adjunct in that function is seen to return in about one third of patients with strokes. As yet, this has not proved therapeutically useful in that regression occurs when the patient is removed from the chamber, which is necessitated to prevent oxygen toxicity. In the future, the physician might expose the fresh stroke patient to hyperbaric oxygen. If improvement occurred, it would mean that reversibility existed and therefore surgery might be beneficial. In this situation, areas of marginal brain might be kept alive by the added oxygen[4] until the revascularization procedure was performed in the chamber.

The optimal time to perform a revascularization procedure is simply not known. The risk of converting an ischemic to a hemorrhagic is generally said to be highest from beyond 24 hours after the stroke up to three or four weeks. The results in the cases which had the shunts performed at a late date following the accident are superior to those in the middle cerebral group but the two most dramatic successes were in patients operated on at 11 and 12 days. No firm conclusion can be drawn.

One of the reasons for presenting this work during its preliminary phase is the hope of stimulating others to pursue it. Once enough general experience has been gained to even propose reasonable hypotheses, a large cooperative study will probably be necessary to arrive at the true facts.

SUMMARY

Utilizing microvascular surgical techniques, the feasibility of achieving patency in middle cerebral artery reconstruction and the creation of extracranial-to-intracranial arterial shunts has been demonstrated. While many of the patients seem to have benefited, the variability of spontaneous improvement in patients with major vascular accidents is so great that the only conclusion drawn is that this preliminary work is worthy of further pursuit.

REFERENCES

1. Chou, S. N.: Embolectomy of middle cerebral artery, J. Neurosurg. **20:** 161, 1963.
2. Donaghy, R. M. P., and Yasargil, M. G.: Micro-vascular surgery, Stuttgart, 1967, Georg Thieme Verlag, St. Louis, 1967. The C. V. Mosby Company, pp. 87-126.
3. Driesen, W.: Erfolgreiche Naht der Linken A.

Cerebri Media Nach Verletzung Durch Tumorresektion, Acta Neurochir. **10:** 462, 1962.
4. Hollin, S. A., Espinosa, O. E., Sukoff, M. H., and Jacobson, J. H.: The effect of hyperbaric oxygenation on cerebrospinal fluid oxygen, J. Neurosurg. **29:** 229, 1968.
5. Jacobson, J. H., and Suarez, E. L.: Microsurgery in anastomosis of small vessels, Surg. Forum **11:** 243, 1960.
6. Jacobson, J. H.: Microsurgical technique, *in* Cooper, Philip, editor: Craft of surgery, Boston, 1964, Little, Brown & Company, vol. I, chap. 67, pp. 799-819.
7. Jacobson, J. H., and Katsumura, T.: Small vein reconstruction, J. Cardiov. Surg. **6:** 157, 1965.
8. Lougheed, W. M., Gunton, R. W., and Barnett, H. J. M.: Embolectomy of internal carotid, middle and anterior cerebral arteries, J. Neurosurg. **22:** 607, 1965.
9. Scheibert, C. D.: Middle cerebral artery surgery for obstructive lesions, presented at the Meeting of Harvey Cushing Society, New Orleans, La., May 2, 1962.
10. Shillito, J., Jr.: Indications for surgery in cerebrovascular accidents, Postgrad. Med. **30:** 537, 1961.
11. Sukoff, M. H., Hollin, S. A., and Jacobson, J. H.: The protective effect of hyperbaric oxygenation in experimentally produced cerebral edema and compression, SURGERY **62:** 40, 1967.
12. Welch, K.: Excision of occlusive lesions of middle cerebral artery, J. Neurosurg. **13:** 73, 1965.
13. Woringer, E., and Kunlin, J.: Anastomose entre la carotide primitive et la carotide intracranienne ou la Sylvienne par greffon selon la technique de la suture suspendue, Neurochir. (Paris) **9:** 181, 1963.
14. Yasargil, M. G.: Microsurgery applied to neurosurgery, Stuttgart, 1969, Georg Thieme Verlag. In press.

DISCUSSION

Chairman Yeager. Dr. Yasargil, I would like to add my personal congratulations on the tremendous step forward in this type of surgery.

I'm sure the enthusiasm from the audience also attests that they feel the same way. You are the first one on this program where the Secretary specifically allowed a participant to complete his presentation. Otherwise, you know, we've cut most people off [laughter] and I think this is a further testimonial to the great contribution that we feel we've been able to listen to today.

I'd like to add my personal congratulations.

Do we have any discussion of Dr. Yasargil's paper?

I think the question is extraneous. I'm sure no one in this audience has the courage to get up and discuss this great contribution [laughter].

Modifications in the technique for femoropopliteal saphenous vein bypass autografts

ROBERT R. LINTON, M.D.
W. LAWRENCE WILDE, M.D.
BOSTON, MASS.
From the Department of Surgery, Massachusetts General Hospital

Reconstructive arterial procedures to restore the circulation of the lower limb in obliterative atherosclerosis continue to remain an enigma of the field of vascular surgery. Excellent short-term results of one to 3 years have been obtained by many surgeons utilizing bypass arterial homografts, synthetic prostheses, and restoration of the arterial lumen in continuity by thromboendarterectomy. Since atherosclerosis obliterans of the lower extremity in the majority of patients is a chronic disease, early failures after one to 3 years with these procedures in the majority of patients has resulted in the abandonment of these methods by many surgeons. Saphenous vein autografts, on the other hand, have proved to give excellent results over a period of 10 years or more in many patients. As a result, they have become established by many surgeons[1, 3, 5, 10] as the best method for the treatment of segmental atherosclerotic occlusive disease of the lower extremities involving the femoral and popliteal arteries, since Kunlin[6] first reported it in 1949. Cumulative patency rates of 75 percent at 5 years and 60 percent at 10 years have been reported by us.[2]

A reversed saphenous vein bypass autograft functions best in the majority of patients when the proximal anastomosis is to the common femoral artery. This optimal type of reconstructive arterial procedure for segmental occlusion of the superficial femoral and proximal popliteal arteries is not always possible because the saphenous vein in about 20 percent of cases is too small to be used as a long graft, especially when it is less than 4 mm. in diameter, or when the segment of good caliber is too short for a bypass graft. Furthermore, it has been our experience that a technically flawless anastomosis, both proximal and distal, is of the greatest importance to insure lasting patency of a vein graft. Thus, early failures have occurred even with vein grafts 5 mm. in diameter when the femoral artery, despite adequate lumen and outflow, had such a thick friable intima that it was impossible to perform a technically satisfactory end-to-side anastomosis with the vein graft. The common femoral artery is the preferred site for the proximal anastomosis because it has a greater blood flow than the superficial femoral artery and as a result gives a better inflow into the graft. It is not uncommon, however, to be confronted with a diseased atherosclerotic common femoral artery with such marked intimal thickening that a satisfactory anastomosis is impossible to accomplish. Another cause of failure has been inadequate inflow into the saphenous vein bypass graft because of severe atherosclerotic occlusive disease in the common femoral and external iliac arteries above the site of proximal anastomosis.

The purpose of this paper is to describe some modifications that have been developed to enable the surgeon to utilize segments of autogenous saphenous veins of smaller caliber and of shorter length as bypass grafts, and to show how to obtain a satisfactory inflow into the graft by endarterectomy of

Presented at the Twenty-third Annual Meeting of the Society for Vascular Surgery, New York, N. Y., July 12-13, 1969.

the common femoral and external iliac arteries, with closure of the femoral arteriotomy with an autogenous vein patch graft to which the proximal end of the vein bypass graft can be anastomosed in a more satisfactory and technically easier fashion.

METHODS

This report comprises 68 operative procedures in 59 patients. Eight patients had two, one on each extremity; and one patient had two of the various anastomoses under study performed at the same operation, one at each end of the graft so that there were a total of 68 anastomotic procedures available for analysis. The period of study includes operations performed from September, 1960, through December, 1965, and includes all patients who underwent these various procedures.

Percutaneous iliofemoral and femoropopliteal arteriograms were performed in all patients with palpable femoral pulses prior to surgery by the method previously reported.[8] In the remainder it was done as part of the operative procedure. The popliteal artery and the outflow tract were graded excellent, good, fair, poor, or none, according to the radiographic findings. "Excellent" included the cases with an essentially normal popliteal artery and outflow vessels. "Good" was applied to those with an almost normal popliteal artery, and two of the three outflow arteries patent. "Fair" indicated a patent popliteal artery with one terminal branch open. "Poor" was applied to cases with a narrow, sclerotic popliteal artery and some outflow through one or two similarly affected outflow arteries. "None" was reserved for those cases where all three major outflow branches of the popliteal were occluded so that the outflow tract was entirely by way of collateral vessels from a short segment of the popliteal artery that was still patent.

There were 41 men and 18 women in the group. Their ages ranged from 39 to 78 years, with an average of 58.9 years. In general, the population in this study was comparable to that in a previous report of saphenous vein bypass grafts with regard to frequency of associated diseases. Operative techniques and general principles of management followed the guidelines previously presented.[2, 8] The saphenous vein in all cases was carefully excised and implanted in the reversed manner.

INDICATIONS FOR RECONSTRUCTIVE ARTERIAL PROCEDURES

The most common indication for reconstructive arterial procedures in this series of 68 extremities was intermittent claudication. It was of moderate severity in 5, or 7.4 percent and severe in 63, or 92.5 percent. The same ratio existed in Groups I and II. In Group I the ischemia was severe enough to cause rest pain in 9 extremities, ischemic ulcerations of the foot or toes in 7, and frank gangrene involving the feet and toes in 5, totaling 21 with the most severe symptoms. In Group II there were 3 extremities so afflicted, 2 with rest pain and 1 with ischemic ulcerations. These figures indicate that the most severely affected were in Group I, and the majority of all of them was in Group IA, since 5 of the ones with rest pain, 6 with ulcers, and 4 with gangrene, totaling 15, or 62.5 per cent, were in Group IA. It is noteworthy that despite this the best results were obtained in this group.

The period of follow-up exceeds 24 months in all living cases. The results were obtained by a personal examination of the patients by the authors, except in three cases where the patient lived at a long distance which precluded re-examination. In 2 of these, written statements by the patients of unlimited exercise tolerance, as compared with their preoperative severe intermittent claudication, were accepted as evidence of a functioning graft. The graft in the third one was known to be occluded by letters received from the patient and the local doctor. A graft was rated successful in all other patients only if distal pulses were unequivocally palpable, and corroborated by sensitive oscillometry, and if the patient had an asymptomatic normal functioning limb on exercise.

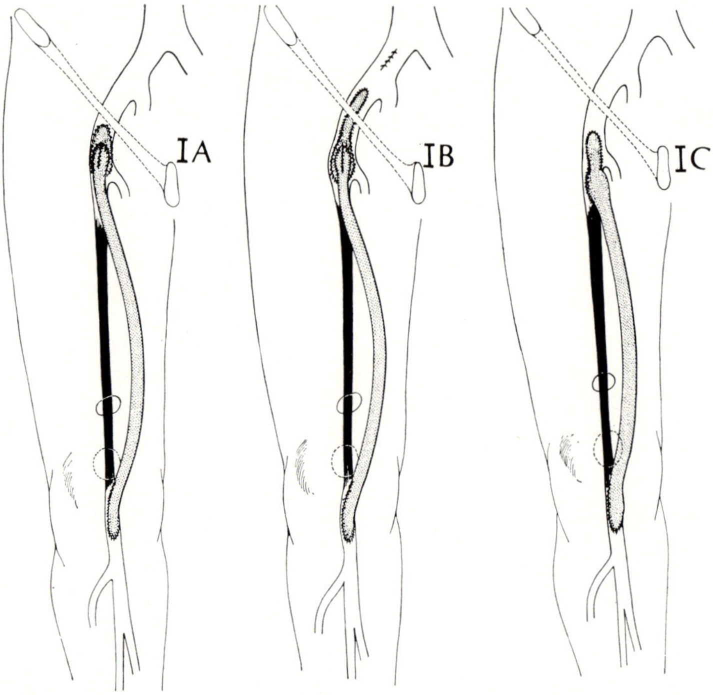

Fig. 1. An artist's drawings to show the three different techniques used in Group I with long autogenous vein bypass grafts.

No patient was lost to follow-up except by death.

The operative procedures were divided into two main groups and each of these into three subdivisions depending on the technique that was employed in the reconstructive procedure.

Group I includes those cases in whom a long autogenous saphenous vein of adequate caliber was available for a bypass graft from the common femoral artery to the distal popliteal artery, and angioplastic procedures were performed to permit the construction of more satisfactory proximal anastomosis. Group II, on the other hand, consisted of composite procedures made necessary because in some extremities only a short segment of the long saphenous vein of sufficient caliber for a graft was found. The reconstructive procedures in these cases consisted of a long endarterectomy of the common and superficial femoral arteries and a short vein bypass graft from the distal end of the endarterectomized superficial femoral artery to the distal segment of the popliteal artery. They were performed in an attempt to utilize autogenous tissues for the reconstructive procedure and avoid the necessity of resorting to plastic prostheses. The results obtained in this series of 68 procedures demonstrates the superiority of those performed in Group I.

Group I. There were 54 procedures in this group characterized by an anastomosis of the saphenous vein bypass graft to a vein patch graft on the common femoral artery at the proximal anastomosis in 45 extremities, and by a vein patch in continuity with the bypass graft in 9 (Fig. 1).

Group IA. Thirty-six operations in this group consisted of a long bypass graft anastomosed proximally to a small patch graft, less than 5 cm. long, usually after a limited local endarterectomy of the common femoral artery and sometimes of the origin of the superficial femoral artery at the site of the arteriotomy (Fig. 1, *A*). In some instances, because of the small caliber of the saphenous

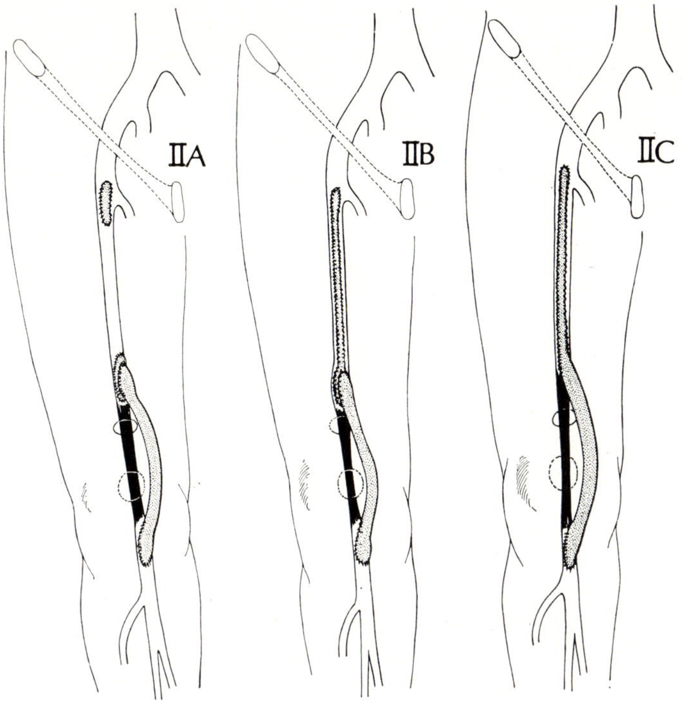

Fig. 2. An artist's drawings to show the three different techniques used in Group II with composite procedures consisting of a long proximal superficial femoral endarterectomy and a short autogenous vein bypass graft.

vein, a wider proximal anastomosis was accomplished by performing an angioplasty between two major branches of the saphenous vein trunk which resulted in a wider cuff of vein with which to construct the anastomosis (Fig. 3). The distal anastomosis in one case also was to a patch graft on the popliteal artery, and in 35 cases a patch graft on the common femoral or the proximal superficial femoral artery. The bypass grafts in this group varied from 31 to 56 cm. in length, with an average of 41.1 cm. Six patients had simultaneous aortoiliac endarterectomies, and one underwent replacement of the diseased aorta with a Dacron prosthesis at the same operation, thereby insuring an adequate outflow from the common femoral artery in each case. The popliteal outflow tracts in these patients were rated excellent or good in 20, and fair, poor, or none, in 16. The distribution of these according to results obtained is described in Table I.

Group IB. Nine procedures in 8 patients of this group consisted of a more extensive proximal endarterectomy of the common femoral artery with a vein patch graft 5 cm. or longer, and a long bypass graft from the patch graft to the distal popliteal artery (Fig. 1, *B*). Three had a partial endarterectomy of the external iliac artery as part of the procedure. The grafts varied from 53 to 36 cm. in length, the average being 44.7 cm. Six extremities had excellent or good outflow tracts and 3 were fair to poor.

Group IC. There were 9 patients in this group characterized by a short proximal vein patch graft in continuity with a long saphenous vein bypass graft applied to the proximal arteriotomy after a local endarterectomy of the proximal end of the superficial femoral artery and the distal end of the common femoral artery (Fig. 1, *C*). These bypass grafts varied between 33 and 49 cm. in length, the average being 42.2 cm. The outflow tracts were rated excellent to good in 5, and fair to poor in 4.

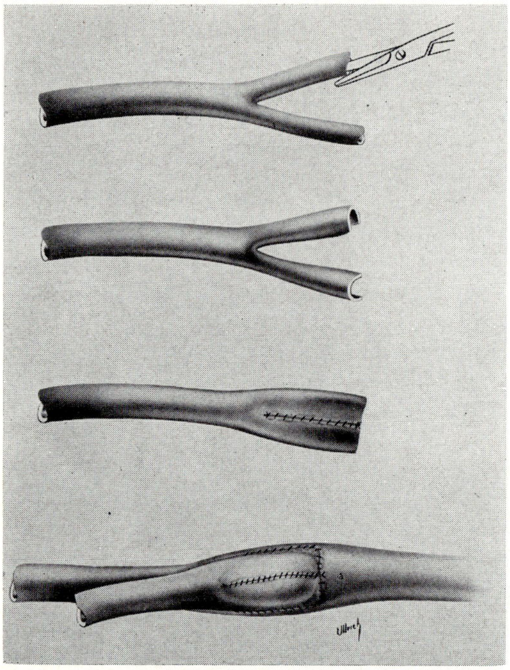

Fig. 3. An artist's drawing to show the angioplastic procedure to increase the width of the proximal end of the reversed saphenous vein autograft. (Courtesy of Maryland State Medical Journal, October, 1965.[7])

Table I. *Correlation of results with quality of outflow tract*

	Excellent or good	*Fair, poor, or none*
Group IA		
Successful	15	11
Failure	4	3
Dead before 24 months (graft not occluded)	1	2
Group IB		
Successful	4	1
Failure	2	2
Group IC		
Successful	5	2
Failure	0	1
Dead before 24 months (graft not occluded)	0	1
Group IIA		
Successful	1	0
Failure	3	2
Group IIB		
Successful	1	1
Failure	2	0
Group IIC		
Successful	2	1
Failure	0	1
Over-all		
Successful	28	16
Failure	11	9

Subdivision IC differed from IA and IB in that a short endarterectomy was performed of the common femoral artery and several centimeters of the superficial femoral artery so that the proximal anastomosis of the vein bypass graft could be made to the distal end of the arteriotomy in the proximal end of the superficial femoral artery. In addition, the proximal part of the arteriotomy was closed with a vein patch graft that was in continuity with the vein bypass graft. This technique was used because in some of the patients the proximal end of the vein grafts were not large enough in caliber to make a satisfactory proximal anastomosis to the common femoral artery, but the narrowed segment could be used as a patch in continuity with the vein graft to close the proximal part of the arteriotomy incision. This permitted the utilization of a shorter vein graft of sufficient caliber to reach from the proximal superficial femoral artery to the distal portion of the popliteal artery.

Group II. There were 14 procedures in this group. It was characterized by a composite procedure consisting of a long endarterectomy of the common and superficial femoral arteries and a short saphenous vein bypass autograft between the distal end of the endarterectomized superficial femoral artery and the distal end of the popliteal artery.

Group IIA. Group IIA consisted of 6 cases of a composite procedure consisting of a long closed type of endarterectomy of the teries, ending just proximal to the adductor common femoral and superficial femoral arhiatus, and with a relative short saphenous vein bypass graft distally. The proximal and distal arteriotomies were closed with short saphenous vein patch grafts (Fig. 2, *A*). Additional patch grafts in a few patients

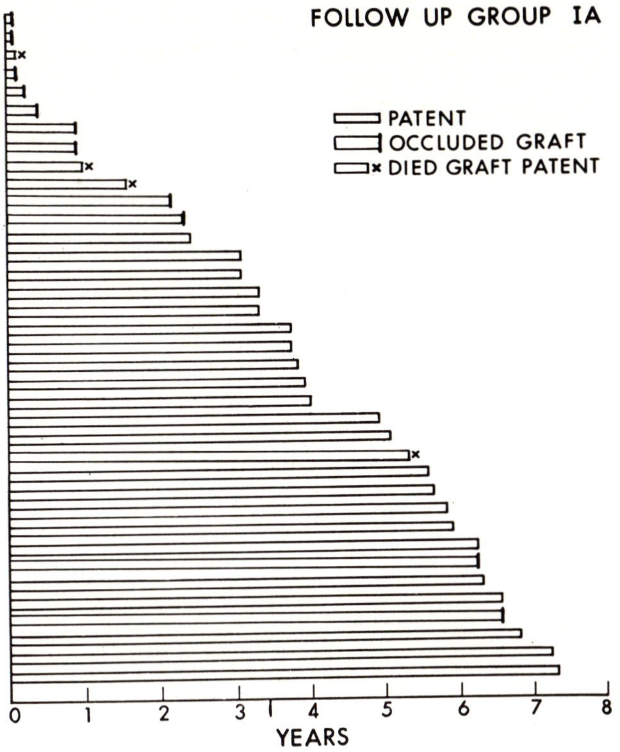

Fig. 4. A graph showing the follow-up results of 36 procedures in Group IA.

were used to close arteriotomy sites in the mid superficial femoral artery that were necessary to complete the endarterectomy. The reconstructive procedure was completed by inserting a short saphenous vein bypass autograft of adequate caliber by the end-to-side technique to the distal patch graft on the superficial femoral artery and distally to the distal segment of the popliteal artery. This method was utilized when the endarterectomy could be accomplished readily and resulted in an adequate arterial lumen that would accept a 20 gauge catheter. Two patients in this group also had endarterectomies of the external iliac arteries to increase the arterial inflow into the reconstructive arterial procedure. The saphenous vein bypass grafts varied from 14 cm. to 30 cm. in length, the average being 21 cm. Three were rated as having excellent to good outflow and 3 were fair to poor.

Group IIB. This group consisted of 4 patients in whom the reconstructive arterial procedure was a long open endarterectomy of the entire length of the superficial femoral artery except the distal few centimeters proximal to the adductor hiatus. This long arteriotomy was closed with an equally long vein patch graft. A short saphenous vein bypass autograft was anastomosed to the distal end of the long vein patch graft and distally to the distal end of the popliteal artery (Fig. 2, *B*). The outflow tracts were rated as excellent to good in 3, and fair to poor in 1. It should be noted that this open type of endarterectomy with a long vein patch graft was used because of the small size of the superficial femoral artery, or because it could not be performed with a loop stripper.

Group IIC. There were 3 patients in this group characterized by a long open endarterectomy of the entire superficial femoral artery, except for the distal few centimeters, as in Group IIB. The reconstructive procedures differed from that group in that the long arteriotomy was closed with a long vein patch graft which was in continuity with a short vein bypass graft from the distal end of the endarterectomy to the distal end of the popliteal artery (Fig. 2, *C*). This procedure was not used more often because of the difficulty in performing a satisfactory proximal anastomosis to the endarterectomized superficial femoral artery. This type of reconstruction was used in reverse in the fourth patient at the distal popliteal anastomosis by using a long vein patch graft in continuity with the vein bypass graft to close a long arteriotomy of most of the popliteal artery. The distal anastomosis was actually at the junction of the superficial femoral and popliteal arteries which was at the proximal end of the in-continuity vein patch. The outflow tract in this group was excellent to good in 2, and fair to poor in 2.

RESULTS

The results obtained in the six types of procedures are represented diagrammatically in Figs. 4, 5, and 6.

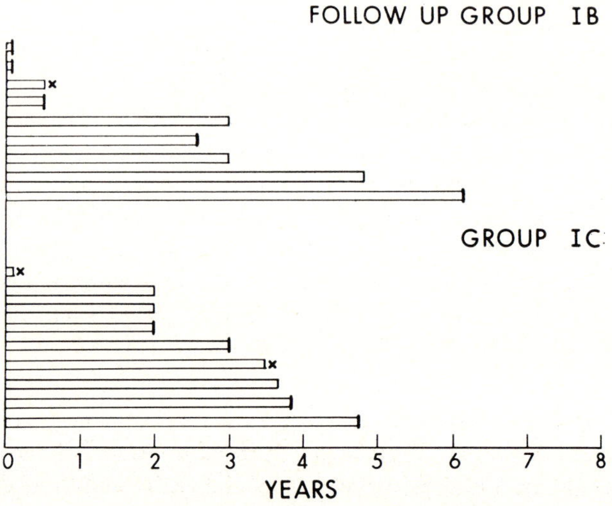

Fig. 5. Graphs showing the follow-up results of 9 procedures each in Groups IB and IC.

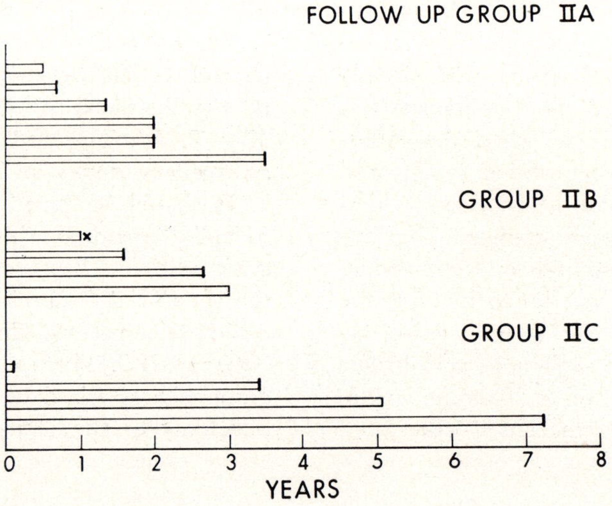

Fig. 6. Graphs showing the follow-up results of 6 procedures in Group IIA, 4 in Group IIB, and 4 in Group IIC.

Experience has shown[2] that the great majority of occlusions of the standard autogenous vein bypass grafts occur within the first 2 years, so that 24 months is probably the earliest time for meaningful analysis of reconstructive vascular surgery in the lower limb. For the purpose of analyzing our results, therefore, a 2 year period of patency from the time of operation was selected as the criterion of a success, whereas if the graft occluded within this 2 year period, it was considered a failure. The time of occlusion was taken as the first time following operation that a graft was noted to be occluded by the criteria previously mentioned.

Group IA. Three of the 36 patients in this group died without occlusion of their grafts at 1 month, 11 months, and 18 months.

Among the 33 remaining cases, there were 7 occlusions before two years, or failures, and 3 late occlusions at 26, 75, and 87 months (Fig. 4). The average period of patency, in the 33 patients who survived their operations, was 47.8 months from the time of operation and in the successful cases who remained patent for 2 years or longer, it was 58 months.

Failure of a graft did not lead to limb amputation in any patient. There was one below-the-knee amputation in a diabetic woman with gangrene of the foot; none of the popliteal outflow arteries was open. The amputation was performed 2½ months after the grafting procedure, which maintained sufficient circulation distally to permit a below-the-knee amputation. The graft remained patent until her death from a massive myocardial infarction 11 months after the graft was implanted.

There were four instances of aneurysm formation of the common femoral artery at the site of the patch graft and the proximal anastomosis, requiring aneurysmorrhaphy and an angioplasty. These procedures were performed at 48, 61, 66, and 75 months. All patients continued to have patent, well-functioning grafts thereafter. The radiographic appearance of such an aneurysm at the site

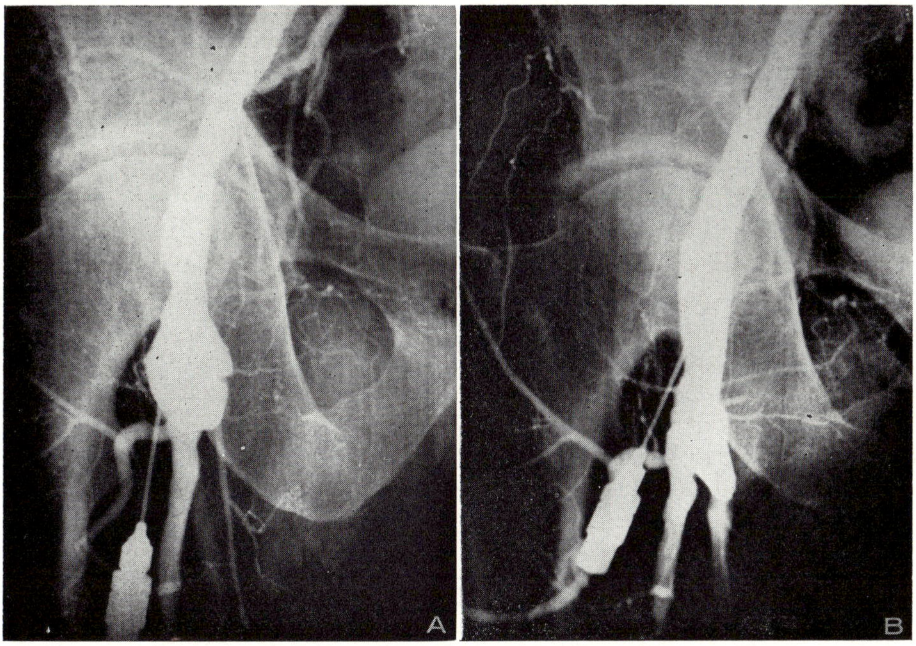

Fig. 7. *A,* A right iliofemoral arteriogram showing aneurysmal dilatation of the femoral artery 4 years following a Type IA procedure. The result of using too large a vein patch graft. *B,* A right iliofemoral arteriogram following an aneurysmorrhaphy of the aneurysm shown in *A* with restoration of normal caliber to the femoral artery and preservation of the vein bypass graft.

of a patch graft and the proximal anastomosis is illustrated in Fig. 7. It should be noted that these 4 patients were early in the group and it is believed that the aneurysms occurred as the result of using too large a vein patch graft, thereby creating a slight aneurysmal dilatation of the femoral artery that was augmented by the end-to-side anastomosis of the vein graft to it. It has been found possible to prevent this complication by implanting the patch graft over an intraluminal stent of a short segment of a polyethylene catheter of the same caliber as the lumen of the common femoral artery. The stent is removed before constructing the end-to-side anastomosis of the vein graft to the patch graft. It is important to note that this technique has another advantage since it permits the removal of any ragged fragments of arterial intima and media at the suture line and can be tailored neatly from within after removing the stent, thereby reducing the incidence of thrombus formation at the proximal anastomosis. There was no correlation between the length of the graft and early occlusion. The 27 successful grafts averaged 43.7 cm. in length and the 6 unsuccessful ones, 46.3 cm. The majority of failures were the result of errors in operative technique.

It is noteworthy also that there was no correlation between the quality of the outflow tract and the success of the graft. Analysis of the figures in Table I by the chi square method reveals that neither among the 33 patients in Group A, nor in the entire group of patients who survived for evaluation, did the outflow tract exert a statistically significant difference between success or failure of the graft. It may be concluded that a saphenous vein autograft is a justifiable procedure even in the presence of a poor outflow tract, providing that an adequate inflow from above is established and also that a patent segment of the popliteal artery is available for a satisfactory distal anastomosis.

Group IB. There were 9 procedures carried out in 8 patients, as one patient had both legs operated upon. There were no postoperative deaths in this group but there were 4 early failures, 2 within 24 hours, and the other 2 at 5 and 6 months. Two of the failures, 1 at 24 hours, and the other at 5 months, were in the two extremities of the same patient (Fig. 5). It is believed that these failures were in part due to technical errors and to hypotension during operation, with the patient's systolic blood pressure at 100 mm. Hg instead of a normal of 140 to 150 mm. The grafts were also unusually long, one measuring 53 cm. and the other 56 cm. in length. In one it was also necessary to excise a portion of the vein graft and reanastomose the two segments, a difficult technical procedure with a venous graft. It is thought all these factors played a role in the failures of the grafts. The third one failed in 24 hours. This also was a long graft of small caliber measuring 51 cm. in length and 3 to 4 mm. in diameter. This failure it is believed was a technical one because of the graft characteristics and the more advanced proximal femoral and iliac artery disease. The fourth one failed at 6 months. It was performed at the same time that an abdominal aortic and bilateral iliac and femoral endarterectomy was performed. It is believed that this much surgery at one time plays a role in graft failures because from the technical point of view they are not done as meticulously as when the surgeon and the patient are in a fresher condition. There were no amputations and no deaths in this group, but a failure rate of 44 percent. The average period of known patency in these patients, even including the two open only for 24 hours each, was 25.7 months. In the remaining 5 successful cases there were two late failures at 31 and 74 months. The average patency rate for these 5 cases was 47 months. The later failures, on the other hand, were probably due to progression of patient's disease. A low-thigh amputation was necessary in the first of the two patients after the graft occluded. It should be noted, however, that the grafting procedure had been performed because of severe rest pain and ischemic ulcers of the foot, which were relieved and healed so that the limb was saved from amputation for 2½ years. It is possible the lower patency rate in this small group of patients may have been due to more extensive atherosclerosis involving the external iliac, common femoral, and proximal superficial femoral arteries necessitating a longer proximal vein patch graft and poorer vein grafts. Technical errors may have played a role as well.

Group IC. There were 9 procedures performed in 8 patients, as one patient had both legs operated upon (Fig. 5). There was one sudden postoperative death, an operative mortality of 11 percent in this small group. It occurred one month after surgery and was due to a massive pulmonary embolism. The operation in this case consisted of a transabdominal external iliac endarterectomy and a femoral popliteal bypass graft. There was one early graft failure in the 8 surviving patients just short of 24 months. In the remaining seven successful cases, there were 4 late occlusions at 36, 42, 46, and 57 months (Fig. 5). The average period of patency in the living patients was 37 months; for the late occlusion cases it was 45 months, and for the unoccluded ones at the time of follow-up, 31 months.

Failure of a graft did not result in amputation in any of the patients. In one patient the procedure failed after 3 years, due to occlusion of the endarterectomized segment of the proximal part of the superficial femoral artery with the in-continuity vein patch. It was possible to salvage the procedure in this case since the long saphenous vein bypass was still patent as a result of a small collateral vessel entering at its proximal end. This was accomplished by inserting another short segment of saphenous vein autograft from the common femoral artery to the proximal end of the previously implanted saphenous vein graft. It remains patent now 2½ years since the second operation.

Group IIA. There were 6 patients in this group without any postoperative deaths (Fig. 6). There were 5 early failures, 83 percent, and 1 late failure after 42 months, which according to our criteria is classified as successful since it was patent longer than 24 months. Two of the early failures are still patent at 36 and 37 months because they were reoperated upon before they became totally occluded. One was done at 6 months and the other at 24 months after the primary procedure. The second operation consisted of inserting additional grafts to bypass the almost occluded endarterectomized segments of the superficial femoral arteries from the common femoral artery to the proximal end of the previously implanted saphenous vein graft. An autogenous vein graft was used in one and in the other a knitted Dacron prosthesis was utilized. Fortunately both of these have been successful to date, but they are considered failures of the primary procedure of this group. The average period of patency in this group of 6 extremities was 20 months. The low patency and high failure rates occurred because of the marked fibrotic changes that developed in and around the endarterectomized segments of the superficial femoral arteries, with resulting occlusion of them. The vein autograft part of these composite procedures continued to function well until the endarterectomized arterial segments occluded.

Group IIB. There were 4 extremities in this group with no postoperative deaths. The results showed that there were 2, or 50 percent early failures at 12 and 18 months, and 2 successes with a late failure of one, at 32 months, the fourth being still patent at 3 years (Fig. 6). It had been hoped that the superficial femoral artery would remain patent after open endarterectomy and closure of the long arteriotomy with an autogenous vein graft to the distal end of which a short vein graft was anastomosed by the end-to-side technique. The results suggest a slight improvement but the number is too small to be statistically significant. The late failure probably could have been salvaged if the patient had followed orders and returned 6 months before the artery occluded. This undoubtedly would have demonstrated some narrowing of the reconstructed femoral artery which could have been reoperated upon, restoring the lumen at those points with short vein patch grafts.

Group IIC. There were 4 extremities in

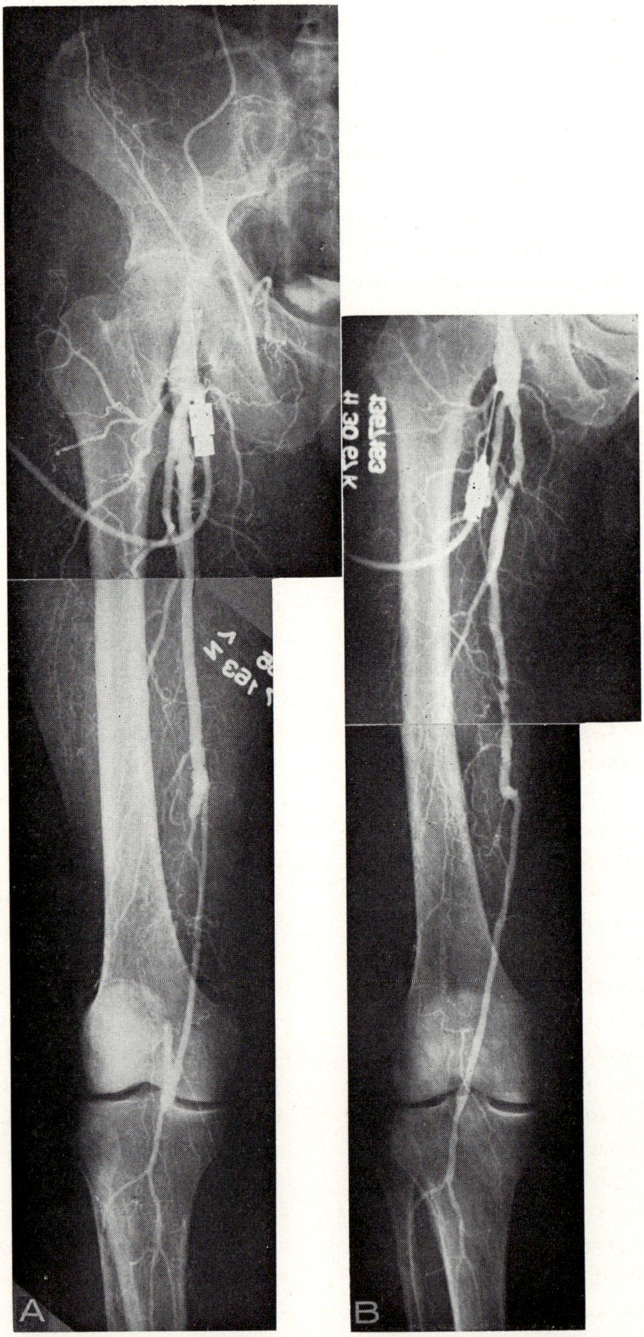

Fig. 8. *A,* A right femoropopliteal arteriogram demonstrating a Group IIA composite procedure performed in a man aged 77 years for severe rest pain. Note the excellent caliber of the endarterectomized superficial femoral artery and the short small-caliber distal saphenous vein bypass graft. *B,* A repeat femoropopliteal arteriogram performed one year after the reconstructive procedure in *A* was performed. Note the excellent condition of our bypass and the marked areas of constriction of the endarterectomized segment of the superficial femoral artery with several areas of almost complete occlusion and return of symptoms. The arterial patency was restored by inserting a knitted Dacron prosthesis from the common femoral artery to the proximal end of the vein bypass, and which is still functioning 20 months later.

this group and no postoperative deaths. There was 1 early failure (25 percent) within an hour of operation that was immediately converted into a Group IIB type. The remaining 3 or 75 percent procedures were successes with 2 late failures at 41 and 87 months (Fig. 6). The other one is patent at 61 months. The average patency rate for these four cases was 47 months and for the three successes 63 months. This type of procedure was similar to IIB except for the fact that the long vein patch graft used to close the arteriotomy incision was left in-continuity with the short vein bypass graft. Despite the apparent superiority of this type of procedure the numbers are too few to be of statistical significance.

COMPLICATIONS

There were three early deaths in Group I, resulting from the operations, an operative mortality of 4.4 percent and a patient mortality of 5.1 percent. One was the result of a myocardial infarction on the fourth postoperative day, one was from pulmonary sepsis on the seventeenth postoperative day secondary to small pulmonary emboli, and the third was from a massive pulmonary embolus on the twenty-fourth postoperative day. In addition, there were four late cardiac deaths in Group I, at 11, 18, 44, and 63 months, and one from this condition in Group II at 18 months. One patient in Group I died of carcinoma of the lung at 24 months. These figures suggest that the poor risk patients were in Group I, since the 3 early deaths and 5 of the 6 late deaths were in this group. There were no instances of wound infection or anastomotic suture line disruption. Four patients developed aneurysms of the common femoral artery at the site of the vein patch grafts, as previously noted. All four underwent successful restorative aneurysmorrhaphy.

Severe stenosis secondary to fibrosis around and involving the walls of the long segments of endarterectomized superficial femoral arteries and atherosclerotic changes in the new intima of these vessels were the causes of failure in the great majority of the cases in Group II (Fig. 8).

DISCUSSION

The surgical techniques presented in this paper were developed to enable the surgeon to utilize autologous saphenous veins of small caliber and of shorter length as bypass grafts when the usual reversed common femoral to distal popliteal artery saphenous vein bypass autograft could not be satisfactorily performed. The two main obstacles encountered were (1) a thick-walled atherosclerotic common femoral artery to which a satisfactory proximal anastomosis with the smaller end of the reversed saphenous vein graft could not be accomplished, and (2) a saphenous vein of insufficient length and adequate caliber to bypass the occluded femoral artery from a point of adequate inflow from the common femoral artery to a suitable place in the distal popliteal artery for the construction of a satisfactory distal anastomosis.

It is believed that an analysis of the results utilizing these methods of arterial reconstruction in the lower limb adds further evidence to the fact that an adequate proximal inflow into the graft from the common femoral artery is one of the most important requirements for a successful graft of long patency.

An analysis of the late success rates in these various groups of the procedures that remained patent for 3 years or longer was made to determine which gave the higher percentage of late patency. The results of this analysis are given in Table II. It is obvious that again the Group IA procedure gave the best results with 70 percent patency. The

Table II. *Percentage late successes over 3 years*

Group	Total No. cases	No. late successes	
		No.	%
I A	33	23	70
I B	9	4	44
I C	9	3	33
Totals	51	30	59
II A	6	0	—
II B	4	1	25
II C	4	1	25
Totals	14	2	14

worst was in Group IIA with no late successes. Comparing all the cases in Group I and Group II it should be noted that in the former there were 30 late successes out of a total of 51 cases, or a late patency rate of 59 percent, whereas in the latter group only 2, or 14 percent out of 14 cases were patent. We believe these results demonstrate that long-term patency can be obtained utilizing Group I procedures, and the best among these is the IA type.

The results obtained in the Group II procedures were a disappointment on the whole because the failures were primarily due to the type of procedure performed rather than a failure of technique. This consisted of a marked fibrotic process that almost invariably involved the entire circumference and length of the endarterectomized segment of the superficial femoral artery. In addition, atheromatous changes were also observed in the pseudointima lining of the previously endarterectomized arteries. The result was an occlusion of this portion of the composite reconstructive procedure despite the fact it was autologous tissue. The best results obtained in this group were in IIC, utilizing a long vein patch graft in continuity with a short vein bypass graft to close the endarterectomized artery. There were too few of these cases, however, to draw any statistically valid conclusions. When combined with the other types of procedures in Group II, the long-term patency was so poor that all the Group II methods have now been abandoned.

In order to salvage these patients for reconstructive procedures in which a portion of the saphenous vein of sufficient caliber for a grafting procedure is too short to extend from the common femoral to the distal popliteal artery, it is suggested that it is worth trying a composite graft of a Dacron prosthesis anastomosed to the short segment of the distal part of the reconstructive procean autogenous vein. The venous segment is dure. It is placed so that it crosses the knee joint and is anastomosed to the distal part of the popliteal artery. The proximal end of the Dacron prosthesis is anastomosed to the common femoral artery. It is too early at this time to determine the success or failure rate of this type of composite graft, since the longest follow-up to date is only 34 months.

SUMMARY

Modifications of the saphenous vein bypass graft technique for the treatment of femoral arteriosclerotic occlusive arterial disease are presented. These were developed because of technical factors due to inadequate length of saphenous vein autografts of suitable caliber, and advanced atherosclerosis of the femoral artery at the point of proximal implantation. The results in a series of 59 patient who underwent 68 operative procedures are reported with long-term follow-up studies from 2 to 8 years. Analysis of the results in relation to the quality of the outflow tract, as evaluated by arteriography, warrants the conclusion that successful grafts of these types can be performed even in the presence of a poor popliteal outflow tract, providing an adequate inflow from the common femoral artery is obtained. Only 3 patients in the group eventually required limb amputation. These were in patients whose limbs were salvaged by the procedures, until arterial reocclusion of them several years later. The results are encouraging and corroborate the desirability of using autogenous vein grafts in dealing with arterial occlusive disease of the lower extremity whenever possible, despite technical difficulties.

REFERENCES

1. Dale, W. A.: Autogenous vein grafts for femoropopliteal occlusion, J. Amer. Med. Ass. **196:** 494, 1966.
2. Darling, R. C., Linton, R. R., and Razzuk, M. A.: Saphenous vein bypass grafts for femoropopliteal occlusive disease: A reappraisal, SURGERY **61:** 31, 1967.
3. De Weese, J. A., Terry, R., Barner, H. B., and Rob, C. G.: Autogenous venous femoropopliteal bypass grafts, SURGERY **59:** 28, 1966.
4. Edwards, W. S.: Venous patch graft reconstruction of chronic femoral-popliteal occlusions, SURGERY **61:** 820, 1967.
5. Gutelius, J. R., Kreindler, S., and Luke, J. C.: Comparative evaluation of autogenous vein bypass grafts and endarterectomy in superficial

femoral artery reconstruction, SURGERY **57:** 28, 1965.

6. Kunlin, J.: Le traitement de l'arterite obliterante par la greffe veineuse, Arch. Malad. Coeur et Vaiss. **42:** 371, 1949.
7. Linton, R. R.: Some recent advances in surgical procedures for treatment of obliterative diseases of the major arteries, Maryland State Med. J., October, 1965.
8. Linton, R. R., and Darling, R. C.: Autogenous saphenous vein bypass grafts in femoropopliteal obliterative arterial disease, SURGERY **51:** 62, 1962.
9. Meade, J. W., Linton, R. R., Darling, R. C., and Menendez, C. V.: Arterial homografts. A long-term clinical follow-up, Arch. Surg. **93:** 392, 1966.
10. Szilagyi, D. E.: Ten years' experience with aorto-iliac and femoropoliteal arterial reconstruction, J. Cardiov. Surg. **5:** 502, 1964.

DISCUSSION

Dr. Makis Tsapogas (Albany, N. Y.). Mr. Chairman, members, and guests:

It is a privilege for me to have the opportunity to discuss the paper by Dr. Linton, who is a pioneer in this field.

The ingenious and painstaking methods described by Drs. Linton and Wilde provide an interesting alternative where the saphenous vein is inadequate. However, I wonder whether these modifications do not prolong the operation when performed by less experienced surgeons and increase the possibility of thrombosis due to the additional angioplastic procedures.

In approximately 25 percent of the patients in our series, the saphenous vein was found unsuitable. In such cases we consider the cephalic vein an alternative graft.

The useful length and diameter of the cephalic vein are frequently adequate for grafting. It withstands high intraluminal pressures and has the advantage of tapering less than the saphenous vein.

We consider that phlebography of the arm in candidates for grafting is useful in assessing the suitability of the cephalic vein. In our view, the first step of the grafting procedure is to explore the saphenous vein at the knee level. If the caliber is inadequate, the cephalic vein is removed by another surgeon, while the common femoral and distal popliteal arteries are being dissected, resulting in shorter operative time.

The short term results of the patients with cephalic vein grafts are promising. It is evident that only by long follow-up the value of the cephalic vein as an arterial graft can be fully assessed.

May I thank the Society for allowing me to participate in this discussion.

Dr. Martin L. Schulman (Great Neck, Long Island, N. Y.). Dr. Yeager, members, and guests:

I was very interested in the techniques described by Drs. Linton and Wilde and I'm sure they will be of value to us on future occasions.

Coincidentally, I also rise to convey my enthusiasm for the use of the cephalic vein as a bypass graft when the saphenous vein is inadequate.

We have used the cephalic vein on three occasions recently and have been most satisfied with the results obtained.

The first patient had a femoral artery occlusion that required a bypass from the common femoral to the distal popliteal. The small saphenous we found led us to use the cephalic vein as a graft.

The second patient had undergone previous vein strippings and a 20 cm. cephalic vein graft was used to bypass his popliteal aneurysm.

In the third patient, the cephalic vein graft was brought from the midsuperficial femoral artery to the posterior tibial artery high in the leg.

All these grafts have been placed in the subcutaneous tissues and a good pulse is palpable in each.

In each of these cases, the cephalic vein has readily admitted a 4 mm. dilator. We have been impressed by the gossamer texture encountered in these veins as contrasted with the thickening and almost fibrotic appearance we have seen in the saphenous veins in these patients. We are all aware that the atherosclerotic process seems to spare the arteries in the upper extremity and it would seem as though the changes of aging in the venous system have likewise spared the upper extremity veins as compared with the saphenous vein.

The long-term patency and integrity of these veins, of course, is still to be determined in a large series. However, the availability of these grafts would seem to offer a solution to many of the problems that we commonly encounter. At future meetings of this Society, it is possible we will hear reports of the use of cephalic vein grafts for axillary-femoral bypass with greatly improved long-term patency and that even in good risk patients, occlusive disease of the aorta and iliac arteries will be treated with operations all performed in subcutaneous tissues.

Dr. Linton (closing). Dr. Yeager, members, and guests:

I've enjoyed the two discussants and would agree that the cephalic vein is possibly a substitute for the saphenous vein. The saphenous vein, fortunately, has been subjected almost to arterial pressure at the ankle level, so that it has already been subjected to a high degree of internal pressure and I just wonder if the cephalic vein is going to hold up since it has not.

I've had one experience using the popliteal vein to replace a popliteal aneurysm and it lasted for about 7 years, then it became aneurysmal and had to be replaced.

So I think the cephalic vein will have to be watched, but I certainly would agree that it's something to utilize if it is large enough, rather than using a prosthesis.

I sometimes think that people have longer arms elsewhere than they do in Boston [laughter] because I'm not sure I can get one quite long enough to go from the common femoral to the distal popliteal artery!

I believe that it is very important to get a good arterial inflow into the graft, whatever type it is, and in my experience it's more difficult to construct a satisfactory proximal anastomosis in severe atherosclerosis than it is to construct the distal one, providing you utilize the popliteal artery distal to the knee where there are no branches and it is usually soft and pliable.

[Slide] These statistics will demonstrate to you why we believe the reverse saphenous vein is a better reconstructive procedure than any of the others.

You will see that there was a total of 31 synthetic prostheses in the lower extremity. At the end of 5 years there were 25 occluded or a failure rate of 81 percent.

Endarterectomy was a great disappointment because I had thought since it was autogenous tissue it might hold up much better, but in our follow-up of 78 procedures, there were 55 failures at the end of 5 years, a failure of 70 percent.

Arterial homografts, surprisingly, were a little better, but not enough so that one would want to utilize them. There were 115 occluded out of 190, a failure rate of 60 percent. The saphenous vein bypass in 295 extremities resulted in 59 failures at the end of 5 years, a 20 percent failure rate or an 80 percent success rate.

[Slide] This demonstrates why I have given up endarterectomy or what the British surgeons call "disobliteration" of the superficial femoral artery because of the poor results.

This patient had one of the composite procedures carried out in Group II. It was a closed endarterectomy from the common femoral down to the distal popliteal artery with a short segment of a saphenous vein bypass graft, from the distal end of the endarterectomized femoral artery to the distal popliteal artery.

This slide shows an arteriogram taken on the operating table after completing the operative procedure. Note the excellent caliber and the smooth contour of the endarterectomized superficial femoral artery.

[Slide] This arteriogram was taken 2 years later. Note the severe changes that have taken place, almost complete occlusion of the endarterectomized artery in several places and marked narrowing throughout.

These changes have been found to be present in almost all the cases. It is mandatory, therefore, if you do an endarterectomy of the superficial femoral artery, repeat arteriograms should be performed within a year. In this way I have been able to salvage some cases by vein patch grafts at the narrowed areas and in others by utilizing a prosthetic graft from the common femoral down to the proximal end of the saphenous vein bypass graft.

[Slide] This arteriogram shows an aneurysm of the common femoral artery at the site of the proximal vein patch graft. This angiogram was performed 5 years after the patch graft and the saphenous vein bypass had been implanted. The aneurysm developed because too large a patch graft had been used, producing a slight dilatation that slowly increased.

[Slide] This arteriogram shows the result of an aneurysmorrhaphy, which was not absolutely satisfactory, but with restoration of the normal lumen and maintenance of the outflow tract.

[Slide] In order to prevent this complication you should use a stent of polyethylene tubing the same size as the lumen of the common femoral artery. The patch graft should be made very taut which will greatly reduce the chance of aneurysmal dilatation.

If this is done the end result with the patch graft should be an artery the same size as the femoral artery. The saphenous vein bypass graft is then anastomosed to the patch graft.

[Slide] This colored operative photograph demonstrates the patch graft in the common femoral artery with the saphenous vein autograft coming off of it, and also showing the angioplastic procedure between two branches of the reverse saphenous vein to facilitate a larger anastomotic opening. By this means we have reduced the twenty percent of patients that do not have a good enough saphenous vein to use as a bypass graft. The cases in Group IA with a small patch graft and a long saphenous vein bypass graft have given excellent results.

Volume 67 *Number* 2 SURGERY

FEBRUARY, 1970

Clinical surgery

Use of diuretic agents during oliguria after renal transplantation

CARL F. ANDERSON, M.D.
HUGH O. O'KANE, M.B., F.R.C.S.
ROY G. SHORTER, M.D.
WILLIAM J. JOHNSON, M.D.
GEORGE A. HALLENBECK, M.D.
ROCHESTER, MINN.
From the Mayo Clinic and Mayo Foundation, Sections of Medicine, Nephrology, and Organ and Tissue Transplantation, and the Mayo Graduate School of Medicine, University of Minnesota

Determining the exact cause of oliguria in the early postoperative period after renal transplantation may be very difficult. If urinary catheter obstruction and fluid depletion are not present, major arterial or venous occlusion, ureteral obstruction or leakage, acute tubular necrosis, and rejection must be considered. Acute tubular necrosis and rejection are the most common causes in our experience. Because some patients (who have not undergone transplantation) with oliguric acute renal failure caused by acute tubular necrosis respond favorably to the intravenous administration of ethacrynic acid according to Maher and Schreiner[5] and Mann and Gilmore[6] or ethacrynic acid and mannitol according to Auger and coworkers,[1] we decided to assess the effects of these drugs in oliguric patients in the early posttransplantation period. This trial was undertaken as a therapeutic measure and for determination of whether the response in urine output might be helpful in the differential diagnosis of the cause of oliguria. This communication describes our observations in five patients in whom oliguria developed during the first 48 hours after renal transplantation.

Supported in part by Research Grant AI-7838 from the National Institutes of Health, United States Public Health Service.

Received for publication March 7, 1969.

METHOD OF TREATMENT

All patients were recipients of renal allografts (three from living related donors and two from cadaveric donors) and each was given horse antihuman–thymus globulin (10 ml. daily, intramuscularly or subcutaneously, for 10 days) in addition to azathioprine and steroids. The immunosuppressive treatment was begun on the day of transplantation in those receiving cadaveric renal allografts and 2 days before transplantation in those receiving allografts from living related donors. There were no major (ABO) blood group incompatibilities between donors and recipients. No preformed lymphocytotoxic antibodies against donor lymphocytes were demonstrated in the sera of any of the recipients prior to transplantation. Bilateral nephrectomy was performed at the time of transplantation in Patients 1, 2, 3, and 5; it had been accomplished 3 months earlier in Patient 4.

Ethacrynic acid (50 mg.) and mannitol (25 Gm.) were administered intravenously to each patient when oliguria appeared during the first 48 hours after renal transplantation. Ethacrynic acid was given without mannitol if extracellular fluid volume excess was suspected. If the urine volume increased during the next 2 hours, an infusion of ethacrynic acid (100 mg.) in 500 ml. of 20 percent mannitol was started to maintain the increased urine output.

CASE REPORTS

The individual cases are summarized in Table I.

In Case 1 at 4 hours after revascularization, the maximal urinary output was only 15 ml. per hour. No fever, renal tenderness, or evidence of extracellular volume depletion was present. A marked, sustained increase in urinary output ensued after the intravenous administration of ethacrynic acid (50 mg.) and mannitol (Fig. 1). By the second postoperative day, the urine volume was 2.9 L. per 24 hours, and the serum creatinine was 2.4 mg. per 100 ml.

In Case 2 the urinary volume averaged 190 ml. per hour for the first 5 hours after revascularization (less than one half the expected volume from patients with an uncomplicated course). Nineteen hours after revascularization, the urinary output had decreased to 30 ml. per hour. No fever, renal tenderness, or evidence of extracellular volume depletion was present, and acute tubular necrosis was suspected. Ethacrynic acid (50 mg.) was administered intravenously; the urinary output increased to 150 ml. per hour within 2 hours and ranged from 90 to 250 ml. per hour for the next 10 hours. The serum creatinine decreased from 7.8 mg. per 100 ml. on the first postoperative day to 1.65 mg. per 100 ml. on the tenth postoperative day.

The third patient underwent bilateral nephrectomy and renal transplantation from a cadaveric donor. Three hours after revascularization, ethacrynic acid (50 mg.) and mannitol (25 Gm.) were administered because of oliguria (Fig. 2). During the first postoperative day, the urinary volume was 1,305 ml. per 24 hours, blood urea 150 mg. per 100 ml., and serum creatinine 11.6

Table I. *Results of infusion of ethacrynic acid and mannitol in cases of oliguria after renal transplantation*

Case	*Age (yr.)*	*Sex*	*Donor*	*Total ischemia time (min.)*	*Urine volume*		*Serum creatinine after dosage (mg./100 ml.)*
					Before dosage	*After dosage*	
1	25	F	Mother	44	15 ml./hr. at 4 hr. postoperatively	At 2 hr. after, 145 ml./hr.	2.4 (postoperative day 2)
2	42	F	Sister	35	30 ml./hr. at 19 hr. postoperatively	At 2 hr. after, 150 ml./hr.; at 10 hr. after 90-250 ml./hr.	7.8 (postoperative day 1)
3	23	M	Cadaver	145	15 ml./hr. at 3 hr. postoperatively	At 2 hr. after, 200 ml./hr.	11.6 (postoperative day 1)
4	32	F	Cadaver	95	O ml./hr. at 1 and 2 hr. postoperatively; 150 ml./hr. at 4 hr. postoperatively; 90 ml./hr. at 8 hr. postoperatively	At 1 hr. after, 240 ml./hr.	8.25 (postoperative day 1)
5	51	M	Sister	45	300-900 ml./hr. on day of operation, then decreased	150 ml./hr. immediately, then 30 ml./hr. at 3 hr.; no response to second dose	

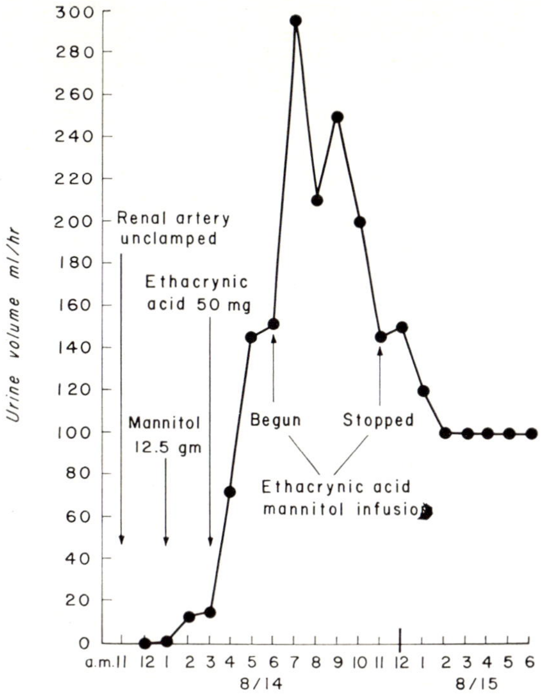

Fig. 1. Case 1—treatment of renal transplant oliguria with ethacrynic acid and mannitol.

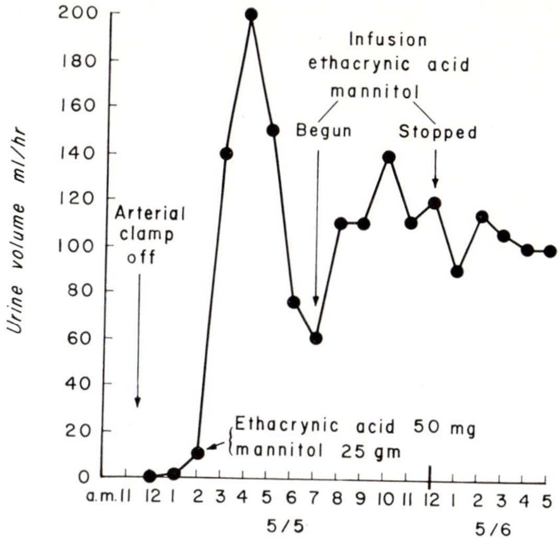

Fig. 2. Case 3—treatment of renal transplant oliguria with ethacrynic acid and mannitol.

mg. per 100 ml. By the second postoperative day, the values were 793 ml. per 24 hours, 192 mg. per 100 ml., and 13.4 mg. per 100 ml., respectively. Prophylactic hemodialysis was performed for 9 hours daily on postoperative days 3 and 5. Ten days after transplantation, the serum creatinine was 1.25 mg. per 100 ml., and the creatinine clearance was 50 ml. per minute per 1.73 M^2.

No urine was produced during the first 2 hours after revascularization in the fourth case. The urinary volume increased to 150 ml. per hour during the fourth hour and then decreased each subsequent hour, to 90 ml. per hour during the eighth hour after revascularization. Ethacrynic acid (50 mg.) and mannitol (25 Gm.) were given intravenously, and the urinary output increased to 240 ml. during the next hour. It averaged 180 ml. per hour during the subsequent 8 hours. On the first postoperative day, the urinary volume was 2,380 ml. per 24 hours, serum creatinine 8.25 mg. per 100 ml., and blood urea 162 mg. per 100 ml. On the next day, the values were 1,190 ml. per 24 hours, 8.0 mg. per 100 ml., and 180 mg. per 100 ml., respectively. Prophylactic hemodialysis was performed on postoperative Days 3 and 5 for 8 hours each day. The urinary volume was 4,540 ml. per 24 hours and serum creatinine 2.8 mg. per 100 ml. on the day of dismissal from the hospital (postoperative day 12).

In the fifth case, urine flow was first noted 30 minutes after revascularization. The output ranged from 300 to 900 ml. per hour on the day of transplantation. A temperature of 102° F. (38.9° C.) was first noted at 2 A.M. of postoperative Day 1, and it increased to 104° F. (40° C.) at 6 A.M. A gradual decrease in urinary output was noted, with no evidence of extracellular volume depletion. Thirty-three hours after revascularization, ethacrynic acid (50 mg.) was administered intravenously, and the urinary output increased from 40 to 150 ml. per hour. However, it decreased to 30 ml. per hour 3 hours later and did not increase in response to a second dose of ethacrynic acid (Fig. 3). Despite intensive antirejection therapy, anuria ensued. When the allograft was removed 19 days after transplantation, complete infarction of the kidney was found in association with complete occlusion of the renal artery by an unorganized thrombus. Because renal arteriography was not performed at the onset of oliguria, we do not know if rejection appeared first or if the renal arterial thrombosis was the initial lesion.

DISCUSSION

During the first 24 hours after transplantation of a renal allograft, it may be difficult to differentiate between acute tubular necrosis and rejection and to differentiate from either the mechanical problems of vascular occlusion or ureteral obstruction. Acute

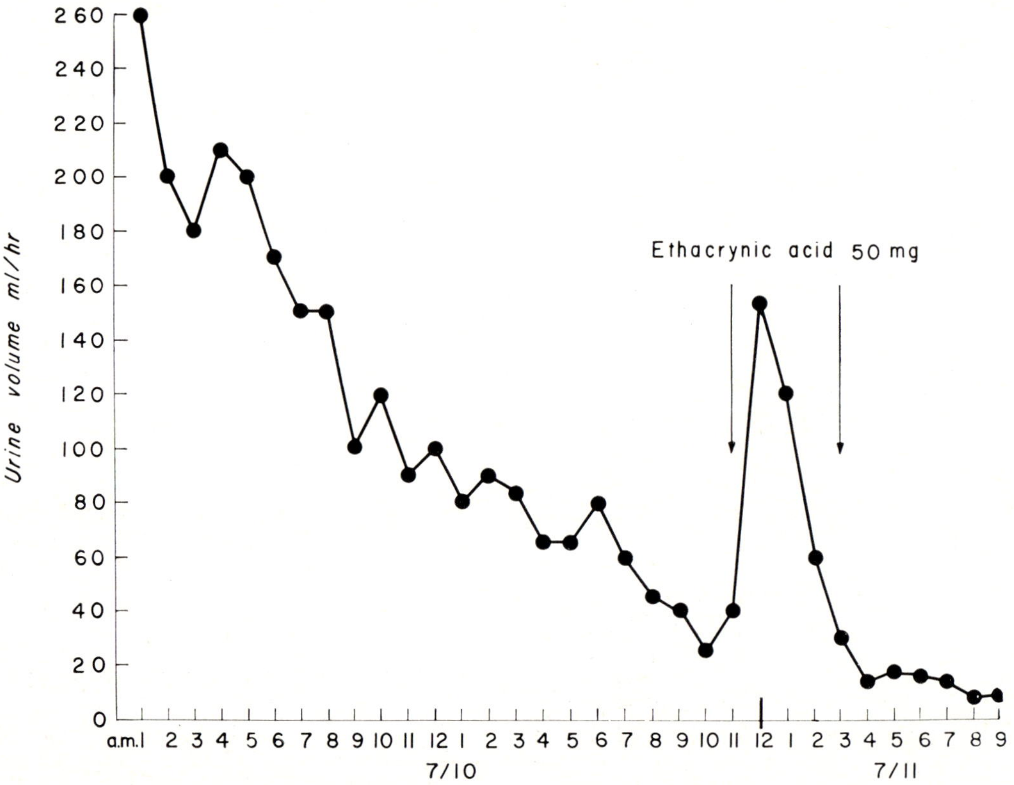

Fig. 3. Case 5—treatment of renal transplant oliguria with two doses of ethacrynic acid.

tubular necrosis is a diagnosis made largely by exclusion, even in patients not undergoing transplantation. Unfortunately, rejection leading to oliguria in the early posttransplantation period also may be a diagnosis made partially by exclusion. Although fever is usually a feature of acute rejection, it is nonspecific, especially in the early posttransplantation period. Leukocytosis is usual in the early posttransplantation period even in patients without complications. Renal tenderness may be difficult to differentiate from wound tenderness, and hypertension is an inconstant feature of early rejection. When the hourly output of urine is used as one of the measurements of kidney function after renal allografting, it is necessary to know what values might be expected from patients without complications. The hourly urinary output was calculated from observations made on 12 other recipients of living-donor renal allografts, in whom no complications were noted during the first week after transplantation (Fig. 4). All of our patients with presumed acute tubular necrosis had urinary volumes less than 200 ml. per hour during the first 5 hours after transplantation, which is less than one half the volume expected during an uncomplicated course.

That the oliguria of acute tubular necrosis may be reversed by the administration of an osmotic diuretic (mannitol) or a potent natriuretic agent or both has been shown in experimental animals by Teschan and Lawson[9] and in some clinical situations by Maher and Schreiner,[5] Mann and Gilmore,[6] and Auger and co-workers.[1] Kjellstrand[3] and Shalhoub and associates[8] found that, if oliguria is reversed at an early stage, renal function may return to normal or to nearly normal. If the oliguria is reversed at an intermediate stage, the oliguric acute renal failure may be converted to a high urinary-output renal failure. This high urinary-output renal failure is often accom-

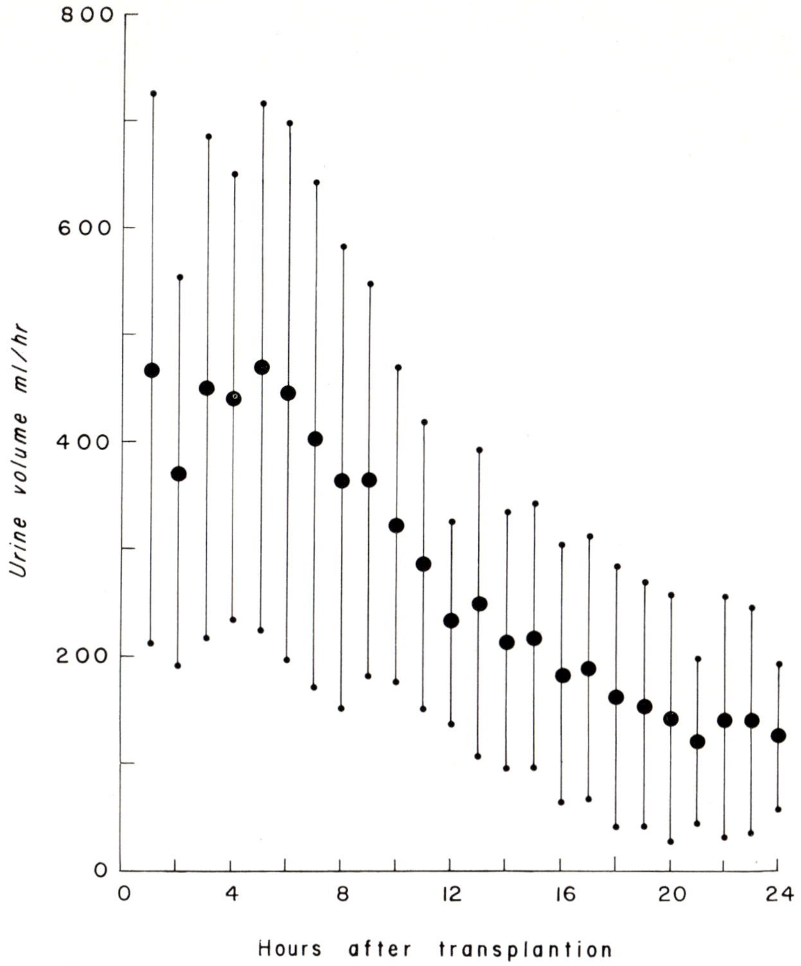

Fig. 4. Hourly urinary volume (mean ± 1 S.D.) in 12 recipients of living-donor renal allografts, with no recognized complications.

panied by increasing blood urea and serum creatinine values. If oliguria continues for a longer period, the urinary output may not increase after the administration of mannitol, as found by Luke,[4] or of ethacrynic acid. The work of Eliahou and Bata[2] suggests that the subdivisions of "incipient" and "irreversible" acute renal failure may merge into one another. Unfortunately, the urine/plasma osmolality ratios which these workers used to differentiate the subdivisions may not be applicable during the early posttransplantation period.

In our first case, the urinary output increased promptly after the administration of ethacrynic acid. Forty-eight hours after revascularization, the renal function (serum creatinine 2.4 mg. per 100 ml.) approached the level expected in the uncomplicated posttransplantation period. This suggests that early oliguric acute renal failure was prevented or reversed. In Cases 2, 3, and 4, despite reversal of oliguria, the serum creatinine value did not decrease as fast as would be expected, suggesting that the oliguric renal failure was transformed into high urinary-output acute renal failure. The increase in urinary volume was transient and unsustained in the fifth patient, which prompted us to consider causes of oliguria other than acute tubular necrosis.

Although ethacrynic acid was used in this group of patients, we have substituted furosemide in equivalent amounts in subsequent trials, with equal success. Because of the report of ototoxicity after the administration of ethacrynic acid in uremia by Mathog and Klein,[7] we now prefer to use furosemide. These findings suggest the merit of the administration of 50 to 100 mg. of furosemide or 50 to 100 mg. of furosemide plus 25 Gm. of mannitol intravenously at the first indication of a low urinary output during the first 48 hours after renal transplantation if a specific mechanical cause is not apparent. The response of the urinary output may serve both as a therapeutic maneuver and as an aid to the differential diagnosis of oliguria. If a marked, sustained increase in urinary output ensues, the diagnosis of acute tubular necrosis is most likely, and an intravenous infusion of 100 mg. of furosemide in 500 ml. of 20 percent mannitol should be given at a rate of 4 ml. per hour to maintain the urinary volume. Such an infusion may be continued for 24 hours; the urinary losses are replaced with 0.45 percent saline containing 20 mEq. of potassium per liter. This replacement solution should be modified if disorders of extracellular volume or abnormalities of sodium or potassium concentration develop.

SUMMARY

Because of the difficulties in determining the exact cause of oliguria in the early postoperative period after renal transplantation, ethacrynic acid and mannitol were administered to five patients with posttransplantation oliguria. The urine output increased from 10 to 90 ml. per hour to 145 to 250 ml. per hour within 2 hours after the administration of these drugs in four patients with presumed acute tubular necrosis. The response was transient and unsustained in a patient with presumed rejection. A trial of both diuretic agents seems indicated in patients with early posttransplantation oliguria if a mechanical cause is not apparent.

REFERENCES

1. Auger, R. G., Dayton, D. A., Harrison, C. E., Jr., Tucker, R. M., and Anderson, C. F.: Use of ethacrynic acid in mannitol-resistant oliguric renal failure, J. A. M. A. **206:** 891, 1968.
2. Eliahou, H. E., and Bata, A.: The diagnosis of acute renal failure, Nephron **2:** 287, 1965.
3. Kjellstrand, C. M.: Ethacrynic acid in acute renal failure, (Abst.) American Society of Nephrology, November, 1968, p. 31.
4. Luke, R. C.: Factors determining response to mannitol in acute renal failure, (Abst.) American Society of Nephrology, November, 1968, p. 38.
5. Maher, J. F., and Schreiner, G. E.: Studies on ethacrynic acid in patients with refractory edema, Ann. Int. Med. **62:** 15, 1965.
6. Mann, J. B., and Gilmore, H. R., III: Ethacrynic acid-induced reversal of mannitol-fast oliguria, (Abst.) Clin. Res. **15:** 364, 1967.
7. Mathog, R. H., and Klein, W. J., Jr.: Ototoxicity of ethacrynic acid and aminoglycoside antibiotics in uremia, New England J. Med. **280:** 1223, 1969.
8. Shalhoub, R. J., Velasquez, M. T., and Antoniou, L. D.: Reversal of surgical oliguric states by furosemide or ethacrynic acid, (Abst.) American Society of Nephrology, November, 1968, p. 60.
9. Teschan, P. E., and Lawson, N. L.: Studies in acute renal failure: Prevention by osmotic diuresis and observations on the effect of plasma and extracelluar volume expansion, Nephron **3:** 1, 1966.

Biliary manometry: Its role in clinical surgery

CLARENCE J. SCHEIN, M.D.
THOMAS C. BENEVENTANO, M.D.
NEW YORK, N. Y.
From the Surgical Division and Division of Diagnostic Radiology of the Montefiore Hospital and Medical Center and the Albert Einstein College of Medicine

This report evaluates the role of biliary manometry in clinical practice. It derives from an intraoperative and postoperative experience with patients undergoing surgery for acute and chronic biliary disease with and without common duct complications. Previous studies from this hospital have established the research value of biliary manometry in recording the cyclic activity of the choledochal sphincter, the pain pattern of the choledochal distention, the mechanism of pancreatic duct filling, and the influences of vagal section and sympathetic block on choledochal dynamics.[5, 7]

Manometric evaluation of the choledochoduodenal junction was initiated in the hope that it would offer more important physiologic data regarding the biliary outflow tract than could be obtained by the gross evaluation of resistance to manual probing, or by endoscopic observation and the morphologic and contour changes observed with conventional hand delivery cholangiography. Could this determination clarify the problem of presumed ampullary obstruction and of the dilated common bile duct encountered in chronic cholecystolithiasis in patients whose small cystic duct diameter would not correlate with the comfortable, but unsupportable, concept of spontaneous passage of calculi? If these expectations could be realized, biliary manometry might point to primary indications for operations in the region of the sphincter that would avoid biliary stasis and postoperative colic that are due to outlet obstruction.

Submitted for publication March 4, 1969; resubmitted April 14, 1969.

METHODS AND MATERIALS

One hundred thirty-seven patients were studied. The initial determinations were made during the surgical procedure. Subsequent determinations were made postoperatively. All intraoperative pressures were obtained under uniform anesthetic conditions. No spasmolytic drugs were employed, no morphine was administered, and meperidine was used in doses of 25 mg. or less. The latter was injected at least 30 minutes prior to manometric determinations. Access to the common bile duct was obtained by either direct intubation of the common bile duct with a catheter or T tube, or by a catheter or cannula inserted through the cystic duct stump. The intraoperative determination was made before open common duct exploration, and repeat determinations were made at the conclusion of the choledochal toilet.

Initial determinations were made with a U-shaped manometer affixed to a saline-primed reservoir. Manometric zero was at the mid-anterior-posterior diameter of the right upper quadrant. All initial determinations have been done under standard conditions with no intracholedochal manipulation, removal of all instruments and abdominal pads, and breathing of the patient on his own without manipulation of the anesthesia apparatus.

The passage pressure is that height of the

saline column that will maintain a continuous flow through the bile duct into the duodenum. Dahl-Iversen and co-workers[2] have termed this the perfusion pressure. The lowest level at which this occurs can be regarded as the opening pressure of the choledochal sphincter. The terms, passage pressure, perfusion pressure, and opening pressure, are, therefore, synonymous. The residual pressure is that at which the column comes to rest after the opening pressure has fallen, and it indicates the highest pressure at which the sphincter is still closed. All common duct pressure measurements are expressed in centimeters of saline and refer to passage pressures unless otherwise stated. The duct was regarded as dilated if it measured 1.2 cm. or more on the film taken at the passage pressure.

After the passage pressure and residual pressures were obtained, the examination was repeated with 50 percent sodium diatrizoate during momentary apnea. One film was obtained at passage pressure and a second at a hypertensive pressure randomly standardized at twice that of passage pressure. Where formal common duct exploration was carried out, the common duct was also evaluated by choledochoscopy. The contrast studies were always repeated postoperatively, 10 to 14 days after common duct exploration. Manometry added no time to that ordinarily required for hand delivery cholangiography.

Postoperative studies were performed in the department of diagnostic radiology on fasted patients who had received no medication for the previous 16 hours. These studies were done by the same perfusion manometric technique with the addition of simultaneous recordings of choledochal morphology on 16 mm. cine strip exposed at 15 frames per second. Except for a group of patients with ampullary fibrosis, all patients had cal-

Table I. *Clinical experience**

Group	*Patients*	*Patients with E.P.†* / *total patients*	*E.P. (percent)*	*Patients with stones* / *total patients*	*With stones (percent)*	*Patients without stones* / *total patients*	*Without stones (percent)*	*Patients with stones & E.P.* / *total patients*	*Patients with stones & E.P. (percent)*
I	19	7/19	54	0/19	0	19/19	100	0	0
II	47	0/47	0	0/47	0	47/47	100	0	0
III	9	9/9	100	0/9	0	9/9	100	0	0
IV	38	10/38	26	10/38	26	28/38	74	2/38	5.2
V	19	19/19	100	8/19	42	11/19	58	8/19	42
VI	5	5	100	0	0	5/5	100	0	0
Total	137	50/137	36	18/137	13	119/137	87	10/137	7.3

*Although 36 percent of all patients had elevated passage pressures, only 7.3 percent of these had associated common duct stones. In the remainder their hypertension remains unclarified or is presumed to be due to ampullary obstructions.

†E.P. = elevated passage pressure (i.e., more than 20 cm. of water).

culus gallbladder disease and were being operated upon for the first time.

RESULTS

The cases are divided by manometric and pathologic diagnosis and are considered in six groups (Table I).

Group 1.

Acute cholecystitis without common duct calculi. Passage pressures were recorded from the cystic duct portal in 19 patients undergoing prompt cholecystectomy for acute obstructive calculus cholecystitis. Twelve of these patients had normal pressures, and seven had elevated pressures ranging between 26 and 35. Five of the latter patients were re-evaluated between the seventh and twelfth postoperative day. In three patients the pressure was in the normal range. In the other two patients it decreased below the final intraoperative determination but remained elevated at 22 and 30.

Group 2.

Chronic cholecystitis with a normal duct and normotensive dynamics. The 47 patients in this group had a normal common bile duct in respect to size, palpation, ease of negotiation of the choledochal sphincter and a normal cholangiogram. Twelve patients had pressures between 6 and 9, and in 35 it ranged between 10 and 20.

Group 3.

Chronic cholecystitis with a normal duct and hypertensive manometrics. These nine patients presented normal ducts, as in Group 2, with the exception that the passage pressures were elevated and ranged between 21 and 26.

Group 4.

Chronic cholecystitis with a presumed choledochopathy as indicated by dilated common bile ducts up to 1.5 cm. in width. Passage pressures were recorded in 38 patients who had an absolute indication for common duct exploration: a dilated duct or a recent history of jaundice. Passage pressures were normal in 28 and elevated in 10 patients. Common duct calculi were present in eight of the former and two of the latter. In those patients without calculi the cause of the choledochal hypertension was not revealed by direct duct exploration, biliary endoscopy, contrast cholangiography, or sphincter resistance to probing.

Group 5.

Ampullary stenosis in the postcholecystectomy syndrome. Nineteen patients were regarded as having fixed choledochoduodenal stenosis as the cause of their persistent or renewed postcholecystectomy pain or dyspepsia. Eight of these patients had free-floating stones; no patient had an impacted stone. Eleven patients had no calculi. In all patients it was difficult to pass a No. 3 Bakes dilator through the sphincter. Passage pressures were obtained before duct exploration and ranged between 27 and 39. All were treated by choledochoduodenostomy; this bypass precludes postoperative manometry.[6]

Group 6.

Chronic cholecystitis with a dilated duct and hypertensive manometrics with presumed hypertensive sphincter. These five patients had greatly dilated ducts, at least 1.6 cm. wide. This differentiates them from the patients in Group 4. There were no cholangiographic abnormalities or calculi, but the passage pressures were 26, 28, 31, 35, and 38. The sphincter area offered resistance to the passage of the dilator which differentiated them from the patients in Group 3. A selective hepatic plexus vagectomy was performed with an immediate decrease in passage pressure in every patient. The average reduction in pressure was 37 percent.[7]

DISCUSSION

Measurements made on the anesthetized patient, at laparotomy, who has already been subjected to the manipulations required for intubation, can hardly be considered as being at physiologic base line. However, because the measurements have been made under standardized intraoperative conditions, comparisons are valid in a single individual.

By accepting a passage pressure of 13 (± 7) cm. of water as being in the normal range, we have reduced the number of patients regarded as having choledochal hypertension or hypotension. We have often encountered normal ducts measuring up to 1 cm. in diameter with pressures between 15 and 20 so that this would appear to be within the upper range of normal. Albot and associates,[1] Hess,[3] and Mallet-Guy[4] regard 15 as the upper limit of normal passage pressure.

It has become apparent that sounding the choledochoduodenal junction with a No. 3 or 4 Bakes dilator can result in sufficient immediate local reaction to elevate the passage pressure above that obtained immediately prior to this maneuver. While this did not occur in all cases it was sufficiently frequent to indicate that postexploratory pressures must be cautiously interpreted. Such elevations range between 20 and 40 percent above that of the initial determination.

When, in the anicteric patient, the contrast material failed to pass through a stone-free duct into the duodenum at a pressure of 15 to 40, further increase of pressure did not alter the roentgen findings or pass the contrast into the duodenum.

Transcystic duct manometry in acute cholecystitis clarified a reason for an elevated serum bilirubin encountered in some patients. It has been our experience that a solitary large nonfacted cholesterol stone in the gallbladder is rarely associated with common duct calculi. Yet some of these patients have bilirubin levels between 2 and 4 mg. percent. We have encountered elevated passage pressures with an enlarged edematous papilla on cholangiograms in some such patients. Postoperative studies 3 weeks later have demonstrated a fall in intraductal pressure and the regression of the ampullary sign. We assume that these changes represent the reversible ampullary and cholangitic reaction to acute cholecystitis. This is one factor responsible for the mild obstructive hyperbilirubinemia sometimes seen in acute obstructive cholecystitis without common duct stones. We have also had choledochoscopic confirmation that ampullary edema is present and not due to a stone, lending further support to the hypothesis that this reversible inflammatory obstruction is due to extrahepatic cholangitis.[8]

A normal passage pressure did not exclude the presence of free-floating nonobstructing intraductal calculi. In the presence of choledocholithiasis an elevated passage pressure cannot be ascribed to intramural sphincter disease. Despite a normal cholangiogram it is not possible reliably to differentiate between outlet obstruction at the sphincter area, and the obstructive effect of the stones. However, a normal passage pressure in the presence of a normal cholangiogram and an adequate cholecystectomy appeared to be strong presumptive evidence against residual biliary disease which could be responsible for postoperative symptoms. At the other extreme of choledochal disease, manometry has proved to be of value in the management of patients having a postcholecystectomy syndrome that is due to ampullary fibrosis. The stenosis at the choledochal-duodenal junction appears to be the result of prior or coexisting biliary lithiasis.

Fixed obstruction was suggested preoperatively by intravenous cholangiography. This study demonstrated delayed contrast excretion from the duct into the duodenum. The stenosis was confirmed intraoperatively by difficulty in passing a Bakes dilator through the distal choledochal segment of the significantly dilated duct. In this group of 19 patients with the roentgen and operative criteria for this diagnosis, manometry did reveal choledochal hypertension. Monometric documentation appears to be a more reliable aid to the diagnosis of ampullary fibrosis than can be obtained from an analysis of the roentgen contour of the distal choledochal segment alone. We have encountered no pathognomonic configuration of the intramural portion of the common duct in cases of proved fibrotic ampullary obstruction. The roentgen patterns encountered in these 19 patients have also been observed in normal individuals and in patients without duct dilation or a time-density delay factor.

In Groups 1, 2, and 6 the manometric

levels conform to and are consistent with other clinical, surgical, and roentgen findings. However, there are instances in Groups 3, 4, and 5 in which the manometric finding cannot be integrated into the other established parameters employed for evaluating the outlet of the common bile duct. The apparent contradictions revolve about the finding of an elevated pressure in the presence of an otherwise completely normal duct, or the demonstration of normal pressures in association with a grossly diseased common bile duct. It is inappropriate to classify chronic cholangitis by the manometric findings alone. The surgeon has to differentiate between reversible ampullary edema, varying degrees of functional but nonanatomic choledochoduodenal junctional stenosis, and the ill-defined entity of the hypertensive choledochal sphincter. This differential diagnosis often cannot be made by single determination manometry. In this problem biliary manometry alone is not as reliable as esophageal manometry in differentiating between functional, hypertensive, and organic outlet obstructions. In part, this is related to the absence of independent peristaltic activity of the common bile duct except at its sphincter. Biliary manometry measures resistance to perfusion flow and sphincter stretch at the end of a nonpropulsive duct. We are unable to extrapolate a therapeutic or clinical implication when ductal hypertension is encountered in an otherwise normal common bile duct. We have not regarded these findings as warranting a surgical approach.

In 1942 Mallet-Guy introduced manometry into operative cholangiography, and by 1952 he was able to report on 1,500 examinations. In a selected series of 100 cases this procedure disclosed another unsuspected pathologic condition in 38 patients. This high incidence is dependent upon the criteria for the diagnosis of biliary hypotonia and obstructive disease of the sphincter of Oddi. He reported on this procedure as a method of deciding whether the duct should be managed by external drainage, primary suture, or bypass as a way of forestalling postcholecystectomy complaints. No clarification of the apparent contradiction between duct size and choledochal pressure is offered. Albot, Olivier, and Libaude[1] employed radio manometry as a way of detecting and evaluating "residual odditis" after the common duct has been cleared of calculi. They arrived at the conclusion that the duct should be drained as long as postoperative studies continue to reveal choledochal hypertension. These authors agree that temporary spastic or permanent organic sphincter changes may occur with cholecystitis. Such dynamic choledochal changes can only be detected by manometry.

This experience suggests that biliary manometry has the following positive aspects: The apparatus is a suitable vehicle for the delivery of contrast material, and there are no disadvantages to its use. The problems are those of interpretation. The presence of a normal passage pressure implies that the choledochoduodenal junction is functionally normal without regard to the presence of calculi. In the presence of choledochal hypertension it is not reasonable to group and classify the common bile duct complications of chronic cholecystitis by the manometric findings alone. The bile duct pressure does not implicate a specific pathogenesis or method of management. An elevated intracholedochal pressure is only one factor in the total evaluation of the common duct, and this determination, of itself, does not differentiate functional reversible inflammatory obstruction from fixed organic stenosis.

SUMMARY

Manometric evaluation of the common bile duct was performed in 137 patients undergoing biliary tract surgical treatment. It was carried out with saline and with contrast material. It has served to confirm the diagnosis of choledochoduodenal junction stenosis in the postcholecystectomy syndrome and to demonstrate a vagally sensitive hypertensive choledochal sphincter.

However, as an adjunct to cholangiography, manometry did not clarify the problem of a dilated duct without choledochal hypertension, nor of the otherwise normal duct with choledochal hypertension.

The data derived from biliary manometry must, therefore, be considered as only one dimension in the total evaluation of the common bile duct.

REFERENCES

1. Albot, G., Olivier, C., and Libaude, H.: Radiomanometric examination of the biliary ducts: Experience with 418 cases, Gastroenterology **24:** 242, 1953.
2. Dahl-Iversen, E., Sorenson, H., and Westengaard, E.: Pressure measurements in the biliary tract in patients after cholecystolithotomy and in patients with dyskinesia Acta chir. scandinav. **114:** 181, 1958.
3. Hess, W.: Die Erkrangungen der Gallenwege and Des Pankreas, Stuttgart, 1961, Georg Thieme Verlag, pp. 260-316.
4. Mallet-Guy, P.: Value of preoperative manometric and roentgenographic examinations in the diagnosis of functional disturbances of the biliary tract, Surg. Gynec. & Obst. **94:** 385, 1952.
5. Schein, C. J., and Beneventano, T. C.: Choledochal dynamics in man, Surg. Gynec. & Obst. **126:** 591, 1968.
6. Schein, C. J., and Beneventano, T. C.: Choledochoduodenal junction stenosis in the postcholesystectomy syndrome, SURGERY **64:** 1039, 1968.
7. Schein, C. J., Beneventano, T. C., Rosen, R. G., Dardik, H., and Gliedman, M. L.: Hepatic plexus vagectomy as an adjunct to cholecystectomy, Surg. Gynec. & Obst. **128:** 241, 1969.
8. Schein, C. J., Stern, W. Z., Hurwitt, E. S., and Jacobson, H. G.: Cholangiography and biliary endoscopy as complementary methods of evaluating the bile ducts, Am. J. Roentgenol. **89:** 864, 1963.

Accelerated rejection of skin grafts in recipients sensitized with extracted human histocompatibility antigens

H. F. SEIGLER*
N. F. MENDES
R. S. METZGAR
DURHAM, N. C.
From the Departments of Microbiology and Immunology and Department of Surgery, Duke University Medical Center, and Veterans Administration Hospital

Recently there have been numerous studies on the extraction, isolation, and characterization of the membrane-associated histocompatibility antigens in mouse, guinea pig, and man. Different methods have been used to extract or separate the transplantation antigens from the membrane. Basically these can be classified as follows: (a) enzymatic digestion, (b) sonication, and (c) detergent treatment.

The in vitro serological and biochemical properties of the enzyme digested alloantigen preparations have been studied in detail, but little is known about their immunogenicity.[2] Kahan and associates,[5-8] who have studied guinea pig alloantigen preparations prepared by sonication,[6, 7] have shown that they are immunogenic,[8] are capable of eliciting a skin test response in immunized guinea pigs,[5] and ilicit a mixed lymphocyte culture reaction.[8] Kandutsch and co-workers[9] have obtained a water soluble H-2 antigen preparation from the detergent soluble material by digestion with snake venom. The yield of active material in the use of this method is relatively high when compared with other methods of extracting antigen, and the detergent-extracted antigen is a good immunogen, producing accelerated graft rejection and hemagglutinating antibodies.[3] The detergent-soluble preparations contain both H-2 and non H-2 antigens and appear to be of a higher molecular weight than the water-soluble preparations since they are excluded from Sephadex G-200.

Our laboratory has studied the serological properties of human alloantigens of the HL-A system extracted by a short treatment with sodium deoxycholate.[11] This paper is concerned with the immunogenic properties of these detergent-soluble human alloantigen preparations.

Supported by National Institutes of Health Grant AM 08054 and United States Public Health Service Contract 43-66-928.

Submitted for publication Feb. 3, 1969; resubmitted April 7, 1969.

*Veterans Administration Clinical Investigatorship.

MATERIALS AND METHODS

Antigen preparation. Approximately 1 ml. packed cell volume of peripheral blood leukocytes, skin fibroblasts, or lymph node cell suspensions were washed three times at 100 × g in cold phosphate buffered saline (PBS) pH 7.2 and resuspended in PBS to a final volume of 10 ml. One milliliter of 5 percent sodium deoxycholate and 1 ml. of pancreatic deoxyribonuclease (0.5 mg. per milliliter) were added to the cell suspension. The mixture was agitated at room temperature for 30 seconds and then incubated at 37° C. for 15 minutes. Three-tenths milliliter of 4M $MgCl_2$ was added and the mixture incubated for an additional 15 minutes at 37° C. The deoxycholate was then precipitated with 3 ml. of 4M MgCl and centrifuged at 100,000 × g for 1 hour. The supernatant was dialyzed overnight at 4° C. against PBS and concentrated four- or fivefold by vacuum dialysis.

Table I. *Summary of results of immunization of human volunteers with extracted human histocompatibility antigens*

	Human recipient			
	E. P.	*B. L.*	*M. H.*	*A. B.*
Tissue or cells used for extraction	3.0 ml. P.C.V.* skin fibroblasts	1.1. ml. P.C.V. skin fibroblasts and 2.2 ml. P.C.V. blood leukocytes	0.5 ml. P.C.V. skin fibroblasts and 2.0 ml. P.C.V. blood leukocytes	4.0 ml. P.C.V. blood leukocytes
Volume of extracted antigen injected intradermally	3.5. ml. in 2 injections over 10 days	3.3 ml. in 4 injections over 4 weeks	10.6 ml. in 9 injections over 9 weeks	11.0 ml. in 11 injections over 15 weeks
Time test skin allograft applied	2 weeks after last injection	1 week after last injection	Same day as last injection	Same day as last injection
Time of allograft rejection	10 days	6 days	3 days	3 days
Results of test for circulating antibody	Negative	Negative	Negative	Negative

*P. C. V. = volume of cell sediment after centrifugation for 10 minutes at 100 × g.

Immunization procedure. The detergent-extracted antigen was sterilized by filtration through a 0.22 μ millipore filter. Each filtrate was tested for sterility and serological activity and was stored at –70° C. until used. The four human volunteers in this study were given intradermal injections of extracted antigen from different individual donors at various time intervals (Table I). Serum samples were collected before each injection.

Skin grafting technique. An 11 mm. trephine was used to cut the grafts. All grafts were full thickness and were sutured with 4-0 black silk, and sterile semipressure dressings were applied. The grafts were photographed daily.

Serological methods. The following techniques were used to detect alloantibodies in the sera of humans immunized with extracted antigen and to test the activity of the extracts.

Leukocyte agglutination. The semimicro method of Amos and Peacocke[1] was used.

INHIBITION OF LEUKOCYTE AGGLUTINATION. From a selected human donor, one volume (0.025 ml.) of antiserum having a titer of 1:4 with cells from the antigen donor was mixed with an equal volume of antigen dilution and incubated for 1 hour at room temperature. Approximately 10^5 leukocytes in 0.025 ml. were then added and the mixture was incubated for 2 hours at room temperature. Agglutination was read microscopically. Titers were expressed as the highest antigen dilution giving complete inhibition of agglutination.

Cytotoxicity. A modification of the semimicro method of Walford and associates[16] was used.

Mixed agglutination. Skin fibroblasts from the antigen donors were grown in monolayers on glass and tested by mixed agglutination using serum from the immunized recipients. The technique of mixed agglutination has been described in detail in previous publications.[10, 12]

INHIBITION OF MIXED AGGLUTINATION. The test for inhibition of this reaction with extracted antigen was performed as follows: Equal volumes (0.5 ml.) of antigen dilutions and isoantiserum were incubated at room temperature for 30 minutes. The standard amount of antiserum used for each inhibition study was three or four times the quantity necessary to produce a positive mixed agglutination reaction. The antigen-antibody mixture in a volume of 1 ml. was added to tube cultures of the appropriate cell line and the remainder of the technique followed as previously described.[10, 12] The inhibition titer was expressed as the highest dilution giving complete inhibition of mixed agglutination. The extracted antigen preparations used in these studies gave inhibition titers from eight to 32 by the two methods described.

RESULTS

Four human volunteers received intradermal injections of detergent-extracted antigen from various cells of individual human donors. The source and amount of cells used for extraction varied considerably, and no effort was made to determine the minimum amount of extracted antigen or donor cells necessary to give accelerated graft rejection. Moreover, because of the limited number of recipients, no attempt was made to determine the optimal antigen dose and route of administration. The primary purpose of the experiments was to determine whether the detergent-extracted human histocompatibility antigens produce an accelerated rejection of donor skin grafts. The immunization procedure, the time of allograft rejection, and the serological findings are given in Table I.

Volunteer E. P. received a total of 3.5 ml. of antigen extracted from 3 ml. of skin fibroblasts (packed cell volume) grown in tissue culture monolayer. The first injection of 0.5 ml. antigen extract was given intradermally and was followed 10 days later with a similar injection of 3 ml. An autograft and two allografts from the donor of the skin were applied 2 weeks later; the allografts were rejected on Day 10 and the autograft healed normally. Ten days after grafting a serum sample was obtained. There was no detectable circulating antibody in the pre- or postgraft serum samples. The recipient received 0.1 ml. of antigen intradermally as a skin test and results were negative at 24, 48, and 96 hours.

Recipient B. L. received a total of 3.3 ml. of extracted antigen intradermally at four different times during a 4 week period. The antigen was extracted from both cultured skin fibroblasts and peripheral blood leukocytes (1.1 ml. and 2.2 ml. packed cell volume, respectively). Two allografts from the antigen donor were applied 1 week after the last injection and were rejected on Day 6; a control autograft healed normally. A serum sample was obtained 9 days after grafting, and again, no antibodies to alloantigens could be detected by any of the serological methods employed.

Volunteer M. H. was given a total of 10.6 ml. of antigen intradermally in nine injections over a 9 week period. This antigen was also extracted from both skin fibroblasts (0.5 ml. packed cell volume) and peripheral blood leukocytes (2.0 ml. packed cell volume). An allograft was applied on the same day as the last injection of antigen and was completely rejected by the third day. No circulating antibody could be detected in any of the nine serum samples taken at various times during the immunization and postgraft period.

Recipient A. B. received only antigen extracted from peripheral blood leukocytes (4.0 ml. packed cell volume). Eleven milliliters of extracted antigen was injected intradermally in 11 divided doses over a 15 week period. Two allografts from the antigen donor and an autograft were applied on the day of the last injection; two addtional autografts were performed. Before being sutured in the graft bed, one graft was allowed to incubate for 30 minutes with extracted antigen from the donor and one with antigen extracted from peripheral blood leukocytes of the recipient. The two allografts and the autograft soaked in donor antigen were rejected by the third day after grafting and had all the usual characteristics of an acute rejection. Microscopic sections of the allografts and the autograft soaked in donor antigen excised in day 3 (Figs. 1 and 2) revealed necrosis of the graft epithelium with mononuclear cell infiltrates with classic perivascular involvement. The untreated autograft and the autograft soaked in autologous antigen healed normally. No circulating anti-

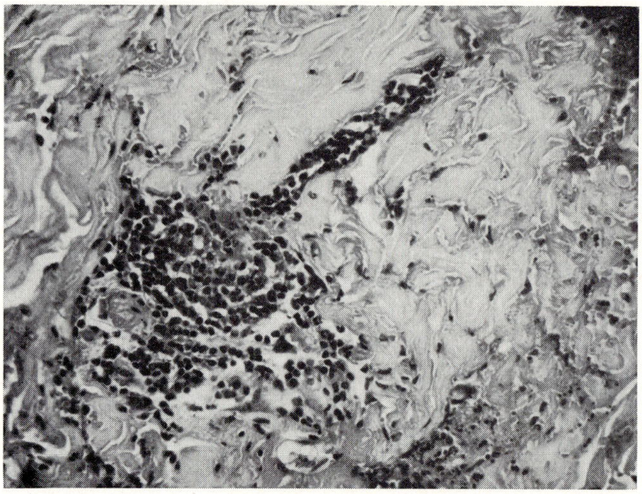

Fig. 1. Allograft from Patient A. B. at Day 3 demonstrating heavy mononuclear cell invasion with perivascular involvement. (Hematoxylin and eosin. Original magnification ×250.)

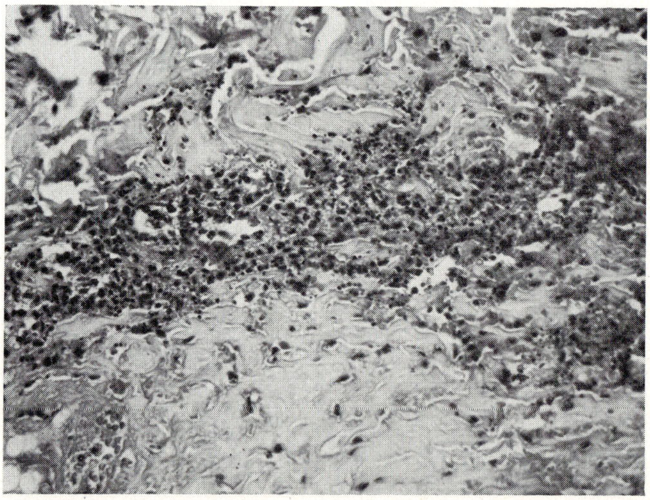

Fig. 2. Base of autograft from Patient A. B. soaked in extracted donor antigen excised on Day 3 demonstrating the same mononuclear cell response as allograft. (Hematoxylin and eosin. Original magnification ×250.)

body was detected in serum samples taken during the course of the immunization, at the time of grafting and 10 days after grafting.

DISCUSSION

The purpose of the experiments reported here was to establish the immunogenicity of the detergent-extracted human alloantigens by determining their ability to elicit accelerated rejection of skin grafts from the antigen donor. It was felt necessary to establish this biological activity with the crude extract before proceeding with separation and purification. The data indicate that under appropriate conditions the extracts are immunogenic. In some instances, skin grafts from the antigen donors were rapidly rejected whereas control autografts remained intact. Several additional experiments could be proposed, e.g., specificity controls, relationship of immunogenicity to current typing or matching procedures, and dosage and route experiments to establish the efficiency or strength of immunogenicity. Specificity controls are difficult to devise for a study of this type of unrelated humans. Although siblings can often be matched for identity of antigens of the HL-A System, unrelated persons cannot be so matched. Moreover, the strength of the individual antigens of this system has not been established. Therefore, it is not possible to choose prospectively an indifferent unrelated donor whose test skin graft should survive longer than a comparable graft from the antigen donor. Similar problems exist for determining the optimal dosage and route of administration of alloantigens. At present, studies of this nature require some sort of genetic uniformity and control which cannot be obtained from an unrelated population by our matching and typing procedures.

The experiments reported here also indicate that the extracted antigens retain their immunogenicity after being stored in PBS at –70° C. for varying periods of time. Most of these human preparations were stored for 1 month or less. The loss of antigenic activity that Rappaport and associates[14] reported with low temperature storage of the subcellular fractions was not encountered.

The markedly accelerated graft rejection (3 days) in two of the human recipients (M. H. and A. B.) in the absence of detectable serum antibody has been encountered with other systems and discussed.[13, 15] The most likely explanations are: (1) Antibody may be present but the serological techniques used for detection are not sensitive enough, (2) the immunoglobulin associated with graft rejection may not be detected by cytotoxicity, leukocyte agglutination, or mixed agglutination, and (3) humoral antibody may not contribute significantly to skin graft rejection.

The rejection of the autograft soaked in the extracted alloantigen is similar to the experiments in mice described by Hellman and Duke.[4] These investigators showed that allogenic skin incubated with syngenic skin altered the syngenic skin so that it behaved as an allogenic graft. It appears that the extracted alloantigens are capable of being absorbed by syngenic graft cells and retained long enough to cause rejection of the graft. However, we have not been able to detect either immediate or delayed skin test hypersensitivity to the detergent-extracted antigen when it was injected intradermally at intervals during immunization and at the time of grafting. Experiments are being conducted to test the skin test activity of the extracted alloantigen absorbed onto the recipients' own lymphocytes.

Little is known about the ability of the various alloantigen extracts to induce accelerated graft rejection, and even less is known about their ability to induce tolerance. The problems of induction of tolerance in humans are formidable for man is not a good species for determining the best dosage, route, form of antigen, genetic combination, and other factors that are necessary to establish reproducible conditions for either immunogenicity or tolerance. If tolerance induction in a random-bred species is to be considered, then a simple, efficient method of antigen extraction from a live donor is desirable; the detergent-soluble alloantigens meet this criterion. It is of paramount importance to establish whether the extracted antigen is in a form which is suitable for induction of tolerance. Although our detergent-solubilized antigen is immunogenic, the strength of the immunogenicity has not been established. The relationship between the degree of immunogenicity of the alloantigen preparation and tolerance induction cannot be predicted. It is quite apparent that more information on tolerance induction with extracted alloantigens in animal models is desirable and probably essential.

SUMMARY

Antigens of the HL-A system can be extracted from human tissues by a short treatment with deoxycholate and deoxyribonuclease. This paper is concerned with the immunogenicity of these detergent soluble human alloantigen preparations. Four volunteers were injected intradermally with antigen extracted from peripheral leukocytes and/or cultured skin fibroblasts of selected donors. After immunization all recipients received full-thickness skin grafts from the antigen donor. Two of the recipients rejected the donor graft as early as 3 days. One of the recipients also received two autografts in addition to the allografts. One of these autografts was incubated with extracted donor antigen for 30 minutes prior to being sutured in the graft bed, the other with extracted antigen from the recipient. The allografts and the autograft incubated with donor antigen were rejected in 3 days. Microscopic sections of the allografts and the autograft incubated with donor antigen excised on Day 3 revealed necrosis of the graft epithelium with mononuclear cell infiltrates and classic perivascular involvement. An untreated autograft and the autograft incubated with autologous antigen healed normally. Sera from the recipients were tested with donor cells by leukocyte agglutination, cytotoxicity, and mixed agglutination. None of the recipients during the course of immunization or 10 days after grafting had antibodies detectable by these techniques.

REFERENCES

1. Amos, D. B., and Peacocke, N.: Leukoagglutination technique, Histocompatibility Testing, Publ. 1229, Nat. Acad. of Sc., National Research Council, 161, 1965.
2. Davies, D. A. L.: Soluble mouse H-2 isoantigens, Transplantation **5:** 31, 1966.
3. Graff, R. J., and Kandutsch, A. A.: Immunogenic properties of purified antigen preparations from a mouse sarcoma, Transplantation **4:** 465, 1966.
4. Hellman, K., and Duke, D. I.: In vitro alteration of skin graft antigenicity, Transplantation **5:** 184, 1967.
5. Kahan, B. D.: Cutaneous hypersensitivity reactions of guinea pigs to proteinaceous transplantation antigen, J. Immunol. **99:** 1121, 1967.
6. Kahan, B. D.: Isolation of a soluble transplantation antigen, Proc. Nat. Acad. Sc. **53:** 153, 1965.
7. Kahan, B. D., and Reisfeld, R. A.: Progress in the purification of a water soluble guinea pig transplantation antigen, Advance in Transplantation, Proceedings of the First International Congress of the Transplantation Society, 395, 1967.
8. Kahan, B. D., Reisfeld, R. A., Epstein, L. B., and Southworth, J. G.: Biologic activities of water soluble guinea pig transplantation antigens, Histocompatibility Testing, 295, 1967.
9. Kandutsch, A. A., Jurgeleit, H. C., and Stimpfling, J. H.: The action of snake venom on an isoantigenic lipoprotein from a mouse sarcoma, Transplantation **3:** 748, 1965.
10. Metzgar, R. S., and Flanagan, J. F.: Mixed agglutination technique for the detection of isoantigens on human kidney cells, Histocompatibility Testing, Publ. 1229, Nat. Acad. of Sc. 183, 1965.
11. Metzgar, R. S., Flanagan, J. F., and Mendes, N. F.: Serological studies of extracted human tissue isoantigens, Histocompatibility Testing, 307, 1967.
12. Metzgar, R. S., Flanagan, J. F., and Zmijewski, C. M.: Detection of tissue isoantigens on primary and serial heteroploid cell lines of human origin by the mixed agglutination technique, J. Immunol. **95:** 494, 1965.
13. Perry, D. Y., Cooper, M. D., and Good, R. A.: Normal second set wottle homograft rejection in agamma-globulinemic chickens, Transplantation **5:** 615, 1967.
14. Rappaport, F. T., Dausset, J., Converse, J. M., and Lawrence, H. S.: Effect of freezing and storage upon the biologic activity of transplantation antigens isolated from human blood leukocytes, Histocompatibility Testing, 315, 1967.
15. Schubert, W. L., Fowler, R., Jr., Martin, L. W., and West, C. D.: Homograft rejection in children with congenital immunological defects: Agamma-globulinemia and Aldrich syndrome, Transplantation Bull. **5:** 615, 1967.
16. Walford, R. L., Gallagher, R., and Troup, G. M.: Human lymphocyte typing with isologous antisera; technical consideration and a preliminary study of the cytotoxic reaction system, Transplantation **3:** 87, 1965.

The influence of thermal burns on gastric acid secretion

JAMES A. O'NEILL, Jr., M.D.*
FORT SAM HOUSTON, TEXAS,
AND COLUMBUS, OHIO
From the U. S. Army Surgical Research Unit, and the Department of Surgery, Children's Hospital and Ohio State University School of Medicine

Gastroduodenal ulceration and gastrointestinal bleeding are commonly associated with thermal injury. Despite the fact that this association has been a recognized clinical entity for many years and despite the fact that many theories have been offered to explain it, the basic etiology is still unknown. Chronic peptic ulcer disease is associated with acid-peptic hypersecretion, but the relationship of hypersecretion to Curling's ulcer has not been established. Previous studies have been contradictory. Friesen[2] was unable to demonstrate hyperacidity in his experimental burn preparations. On the other hand, Hummel and co-workers[3] reported elevated uropepsin levels in burned patients, especially if their injuries were more extensive than 35 percent of body surface. However, these elevated uropepsin levels were not associated with increases in gastric acidity.

Since indirect indications of gastric activity such as uropepsin output are subject to error, and since they do not necessarily reflect the gastric functional state at the time of collection, direct measurements of gastric secretory activity seemed to be warranted. Little or no information of this sort is available.

Presented at the first annual research session of The American Burn Association, Atlanta, March 14-15, 1969.

Received for publication March 20, 1969.

Reprint address: U. S. Army Institute for Surgical Research, Brooke Army Medical Center, Fort Sam Houston, Texas 78234.

*Present Address: Department of Surgery, Louisiana State University School of Medicine, 1542 Tulane Avenue, New Orleans, La. 70112.

Several methods for the estimation and direct measurement of gastric acid output are currently available.[9] Direct measurement is the only method which gives some idea of the net effect in the patient or experimental subject. Much information is available on levels of total and free acidity in nocturnal collections from normal individuals and from those with peptic ulcer. Hence, this would appear to be a satisfactory basis for comparison with other disease states which are associated with gastric secretory changes. In addition, the augmented histamine test has proved to be valuable in the estimation of total secretory potential.[4]

METHODS

Experimental studies. Isolated innervated (Pavlov) and denervated (Heidenhain) gastric pouches were constructed in two groups of four dogs. The presence or absence of vagal innervation was verified by insulin stimulation. After a 1 month recovery period, standard fasted 3 hour collections were made in specially constructed cages to which the animals were accustomed. The 3 hour collection was followed by an augmented histamine stimulation test daily for 2 weeks. The dogs were then subjected to 20 percent full-thickness burns inflicted by sequential applications of an iron with known surface area heated to 350° C. Gastric secretory studies were then continued for 2 weeks after burning. The collected gastric juice was analyzed for volume, pH, total titratable acidity (pH 7.0), and free

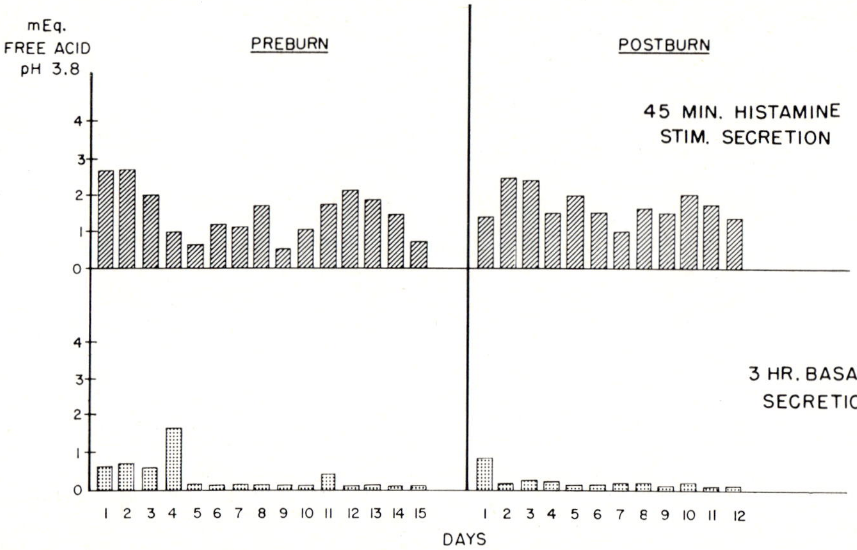

Fig. 1. The mean response of three dogs with denervated Heidenhain pouches to burn injury. No increase in gastric acid secretion was found.

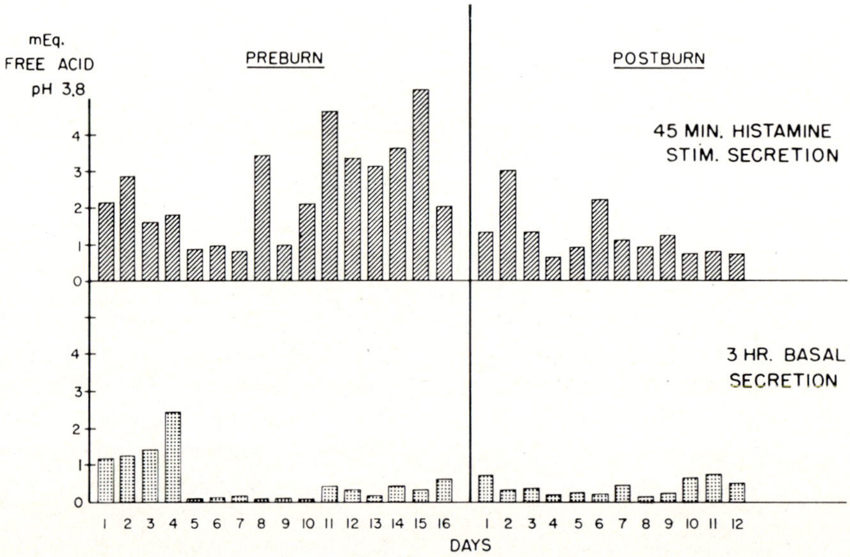

Fig. 2. The mean response of three dogs with innervated Pavlov pouches to burn injury. No increase in secretion was seen following burning.

acid (titrated to pH 3.8 with a pH meter).

Clinical studies. Patients with varying-sized burns were studied. Patients with sepsis, a past history of ulcer, or evidence or suspicion of current gastrointestinal bleeding were included. Collections of 12 hour nocturnal gastric secretory output were made, with special attention given to technical considerations such as tube placement, patient position, tube patency, and fractionation of collection periods. Although augmented histamine tests were originally planned for patient study, it was not proved feasible to stimulate acutely ill patients in this fashion, so these studies were not performed. The nocturnal collections were analyzed for vol-

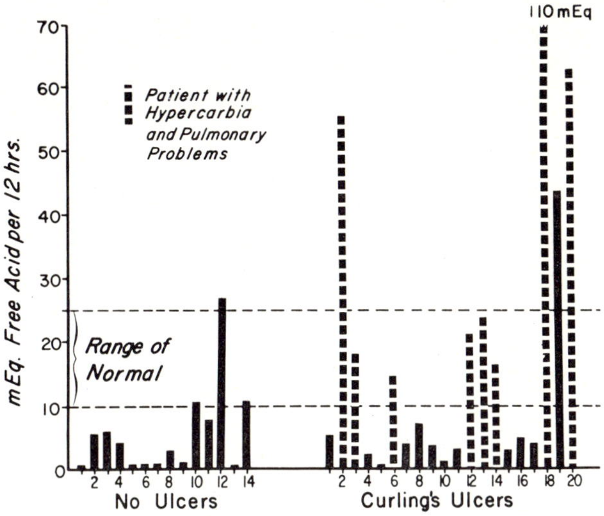

Fig. 3. Twelve-hour nocturnal gastric analyses in 14 mafenide–treated burned patients without any evidence of Curling's ulcer and 20 patients with ulceration. Note that there was no pattern of hyperacidity unless respiratory acidosis was present. Also, note the general trend of higher acid levels in those with ulcers.

ume, pH, bile, blood, total titratable acidity, and free acid, utilizing a pH meter as with the dog studies.

The first group of patients studied at the U.S. Army Surgical Research Unit were treated with mafenide (Sulfamylon) topical therapy. Since mafenide has a carbonic anhydrase inhibiting effect, which might at least initially depress gastric acidity, similar studies were carried out at the Columbus Children's Hospital in a second group of patients, treated with 0.5 percent silver nitrate topical therapy.[7]

RESULTS

Experimental studies (Figs. 1 and 2). One animal in each group had early problems with cannula maintenance and was excluded from the study. Hence, two groups of three animals with Heidenhain and Pavlov pouches were studied according to the protocol. In neither the animals with innervated nor those with denervated gastric pouches could a pattern of hyperacidity in response to burn injury be demonstrated either in basal or histamine-stimulated secretory studies.

Patient studies (Figs. 3 and 4). Forty-

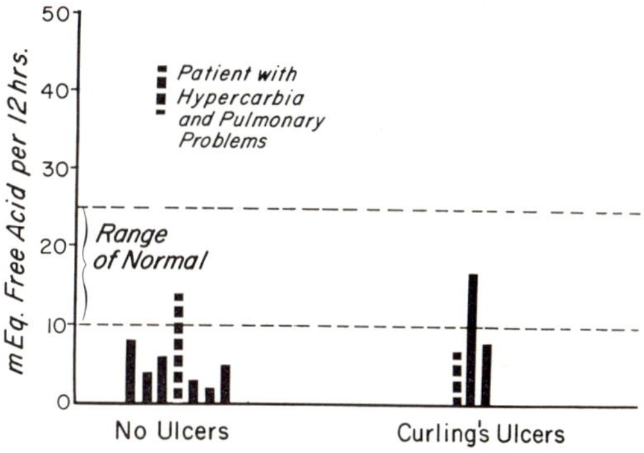

Fig. 4. Twelve-hour nocturnal gastric analyses in seven silver nitrate–treated patients without ulcers and three with ulcers. No hyperacidity was found in any of these patients.

four patients were studied. Thirty-four patients treated with mafenide topical therapy had 12 hour nocturnal collections of gastric secretory output made. The patients ranged from 9 months to 75 years in age with an average of 25 years. The total extent of burn ranged from 7 to 95 percent, with a mean of 49 percent. The mean burn index* was

*Burn index = total amount of third degree burn plus one half the total second degree burn. This puts patients on an equal basis with respect to extent and depth of injury.

40 percent. Twenty of the 34 patients had a diagnosis of Curling's ulcer made either at the time of postmortem examination, at the time of operation, or on the basis of massive hemorrhage. The 20 patients with ulcers had an average total burn of 60 percent (burn index, 43 percent), and the 14 without evidence of ulceration had an average total burn of 45 percent (burn index, 36 percent).

If 18 mEq. of free acid in a 12 hour collection of gastric secretions is considered to be the upper limit of normal, only five of these patients can be considered to have hypersecretion. One patient with a 12 hour output of 55.4 mEq. was 28 years old, had a 24 percent total body burn and a crushed chest, and bled massively on the third day after the burn. A second patient with a 12 hour output of 110 mEq. of free acid was 37 years old, had a 61 percent total body burn, severe bilateral pneumonia, and multiple gastric and duodenal ulcers at postmortem examination. The third patient with hypersecretion put out 43.2 mEq. of free acid in 12 hours. He was 20 years old, had a 63.5 percent total body burn, had no pulmonary problems, and bled massively enough from a duodenal ulcer to require operative intervention. A fourth patient with hypersecretion of 62.6 mEq. of free acid in 12 hours was 49 years old and had a 45 percent total body burn and severe pneumonia. He bled massively and required operation, at which time multiple gastric and duodenal ulcers were found. The last patient with hypersecretion had 26.8 mEq. of free acid output in 12 hours. He was 22 years old and had a 32 percent body burn. He had no pulmonary difficulties and no evidence of Curling's ulceration. The remainder of the patients had no evidence of hypersecretion. In an analysis of the pattern of secretion in the 14 patients without ulcers and the 20 patients with ulcers, there is a tendency towards higher secretory levels in the ulcer group; however, most determinations were still within the range of normal.

Ten patients treated with 0.5 percent silver nitrate soaks had 12 hour gastric secretory studies performed. The patients ranged from 3 to 12 years in age with an average of 8 years. The total extent of burn ranged from 10 to 70 percent with a mean of 35 percent. The mean burn index was 30 percent. Three of the ten patients had a diagnosis of Curling's ulcer made on the basis of excessive bleeding. None of these patients had more than 18 mEq. of free acid output in 12 hours.

COMMENT

Animals prepared with isolated innervated and denervated gastric pouches were not shown to respond to burn injury with hypersecretion. In fact, the tendency in animals with innervated pouches was a pattern of hyposecretion, especially in stimulated secretory studies.

The patients displayed a pattern of secretion not unlike that seen in the experimental animals. Of significance is the finding that not only is there not a pattern of hypersecretion in patients with burn injury alone, but also there is no evidence for acid hypersecretion in burned patients with known Curling's ulcer. One patient in the group without ulcers had evidence of hypersecretion, and only one patient in the ulcer group had evidence of hypersecretion unassociated with any other factor which might predispose to hypersecretion. Three of the patients with ulcers and gastric hypersecretion had severe pulmonary difficulties with hypercarbia. It is known that both acute and chronic hypercarbia are associated with hypersecretion, so the hypersecretion seen in these patients may not necessarily be related to their burns.[8]

The first group of patients were treated with topical mafenide therapy. This drug is a carbonic anhydrase inhibitor and theoretically might cause a decrease in gastric acid output and, in that manner, mask the effect of the injury itself.[1, 7] However, this consideration is probably of little importance since more powerful carbonic anhydrase inhibitors such as acetazolamide only temporarily reduce gastric acidity when given in massive doses, and not at all in the presence of metabolic acidosis.[1] In support of this is the fact that none of the silver nitrate–treated patients had hypersecretion either.

It has been shown in other studies that burn injury is associated with marked decreases in the rate of renewal of the gastric mucous barrier in experimental animals.[6] If this is true in patients, it would seem reasonable to assume that those patients who developed Curling's ulcer had a greater deficit in the mucous protective layer of their stomachs. Since gastric mucus also has a known buffering capacity of approximately 50 mEq. of HCl per liter of gastric mucus, those patients who developed ulcers would be expected to have higher acid levels than those patients who did not. It is interesting to note that this is exactly the pattern observed. It may be that even though absolute hyperacidity could not be demonstrated to be a factor in Curling's ulceration, "relative hyperacidity" may be a factor in those patients with Curling's ulceration who have a decrease in the rate of renewal of gastric mucus.

SUMMARY

Studies in experimental animals with both innervated and denervated gastric fundic pouches and also studies of nocturnal gastric secretory output in burned patients, half of whom had Curling's ulcer, give no support to the theory that absolute acid-peptic hypersecretion is related to this entity. It may well be that relative hyperacidity may be present on the basis of a decrease in the amount of gastric mucus present.

REFERENCES

1. Davenport, H. W.: Physiology of the digestive tract, Chicago, 1966, Year Book Medical Publishers, p. 109.
2. Friesen, S. R.: The genesis of gastroduodenal ulcer following burns. An experimental study, SURGERY **28:** 123, 1950.
3. Hummel, R. P., Lanchantin, G. F., and Artz, C. P.: Clinical experiences and studies in Curling's ulcer, J. A. M. A. **164:** 141, 1957.
4. Kay, A. W.: Effect of large doses of histamine on gastric secretion of HCl. An augmented histamine test, Brit. M. J. **2:** 77, 1953.
5. Newman, S. F., Silbergleit, A., and Thal, A. P.: Stimulation of gastric secretion by hypercarbia, SURGERY **57:** 285, 1965.
6. O'Neill, J. A., Jr., Ritchey, C. R., Mason, A. D., Jr., and Villarreal, Y.: Influence of thermal burns on gastric mucous production, S. Forum **17:** 293, 1966.
7. Pruitt, B. A., Jr., O'Neill, J. A., Jr., Moncrief, J. A., and Lindberg, R. B.: Successful control of burn wound sepsis, J. A. M. A. **203:** 1054, 1968.
8. Ridgen, B. G.: Chest disease and peptic ulcer, Gut **2:** 89, 1961.
9. Rovelstad, R. A.: Gastric analysis, Gastroenterology **45:** 90, 1963.

Long-term sequelae of common femoral vein ligation in the treatment of thromboembolic disease

ROBERT A. NABATOFF, M.D.
LESTER BLUM, M.D.
ARTHUR S. W. TOUROFF, M.D.
NEW YORK, N. Y.
From the Department of Surgery, The Mount Sinai Hospital

Despite extensive research and excellent clinical studies,[8] thromboembolic disease continues to produce considerable morbidity and a rather high mortality rate. The short-term effects of femoral vein ligation have been amply described. Little, however, has been reported concerning the late sequelae of this procedure when performed either prophylactically or in the presence of obvious thromboembolic disease. Agrifoglio and Edwards[1] investigated the manifestations of venous stasis after vein ligations for thromboembolic disease in 195 patients who survived the operation from 1 to 10 years. The common femoral vein was ligated immediately above its formation but below the circumflex and saphenous veins. "Stasis effects were more severe and long lasting after ligation of the superficial femoral vein than of the common femoral vein." However, according to Crane,[2] "Almost all observers agree that postligation sequelae are most frequent after common femoral vein division than when the profunda femoris vein is left open." This latter conclusion was also arrived at by Robinson and Moyer[11] who performed 31 ligations of the common femoral vein and 43 ligations of the superficial femoral vein. There was an 8 year follow-up period. "Within one to eight years after ligation and division of the common femoral vein incapacitating sequelae appear in more than three-fourths of the persons operated upon; however, ligation and division of the superficial femoral vein are attended by the same sequelae, with a frequency of less than one in ten."

The majority of pulmonary emboli probably originate in the veins of the lower extremity and proceed upward via the superficial femoral vein to the lungs. When femoral vein ligation is performed, many surgeons interrupt the superficial femoral vein. However, a communication between the deep and superficial veins has been demonstrated in 10 percent of autopsy specimens.[3] In these patients, thrombi could pass upward along the distal part of the superficial femoral vein into the deep femoral vein and then to the lungs. Thus, pulmonary embolization could occur despite superficial femoral vein ligation.

MATERIAL AND METHODS

This report describes 73 patients in whom a total of 109 common femoral vein ligations have been performed. The operation was carried out in patients with thromboembolic disease to prevent pulmonary embolization. Phlebography was routinely performed as soon as the diagnosis of thrombophlebitis or pulmonary embolism was suspected. The femoral vein ligation was not performed unless definite evidence of phlebitis or embolism was demonstrated clinically, or visualized by x-rays or phlebograms. The patient was taken to the operating room as soon as a definite diagnosis was made. The femoral vein was ligated immediately below the inguinal ligament, prox-

Received for publication March 13, 1969.

imal to the entrance of the saphenous and deep femoral veins. This high ligation site was chosen to prevent embolization via the deep femoral vein. For comparison, a study was made of 33 patients who developed thrombophlebitis but who were not subjected to femoral vein ligation. The period of observation in both series ranges from 6 months to 15 years.

Common femoral vein ligation. Seventeen of the patients in this group were between 20 and 40 years of age and the remainder were 40 to 60 years old. There were 35 men and 38 women. Only seven patients had a previous history of varicose veins. In 38 instances the thromboembolic process occurred as a postoperative complication. The other 35 patients developed their first symptoms on the medical ward. In the "postoperative group" symptoms first developed 5 to 10 days after operation in 15 patients, 10 to 15 days in 18, and 15 to 20 days postoperatively in 5. At the time of common femoral vein ligation, thrombi were found in the femoral vein in 32 of 103 extremities. The external iliac vein was always aspirated through the proximal end of the divided femoral vein until there was a free flow of blood. Intravenous heparin was begun several hours after operation and was continued for 3 days.

The patients subjected to common femoral vein ligation were divided into four groups (Table 1): (1) patients with findings indicating pulmonary embolization but no symptoms referable to the lower extremities, (2) patients whose only manifestation was calf tenderness, (3) those with definite evidence of thrombophlebitis of the lower extremity but without edema, (4) those with definite phlebitis and edema. There were 20 extremities in which there were no symptoms of phlebitis at the time of pulmonary embolization. Following common femoral vein ligation, five have remained asymptomatic, eight manifest slight-to-moderate edema but are asymptomatic, six have slight-to-moderate edema, associated with intermittent pain, and one exhibits moderate edema, associated with pain, pigmentation, and intermittent ulceration.

There were 56 extremities in which only calf tenderness was present at the time of vein ligation. In this group, four have remained completely asymptomatic, 33 have slight-to-moderate edema without significant symptoms, 16 have moderate edema associated with significant pain, and three have moderate edema, associated with pain, pigmentation, and intermittent ulceration of the leg.

In the third group, there were 25 extremities with definite thrombophlebitis but no edema prior to vein ligation. One has remained completely asymptomatic, four have slight-to-moderate edema without significant

Table I. *Sequelae following common femoral vein ligation*

Group	*No. of extremities*	*Physical signs*	*Asymptomatic*	*Slight-to-moderate edema without significant symptoms*	*Moderate edema plus significant symptoms*	*Marked edema, pain, and ulceration*
1	20	None, ligation performed because of occurrence of pulmonary emboli	5	8	6	1
2	56	Only calf tenderness	4	33	16	3
3	25	Calf and thigh tenderness, no edema	1	4	16	4
4	2	Calf and thigh tenderness plus edema	0	0	1	1
Total	103		10	45	39	9

symptoms, 16 have moderate edema associated with intermittent pain, and four manifest edema, pigmentation, and ulceration.

In the fourth group the extremities with phlebitis also had definite edema prior to operation. One extremity is now moderately edematous and markedly pigmented, and the other is edematous, painful, pigmented, and ulcerated.

Thus, of the entire group only 10 have no sequelae. In 45 instances, there is slight-to-moderate edema but no functional disturbance thus far. However, these patients have to wear elastic bandages to prevent complications. Thirty-nine extremities are edematous and painful, and nine are markedly affected as a result of the edema, pain, and intermittent ulceration that are due to impaired venous return. Thus, 93 of the 103 lower extremities manifest some degree of chronic venous insufficiency.

Patients with thromboembolic disease treated conservatively. The second aspect of this study concerned patients who were not subjected to femoral vein ligation. There were 33 patients in this group, representing a total of 46 lower extremities. There were 18 men and 15 women. In four of the involved extremities there was a previous history of varicose veins. Thirteen of the 33 patients in this group developed thromboembolic complications following surgical procedures. The time interval from the date of operation to the onset of symptoms was 10 to 14 days in 10 patients and 15 to 17 days in three. Follow-up observations ranged from 6 months to 2 years in 10 patients, 2 to 5 years in 11, 5 to 10 years in 7, and 10 to 15 years in 5.

These patients were also divided into four groups (Table II): (1) those patients with only calf tenderness, (2) patients with calf and thigh tenderness without edema, (3) those with calf and thigh tenderness with slight-to-moderate edema, (4) patients with severe thrombophlebitis and marked edema.

In those five extremities in which there was only calf tenderness, there were no sequelae. Of the 14 extremities with phlebitis but no edema, 12 have remained asymptomatic and two have slight edema. Of the 13 extremities with phlebitis plus edema, 12 have remained asymptomatic and one is markedly edematous and has a healed ulcer. Of the 14 extremities with severe thrombophlebitis, one has remained asymptomatic, two have slight edema, and 11 have moderate-to-marked edema and are painful, pigmented, and intermittently ulcerated.

DISCUSSION

It is apparent that patients develop edema, pigmentation, and ulceration of the legs if there is sufficient impairment of venous return, whether or not a vein ligation

Table II. *Sequelae following thrombophlebitis, no vein ligation performed*

Group	*No. of extremities*	*Physical signs*	*Asymptomatic*	*Slight-to-moderate edema without significant symptoms*	*Moderate edema plus significant symptoms*	*Marked edema, pain, and ulceration*
1	5	Only calf tenderness	5			
2	14	Calf and thigh tenderness without edema	12	2		
3	13	Calf and thigh tenderness plus slight-to-moderate edema	12			1
4	14	Calf and thigh warm and tender, bluish discoloration of leg	1	2		11
Total	46		30	4		12

is performed. The vein ligation naturally increases the possibility of subsequent sequelae. In contradistinction to patients with peripheral arterial disease, individuals with venous stasis develop symptoms at rest. There is relief as soon as exercise or massage is performed. If the superficial femoral vein is interrupted, there is little chance of postphlebitic sequelae if there has not been extensive venous thrombosis prior to vein ligation. However, if only the superficial femoral vein is interrupted, it is possible that the thrombus will propagate via the deep femoral vein.[5]

An important deterrent to the development of sequelae following thrombophlebitis or vein ligation is the prompt use of anticoagulants. Since the occurrence of sequelae depends upon the number of veins damaged as a result of thrombophlebitis and/or vein ligation, the more prompt and adequate the anticoagulant therapy, the less likelihood there is of progressive thrombosis and subsequent complications. Heparin can dissolve recent thrombi, if given before organization occurs.[9] It has been demonstrated experimentally that the " . . . combined administration of heparin and penicillin will cause the solution or disappearance of a clot in a fairly large number of cases of thrombophlebitis, and especially if given in the early stages of the clot formation."[10] In another study,[4] the use of anticoagulants reduced the incidence of secondary embolism from an expected 30 percent to 2.17 percent. It reduced the rate of secondary fatal embolism from an expected 25 percent to zero. The incidence of postphlebitic edema is strikingly diminished in those patients who are adequately treated with anticoagulants. In those cases with the process confined to the leg, the incidence of postphlebitic edema is less then 5 percent whereas in those having thrombus in the iliofemoral region, there is minimal-to-moderate edema after a follow-up of 1 to 2 years.

Thus, anticoagulants decrease the incidence of progressive thrombosis and subsequent pulmonary embolization without producing the additional venous obstruction which is inevitable with a vein ligation.

If anticoagulants are contraindicated or if pulmonary emboli occur despite their use, a vein ligation is indicated. If there is marked venous thrombosis, subsequent complications will develop whether or not the vein interruption is performed. If the common femoral vein is ligated, some degree of edema, pain, pigmentation, or ulceration will develop in the majority of patients. The edema resulting from vein ligation is seldom as pronounced when the iliac veins are tied off as compared with when the common femoral vein is interrupted.[6, 7] This is because of the greater availability of collateral vessels following the former procedure. If the superficial femoral vein is ligated, there is little chance of subsequent edema, pain, and ulceration, but there is a possibility of embolization via the deep femoral vein. If a vein ligation is mandatory to prevent pulmonary emboli, it is probably advisable to ligate the inferior vena cava. A ligation at this level effectively prevents embolization, and there is a large amount of available collateral circulation. The patient should be ambulatory practically immediately following operation to minimize venous thrombosis and promote the development of collateral circulation.

SUMMARY

1. This report describes follow-up observations after common femoral vein ligation in 103 lower extremities.

2. In only 10 instances were there no sequelae whatever. In the remaining 93 extremities there was some evidence of venous stasis. This was manifested by minimal edema in some cases, but other patients developed marked edema, pain, pigmentation, and intermittent ulceration of the leg.

3. In patients with marked venous stasis, the symptoms and physical signs of venous impairment often became apparent immediately. Long-term studies are essential since the postphlebitic or postligation effects often appeared, for the first time, several years or longer after the acute phlebitis or vein ligation. Once symptoms start they frequently become gradually worse, especially if the

edema is not completely controlled with proper elastic supports. In severe cases, the ankle ulceration and other sequelae of chronic venous stasis can produce marked disability.

4. In view of the great frequency of postoperatively sequelae, common femoral vein ligation is not indicated as a routine procedure for the prevention of pulmonary embolization from the lower extremities.

REFERENCES

1. Agrifoglio, G., and Edwards, E. A.: Venous stasis after ligation of femoral veins or inferior vena cava, J. A. M. A. **178:** 101, 1961.
2. Crane, C.: Deep venous thrombosis and pulmonary embolism, New England J. Med. **257:** 147, 1957.
3. Edwards, E., and Robuck, J.: Applied anatomy of the femoral vein and its tributaries, Surg. Gynec. & Obst. **85:** 547, 1947.
4. Felder, D.: Evaluation of the various clinical signs of thrombophlebitis and experience in therapy with anticoagulants, Surg. Gynec. & Obst. **88:** 337, 1949.
5. Fine, J., Frank, H., and Starr, A.: Recent experiences with thrombophlebitis of the lower extremity and pulmonary embolism, Ann. Surg. **116:** 574, 1942.
6. Fine, J., and Starr, A.: The surgical therapy of thrombosis of the deep veins of the lower extremities, Surgery **17:** 232, 1945.
7. Homans, J.: Deep quiet venous thrombosis in the lower limb. Preferred levels for interruption of veins, Surg. Gynec. & Obst. **79:** 70, 1944.
8. Ochsner, A., De Bakey, M. E., De Camp, P. T., and da Rocha, E.: Thromboembolism: Analysis of cases at Charity Hospital in New Orleans over 12-year period, Ann. Surg. **134:** 405, 1951.
9. Rabinovitch, J., and Pines, B.: The effect of heparin on experimentally produced venous thrombosis, Surgery **14:** 669, 1943.
10. Rabinovitch, J., and Pines, B.: Effect of heparin and penicillin on experimentally produced thrombophlebitis, Arch. Surg. **58:** 163, 1949.
11. Robinson, J. R., and Moyer, C. A.: Comparison of late sequelae of common and superficial femoral vein ligations, Surgery **35:** 690, 1954.

The duplicated saphenous vein in femoropopliteal bypass grafting

H. GAYLIS, Ch.M., F.R.C.S. (Eng.)
JOHANNESBURG, SOUTH AFRICA
From the Department of Surgery, University of the Witwatersrand and the General Hospital

Autogenous saphenous vein seems to be the best available material as a graft for femoropopliteal arterial occlusions.[2, 3, 5] The long saphenous vein, however, is not always obtainable and for one reason or another may not be so in 10 to 15 percent of cases. For example, the vein may be too small or too dilated, not of sufficient length, fibrosed from previous thrombophlebitis, or absent, having been previously removed by stripping. The saphenous vein may be duplicated, the two limbs of the vein joined to form a loop. Some consider this anomaly a contraindication to its use.[4] Others have recommended that if this anomaly is present, the two limbs should be converted into one by incising the opposing borders of the vein and resuturing the edges so that the two are converted into a single channel.

This report embodies experience of six duplicated saphenous veins encountered during bypass grafting in the thigh. As a result, it is contended that duplication of the saphenous vein is not necessarily a contraindication to its use; neither are complicated plastic procedures necessary to convert the two channels into a single lumen. The main purpose of this paper, however, is to draw attention to a means of recognizing this anomaly so as to prevent accidental ligation of one of the limbs of the vein, during dissection of the saphenous vein prior to grafting.

The incidence of duplication of the saphenous vein varies and, according to Allan,[1] who dissected 165 limbs, 86 percent of limbs had a loop somewhere along the course of the long saphenous vein, but most were situated below the knee. The loops varied in number and length. Eighteen percent had loops in the thigh, 15 percent had a loop at the knee, and 43 percent had a loop in the leg part.

Received for publication March 13, 1969.

RECOGNITION OF THE DUPLICATED SAPHENOUS VEIN

The duplicated saphenous vein may be recognized clinically before operation or at the time of operation by the following methods:

By careful preoperative inspection and palpation of the medial aspect of the thigh and leg, with the patient standing, it is sometimes possible to recognize a duplicated vein and to mark its course on the skin. In any event it is good practice to chart the course of the long saphenous vein before operation as this can prevent unnecessary undermining of the skin flaps with the possibility of flap necrosis if the vein lies in an unexpected position. At operation, the duplicated vein may be easily recognized if the two limbs run close to each other. However, if they course at some distance from each other, or if they lie in two different planes, the unwary or inexperienced surgeon may divide one limb of the loop mistaking it for a branch. This error can be avoided by considering the junction of normal veins.

At the junction of two veins the lumen of the common or proximal formed vein is larger in diameter than either the distal or two entering veins forming the junction. This is physiological considering that the newly formed channel has to accommodate an increased volume of blood. However,

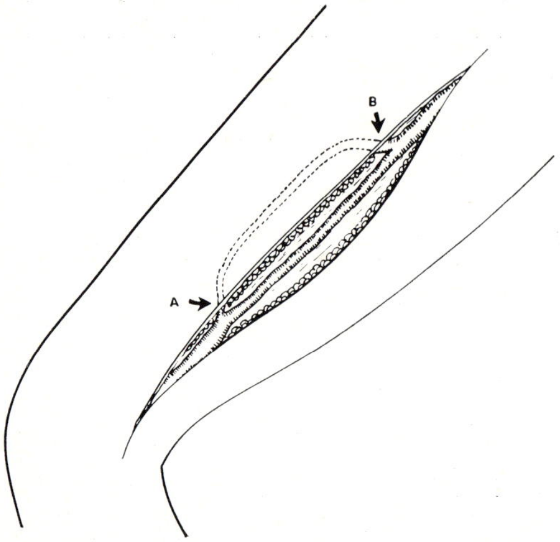

Fig. 1. Diagram to illustrate a duplicated long saphenous vein in the thigh. At (*A*), the junction of two veins, the common or proximal vein is smaller in diameter than the two entering veins. This should immediately arouse the suspicion of a duplicated vein (interrupted lines). At (*B*), the two limbs join and the common vein is wider in diameter than that of the two limbs.

when a vein junction is seen and the common or proximal vein is smaller in diameter than either of the tributary veins, duplication should be immediately suspected (Fig. 1). If this is encountered, the entering vein should not be ligated and cut but dissected under the flap to confirm the presence or absence of duplication. If a duplicated vein is found, both limbs of the loop should be dissected free and their branches tied and divided. Such a double-channeled vein may be used as a bypass graft in the same way as a normal saphenous vein.

DISCUSSION AND CONCLUSION

In this series of cases, duplicated veins were used on six occasions. The length of the duplication varied from 2 to 25 cm., and the early results in all cases were successful. One duplicated vein which extended from just above the knee to the groin occluded after a period of 6 years. The long-term follow-up of the remaining grafts is not yet available, but there is no reason to suspect that the behavior of these will be any different from that of single-channel saphenous vein bypass grafts.

There is no need to reject a duplicated or looped vein as a graft unless the length exceeds that which is required. Further, there is no need to convert the two limbs into a single channel by an extensive and time-consuming plastic procedure. If a duplicated vein conducts blood satisfactorily with the slow velocity of the venous system it should, and does, perform well with the fast moving arterial blood.

SUMMARY

1. Duplication of the saphenous vein is not a contraindication to its use as a bypass graft in femoropopliteal arterial occlusions. Neither is it necessary to convert the two limbs into a single channel by extensive and time-consuming plastic procedures.

2. The surgeon should anticipate this anomaly as the unwary may accidentally divide one of the limbs with the possibility that the vein will be discarded.

3. Methods for recognition of the duplication of the saphenous vein are discussed.

Gratitude is expressed to Professor D. J. du Plessis of the Department of Surgery and Mr. J. C. Allen of the Department of Anatomy for their comments.

REFERENCES

1. Allan, J. C.: Personal communication, 1968.
2. Dale, W. A., and Mavor, G. E.: Brit. J. Surg. **46:** 305, 1959.
3. Edwards, W. S.: Composite reconstruction of small leg arteries after endarterectomy, SURGERY **51:** 58, 1962.
4. Kakkar, V. V.: Use of the cephalic vein as a peripheral vascular graft, Presented at the Seventeenth International Congress of the European Society of Cardiovascular Surgery, London, 1968.
5. Linton, R. R., and Darling, R. C.: Autogenous saphenous vein bypass grafts in femoropopliteal obliterative arterial disease, SURGERY 51: 62, 1962.

Venous pressure monitor

BERNARD VIDNE, M.D.
SHAUL LEVINSON, Eng.
MORRIS J. LEVY, M.D.
TEL AVIV, ISRAEL
From the Thoracic and Cardiovascular Surgery Department, Beilinson Hospital, and University of Tel Aviv Medical School

Central venous pressure monitoring has, in recent years, received attention as a guide in determining the relationship between venous return and cardiac output, that is, as an indicator of myocardial performance.[1] Subject to careful interpretation in dynamic situations, this type of monitoring provides valuable information that enables us to apply proper therapy to the patients' blood losses as well as to problems related to the heart function.

Although continuous central pressure monitoring is not the sole source of such information, it has become an adjunct in a variety of surgical and medical patients with shock problems, hypovolemia, and/or circulatory failure.

Two problems bar such monitoring from wider use in these patients: The first has been the lack of ease in placing the catheter in a central vein or atrium, and the second is the maintenance of a steady base line for the water manometer when the position of the patient is changed.

The purpose of this communication is to describe a simple central vein pressure monitor and the technique for its clinical application.

The venous pressure monitor consists of a plastic tube attached to an intravenous catheter by a 4 way stopcock. The column measuring the central venous pressure is attached to a graduated scale, 40 cm. long. The distal end of this column terminates in a small plastic bag closed to the atmosphere. In the lower part of the scale there is a small telescope through which the zero line can be easily adjusted, with the sternal level, or the thoracic wall when the patient is turned on his side, as a guide. The scale is movable and fixed readily when attached to the bedside. With the aid of the telescope control it is easy to move the graduated scale up and down until the zero line is attained.

The 4 way stopcock connected with the catheter, proximal to the venous pressure line, facilitates measurement of the central venous pressure as well as the administering of two different fluids simultaneously if necessary. Drugs can also be administered intravenously through a separate channel without disconnecting the line (Fig. 1).*

The plastic bag topping the venous pressure column prevents direct contact between the fluid in the column and the atmosphere, thus diminishing possible contamination when the pressure is monitored for hours or days.

In all our open-heart cases for which there is need for a groin incision, the catheter has been routinely inserted through the great saphenous vein into the inferior vena cava and left there as long as necessary, occasionally up to 4 or 5 days after operation (Fig. 2). In other surgical or medical cases in which there was an indication for central venous pressure to be continuously measured for several days, a central vein

Received for publication March 21, 1969.

*This set, scale, and stopcock will be marketed by the Sherwood Medical Industries, St. Louis, Mo.

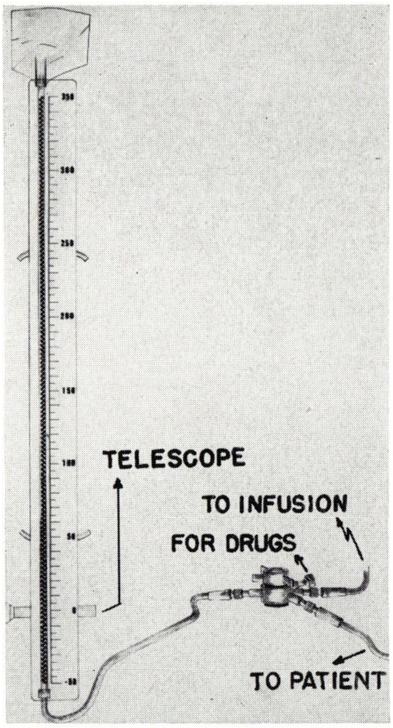

Fig. 1. Schematic representation of the venous pressure monitor connected to the 4 way stopcock. The venous pressure monitor terminates in a plastic bag. At the bottom of the scale there is a small telescope for adjusting the level of the scale to the zero line of the patient.

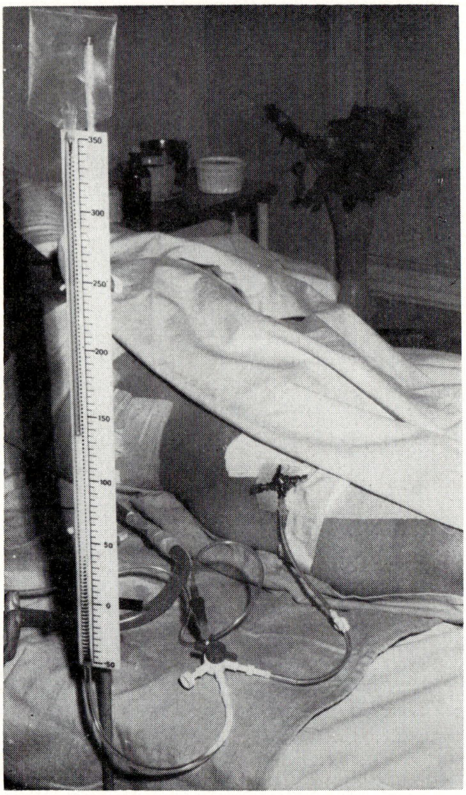

Fig. 2. Photograph of the patient after termination of an open-heart procedure in which a catheter has been placed in a central vein via the saphenous vein at the beginning of the operation. The catheter is connected to the central venous pressure monitor by the 4 way stopcock.

was approached through the femoral or subclavian vein percutaneously. The vein was punctured by a large number 14 gauge needle, and the catheter was inserted through the needle into the vein and advanced as far as necessary, followed by removal of the needle.[2]

In no case so far have we encountered thromboembolic problems related to the catheter tip or infection around the catheter entrance.

REFERENCES

1. Longerbeam, J. K., Vannix, R., William, W., and Joergenson, E.: Central venous pressure monitoring: A useful guide to fluid therapy during shock and other forms of cardiovascular stress, Am. J. Surg. **110:** 220, 1965.
2. Mogil, R. A., De Laurentis, D. A., and Rosemond, G. P.: The infraclavicular venipuncture: Value in various clinical situations including central venous pressure monitoring, Arch. Surg. **95:** 320, 1967.

Carcinoma of thyroglossal duct cyst: Case reports and review of the literature

BELUR S. BHAGAVAN, M.B., B.S.*
D. R. GOVINDA RAO, M.B., B.S.
TOBIAS WEINBERG, M.D.
BALTIMORE, MD.
From the Departments of Pathology, Sinai Hospital and St. Joseph's Hospital

Carcinoma arising from a thyroglossal duct remnant is rare. In a study of 128 cases of thyroglossal duct cysts, Nachlas[27] reported one case of malignant tumor. In 130 patients surgically treated for thyroglossal duct cysts at the University of California Hospital, two cases of papillary carcinoma were found.[8] Doubt has been expressed regarding the occurrence of these tumors, and their origin from the thyroglossal duct has been viewed with skepticism.[20, 28] A survey of the literature reveals 40 cases of carcinoma arising within the thyroglossal duct remnants. The purpose of this paper is (1) to report three additional cases, (2) to review the available literature, and (3) to examine the validity of the skepticism expressed concerning the occurrence and origin of these tumors.

CASE REPORTS

Case 1. L. M. (U No. 97249), a 66-year-old Caucasian man, was admitted to Sinai Hospital for removal of a small, painless, midline mass that had been present in the neck for 1 year. The mass had gradually increased in size during the past year, but had produced no discomfort. A roughly spherical 4 cm. firm nodule was located immediately below the hyoid bone. At operation, the mass was found to lie immediately beneath the strap muscles and was removed along with the central portion of the hyoid bone. Gross examination of the specimen revealed a biloculated intercommunicating cystic mass measuring 3.5 by 4 by 3 cm. The wall of the cyst showed a tannish-gray granular and papillary tumor mass measuring up to 0.8 cm. in thickness (Fig. 1). The loculi of the cyst contained a brownish, shimmering, viscid fluid. Microscopically, the cyst had a fibrous wall with no recognizable internal-lining epithelium. Focal areas of hemorrhage and cholesterol granulomas were noted. The infiltrating tumor was a papillary adenocarcinoma, similar to those seen in the thyroid gland (Fig. 2). No normal thyroid tissue was found in the sections examined. Twenty-two days after discharge, he died, at another hospital because of cardiac arrhythmia, with cardiac arrest. Postmortem examination was not performed.

Case 2. P. S. (U No. 358193), a 38-year-old man, was admitted with the chief complaint of an asymptomatic lump in the midline of the neck which had been present for 3 years and had steadily grown in size. The mass was smooth surfaced, hard, partly mobile, and nontender; it measured 6 cm. in diameter and was located slightly to the left of the midline at the suprahyoid level. A thyroid scan demonstrated a normally outlined gland. The mass was removed by Sistrunk[36] procedure. The thyroid gland was normal. Gross examination of the specimen revealed a tubular tract measuring 0.8 cm. in length. The mass was yellowish-pink and soft, and measured 4 by 2.2 by 1.5 cm. The cut surface of the mass was pinkish-red and partly cystic with multiple loculi with intervening areas of trabecular fibrous tissue in broad bands. The inner surface of the largest loculus showed a papillary growth measuring 0.8 cm. in diameter (Fig. 3). Microscopically, the sections revealed complex papillary structures covered by a relatively well-preserved one to two layers of cuboidal to columnar epithelium with focal cellular atypism (Fig. 4). Calcerospheroids were seen in and around the tumor. Normal thyroid tissue was not seen either in the tract or in the mass itself. The pathologic diagnosis was papillary carcinoma arising in a thyroglossal duct cyst. He

Submitted for publication March 10, 1969; resubmitted March 24, 1969.

*Reprint Address: Department of Pathology, Sinai Hospital of Baltimore, Inc., Baltimore, Md. 21215.

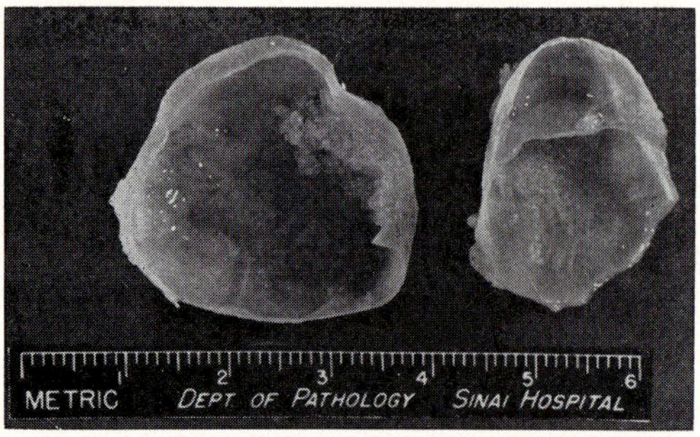

Fig. 1. Papillary carcinoma of the thyroglossal duct cyst from Case 1. Biloculate cyst with the papillary tumor partly projecting into the lumen.

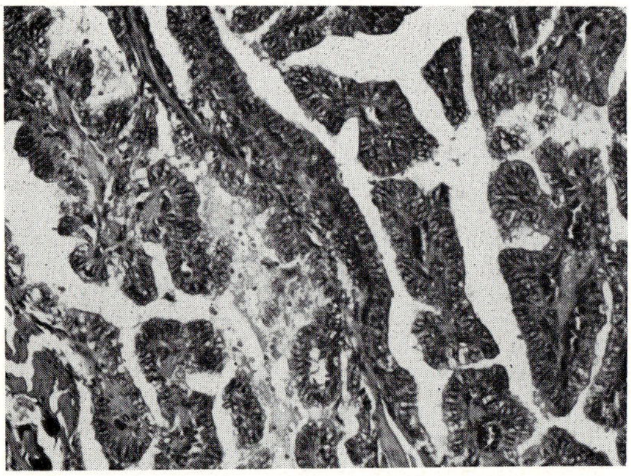

Fig. 2. Papillary carcinoma of the thyroglossal duct cyst from Case 1. Calcerospheroids are seen in lower left. (Hematoxylin and eosin. Original magnification ×340.)

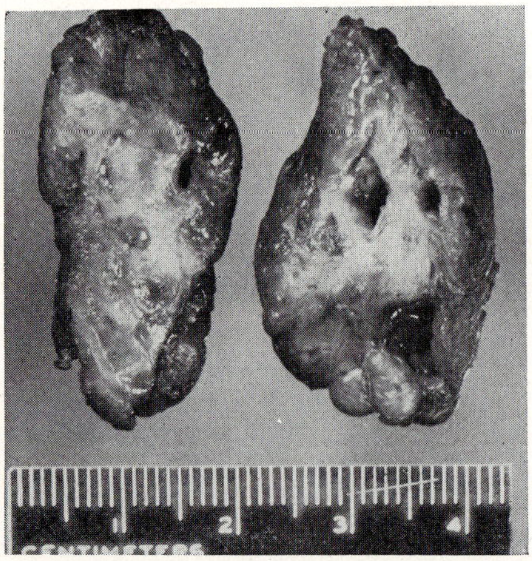

Fig. 3. Papillary carcinoma of the thyroglossal duct cyst from Case 2. The mass is generally solid with several cystic loculi.

was discharged and has remained asymptomatic and well during a 26 month follow-up period.

Case 3. A 26-year-old Caucasian man was admitted for a submental mass present in the neck for 6 months. Physical examination revealed a midline, rounded, firm-to-hard mass in the submental region measuring about 6 cm. in diameter. A scan of the thyroid showed both lobes to be of normal size, shape, and configuration. At operation, the mass was found to be adherent to the strap muscles; its wall was thick and fibrous and was removed intact without resection of the hyoid bone. Dissection of the neck with resection of all the submental and anterior cervical nodes was done. Grossly, the mass measured 6.5 cm. in its greatest diameter. There was a central cystic area about 1.5 cm. in diameter containing a pinkish-tan papillary tumor. The thick cyst wall was extremely firm and fibrous and measured up to 1.2 cm. At one pole there was another slightly elongated cystic area containing papillary excrescences (Fig. 5). No connection with the central cyst was demonstrable. Microscopically, it was an infiltrating cystic papillary carcinoma (Fig. 6). The regional lymph nodes contained metastatic papillary tumor. No normal thyroid tissue was present in the cystic mass. The postoperative course was uneventful for a period of 18 months when a solitary lymph node became palpable in the right side of the neck and was found to contain metastatic tumor. A radical neck dissection was done. The patient has been doing well for 6 months after this second surgical procedure.

DISCUSSION

Embryologically, the anlage of the thyroid gland projects downward from the region of the foramen cecum of the tongue in the 2 to 2.5 mm. human embryo and with development progressive descent occurs to its ultimate location in the anterior cervical region. In normal development, the connection between the cervical thyroid gland and the point of origin from the foramen cecum is obliterated. Persistence and incomplete obliteration of this connection results in a thyroglossal duct characterized by a tubular structure lined by a definite epithelial membrane. This tract passes through or close to the midportion of the second branchial arch which is destined to become the hyoid bone. The persistent duct might end blindly in the vicinity of the hyoid bone. However, because the hyoid bone anlagen fuse in the midline, the thyro-

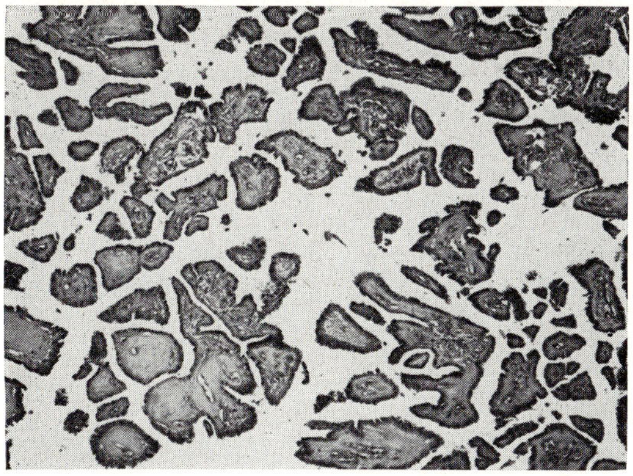

Fig. 4. Papillary carcinoma of the thyroglossal duct cyst from Case 2. The epithelium lining the complex papillary fronds is generally a layer one to two cells thick. (Hematoxylin and eosin. Original magnification ×172.)

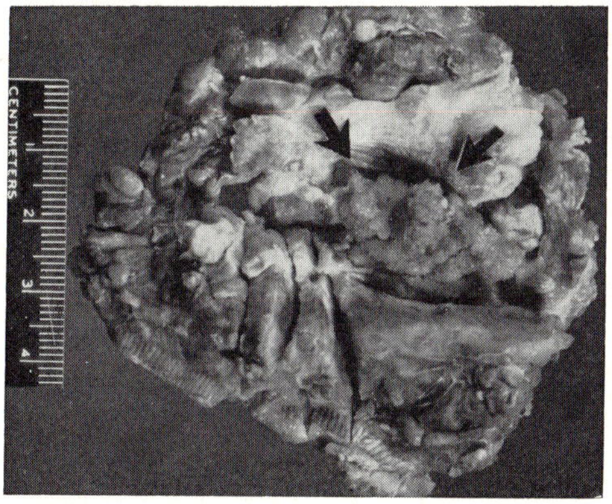

Fig. 5. Papillary carcinoma of the thyroglossal duct cyst from Case 3. Note the papillary tumor in the central cystic area.

glossal duct might get entrapped in the bone. Dilatation of the thyroglossal duct at any point evidently produces a cyst. The great majority of the cysts are located in the subcutaneous position. Since the sinus tract when persistent is likely to pass through, or is extremely close to, the hyoid bone, it is necessary to remove the midportion of the hyoid bone for total eradication, as Sistrunk[36] emphasized.

When there is cyst formation, of whatever size, a moderate-to-extreme degree of surrounding inflammatory reaction is frequent.

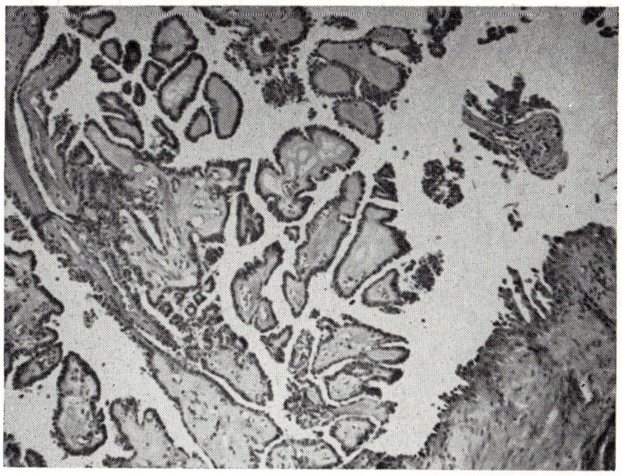

Fig. 6. Papillary carcinoma of the thyroglossal duct cyst from Case 3. The cyst wall with atypical stratified epithelium is in the lower right. (Hematoxylin and eosin. Original magnification ×172.)

The cysts vary in size from 2 to 4 cm. in diameter, but a 10 cm. size is not unusual.

The microscopic appearance of the mucosal epithelial lining of the cyst, and often the entire sinus tract is characteristic. Wide variations are reported in the types of epithelium encountered—stratified squamous, respiratory, and simple cuboidal, the first two types being more frequent. Typical mucous or seromucinous salivary type glands and rarely even sebaceous glands have been noted in the cyst wall.[12, 44] When sebaceous glands and hair follicles are present, they throw considerable doubt on the validity of designating these lesions as thyroglossal duct cysts. Lymphoid tissue, with or without germinal centers in the wall of the duct and cyst, has been noted, but is inconstant.[23, 42, 44] Long-standing inflammation may obliterate the mucosal elements entirely, and in such cases only an inflamed fibrous cyst wall persists and diagnosis can only be presumptive.

A survey of the literature reveals 40 cases of carcinoma of thyroglossal duct origin reported to date. It is possible that the case reported by Marshall and Becker[24] is the same one mentioned by Clute and Cattell,[10] both reporting from the Lahey Clinic. With the addition of our own 3 cases, a total of 43 cases became available for analysis (Table I).

Clinically, a mass was the presenting

Table I. *Forty-three cases of thyroglossal duct cyst carcinoma*

No.	Year	Authors	Age (yr.)	Sex	Race	Duration of mass	Mass
1	1911	Brentano[6]	42	F	N.A.*	9 years	"Small"
2	1927	Owen and Ingelby[31]	45	F	N.A.	3 years, rapid growth for 1 year	"Hen's egg size"
3	1930	Clute and Cattell[10]	6½	M	N.A.	4 weeks	Marble size
4	1949	Marshall and Becker[24]	N.A.	N.A.	N.A.	N.A.	N.A.
5	1950	Nachlas[27]	N.A.	N.A.	N.A.	N.A.	N.A.
6	1952	Aronoff[2]	48	F	N.A.	1 year	3.5 cm.
7	1952	Byrne[7]	44	F	Negro	15 years	4 cm.
8	1953	O'Kane and Straus[30]	75	F	Caucasian	3 months	2.5 cm.
9	1953	Rees and Brown[33, 8]	41	F	N.A.	Several years	4 cm.
10	1956	Dalgaard and Wetteland[12]	44	F	N.A.	10 years	Cystic
11	1959	Keeling and Ochsner[22, 29]	9	F	Caucasian	7 years	2.5 cm.
12	1959	Keeling and Ochsner[22, 29]	41	M	Caucasian	3 weeks	2 cm.
13	1960	Maxwell and Marchetta[25, 26]	60	M	N.A.	N.A.	4 cm.
14	1960	Ghent and Waugh[16, 17]	41	F	Caucasian	2 months	Small
15	1961	Hill[19]	73	M	Caucasian	N.A.	2.6 cm.

*N.A. = not available.

Treatment	*Follow-up*	*Pathologic diagnosis*	*Findings in the thyroid gland*
Incomplete removal followed by recurrent tongue lesion, bilateral cervical lymphadenectomy and complete excision of tongue tumor	Well for 6 months	Malignant struma	N.A.
Cyst incompletely removed, recurrence 5 months later, 2 tumors removed	Well for 21 years	Papillary adenocarcinoma	Grossly normal
Radical operation followed 16 days later by more radical removal of muscular planes	N.A.	Adenocarcinoma	Grossly normal
Radical removal of cyst	Well for 17 years	Adenocarcinoma	N.A.
N.A.	N.A.	Epidermoid carcinoma of thyroglossal remnant	N.A.
Sistrunk[36]	Well for 11 years	Papillary cystadenocarcinoma	N.A.
Sistrunk,[36] admitted second time for further surgical treatment	Sudden death 37 days after initial operation from undetermined cause, no autopsy	Papillary cystadenocarcinoma	Grossly normal
Sitsrunk[36] with removal of the pyramidal lobe	Well for 1½ years	Papillary adenocarcinoma	Pyramidal lobe, no tumor microscopically, rest of the thyroid grossly normal
Sistrunk,[36] radical thyroidectomy and bilateral lymph node dissection of neck with irradiation 2 months later	Well for 10 years	Papillary adenocarcinoma	Papillary carcinoma of right lobe and isthmus, small foci
Local excision, a slow-growing tumor recurring in the same place 13 years later, extirpated completely	Well for 28 years	Low-grade carcinoma probably arising in a thyroglossal cyst, solid cellular epithelioma, possibly basal cell type	Grossly normal
Cyst removal, right radical neck dissection 17 days later on basis of pathologic report, no evidence of metastases, biopsy of lymph node 13 months later showing metastatic carcinoma, left neck dissection	Died 8 hours postoperatively, autopsy done	Papillary adenocarcinoma	No tumor in thyroid gland at autopsy
Radical local excision	Well for 11 years	Papillary adenocarcinoma	Grossly normal
Sistrunk[36] with removal of pyramidal lobe and isthmus	Well for 12 years	Papillary adenocarcinoma	Thyroid scan, negative 3 times
Excision of mass and remnants of thyroglossal cyst and pyramidal lobe of thyroid	Well for 9 years	Well-differentiated adenocarcinoma, follicular	Grossly normal
Nil	Incidental finding at autopsy	Papillary carcinoma of thyroid	Examined at autopsy, no evidence of tumor

Continued on next page.

Table I. *Cont'd*

No.	*Year*	*Authors*	*Age (yr.)*	*Sex*	*Race*	*Duration of mass*	*Mass*
16	1961	Bergera and Horwitz[3]	58	M	Caucasian	1 year	3 cm.
17	1962	Bochetto, Montoya, and Sunde[4, 5]	36	F	Caucasian	6 months	2 cm.
18	1962	Bochetto, Montoya, and Sunde[4, 5]	22	F	Caucasian	5 months	2 cm.
19	1962	Clawson and Kimball[9]	18	F	Mexican	2 months	4 cm.
20	1962	Guraieb and Vieta[18, 41]	52	M	N.A.	2 years	3 cm.
21	1962	Werner[45]	55	M	N.A.	40 years	N.A.
22	1962	Werner[45]	N.A.	M	N.A.	Short	N.A.
23	1962	Werner[45]	N.A.	M	N.A.	N.A.	N.A.
24	1962	Werner[45]	N.A.	M	N.A.	N.A.	N.A.
25	1963	Fish and Moore[15]	33	F	Caucasian	8 years	10 cm.
26	1963	Tanaka and Civin[40]	37	F	Filipino	5 years	N.A.
27	1964	Choy, Ward, and Richardson[8]	56	F	N.A.	10 days	3.5 cm.
28	1964	Choy, Ward, and Richardson[8]	22	F	N.A.	1 year	3 cm.
29	1964	Choy, Ward, and Richardson[8]	23	F	N.A.	3 weeks	3 cm.
30	1965	Snedecor and Groshong[37, 38]	9	F	Caucasian	4½ years, recent rapid growth	5 cm.
31	1965	Snedecor and Groshong[37, 38]	35	F	Caucasian	3 years and 9 months	3 cm.
32	1965	Snedecor and Groshong[37, 38]	46	F	Caucasian	7 years	3 cm.
33	1965	Snedecor and Groshong[37, 38]	16	M	Caucasian	1 month	N.A.

Treatment	*Follow-up*	*Pathologic diagnosis*	*Findings in the thyroid gland*
Sistrunk[36]	Well for 7 years and 2 months	Papillary adenocarcinoma	N.A.
Sistrunk[36]	Well for 8 years	Papillary adenocarcinoma	Grossly normal
Sistrunk,[36] excision of the tumor and a small nodule medial to the cyst, recurrent nodule 2 months later (suture granuloma), treated by local bloc excision including right submaxillary gland	Well for 7 years	Papillary adenocarcinoma with infiltration	Thyroid scan normal
Radical excision of tumor, 14 days later a wider local excision, left radical neck dissection, and removal of left lobe and isthmus of thyroid, 6 months following 3 firm nodules of unknown nature at left anterior border of trapezius	Well for 8 months	Papillary adenocarcinoma	Microscopically examined left lobe and isthmus normal, right lobe grossly normal
Sistrunk[36]	Well for 8 years	Papillary adenocarcinoma	N.A.
N.A.	Well for 1 year	Papillary carcinoma	N.A.
N.A.	Well for 1 year	Papillary carcinoma	N.A.
N.A.	Well for 1 year	Papillary carcinoma	N.A.
N.A.	Well for 4½ years	Papillary carcinoma	N.A.
Sistrunk[36] and removal of 4 nodes in the area of the mass, one week later removal of right submaxillary lymph nodes containing metastatic carcinoma	Well for 1 year	Papillary adenocarcinoma of thyroid tissue	Grossly normal
Sistrunk[36]	Well for 3 months	Papillary adenocarcinoma	Grossly normal
Sistrunk[36]	Well for 8½ years	Papillary adenocarcinoma	N.A.
Sistrunk,[36] 7 weeks later total thyroidectomy with removal of anterior strap muscles, 1 year, 1 month later a single enlarged lymph node in right neck with metastatic tumor, enlarged right neck tumor removed, 1 month later radical right neck dissection, no metastasis	Well for 7 years	Papillary adenocarcinoma with metastasis to a single right cervical lymph node	Thyroid, 35 random sections examined, no tumor found
Sistrunk[36] initially, 6 days later a total thyroidectomy and bilateral suprahyoid neck dissection	Well for 15 months	Papillary adenocarcinoma	Serial sections of the thyroid gland showed no carcinoma
Sistrunk[36]	Well for 5 years	Papillary carcinoma	Grossly normal
Sistrunk,[36] thyroidectomy	Well for 14 years	Papillary carcinoma	Thyroid gland examined microscopically and found normal
Sistrunk[36]	Well for 6 years	Papillary carcinoma	Grossly normal
Excision, excision of an enlarged cervical lymph node, no evidence of metastasis	Well for 5 years	Papillary carcinoma	N.A.

Continued on next page.

Table I. *Cont'd*

No.	*Year*	*Authors*	*Age (yr.)*	*Sex*	*Race*	*Duration of mass*	*Mass*
34	1965	Coon[11]	16	F	N.A.	As long as she could remember	3 cm.
35	1966	Kalderon and Cohn[21]	46	M	Chinese	10 years	3.5 cm.
36	1966	Falkinburg, Hoey, and Stuart[14]	44	F	Caucasian	11 months	5 cm.
37	1966	Ruppmann and Georgsson[34]	50	F	N.A.	4 years	N.A.
38	1967	Akbari, Richter, and Papadakis[1]	35	F	Negro	5 months	3 cm.
39	1968	Shepard and Rosenfeld[35]	55	M	Caucasian	2 months	2 cm.
40	1968	Shepard and Rosenfeld[35]	28	F	Caucasian	3 years	2.5 cm.
41	1968	Bhagavan, Rao, and Weinberg	66	M	Caucasian	1 year	4 cm.
42	1968	Bhagavan, Rao, and Weinberg	38	M	Caucasian	3 years	6 cm.
43	1968	Bhagavan, Rao, and Weinberg	26	M	Caucasian	8 months	6 cm.

symptom in almost all cases. A history of recent sudden enlargement of a relatively stationary or slowly growing mass was occasionally forthcoming. Sudden increase in size is not necessarily an indication of malignancy in a thyroglossal duct cyst since sudden enlargement and even spontaneous first appearance of benign cysts have occurred during acute infections, e.g., common cold, angina, tonsillitis, mumps, measles, and pertussis.[12] Pain was a rare symptom being noted only in three cases. Other uncommon symptoms include hoarseness, dysphagia, weight loss, choking, and draining sinus. Tenderness was uncommon and was noted in six cases. Twenty-seven masses were located in the midline, and eight were located slightly off the midline. In eight cases, the location was not mentioned. When the mass was lateral, it tended to be off to the left more frequently, this being noted in seven cases. This is in keeping with the previous observation that 21 percent of thyroglossal duct cysts are lateral with the swelling more commonly on the left.[27] In the vertical plane, 11 were suprahyoidal, 13 infrahyoidal, and 7 were at the level of the hyoid bone, the exact location being unknown in the others. The malignant character of these masses was only rarely suspected clinically.[1, 8, 30] Metastases to the regional lymph nodes had occurred in only six. Metastases to the lungs and liver had occurred in a single instance, that of a 7-year-old boy reported by Keeling and Ochsner.[22] Local extension and infiltration occurred in eight cases.

A variety of concurrent and apparently unrelated diseases have been noted: auric-

Treatment	*Follow-up*	*Pathologic diagnosis*	*Findings in the thyroid gland*
Local excision and total thyroidectomy, 11 months later an increase in radioactive iodine uptake in the midline above cricoid cartilage, treated with radioactive iodine	Well for 11 months	Papillary carcinoma	Thyroid examined microscopically, no tumor found
Sistrunk[36]	Well for 3 months	Papillary adenocarcinoma	N.A.
Excision	Well for 3 years	Papillary adenocarcinoma	N.A.
Radical removal following 3 previous local operations	N.A.	Squamous cell carcinoma	N.A.
Radical excision of mass	Well for 2½ years	Follicular and papillary adenocarcinoma	Grossly normal
Radical excision of mass, 6 months later a scar nodule removed	Well for 2 years	Papillary carcinoma	N.A.
Excision in another hospital 4½ months before with irradiation; recurrent mass 8 by 6 cm. invading epiglottis, tongue, and neck; laryngectomy; feeding gastrostomy	Died 1 year later	Squamous cell carcinoma	N.A.
Sistrunk[36]	Died 27 days after operation, no autopsy	Papillary carcinoma	Grossly normal
Sistrunk[36]	Well for 26 months	Papillary carcinoma	Grossly normal
Excision with bilateral lymph node dissection, solitary lymph node of right neck with metastatic tumor, radical neck dissection	Well for 2 years	Papillary carcinoma	Grossly normal

ular fibrillation with decompensation,[8] carcinoma of the ovary,[9, 31] cerebral vascular thrombosis,[19] psychosis,[7] obesity,[14] and coronary insufficiency each once and hypertension[14, 19] in two cases. Carcinoma of the breast was noted in two cases.[2, 8] In two cases the mass had been first noted during the last trimester of pregnancy.[5, 15] In one, a small mass, that had been noted 8 years previously following delivery of her first child at age 25, had enlarged slowly with each yearly pregnancy during the first 4 years.[15] The tumor had exhibited accelerated growth with her last four pregnancies, ultimately being excised; it measured 10 by 8.2 by 3 cm.

The pathologic diagnoses were papillary adenocarcinoma in 34 cases, adenocarcinoma in two, epidermoid carcinoma in three, malignant struma in one, follicular carcinoma in one, and mixed follicular and papillary adenocarcinoma in one. The case reported by Dalgaard and Wetteland[12] appears to be solid undifferentiated carcinoma and bears resemblance to the recently recognized medullary carcinoma with amyloid stroma.

Judd[20] believes that thyroid tissue in and around the thyroglossal duct is rarely encountered and that the occasional recording of papillary carcinoma of thyroglossal duct cyst or sinus is erroneous. He contends that when a papillary carcinoma is encountered in this region, the thyroid gland is always incriminated as the source, and that if there were a true carcinoma of thyroglossal duct or sinus origin, it would be expected to be of the squamous cell variety. Thyroid tissue has been found with thyroglossal duct remnants in widely varying frequency, the range being 3 to 36.5 percent.[8, 13, 32, 39, 43, 44] Whether the presence of thyroid tissue in and around the thyroglossal duct cysts and sinuses is a prerequisite for the origin of these carcinomas is a moot point. It should be pointed out that six of seven total thyroid glands removed from patients with thyroglossal duct carcinomas and examined microscopically did not contain a primary tumor. Indeed, three cases of squamous cell carcinoma arising from the thyroglossal duct are recorded. Furthermore, it is not hard to conceive that the stomodeal epithelium of the thyroglossal duct with its embryologic potential of thyroidogenesis could produce a neoplasm resembling that of thyroid origin.

In support of his belief that thyroglossal duct cyst carcinomas are metastatic in nature, Nuttall[28] points out an apparently incongruous fact that while almost all cases of carcinoma presumably originating in a thyroid rest in the wall of a thyroglossal duct remnant are histologically papillary, contrastingly, carcinomas found in lingual thyroid rests have been of a varied histologic type similar to those found in the thyroid gland itself. This conclusion appears to have been drawn from Fish and Moore's[15] 21 collected cases in which the precise histologic characterization of the tumors is entirely inadequate. In our review, although we have found the great majority of thyroglossal duct cyst carcinomas to be papillary, other histologic types labeled as adenocarcinoma, malignant struma, low-grade thyroid carcinoma (solid cellular epithelioma possibly basal cell type), follicular and mixed papillary and follicular carcinomas, and squamous cell carcinomas have been recorded. Nine out of 43 tumors (21 percent) were nonpapillary. Further, it is not surprising that a great majority of all carcinomas of the thyroglossal duct cyst are papillary in type. Papillary carcinomas tend to be the largest single type of thyroid cancer occurring in the thyroid gland itself. In a series of 885 cases of thyroid cancers[46] observed over a 30 year period, 61.1 percent were papillary.

Analysis of the information on the thyroid status reveals that in 17 patients from Group I, information regarding the state of the thyroid gland is not available. Follow-up reveals that those patients were well for periods ranging from a few months to 17 years.

In 17 others from Group II, where the thyroid was considered to be normal grossly and/or by scan, the follow-up shows that they were well for periods ranging from a few months to as long as 28 years.

In nine cases from Group III, microscopic examination of the thyroid gland was done, and no tumor was demonstrable in eight of these. In two of these cases however, only part of the thyroid gland was examined. Papillary adenocarcinoma was found in a single instance.

While nothing is mentioned about the state of the thyroid gland in Group I, it appears reasonable to presume that the thyroid was grossly normal for had it been otherwise, either the abnormal condition would have been mentioned or operation would have been performed. The follow-up data in Groups I and II are similar, the patients being well from one to several years and as long as 28 years.

Group III reveals the absence of tumor in thyroid in eight cases, giving strong support to the de novo origin of carcinoma in the thyroglossal duct. We know of another case[37] in which thyroidectomy following removal of thyroglossal duct cyst carcinoma was done finding no evidence of primary tumor in the thyroid gland itself.

The skepticism as to whether some of the carcinomas associated with thyroglossal ducts and cysts may not, in fact, represent metastases from a small primary tumor of the thyroid gland deserves consideration. In only one case from Group III, tumor was found in the thyroid gland on microscopic examination.[8, 33] This could be interpreted in three ways: namely, (a) primary carcinoma of the thyroid with metastases to the thyroglossal duct cyst, (b) primary carcinoma of the thyroglossal duct with metastasis to the thyroid gland, and (c) two independent primary foci of multicentric origin. While we are fully convinced about the occurrence of primary carcinoma of the thyroglossal duct, the fact that in a single instance there was microscopically demonstrable carcinoma in the thyroid gland makes one wonder what the 34 cases from Groups I and II might have revealed if the thyroid glands were available for microscopic examination. Surgical criteria for diagnosis of thyroglossal duct cysts are not enough in many instances, and it is possible that cystic metastases from a primary carcinoma of the thyroid could be mistaken for thyroglossal duct carcinoma. Six cases of occult papillary carcinoma of the thyroid erroneously diagnosed as thyroglossal duct cysts in the review of Woolner and associates[46] as well as Case 1 reported by Nuttall[28] illustrate this point. It is, therefore, imperative to convince oneself that the carcinoma of the thyroglossal duct cyst is primary and that the thyroid itself is free of tumor. Removal of the thyroid and thorough gross and microscopic examination are the only ways to be absolutely certain that there is no tumor lurking in the organ. Though the possibility of a primary or metastatic tumor in the thyroid does exist, the probability does not appear to be high. This raises the question as to whether thyroidectomy should be considered in cases in which a diagnosis of thyroglossal duct carcinoma is made. In those cases in which the thyroid gland is not removed, careful clinical follow-up including scintiscan studies over many years is necessary.

The factual, supportive, and theoretical evidences in favor of de novo occurrence of these tumors are: (1) absence of primary carcinoma in the thyroid glands microscopically examined, (2) occurrence of squamous cell carcinoma in thyroglossal duct cysts, (3) the long periods of survival in many instances after removal of the thyroglossal duct cyst cancer, (4) the presence of histologically convincing and characteristic epithelium of thyroglossal duct cysts with the tumor, and (5) the embryologic thyroidogenic potential of the thyroglossal duct epithelium.

SUMMARY

Three cases of surgically treated thyroglossal duct cyst carcinoma are presented, and the literature is reviewed. There are 40 reported cases to date. In nearly all cases the clinical diagnosis was thyroglossal cyst, and when malignancy was suspected there appears to be no unique feature which helps establish a clinical diagnosis. Although a great majority of the tumors were papillary adenocarcinomas, 21 percent were of other histologic types. The treatment has been quite variable, the most common initial treatment being the radical excision of Sistrunk.[36] Thyroidectomy done in several cases failed to show any evidence of malignancy in most cases which establishes firmly the de novo origin of these malignant tumors from the thyroglossal duct remnants. The tumor had disseminated to distant organs, the lungs and liver in a solitary instance. The skepticism as to whether some of the carcinomas associated with thyroglossal duct remnants may not in fact represent metastases from a small primary tumor of thyroid gland is examined. It appears that though a distinct possibility of a primary or metastatic tumor in the thyroid does exist, the probability does not appear to be high. It is suggested that the surgeon might consider the advisability of a thyroidectomy after the diagnosis of a thyroglossal duct carcinoma has been made.

The authors wish to express their thanks to Drs. Mark E. Gann, Jerel I. Katz, and William A. Rodgers for permitting them to publish these cases.

REFERENCES

1. Akbari, Y., Richter, R. M., and Papadakis, L. E.: Thyroid carcinoma arising in thyroglossal duct remnants, Arch. Surg. **94:** 235, 1967.
2. Aronoff, B. L.: Papillary thyroid cancer originating in the thyroglossal cyst, Am. Surgeon **18:** 362, 1952.
3. Bergera, J. J., and Horwitz, A.: Papillary adenocarcinoma arising in a thyroglossal duct cyst, Am. Surgeon **27:** 759, 1961.
4. Bochetto, J. F.: Personal communication, 1968.
5. Bochetto, J. F., Montoya, A., and Sunde, E. A.: Papillary carcinoma of the thyroid in thyroglossal duct cysts, Am. J. Surg. **104:** 773, 1962.
6. Brentano, H.: Struma aberrata linguae mit Drüsenmetastasen, Deutsche med. Wchnschr. **37:** 665, 1911.
7. Byrne, J. J.: Carcinoma in a thyroglossal cyst:

Report of a case, Boston M. Quart. **3:** 86, 1952.
8. Choy, F. J., Ward, R., and Richardson, R.: Carcinoma of the thyroglossal duct, Am. J. Surg. **108:** 361, 1964.
9. Clawson, J., and Kimball, H.: Papillary adenocarcinoma of the thyroglossal duct cyst, Arizona Med. **19:** 80, 1962.
10. Clute, H. M., and Cattell, R. B.: Thyroglossal cysts and sinuses, Ann. Surg. **92:** 57, 1930.
11. Coon, W. W.: Thyroid carcinoma—three unusual problems in diagnosis and management, Am. J. Surg. **109:** 629, 1965.
12. Dalgaard, J. B., and Wetteland, P.: Thyroglossal anomalies, Acta chir. scandinav. **111:** 444, 1956.
13. Dische, S., and Berg, P. K.: An investigation of the thyroglossal tract using the radioisotope scan, Clin. Radiol. **14:** 298, 1963.
14. Falkinburg, L. W., Hoey, W. O., and Stuart, J. R.: Papillary adenocarcinoma arising in a thyroglossal duct cyst, Oral Surg. **21:** 358, 1966.
15. Fish, J., and Moore, R. M.: Ectopic thyroid tissue and ectopic thyroid carcinoma; a review of the literature and report of a case, Ann. Surg. **157:** 212, 1963.
16. Ghent, W. R.: Personal communication, 1968.
17. Ghent, W. R., and Waugh, D.: Carcinoma in a thyroglossal remnant, Canad. J. Surg. **4:** 79, 1960.
18. Guraieb, S. R., and Vieta, L. J.: Carcinoma in thyroglossal cyst. Report of a case, Arch. Otolaryng. **75:** 89, 1962.
19. Hill, D. P.: Papillary carcinoma arising in a thyroglossal tract, Canad. M. A. J. **85:** 791, 1961.
20. Judd, E. S.: Thyroglossal duct cysts and sinuses, S. Clin. North America **43:** 1023, 1963.
21. Kalderon, A. E., and Cohn, J. D.: Papillary adenocarcinoma in a thyroglossal cyst, Cancer **19:** 839, 1966.
22. Keeling, J. H., and Ochsner, A.: Carcinoma in thyroglossal duct remnants, Cancer **12:** 596, 1959.
23. Krarup, B.: Congenital cervical cysts and fistulas, Acta oto-laryng. **158:** 173, 1960. (Suppl.)
24. Marshall, S. F., and Becker, W. F.: Thyroglossal cysts and sinuses, Ann. Surg. **129:** 642, 1949.
25. Maxwell, W. T.: Personal communication, 1968.
26. Maxwell, W. T., and Marchetta, F. C.: Papillary adenocarcinoma of the thyroglossal duct tract, Arch. Surg. **80:** 224, 1960.
27. Nachlas, N. E.: Thyroglossal duct cysts, Ann. Otol. Rhin. & Laryng. **59:** 381, 1950.
28. Nuttall, F. Q.: Cystic metastases from papillary adenocarcinoma of the thyroid with comments concerning carcinoma associated with thyroglossal remnants, Am. J. Surg. **109:** 500, 1965.
29. Ochsner, A.: Personal communication, 1968.
30. O'Kane, C. R., and Straus, F. H.: Papillary adenocarcinoma arising in association with a persistent thyroglossal duct, Ann. Surg. **138:** 805, 1953.
31. Owen, H. R., and Ingelby, H.: Carcinoma of the thyroglossal duct, Ann. Surg. **85:** 132, 1927.
32. Pollack, W. F., and Stevenson, E. O.: Cysts and sinuses of the thyroglossal duct, Am. J. Surg. **112:** 225, 1966.
33. Rees, C. E., and Brown, M. J.: Cysts of the thyroglossal duct, Am. J. Surg. **85:** 597, 1953.
34. Ruppmann, E., and Georgsson, G.: Squamous carcinoma of the thyroglossal duct, German M. Monthly **11:** 442, 1966.
35. Shepard, G. H., and Rosenfeld, L.: Carcinoma of thyroglossal duct remnants, Am. J. Surg. **116:** 125, 1968.
36. Sistrunk, W. E.: Technique of removal of cysts and sinuses of the thyroglossal duct, Surg. Gynec. & Obst. **46:** 109, 1928.
37. Snedecor, P. A.: Personal communication, 1968.
38. Snedecor, P. A., and Groshong, L. E.: Carcinoma of the thyroglossal duct, SURGERY **58:** 969, 1965.
39. Stahl, W. M., and Lyall, D.: Cervical cysts and fistulae of thyroglossal tract origin, Ann. Surg. **139:** 123, 1954.
40. Tanaka, K., and Civin, W. H.: Cancer arising in thyroglossal duct remnant, Arch. Surg. **86:** 466, 1963.
41. Vieta, L. J.: Personal communication, 1968.
42. Ward, G. E., and Hendrick, J. W.: Tumors of the head and neck, Baltimore, 1950, The Williams & Wilkins Company, p. 633.
43. Ward, G. E., Hendrick, J. W., and Chambers, R. G.: Thyroglossal tract abnormalities—cysts and fistulae, Surg. Gynec. & Obst. **89:** 727, 1949.
44. Webb, R.: Thyroglossal cyst, Australian & New Zealand J. Surg. **22:** 211, 1953.
45. Werner, S. C., editor: The thyroid, ed. 2, New York, 1962, Harper & Row, Publishers, p. 342.
46. Woolner, L. B., Beahrs, O. H., Black, M. B., McConahey, W. M., and Keating, F. R., Jr.: Classification and prognosis of thyroid carcinoma: A study of 885 cases observed in a 30 year period, Am. J. Surg. **102:** 354, 1961.

Management of malignant esophagobronchial fistula

G. B. ONG
K. H. KWONG
HONG KONG
From the Department of Surgery, University of Hong Kong

It is generally agreed that when esophagobronchial fistula has developed as a result of malignancy arising from the bronchus or esophagus, curative treatment is not possible. Terracol and Sweet[14] stated that when a malignant fistula had occurred between the esophagus and bronchus, only a rare case had been known to survive for a period longer than 1 month.

While it is true that curative therapy is out of the question, there is still the desirability of relieving the patient of his distressing spasm of productive cough whenever he swallows. This paper describes the various methods we have employed in giving relief to these cases.

SUBJECTS

From 1964 to 1968, 18 patients with malignant esophagobronchial fistula were admitted to the University Surgical Unit at the Queen Mary Hospital, Hong Kong. There were 16 men and 2 women. The age range was from 44 to 66, with an average of 54.

Symptoms. All of them were admitted because of dysphagia of varying duration. The longest history was in a 49-year-old man who was found to have carcinoma of the esophagus a year prior to admission. The shortest period of dysphagia was 2 months. The average duration of dysphagia in the 18 cases was 6 months.

There was marked loss of body weight in each case, and the most dramatic one was of a female patient who lost more than 20 pounds of body weight within a period of 5 months.

The amount of sputum expectorated daily varied between 5 and 12 ounces. The paroxysm of cough and choking was especially severe when the patient swallowed. This paroxysmal cough was also severe at night so much so that sleep was disturbed.

In four of them radiotherapy had been instituted for the control of their malignant condition. In addition to the above symptoms, these four patients also complained of substernal pain radiating to the back.

Site of the fistula. The site of the fistula depended on the level of the growth. As most of the growths arose at the level where the esophagus crossed the left bronchus, most of the fistulous connections were between the left main bronchus and the esophagus. Growths lower down might involve the lung parenchyma, and here the right lower lobe was more commonly invaded than the left.

Of the 18 cases, 17 were growths arising from the esophagus. In three of these the fistula was located between the right lower lobe and the esophagus, in nine at the left main bronchus, in two at the bifurcation of the trachea, and in four at the right main bronchus. In one case, the cause of the fistula was a carcinoma arising from the left main bronchus which had invaded the esophagus. This patient developed fistula while undergoing radiotherapy.

Preoperative management. As most of these patients were in a dehydrated state,

Submitted for publication March 10, 1969; resubmitted April 16, 1969.

Table I

Case No.	*Type of operation*	*Time of death following operation*	*Relief of symptoms*	*Postmortem findings*
1. J. K. M. (19054/64) man, 56	Esophagectomy with excision of fistula and repair of bronchus with pericardium	9 months	Complete	No postmortem examination, died somewhere else
2. H. S. Y. (18284/65)	Esophagectomy with excision of fistula and repair of bronchus with pericardium	6 months	Complete	Ulcer of stomach eroding a main branch of pulmonary artery
3. C. C. F. (3112/65) man, 44 woman, 57	Esophagectomy and lobectomy	8 hours	Nil	Shock, inadequate blood replacement
4. W. Y. (14843/66) man, 66	Esophagectomy and lobectomy	1 month	Nil	Leakage of anastomosis and breakdown of bronchial stump
5. L. C. (6345/67) man, 60	Esophagectomy and lobectomy	11 months	Complete	Extensive metastases, died suddenly
6. C. T. (21494/66) man, 45	Gastrostomy, tracheostomy, and intercostal drainage	4 days after admission	Nil	Growth ruptured through pleural cavity, growth from lower middle third of esophagus, with fistula in right lower lobe of lung
7. L. T. (14690/65) man, 50	Escophagectomy— first operation: repair of fistula with pericardial flap, cervical esophagostomy and gastrostomy; Second operation: lobectomy and repair of fistula	18 days 11 hours	For 17 days Nil	Left pleural cavity containing slight amount of sanguineous fluid, second bronchial repair intact
8. L. T. (14690/65) man, 50	Esophagectomy, repair of fistula with pericardial flap, cervical esophagectomy and gastrostomy	36 hours	Nil	Left pleural cavity containing 200 ml. of blood clot, fibrinopurulent material in diaphragmatic visceral pleural surface, no leakage of bronchial repair
9. C. Y. S. (12471/65) man, 49	Jejunal bypass and esophagocardiogastrostomy	2 months	Condition worse than before operation	Excoriation of abdominal wall, lungs showed consolidation, fistula between bronchus and esophagus, large lymph nodes in left supraclavicular fossa
10. C. S. (22029/69) man, 55	Double jejunal bypass	4 months	Complete	Large carcinoma with multiple seedlings in pericardium and infiltration of aorta, esophagobronchial fistula
11. C. C. (9266/66) man, 57	Double jejunal bypass	8 months	Complete	Extensive metastases in bones and viscera
12. L. K. K. (3479/66) man, 45	Double jejunal bypass	5 months	Complete	No postmortem examination, circumstances of death unknown
13. M. L. F. (11935/66) man, 45	Double jejunal bypass	6 hours	Nil	Shock and hemorrhage, site of hemorrhage not found

Table I. *Cont'd*

Case No.	*Type of operation*	*Time of death following operation*	*Relief of symptoms*	*Postmortem findings*
14. L. P. (9339/66) man, 60	Double jejunal bypass	1 month	Nil	Leakage of anastomosis, extensive bronchopneumonia
15. L. Y. (5098/67) man, 46	Double jejunal bypass	1 month	Temporary	Disruption of neck anastomosis, extensive bronchopneumonia
16. L. Y. (250/68) woman, 66	Double jejunal bypass	1 month	Temporary	Extensive tumor invasion, rupture of esophagus into right pleural cavity
17. L. H. S. (21611/67) man, 51	Double jejunal bypass	5 months	Complete	Postmortem examination refused
18. T. H. C. (9340/68) man, 54	Double jejunal bypass	2 months since operation	Complete	Still alive and well

intravenous therapy had to be instituted soon after admission to the hospital. Anemia was corrected, if necessary, with blood transfusion.

When the general condition was extremely poor, gastrostomy was done at the same time that esophagoscopy and bronchoscopy were performed. We were convinced that intravenous fluid replacement could not take the place of oral or gastric alimentation in these chronically starved patients. After a week or so of such management, the patients would become sufficiently well to withstand a major operation.

X-ray investigation. Barium swallow was done in every case of esophageal cancer admitted under our care, but when there was profuse sputum and a fistulous tract between the esophagus and bronchus was suspected, 40 percent oral Hypaque (Winthrop, U.S.A.) was used instead. This not only demonstrated the fistula better, but unlike barium it was not irritating to the lungs. By this method of investigation, in 14 out of the 18 cases, the fistula could be demonstrated.

Esophagoscopy and bronchoscopy. Both these procedures were carried out under general anesthesia. Esophagoscopy not only allowed histologic confirmation of the malignant nature of the lesion, but also was a useful method of removing the accumulated and putrid food; this infected material would otherwise drain into the bronchus.

Bronchoscopy was done mainly for promoting bronchial toilet as the fistula could be demonstrated by this means in only nine cases.

Treatment. Reference to Table I shows that of the 18 cases, one was admitted in a moribund state. He was a man aged 45 who had a gastrostomy performed in another hospital. While in that hospital he also developed hydropneumothorax, for which intercostal drainage was done. As the sputum was profuse and he was too weak to expectorate, tracheostomy as well was carried out. It was at this stage that he was transferred under our care. No further treatment was possible, and he died 4 days after admission. For the remaining 17 cases some form of surgical treatment was possible.

Esophagectomy with pulmonary lobectomy. In three cases in which the carcinoma had infiltrated a pulmonary lobe, but had not infiltrated any other structures, esophagectomy with lobectomy was carried out.

The technique of esophagectomy employed in the treatment of these cases has been previously described.[9, 10, 12] Briefly this

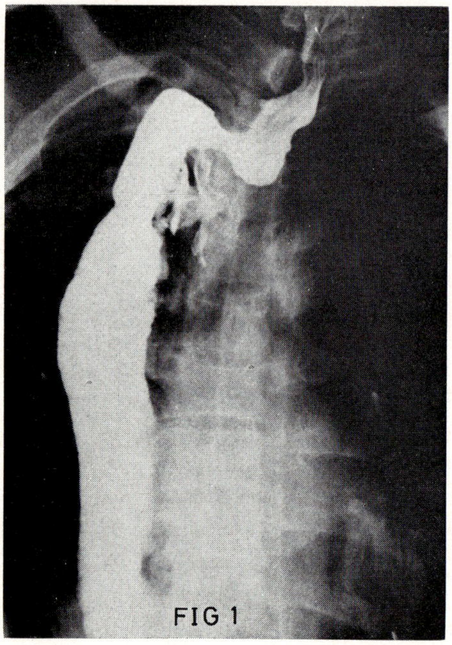

Fig. 1. Barium swallow showing slightly narrowed stoma of esophagogastric anastomosis made at the apex of the right pleural cavity.

consists of exploration of the growth, which is carried out at laparotomy with the hand introduced into the right pleural cavity through the esophageal hiatus. If the growth is found to be resectable, the stomach is mobilized, pyloromyotomy and Kocher's maneuver done, and the abdomen closed. The right side of the chest is now opened through the fifth intercostal space, and esophagectomy with resection of the involved lung is performed.

The anastomosis between the fundus of the stomach and the resected esophagus is made either in the right side of the chest or in the neck (Fig. 1). If at laparotomy the growth is found to be nonresectable, an alternative method can be carried out. Exploration of the growth through the esophageal hiatus is a fairly accurate means of assessing its resectability. But it is not always possible to carry out the maneuver for often, as a result of old plastic pleurisy, the right pleural cavity is obliterated. It is also not possible to know whether the growth has invaded the bronchus by feeling the tumor with the hand in the right pleural cavity. This is because the bronchus is normally mobile. Any manipulation of the esophageal growth will cause the bronchus to move with it even if the latter is heavily infiltrated. On the other hand, infiltration of the esophageal growth into the vertebral column or aorta is easily assessed. These latter two structures are fixed, and if there is any infiltration the esophageal growth will also be immobile.

It is not often that the growth infiltrates the aorta. This is probably due to the fact that constant movement of the aorta at each systole and diastole prevents infiltration of the growth into its wall. Very often what seems to be a nonresectable growth will be found to be easily removed if the dissection is carried along the plane between the adventitia and media of the vessel.

Esophagectomy with cuff resection of the involved bronchus. In Cases 1 and 2, the growth was found to have invaded the main bronchus, but this was not too extensive. Esophagectomy with resection of a cuff of the invaded bronchus was therefore done. The defect was repaired with a pericardial flap. The two cases treated thus had smooth convalescence. One of them subsequently showed a slight stenosis but this did not produce any adverse effect (Fig. 2). A longer survival of more than 6 months might have been the result if it were not for the fact that an ulcer of the displaced stomach had perforated a main branch of the pulmonary artery (Fig. 3). The nature of the ulceration was not known. There was no evidence that it developed as a result of stasis. There was also no evidence that it was a malignant ulcer. But active pulmonary tuberculosis, proved by histologic section, was an associated finding. It was possible that the ulceration could have resulted from a ruptured tuberculous abscess into the main pulmonary artery and stomach. These two structures were in close proximity.

These two cases show that the defects in the bronchus, after esophagectomy with excision of the esophagobronchial fistula, can be effectively repaired by pericardial flaps.

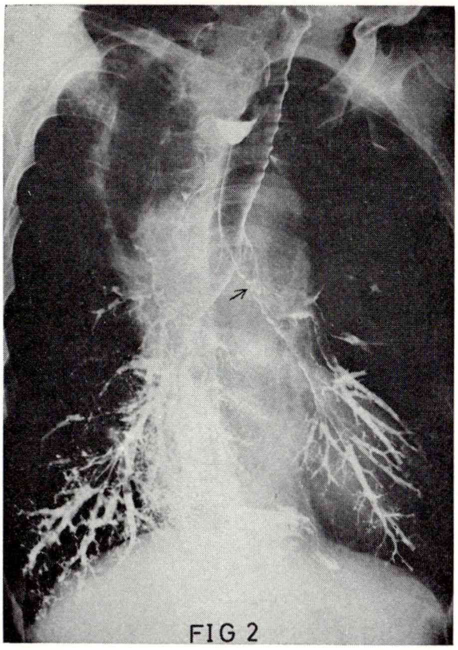

Fig. 2. Bronchogram showing narrowing of the left main bronchus (arrow).

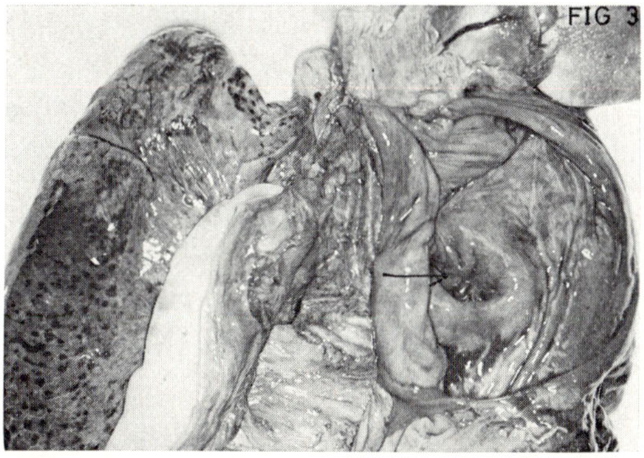

Fig. 3. Postmortem specimen of lung and intrathoracic stomach. Arrow points to the ulcer in the stomach.

However, when esphagobronchial fistula develops following radiotherapy, such a procedure is doomed to failure. Cases 7 and 8 are such examples. Both had excision of the esophagus with free pericardial patches to the bronchial defects. No reconstruction of the esophagus was attempted as it was considered to be too major a surgical undertaking. Both died in the immediate postoperative period.

Bypass operation with isolation of the fistula from the upper alimentary tract. As a result of failure in the treatment of the two patients who had undergone radiotherapy, it was felt that considerable palliation might be achieved if the bronchoesophageal fistula could be completely isolated from the upper alimentary tract. This isolation could be accomplished by using the jejunum and performing a subcutaneous bypass of the esophageal obstruction. The anastomosis is made between the proximal divided end of the cervical esophagus and the proximal end of the prepared jejunal loop. The distal severed end of the cervical esophagus is closed. The distal end of the jejunal loop is now implanted into the stomach. However, the fistula is still in communication with the lower esophagus and stomach. If there is any regurgitation of stomach contents into the esophagus, the bronchus can still be flooded. This can be avoided if the lower esophagus or cardia is transected and brought out through the abdominal wall (Fig. 4). Only one case (Case 9) was thus treated. The treatment was a total failure for whenever he swallowed, acid secretion from the esophagocardiogastrostomy caused considerable excoriation of the surrounding skin. A sudden hemorrhage through this cardiogastrostomy caused his death.

Double bypass of the lesion with complete isolation of the fistula. It occurred to us that, if instead of an esophagocardiogastrostomy, a Roux-en-Y anastomosis were made to the divided cardioesophageal junction, then complete isolation of the fistula from the alimentary tract could be accomplished. This was accordingly carried out in patients with esophagobronchial fistulas which were deemed to be nonresectable. The operation was carried out under general anesthesia. A midline upper abdominal incision was made extending from the xiphisternum to about an inch below the umbilicus. A long jejunal loop was isolated with division of several (usually four) main jejunal vessels. This loop was measured and should reach the

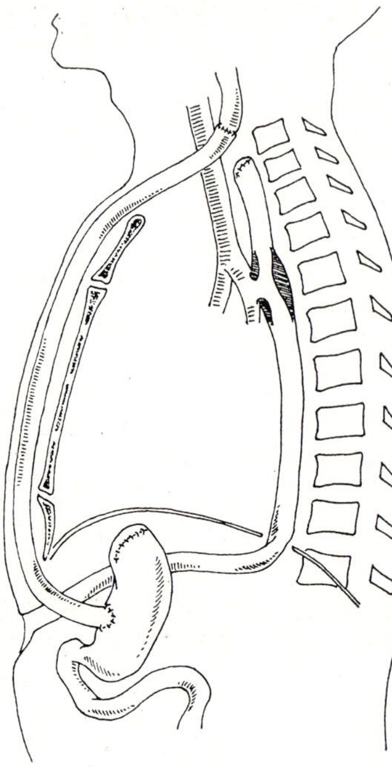

Fig. 4. Diagram to show the operation where the cardia was brought to the anterior abdominal wall.

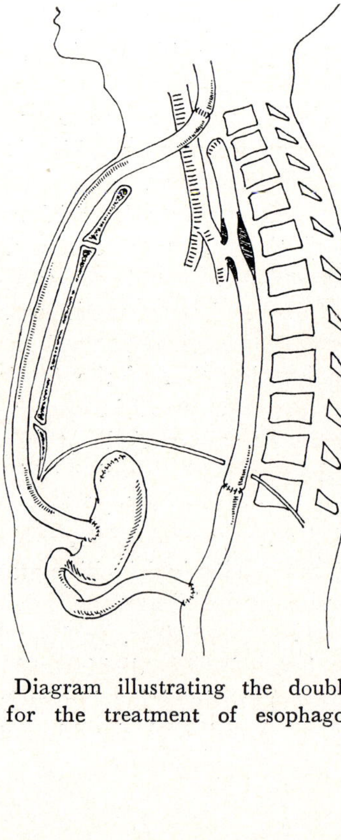

Fig. 5. Diagram illustrating the double jejunal bypass for the treatment of esophagobronchial fistula.

neck without difficulty. The whole loop was then threaded through a window made in the transverse mesocolon and out through the lesser omentum. Thus the vascular pedicle came to lie in the lesser sac. A subcutaneous tunnel was made and the loop brought up to the neck of anastomosis to the proximal divided end of the cervical esophagus. The distal divided end of the esophagus was closed in two layers. The wound at the neck was closed with drainage.

Attention was then paid to the abdominal part of the operation. The distal end of the isolated jejunal loop was implanted into the stomach while the lower esophagus was transected above the cardia which was closed with two layers of continuous catgut. The distal divided loop of the jejunum was brought up to be anastomosed to the lower esophagus. Continuity of the upper intestinal tract was established by joining the upper divided jejunum to this vertical limb (Fig. 5).

This operation was carried out in 9 cases. The last patient (Case 18) was extremely happy with the result. He could eat normal diet, and barium studies showed a good functioning jejunal loop (Fig. 6). The paroxysms of cough which he experienced whenever he swallowed had disappeared. Although he was conscious of the peristalsis, the subcutaneous esophagoplasty did not bother him and within a period of 3 months he had gained 6 pounds in body weight (Fig. 7).

RESULTS

Mortality ratc. Considering the poor general condition of these patients, the operative mortality rate would understandably be expected to be high. Two patients died of shock, while two died as a result of anastomotic leakage.

The two patients who received extensive radiotherapy were really nontreatable. Perhaps a better form of treatment for them would have been a double jejunal bypass rather than excision and repair with pericardial flap.

The mortality rate, however, has dropped as a result of better preparation and post-

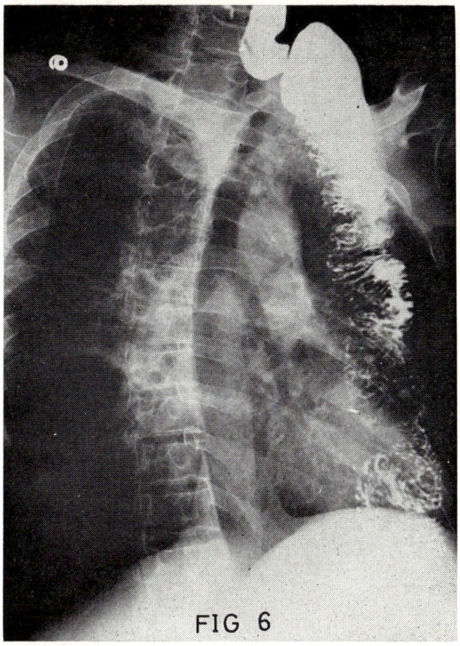

Fig. 6. Barium swallow shows easy passage of the medium.

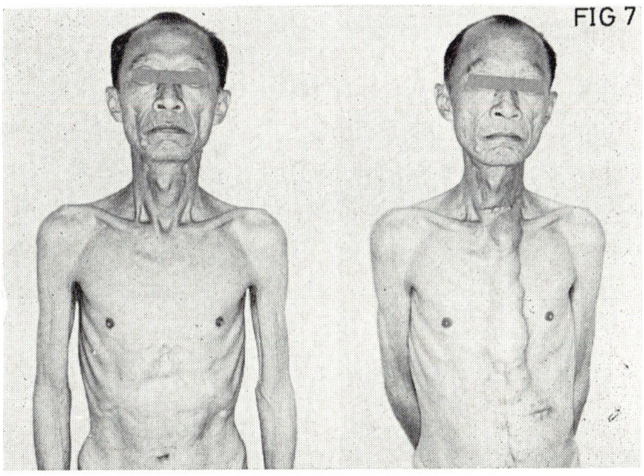

Fig. 7. The patient before and after undergoing the "double bypass" operation.

operative care. With an improvement in the selection of operation and technique, it should reach an acceptable level.

Relief of symptoms. The desired result of any treatment in malignant esophagobronchial fistula is to get rid of the severe paroxysm of cough and to enable the patient to swallow normally. The ideal treatment would be to excise the esophagus with the fistula which in three cases was possible as it occurred between the esophagus and a lobe of the lung. Two patients died as a result of the operation. Both deaths could have been avoided if in the one case anastomosis between the esophagus and stomach had not broken down, and if in the other, blood loss resulting in shock had been adequately replaced. The one successfully treated patient had complete relief of symptoms but died suddenly of extensive malignant disease. He was able to eat normal solid diet up to the last moment of his life and had no cough.

The two cases that had wedge excision of the involved bronchus also had complete relief of cough and dysphagia. There was a possibility that in one of them, a longer survival could have taken place if an ulcer from the stomach had not eroded a main branch of the pulmonary artery.

DISCUSSION

Use of the plastic tube in treatment of esophagotracheal fistula. The introduction of the plastic esophageal tube has touched off a wave of enthusiasm in its use for the treatment of malignant lesion of the esophagus.[2, 5, 6] Judd and Codd[7] applied the Mousseau-Barbin esophageal tube for the treatment of esophagotracheal fistula. They reported three cases, but none of the patients lived longer than 4 months. Kovarik[8] utilized a de Pezzer catheter and by cutting the bulb produced a serrated flange. He then inserted the modified catheter under endoscopy. His patient survived for only 17 days and during this period was able to eat only "Jello, cereal, and puree foods."

The argument in favor of its use is its simplicity of application. But no account has been taken of the failure to eat normal solid diet and of its temporary nature. Its use is not without danger, for perforation of the esophagus can easily take place. Moreover, in the treatment of the esophagobronchial fistula, its tamponade effect does not seem to last very long for it can produce pressure necrosis of the tumor and thus enlarge the opening. Even in successful cases only a puree type of food can be taken.

Its use for the relief of obstruction in carcinoma of esophagus, followed by radiotherapy, can sometimes cause the most intractable esophagobronchial fistula. This happened in two of our cases. Radiotherapy with mego-voltage deep x-ray can literally melt the sensitive tumor. Hence when the tumor has invaded the bronchus but has not undergone necrosis, radiotherapy will cause the development of such a fistula.

Repair of fistula. In a malignant lesion, excision of the fistula with repair of the bronchus is not always possible. Of the 18 cases in only two cases was this practicable. Taffel[12] and Belsey[1] utilized free fascia graft to repair tracheal defects, while in a discussion on a paper read by Bryant,[3] Brantigan stated that he had considerable success in using pedicle intercostal grafts for repair of bronchial defects. This type of repair, we believe, would be useful in effecting a large circumferential defect. In order to replace the rigid cartilaginous rings, the rib could be split longitudinally and its inner portion included in the intercostal flap.

In the laboratory, Bryant[4] utilized the pericardium for repair of tracheobronchial defects. He had shown that even in circumferential defects he was successful in repairing it with pericardial flap, provided that it was not longer than 2.5 cm. Weisel, Lepley, and Watson[16] were successful in treating four cases of respiratory adenomas for which they had done sleeve resections.

For repair of tracheobronchial defects that is a very convenient maneuver as the membrane is tough and fibrous and it can be easily rendered airtight. As most of the fistulas are posterior to the tracheobronchial tree, the cartilaginous portion can be preserved and this gives the rigidity required of the respiratory tract.

The bypass operation. In the majority of esophagobronchial fistulas which are not resectable, some form of bypass is a desirable mode of treatment. By a bypass operation, utilizing the colon, stomach, or jejunum, the patient will be able to swallow normal solid food rather than the puree form. Such an operation, however, ought to prevent a regurgitation of gastric contents. Papaioannou[11] performed a cervical esophagostomy and gastrostomy and tied the lower end of the esophagus. His patient survived 4 weeks. In this operation, no reconstruction of upper alimentary tract was considered and the patient had to be fed through a gastrostomy tube. However, he showed that by ligating the lower esophagus with heavy silk he was able to prevent gastric regurgitation. Whether this would be true if his patient had survived for a longer period is uncertain. Van De Water, Katz, and Hughes[15] went a step further when they performed a substernal colonic bypass and closed the lower esophagus with heavy silk ligature. They treated two patients in this way, and their survival times were only 2 weeks and 4 weeks, respectively.

Again it is not known whether the ligatured esophagus will stay closed, as their period of survival is too short. In one of their cases, "occasional episodes of coughing believed to be due to aspiration of mucus" was found at autopsy. Their other case was found to show "chronic pulmonary infection" on postmortem examination.

On the other hand, after performing a bypass, if the lower esophagus were excluded from the gastrointestinal tract, the patient would be able to eat normal diet and yet escape the paroxysmal bouts of coughing. We first thought that exclusion of the lower esophagus could be achieved by exteriorizing it. However, we found that it was not possible to do so without including the cardiac portion of the stomach. In one such case, acid secretion was profuse during deglutition and produced excoriation of the skin which caused him more misery than relief. It was an ill-conceived operation and should not have been done. On the other hand, good result with complete relief of symptoms could be obtained by performing a Roux-en-Y anastomosis to the abdominal esophagus.

This operation was done in nine cases with complete relief of symptoms in five, partial relief in two, and no relief in two cases. The failures already referred to in the table should not be a reflection on the success of the operation for in each case there was a complication that caused it.

SUMMARY AND CONCLUSION

Malignant esophagobronchial fistula is a difficult condition to treat. With the application of mega-voltage deep x-ray therapy for the treatment of esophageal cancer, more cases can be expected.

From 1964 to 1968, 18 cases came under our care. In one case no treatment was possible, while in the other 17 cases some form of operative treatment was undertaken.

Whenever the fistulous tract was between the esophagus and a pulmonary lobe, resection of the lung with esophagectomy, if possible, was carried out. In two cases the fistula and the esophagus could be excised with a cuff of the bronchial wall, and the defect left in the respiratory apparatus was repaired with pericardial flap. For those cases in which no resection was possible, a double bypass of the lesion was undertaken. There was complete relief of symptoms in the successful cases. In one case a single bypass with exteriorization of the lower esophagus and cardia ended disastrously, while in two cases repair with pericardial flaps was unsuccessful. The failure we believe was due to irradiation and infection.

REFERENCES

1. Belsey, R.: Resection and reconstruction of the intrathoracic trachea, Brit. J. Surg. **38:** 200, 1950.
2. Bestler, J. M., Frazer, J. P., and Yarington, C. T., Jr.: A comparative study of the palliative results of the indwelling esophageal tube, Laryngoscope **76:** 651, 1966.
3. Bryant, L. R.: Experimental evaluation of intercostal pedicle grafts in esophageal repair, J. Thoracic & Cardiovas. Surg. **50:** 626, 1965.
4. Bryant, L. R.: Replacement of tracheobronchial defects with autogenous pericardium, J. Thoracic & Cardiovas. Surg. **48:** 733, 1964.
5. Celestin, L. R.: Permanent intubation in inoperable carcinoma of esophagus and cardia; a new tube, Ann. Roy. Coll. Surgeons England **25:** 165, 1959.
6. Fortin, C. L., and Menzies, T.: Inoperable carcinoma of the esophagus and cardia: Permanent intubation with the Celestin tube, Canad. J. Surg. **8:** 276, 1965.
7. Judd, D. R., and Codd, J.: Palliation for malignant esophagotracheal fistula, J. Thoracic & Cardiovas. Surg. **54:** 751, 1967.
8. Kovarik, J. L.: Palliative treatment of a bronchoesophageal fistula, J. Thoracic & Cardiovas. Surg. **46:** 252, 1963.
9. Lewis, I.: The surgical treatment of carcinoma of the esophagus, Brit. J. Surg. **34:** 18, 1946.
10. Ong, G. B., and Kwong, K. H.: The Lewis-Tanner operation, J. Roy. Coll. Surgeons Edinburgh **1:** 1, 1969.
11. Papaioannou, A. N.: A sample operation for the palliative treatment of tracheal esophageal fistula due to cancer, J. Thoracic & Cardiovas. Surg. **49:** 881, 1965.
12. Taffel, M.: The repair of tracheal and bronchial defects with free fascia grafts, SURGERY **8:** 56, 1940.
13. Tanner, N. C.: The present position of carcinoma of the esophagus, Postgrad. M. J. **23:** 109, 1947.
14. Terracol, J., and Sweet, R. H.: Diseases of the esophagus, Philadelphia, 1958, W. B. Saunders Company.
15. Van De Water, J. M., Katz, R. I., and Hughes, R. K.: Management of patients with acquired malignant esophagorespiratory fistulas, Am. Surgeon **31:** 629, 1965.
16. Weisel, W., Lepley, D., Jr., and Watson, R. R.: Respiratory tract adenomas: A ten year survey, Ann. Surg. **154:** 898, 1967.

Elevation of serum creatine kinase following amputation of the leg

RAYMOND PENNEYS, M.D.
J. HENRY WILKINSON, D.Sc., Ph.D.
PHILADELPHIA, PA.
From the Vascular Section, Department of Medicine, and Pepper Laboratory of Clinical Medicine, Hospital of the University of Pennsylvania, and the Peripheral Vascular Section, Heart Station, Philadelphia General Hospital

The question as to whether surgical severance of normal, healthy skeletal muscle damages the muscle to the extent that its enzymes are released into the circulation has arisen during the course of past investigations on the ischemic limb. In the one patient studied, amputation of a leg failed to alter the serum enzyme pattern, including that of the isoenzymes of lactate dehydrogenase (LDH),[11] indicating that severance of the muscle of the leg produced no release of its enzymes.

Creatine kinase (CK) determination has since been added to the armamentarium of commonly available enzyme tests. This enzyme has proved to be highly sensitive to muscle ischemia, i.e., of the myocardium, and is present in abundance in skeletal muscle, so our studies on the amputated leg have been extended to include CK, along with glutamate-oxalacetate transaminase (GOT), glutamate-pyruvate transaminase (GPT), lactate dehydrogenase (LDH) (total and isoenzymes), and alpha-hydroxybutyrate dehydrogenase (HBD).

Received for publication March 17, 1969.

METHOD

Six patients were studied, five of whom had an amputation of a leg for arteriosclerotic gangrene, or pregangrene, and the sixth for osteomyelitis. Five of the amputations were done below the knee and the sixth, above. No delay in healing of the surgical site and no postoperative complications occurred in any of these patients.

Blood samples were obtained by venipuncture. A single preoperative sample was taken from each patient on the day the operation was performed. Daily postoperative specimens were collected as far as possible, but this was not always practicable.

Serum enzyme activities were determined

Table I. *Serum enzyme activities (I.U./liter at 25°) before and after operation**

Patient	Sex	GOT Before	GOT After	GPT Before	GPT After
J. A.	M	17	15	14	21
J. D.	M	12	20, 12, 7	17	15, 11, 22
E. G.	F	12	6, 10, 11	10	12, 20, 23
D. G.	F	11	14, 5, 13	14	10, 15, 22
M. L.	M	12	10, 12	12	10, 12
G. F.‡	M	8	8, 8	9	7, 7

*The days on which the postoperative samples were obtained are indicated in Fig. 1.
†LDH isoenzyme studies were also performed on these samples. The preoperative patterns were all normal. Minor changes only wer
‡G. F. is the only patient whose leg was amputated for osteomyelitis.

at 25° ± 0.2° by methods described in the literature: GOT,[4] GPT,[4] LDH,[17] HBD,[16] and CK.[15] The results are expressed as international (micromolar) units per liter. The upper limits of normal values are GOT, 19; GPT, 19; LDH, 200; HBD, 130; CK, 45 (males), 35 (females).

LDH isoenzymes were separated by acrylamide-gel electrophoresis.[13]

RESULTS

The results of the serum enzyme tests are listed in Table I, which shows that only in the case of CK was there a definite elevation after operation. For statistical analysis the postoperative observations were subdivided into three 2 day periods. (In the case of one patient, E.G., seen on both days of a single 2 day postoperative period, the value of the first day only was used.) Differences between the preoperative values and those for each postoperative period were then used to calculate the mean changes shown in Table II.

Student's t test for paired differences showed the mean change in the CK to be statistically significant ($p < 0.05$) on each of the first two postoperative periods. The changes in the serum CK of each patient are illustrated in Fig. 1.

DISCUSSION

There is substantial evidence in the literature indicating that elevation of the serum CK is specific for skeletal or cardiac muscle disease or trauma.[2, 3, 5, 9, 10, 14] This also applies in the stress situations resulting from acute and chronic alcoholism,[7, 8, 12] epilepsy,[1] and acute psychoses,[6] and electrophoretic studies have shown the serum enzyme to be of the muscle rather than of brain type.[6] The most likely explanation of

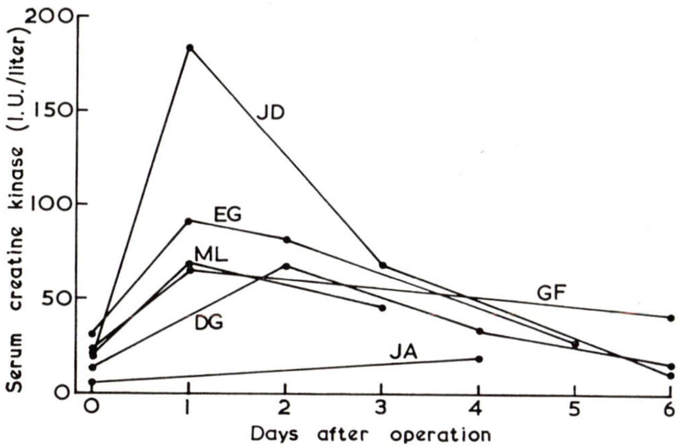

Fig. 1. Serial serum CK values. The values on Day 0 are the preoperative control levels.

LDH		HBD		CK	
Before	After	Before	After	Before	After
125†	105†	58	48	3	19
125†	96,† 155,† 105	87	87, 135, 68	19	182, 68, 11
145†	145,† 115, 190	96	96, 87, 106	31	91, 82, 27
135†	155,† 125, 210	77	87, 87, 154	14	68, 34, 17
270†	160,† 220	203	116, 111	20	70, 46
120†	115,† 160	97	77, 125	23	67, 42

observed in the postoperative specimens.

Table II. *Serum enzymes; statistical analysis*

Preoperative		*Postoperative*								
		1 to 2 days			*3 to 4 days*			*5 to 6 days*		
Enzyme	*Value (mean)*	*No. of patients*	*Mean change**	*S.E.†*	*No. of patients*	*Mean change*	*S.E.*	*No. of patients*	*Mean change*	*S.E.*
GOT	25	5	1.8	4.8	4	-4.25	3.1	4	-2.0	3.2
GPT	27	5	-5.4‡	1.2	4	0.75	5.5	4	11.5	6.7
LDH	318	5	-52.0	47.3	4	-27.5	35.0	4	75.0	41.9
HBD	213	5	-40.0	36.3	4	-22.5	61.2	4	50.0	42.0
CK	18	5	74.2‡	22.4	4	27.8‡	7.4	4	2.5	6.0

*Mean changes are in enzyme units.

†S.E. = standard error of the mean.

‡Statistically significant at the 5 percent level.

the elevation after amputation observed in the present study is therefore the release of the enzyme from skeletal muscle severed during operation. It is noteworthy that this enzyme test can detect a degree of damage to skeletal muscle not discernible by the GOT or LDH procedures or by LDH isoenzyme studies.

This elevation of the serum CK is of practical importance since it might obscure a simultaneous increase due to acute ischemic damage elsewhere, e.g., in the myocardium or in another extremity. No evidence of such complications was detected in any of the patients studied during the present investigation.

The authors wish to thank Miss Kathryn D. Schiffelbian for her valued assistance. Gratitude is also expressed to Dr. Stanley Schor, Department of Biometrics, Temple University School of Medicine, for the statistical analyses presented in Table II.

REFERENCES

1. Belton, N. R., Backus, R. E., and Millichap, J. G.: Serum creatine phosphokinase activity in epilepsy. Clinical and experimental studies, Neurology **17:** 1073, 1967.
2. Dreyfus, J.-C., Schapira, G., Resnais, J., and Scebat, L.: La créatine kinase sérique dans le diagnostic de l'infarctus myocardique, Rev. Franç. Etud. Clin. et Biol. **5:** 386, 1960.
3. Ebashi, S., Toyokura, Y., Momoi, H., and Sugita, H.: High creatine phosphokinase activity of sera of progressive muscular dystrophy, J. Biochem. **46:** 103, 1959.
4. Henry, R. J., Chiamori, N., Golub, O. J., and Berkman, S.: Revised spectrophotometric methods for the determination of glutamic-oxalacetic transaminase, glutamic-pyruvic transaminase and lactic acid dehydrogenase, Am. J. Clin. Path. **34:** 381, 1960.
5. Hughes, B. P.: A method for the estimation of serum creatine kinase and its use in comparing creatine kinase and aldolase activity in normal and pathological sera, Clin. chim. acta **7:** 597, 1962.
6. Meltzer, H.: Creatine kinase and aldolase in serum: Abnormality common to acute psychoses, Science **159:** 1368, 1968.
7. Nygren, A.: Serum creatine phosphokinase activity in chronic alcoholism in connection with acute alcohol intoxication, Acta med. scandinav. **179:** 623, 1966.
8. Nygren, A.: Serum creatine kinase in chronic alcoholism, Acta med. scandinav. **182:** 383, 1967.
9. Okinaka, S., Sugita, H., Momoi, H., Toyokura, Y., Watanabe, T., Ebashi, F., and Ebashi, S.: Cysteine-stimulated serum creatine kinase in health and disease, J. Lab. & Clin. Med. **64:** 299, 1964.
10. Pearce, J. M. S., Pennington, R. J. T., and Walton, J. N.: Serum enzyme studies in muscle disease. Part II. Serum creatine kinase activity in muscular dystrophy and in other myopathic and neuropathic disorders, J. Neurol. Neurosurg. & Psychiat. **27:** 96, 1964.
11. Penneys, R.: Serum lactic dehydrogenase (LDH) isozymes with ischemic damage of skeletal muscle of the human limb, Angiology **18:** 678, 1967.
12. Perkoff, G. T., Hardy, P., and Velez-Garcia, E.: Reversible acute muscular syndrome in chronic alcoholism, New England J. Med. **274:** 1277, 1966.
13. Raymond, S., and Weintraub, L.: Acrylamide gel as a supporting medium for zone electrophoresis, Science **130:** 711, 1959.
14. Richterich, R., Rosin, S., Aebi, U., and Rossi, E.: Progressive muscular dystrophy. V. The identification of the carrier state in the

Duchenne type by serum creatine kinase determination, Am. J. Human Genet. **15:** 133, 1963.

15. Rosalki, S. B.: An improved procedure for serum creatine phosphokinase determination, J. Lab. & Clin. Med. **69:** 696, 1967.
16. Rosalki, S. B., and Wilkinson, J. H.: Reduction of α-ketobutyrate by human serum, Nature **188:** 1110, 1960
17. Wróblewski, F., and LaDue, J. S.: Lactic dehydrogenase activity in blood, Proc. Soc. Exper. Biol. & Med. **90:** 210, 1955.

A technique for prolonged splenic perfusion

ROBERT ATKINS, M.B., M.R.A.C.P.*
CLEVE TRIMBLE, M.D.
BEN EISEMAN, M.D.
DENVER, COLO.
From the Department of Surgery, University of Colorado Medical Center

The isolated spleen perfused and oxygenated at normal temperature can provide a potential source of antibodies produced under highly controlled conditions. As such, this preparation is of importance as a model to study the immunologic response and as a potential source of antibodies for clinical use during infection or in tumor immunotherapy. To be of more value than simple lymphocyte culture, the spleen must maintain its viability for at least a week.

This paper describes a technique for maintaining the function of an excised spleen with oxygenated perfusion. Subsequent papers concerning this technique will detail metabolic and immunologic functions of this preparation.

PREPARATION OF THE SPLEEN

Splenectomy was performed under sterile operating conditions on 12 to 16 kilogram heparinized (3 mg. per kilogram) Hampshire pigs. The spleen was weighed (35 to 70 grams), and the hilar artery and vein were cannulated with 10 and 13 gauge beveled needles which were incorporated into the top of the splenic container (Fig. 1). Splenic washout was performed with 1 to 2 L. of 0.9 percent sodium chloride containing 100 mg. of heparin, 60 mg. of procaine hydrochloride, and 7 mEq. of sodium bicarbonate per liter. Washout pressure was 120 mm. Hg (Fig. 2).

Perfusion circuitry (Fig. 3). The main elements of the circuit are a fluid-filled perfusion chamber containing the cannulated spleen, a membrane oxygenator, and a roller pump.

The perfusion chamber (Fig. 4) is a 13 by 2½ inch plexiglass cylinder, one end of which accommodates the splenic arterial and venous cannulas (Fig. 1). A dependent effluent connected the fluid within the chamber to the venous line. A stopcock in the top of the chamber permitted air removal. A thermistor probe was passed through one end plate into the perfusing medium surrounding the spleen.

The membrane oxygenator (Figs. 5A to 5D) is of our own design as previously de-

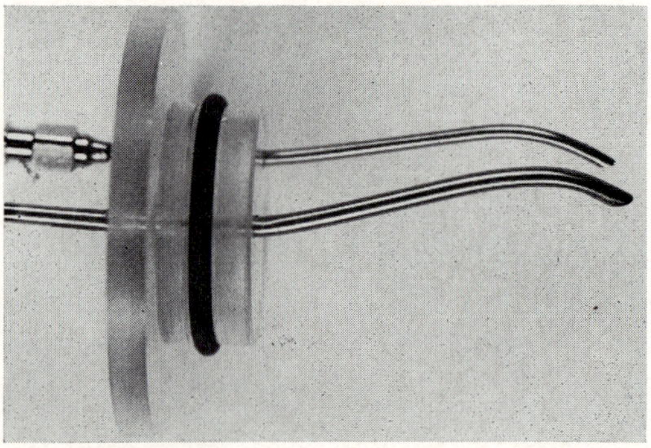

Fig. 1. Photograph of the splenic container top which incorporates the beveled arterial (13 gauge) and venous (10 gauge) stainless steel cannulas.

Supported by a grant from the Hartford Foundation.
Received for publication Jan. 3, 1969.
*Research Fellow in Surgery.

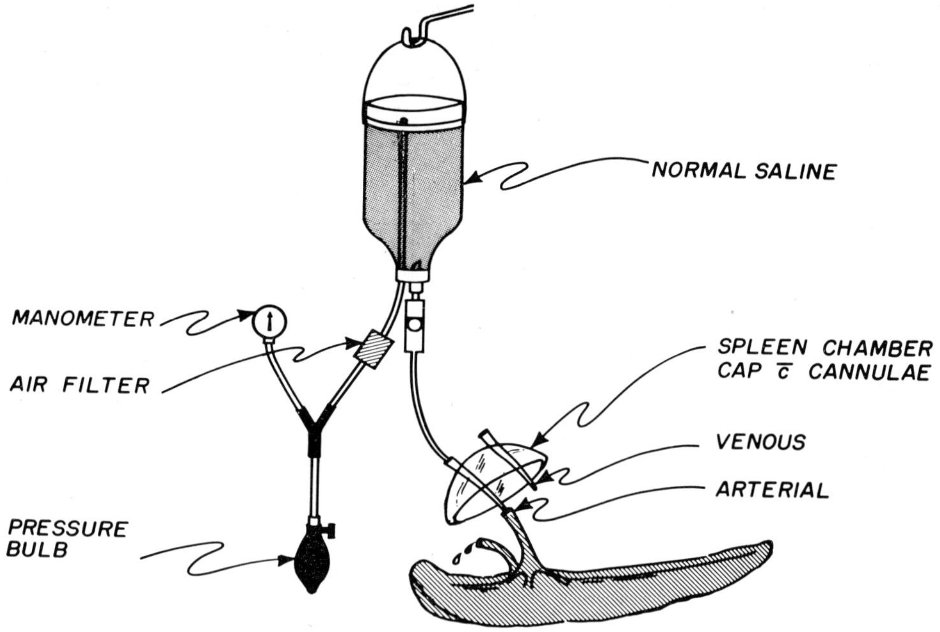

Fig. 2. Diagram of splenic washout apparatus. Pressure of 120 mm. Hg was maintained by pumping aid with a sphygmomanometer bulb through a sterilizing cotton filter into the reservoir.

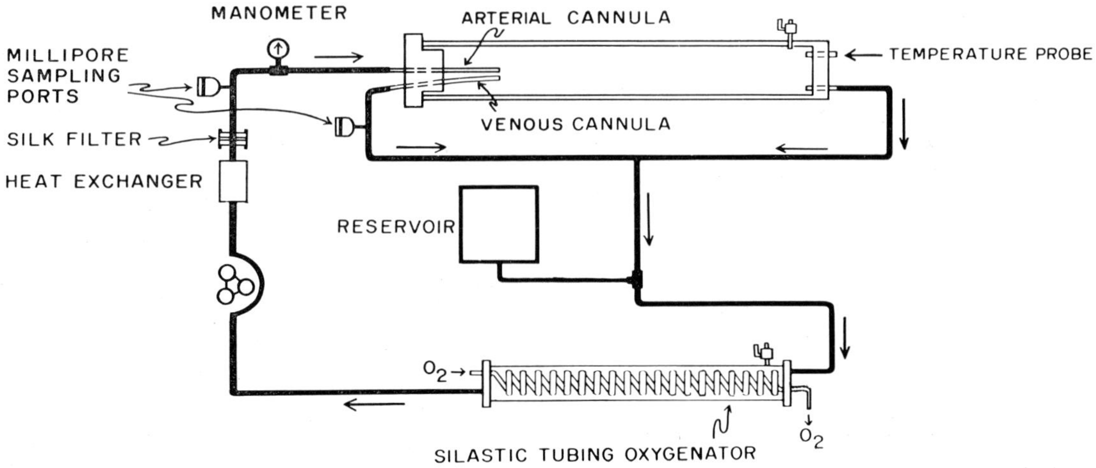

Fig. 3. Diagram of the splenic perfusion circuit.

scribed.[1] Pig spleen perfusion requires 50 feet of 0.125 O.D. (outside diameter) by 0.078 inch I.D. (inside diameter) Silastic tubing contained in a 14 by 4 inch cylindrical oxygenator. Oxygen flows within the Silastic tubing and diffuses through the wall into the surrounding perfusate. Perfusate oxygen tension was regulated by submersion of the oxygen outlet at varying depths beneath a 25 cm. column of mercury.

Perfusion at 0.5 to 3 ml. per gram of splenic weight per minute was by Model

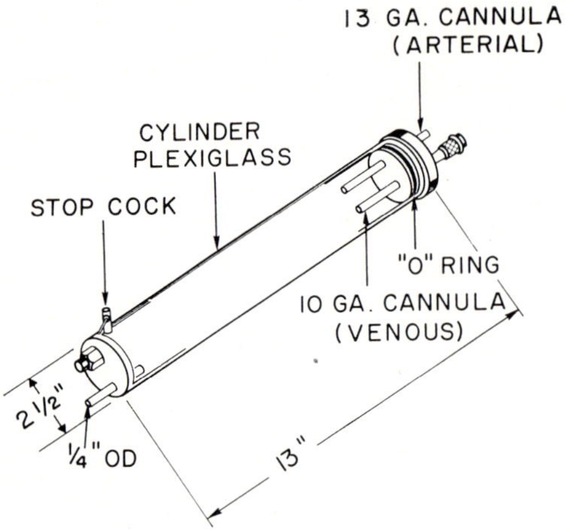

Fig. 4. Splenic perfusion chamber.

7015 Cole-Parmer constant-flow pump.* All perfusion lines were of 5/8 O.D. by 3/8 inch I.D. Silastic tubing. Y-connectors were of polypropylene and stainless steel. All elements were siliconized and steam or gas sterilized prior to use.

A reservoir consisting of a commercially available distensible plastic bag† replenished perfusate volume after samples were withdrawn. The reservoir also adjusted to pressure changes throughout the system. Since the reservoir was attached to the splenic venous line, regulation of its height suitably changed splenic venous pressure.

Sampling ports were protected from bacterial contamination by Millipore filters (0.45 μ).‡ A silk filter of heavy weave§ silk within a reusable plastic casing was used to prevent tissue debris from causing small vessel obstruction. A heat exchanger of stainless steel maintained normothermia in association with a constant temperature water bath. The perfusate (900 ml.) was Medium 199. The perfusate composition is shown in Table I, and the perfusate electrolyte final concentrations are given in Table II. The fetal calf serum was frozen, thawed, and

*Cole-Parmer, Chicago, Ill.
†Fenwall, Denver, Colo.
‡Millipore Corporation, Bedford, Mass.
§Sargent—Type A, Chicago, Ill.

Table I. *Perfusate composition*

Constituent	*Quantity (to 500 ml.)*	*Final concentration*
Medium 199*	450 ml.	90%
Fetal calf serum*	50 ml.	10%
Glucose 50%	2 ml.	300 mg.%
Sodium bicarbonate	5 mEq.	pH 7.45
Penicillin	62,500 U.	125 U./ml.
Neomycin	20 mg.	40 μg/ml.

*Supplied by Colorado Serum Company, Denver, Colo.

Table II. *Perfusate electrolyte final concentrations*

	Values
Na+	170 mEq./L.
K+	6.4 mEq./L.
Ca++	2.1 mEq./L.
Cl−	150 mEq./L.
Glucose	300 mg.%
pH	7.45
Osmolarity	360 mOsm./Kg.

filtered (Millipore 0.22 μ) to remove lipoprotein[3] prior to use.

PERFUSION TECHNIQUE

Compulsive attention to sterility was observed throughout perfusion. Perfusion flow rate was adjusted between 0.5 to 3 ml. per gram of splenic weight per minute. Vascular resistance (mm. Hg per cubic centimeter per minute) was determined by arterial pressure divided by flow rate.

Glucose was added intermittently throughout the perfusion to maintain concentrations of 300 mg. percent. The pH of the perfusing medium was maintained between 7.1 and 7.3 by the addition of sodium bicarbonate as required. The temperature was constant at 37° C.

RESULTS

Fig. 6 graphically illustrates the vascular resistance of spleens asanguinally perfused at various flow rates. Vascular resistance is not appreciably altered by rates of flow within physiologic range. Indeed, spleens with the

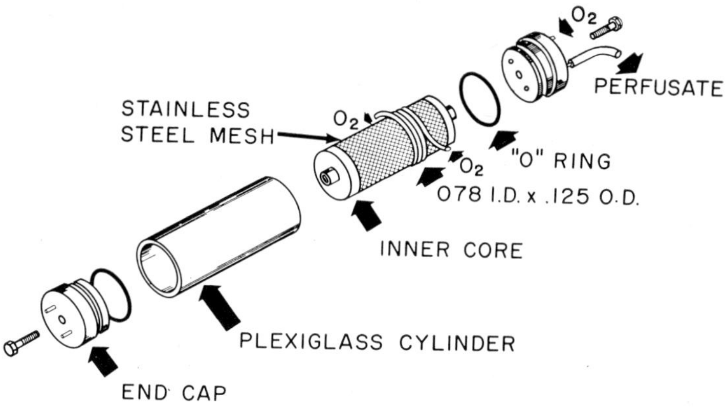

Fig. 5A. Diagrammatic exploded view of the membrane oxygenator.

higher perfusate flow had the lowest vascular resistance.

In contrast, when perfused with homologous blood and a disc oxygenator, splenic vascular resistance averaged 12 mm. Hg per cubic centimeter per minute, after only 6 hours of perfusion.[4] In vivo pig spleen vascular resistance is 3 mm. Hg per milliliter per minute.[12]

An angiogram of a typical spleen after 3 days of normothermic perfusion is shown in Fig. 7. Small vessel integrity is apparent.

Weight change during perfusion is recorded in Table III. There was no significant weight increase during perfusion in any of the flow groups studied. Belzer and coworkers[3] suggest that a 5 percent organ weight gain following perfusion indicates tissue destruction and cellular death.

DISCUSSION

This perfusion technique maintains splenic viability and function for up to a week. Previously, in splenic perfusions using a sanguinous perfusate and disc oxygenator, development of increased vascular resistance stopped perfusion after 4 or 6 hours.[4, 12] The hallmarks of increased vascular resistance, rising arterial pressure, falling perfusate flow, and organ edema have been overcome. Contributing factors have been the following: use of an asanguinous, afibrinous perfusate; partial lipoprotein removal; hyper-

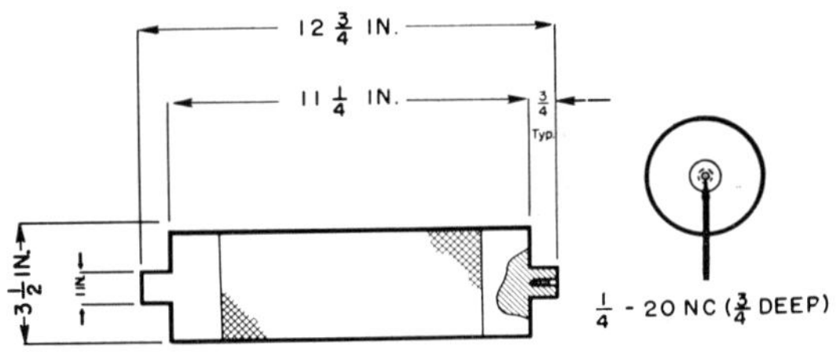

Fig. 5B. Plexiglass inner core of the oxygenator.

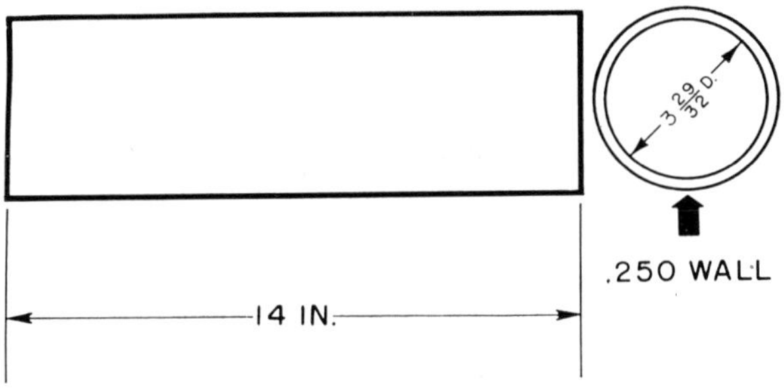

Fig. 5C. Plexiglass outer casing of the oxygenator.

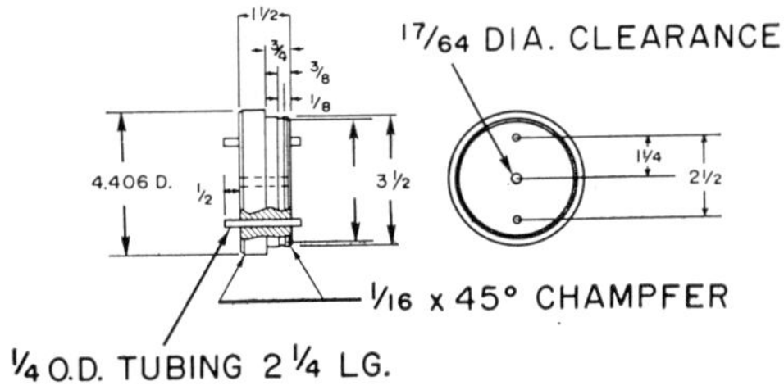

Fig. 5D. Detail of the plexiglass end cap of the oxygenator.

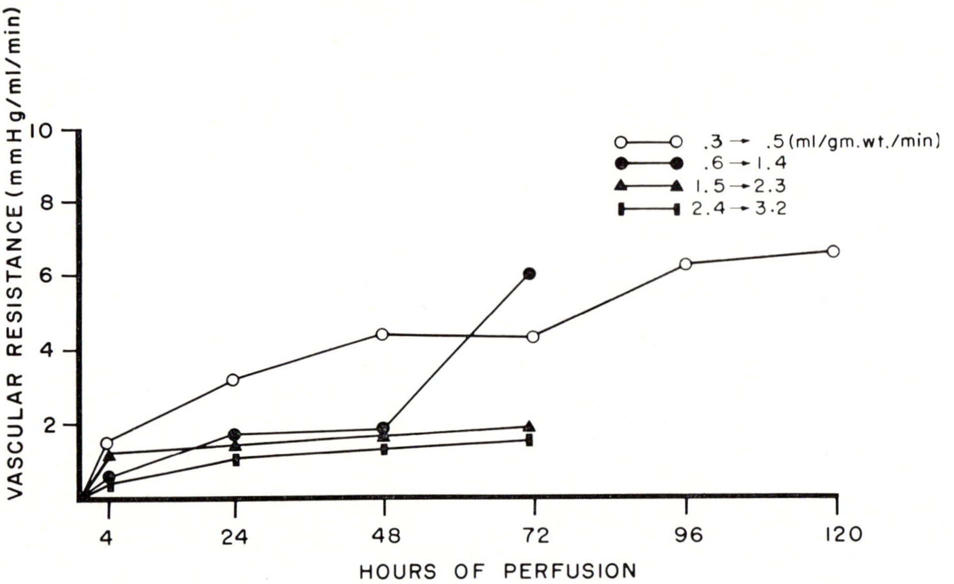

Fig. 6. Splenic vascular resistance of groups of spleens perfused at varying asanguinous perfusate flows: 0.3 to 0.5 ml. per gram of weight per minute (average 8 spleens); 0.6 to 1.4 ml. per grams of weight per minute (average 3 spleens); 1.5 to 2.3 ml. per grams of weight per minute (average 6 spleens); 2.4 to 3.2 ml. per grams of weight per minute (average 3 spleens).

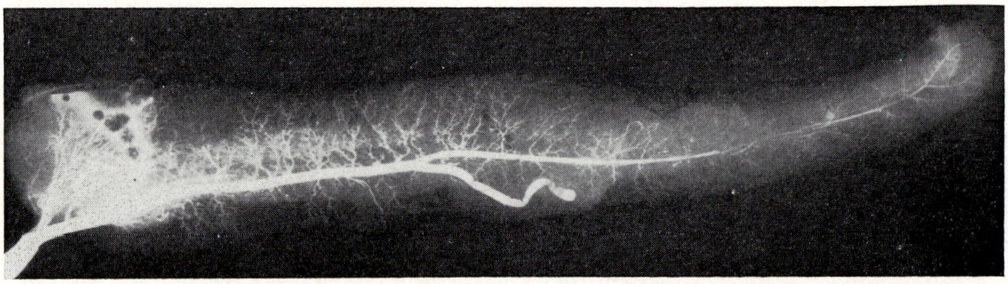

Fig. 7. Typical angiogram of a spleen after 3 days of normothermic perfusion. The area in the head represents a splenic biopsy taken prior to angiograph. Small vessel integrity is apparent.

osmolarity, an entirely closed system with membrane oxygenation; and siliconized apparatus.

The concept of an asanguinous perfusate was first introduced by Carrel and Lindbergh.[5] Recently Folkman and associates[7] also using an acellular perfusate have perfused thyroids for up to 30 days. Belzer and coworkers[2] and Humphries[8] have had success in kidney transplantation following asanguinous perfusion-preservation for 72 hours. Humphries[8] feels that an acellular perfusate is mandatory for prolonged perfusion. He maintains increased vascular resistance with cellular perfusates is due to mechanical blockage. Schneider and Swank[16] incriminate platelets in capillary plugging.

Membrane oxygenation is an important feature and enables a totally closed system (no air-fluid interface). Lee and associates[9] demonstrated damage to blood elements, especially protein, during bypass procedures

Table III. *Weight change in spleens after 3 day perfusions at varying flow rates**

Perfusate flow rate (ml./Gm. splenic wt./min.)	*Weight before treatment (Gm.)*	*Weight after (Gm.)*	*Weight change (%)*
0.3 to 0.5 (average 5 spleens)	52	50	- 3.7
0.6 to 1.4 (average 3 spleens)	78	48	-39
1.5 to 2.5 (average 4 spleens)	44.5	46	+ 1.6
2.4 to 3.2 (average 2 spleens)	44	44	0

*There was no significant weight increase in any of the flow groups studied.

with oxygenators incorporating air-fluid interfaces. Owens and co-workers[14] showed fat embolization in dogs following bypass with a bubble oxygenator being used but not with a membrane oxygenator being used.

Perfusate hyperosmolarity is utilized in Folkman and associates'[7] prolonged organ perfusions. He feels that hyperosmolarity keeps the intravascular compartment replete and allows faster perfusate flows to be tolerated.

Oxygen toxicity has been shown in whole animals,[17] tissue culture,[6] and in isolated organs,[15] to be of importance in cellular integrity. Thus with an asanguinous perfusate a compromise between flow and PO_2 must be obtained. Too high a PO_2 might result in oxygen poisoning. Too high a flow results in tissue disruption. For splenic perfusion we found optimal glucose metabolism at a perfusate flow of 2 ml. per gram splenic weight per minute with an arterial PO_2 of 250 to 300 mm. Hg.[15]

Nutrients are necessary to maintain metabolic integrity. Tissue culture Medium 199 contains all the essential amino acids, minerals, and vitamins needed for cell growth in isolated tissue culture.[13] With the addition of 10 percent fetal calf serum, minute amounts of ill-defined yet indispensable serum factors are incorporated. We have not found cortisone, insulin, or other hormones necessary. Although regular change of perfusing medium may be important if the organ weight to perfusate volume ratio is low, accumulation of metabolic end products has not necessitated medium exchange or incorporation of a dialysis unit. Carbon dioxide is removed by the membrane oxygenator. The only required additives are intermittent glucose and sodium bicarbonate.

Infection, an enormous hazard in prolonged normothermic perfusion, has been completely overcome by compulsive attention to sterility, bactericidal perfusate antibiotic levels, a closed system, and Millipore protection of sampling ports.

The question of pulsatile versus nonpulsatile flow is a disputed one. Many investigators advocate pulsatile flow.[8, 10, 11] We use a constant perfusate flow. However, with its stagnant sinusoidal system, the spleen may not be as dependent on pulsatility as other organs.

A system capable of maintaining splenic viability and function for up to a week has been described. Subsequent papers will show that spleens thus perfused maintain their metabolic activity and immunologic function.

SUMMARY

A plastic perfusion apparatus has been described which has enabled normothermic, asanguinous pig spleen perfusion for up to a week. Features include a completely closed, siliconized system, membrane oxygenation, and an asanguinous tissue culture medium perfusate. Increase in vascular resistance was minimal throughout perfusion.

REFERENCES

1. Atkins, R. C., Trimble, C., and Eiseman, B.: B.: A countercurrent membrane oxygenator for prolonged preservation of ex vivo organs, S. Forum **19:** 356, 1968.
2. Belzer, F. O., Ashby, B. S., and Dunphy, J. E.: 24-hour and 72-hour preservation of canine kidneys, Lancet. **2:** 536, 1967.
3. Belzer, F. O., Ashby, B. S., Huang, J. S., and Dunphy, J. E.: Etiology of rising perfusion pressure in isolated organ perfusion, Ann. Surg. **168:** 382, 1968.
4. Boxall, T. A., Hirose, S., and Eiseman, B.: Experimental evaluation of heterologous ex vivo spleen perfusion, Ann. Surg. **166:** 118, 1967.
5. Carrel, A., and Lindbergh, C. A.: The culture of organs, New York, 1938, Paul B. Hoeber, Inc., Medical Book Division of Harper & Row, Publishers.
6. Cooper, P. D., Burt, A. M., and Wilson, J. N.: Critical effects of oxygen tension on rate and growth of animal cells in continuous suspended culture, Nature **182:** 1508, 1958.
7. Folkman, J., Cole, P., and Zimmerman, S.: Tumor behavior in isolated perfused organs: In vitro growth and metastases of biopsy material in rabbit thyroid and canine intestinal segment, Ann. Surg. **164:** 491, 1966.
8. Humphries, A. L.: Problems of organ preservation. Organ preservation: A review, Transplantation **5:** 1138, 1967.
9. Lee, W. H., Krumhaar, D., Fonkalsrud, E. W., Schjeide, O. A., and Maloney, J. V.: Denaturation of plasma proteins as a cause of morbidity and death after intracardiac operations, SURGERY **50:** 29, 1961.
10. McLaughlin, E. D., and Austen, W. G.: Perfusion of the isolated canine liver in vivo and in vitro, Tr. Am. Soc. Artif. Intern. Organs **12:** 259, 1966.
11. Mandelbaum, I., and Burns, W. H.: Pulsatile and nonpulsatile blood flow, J. A. M. A. **191:** 121, 1965.
12. Moore, A. R., Mieny, C., and Eiseman, B.: Vascular resistance in splenic perfusion. In press.
13. Morgan, J. F.: Tissue culture nutrition, Bact. Rev. **22:** 20, 1958.
14. Owens, G., Adams, J., and Scott, H. W.: Embolic fat as a measure of adequacy of various oxygenators, J. Appl. Physiol. **15:** 999, 1960.
15. Ruble, R. T., Atkins, R. C., Bielanski, E., and Eiseman, B.: The effect of perfusate oxygen tension and flow rate on glucose metabolism of the isolated perfused pig spleen, Arch. Surg. In press.
16. Schneider, M., and Swank, R. L.: Blocks in lung capillaries linked to transfusion, Med. World News **7:** 41, Sept. 2, 1966.
17. Stadie, W. C., Riggs, B. C., and Haugaard, N.: Oxygen poisoning, Am. J. M. Sc. **207:** 84, 1944.

Arteriography as an adjunct to the diagnosis of splenic injury*

STANTON G. POLIN, Commander, MC, USNR
WILLIAM D. WALKLETT, Commander, MC, USN
OSBEY L. SAYLER, Lieutenant Commander, MC, USN
PORTSMOUTH, VA.
From the Departments of Surgery and Radiology, Naval Hospital

Undiagnosed, and therefore untreated, rupture of the spleen is associated with a very high mortality rate. The magnitude of the problem becomes apparent when one recognizes that the spleen is the most frequently injured organ in cases of blunt trauma.[13] In classic cases of splenic rupture the diagnosis is readily made and splenectomy performed.

However, all too frequently the diagnosis cannot be made and treatment is postponed. In the latter case the patient is usually hospitalized for an indefinite period for observation. If the diagnosis is in doubt, but there is strong suggestive evidence, then exploratory laparotomy is justified.

A reliable, safe method is hereby presented to confirm the diagnosis of splenic injury and obviate the period of hospitalization for observation or the need for "negative" exploratory laparotomies.

METHOD

On the basis of a small, but growing, popularity of arteriography as an adjunct to identifying organs involved in abdominal trauma, a laboratory study was undertaken to determine the degree of accuracy that arteriograms have in diagnosing splenic injury. Also, an investigation was made of the degree and severity of injury that is detectable by arteriography.

Seventeen mongrel dogs were operated on under general anesthesia. In each case the splenic artery was cannulated near its origin at the celiac axis. A hand-injection splenic arteriogram was performed with 10 c.c. methylglucamine diatrizoate* 60 percent, and a single film was exposed near completion of the injection. This film then became the control for the subsequent study.

The spleen was then injured in any of a number of ways. The spleen was compressed to simulate blunt trauma. Different patterns of injury could be made this way and were reproducible. Blunt types of injury are outlined as follows:

A. Capsule intact
   1. Superficial subcapsular hematoma of any size
   2. Deep disruption of parenchyma with deep hematoma
   3. Possible intrasplenic arteriovenous fistula

B. Capsule broken with resultant extravasation of blood
   1. Superficial injury
   2. Large fracture of spleen.

Received for publication Jan. 14, 1969.

*The opinions or assertions contained herein are those of the authors and are not to be construed as official or reflecting the views of the Navy Department or of the Naval Service at large.

*Renografin: E. R. Squibb & Sons, Inc., New York, N. Y.

Table I. *Summary of the type of injury and arteriographic findings*

Dog No.	Type of injury	*Arteriographic finding* Contrast pooling	Contrast leakage
1	1 inch subcapsular hematoma, middle ⅓	+	
2	1 inch subcapsular hematoma at hilum	+	
3	2 stabs in middle ⅓ of spleen (¼ inch depth, ¼ inch length)	+	+
4	Extensive subcapsular hematoma on middle ⅓	+	
5	Blunt crush upper ½	+	
6	A. Stab near hilum,		+
	B. Blunt trauma to upper ½	+	
7	1 inch compression of midportion lateral surface	Cleft seen on arteriogram	
8	A. ½ inch stab at hilum	+	+
	B. ½ inch deep hematoma upper pole	+	
	C. Superficial hematoma lateral surface	+	
9	A. ½ inch hematoma edge of midportion	+	
	B. 1 inch laceration lower pole		+
10	A. Blunt trauma entire spleen	+	
	B. Stellate superficial laceration lateral surface middle ⅓		+
11	A. 2 inch cut upper pole	+	+
	B. ½ inch deep hematoma lower pole	+	
12	A. ½ inch hematoma lower ⅓	+	
	B. blunt crush middle ⅓	+	
13	A. Stab upper pole	+	+
	B. Pinpoint stab lower pole with deep hematoma		+
14	A. 1 inch hematoma in middle ⅓	+	
	B. Stab lower pole		+
15	2 adjacent 1 inch hematomas in middle ⅓	+	
16	Massive contusion of spleen with small capsular tear on back surface	+	+
17	A. ½ inch hematoma upper pole	+	
	B. Stab at hilum	+	+
	C. Deep hematoma lower ½	+	

The spleen was also punctured to simulate penetrating injuries. The depth and extent of the puncture could be controlled. On some spleens more than one type of trauma was induced. Immediately after the wound was made another single exposure arteriogram was made. On some dogs 30 seconds after the injury another similar arteriogram was made. A splenectomy was then performed and the laparotomy incision closed.

Table I shows that there were 28 distinct injuries in the 17 spleens. In each area of injury the arteriographic pattern was different from the control. Certain patterns occurred commonly and were detectable by the single film arteriogram. It is possible that finer radiologic interpretation could be made from rapid, serial arteriograms.

DISCUSSION

Since the spleen is a veritable vascular sponge, it should be possible to detect dis-

A

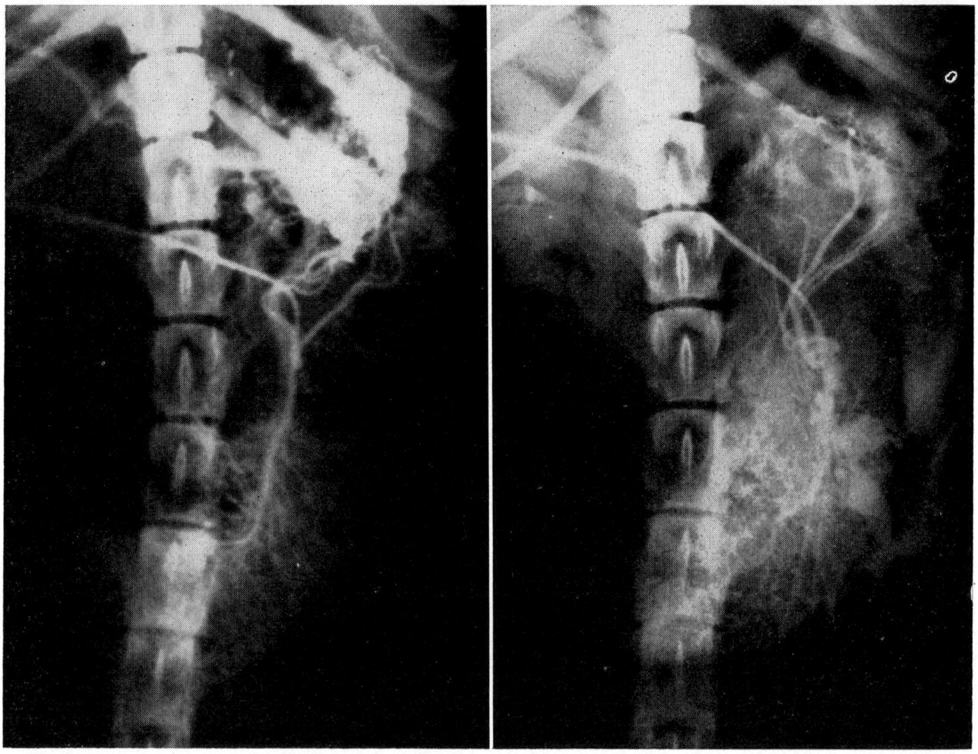

B

Fig. 1. *A,* Preliminary arteriogram of Dog 3 demonstrates the usual configuration of the splenic artery and vein and pulp opacification. The radiopaque vessels over the upper pole represent gastric vessels that were incompletely ligated. *B,* Following trauma the spleen is somewhat smaller in this case. Extravasation is the primary pattern. It outlines the lateral peritoneal wall and loops of bowel. The tracts of two stab wounds are evident in the midlateral portion of the spleen. No parenchymal hematoma is evident.

ruption of the capsule or subcapsular hematoma by means of angiography. Indeed, Norell[8] in 1957 gave the first description of angiographic findings in a case of traumatic rupture of the spleen. In the next decade only four cases[2, 7, 9, 12] have appeared in American medical journals. Aakhus and Enge[1] described angiographic patterns in five cases of traumatic rupture of the spleen in 1967. The 1968 literature reveals three articles[3, 4, 6] by one group of authors describing angiographic findings and another paper[10] that mentions the subject briefly.

Therefore, a review of the literature failed to indicate that arteriography is a popular diagnostic method for investigating splenic trauma. This lack of popularity is not warranted in view of the clinical experience of others and the quantitative laboratory results presented here.

Little has been said about the incidence of false negative arteriograms or the potential value of a negative study in allowing earlier discharge of patients. This study was designed to help ascertain these two highly significant features.

No false positive arteriograms were found in the control studies. All injuries produced on the spleens were matched by abnormal angiograms. The angiograms even showed small wounds such as stab wounds ¼ inch deep and ¼ inch long (Dog 3, Fig. 1) or superficial hematomas ¼ inch square (Dogs 9, 12, and 17). Small, deep wounds were also detectable and not masked by the surrounding intact vascular pattern, e.g., ¼

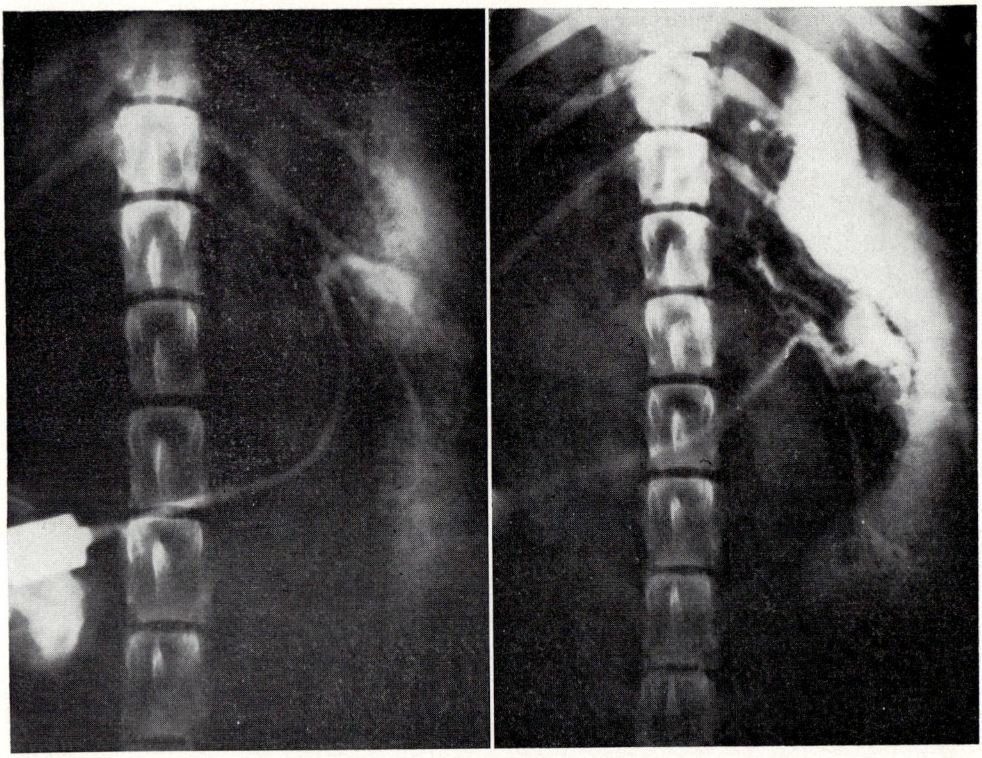

A B

Fig. 2. *A,* Control arteriogram in Dog 6 is shown for spleen size. *B,* Following trauma the upper pole has enlarged and shows the uniform radiopaque pattern associated with parenchymal hematoma. No subcapsular extension is present. A small extrasplenic collection of contrast medium is seen in the hilum. This represents the separate effect of a stab wound near the hilum.

inch square hematoma deep in the parenchyma of the spleen (Dog 8). Massive hematomas left unquestioned angiographic abnormalities. Thus, no false negative arteriograms were seen.

The types of arteriographic findings have been classified in Table I. It should be noted that arteriovenous shunts were not seen in this study although they were reported by Love and associates[6] and Aakhus and Enge.[1] This is possibly because the single exposure arteriogram employed here could not record such detail. Splenic enlargement was detected occasionally as it was by Love and associates.[6] Localized enlargement due to hematoma was seen more commonly than diffuse enlargement. Significant enlargement was probably not seen in all our cases because the experiment did not always allow sufficient time for the hematoma to expand.

Two arteriographic patterns that appear most frequently are pooling of the contrast medium in a hematoma (Fig. 2) and leakage of contrast medium (Fig. 3). The former occurs commonly rather than the expected parenchymatous filling defect because the hematoma is actively enlarging during the time of these early posttrauma arteriograms so contrast medium "bleeds" into the injured area. This situation is unlike the finding of Aakhus and Enge[1] where hematomas were represented by parenchymatous filling defects. In their cases the arteriography was performed long after the hematomas stopped enlarging so no contrast medium accumulated in the areas. Leakage of the contrast medium occurred in all of the capsular tears in the dog cases. This high incidence may also be due to the active bleeding that takes place during the arteriogram performed so shortly after trauma.

It is imperative to diagnose trauma to the

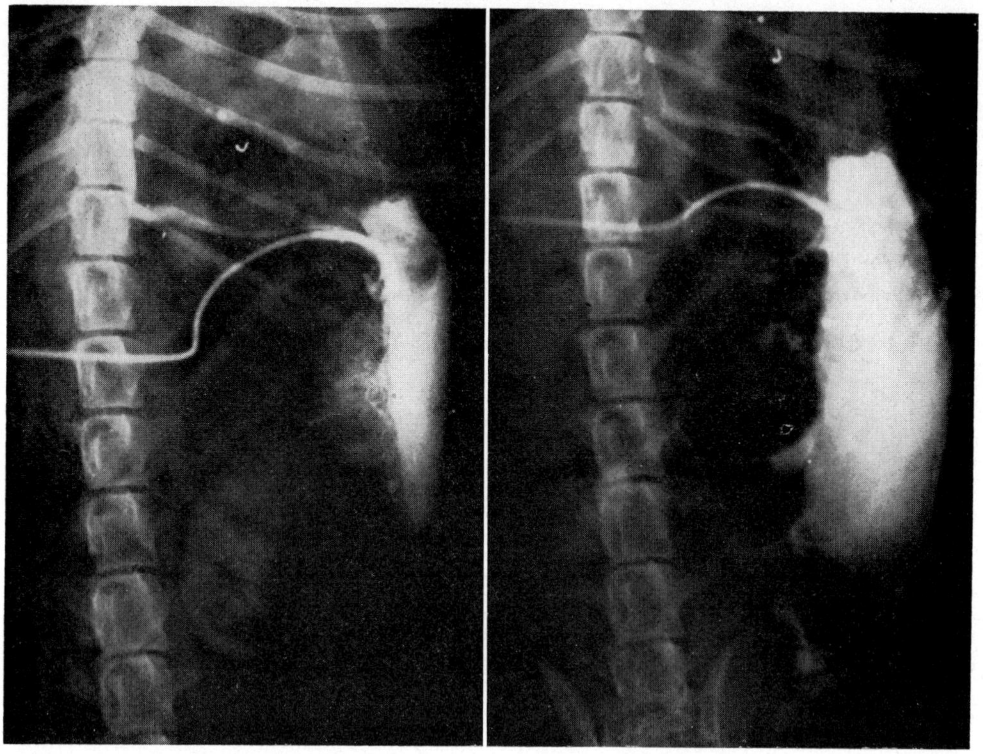

Fig. 3. *A,* Control arteriogram in Dog 10 is shown for spleen size and pulp opacification. *B,* The entire spleen is enlarged. The pulp is diffusely opacified, and extravasated contrast material outlines loops of bowel. The entire spleen was bluntly traumatized producing a diffuse hematoma. A stellate laceration on the lateral surface causes a leak of contrast material into the peritoneal cavity.

spleen because neglected injury of this organ may result in a mortality rate of 90 to 95 percent.[11] Many nonspecific physical diagnostic, laboratory, and radiographic techniques are available to assist in finding most cases. Radioisotopic detection is being evaluated as a reliable measure of making the diagnosis,[5] but angiography seems to be capable of finding recent as well as older splenic injuries of even minute proportions. It is important to find the patients even with small splenic injuries because these injuries, too, result in fatal bleeding.

SUMMARY

A laboratory study on dogs was undertaken to test the reliability of angiography as a means of diagnosing injuries to the spleen. A wide variety of wounds was produced on spleens, and angiography was performed. Every injury, regardless of how small, was associated with an abnormal arteriogram. An interpretation of the angiographic findings is given.

REFERENCES

1. Aakhus, T., and Enge, I.: Angiography in traumatic rupture of the spleen, Brit. J. Radiol. **40:** 855, 1967.
2. Baum, S., Nusbaum, M., Blakemore, W. S., and Tinkelstein, A. K.: The preoperative radiographic demonstration of intra-abdominal bleeding from undetermined sites by percutaneous selective celiac and superior mesenteric arteriography, SURGERY **58:** 797, 1965.
3. Freeark, R. J., Love, L., and Baker, R. J.: The role of aortography in the management of blunt abdominal trauma, J. Trauma **8:** 557, 1968.
4. Freeark, R. J., Shoemaker, W. C., and Baker, R. J.: Aortography in blunt abdominal trauma, Arch. Surg. **96:** 705, 1968.
5. Jackson, G. L., and Albright, D.: Splenic rupture: Application of radioisotopic tech-

niques in diagnosis. J. A. M. A. **204:** 930, 1968.
6. Love, L., Greenfield, G. B., Braun, T. W., Moncada, R., Freeark, R. J., and Baker, R. J.: Arteriography of splenic trauma, Radiology **91:** 96, 1968.
7. Nelson, J. F.: The roentgenologic evaluation of abdominal trauma, Radiol. Clin. North America **4:** 415, 1966.
8. Norell, H. G.: Traumatic rupture of the spleen diagnosed by abdominal aortography: Report of a case, Acta radiol. **48:** 449, 1957.
9. Pollard, J. J., and Nebesar, R. A.: Splenic rupture demonstrated by selective splenic artery angiogram, J. A. M. A. **187:** 944, 1964.
10. Ranniger, K., and Saldino, R. M.: Abdominal angiography, *in* Current problems in surgery, Chicago, March, 1968, Year Book Medical Publishers, Inc., p. 1.
11. Shires, G. T.: Care of the trauma patient, New York, 1966, McGraw-Hill Book Company, p. 398.
12. Steinberg, I., and Karl, R. C.: Diagnosis of rupture of the spleen by intravenous abdominal aortography: Report of a case, Am. J. Roentgenol. **84:** 902, 1960.
13. Stivelman, R. L., Glaubitz, J. P., and Crampton, R. S.: Laceration of the spleen due to nonpenetrating trauma. One hundred cases, Am. J. Surg. **106:** 888, 1963.

The effect of liver disease on the need for venous decompression during the anhepatic phase of canine orthotopic liver transplantation

REGINALDO S. PICACHE, M.D.
BRIJ M. L. KAPUR, F.R.C.S.
THOMAS E. STARZL, Ph.D., M.D.
DENVER, COLO.
From the Department of Surgery, University of Colorado School of Medicine and the Veterans Administration Hospital

In at least one important way, an erroneous conclusion was reached from animal experimentation about the technical requirements for successful orthotopic transplantation of the human liver. During the anhepatic phase, it is necessary to cross-clamp the great veins which drain the intestine and the lower half of the body. It was soon learned that normal dogs rapidly developed shock and almost inevitably failed to survive operation if the stagnant venous pools were not decompressed. Eventually, methods were developed in which external plastic catheters were used to temporarily permit runoff from the occluded inferior vena caval and splanchnic systems into the cervical veins, bypassing the obstruction.[1, 3] The same precaution was taken in the first clinical attempts at liver replacement.[5]

Subsequent experience has proved that simultaneous occlusion of the portal vein and inferior vena cava can be tolerated in human subjects for a long enough time to permit recipient hepatectomy and the insertion of a new liver.[2, 4] It has been suggested that the relative safety with which this could be done was due to the presence of venous collaterals secondary to the underlying hepatic disease.[2]

In the present study, this hypothesis has been tested in dogs. Liver injury was produced by ligation of the common duct. Several months later, orthotopic homotransplantation was performed without any provision for venous decompression.

Supported by United States Public Health Service Grants AM-06344, HE-07735, AM-07772, AI-04152, FR-00051, FR-00069, AM-12148, and AI-AM-08898.

Received for publication Jan. 9, 1969.

METHODS

Twelve mongrel dogs weighing 10 to 25 kilograms were subjected to cholecystectomy and ligation and division of the common duct. In addition, all periportal tissue was also divided sparing only the skeletonized hepatic artery and portal vein. Portal pressure was measured.

Two to 3 months later, the animals were re-explored and the portal pressure was determined again. Orthotopic hepatic transplantation was then carried out with nonrelated mongrel donors of approximately matching size. The vascular structures entering and leaving the liver were all reconnected with end-to-end anastomoses. During the anhepatic phase external bypasses were not used. Postoperatively, the animals were treated with azathioprine, prednisolone, and horse anticanine-lymphocyte globulin.

RESULTS

At the time of the first operation, the portal pressures ranged from 7 to 13 cm. of water. Postoperatively, the stools became acholic. The serum bilirubins rose to 4 to 13 mg. percent along with marked rises in the alkaline phosphatase, serum glutamic oxalacetic transaminase, and serum glutamic pyruvic transaminase. Eventually, the animals became wasted and had prolonged prothrombin times. The serum protein concentrations fell from about 6 Gm. percent to an average of 3.5 Gm. percent. Half the dogs developed ascites, and in two of these there was over 5 L. of intraperitoneal fluid at the time of re-exploration; the latter two animals had become azotemic by this time. Death terminated two of the 12 experiments before transplantation could be attempted.

The 10 remaining dogs were subjected to orthotopic liver transplantation despite the fact that they were all seriously ill by this time. Upon reopening the abdomen, portal pressures were measured at 27 to 35 cm. of water. Extensive venous collaterals were found in the abdominal wall, the retroperitoneal space, and in all the viscera. The presence of large and thin-walled veins in the gastrohepatic ligament made dissection of the portal triad unusually difficult. During the anhepatic phase when the portal vein and inferior vena cava were cross-clamped for 45 to 60 minutes, the intestines remained pink and motile.

One of the dogs was lost intraoperatively because of a technical accident. Two more died 1 day later without having regained consciousness. The other seven recovered promptly from anesthesia and were able to walk around on the following day; several began to eat. There was invariably a prompt alleviation of the hyperbilirubinemia and usually the depressed prothrombin times were restored toward normal. However, all seven animals which survived operation died after 3 to 10 days. Their extremely debilitated state seemed to be the most important factor. Pneumonitis was regularly found. None of the dogs had secondary rises in serum bilirubin before death, although some of the livers had pathologic findings suggestive of early rejection.

DISCUSSION

When the portal vein and suprarenal inferior vena cava are abruptly cross-clamped in normal dogs, a dramatic and rapidly evolving lethal syndrome is produced. Within a few minutes the intestines become first deeply cyanotic and then black. The kidneys and the other contents of the retroperitoneal space undergo similar changes. The blood pressure falls precipitously, and death usually follows within 20 to 30 minutes.

None of these events in the present study were observed in the animals which had been conditioned by long-term extrahepatic biliary obstruction. These dogs had developed extensive venous collaterals and moderate portal hypertension. Obstruction of the great veins draining the splanchnic bed and the lower portion of the body for as long as 1 hour did not cause grave cardiodynamic consequences. The intestines did not change color at all. These observations support the hypothesis that the presence of hepatic disease eliminates or reduces the need for decompressing bypasses during the anhepatic phase of orthotopic liver transplantation.

SUMMARY

After common duct ligation in dogs, it is possible within 2 to 3 months to safely cross-clamp the portal vein and suprarenal inferior vena cava for at least 1 hour during the course of orthotopic liver replacement. The lack of serious hemodynamic consequences under these circumstances as opposed to those in normal animals is apparently explained by the increased venous collaterals that develop in the course of liver disease.

REFERENCES

1. Moore, F. D., Wheeler, H. B., Demissianos, H. V., Smith, L. L., Balankura, O., Abel, K., Greenberg, J. B., and Dammin, G. J.: Experimental whole organ transplantation of the liver and of the spleen, Ann. Surg. **152:** 374, 1960.
2. Starzl, T. E., Groth, C. G., Brettschneider, L., Moon, J. B., Fulginiti, V. A., Cotton, E. K., and Porter, K. A.: Extended survival in 3 cases of orthotopic homotransplantation of the human liver, SURGERY **63:** 549, 1968.
3. Starzl, T. E., Kaupp, H. A., Brock, D. R., Lazarus, R. E., and Johnson, R. U.: Reconstructive problems in canine liver homotransplantation with special reference to the post-

operative role of hepatic venous flow, Surg. Gynec. & Obst. **111:** 733, 1960.

4. Starzl, T. E., Marchioro, T. L., Huntley, R. T., Rifkind, D., Rowlands, D. T., Jr., Dickinson, T. C., and Waddell, W. R.: Experimental and clinical homotransplantation of the liver, Ann. New York Acad. Sc. **120:** 739, 1964.
5. Starzl, T. E., Marchioro, T. L., von Kaulla, K., Hermann, G., Brittain, R. S., and Waddell, W. R.: Homotransplantation of the liver in humans, Surg. Gynec. & Obst. **117:** 659, 1963.

Effects of phytohemagglutinin on humoral antibody response, delayed hypersensitivity, and homograft rejection

KEIJI ONO, M.D.
HERVE BLANCHARD, M.D.
NOBORU KASHIWAGI, M.D.
RODERICK N. M. MacSWEEN, M.B.
HENRY N. CLAMAN, M.D.
THOMAS E. STARZL, M.D.
DENVER, COLO.
From the Departments of Surgery, Pathology, and Medicine, The University of Colorado School of Medicine and the Veterans Administration Hospital

Phytohemagglutinin (PHA), a mucoprotein derived from the red kidney bean, *Phaseolus vulgaris,* has erythroagglutinating and leukoagglutinating properties and stimulates the small lymphocytes of the peripheral blood to transform into large blast cells.[4, 5, 16, 18] When administered parenterally, it can suppress the immune response in animals, if treatment is started several days before the antigenic stimulation.[7, 8, 10, 12, 15, 18, 19]

To our knowledge 6 studies have been reported concerning the effect of PHA on the survival of skin or renal homografts, with conflicting results.[2, 3, 6, 13, 14, 17] Calne and associates[2] and Casciani and Cortesini[3] treated canine recipients of renal allografts solely with PHA and found a slight immunosuppressive activity; the effect was additive to that of azathioprine if the 2 agents were given together. Two of 4 publications concerned with skin grafts in rodents and rabbits reported no detectable effect of PHA,[6, 13] but the other 2 claimed slight prolongation of skin viability.[15, 17]

In our laboratory the immunosuppressive qualities of a particular batch of PHA were evaluated by the ability of this agent to blunt humoral antibody formation in rabbits, to suppress the development of delayed hypersensitivity reactions in guinea pigs, and to mitigate the rejection of renal homografts in dogs. In addition the effect of red cell absorption on the biologic activity of PHA was assessed.

METHODS

Effect of absorption. The preparation and characteristics of this PHA batch* were described by Hurn,[11] who reported that it was able to agglutinate both red and white blood cells. An attempt was made in the present study to remove the hemagglutinins by doubly absorbing 1 volume of reconstituted PHA solution with 1.5 volumes of packed canine red blood cells. On both occasions the mixture was incubated at 4° C. for 30 minutes.

The effect of the procedure was quantitated in 2 ways. The first was by measurement of the hemagglutinin and leukoagglutinin titers of the PHA solution before and

Supported by United States Public Health Service Grants AM-06344, HE-07735, AM-07772, FR-00051, AI-04152, FR-00069, AM-12148, and AI-AM-08898.
Received for publication Jan. 20, 1969.

*The desirability of performing this study was suggested to us by Dr. Maurice Landy of Bethesda, Md. He also assisted in formulating the experimental protocol. The PHA used, Phytoclin Batch E313, was obtained by Dr. George Hitchings from the Wellcome Research Laboratories, Beckenham, England. The desiccated PHA was reconstituted by adding 1 ml. normal saline to 10 mg. of the powder before use.

after absorption with red blood cells, making use of standard twofold dilution techniques. For both examinations 0.1 ml. reconstituted PHA was the original volume from which dilution was begun; 0.1 ml. of a 2 percent suspension of triply washed canine red blood cells or, alternatively, 0.1 ml. of a canine leukocyte suspension (corrected to 5,000 per cubic millimeter) was added at each dilution and the presence of agglutination determined microscopically.

Second, both the absorbed and unabsorbed PHA solutions were tested for their mitogenic effect on the lymphocytes of human peripheral blood. Human instead of canine white blood cells were used because they are so much more easily grown in culture. The cultures were adjusted to contain 10^6 lymphocytes and various doses of the PHA solution were instilled. After 69 hours, ^{3}H-thymidine (2 μc per tube) was added. The cells were harvested 3 hours later. The results of thymidine uptake were expressed as mean counts per minute per tube.

Tests of immunosuppression.

Humoral antibody. Four rabbits of about 2.5 kilograms were immunized with 1 ml. per kilogram of 20 percent sheep red blood cells (SRBC) intravenously on Day 0. They were treated daily with 1 ml. per kilogram unabsorbed PHA intraperitoneally from Day –2 to Day 4. Another 4 rabbits of similar weight were immunized with the same amount of SRBC on Days 0 and 10 and were treated with PHA for 7 days starting on Day 8. As control animals 5 rabbits were immunized with SRBC on Days 0 and 10 and received no treatment. In all 3 groups hemagglutinin titrations were performed every other day beginning Day –2.

Delayed hypersensitivity. Twenty-five guinea pigs weighing 600 to 700 grams were immunized subcutaneously on Days 0 and 7 with a 0.25 mg. water-in-oil suspension of killed tubercle bacilli.* Thirty-four days after the initial immunization, the guinea pigs were divided into 4 groups for single intraperitoneal injections as follows: 5 animals, 10 mg. unabsorbed PHA; 5 animals, 5 mg. unabsorbed PHA; 4 animals, 2.5 mg. unabsorbed PHA; and 7 animals, 2.5 mg. absorbed PHA. A fifth group consisted of 4 animals which were untreated control animals.

Two days after the injections, each of the guinea pigs was challenged intracutaneously with 0.1 ml. of the standard strengths of purified protein derivatives (PPD). Induration at the PPD inoculation sites was measured after 24 to 48 hours.

Canine renal transplantation. Pelvic renal transplantation was performed in adult unrelated mongrel donors and recipients with concomitant removal of both kidneys of the recipient. Five experiments were discarded because of vascular thromboses within the first 6 days. The animals had biweekly determinations of the leukocyte count, peripheral smear, hematocrit, and BUN. At autopsy, the renal homograft, spleen, liver, lung, heart, and mesenteric lymph nodes were examined. In the test animals, the PHA was given subcutaneously each day beginning on Day –2 and continuing for at least 2 weeks in animals which survived that long. There were 4 experimental groups. Eleven animals received no treatment; 8 animals, 2.5 mg. per kilogram unabsorbed PHA per day; 6 animals, 2.5 mg. per kilogram absorbed PHA per day; and 6 animals, 5.0 mg. per kilogram absorbed PHA per day.

RESULTS

Effects of absorption.

Titers. The unabsorbed PHA solution (10 mg. per milliliter) had hemagglutinin and leukoagglutinin titers of 1:256 and 1:512. After double absorption with red blood cells, these declined to 1:8 and 1:256, respectively.

Mitogenic activity. The unabsorbed PHA killed all cells at a dose of 1 mg., whereas the same quantity of the absorbed material both killed and stimulated (Table I). In smaller amounts (particularly well seen with 0.001 mg.), the unabsorbed PHA was many times more potent in stimulating blast transformation. Thus the absorption process had

*Three other control animals were inoculated with a water-in-oil suspension without killed tubercle bacilli. They did not become purified protein derivative–positive.

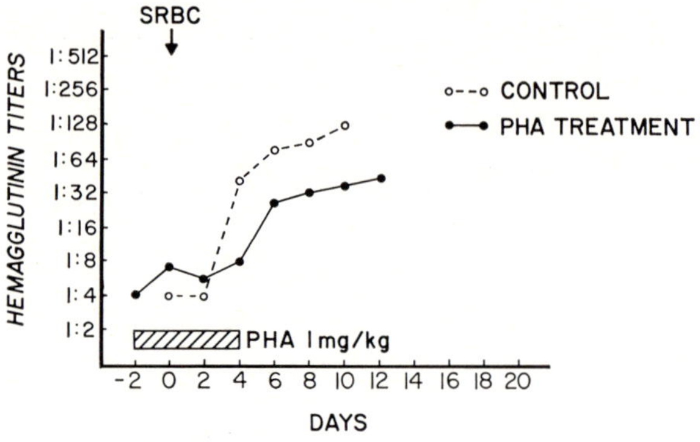

Fig. 1. The suppressive effect of unabsorbed PHA on the hemagglutinin response of rabbit immunized intravenously with sheep red blood cells (SRBC). The results in the 2 groups were pooled from 4 PHA-treated and 5 control animals.

Table I. *^{3}H-thymidine uptake of tissue-cultured human peripheral lymphocytes*

Dose of PHA in mg./tube	*Control (c.p.m.)*	*Nonabsorbed (c.p.m.)*	*Absorbed (c.p.m.)*
0	865		
1.0		87	24,690
0.1		6,335	90,230
0.01		76,950	118,780
0	1,070		
0.01		50,350	72,020
0.001		58,760	4,700
0.0001		1,645	1,245

Table II. *The toxicity and immunosuppressive effect of PHA in guinea pigs previously immunized with killed tubercle bacilli*

Group	*48 hour mortality rate of PHA*	*Frequency of positive PPD skin tests (intermediate strength)**	
		24 hours	*48 hours*
10 mg.†	3/5	0/2	0/2
5 mg.†	3/5	0/2	0/2
2.5 mg.†	0/4	0/4	0/4
2.5 mg.‡	0/7	0/7	0/7
Control animals		3/4	3/4

*A positive skin test was defined as induration of 5 mm. or greater At full strength PPD, 3 of the 15 PHA-treated animals had positive skin tests as did all 4 of the control animals.

†Unabsorbed.

‡Absorbed.

significantly reduced the mitogenic quality.

Tests of immunosuppression.

Humoral antibody. In the rabbits the unabsorbed PHA suppressed but did not abolish the primary hemoagglutinin response to intravenous SRBC (Fig. 1). However, there was no effect whatever on the response to rechallenge when PHA was started 2 days before a supplementary dose of SRBC was given to a previously exposed animal.

Delayed hypersensitivity. Unabsorbed PHA in single 10 and 5 mg. injections intraperitoneally caused a 60 percent mortality rate within 48 hours (Table II). With 2.5 mg. no deaths occurred with either the absorbed or unabsorbed PHA. At all the PHA dose levels, the expression of delayed hypersensitivity to tuberculin was blunted or blocked compared with that in the control animals (Table II). There were no significant tuberculin reactions with the first and second strength PPD injections, although 3 of the 15 PHA-treated animals developed skin induration of 5 mm. or more at the site of the full strength PPD inoculation.

Canine renal transplantation. The PHA was toxic. Anorexia, diarrhea (often bloody), and weight loss were seen in most of the dogs. Some of the animals had remarkable swelling of the extremities in which the subcutaneous injections were given. Anemia was almost universal (Fig. 2). All the foregoing side effects were most severe and common in the dogs treated with unabsorbed PHA.

Table III. *The effect of absorbed and unabsorbed PHA on survival after canine renal transplantation*

Group	No. of dogs	Survival (days)	Range (days)	p
Control animals	11	9.0 ± 1.7 (S.E.)	4 to 21	
2.5 mg./kg.*	8	16.3 ± 2.3 (S.E.)	8 to 27	< 0.01
2.5 mg./kg.†	6	10.2 ± 1.3 (S.E.)	6 to 14	
5.0 mg./kg.†	6	25.4 ± 7.8 (S.E.)	5 to 52	< 0.01

*Unabsorbed.
†Absorbed.

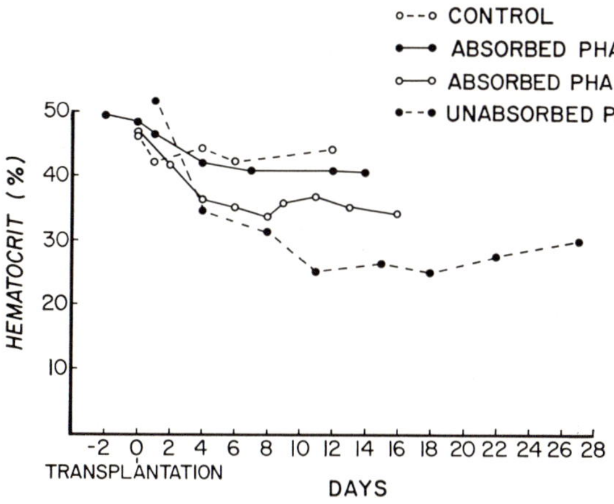

Fig. 2. The anemia seen in dogs subjected to renal homotransplantation and treated with either absorbed or unabsorbed PHA. Note that the hematocrit falls were most pronounced in the animals injected with unabsorbed PHA. The animals that contributed to each study group are the same as in Table III.

Treatment with PHA invariably induced a leukocytosis in the pretransplantation period, with the appearance of immature forms of all cell types. After transplantation there was no significant difference in the lymphocyte counts in the control animals as compared with those treated with PHA.

The results in these experiments are summarized in Table III. At doses of 2.5 mg. per kilogram per day, the animals receiving the unabsorbed PHA had a significantly prolonged survival ($p < 0.01$) whereas those treated with the absorbed material did not. The best results were with 5 mg. per kilogram per day of absorbed PHA (Table III). It was necessary to stop the injections in 3 dogs in the latter group 16, 23, and 32 days after transplantation because of a shortage of PHA. The dogs died of uremia 17, 29, and 8 days later (Fig. 3). On histologic examination, there were no distinguishing features of the homografts retrieved from the treated dogs as compared with those from the control animals. Both had classical evidence of rejection.

In the spleens of the animals treated with PHA, there was generally a reduced cellularity in the red pulp. Contrary to what has been reported in mice,[9] the white pulp was not hyperplastic and, if anything, seemed reduced in mass; this was particularly true if unabsorbed PHA had been given.

Extramedullary hematopoiesis in both the spleen and liver was common in the PHA-treated animals, especially prominently in those which had received the unabsorbed material and had developed severe anemia. Mild intrahepatic cholestasis was pres-

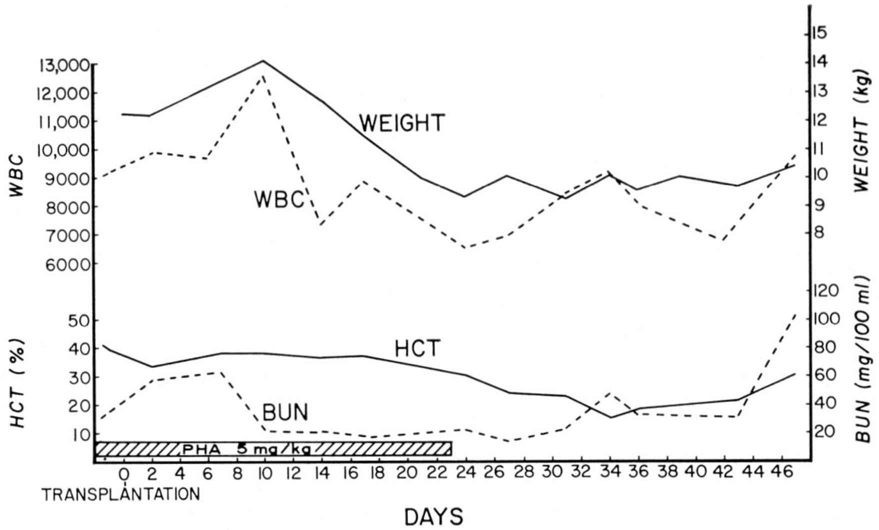

Fig. 3. The course of a dog after a renal homotransplantation from a nonrelated mongrel donor. Treatment was with 5 mg. per kilogram per day absorbed PHA; injections were stopped after 23 days. The dog developed rejection and died 52 days after operation. Note the progressive anemia and weight loss.

ent in the livers of several of the same dogs.

The most disquieting extrarenal finding was myocardial necrosis in 3 of the 12 PHA-treated animals from which the heart was examined histologically. The infarctions were of moderate size, were not transmural, and appeared to be 3 or 4 days old. The significance of these abnormalities is obscured by the fact that similar lesions can be caused in dogs by other kinds of trauma.[20]

DISCUSSION

The results of the present study add to the growing body of evidence that PHA is an immunosuppressive agent of intermediate effectiveness. Its ability to suppress a humoral antibody response has been most widely accepted[7, 8, 10, 12, 15, 18] and has been confirmed in our experiments. The striking way in which PHA partially or completely prevents the expression of a pre-existing state of delayed hypersensitivity has not been generally appreciated, the only other description of this effect being that of Stevens and Willoughby.[19]

Unfortunately, the side effects of the relatively unrefined PHA used in the present study were too severe to permit its use in clinical medicine. A number of deaths were caused in average-sized guinea pigs with a single intraperitoneal injection of 5 or 10 mg. In dogs given 2.5 or 5 mg. per kilogram, severe local reactions at the sites of injection were common. With continued treatment the animals became clinically ill. Anemia was often severe.

Hope that an improved PHA might be developed derives from the fact that some of the toxic properties can be largely removed by simple absorption technique. The investigations of Barkhan and Ballas[1] suggested that the leukoagglutinating and hemagglutinating activities of PHA were not closely interrelated. This observation was exploited in the present experiments by absorbing most of the hemagglutinating properties with red blood cells.

In doing so, there was a concomitant loss of some of the leukoagglutinating and mitogenic potential of the PHA solution as judged by both in vitro and in vivo testing. This necessitated upward dose adjustments in the transplantation experiments. Nevertheless, the absorbed PHA seemed to have an improved therapeutic index.

SUMMARY

Phytohemagglutinin (PHA) has been shown to inhibit the hemagglutinin response of rabbits to intravenous sheep red blood cells, to suppress the expression of pre-existing tuberculin sensitivity in guinea pigs, and to prolong the functional survival of renal homograft in dogs. Concomitant with these desired effects are a number of side reactions; sudden death can be caused in guinea pigs and in dogs, and anemia and wasting can be induced. The toxicity of PHA can be partly reduced by preliminary absorption with red cells.

REFERENCES

1. Barkhan, P., and Ballas, A.: Phytohaemagglutinin: Separation of haemagglutinating and mitogenic principles, Nature **200:** 141, 1963.
2. Calne, R. Y., Wheeler, J. R., and Hurn, B. A. L.: Combined immunosuppressive action of phytohaemmagglutinin and azothioprine (Imuran) on dogs with renal homografts, Brit. M. J. **2:** 154, 1965.
3. Casciani, C., and Cortesini, R.: Phytohemagglutinin action of renal homograft survival, *in* Curtoni, E. S., editor: Histocompatibility testing, 1967, Baltimore, 1967, The Williams & Wilkins Company, p. 83.
4. Claman, H. N., and Brunstetter, F. H.: Effects of antilymphocyte serum and phytohaemagglutinin upon cultures of human thymus and peripheral blood lymphoid cells. I. Morphologic and biochemical studies of thymus and blood lymphoid cells, Internat. Acad. Path. **18:** 757, 1968.
5. Cooper, H. L., and Rubin, A. D.: RNA metabolism in lymphocytes stimulated by phytohemagglutinin: Initial responses to phytohemagglutinin, Blood **25:** 1014, 1965.
6. Elves, M. W.: The in vivo effect of phytohemagglutinin on homograft reactions, Transplantation **5:** 1532, 1967.
7. Elves, M. W.: On the mechanism of action of phytohaemagglutinin on immunological reactions, Internat. Arch. Allergy **33: 353,** 1968.
8. Elves, M. W.: Suppression of antibody production by phytohaemagglutinin, Nature **213:** 495, 1967.
9. Gamble, C. N.: The effects of PHA on mouse spleen cells in vivo, Blood **28:** 175, 1966.
10. Gengozion, N., and Huebner, K. F.: Effect of phytohemagglutinin (PHA) on an antibody-forming system, J. Immunol. **99:** 184, 1967.
11. Hurn, B. A. L.: Preparation and partial characterisation of the mitogenic principle from *Phaseolus vulgaris* seeds, *in* Elves, M. W., editor: Proc. Symposium, The biological effects of phytohaemagglutinin, Oswestry, England, 1967, The Robert Jones and Agnes Hunt Orthopaedic Hospital Management Committee, p. 83.
12. Jennings, J. F., and Oates, C. M.: The effect of phytohaemagglutinin on the immune response in vivo, Clin. Exper. Immunol. **2:** 445, 1967.
13. Kehn, B., and Rigby, P.: Effects of phytohaemagglutinin on homograft rejection, Nature **217:** 182, 1967.
14. Markley, K., Evans, G., and Smallman, E.: Prolongation of skin allograft survival time by phytohaemagglutinin, Transplantation **5:** 1535, 1967.
15. Markley, K., Smallman, E., and Evans, G.: Decreased mouse circulating antibodies to sheep erythrocytes by phytohaemagglutinin, Internat. Arch. Allergy **32:** 482, 1967.
16. Nowell, P. C.: Phytohemagglutinin: An initiator of mitosis in cultures of normal human leukocytes, Cancer Res. **20:** 462, 1960.
17. St. Pierre, R. L., Younger, J. B., and Zmijewski, C. M.: Effect of phytohemagglutinin on skin allograft survival in mice, Proc. Soc. Exper. Biol. & Med. **126:** 687, 1967.
18. Spreafico, F., and Lerner, E. M., II: Suppression of the primary and secondary immune response on the mouse by phytohaemagglutinin, J. Immunol. **98:** 407, 1967.
19. Stevens, J. E., and Willoughby, D. A.: Phytohaemagglutinin and cell mediated hypersensitivity reactions in rat, Nature **215:** 967, 1967.
20. Tanturi, C., Mejia, R. H., Canepa, J. F., and Gomez, O. T.: Electrocardiographic and humoral changes in transient occlusion of the portal vein in the dog, Surg. Gynec. & Obst. **110:** 537, 1960.

Demonstration of humoral immunity against aortic leaflet heterografts

GEORGE E. PIERCE, M.D.
INGEGERD E. HELLSTRÖM, M.D., Ph.D.
HITOSHI MOHRI, M.D., D.M.Sc.
DENNIS D. REICHENBACH, M.D.
K. ALVIN MERENDINO, M.D., Ph.D.
SEATTLE, WASH.
From the Departments of Surgery, Microbiology, and Pathology and the First Surgical Service of the University Hospital, University of Washington School of Medicine

Aortic valve replacement with allogenic (homologous) leaflet grafts offers at least one advantage over currently available prostheses, i.e., an extremely low incidence of thromboembolism even without anticoagulation.[2, 4]

Because of difficulties inherent in the procurement of human leaflets there has been some recent interest in the use of xenografts (heterografts).[3, 16] The use of such grafts has been encouraged by the observation that allograft leaflets incite only a weak, if any, immune reaction.[10, 13, 14] Viable donor leaflet cells have been found as late as 1 year following the transplantation of aortic leaflets in the subcoronary position in dogs.[14] It has been assumed that either the relatively hypocellular valves are nonantigenic or that the subcoronary position is an "immunologically privileged site."

The data currently available on the immunogenicity of leaflet xenografts are inconclusive. The problem has been complicated by the use of nonsterile leaflets[9]; the inflammation present in some of these transplants may be secondary to bacterial contamination. The present study, therefore, was designed to determine whether xenograft leaflets placed in the subcoronary position can incite a specific immunologic response. Fresh, sterile aortic valve leaflets from sheep were transplanted to the subcoronary position in dogs. A search was made in the recipients for serum antibodies directed against sheep valve cells with an in vitro assay.[7]

METHODS AND MATERIALS

Single cusp replacement with a xenogenic aortic leaflet was performed in eight adult male mongrel dogs which weighed 15 to 20 kilograms; total circulatory arrest was used with the aid of surface-induced deep hypothermia.[11]

Fresh valves were obtained from female sheep under sterile conditions and preserved in lactated Ringer's solution for periods of 60 minutes or less. One leaflet was preserved for tissue culture as described subsequently. Another was prepared as a single cusp graft consisting of the leaflet, adjacent aortic wall, and a thin margin of myocardium below the cusp. The noncoronary leaflet of the recipient was excised and the single cusp graft inserted with two rows of continuous suture.[1, 12]

Postoperatively, the dogs received tetracycline and penicillin for 14 days; no immunosuppressive drugs or anticoagulants were administered.

The sheep leaflet used for tissue culture

Aided in part by funds accruing from United States Public Health Service Grants HE-03379-10 and 11-6165 and GM-13543 and a grant from the Washington State Heart Association.

Received for publication Feb. 3, 1969.

was cut into fine pieces, sandwiched between two coverslips, and placed in Leyton tubes partially filled with Waymouth's medium. The tubes were incubated at 37° C., and the pH was maintained with variable inflow of carbon dioxide. After approximately 2 weeks the leaflet fibroblasts were removed from the coverslips by trypsinization and transferred as single cell suspensions to 6 ounce culture bottles filled with Waymouth's tissue culture media containing 20 percent newborn calf serum.

The dog sera were obtained from the experimental group just prior to operation and at different times following insertion of the leaflets. Samples were also obtained from control dogs which had undergone other thoracic or abdominal operations within 2 weeks to 2 months prior to serum sampling. The sera were extracted from clotted blood obtained by venipuncture, heated at 56° C. for 30 minutes, and stored at –20° C.

When the sheep fibroblasts had grown in sufficient amounts (i.e., usually within 2 weeks), the cells were trypsinized and then suspended in conditioned Waymouth's medium containing 40 percent fetal calf serum. A volume of 0.1 ml. of cell suspension containing 2 or 4 $\times 10^5$ cells per milliliter was added to each of a series of tubes containing 0.1 ml. of the recipient dog's sera in various dilutions.

The mixtures were then incubated for 20 minutes at 37° C. after which 0.8 ml. of a pool of previously tested rabbit complement (C'_1) diluted 1:6 or 1:10 was added. After another 60 minutes of incubation, the content of each tube was diluted with 15 ml. of Waymouth's medium containing 40 percent fetal calf serum and plated into 50 mm. plastic Petri dishes in aliquots of 4 ml. containing either 500 or 1,000 cells. Control groups were usually included with complement inactivated by heating at 56° C. for 30 minutes.

The dishes were incubated for 7 days, then gently washed with phosphate-buffered saline, and stained with crystal violet. The cell colonies were counted under a stereomicroscope.

Three or four Petri dishes were included for each group and the mean colony counts ± the standard errors of the means were calculated for each group. The percentage reduction in colony counts obtained with postoperative sera compared with preoperative sera was then determined, and the statistical significance of these reductions was calculated with Student's t test.

RESULTS

The percentage reductions obtained from seven different experiments comparing pre- and postoperative sera from six different leaflet recipients are given in Table I. Counts ranged from 30 to 70 colonies per dish (varying with different experiments) in the groups treated with preoperative or control sera.

From each of the six experimental dogs, serum samples obtained within 10 days to 2 months following implantation of a sheep leaflet were highly toxic to sheep fibroblasts when compared with peroperative samples. The percentage reductions ranged from 64 to 100 percent, and, in most cases, these reductions were highly significant, i.e., $p \leqq 0.001$. Even with serum dilution of 1:32 there was marked inhibition of sheep fibroblast growth. (See Experiments 5, 6, and 7 in Table I.)

The reductions were completely complement dependent except for postoperative serum from R25 (Experiments 4 and 6) which was toxic at a dilution of 1:8 in the absence of complement.

None of the sera from five control dogs was toxic when compared with the preoperative samples from the experimental animals.

DISCUSSION

The colony inhibition assay was first developed by one of the authors (I. H.) as an in vitro technique for the demonstration of immune reactions against tumor-specific transplantation antigens.[7] In this assay death or growth inhibition of the target cells is reflected by a decrease in the number of colonies formed by the cells when exposed to experimental sera in the presence of com-

Table I. *Percent of reduction in colony counts of sheep fibroblasts when exposed to preoperative as compared with postoperative dog sera*

Recipient No.	Experiment No.	Time interval between operation and serum sampling	Active pooled rabbit complement C'₁ — Serum dilutions 1:8 (%)	1:16 (%)	1:32 (%)	Heat-inactivated pooled rabbit complement C'₁ — Serum dilutions 1:8 (%)	1:16 (%)	1:32 (%)
R15	2	1 month	85			0		
R16	1	1 month	100					
R20	3	10 days	68			0		
R22	4	2 months	100	100		0	0	
R22	5	2 months	100	97	88	0	0	
R22	6	2 months	94*	74	64*	0	0	
R25	4	18 days	100	100		62†	0	
R25	6	18 days	100*	100	100	82	0	
R27	5	2 months	100	100	100	0	0	
R27	6	2 months	100*	100	100	0	0	
R27	7	2 months	100	100	100	0	0	

All reductions significant at $p \leq 0.001$ unless otherwise noted.
*Significant at $p \leq 0.01$.
†Significant at $p \leq 0.02$.

plement. The technique has also been modified to detect lymphocyte-mediated immune reactions and has been used extensively in a number of tumor systems.[5, 6, 8] The present experiments suggest that the colony inhibition assay may also be applied to the study of certain problems related to transplantation of normal tissues.

When tested with serum dilutions of 1:8 and 1:16, the sera from all six dogs obtained from 10 days to 2 months following implantation of a sheep leaflet were highly toxic to sheep fibroblasts grown in tissue culture. When tested in the absence of active complement the toxicity of postoperative serum compared with preoperative serum samples was generally abolished. Thus, this toxicity was specific and appears to represent an immune reaction mediated by dog serum antibodies directed against sheep fibroblasts.

The possibility cannot be excluded that the operation nonspecifically stimulated a rise in pre-existing heteroantibodies which were toxic for sheep cells. However, none of five different control sera obtained following several different thoracic and abdominal operations was toxic when compared with the preoperative sera of the experimental group. Therefore, it appears likely that the immune reactions demonstrated in these experiments are specific, i.e., induced by the transplanted sheep leaflets.

On the basis of the present in vitro findings, death of the sheep cells would be expected within a few weeks following transplantation. Parallel studies that were done with sex chromatin markers confirm this prediction and are the basis of another report.[15]

To what extent, if any, the functionally important properties of leaflet connective tissue are dependent upon the presence of viable fibroblasts is unknown. Neither is it known what degree of inflammation accompanies immune destruction of the fibroblasts and whether this inflammation, if any, affects the mechanical properties of the leaflet. It can only be stated that transplantation of xenograft leaflets does incite a humoral immune response which is toxic to the donor fibroblasts. The practical effects that this immunity might have on long-term function of the leaflets remain unknown.

SUMMARY

Serum samples obtained from dogs within 10 days to 2 months following subcoronary implantation of sheep aortic leaflets were cytotoxic to sheep fibroblasts grown in tissue culture. This toxicity or growth inhibition was complement dependent, a finding which suggests that the dogs developed a specific humoral immune response directed against the sheep fibroblasts.

REFERENCES

1. Barnes, R. W., Mohri, H., and Merendino, K. A.: Experimental aortic valve homotransplantation without cardiopulmonary bypass, Surgery **64:** 647, 1968.
2. Barratt-Boyes, B. G., Lowe, J. B., Cole, D. S., and Kelly, D. T.: Homograft valve replacement for aortic valve disease, Thorax **20:** 495, 1965.
3. Binet, J. P., Carpentier, A., and Langlois, J.: Clinical use of heterografts for replacement of the aortic valve, J. Thoracic & Cardiovas. Surg. **55:** 238, 1968.
4. Davies, H., Missen, G. A. K., Blandford, G., Roberts, C. I., Lessof, M. H., and Ross, D. N.: Homograft replacement of the aortic valve: A clinical and pathologic study, Am. J. Cardiol. **22:** 195, 1968.
5. Hellström, I., Hellström, K. E., and Pierce, G. E.: In vitro studies of immune reactions against autochthonous and syngenic mouse tumors induced by methylcholanthrene and plastic discs, Internat. J. Cancer **3:** 3467, 1968.
6. Hellström, I., Hellström, K. E., Pierce, G. E., and Bill, A. H.: Demonstration of cell-bound and humoral immunity against neuroblastoma cells, Proc. Nat. Acad. Sc. **60:** 1231, 1968.
7. Hellström, I., and Sjögren, H. O.: Demonstration of H-2 isoantigens and polyoma specific tumor antigens by measuring colony formation in vitro, Exper. Cell Res. **40:** 212, 1965.
8. Hellström, I., and Sjögren, H. O.: In vitro demonstration of humoral and cell-bound immunity against common specific transplantation antigen(s) of adenovirus 12-induced mouse and hamster tumors, J. Exper. Med. **125:** 1105, 1967.
9. Kwong, K. H., Paton, B. C., and Hill, R. B., Jr.: Experimental use of immunosuppression in aortic valve homografts and heterografts, J. Thoracic & Cardiovas. Surg. **54:** 199, 1967.
10. Lower, R. R., Pillsbury, R. C., Angell, W. W., and Kosek, J. C.: Homograft heart valves, Circulation **33:** 135, 1966. (Suppl.)
11. Mohri, H., Hessel, E. A., II, Nelson, R. J., Matano, I., Anderson, H. N., Dillard, D. H., and Merendino, K. A.: The use of rheomacrodex and hyperventilation in prolonged circulatory arrest under deep hypothermia induced by surface cooling: A method for open heart surgery in infants, Am. J. Surg. **112:** 241, 1966.
12. Mohri, H., Reichenbach, D. D., Barnes, R. W., and Merendino, K. A.: A biologic study of the homologous aortic valve in dogs, J. Thoracic & Cardiovas. Surg. **54:** 622, 1967.
13. Mohri, H., Reichenbach, D. D., Barnes, R. W., and Merendino, K. A.: Homologous aortic valve transplantation: Alterations in viable and nonviable valves, J. Thoracic & Cardiovas. Surg. **56:** 767, 1968.
14. Mohri, H., Reichenbach, D. D., Barnes, R. W., Nelson, R. J., and Merendino, K. A.: Studies of antigenicity of the homologous aortic valve, J. Thoracic & Cardiovas. Surg. **54:** 564, 1967.
15. Mohri, H., Reichenbach, D. D., Barnes, R. W., Pierce, G. E., Hellström, I. E., and Merendino, K. A.: Viable aortic valve heterotransplantation, Presented at the Meeting of the American Heart Association, Miami, Fla., Nov. 23, 1968.
16. O'Brien, M. F., and Clarebrough, J. K.: Heterograft valve transplantation for human valve disease, Australian M. J. **2:** 228, 1966

Autoradiographic studies on the incorporation of foreign DNA and RNA into kidney allografts

GOTTFRIED LEMPERLE
WOLF MICHAELIS
ULF WIECZOREK
FREIBURG, GERMANY
From the Department of Surgery, University of Freiburg

Since transplantation antigens are specific, they probably receive their characteristics from the template of the DNA and RNA existent in the cells. Therefore, a lasting change of antigenicity can possibly be obtained by changing the structure or the amount of the responsible nucleic acids. While for bacteria a genetic transformation through foreign DNA or RNA has been confirmed, this possibility for mammalian cells can only be assumed from various observations in tissue cultures.[1, 2, 4, 11] Our own experiments with skin allografts in inbred mice which had been incubated with recipient specific RNA or DNA showed a significant prolongation of survival time, indicating a certain effect of foreign nucleic acids on complete organs also.[8] Moreover, pilot studies on kidney allografts in dogs resulted in a significantly prolonged survival up to 52 days without immunosuppression when the kidneys were perfused with recipient RNA[6] or DNA[9] prior to transplantation.

In order to gain an insight into the fate of foreign nucleic acids in the different organs, first we perfused rat and rabbit kidneys with in vivo–labeled RNA or DNA and demonstrated their incorporation with the help of autoradiographies. Since there are no exact criteria besides the biologic proof of a genetic alteration through foreign nucleic acids, the value of autoradiography is limited to the study of optimal perfusion conditions.

Supported by the Wissenschaftliche Gesellschaft Freiburg.
Received for publication Feb. 8, 1969.

MATERIAL AND METHODS

Thymidine (methyl-H3) was injected intraperitoneally into four young Sprague-Dawley rats, which weighed about 50 grams, in rising doses every 8 hours up to a total of 1,080 μc for each animal. DNA was extracted from livers and spleens 8 hours after the last injection with the method of Marmur[10] with the aid of laurylsulfate and isoamyl alcohol.

Uridine (methyl-H3) was injected according to the same schedule into newborn rabbits, which weighed about 120 grams, up to a total of 1220 μc radioactivity. RNA was extracted from livers and spleens 1 hour after the last injection with the aid of acridine orange and ion exchange resin.[8]

The kidneys of 10 adult rats were then perfused in vivo with a standard perfusion solution[7] containing 5 percent dextran, heparin, procaine, tris buffer, and an optimal oxygen pressure. The labeled DNA was dissolved in this standard solution in concentrations of 40 or 80 μg per milliliter and perfused over 15 or 30 minutes at temperatures of 4, 20, and 37° C.

The same variations were used for the perfusion of 50 or 100 ml. of RNA (180 μg per milliliter) through the kidneys of eight adult rabbits. Control kidneys were perfused with 100 ml. of a 3H-thymidine (2.9 μc per milliliter) or a 3H-uridine (1.25 μc per milliliter) containing standard solution or of an unlabeled RNA or DNA solution of similar concentration.

After repeated rinsing, the kidneys were subsequently fixed in Bouin's fluid and histologically examined. The thickness of the sections was 1.5 to 3.0 μ. The autoradiographic work-up was made with the stripping film "Kodak AR 10" during 24 days. Homogenates of kidneys, livers, and spleens as well as samples of the in- and outflow were examined for content of labeled material in a liquid scintillation counter.

RESULTS

The autoradiographic sections of organs of those animals into which radioactive nucleosides had been injected showed, for example, a nuclear marking of only 42 percent of the spleen cells and 83 percent of the liver cells after 3H-thymidine injection, while only 25 percent of the spleen cells and 56 percent of the liver cells were clearly labeled after 3H-uridine injections. Since both extraction methods revealed approximately 80 percent of the total RNA or DNA, it can be assumed that less than 1 percent of the nucleic acids in the perfusion media were labeled.

The autoradiographies show in all experiments a relatively strong labeling of most cells after perfusion of DNA and RNA (Fig. 1). There were no labels found within the glomeruli, the endothelial cells of the vessels, and in the lumen of the tubuli. In general, the cytoplasm near the basement membrane showed a stronger radioactivity than the cytoplasm next to the lumen. The amount of incorporated labeled material after RNA perfusion was similar to that after DNA perfusion, even if there were obvious differences in the intracellular localization (Fig. 2).

After RNA perfusion, the greater amount of labels was found in the cytoplasm and only a few within the nucleus and there mainly within the nucleolus. In contrast, after DNA perfusion, a concentration of radioactive markers was obvious within the nuclei of the tubular cells. Figs. 3 and 4 demonstrate the amount of incorporated labeled material into tubular cells under various conditions. In each histologic section 200 tubules of the renal cortex with 1,500 to 2,000 cells were enumerated. Only those cells have been valued whose markings definitely exceeded the background. In DNA experiments, an optimal labeling was attained at 20° C. and a perfusion time of 30 minutes; in RNA experiments, at 37° C. after 15 minutes. As it has been demonstrated in RNA- or DNA-incubated skin allografts,[8] concentration of nucleic acids seems to be important for the

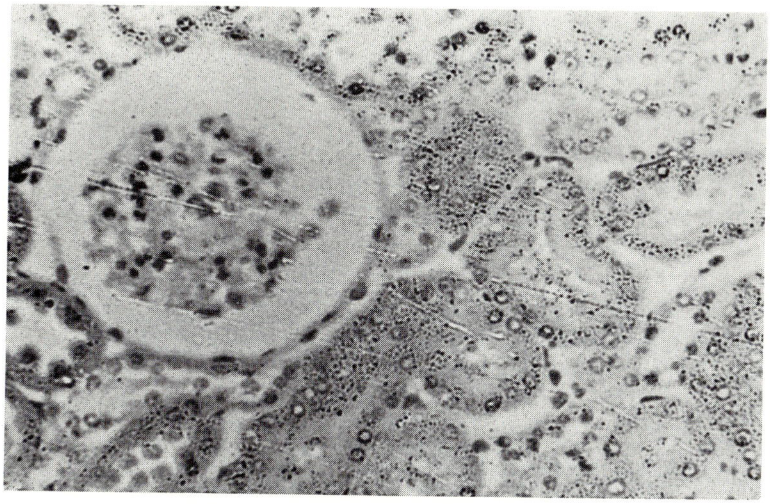

Fig. 1. Rat kidney after perfusion of 4 mg. of allogenic DNA at 20° C. 3H-labels are found within the nuclei and the cytoplasm of the tubular cells; the glomeruli are free of radioactive material. (Original magnification ×400.)

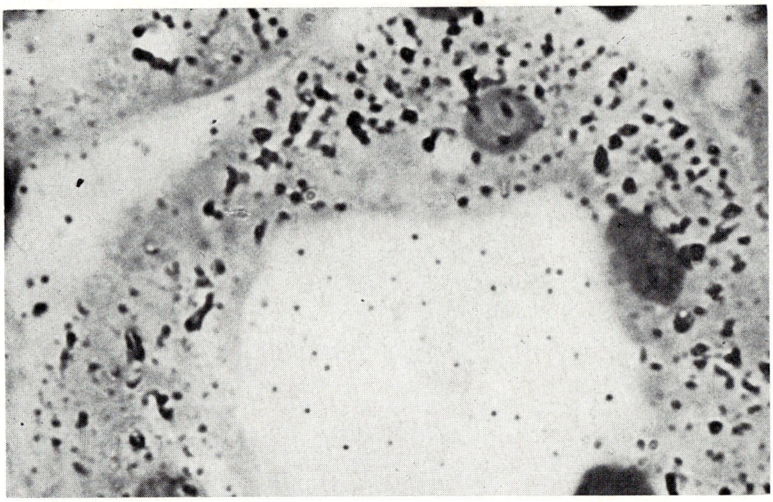

Fig. 2. Tubule of a rabbit kidney after perfusion of 18 mg. of RNA at 37° C. The labels are found preferably within the cytoplasm. (Original magnification ×1,600.)

incorporation. Since nucleic acids may be toxic in higher concentrations, studies on optimal perfusion conditions have to be subject to further investigation.

After the incorporation of foreign DNA or its breakdown products into the kidney tissue, an alteration of the cell nuclei follows. They swell, loosen centrally, and show a clearly recognizable nucleolus (Fig. 5). These alterations are not an effect of irradiation but of the DNA uptake itself, since the nuclei of kidney cells perfused with 3H-thymidine only had a normal homogeneous structure. In all histologic sections, three kinds of labeling were found; there were (1) a diffuse and uncharacteristic distribution of labels within the nuclei, (2) a concentration of labels in the periphery of the nuclei, and (3) a pronounced accumulation of 3H-labels around the nucleolus in the shape of a rosette. These findings probably are due to the 1.5 to 3 μ thin section out of a three dimensional 10 μ thick nucleus.

According to the radioactive counts in the in- and outflow as well as in the homogenized renal parenchymal tissue, an uptake of 2 to 4 percent of the labeled DNA and an uptake of 1 to 2 percent of the labeled RNA at a temperature of 20° C. could be calculated from the results of the liquid scintillation counter. Here too, the amount of incorporated DNA, RNA, or their breakdown products was proportional to the perfusion time, temperature, and concentration and reached a limit after 15 to 30 minutes. As it may be stated from the graphs (Figs. 3 and 4), there exists a marked difference in cell labeling after perfusion of labeled nucleic acids and the perfusion of pure 3H-thymidine or 3H-uridine, whose radioactivity was approximately tenfold higher.

DISCUSSION

The informative results of the autoradiographic studies on the uptake of 3H-labeled DNA and RNA in kidney parenchymal cells give only a clue in regard to optimal perfusion conditions. They permit no conclusions on the mechanism of incorporation. It must be assumed that a large part of DNA and RNA was degraded by intra- and extracellular DNase or RNase, respectively. Another part may enter the cells undegraded, either through active penetration similar to a viral infection or through passive incorporation by way of pinocytosis. Since the informative character of nucleic acids will not be altered essentially by extracellular destruction of the integrity of the molecules,[2] it seems to be of secondary significance whether whole DNA

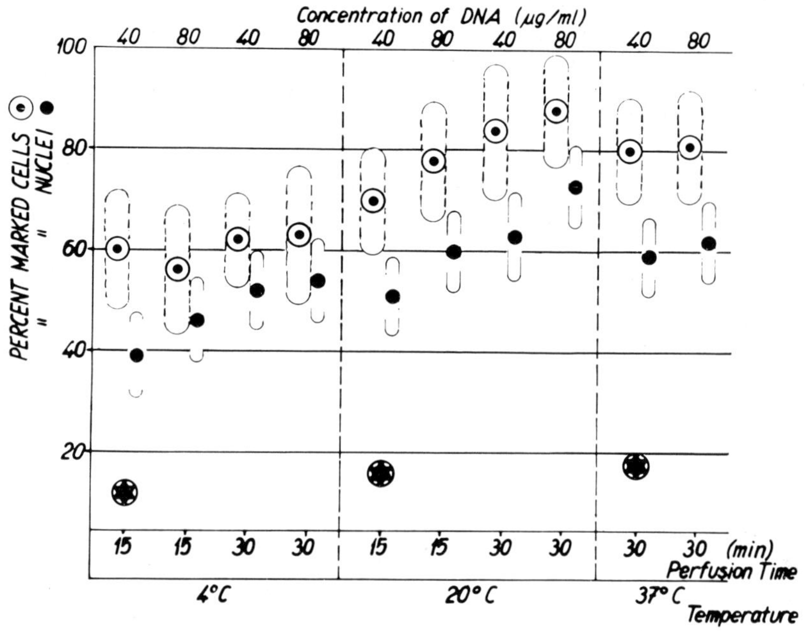

Fig. 3. The amount of labeling after DNA perfusion at various temperatures, concentrations, and perfusion times. The stars at the bottom express the labeled cells after perfusion with 150 μc 3H-thymidine solution.

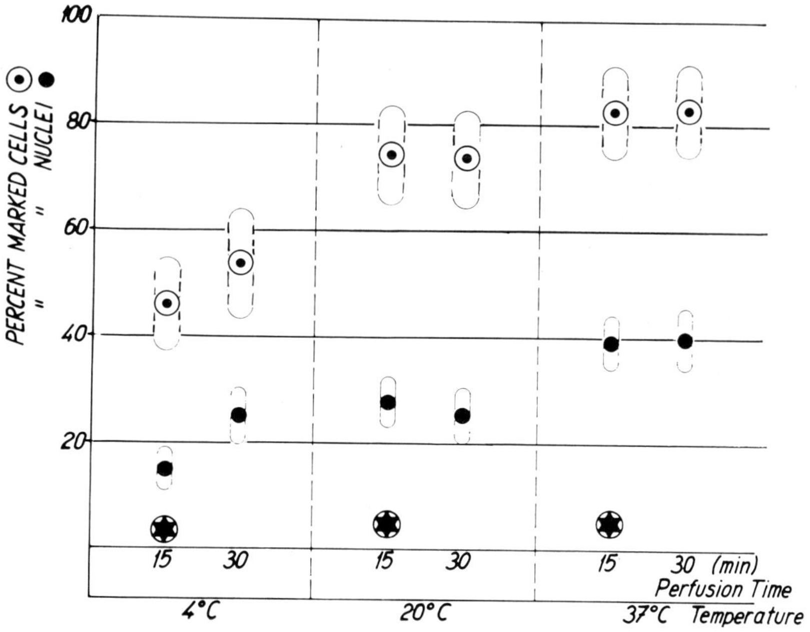

Fig. 4. The percentage of labeled cells and nuclei after perfusion with 9 or 18 mg. of allogenic RNA. The ellipsoids express the standard deviations. The differences between 4° C. and 37° C. perfusion temperature are statistically significant ($p < 0.01$).

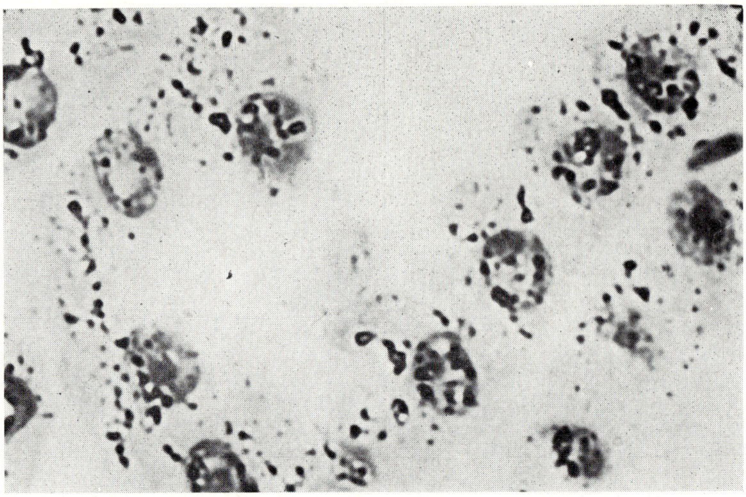

Fig. 5. Rat kidney tubule after 3H-thymidine–labeled DNA perfusion at 20° C. Note the swelling of the nuclei. (Original magnification ×1,200.)

or RNA molecules or their fragments pass the cell membrane. The assumed infectivity of nucleic acids might be increased, furthermore, by coating with simple proteins, as, for example, experiments with the addition of protamine to the incubation media have shown.[8, 12] According to the spectrophotometric biuret reaction, we expect a protein contamination of 0.5 to 1 percent of the DNA extracted after the method of Marmur[10] and the RNA extracted after our own method.[8]

From the results of transplantation experiments on skin[8] and kidneys,[6, 9] one can conclude that the used nucleic acids or its fragments are "biologically active," e.g., incubation or perfusion of allografts prior to the grafting procedure with nucleic acids diminished antigenicity significantly. Whether this effect is a specific or unspecific one, and whether exogenous nucleic acids affect the antigen production by a mere injury of the protein synthesis, by covering antigen recognition areas, or through actual genetic transformation, must be left undecided at this time.

SUMMARY

Pilot studies on kidney allografts in dogs resulted in a prolonged survival time up to 52 days without immunosuppression when the kidneys were perfused with recipient RNA or DNA prior to transplantation. In order to establish optimal perfusion conditions, the fate of tritium-labeled RNA and DNA was studied in kidneys from rabbits and rats. After perfusion with in vivo–labeled nucleic acids under certain conditions, kidney specimens were subjected to autoradiographic examinations and tested for tritium content in a liquid scintillation counter. After perfusion of DNA at 20° C. almost 100 percent of the tubular cells were labeled, preferably in the nuclear area. After perfusion with RNA most labels were found within the cytoplasm. The amount of incorporated RNA and DNA or their breakdown products was directly proportional to perfusion time, temperature, and concentration and reached a limit after 15 to 30 minutes. No labeled material was found within the glomeruli, blood vessels, and lumina of the tubules. Approximately 2 to 4 percent of the DNA labels and 1 to 2 percent of the RNA labels were incorporated by the kidneys at 20° C. or 37° C., respectively.

We are obliged to Priv. Doz. Dr. D. Hammer, Max-Planck-Institut für Immunbiologie, Freiburg, for his valuable assistance in preparing the autoradiographs.

REFERENCES

1. Bensch, K. G., and King, D. W.: Incorporation of heterologous deoxyribonucleic acid into mammalian cells, Science **133:** 381, 1961.
2. Bradley, T. R., Roosa, R. A., and Law, L. W.: DNA transformation studies with mammalian cells in culture, J. Cell & Comp. Physiol. **60:** 127, 1962.
3. Chorazy, M., Wilczok, T., Jergovic, D., and Mendecki, J.: Studies on adsorption of deoxyribo- and ribonucleic acids by neoplastic cells, Acta Unio internat. contra cancrum **20:** 1003, 1964.
4. Cohen, E. P., and Parks, I. P.: Antibody production by nonimmune spleen cells incubated with RNA from immunized mice, Science **144:** 1012, 1964.
5. Floersheim, G. L.: Aufnahme von vital H3-markierter Desoxyribonukleinsäure in Milz und Knochenmarkzellen in vitro, Nuclear-Medizin **2:** 295, 1962.
6. Groth, C. G., Porter, K. A., Daloze, P. M., Huguet, C., Smith, G. V., Brettschneider, L., and Starzl, T. E.: Effect of ribonucleic acid perfusion on canine kidney and liver homograft survival, SURGERY **64:** 31, 1968.
7. Largiadèr, F.: Organ transplantation, Stuttgart, 1966, Georg Thieme Verlag, p. 58.
8. Lemperle, G.: Prolonged survival of skin allografts after incubation with recipient DNA or RNA, J. S. Res. **8:** 511, 1968.
9. Lemperle, G., Hauptmann, A., Michaelis, W., Wieczorek, U., and Gaca, A.: Die Perfusion homologer Nieren mit Nucleinsäuren des Empfängers, Arch. klin. Chir. **322:** 1163, 1968.
10. Marmur, J.: A procedure for the isolation of deoxyribonucleic acid from micro-organisms, J. Molec. Biol. **3:** 208, 1961.
11. Niu, M. C.: The mode of action of ribonucleic acid, Develop. Biol. **7:** 379, 1963.
12. Yoon, C.: Incorporation of exogenous RNA into Nelson's ascites cells in vitro, Exper. Cell Res. **38:** 386, 1965.

The role of vasoconstriction in the suppression of hemorrhage from arteries. I. The completely severed artery

STEPHEN L. WANGENSTEEN, M.D.
STEPHEN F. KIECHEL, B.A.
ROBERT M. LUDEWIG, M.D.
JAMES J. MADDEN, JR., M.D.
CHARLOTTESVILLE, VA.
From the Department of Surgery, University of Virginia Medical Center

The thesis that the completely severed artery has the ability to constrict and thereby suppress the severity of hemorrhage has been accepted for many years. John Hunter[3] described the phenomenon of vasospasm and believed the contractile properties of the severed artery were natural mechanisms that reduced bleeding. In 1919 in a monograph entitled *Gunshot injuries to the blood-vessels,* Makins[5] discussed the retraction and spasm of the free ends of the completely divided artery which spontaneously stopped hemorrhage. In 1940 Cohen[1] examined traumatic spasm and postulated that the elastic recoil of the divided artery acted as a stimulus for initiating vasoconstriction which sealed the lumen of the vessel and stopped bleeding. More recently Saletta and Freeark,[6] in discussing partially severed arteries in man, assumed that vasoconstriction across the open lumen of a completely severed artery was one of the primary mechanisms that decreased the severity of hemorrhage. Decreased bleeding by vasoconstriction was not observed for the partially severed artery.

Makins[5] and Cohen[1] both observed that an artery which was divided with a blunt instrument often bled less than an atraumatic transection of an artery. Cohen[1] believed that this was a function of the amount of traumatic displacement of the vessel by the blunt instrument.

The purpose of the present study was to assess quantitatively the role of vasoconstriction in the control of hemorrhage from the completely severed femoral artery in the anesthetized dog.

MATERIALS AND METHODS

Twenty-seven mongrel dogs weighing 10 to 18 kilograms were anesthetized with sodium pentobarbital 25 to 30 mg. per kilogram intravenously. The dogs were divided into four groups: Group I—control; Group II—norepinephrine, maximal vasoconstriction; Group III—acetylcholine, maximal vasodilation; Group IV—blunt trauma. In all four groups, the superficial femoral artery was exposed as atraumatically as possible. In Groups I, II, and III, the superficial femoral artery was completely transected between the most distal muscular branch and the saphenous artery, with atraumatic technique, within 30 seconds after the topical administration of the specified solution. The transection was carefully positioned away from arterial branches to allow retraction of the artery. A double-edged, clefted cutting surface consisting of two overlapping No. 11 scalpel blades was used to transect the artery. In Group IV, the artery was initially traumatized by stretching and was transected with a blunt instrument—household wire clippers. In all dogs hemorrhage from the proximal end of the divided vessel

Supported by the United States Army Medical Research and Development Command, Department of the Army, under Research Contract 17-67-C-7039 and Grant HE-02038 from the National Institutes of Health.
Received for publication Feb. 3, 1969.

was allowed to occur for 2 minutes after transection.

Total blood volume was measured at the beginning of each experiment with radioactive iodinated serum albumin (RISA) and a Picker Hemoliter apparatus. The amount of bleeding in the 2 minute interval was determined by the sponge-weighing method. Arterial blood pressure was obtained by passing a polyethylene catheter from the carotid artery into the aortic arch. Blood pressure was monitored with an electronic transducer and was recorded on a multichannel recorder. All dogs were heparinized (1 mg. per pound) to eliminate coagulation factors which could influence the amount of hemorrhage.

Group I—control. The arteries of six dogs were treated topically over a 3 to 5 cm. length of superficial femoral artery with 2 ml. normal saline solution prior to atraumatic transection.

Group II—maximal vasoconstriction. The arteries of six dogs were treated topically over a 3 to 5 cm. length of artery with 2 ml. of a 10^{-3} solution of norepinephrine in normal saline prior to transection.

Group III—maximal vasodilation. The arteries of ten dogs were treated topically over a 3 to 5 cm. length of artery with 2 ml. of a 1 mg. per milliliter solution of acetylcholine in normal saline prior to transection.

Group IV—trauma. The arteries of five dogs were traumatically stretched and tented before transection with wire clippers which crushed the intima of the superficial femoral artery.

In four dogs, the topical effect of solutions of saline, norepinephrine, and acetylcholine on the rate of blood flow in the superficial femoral artery was measured with electronic blood flow transducers and an electromagnetic blood flowmeter. The arteries were not transected in these animals.

RESULTS

All results are summarized in Table I.

Group I—control. The mean blood loss from superficial femoral arteries pretreated with normal saline solution was 45.8 percent of the measured blood volume in 2 minutes (S.E. = 3.9). The mean decrease in arterial blood pressure was 70.1 percent (S.E. = 4.9) in 2 minutes. The average initial mean blood pressure of these dogs was 149 mm. Hg.

Group II—norepinephrine, maximal vaso-

Table I. *Blood loss and fall in blood pressure after artery transection in all groups*

	Group I—controls		*Group II—norepinephrine*		*Group III—acetylcholine*		*Group IV—trauma*	
Dogs in each group	*Blood loss (%)*	*Blood pressure loss (%)*	*Blood loss (%)*	*Blood pressure loss (%)*	*Blood loss (%)*	*Blood pressure loss (%)*	*Blood loss (%)*	*Blood pressure loss (%)*
1	34.5	77.8	4.9	12.5	37.2	88.6	26.7	57.0
2	38.0	47.7	35.2	84.2	44.0	93.3	35.5	49.0
3	40.0	82.0	19.5	25.8	22.0	17.0	24.4	35.1
4	58.8	68.7	24.7	72.0	36.0	75.0	45.0	88.8
5	53.3	75.0	20.7	29.2	47.2	81.0	35.0	91.0
6	49.3	70.3	33.0	73.5	36.9	64.4		
7					49.1	68.0		
8					32.7	54.0		
9					28.7	67.0		
10					26.9	77.0		
Mean % $\bar{x}$	45.8	70.1	23.0	47.9	36.2	68.7	33.3	64.2
Standard error	3.9	4.9	4.5	12.5	2.6	6.8	3.7	11.1
Average initial blood pressure	149		161		142		156	

constriction. The mean blood loss from arteries pretreated with norepinephrine was 23 percent in 2 minutes (S.E. = 4.5). The mean decrease in blood pressure was 47.9 percent in 2 minutes (S.E. = 12.5). The average and initial mean blood pressure of these dogs was 161 mm. Hg.

Group III—acetylcholine, maximal vasodilation. The average blood loss from arteries pretreated with acetylcholine was 36.2 percent in the 2 minute period (S.E. = 2.6). The average decrease in blood pressure was 68.7 percent in 2 minutes (S.E. = 6.8). The average initial mean blood pressure was 142 mm. Hg.

Group IV—trauma. The average blood loss was 33.3 percent in the 2 minute period of bleeding (S.E. = 3.7). The average decrease in blood pressure was 64.2 percent in 2 minutes (S.E. = 11.1). The average initial mean blood pressure of these dogs was 156 mm. Hg.

The local application of a 10^{-3} solution of norepinephrine decreased the average blood flow in the superficial femoral artery from 120 to 20 ml. per minute. A 1 mg. per milliliter solution of acetylcholine increased the average rate of blood flow from 120 to 400 ml. per minute. Normal saline produced no change in the rate of blood flow. The 1 mg. per milliliter solution of acetylcholine decreased the arterial blood pressure approximately 20 mm. Hg within 1 to 2 minutes after topical application. No change was observed in the arterial blood pressure following norepinephrine application.

DISCUSSION

Solutions of norepinephrine and acetylcholine were selected to establish the pharmacologic limits of vasomotor activity. It was believed that the topical application of norepinephrine would effect near maximal vasoconstriction and reduced blood flow and that the application of acetylcholine would cause near maximum vasodilation and increased blood flow. The results of blood flow studies on the superficial femoral artery with the use of blood flow transducers indicated that these pharmacologic agents did alter vasomotor tone on the intact blood vessel.

The control dogs in Group I and the dogs treated with acetylcholine in Group III bled significantly more during the 2 minute period of hemorrhage than the dogs treated with norepinephrine in Group ($p < 0.01$). In the present experiments the control dogs were observed to bleed more than the dogs treated with acetylcholine ($p < 0.05$). This observation possibly may be explained by blood pressure differences: (1) The topical application of acetylcholine lowered the systemic arterial blood pressure approximately 20 mm. Hg within 1 to 2 minutes, and (2) the mean initial blood pressure of the control dogs was slightly higher than the mean pressure for acetylcholine dogs. Prior studies from this laboratory using an ex vivo model system indicated that the rate of bleeding from an arterial laceration was related to the transmural pressure gradient by a derivation of the Bernoulli equation[2]:

$$Q = A \cdot \sqrt{\frac{2\ \Delta P}{\rho} + v^2}$$

where Q = rate of bleeding, A = area of the laceration, ΔP = transmural pressure gradient, ρ = density of fluid (blood), and v = mean velocity of flow. Therefore, as the arterial blood pressure is lowered the transmural pressure gradient (intraluminal pressure minus extraluminal pressure) is reduced and bleeding is retarded.

The dogs in Group IV that had blunt trauma to the arteries bled less than the control dogs in Group I ($p < 0.05$). However, the dogs in Group II that had topical application of norepinephrine bled less than the dogs given trauma to the arteries ($p < 0.1$).

The results of these studies in anesthetized dogs indicated that active vasoconstriction across the lumen of the transected superficial femoral artery as measured by blood loss did not occur to an extent to suppress hemorrhage significantly during a 2 minute period of observation. Further, blunt trauma and transection of an artery that included crushing of the intima did not result in the degree of suppression of hemorrhage that was achieved with pharmacologically induced vasoconstriction. In view of these findings, the long-held tenet that complete division of an artery results in the immediate retraction and vasospasm of the vessel sufficient to control hemorrhage must be seriously questioned.

SUMMARY

The role of vasoconstriction in the suppression of hemorrhage was studied in the completely severed artery. Twenty-seven mongrel dogs were divided into groups: Group I—control; Group II—norepinephrine, maximal vasoconstriction; Group III—acetylcholine, maximal vasodilation; Group IV—blunt trauma. Solutions of norepinephrine and acetylcholine were topically applied to an exposed segment of the superficial femoral artery to establish the limits of vasomotor activity. The superficial femoral artery was transected in a standardized manner with atraumatic technique. In Group IV, the artery was traumatized by stretching and was transected with a blunt instrument. Bleeding was allowed to continue for 2 minutes.

The control animals' arteries (Group I) bled as much as arteries treated with acetylcholine (Group III). The control animals' arteries and arteries pretreated with acetylcholine bled significantly more than the arteries of the dogs in the norepinephrine Group II. The dogs with traumatized arteries (Group IV) bled less than the control group ($p < 0.05$) but more than the norepinephrine group. Under the conditions of the experiment, active vasoconstriction across the lumen of the transected artery as measured by blood loss did not occur to a degree to suppress hemorrhage significantly unless the vessel was intentionally traumatized.

REFERENCES

1. Cohen, S. M.: Vasospasm, Guy's Hosp. Rep. **90:** 201, 1940.
2. Eddy, D. M., Wangensteen, S. L., and Ludewig, R. M.: The kinetics of fluid loss from leaks in arteries tested by an experimental ex vivo preparation and external counterpressure, SURGERY **64:** 451, 1968.
3. Hunter, J.: A treatise on the blood, inflammation, and gunshot wounds, Philadelphia, 1796, Thomas Bradford.
4. Kinmouth, J. B.: Traumatic vasospasm, Brit. M. J. **1:** 59, 1952.
5. Makins, G. H.: Gunshot injuries to bloodvessels, New York, 1919, W. Wood and Co.
6. Saletta, J. D., and Freeark, R. J.: The partially severed artery, **97:** 198, 1968.

Blood viscosity in the normal man

MARTIN S. LITWIN, M.D.*
KENNETH CHAPMAN, B.S.
J. BRUCE STOLIAR, M.D.**
NEW ORLEANS, LA.
From the Shock and Trauma Laboratory, Department of Surgery, Tulane University Medical School

Experimental studies in animals indicate that blood viscosity is an important determinant of peripheral blood flow and tissue perfusion. When blood viscosity is increased, tissue perfusion decreases and a tissue oxygen debt develops. Conversely, a decrease in blood viscosity leads to tissue perfusion increase and an increase in oxygen consumption.[3, 4]

Because of recent advances in instrumentation, blood viscosity determinations can now be performed practically in the clinical laboratory.[11] These may prove of use as guides to the peripheral circulatory status of certain patients and the clinical effectiveness of certain therapeutic regimens. Extensive research has been conducted in animals and certain limited experiments have been performed with reconstituted human blood specimens[1, 3, 4, 6-11]; however, the standard range of blood viscosity in the normal human has not been defined.

It was the purpose of this investigation to define blood viscosity range in the normal human and to correlate these standards with other parameters known to be of importance in the determination of blood viscosity.

Supported by contract DADA17-67-C-7049, Surgical Research Branch, United States Army Medical Research and Development Command, Office of the Surgeon-General.

Received for publication Feb. 3, 1969.

*Associate Professor of Surgery and Public Health Service Research Career Program Awardee 1-K3-HE-38, 604-01 from the National Heart Institute.

**Formerly Surgical Research Fellow.

METHODS

Fifty normal healthy adults, 39 men and 11 women, were studied. Excluded were those individuals with a history of either minor or major illness during the preceding 3 months, those with a possible history of chronic disease and menstruating women. When the investigators were satisfied that past history and physical examination were negative, a blood sample was obtained by venipuncture in a syringe lubricated with the minimal amount of heparin needed to prevent clotting.

Whole blood (WB) viscosity was measured immediately after withdrawal at varying shear rates and at 37.5° C. in a Wells-Brookfield synchrolectric viscometer for microsamples. While WB viscosity was being determined, the red cells in an unused portion of this sample were being separated by centrifugation for 30 minutes at 3,000 r.p.m. Supernatant plasma in this specimen was removed at once and packed cell (PC) and plasma (P) viscosities determined at varying rates of shear under the same conditions as when WB viscosity had been determined.

Hematocrit and corrected erythrocyte sedimentation rate (ESR) were determined by standard methods. Total red blood count was determined by counting the number of cells present in a cubic milliliter of blood in a microscope blood cell counting chamber or by counting in a Coulter counter. Total plasma protein, albumin, globulin, and fibrinogen concentrations were determined

Table I. *Blood viscosity determinants in normal humans*

Data	Composite average	Average by sex: Male	Average by sex: Female
Hematocrit (%)	45.9	46.4	41.9
Erythrocyte sedimentation rate (corrected—mm./hr.)	10.1	9.4	10.8
Red blood cell count (million cells/mm.^{3})	4.67	4.83	4.27
Total plasma protein (Gm. %)	7.3	7.4	7.2
Albumin (Gm. %)	4.3	4.4	4.2
Globulin (Gm. %)	3.0	3.0	3.0
Fibrinogen (mg. %)	220	240	200

Table II. *Whole blood viscosity curve in the normal human*

	Composite average		Average by sex: Male		Average by sex: Female	
Shear rate (sec.$^{-1}$)	Viscosity (cps)	S.D.	Viscosity (cps)	S.D.	Viscosity (cps)	S.D.
5.80	11.4	± 2.5	12.3	± 2.1	8.9	± 1.6
11.50	8.5	± 1.8	9.1	± 1.5	6.7	± 1.4
23.00	6.7	± 1.1	7.0	± 0.9	5.5	± 0.6
46.00	5.6	± 0.8	5.9	± 0.7	4.8	± 0.6
115.00	4.6	± 0.6	4.8	± 0.6	4.0	± 0.4
230.00	4.1	± 0.6	4.3	± 0.5	3.6	± 0.6
Average hematocrit	45.9%		46.4%		41.9%	

Table III. *Packed red cell viscosity curve in the normal human*

	Composite average		Average by sex: Male		Average by sex: Female	
Shear rate (sec.$^{-1}$)	Viscosity (cps)	S.D.	Viscosity (cps)	S.D.	Viscosity (cps)	S.D.
1.15	280.5	± 61.4	283.0	± 67.2	273.3	± 32.6
2.30	194.7	± 30.6	198.0	± 32.6	185.4	± 22.2
5.80	134.2	± 21.9	136.2	± 22.8	128.5	± 18.9
11.50	110.6	± 18.6	112.1	± 19.9	106.2	± 13.9
23.00	85.2	± 7.5	86.1	± 8.0	82.5	± 7.1

by the Howe[2] sodium sulfate system and checked for percent distribution of fractions on Sepraphore III strips in Gelman chambers.[5]

RESULTS

Average hematocrit, corrected ESR, red blood cell count, and total plasma protein, albumin, globulin, and fibrinogen concentrations for the composite group and for male and female subjects separately are shown in Table I. Average WB viscosities at varying shear rates ranging from 5.8 through 230 sec.$^{-1}$ for the composite group and separated by sex and their standard deviations (S.D.) are shown in Table II. Included in this chart is the average hematocrit. Average PC viscosities at varying shear

Table IV. *Plasma viscosity curve in the normal human*

	Composite average		*Average by sex*			
			Male		*Female*	
Shear rate ($sec.^{-1}$)	*Viscosity (cps)*	*S.D.*	*Viscosity (cps)*	*S.D.*	*Viscosity (cps)*	*S.D.*
23.00	1.8	± 0.4	1.8	± 0.5	1.7	± 0.4
46.00	1.6	± 0.5	1.6	± 0.5	1.5	± 0.4
115.00	1.4	± 0.1	1.4	± 0.2	1.4	± 0.2
230.00	1.4	± 0.1	1.4	± 0.1	1.4	± 0.1

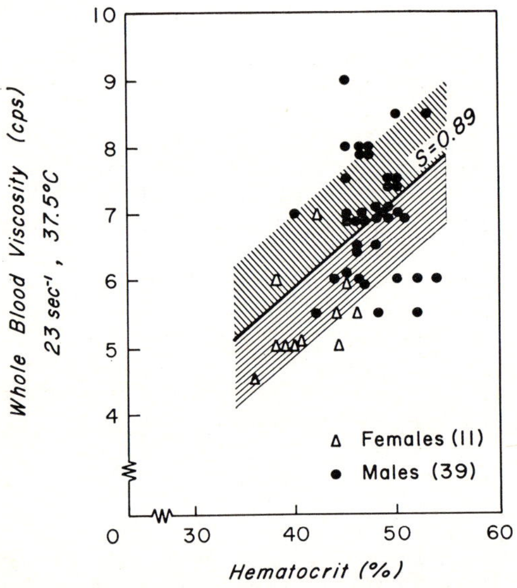

Fig. 1. Relation of whole blood viscosity at 23 $sec.^{-1}$ to hematocrit in the normal human. Hematocrit is the most important determinant of blood viscosity in the normal human; an almost direct relationship appears to exist. Correlation of the two is 78 percent, and the slope of the line is 0.890.

rates ranging from 1.15 through 23 $sec.^{-1}$ for the composite group and separated by sex and their S.D. are shown in Table III. Average P viscosities at varying shear rates ranging from 23 through 230 $sec.^{-1}$ for the composite group and separated by sex and their S. D. are shown in Table IV.

Coefficients of variation ($\underline{V}$) for whole blood at 23 $sec.,^{-1}$ that rate of shear which could be read out directly from the viscometer in centipoise (cps), were 16 percent for the composite sample, 13 percent for the men, and 11 percent for the women. When the composite sample was considered in determination of PC viscosity at this same shear rate, $\underline{V}$ were even less, 9 percent for the composite sample, 9 percent for the men and 9 percent for the women. P viscosity could be determined with only limited accuracy at 23 $sec.^{-1}$; $\underline{V}$ were 22 percent for the composite group, 28 percent for the men and 24 percent for the women. When shear rate was increased to 230 $sec.^{-1}$, $\underline{V}$ were only 7 percent for the composite group and 7 percent for each of the separate groups.

DISCUSSION

Hematocrit is the most important factor in the determination of WB viscosity in the normal human. In fact, an almost inverse relationship appears to exist between the two as shown in Fig. 1, where the slope of the line relating WB viscosity at 23 $sec.^{-1}$ to hematocrit is approximately 0.890, and there is a 78 percent correlation of the two.

When red blood count in millions was related to WB viscosity, correlation was only 38 percent and the slope of the line was 0.348. This was undoubtedly due to the fact that red blood counts in most of these experiments were performed visually in a counting chamber rather than in a more accurate electronic Coulter counter. Correlation with plasma albumin concentration was 4 percent, with globulin 2.8 percent and with fibrinogen 2.3 percent.

Together with platelets, the concentration of which cannot be determined with great accuracy by present methods, the parameters studied here are considered to be the most important affecting blood viscosity. Other factors, however, may also be of importance in producing blood viscosity changes. In Waldenstrom's macroglobulinemia, for instance, blood viscosity may be greatly increased by the accumulation in plasma of high molecular weight protein fractions. This is similar to the effect observed in animal experiments when high molecular weight dextran was infused.[4] The physiologic effect in these circumstances is the same as that observed when hematocrit is abnormally high, as in polycythemia vera. In the present studies the authors did not attempt to define these abnormal parameters or their effects but sought to set down certain normal standards by which future clinical and experimental judgments may be made in the human.

As can be noted in Tables II, III and IV, normal human whole blood, packed cell, and plasma viscosities could be determined with a fair degree of accuracy at varying shear rates. These measurements may be done practically in the clinical laboratory utilizing currently available instrumentation.

SUMMARY

Whole blood (WB), packed cell (PC), and plasma (P) viscosities and various parameters in blood felt to be most influential in these determinations have been measured in 50 normal adult human subjects. Average normal WB viscosity at 23 $sec.^{-1}$ was 6.7 cps (S.D. ± 1.1) for the composite group, 7.0 cps (S.D. ± 0.9) for the men, and 5.5 cps (S.D. ± 0.6 for the women. Average PC viscosity at the same shear rate was 85.2 cps (S.D. ± 7.5) for the composite sample, 86.1 cps (S.D.) ± 8.0) for the men, and 82.5 cps (S.D.) ± 7.1) for the women. Average P viscosity at 230 $sec.^{-1}$ was 1.4 cps (S.D. ± 0.1) for the composite group, for the men, and for the women.

REFERENCES

1. Chien, S., Usami, S., Taylor, H. M., Lundberg, J. L., and Gregersen, M. I.: Effects of hematocrit and plasma proteins on human blood rheology at low shear rates, J. Appl. Physiol. **21:** 81, 1966.
2. Howe, P. E.: Use of sodium sulfate as the globulin precipitant in the determination of protein of the blood, J. Biol. Chem. **49:** 93, 1921, and **57:** 235, 1923.
3. Litwin, M. S.: Blood viscosity changes following surgical procedures, S. Forum **19:** 51, 1968.
4. Litwin, M. S., Bergentz, S.-E., Carlsten, A., Gelin, L.-E., Rudenstam, C.-M., and Söderholm, B.: Hidden acidosis following intravascular red cell aggregation in dogs, Ann. Surg. **161:** 532, 1965.
5. Milne, J.: Serum protein fractionation: Comparison of sodium sulfate precipitation and electrophoresis, J. Biol. Chem. **169:** 595, 1947.
6. Putnam, T. C., Kevy, S. V., and Replogle, R. L.: Factors influencing the viscosity of blood, Surg. Gynec. & Obst. **124:** 547, 1967.
7. Rand, P. W., and Lacombe, E.: Hemodilution tonicity and blood viscosity, J. Clin. Invest. **43:** 2214, 1964.
8. Rand, P. W., Lacombe, E., Hunt, H. E., and Austin, W. H.: Viscosity of normal human blood under normothermic and hypothermic conditions, J. Appl. Physiol. **19:** 117, 1964.
9. Reemtsma, K., and Creech, O.: Viscosity studies of blood, plasma and plasma substitutes, J. Thoracic & Cardiovas. Surg. **44:** 674 and 695, 1962.
10. Replogle, R. L., and Merrill, E. W.: Hemodilutin: Rheologic hemodynamic and metabolic consequences in shock, S. Forum **18:** 157, 1967.
11. Wells, R. E., Denton, R., and Merrill, E. W.: Measurement of viscosity of biologic fluids by cone plate viscometer, J. Lab. & Clin. Med. **57:** 646, 1961.

Cholesterol excretion following chronic ileal bypass

MARSHALL Z. SCHWARTZ, B.S.
RICHARD B. MOORE, M.D.
HENRY BUCHWALD, M.D., PH.D.*
MINNEAPOLIS, MINN.
From the Departments of Surgery and Medicine, The University of Minnesota Medical School

Today it is generally accepted that an elevated circulating cholesterol level is frequently associated with atherosclerosis. In recent years various approaches have been utilized to attempt to lower the blood cholesterol. One approach that has been shown to be effective is surgical exclusion of the distal ileum from continuity with the rest of the small intestine.[5] Two methods of accomplishing this have been experimentally studied: partial ileal bypass and partial ileal excision.[2, 4] It was shown that partial ileal bypass in the rabbit results in essentially twice the reduction in the blood cholesterol concentration as excision of an identical ileal segment. This finding has been confirmed by Welborn and associates[7] in the dog. In another study, in which an acute rabbit gastrointestinal tract preparation was used, we have previously shown that 24 hours after an intravenous injection of cholesterol-4-C^{14} 40 percent of the excreted radioactivity was recovered from the small intestine (with 20 percent from the jejunum and the other 20 percent from the ileum) and the remaining 60 percent was recovered from the bile.[3] Whether this acute cholesterol excretion ability is operative in the chronically bypassed ileal loop remained to be tested.

The purpose of the present experiment was: (1) to determine if the chronically bypassed ileum retains its cholesterol excretory ability and (2) to determine if the cholesterol excreted from the bypassed loop is a factor in accounting for the greater hypocholesterolemic effect of ileal bypass in comparison with ileal excision.

DESIGN OF EXPERIMENT

Control blood and feces samples were collected from white New Zealand rabbits averaging 7 to 8 pounds each. The rabbits were then injected intravenously via a superficial ear vein with 10 μc of cholesterol-4-C^{14}. Blood and 24 hour feces collections were obtained at daily intervals for 3 days. Following the sample collections the distal half of the small intestine was bypassed in each of the animals by placing an umbilical tape tie around the small bowel at its approximate midpoint and constructing a side-to-side ileocecostomy just proximal to the tie (Fig. 1).

After a minimum of 6 weeks following ileal bypass, collection catheters were placed in the proximal and distal ends of the bypassed segment. Placement of the distal catheter was accomplished by making a stab incision into the cecum distal to the ileocecal valve, threading a polyethylene tube retrograde through the valve into the ileum, and anchoring it with an umbilical tape tie. The stab incision was closed with a purse-string suture followed by a Witzel closure (Fig. 2). The proximal polyethylene catheter was inserted through a longitudinal incision made

Supported by United States Public Health Service Grant No. HE-11901 and the American Heart Association Grant No. 67825.

Received for publication Feb. 6, 1969.

*Established Investigator, American Heart Association.

in the afferent end of the bypassed ileal loop and anchored in place with an umbilical tape ligature (Fig. 2). Two stab incisions were then made in the abdominal wall and the catheters brought to the outside. The cecum in the area of the efferent catheter was fixed to the abdominal wall by four sutures. The afferent ileal incision was converted to an ileostomy and the abdominal incision closed (Fig. 3). Placement of these catheters in this fashion allowed the use of a washout technique for collecting the ileal excretions.

At least 5 days after the catheter implantation, blood, feces, and ileal excretions were collected in order to measure the residual radioactivity. This was followed by a second intravenous injection of 10 μc of cholesterol-4-C^{14} and the collection of blood, 24 hour feces, and 24 hour ileal excretions at daily intervals for 5 days.

The animals used in the study were in optimum health throughout the experiment and were feeding normally except for brief periods after operation. Other rabbits who were not feeding normally or whose catheters failed to function adequately were eliminated from the study. The over-all animal mortality rate for the entire period of study was 79 percent (48 rabbits were required to allow for 10 rabbits suitable for physiological evaluation).

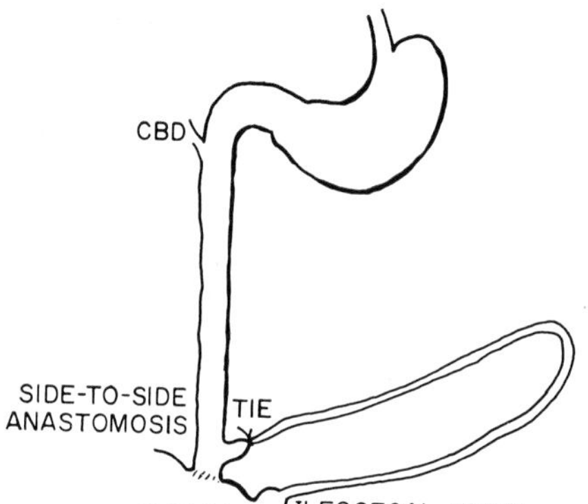

Fig. 1. Schematic representation of ileal bypass procedure.

METHODS OF ANALYZING SAMPLES

The total radioactivity of the feces and ileal excretions was measured by wet com-

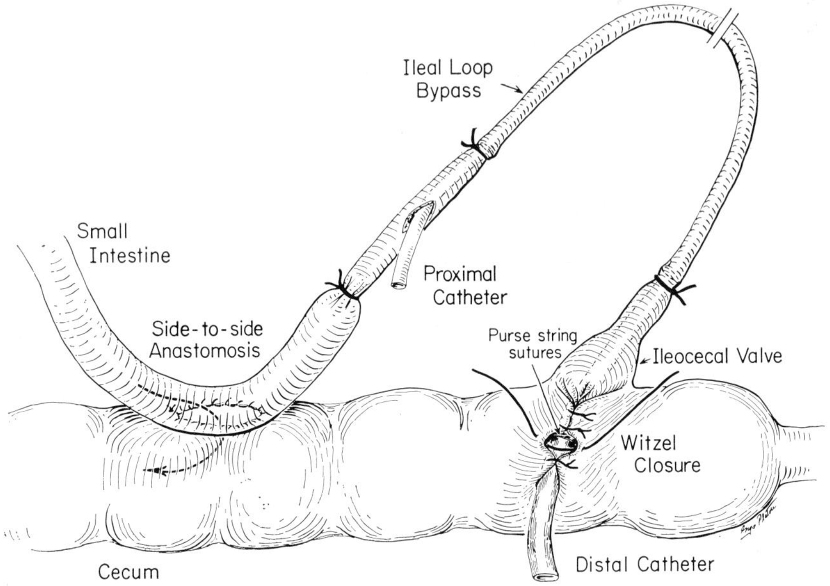

Fig. 2. Diagram showing the area of the ileocecal junction in the rabbit, illustrating the ileocecostomy and the technique for placement of the polyethylene catheters.

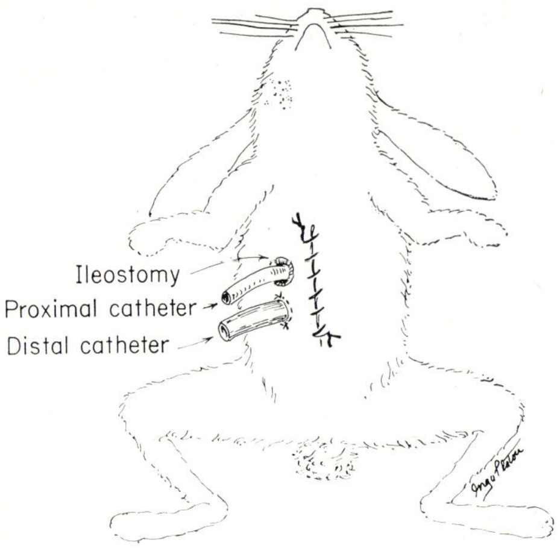

Fig. 3. Diagram of animal after placement of catheters.

Table I. *Average daily fecal cholesterol excretion (in milligrams) before and after partial ileal bypass*

Rabbit No.	*Before bypass (mg.)*	*After bypass (mg.)*	*Increase*
1	78	262	+3.4×
2	22	122	+5.5×
3	36	71	+2.0×
4	33	31	0
5	23	77	+3.3×
6	37	104	+2.8×
7	20	116	+5.8×
8	19	34	+1.8×
9	38	37	0
10	62	160	+2.6×
Average	37	100	+2.7×

bustion of a weighed aliquot, combination of the evolved $C^{14}O_2$ with phenethylamine, and liquid scintillation counting of C^{14}.[6]

The specific activity of the whole blood cholesterol was determined by liquid scintillation counting of the C^{14} radioactivity of the cholesterol extracted by the method of Abell, Levy, Brodie, and Kendall[1] and by the colorimetric measurement of the cholesterol concentration in the same sample with the use of the Liebermann-Burchard reagent. To rule out de novo synthesis and unilateral flux of cholesterol into the bypassed ileal lumen, the specific activity of the cholesterol in the ileal excretions was also determined in a similar manner.

RESULTS

Table I represents a comparison of daily fecal cholesterol excretion (in milligrams) before and after ileal bypass. The average 24 hour excretion before bypass was 37 mg. per day and after bypass it was elevated to 100 mg. per day, thus producing a 2.7 fold increase in fecal cholesterol excretion.

The percent of the total (feces plus bypassed segment) radioactivity excreted in the bypassed ileal loop of each rabbit for each 24 hour time period is illustrated in Table II. The average percent of the total radioactivity coming from the bypassed loop for each rabbit is shown on the right side of Table II. The over-all average for the group of ten rabbits was 1.01 percent. Thus only 1 percent of the total radioactivity excreted per day was contributed by the bypassed ileal segment.

The cholesterol specific activity of the bypassed ileal loop contents was found to be the same as the blood specific activity in a given rabbit. This demonstrated that the ileal loop cholesterol was derived from the circulating blood cholesterol only and that a mechanism of local intestinal de novo cholesterol synthesis with unidirectional flux secretion into the lumen was not present.

DISCUSSION

It has previously been shown that both ileal bypass and ileal excision produce a fourfold increase in the rate of cholesterol synthesis and that there is no statistically significant difference between the synthesis rates in these two preparations.[2, 4] As previously stated, the ileum, in an acute situation, excretes 20 percent of the total radioactive cholesterol excreted during a given test period.[3] Thus the most logical explanation for the twofold greater cholesterol-lowering efficacy of ileal bypass in comparison with ileal excision would be that the chronically bypassed ileum continues to produce a significant net excretion of endogenous cholesterol. However, the data from the

Table II. *Percent of total radioactivity excreted by the bypassed ileal segment**

Rabbit No.	Time after injection of cholesterol-4-C^{14} 24 hr.	48 hr.	72 hr.	96 hr.	120 hr.	Average value
1	0.46	—	0.35	0.28	0.25	0.34
2	11.21	0.12	0.74	0.72	0.68	2.69
3	0.33	0.52	0.49	0.45	0.47	0.45
4	1.25	0.01	—	5.32	1.28	1.97
5	—	0.73	0.62	0.41	0.98	0.69
6	—	1.16	0.31	0.54	0.55	0.64
7	0.59	1.28	0.31	0.39	0.73	0.66
8	—	6.87	0.69	0.27	0.17	2.00
9	—	0.35	0.32	0.56	0.34	0.39
10	0.64	0.19	0.11	0.11	0.08	0.23
Group average						1.01%

$$*\%\ C^{14}\ \text{in loop} = \frac{\text{loop d.p.m./24 hr.}}{\text{total (feces + loop) d.p.m./24 hr.}} \times 100.$$

present experiment are not in accord with this hypothesis. We are, therefore, inclined to look for another, and possibly more subtle, metabolic explanation for the greater effectiveness of ileal bypass in comparison with ileal excision in lowering the blood cholesterol concentration in the rabbit.

SUMMARY

This experiment was designed to determine if the chronically bypassed ileum retains the cholesterol excretory ability found in an earlier acute rabbit study and to determine if the cholesterol excreted by the bypassed loop is a factor in accounting for the known greater hypocholesterolemic effect of ileal bypass in comparison with ileal excision in the rabbit. From the data obtained in this experiment it can be shown that: (1) Ileal bypass in the ten rabbits studied resulted in a 2.7 fold increase in total fecal cholesterol excretion; (2) cholesterol excretion in the chronically bypassed ileal loop was approximately 1 percent of the total fecal cholesterol excretion; and (3) cholesterol excretion in the chronically bypassed ileal loop was 5 percent (1/20) of that measured in an acutely bypassed ileal loop.

The authors wish to express their gratitude to Mrs. Josephine Bertish, Miss Laurie Fitch, and Miss Karen Settevig for their dedicated assistance.

REFERENCES

1. Abell, L. L., Levy, B. B., Brodie, B. B., and Kendall, S. E.: A simplified method for the estimation of total cholesterol in Serum and demonstration of its specificity, J. Biol. Chem. **195:** 357, 1952.
2. Buchwald, H., Frantz, I. D., Jr., Gebhard, R. L., and Moore, R. B.: The effect of ileal bypass versus ileal excision on cholesterol synthesis and whole blood cholesterol concentrations in the rabbit, SURGERY **64:** 126, 1968.
3. Buchwald, H., and Gebhard, R. L.: Cholesterol excretion into the small intestine, SURGERY. Accepted for publication.
4. Buchwald, H., Gebhard, R. L., Frantz, I. D., Jr., and Moore, R. B.: Ileal bypass versus ileal excision; Effect on cholesterol concentrations in the rabbit, preliminary report, S. Clin. North America **49:** 1353, 1967.
5. Buchwald, H., Moore, R. B., Lee, G. B., Frantz, I. D., Jr., and Varco, R. L.: Combined dietary, surgical, and bile salt binding resin therapy in the treatment of hypercholesterolemia, Arch. Surg. **97:** 275, 1968.
6. Moore, R. B., Crane, C. A., and Frantz, I. D., Jr.: An apparatus and a method using phenethylamine for liquid scintillation counting of $C^{14}O_2$ obtained by wet oxidation of biological materials, Anal. Biochem. **24:** 545, 1968.
7. Welborn, M. D., Jr., Wimberly, J. E., Younger, R. K., Stephenson, S. E., Jr., and Scott, H. W., Jr.: Comparison of the protective effects of ileal resection and bypass in experimental atherosclerosis, S. Forum **19:** 299, 1968.

Potassium vasoactivity—a biphasic effect

SCOTT J. BOLEY, M.D.
NEIL KAMIL, B.S.
BERNARD S. LEVOWITZ, M.D.
WILLIAM F. TREIBER, Jr., B.S.
GIRHAR P. AGRAWAL, M.D.
FRANK J. VEITH, M.D.
NEW YORK, N. Y.
From the Departments of Surgery, Montefiore Hospital and Medical Center, Jewish Hospital of Brooklyn, and Albert Einstein College of Medicine

The effect of altered potassium ion concentrations on vascular smooth muscle and thus on blood flow has been studied by physiologists for many years. The possible role of this cation in work hyperemia, autoregulation, and hypertension has stimulated numerous experimental approaches that have produced confusing and often contradictory conclusions. Vasoconstriction[3, 14] and vasodilation[6, 12] have been reported with elevated potassium levels, and some investigators found both responses, depending upon the degree of increase in potassium concentration.[13]

Recently, the finding of small intestinal ulcerative lesions after ingestion of enteric-coated potassium chloride[2, 11] has raised speculation that the vasoactive effects of potassium may cause tissue damage. Experimental and clinical investigations[1, 4] have suggested that these lesions are venous infarctions which occur in response to high levels of potassium in the veins of a short segment of intestine. This situation presumably results from the sudden release of potassium chloride from the enteric-coated tablet with absorption over a limited length of bowel.

Supported in part by grants from the United States Public Health Service (HE 11567), the James Picker Foundation, and the Research Department of Ciba Pharmaceutical Company.

Received for publication Feb. 19, 1969.

The present work was undertaken to study the vasoactivity of increased serum potassium. Experiments were performed to evaluate the effects of elevated potassium concentrations on renal, mesenteric, and limb blood flows. The results appear to clarify some of the previous conflicting observations.

METHODS

The effects of acute local elevations of serum potassium concentration were studied in the renal, limb, and mesenteric vascular beds of 30 animals. All studies were performed on adult mongrel dogs under pentobarbital anesthesia. Arterial blood flows to the kidney, limb, or a portion of intestine were measured by noncannulating probes and a square-wave or pulsed-logic electromagnetic flowmeter.* Potassium chloride (1 to 2 mEq. per milliliter) was continuously infused through a catheter introduced via a side branch of the artery peripheral to the probe (Fig. 1). Based upon the control blood flow, potassium chloride was infused at a rate calculated to elevate the serum potassium of the blood flowing to the vascular bed under study to 6 to 16 mEq. per liter. Usually the initial infusion rate was maintained regardless of subsequent alter-

*Carolina Medical Electronics, Inc., Winston-Salem, N. C., or Biotronex Laboratory, Inc., Silver Springs, Md.

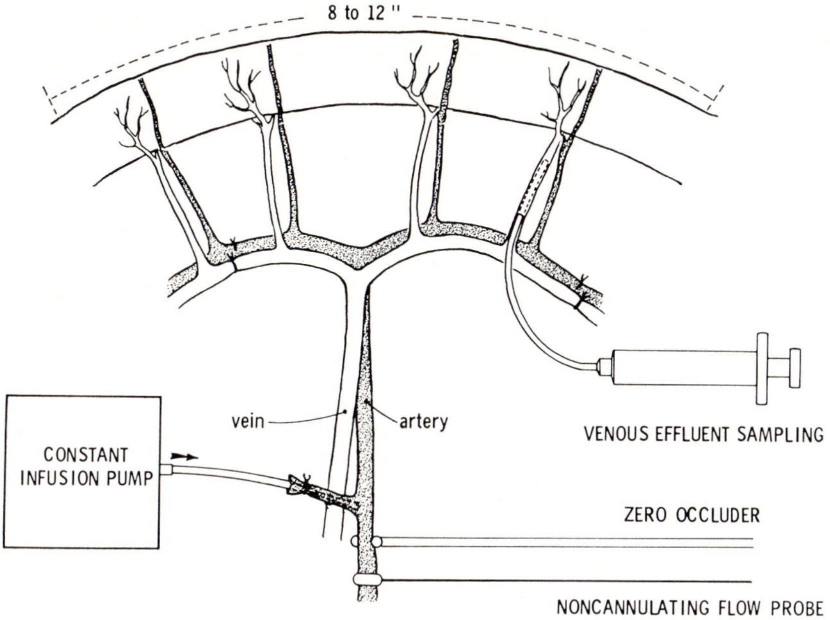

Fig. 1. Diagram of experimental technique as used in mesenteric vascular bed. Flow probe is connected to an electromagnetic flowmeter. Rate of infusion and potassium concentration of infusate are both varied to add selected amounts of potassium to blood flowing to the segment being studied.

ations in blood flow, but in several experiments the infusion rate was continuously altered so as to maintain the potassium at a constant level despite changes in blood flow. In two groups of five animals each, the effects of potassium infusion into the kidney or extremity were simultaneously determined in the infused and contralateral sides. Systemic arterial pressure was measured with a strain-gauge transducer via a catheter in a femoral artery.

RESULTS

In all three vascular beds studied a similar biphasic response was observed, although it varied in degree and rapidity of onset. In 42 of 45 determinations an immediate initial increase in blood flow occurred regardless of the concentration of potassium, but appeared to vary quantitatively from 20 to 200 percent in direct proportion to the potassium concentration. This was followed in 2 to 60 minutes by a marked fall in flow below the control level, and, if the infusion of potassium chloride was continued unaltered, thus creating a rising concentration as blood flow diminished, the blood flow approached zero (Fig. 2). If the potassium infusion was continuously corrected to maintain a constant blood concentration, blood flow leveled off at approximately 20 to 50 percent of control values (Fig. 3). If the potassium infusion was discontinued promptly after the maximum fall in blood flow a transient increase in blood flow occurred to well above control levels (Fig. 2). However, if blood flow was maintained at zero for more than 30 minutes, stopping the potassium infusion did not restore blood flow. When potassium concentrations were elevated above 10 mEq. per liter a marked increase in flow occurred followed in 5 to 30 minutes by a marked decrease to below control levels. Concentrations of approximately 8 mEq. per liter produced the vasoconstrictive effect only after maintenance at this level more than 60 minutes.

Systemic arterial pressure varied little or not at all during the phasic alteration in local blood flow, and no evidence of systemic vasoconstriction occurred even when

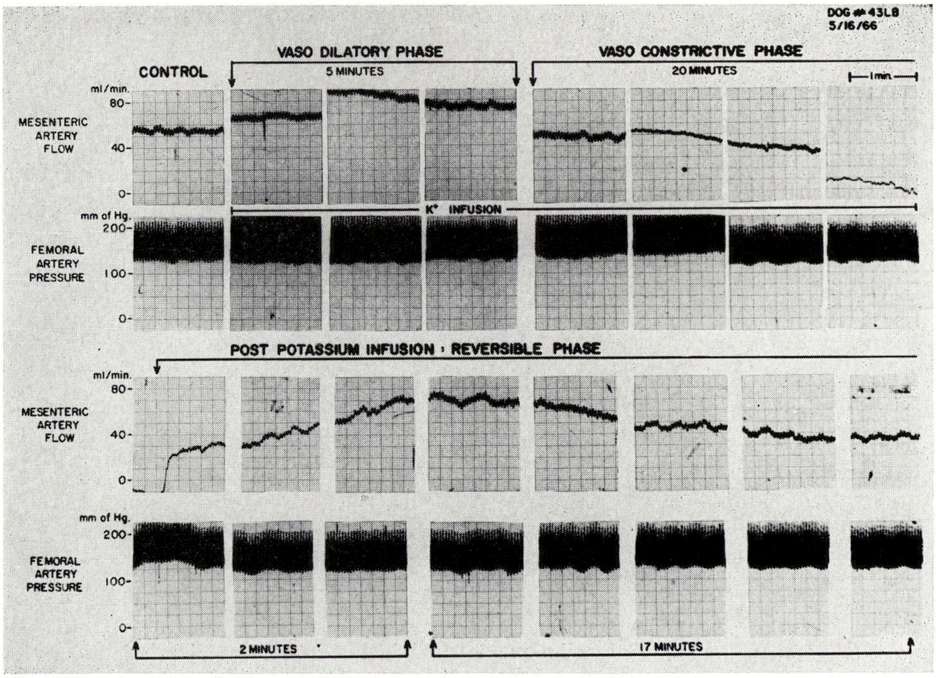

Fig. 2. Effect of local arterial potassium chloride (0.38 ml./mm. = 0.38 mEq./min.) infusion on mesenteric blood flow. Based on the control blood flow, potassium was infused at a constant rate calculated to elevate arterial potassium to 8 mEq. per liter. The typical biphasic response is shown followed by a rise in flow to above control when the potassium infusion was stopped.

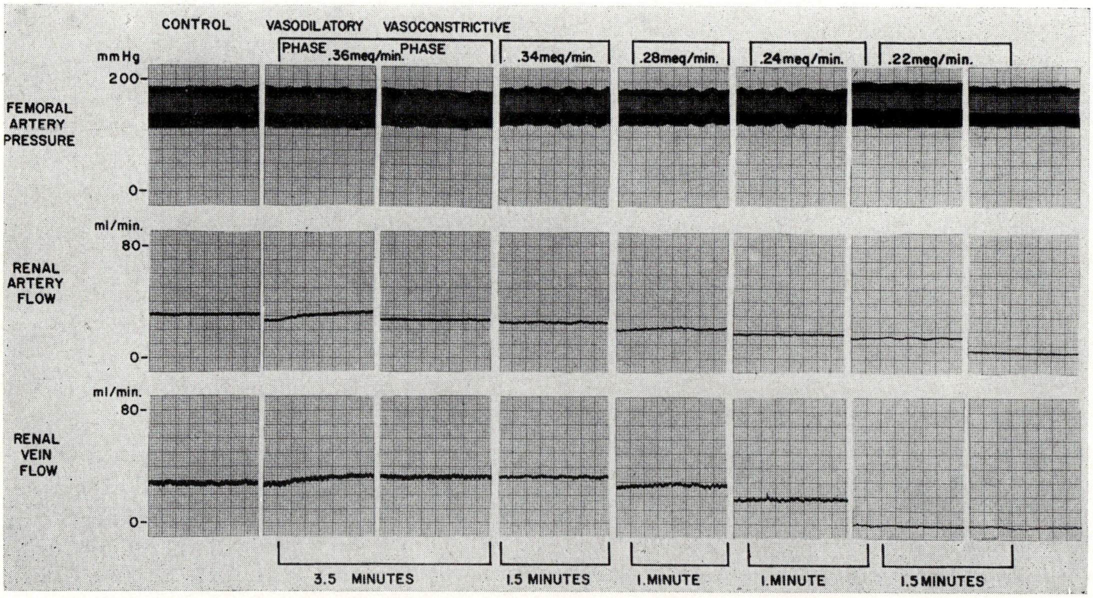

Fig. 3. Effect of local arterial potassium chloride infusion on renal arterial and venous blood flow. Flow probes were placed around both renal vessels in this experiment. Potassium infusion was continuously varied to maintain K^+ level in blood to kidney at 16 mEq. per liter.

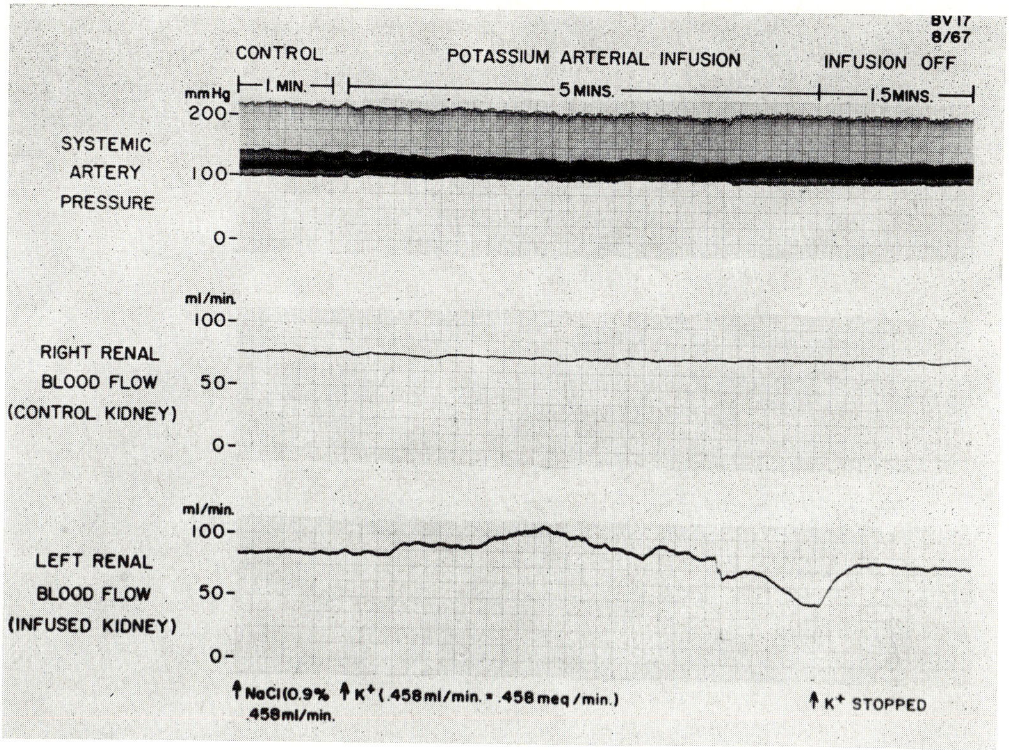

Fig. 4. Effect of local arterial potassium chloride infusion upon blood flow to the infused and the contralateral kidney. Based upon control flow, potassium was infused at a constant rate to elevate arterial potassium to 10 mEq. per liter. In the infused kidney the typical biphasic response is seen while flow to the contralateral kidney and the systemic blood pressure are unaltered.

local flow fell to zero. Simultaneously measured contralateral renal and limb flows showed no change while blood flow to the infused side was increasing, and either no change or a paradoxical increase when flow to the infused bed was decreasing (Fig. 4).

DISCUSSION

Other investigations of the effect of potassium on smooth muscle have utilized muscle strip techniques,[3] isolated perfusion,[6] direct visualization of capillaries,[14] and measurements during injection in conscious human volunteers.[12] Haddy and his co-workers[8] have measured resistance changes while maintaining a constant blood flow and have correctly described both vasoconstrictive and vasodilatory responses. Their conclusion that the nature of the response is dependent on concentration does not coincide with our findings, but may be explained by their technique of measuring the effects of increasing concentrations in sequential order for periods as brief as 30 seconds. Our results suggest that an initial vasodilatation occurs with any increase in potassium concentration and as the vascular smooth muscle continues to be exposed to these higher levels vasoconstriction occurs. While the mechanism of potassium vasoactivity has not been elucidated, it has been suggested that changes in the ratio of intracellular and extracellular potassium affect the membrane potential of vascular smooth muscle.[9] Slowly rising concentrations of the intracellular potassium ion might then reverse the initial response of the cell to high extracellular potassium concentrations. The more rapid completion of the sequence of dilatation and constriction with higher concentrations of potassium supports this mechanism. The transient increased flow when potassium infusion is stopped promptly after the maximal fall may represent compensatory vasodilatation or a third phase in membrane potential alteration.

Other authors have implicated an adrenal medullary discharge in response to elevations in blood potassium as the mechanism for vasoconstriction.[7, 9] In our study the lack of any systemic arterial pressure rise and the paradoxical increase in blood flow in contralateral beds fails to support this mechanism. The present studies suggest that the potassium ion exerts its effect locally on vascular smooth muscle.

Enteric-coated potassium chloride is believed to produce small intestinal lesions through a vasoconstrictive effect on intramural veins.[5] While the present observations are based on intra-arterial infusions, they do indicate that high potassium concentrations cause contraction of vascular smooth muscle. Concentrations of potassium as high as 20 mEq. per liter have been found in the venous effluent from 8 inch segments of small intestine filled with 20 ml. of saline containing 10 mEq.[10] These levels far exceed those that might produce contraction of venous smooth muscle.

The biphasic, or possibly triphasic, response to acute local hyperkalemia demonstrated with this simple experimental model may clarify the conflicting results of other studies of potassium vasoactivity. At least some of the confusion lies in the need for prolonged observation of elevated local levels as well as monitoring of adequate parameters to identify or exclude systemic factors.

SUMMARY

Acute local elevations of serum potassium in blood flowing to the mesenteric, renal, and limb vascular beds were produced by continuous infusion of potassium chloride into the respective arterial supply. Calculated potassium concentrations of 8 to 16 mEq. per liter produced transient increases in flow followed by prolonged marked decreases to well below control levels. This biphasic response occurred at all concentrations and in all three vascular beds. Simultaneously monitored systemic blood pressures and blood flow to contralateral vascular beds were unaltered. Potassium appears to exert a local effect on vascular smooth muscle.

REFERENCES

1. Allen, A. C., Boley, S. J., Schultz, L., and Schwartz, S.: Potassium-induced lesions of the small bowel. II. Pathology and pathogenesis, J.A.M.A. **193:** 1001, 1965.
2. Baker, D. R., Schrader, W. H., and Hitchcock, C. R.: Small-bowel ulceration apparently associated with thiazide and potassium therapy, J.A.M.A. **190:** 586, 1964.
3. Bohr, D. F., Brodie, D. C., and Cheu, D. H.: Effect of electrolytes on arterial muscle contraction, Circulation **17:** 746, 1958.
4. Boley, S. J., Allen, A. C., Schultz, L., and Schwartz, S.: Potassium-induced lesions of the small bowel. I. Clinical aspects, J.A.M.A. 193: 997, 1965.
5. Boley, S. J., Schultz, L., Krieger, H., Schwartz, S., Elguezabel, A., and Allen, A. C.: Experimental evaluation of thiazides and potassium as a cause of small bowel ulcers, J.A.M.A. **192:** 763, 1965.
6. Dawes, G. S.: The vaso-dilator action of potassium, J. Physiol. **99:** 224, 1941.
7. Fenn, W. O.: Role of potassium in physiologic processes, Physiol. Rev. **20:** 377, 1940.
8. Haddy, F. J., and Scott, J. B.: Effects of electrolytes and water upon resistance to blood flow through intact vascular beds, *in* Bajusz, E., editor: Electrolytes and cardiovascular diseases, Basel, 1965, S. Karger AG, pp. 383-400.
9. Laszt, L.: Effect of potassium on muscle tension, especially on that of vascular muscle, Nature **185:** 696, 1960.
10. Levowitz, B. S., Boley, S. J., Agrawal, G. P., Glotfelty, E., Kamil, N., and Allen, A. C.: Vascular basis of the potassium ulcer and its reversal by magnesium ion, S. Forum **18:** 315, 1967.
11. Lindholmer, B., Nyman, E., and Raf, L.: Non-specific stenosing ulcerations of the small bowel: A preliminary report, Acta chir. scandinav. **128:** 310, 1964.
12. Lowe, R. D., and Thompson, J. W.: The effect of intra-arterial potassium chloride infusion upon forearm blood flow in man, J. Physiol. **162:** 69, 1962.
13. Scott, J., Emanuel, D., and Haddy, F.: Effect of potassium on renal vascular resistance and urine flow rate, Am. J. Physiol. **197:** 305, 1959.
14. Sudak, F. N., and Fulton, G. P.: Peripheral vasoconstriction associated with hyperpotassemia, Circulation Res. **10:** 587, 1962.

A new type subcutaneous arteriovenous fistula for chronic hemodialysis in children

JUAN J. PÉREZ ALVAREZ, M.D., F.A.C.C.
RUBÉN VARGAS-ROSENDO, M.D.
RAMÓN GUTIÉRREZ-BOSQUE, M.D.
MANUEL MATOS DÍAZ-ORDAZ, M.D.
DAVID SANTOS-ATHERTON
MEXICO CITY, MEXICO

From the Departments of Cardiovascular Surgery and Nephrology, Hospital de Pediatría, Centro Médico Nacional, Instituto Mexicano del Seguro Social

The use of chronic hemodialysis in children is hindered by the small size of their vessels which prevents, or make very difficult, the insertion of catheters of adequate size to establish a functional external Silastic-tubing arteriovenous fistula.[4] In addition, it involves the risks of infection[5] and of potentially fatal accidental or purposeful disconnection.

The performance of a direct side-to-side anastomosis between the radial artery and one of the neighboring veins in the wrist is an alternate procedure,[1] but it is technically difficult. The anastomosis can easily thrombose,[3] and it may be necessary to wait until the arteriovenous shunt produces enough enlargement of the veins in the forearm to allow their cannulation with trocars of a sizeable caliber to permit an adequate blood flow.

Flores-Izquierdo[2] has recently devised a new technique which he and his associates have successfully applied on a number of adult patients subjected to chronic hemodialysis.

The technique consists of the subcutaneous implantation in the forearm of a long free loop of one of the patient's own saphenous veins which is sutured at one end to a good-sized opening in the brachial artery, slightly above its bifurcation in an end-to-side fashion, and at the other end to either the cephalic or basilic veins, whichever is bigger.

SURGICAL TECHNIQUE

Preferably the patient is under general anesthesia while two surgical teams work simultaneously. The first team removes the entire length of the internal saphenous vein, starting at the Scarpa triangle, through a 10 cm. incision made parallel to the femoral vessels, taking special care not to injure the saphenous vein at any level (Fig. 1).

The saphenous-femoral junction is carefully dissected and a heavy ligature tied flush to the femoral vein. A hemostat is applied distally to the saphenous vein which is then cut between the ligature and the clamp. Dissection of the saphenous vein is then carried down as far distally as possible through the same skin incision, meticulously tying off with nonabsorable fine suture material every branch found on the way. Two or three more skin incisions 2.5 to 3 cm. long are made along the inner aspect of the thigh, down to the knee level, following the

Received for publication July 9, 1969.

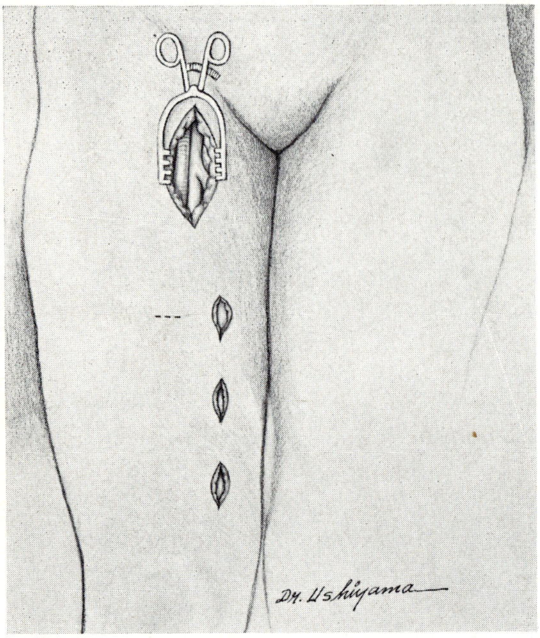

Fig. 1. Obtention of autogenous saphenous vein graft (see text).

trajectory of the saphenous vein which is bluntly dissected between one incision and the next; every branch as well as the distal end of the main vein is tied off and cut, and the entire vein is removed.

The free graft thus obtained is prepared first by filling it up with heparin solution (10 mg. in 10 ml. of saline), making certain that the proximal and distal ends are conveniently identified and marked. The adventitia of the graft is carefully removed with fine scissors, especially at the places where it produces strictures when the graft is fully distended with heparin solution. The entire length of the vein, and especially every stump of a ligated branch, are checked for leaks, and care is taken not to produce strictures of the vein when applying extra ligatures at the leaking points.

Meanwhile, the other surgical team makes a 10 to 12 cm. long Z-type incision along the inner aspect of the arm, the antecubital fossa, and the anterior aspect of the forearm to expose the brachial artery and its bifurcation, as well as the biggest subcutaneous vein available (Fig. 2). Heavy threads are passed around the dissected vessels. The brachial artery is then temporarily occluded both proximally and distally with atraumatic clamps; an incision 8 mm. in length is made on its anterior wall, and the edges are trimmed in order to make an oval-shaped orifice. Through this orifice, a fine plastic catheter is introduced distally and 10 to 20 ml. of heparin solution (depending on the patient's size) are injected. The temporarily occluding distal clamp is then reapplied.

The distal end of the saphenous vein graft is tailored by cutting it transversely, then enlarging its orifice by means of a small longitudinal incision and trimming of the resulting angles, thus making a beveled orifice equal in size to the one in the brachial artery. The two orifices are sutured together by a continuous stitch of very fine (No. 6-0) suture material.

The distal clamp on the brachial artery is first removed and then also the proximal one in order to test for leaks at the suture line, while the opposite end of the vein graft is kept occluded with an atraumatic vascular clamp. Extra stitches are placed if necessary. Again the vein graft is clamped, this time near the anastomosis, and it is flushed with heparin to wash out the blood contained in it. A loop is formed with the graft over the skin to determine its position when the venous anastomosis will be completed, and two 15 mm. long skin incisions are made transversely at the appropriate level on the forearm, separated from each other by 3 to 4 cm. By the use of a long hemostat, two tunnels are made right under the skin to connect the proximal incision to each of the two small distal ones and these two to each other. It is inconvenient to make one single tunnel for both arms of the venous loop because they will stay too close together and make its puncture hazardous later on.

By the use of the same long hemostat, the vein graft is drawn first down, then across, and finally up again under the skin to bring it into the proximal incision near the place selected to make the venovenous anastomosis, which is performed in a way similar to the one described for the arterial side (Fig. 3).

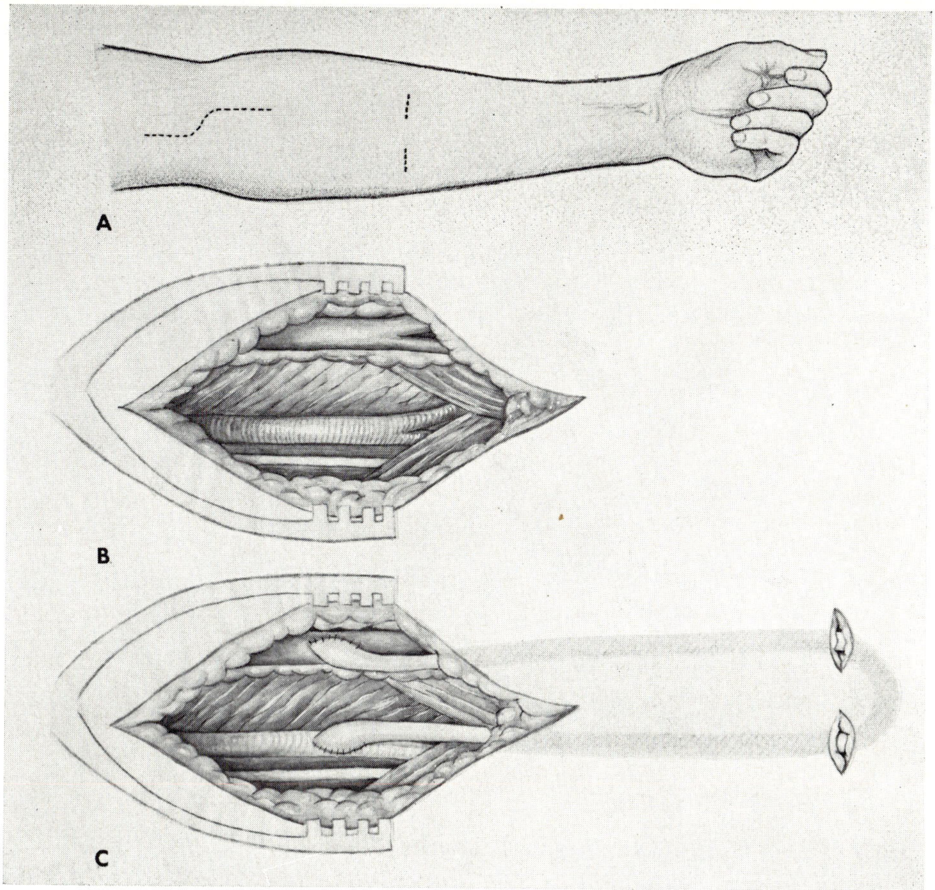

Fig. 2. *A,* Site of incisions for a forearm fistula. *B,* Dissection of brachial artery and cephalic vein. *C,* Fistula completed (see text).

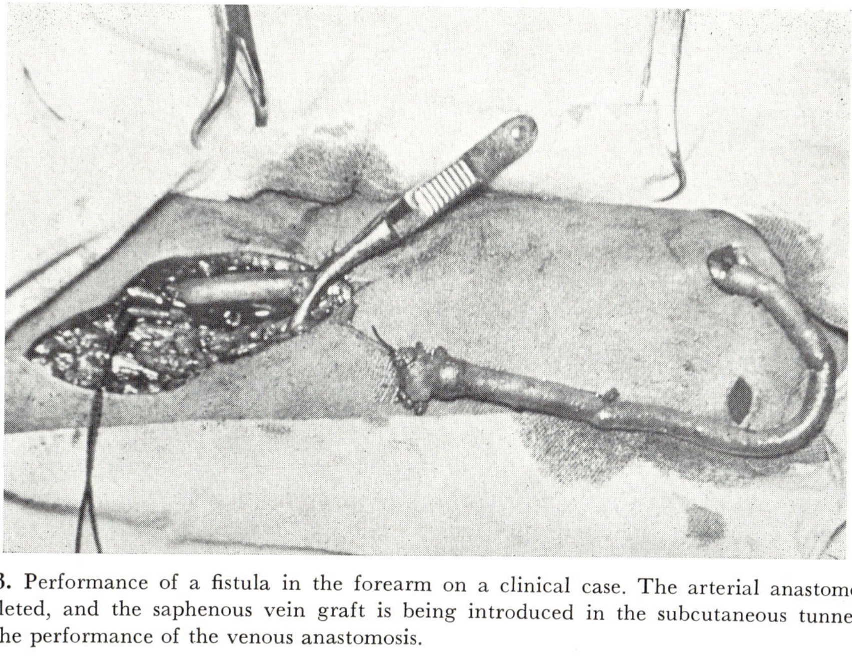

Fig. 3. Performance of a fistula in the forearm on a clinical case. The arterial anastomosis is completed, and the saphenous vein graft is being introduced in the subcutaneous tunnels before the performance of the venous anastomosis.

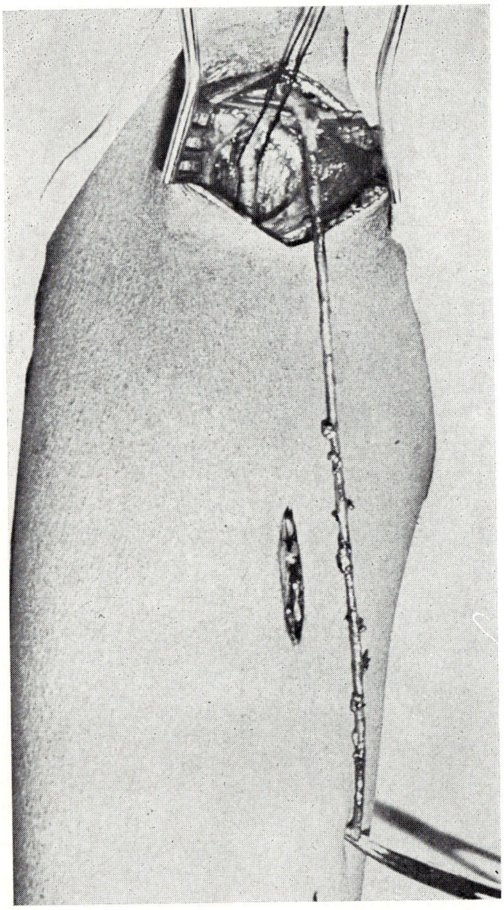

Fig. 4. Preparation of the saphenous vein—leaving its femoral junction untouched—to perform a fistula in the thigh. The femoral artery has been dissected free.

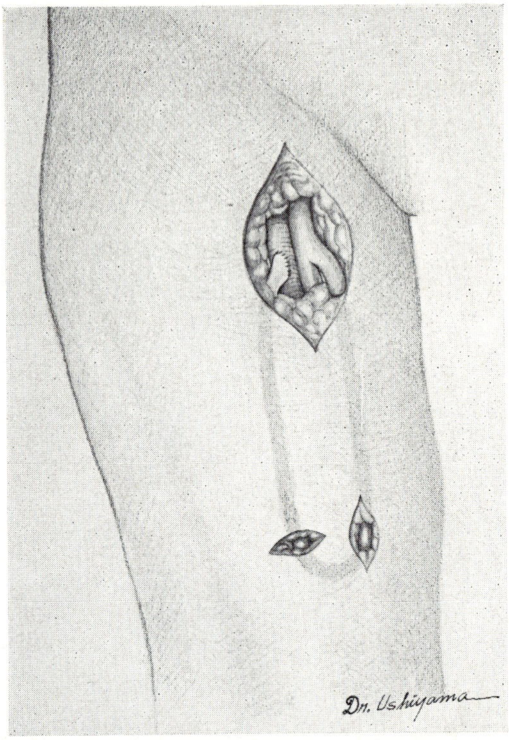

Fig. 5. Arteriovenous fistula in the thigh (see text).

In drawing the graft under the skin, care must be taken not to produce any torsion of the vein along its longitudinal axis. The skin incisions are sutured together while it is made sure that neither the anastomoses nor the graft are compressed. Dressings are applied and the arm is immobilized in a posterior plaster splint with the elbow flexed at a 60° angle during the following 3 or 4 days. A continuous machinery murmur and thrill will be present along the inner aspect of the arm if the fistula is working satisfactorily. On the seventh or eighth postoperative day, the skin sutures are removed and the fistula can be used for hemodialysis.

A variant of this technique, which we found useful when the arm veins are too small, consists of the complete dissection of the entire length of the saphenous vein in the thigh but leaving the saphenous junction to the femoral vein untouched, turning the vein up to form a loop which is buried in a tunnel right under the skin, and anastomosing it end-to-side to the femoral artery, thus requiring only one suture line (Figs. 4 and 5).

Characteristic of either type of fistula is that there remains a good-sized vessel immediately underneath unscarred skin which protects it well and can be punctured even on both arms of the loop if veins are unavailable anywhere else in the body for reinfusion of the dialyzed blood (Fig. 6).

From September, 1968, to the date of this writing, a total of 130 hemodialyses have been performed on 3 patients aged 15, 13, and 7 years with the type of fistula described first and on 2 patients aged 13 and 12 years

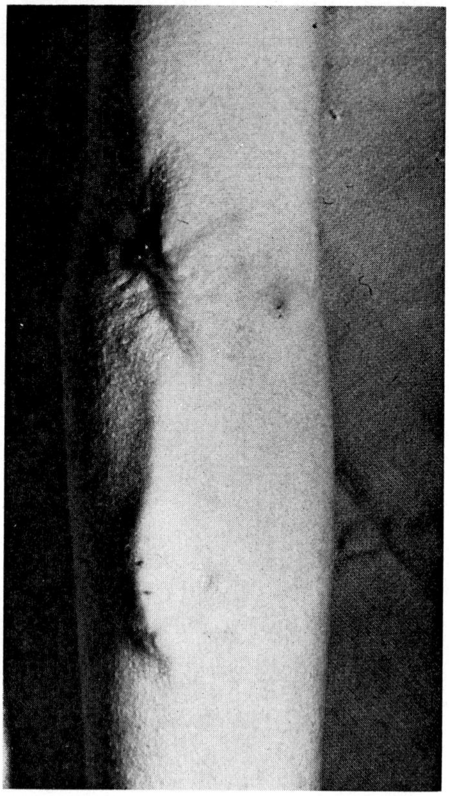

Fig. 6. Late postoperative appearance of an arteriovenous fistula in the forearm. Notice the recent puncture sites.

with the second one, with the use of flows that have ranged from a minimum of 100 to a maximum of 300 ml. per minute.

Results have been excellent thus far. There have been no infectious complications; cardiac failure has not been produced in any of the patients; the presence of the fistula does not disturb them; and they perform normally with the limitations imposed by their original illness.

SUMMARY AND CONCLUSIONS

A description has been given of a new type of subcutaneous arteriovenous fistula for hemodialysis to be used particularly in children. This technique uses an autogenous free saphenous vein graft placed subcutaneously in the forearm, forming a U whose ends are anastomosed to the brachial artery and either the cephalic or basilic brachial veins.

A variant of this technique is also described, which consists of the anastomosis of the totally dissected long saphenous vein to the femoral artery to form also a subcutaneous U in the thigh.

By the use of either one of these techniques, percutaneous puncture of the graft is feasible with a fair-sized trocar to permit a satisfactory flow.

A preliminary report is made of 5 patients whose ages varied from 7 to 15 years, and on whom 130 hemodialyses have been performed without complications with the use of this type of fistula.

Recognition is gratefully acknowledged to Dr. G. Flores-Izquierdo and the Vascular Surgery Team of Hospital General, Centro Médico Nacional, Instituto Mexicano del Seguro Social, for their advice and assistance to initiate the performance of this type of fistula at our institution.

REFERENCES

1. Brescia, M. J., Cimino, J. E., Appel, K., and Hurwich, B. J.: Chronic hemodialysis using venipuncture and a surgically created arteriovenous fistula, New Eng. J. Med. **275:** 1089, 1966.
2. Flores-Izquierdo, G., Ronces-Rivero, R., Exaire, E., Hernández-Chávez, A., and Gómez de los Ríos, J.: Autoinjerto venoso para hemodiálisis (técnica original). Comunicación preliminar, Arch. Inst. Cardiol. Mex. **39:** 259, 1969.
3. Mustard, W. T.: Personal communication.
4. Quinton, W. E., Dillard, D., and Scribner, B. H.: Cannulation of blood vessels for prolonged hemodialysis, Trans. Amer. Soc. Artif. Intern. Organs. **6:** 104, 1960.
5. Starzl, T. E.: Experience in renal transplantation, Philadelphia, 1964, W. B. Saunders Company, p. 20.

Gastric secretion in the canine fetus following maternal stimulation: Experimental studies on placental transfer of insulin, histamine, and gastrin

WALTER L. BRUCKNER, M.D.
HAROLD D. SNOW, D.V.M.
ERIC W. FONKALSRUD, M.D.
LOS ANGELES, CALIF.
From the Department of Surgery, UCLA School of Medicine

Spontaneous gastric perforation and peptic ulcer in the newborn have been known for 140 years,[2, 15, 21] and some research has been done in an attempt to clarify the cause. The development of gastric epithelial cells has been examined histologically in the fetus and newborn of several species.[8, 11, 18] Gastric secretion in the newborn period has been studied by several investigators.[9, 12, 17] but little information concerning gastric secretion in the fetus has been available until recently.[7, 20] In a previous communication, it was demonstrated that the gastric mucosa of the canine fetus may be stimulated during the last week of gestation.[3] Following direct fetal stimulation with histamine, insulin, and gastrin, a significant increase in acid and pepsin output was observed.

The present study was carried out to determine whether histamine, insulin, and gastrin, given to the mother, are able to cross the placenta and stimulate secretion in the gastric mucosa of the canine fetus.

MATERIALS AND METHODS

Fifteen fasting pregnant dogs (near term) were placed under light general anesthesia with intravenous secobarbital. A hysterotomy was performed on each bitch with no attempt made to retain amniotic fluid. The abdomen was opened in each fetus by a left subcostal incision, and care was taken to avoid injury to the umbilical vessels. The pylorus was mobilized and occluded in its midportion with a No. 2-0 silk ligature (Shay procedure[19]) without interrupting the gastric vascular supply. The abdomen of each fetus was then closed to restore normal intra-abdominal pressure. All fetuses were placed in the peritoneal cavity of the mother under a heat lamp and moistened frequently to simulate an extrauterine pregnancy. Care was taken not to stretch or kink the umbilical cord and a good fetal heartbeat and circulation were maintained. Four hours after pyloric ligation, the abdomen of each fetus was reopened, the esophagocardiac junction was occluded, and the entire stomach was excised. The fetus then was killed with an overdose of secobarbital after the umbilical cord had been severed. Baseline gastric secretion was studied in the fetuses of four bitches (27 pups). Protamine zinc insulin (Squibb) (0.5 units per kilogram of body weight per hour) was given subcutaneously to five bitches (41 pups). Four bitches (30 pups) received histamine phosphate (0.1 mg. per kilogram per hour) and three (21 pups) received human gastrin I* intravenously for two hours (25 μg per

Supported by United States Public Health Service Grant No. HE 11695-01.
Received for publication May 26, 1969.

*Imperial Chemical Industries, Ltd., Alderley Park, Macclesfield Cheshire, England.

kilogram per hour in 0.09 per cent NaCl solution). After the fetal stomach was excised four hours later, each was examined for total fluid volume, pH, total acidity, pepsin content, and electrolytes.

RESULTS

One hundred and nineteen fetuses were studied; three died prior to completion of the experiment. The average base-line gastric secretion (27 pups) one week before term was 0.73 ml. after four hours (Fig. 1). The average pH was 7.06 (Fig. 2). Following maternal stimulation with insulin, the average fetal gastric secretion (25 pups) one week before term was 1.716 ml., and the average pH was 6.00. When histamine was given to the mother, the average fetal gastric secretion after four hours was 2.16 ml. (19 pups) one week before term. The average pH was 5.92. Following maternal stimulation with gastrin, the average gastric secretion of the fetus (14 pups) one week before term was 0.74 ml. and the average pH was 4.88. The fetal gastric mucosa in fetuses that were two or more weeks before term was stimulated by administration of secretagogues to the mother. Fig. 2 shows the response of gastric pH in each fetus following maternal stimulation one week before term. The average pepsin content was 0.021 mg. total in the controls. Following maternal stimulation with histamine, insulin, or gastrin, no significant changes in pepsin output were observed. Significant changes, however, were detected in potassium and chloride output (Table I).

DISCUSSION

The age of the fetuses in the present study was determined by estimating the stage of pregnancy or by examining the signs of fetal maturity, as described previously.[3] The fetal gastric mucosa did not respond to stimuli when the fetuses were two or more weeks

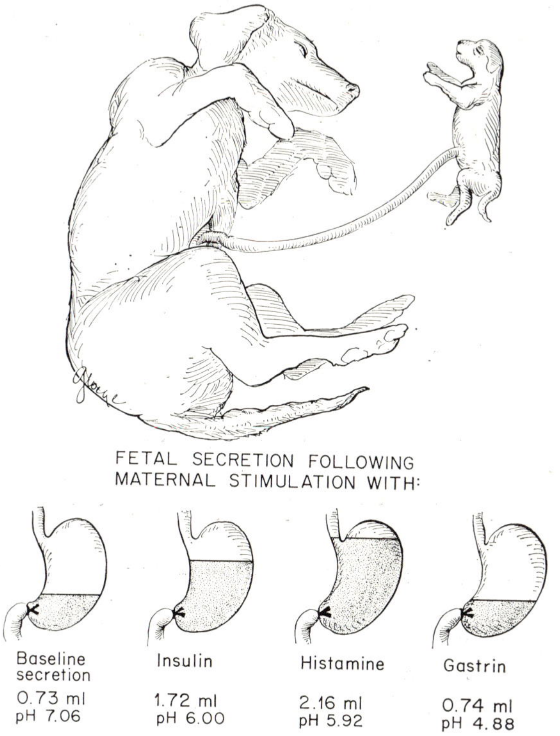

Fig. 1. Fetal (one week before birth) gastric pH values following maternal stimulation. Comparison of gastric volume and pH in canine fetuses. Baseline values were measured in 27 pups from 4 bitches. The effects of insulin stimulation were measured in 41 pups from 5 bitches. The effects of histamine stimulation was studied in 4 bitches (30 pups). Three bitches (21 pups) received human gastrin I.

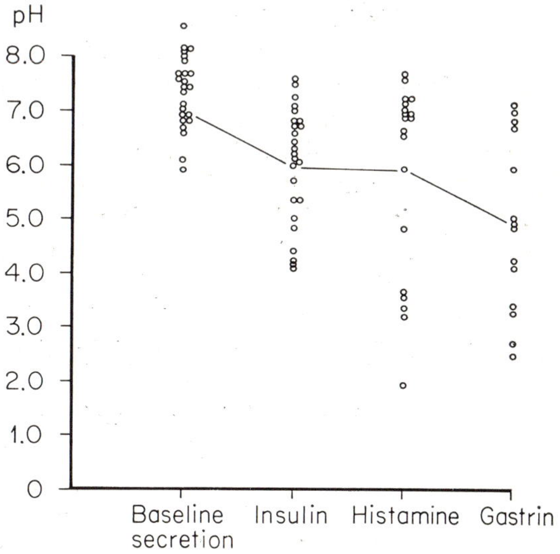

Fig. 2. Individual gastric pH values in fetuses following material stimulation with insulin, histamine, or gastrin.

Table I. *Electrolyte composition of fetal gastric juice following maternal stimulation*

Type of stimulation	Fetal gastric juice composition: Potassium (mEq./L.)	Fetal gastric juice composition: Chloride (mEq./L.)
Base-line secretion (27 pups)	3.24	81.96
Maternal stimulation with		
Gastrin (14 pups)	3.97	138.20
Insulin (25 pups)	8.51	227.95
Histamine (19 pups)	11.94	482.48

Table II. *Significance of increase in canine fetal acid output following maternal stimulation*

Maternal stimulation with	*t value*	*P value*
Histamine	2.5099	<0.02
Insulin	3.2605	<0.01
Gastrin	4.456	<0.01

before term. During the last week of gestation, however, a significant increase in acid output was observed in fetuses following maternal stimulation with histamine, insulin, or gastrin (Table II).

The classic concept of the placenta as a simple, passive, semipermeable filter is no longer tenable in the light of present knowledge.[13] In general, compounds of small molecular size diffuse more rapidly across the placenta than those with larger molecules. Substances above the molecular weight of 1,000 cross the placental membranes only when special metabolic or oncotic pressures are present.[1] Labeled amino acids cross the placenta rapidly; however, the placenta does appear to allow passage of amino acids with certain configurations more rapidly than others. Experiments in monkeys and guinea pigs indicate that all of the maternal serum protein fractions are transferred, although in different amounts.[4] Gelfand and associates[5] found no relationship between the rate of transfer and the molecular weight or the molecular size of the constituents. Page[14] postulated that all substances can cross the placenta slowly and in the same direction provided that they are not destroyed or "trapped" during passage. For any given placenta at any given time, relative rates of passage are dependent upon constants peculiar to the substances to be transported. Dancis and Shafran[4] concluded that other plasma proteins in addition to gamma globulins are transferred in large volumes to the fetus. Studies in vitro failed to demonstrate any specific proteolytic powers in the placenta which degrade maternal plasma proteins. Presumably for the protection of the fetus, the placenta is able to deaminate usual volumes of amines, such as tyramine, 5-hydroxy-tryptamine, and probably histamine. It has been demonstrated that the placenta contains monoamino oxidase and diamino oxidase. According to Barnes,[1] the important polypeptide hormones cross the placenta slowly or not at all. Two hours after administration, the fetal blood concentration of insulin reaches only one tenth the maternal level. When histamine does pass the barrier of the placenta, a large proportion still has to pass the fetal liver. A certain amount will bypass the liver through the ductus venosus. Lick and associates[10] demonstrated that over 90 per cent of histamine injected into the portal system is inactivated in the liver.

As previously reported,[3] an increase in fetal gastric secretion was not universally observed following stimulation with insulin. In that study no response to direct stimulation was found in 4 of 19 fetuses. It is believed that the fetal vagus centers may not be stimulated in all instances before birth.

The gastrin used in the present study was synthetic human gastrin I. The best response to gastrin was observed when it was given over a period of two hours in a constant infusion of normal saline (100 ml. per hour). This is recommended because the biological half-life of gastrin is only 5 minutes. The possibility of hormonal catabolism and subsequent fetal resynthesis to an active component (tetrapeptide or pentapeptide) cannot be excluded. The role of labeled (tagged) gastrin or labeled tetrapeptide is questionable, because the radioactivity measured in the fetal circulation may not be identical with the actual enzyme activity.

CONCLUSION

From the present study, it is apparent that insulin, histamine, and gastrin, given to a pregnant dog, are able to cross the placental barrier to a certain extent and stimulate gastric secretion in the fetus. The fetal gastric response following maternal stimulation with gastrin is similar to that observed following direct fetal stimulation. The fetal response following maternal stimulation with histamine or insulin is significant, but not as great as that observed following direct fetal stimulation. Further long-term studies will be necessary to demonstrate if the gastric mucosa of the fetus will respond in the same way following chronic stimulation of the mother. Additional studies with different secretagogues will shed more light on the cause of peptic ulcer in the newborn.

SUMMARY

Gastric secretion was studied in the fetuses of 15 pregnant dogs (116 pups) near term. Base-line secretory values were determined and fetal gastric secretion was observed following maternal stimulation with insulin, histamine, and gastrin. The placental transfer of insulin, histamine, and gastrin are demonstrated.

The authors gratefully acknowledge the technical assistance of Bonifacio Renardo in carrying out this investigation.

REFERENCES

1. Barnes, A. C.: Intrauterine development, Philadelphia, 1968, Lea & Febiger, Publishers.
2. Bisset, A. G.: A case of perforated gastric ulcer with fatal hemorrhage from the bowel in an infant 45 hours old, Lancet **2:** 78, 1905.
3. Bruckner, W. L., Snow, H. D., Davidson, T., and Fonkalsrud, E. W.: Normal and augmented gastric secretion in the canine fetus, J. Surg. Res. In press.
4. Dancis, J., and Shafran, M.: The origin of plasma proteins in the guinea pig fetus, J. Clin. Invest. **37:** 1093, 1958.
5. Gelfand, M. M., Strean, G. J., Pavilanis, V., and Sternberg, J.: Studies in placental permeability, Amer. J. Obstet. Gynec. **79:** 117, 1960.
6. Hagerman, D. D., and Villee, C.: Transport functions of the placenta, Physiol. Rev. **40:** 313, 1960.
7. Hartmann, J. F., and Wells, L. J.: Fate of food introduced directly into the fetal stomach, Proc. Soc. Exp. Biol. Med. **68:** 327, 1948.
8. Hayward, A. F.: The ultrastructure of developing gastric parietal cells in the foetal rabbit, J. Anat. **101:** 69, 1967.
9. Hess, A. F.: The gastric secretion of infants at birth, Amer. J. Dis. Child. **6:** 264, 1913.
10. Lick, R. F., Welsch, K. H., Hart, W., Bruckner, W., Balser, D., and Gurthner, T. H.: On the secretory function of the stomach after injection of histamine, gastrin, and synthetic tetrapeptide into the systemic and portal circulation, Z. Gastroent. **5:** 7, 1967.
11. Menzies, G.: Observations on the development of certain cell types in the fundic region of the rabbit's stomach, Quart. J. Micr. Sci. **105:** 449, 1964.
12. Miller, R. A.: Observations on the gastric acidity during the first month of life, Arch. Dis. Child. **16:** 22, 1941.
13. Moya, F., and Thorndike, V.: Passage of drugs across the placenta, Amer. J. Obstet. Gynec. **84:** 1778, 1962.
14. Page, E. W.: Transfer of materials across the human placenta, Amer. J. Obstet. Gynec. **74:** 705, 1957.
15. Pertsemlidis, D.: Neonatal perforation, J. Mount Sinai Hosp. **31:** 97, 1964.
16. Raffensberger, J. G., Condon, J. B., and Greengard, J.: Complications of gastric and duodenal ulcers in infancy and childhood, Surg. Gynec. Obstet. **123:** 1269, 1966.
17. Rodbro, P., Krasilnikoff, P. A., and Christiansen, P. M.: Parietal cell secretory function in early childhood, Scand. J. Gastroent. **2:** 209, 1967.
18. Salenius, P.: On the odontogenesis of the human gastric epithelial cells, Acta Anat. Suppl. **46:** 1962.
19. Shay, H., Sun, D. C. H., and Gruenstein, M.: A quantitative method for measuring spontaneous gastric secretion in the rat, Gastroenterology **26:** 906, 1954.
20. Sutherland, G. F.: Contributions to the physiology of the stomach. LVII. The response of the stomach glands to gastrin before and shortly after birth, Amer. J. Physiol. **55:** 398, 1921.
21. Von Siebold, A. E.: Brand in der kleinen Curvatur des Magens eines atrophischen Kindes, J. Geburtshulfe, Frauenz.-und Kinderkrankheiten **5:** 3, 1826.

Jejunoileocolic intubation and plication for intestinal obstruction caused by massive adhesions in infancy

THOMAS C. MOORE, M.D.*
ARNOLD M. SALZBERG, M.D.
E. ARMISTEAD TALMAN, M.D.
RICHMOND, VA., AND LOS ANGELES, CALIF.
From the Surgical Services of the Medical College of Virginia and the Johnston-Willis Hospitals, and the Departments of Surgery, the University of California, Los Angeles, and the Medical College of Virginia

Postoperative intestinal obstruction may prove to be a difficult problem to manage in any age group. It is especially troublesome in infancy. Devens,[1] in 1963, reported a mortality rate of 71 percent in 24 patients who developed recurrent intestinal obstruction following an initial operation for intestinal obstruction in the newborn period. Raffensperger and Baker,[8] in 1966, reviewed an experience with 47 episodes of postoperative mechanical intestinal obstruction in 43 infants and children. These obstructions had occurred from 3 days to 11 years after operation and were due to adhesions in 39 of the 47 obstructions (83 percent). A single obstructing band was encountered in only three of the 31 patients managed by lysis of adhesions. The remaining 28 patients had extensive adhesions between loops of intestine, mesentery, and the abdominal wall. Four additional patients had gangrene in association with adhesions, and bowel resection was required in all. Nonoperative management with intubation and suction was successful in only three episodes of obstruction in two children. This finding and the high incidence of intussusception (six cases) led Raffensperger and Baker[8] to recommend early operative intervention in cases of postoperative intestinal obstruction in infancy and childhood.

It is of interest that seven of the eight deaths reported by Raffensperger and Baker[8] occurred in infants under 1 year of age and that three of the eight deaths involved infants with omphalocele or gastroschisis. The difficulty in all three cases of omphalocele or gastroshcisis resulted from massive adhesions. In the series of Raffensperger and Baker,[8] an attempt was made in two patients to prevent further adhesive obstruction by antegrade or retrograde intubation of the entire small intestine. The tubes were brought out through the abdominal wall in the cecal area.[7] Both patients died. The use of intestinal intubation to prevent recurrence of midgut volvulus has been reported recently by Ravitch and Cherry.[9]

The use of intestinal plication was described by Noble[5] in 1937. Poth[6] has recommended intestinal plication when extensive serosal damage has occurred; he has utilized this procedure in 132 patients. Eight of his patients were under 10 years of age. Lance and Prochiantz,[3] in 1958, described the successful use of plication for recurrent intestinal obstruction in a 4-month-old infant whose initial operation had been at 2 months of age for malrotation of the intestines with volvulus. Hartl,[2] in 1961, reported the successful use of this procedure in five children from 4 to 12 years of age.

Received for publication July 22, 1969.

*Present address: UCLA–Harbor Medical Center, 1000 W. Carson St., Torrance, Calif.

The purpose of this paper is to record the use of the combination of intestinal plication and intubation for postoperative intestinal obstruction caused by extensive adhesions in a 5 pound infant. The initial operation had been for ileal atresia and perforation in a newborn infant with an omphalocele.

CASE REPORT

The patient, D. C., was born at the Johnston-Willis Hospital in Richmond, Virginia, on August 29, 1967, at the termination of a normal pregnancy. His birth weight was 5 pounds, 10 ounces. The father was 30 years of age and the mother was 26. One sibling was living at 13 months of age, and there was no family history of congenital malformations.

At birth, the infant was found to have an omphalocele with a 3 cm. defect. He was operated on shortly after birth. The omphalocele was opened and multiple loops of small intestine were found to be adherent densely to the sac from meconium peritonitis that was due to perforation of the ileum at the omphalomesenteric duct junction. The perforation was immediately proximal to an atretic segment of ileum. The adherent loops of small intestine were mobilized and a 6 cm. segment of ileum, including the perforation and atresia, was resected. Small intestinal continuity was re-established by means of an end-to-end anastomosis. The omphalocele opening had been enlarged as a transverse opening and this was closed. The infant had good bowel sounds following operation, and nasogastric suction was discontinued 72 hours after operation. Eleven days later the infant was released from the hospital weighing 5 pounds, 3 ounces.

The patient did well until November 2. At this time, the infant started to vomit, and two episodes of diarrhea were observed with abdominal distention. Some loss of weight had been observed prior to this time. On November 3, he was admitted to the Hospital of the Medical College of Virginia (No. 5-22-42-18). His abdomen was distended and he weighed 5 pounds, 4 ounces. His blood study revealed a hematocrit of 29 percent, a hemoglobin of 9.5 Gm. and a white blood count of 21,000. Intermittent vomiting and diarrhea continued. There was roentgen evidence of colonic malrotation. Increased vomiting and distention were noted on December 4. On December 5, a gastrostomy with a No. 18 Foley catheter for controlled decompression and feeding was carried out. The infant's vomiting diminished following gastrostomy. By December 23 he weighed 6 pounds, 5 ounces. His face, thorax, and extremities appeared cachectic, and there was marked abdominal distention. By December 28 the partial

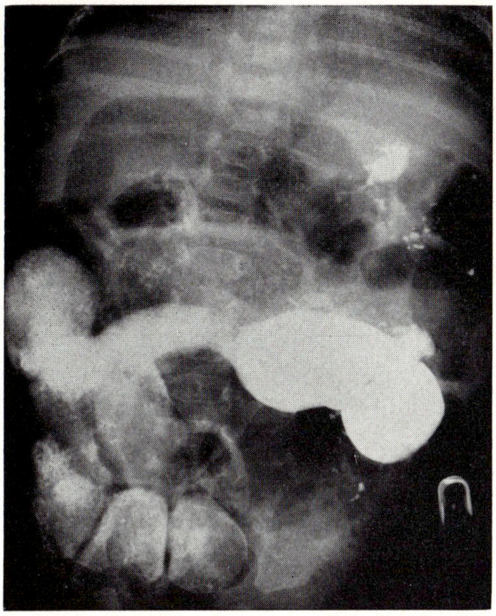

Fig. 1. Roentgenogram of the abdomen after oral administration of a small amount of barium. Delayed passage of the barium, multiple areas of near complete small bowel obstruction, and considerable distention of the small intestine were observed. The infant's abdomen was greatly distended.

small bowel obstruction had become more complete, and there was radiologic evidence of marked small intestinal distention with multiple areas of near complete obstruction (Fig. 1). On this day his weight was 6 pounds, 8 ounces, but it was apparent that a significant portion of this weight gain was due to the marked abdominal distention rather than to a gain in nutritional well-being. At this time, his hemoglobin was 9.9 Gm. and his hematocrit was 26 percent. His white blood count was 17,000.

Because of his progressively cachectic state and the increasing completeness of his partial and chronic small bowel obstruction, he was taken to the operating room for exploration by the senior author on December 30. The peritoneal cavity was entered by means of a long right rectus muscle–retracting incision. The entire small intestine and approximately one third of the large intestine were found to be one massive ball of adhesions and distended intestine. This mass was densely adherent to the anterior abdominal wall in one area and was surrounded by clear ascitic fluid. The entire small intestine and the involved portion of the colon were dissected free from the massive ball of adhesions by sharp and blunt dissection. Multiple areas of near complete obstruction were encountered. There also were some edema and obstruc-

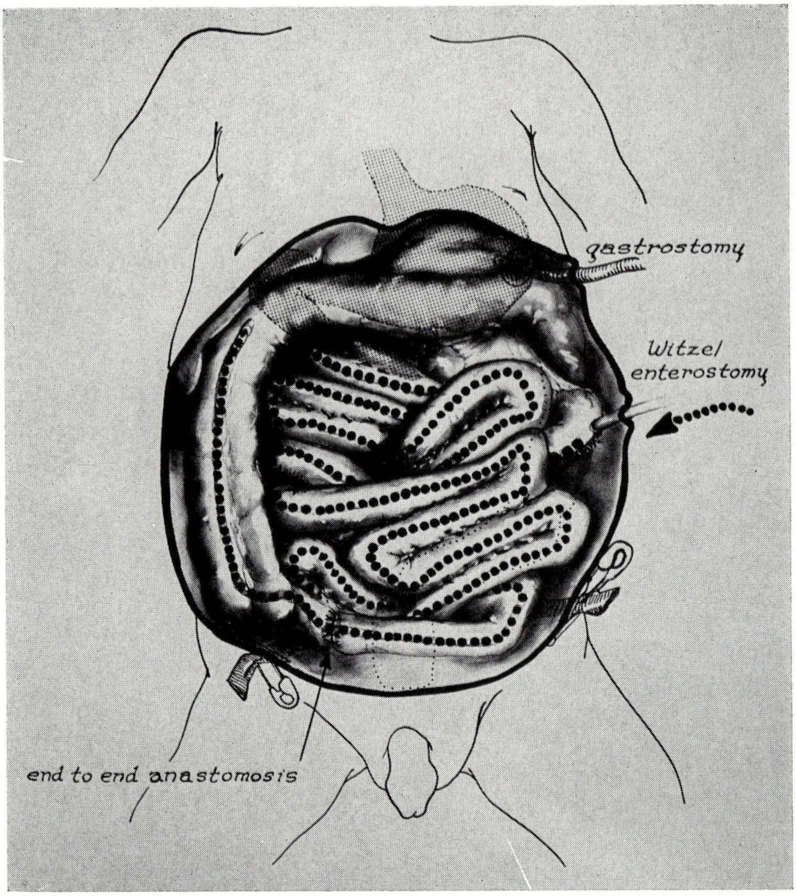

Fig. 2. Drawing illustrating the intubation of the small intestine and proximal colon with a long tube (dotted line) from a Witzel jejunostomy just distal to the ligament of Treitz. The end of the long tube was left free in the lumen of the colon. The plication of the entire small intestine distal to the Witzel jejunostomy, the gastrostomy, and the site of distal ileal end-to-end anastomosis also are shown. The long tube passes through the area of noninverting ileal anastomosis. (Drawing by Mrs. Willard E. Goodwin.)

tion at the area of distal ileal resection and anastomosis. The small intestine, greatly distended with air and fluid, was decompressed by an ileostomy and the passage in both directions of a sheathed Poole suction device as described by one of us (T. C. M.) in 1957.[4] The pediatric-size Poole suction device could not be passed beyond the old anastomotic area in the distal ileum. This area of narrowing and reduction in ileal lumen was resected, and continuity was re-established by means of a noninverting type of end-to-end anastomosis. A running suture of 5-0 chromic catgut was used and reinforced with interrupted sutures of 5-0 arterial silk. Inspection of the resected ileal segment revealed granulation tissue and edema at the site of the prior inverting anastomosis. There had been significant kinking with adhesions at this point.

Because of the massive character of the adhesions, the degree of intestinal inflammation and edema encountered, and the bowel resection which had been carried out, serious thought was given to measures for preventing the recurrence of obstruction. A method used with success by the senior author in selected adult cases in the prior 7 years was decided upon. It consisted of a combination of intubation of the entire small intestine and proximal colon via a proximal Witzel jejunostomy and plication of the small intestine from the ligament of Treitz to the ileocecal valve. A sterile, No. 10 soft red-rubber nasogastric tube was inserted into the jejunum just beyond the ligament of Treitz and was passed intraluminally through the entire small intestine, including the new ileoileal anastomosis, and into the midtransverse colon. The end of the nasogastric tube was left lying free in

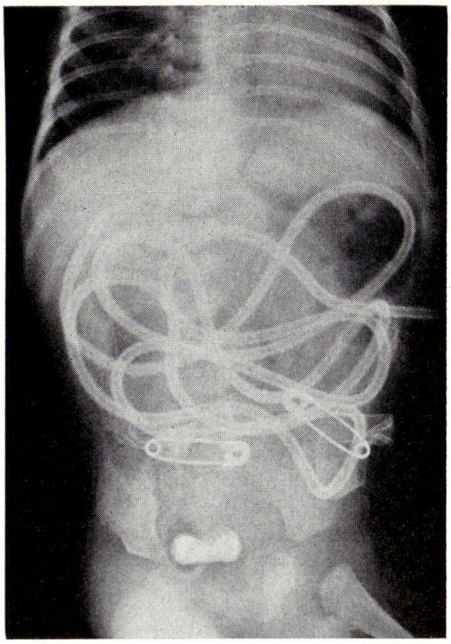

Fig. 3. Postoperative abdominal roentgenogram showing correction of the marked abdominal distention and intubation of the plicated small intestine. The tip of the long tube which was left free in the lumen of the middistal transverse colon at operation has come back to the hepatic flexure area of the colon in this study done in the early postoperative period.

the lumen of the transverse colon. The jejunal opening was closed about the nasogastric tube in the manner of a Witzel jejunostomy and was secured with sutures to the anterior abdominal wall of the infant at the right upper quadrant site where the tube was brought through a stab wound in the abdominal wall. The major purpose in the placement of the tube was that it should serve as an intraluminal intestinal scaffold to minimize the likelihood of recurrence of obstruction. The tube also could serve for suction and the instillation of intestinal antimicrobial fluids if needed. As an added precaution, the entire small intestine was plicated with continuous sutures of fine chromic catgut (Fig. 2). Two small Penrose drains were inserted into the peritoneal cavity through left and right lower quadrant stab wounds, and the patient's incision was closed with interrupted nonabsorbable sutures.

Except for a brief period of electrolyte imbalance 1 week after operation, the postoperative course was uncomplicated. Bowel sounds returned in 24 hours and gastrostomy feeding was resumed in 72 hours. Roentgen study of the abdomen revealed that the nasogastric tube tip had come back into the right lower quadrant of the abdomen from its intraoperative position in the transverse colon (Fig. 3). Gravity drainage of the long tube was maintained for 72 hours. The infant continued to gain weight and to improve. On January 26, he weighed 6 pounds, 10 ounces. He was discharged from the hospital on January 26. The staged removal of long tube through the Witzel jejunostomy was completed 18 days after operation. The gastrostomy tube was removed after 3 months. He has continued to do well and has experienced no recurrence of intestinal obstruction.

DISCUSSION

The use of intubation and plication of the entire small intestine should be considered in the management of carefully selected cases of recurrent and postoperative intestinal obstruction that is due to massive adhesions in infancy and childhool. This type of obstruction appears to occur more often in infants whose peritoneal cavity has been contaminated extensively by intestinal perforation, especially in the neonatal period, and in those born with omphalocele or gastroschisis. The intubation provides an internal support for the plicated intestine and may be left in place for many days after the infant has been returned to normal oral or gastrostomy feedings. The tube also may be employed for intestinal decompression by suction or gravity drainage and may provide a means for the local instillation of intestinal antibiotics. The intubation was especially useful in the case reported here in which distal ileal resection and anastomosis also were required. The plication gave an added measure of assurance that the serosally denuded loops of intestine would become fixed by adhesions in an orderly rather than a potentially hazardous, irregular pattern. The noninverting ileal anastomosis seemed to be a suitable measure for diminishing the likelihood of luminal occlusion in this situation.

The infant in the case reported here was markedly cachectic with massive abdominal distention. It is probable that a modest portion of this infant's 6 pounds and 8 ounces of weight at the time of the operation was due to edema of the obstructed intestines and mesentery and to the large amount of fluid in the distended loops of bowel. It also is likely that the gastrostomy delayed the clear need to operate upon this infant for recurrent obstruction. In some cases it is possible that gastrostomy decompression may lessen the need for urgent operation for recurrent obstruction caused by adhesions.

The value of decompression of greatly distended and obstructed small intestine, through an ileotomy in infancy by means of a sump-type Poole suction device again was demonstrated. This is of especial value when an intestinal resection and anastomosis also may be required.

It is probable that leaving the tip of the long tube used for intubation in the lumen of the distal ileum or proximal colon may be less hazardous than attempting to bring it out through an opening in the cecum.

SUMMARY

A case of postoperative intestinal obstruction caused by massive adhesions in a markedly cachectic 4-month-old infant who weighed 5 pounds is reported. The recurrent obstruction was managed successfully after lysis of the adhesions by plication and intubation of the entire small intestine. Resection of a portion of distal ileium was required and an end-to-end, noninverting anastomosis was carried out. The long tube was introduced into the small intestine through a Witzel jejunostomy just distal to the ligament of Treitz, and its end was left free in the lumen of the transverse colon. The original operation had been performed at birth for omphalocele with ileal atresia and perforation. The suitability of this approach to the management of recurrent neonatal intestinal obstruction that is due to extensive adhesions is suggested.

REFERENCES

1. Devens, K.: Recurrent intestinal obstruction in the neonatal period, Arch. Dis. Child. **38:** 118, 1963.
2. Hartl, H.: Plikation nach Noble bei rezidivierendem Adhäsionsileus des Kindesalters, Wien Med. Wschr. **111:** 453, 1961.
3. Lance and Prochiantz: A propos de l'operation de Noble; un cas opéré chez un nourrisson, Mem. Acad. Chir. **84:** 972, 1958.
4. Moore, T. C.: Transmesenteric hernia in infancy, with a note on operative intestinal decompression in infancy, SURGERY **41:** 438, 1957.
5. Noble, T. B., Jr.: Plication of small intestine as a prophylaxis against adhesions, Amer. J. Surg. **35:** 41, 1937.
6. Poth, E. J.: Plication in the surgical treatment of chronic recurrent intestinal obstruction, Amer. J. Surg. **104:** 413, 1962.
7. Raffensperger, J. G.: Personal communication.
8. Raffensperger, J. G., and Baker, R. J.: Postoperative intestinal obstruction in children, Arch. Surg. **94:** 450, 1967.
9. Ravitch, M. M., and Cherry, J.: Intestinal intubation to prevent recurrence of midgut volvulus, Amer. J. Surg. **116:** 101, 1968.

Infections: Prophylaxis and management—a symposium*

WILLIAM A. ALTEMEIER, M.D.**
BENJAMIN A. BARNES, M.D.
EDWIN J. PULASKI, M.D.
WILLIAM R. SANDUSKY, M.D.***
JOHN F. BURKE, M.D.
GEORGE H. A. CLOWES, JR., M.D.
CINCINNATI, OHIO

Prophylactic use of antibiotics

BENJAMIN A. BARNES, M.D.
BOSTON, MASS.

From the Department of Surgery, Harvard Medical School

Prophylactic use of antibiotics will be considered under three headings: principles of prophylactic antibiotic therapy, misuses of prophylactic antibiotic therapy, and examples of prophylactic antibiotic therapy.

PRINCIPLES

The use of antibiotics for the purpose of prophylaxis has been confined to four major situations: (1) protection of healthy individuals against specific organisms as in the use of penicillin G for prevention of gonorrheal or meningococcal infections in military establishments, (2) protection of acutely or chronically ill individuals from becoming victims of secondary invaders as in the use of penicillin G for prevention of respiratory tract infections in the aged, (3) protection of a patient against the spread of an infection from a known source as in the use of isoniazid and para-aminosalicylic acid during and after pulmonary resections for tuberculosis, and (4) protection of patients recovering from trauma or undergoing surgical operations with a recognized increased risk of infection. Of these four major indications for prophylaxis with antibiotic therapy only the indications related to surgery will be considered (2 and 3).

MISUSES

Improper dose and duration of therapy. High dosage for a short period is the recommended procedure. Superinfection with *Pseudomonas aeruginosa, Proteus mirabilis, Candida albicans,* and *Staphylococcus aureus* are facilitated by a long course of therapy altering the bacterial ecologic condition of the patient. Likewise, the emergence of resistant strains is favored particularly with the tubercle bacillus and staphylococcus.

Improper use of antibiotics in the presence of localized abscesses, foreign bodies with infection, obstruction of an excretory organ with infection, or ischemic tissue with infection. The presence of these conditions does not warrant prophylactic antibodies for the protection of a patient against the spread of an infection unless the particular surgical condition is remedied directly.

Received for publication May 1, 1969.

*A program presented at the Postgraduate Course on Pre- and Postoperative Care at the Fifty-fourth Annual Clinical Congress of the American College of Surgeons at Atlantic City.

**From the Department of Surgery, University of Cincinnati.

***The material was compiled and edited by Dr. Sandusky.

EXAMPLES

Clean surgical procedures. Thyroidectomy, thymectomy, cholecystectomy for cholelithiasis, excision of ovarian cyst, removal of subcutaneous lipoma, biopsy of subcutaneous skin nodules, and so forth have no recognized increased risk of infection and do not require any prophylactic antibiotics.

Potential contamination of surgical procedure. Oral surgery, esophagectomy, lobectomy, bronchial reconstructions, gastrectomy, small and large bowel resections, vaginal surgery, urinary bladder resections, and others have a recognized increased risk of infection, and prophylactic systemic antibiotics are indicated if local cleansing or topical therapy cannot be effective.

Infectious process treated by surgical procedure. Excision of tuberculous lymph nodes, excision of pulmonary abscess, drainage of major abscess across uncontaminated tissue planes as incision and drainage of a subdiaphragmatic abscess, cholecystectomy for a gangrenous cholecystitis, operation for perforation of the colon from carcinoma, diverticulitis, or trauma are procedures or conditions which invariably justify prophylactic antibiotic therapy against the spread of an infection from a known source. The disease, the patient, and the operation each influence choice of antibiotic drug.

Traumatic contaminated wounds treated by surgical procedure. Superficial wounds, seen early, not grossly contaminated, not involving joints, and not ischemic do not require any prophylactic antibiotics. Deep wounds with contused tissue seen late (after more than 2 hours), grossly contaminated, involved with tissues with poor resistance to infection, and associated with ischemia caused by prior arterial disease or concomitant arterial injury justify the use of prophylactic systemic antibiotics. Tetanus prophylaxis with antitoxin or toxoid is mandatory.

Vascular surgical procedures. Cardiac valve operations, resection of aortic aneurysms, peripheral reconstructive vascular surgery, and extracorporeal circulation have in common periods of poor tissue perfusion, manipulation of tissues with relatively poor resistance to infection, and disastrous morbidity, perhaps leading to death associated with septic complications. Prophylactic systemic antibiotics are justified in these cases.

REFERENCES

1. Altemeier, W. A., Hummel, R. P., and Hill, E. O.: Prevention of infection in colon surgery, Arch. Surg. **93:** 226, 1966.
2. Bernard, H. R., and Cole, W. R.: The prophylaxis of surgical infection: The effect of prophylactic antimicrobial drugs on the incidence of infection following potentially contaminated operations, SURGERY **56:** 151, 1964.
3. Bernard, H. R., Cole, W. R., Gravens, D. L., et al.: Chemoprophylaxis of postoperative surgical infection: The effect upon nasal carriage of Staphylococcus aureus, Arch. Surg. **96:** 476, 1968.
4. Campbell, P. C.: Large doses of penicillin in the prevention of surgical wound infection, Lancet **2:** 805, 1965.
5. Johnstone, F. R. C.: An assessment of prophylactic antibiotics in general surgery, Surg. Gynec. & Obst. **116:** 1, 1963.
6. Kunin, C. M., and Finland, M.: Persistence of antibiotics in blood of patients with acute renal failure. III. Penicillin, streptomycin, erythromycin and kanamycin, J. Clin. Invest. **38:** 1509, 1959.
7. Kunin, C. M., Glazko, A. J., and Finland, M.: Persistence of antibiotics in blood of patients with acute renal failure. II. Chloramphenicol and its metabolic products in the blood of patients with severe renal diseases and hepatic necrosis, J. Clin. Invest. **38:** 1498, 1959.
8. Kunin, C. M., Rees, S. B., Merrill, J. P., and Finland, M.: Persistence of antibiotics in blood of patients with renal failure. I. Tetracycline and chlortetracycline, J. Clin. Invest. **38:** 1487, 1959.

Newer antibiotics and hospital-acquired infections

EDWIN J. PULASKI, M.D.
MORTON GROVE, ILL.

From the Department of Clinical Research, Travenol Laboratories, Inc.

The increasing incidence of hospital-acquired infection has become a problem of growing dimensions. Bacteriologically, this problem involves not only the patient but the hospital staff and the environment. The rate of infection has been paralleled by research efforts aimed at developing newer antibiotics which would improve the safety and efficacy of the older ones. Biosynthetic penicillins were sought which would achieve acid resistance for oral therapy, overcome the inhibitory effects of penicillinase-producing staphylococci, broaden the activity of the drug to include the pathogenic gram-negative bacteria, and avoid hypersensitive reactions in patients allergic to the natural penicillins.

Hospital-acquired organisms tend to be resistant to the commonly employed antimicrobials. Fortunately, the isolation of the 6-amino-penicillanic acid molecule (6-APA) in 1959 led to the discovery and exploration of new classes of semisynthetic penicillin which has increased their therapeutic spectrums.

NEWER PENICILLINS

The newer penicillins are: (1) the phenoxymethyl derivatives (phenoxypenicillin and phenethicillin), with substitution of a gamma-carbon, resulting in acid stability and good absorption from the gastrointestinal tract; (2) the variety of semisynthetic penicillins active against penicillinase-producing staphylococci, including methicillin, nafcillin, and the isoazolyl group (oxacillin, cloxacillin, and dicloxacillin); and (3) other penicillin derivatives, made by the addition of functional groups to the basic penicillin molecule, such as ampicillin, hetacillin, and carbenicillin. With a broader spectrum than benzylpenicillin, ampicillin is the most effective of the penicillins against *E. coli, Haemophilus influenzae,* and certain strains of Proteus. Hetacillin has essentially the same antimicrobial activity as ampicillin but persists in the body longer than ampicillin. Carbenicillin, one of the newest antibiotics, has shown good activity against *Pseud. aeruginosa* in man.

These penicillin compounds are active against so many pathogens that it is perhaps simpler to discuss the contraindications to their use rather than the indications themselves. Infections caused by certain resistant gram-negative or gram-positive bacilli (Aerobacter, *Prot. morganii, Prot. rettgeri, Staph. albus*) are not influenced by the penicillins. Infections normally sensitive to one or more forms of natural penicillin, such as *E. coli,* Proteus, and certain staphylococci, need not and should not be treated with semisynthetic penicillins. Penicillin G is contraindicated in all Rickettsia, all Mycoplasma, all fungi but Actinomyces, and all virus diseases but psittacosis.

OTHER NEWER ANTIBIOTICS

Other newer antibiotics of value include the following. (1) Lincomycin is primarily effective against gram-positive organisms. (2) Colistin is active against a number of gram-negative bacilli (Pseudomonas, Escherichia, Klebsiella, Aerobacter, Salmonella, Shigella, and Haemophilus species), but not against Proteus or gram-positive bacteria. (3) Cephalothin has a broad antibacterial spectrum comparable to that of certain penicillins. Cephalothin has shown efficacy against penicillinase-producing staphylococci, certain other gram-positive cocci, gram-negative bacilli, and most penicillin-sensitive bacteria. (4) Cephaloridine, related in structure to cephalothin, has been reported to possess antibacterial activity against gram-positive organisms as well as effectiveness against benzylpenicillin-sensitive and resistant *Staph. aureus* and certain gram-negative bacilli. (5) Gentamicin, chemically related to the neomycin-kanamycin-streptomycin group of antibiotics, is effective against both gram-positive and gram-negative bacteria some of which are resistant to other drugs. (6) Most gram-negative bacilli are susceptible to the activity of nalidixic acid, a synthetic derived from naphthyridine. With the exception of *Pseud. aeruginosa,* this drug is bacteriocidal against these organisms, including *E. coli, Aerobacter aerogenes,* Proteus, and Paracolobactrum.

The agent selected must be based on careful bacteriologic screening followed by determination of susceptibility to various antibiotics. A well-chosen, narrow-spectrum antibiotic is more desirable than a less precise broad-spectrum one. The patient must be evaluated for possible factors (hepatic, renal, neurologic) which might alter the dose-response relationships and for any state which might interfere with the absorption, distribution, or excretion. In addition sufficient blood concentrations must be obtained so that upon reaching the site of pathogenic activity the antimicrobial agent may be introduced readily and effectively.

REFERENCES

1. Barrett, F. F., Casey, J., and Finland, M.: Infections and antibiotic use among patients at Boston City Hospital, February, 1967, New England J. Med. **278:** 5, 1968.
2. Beaty, H., and Petersdorf, R.: Iatrogenic factors in infectious disease, Ann. Int. Med. **65:** 641, 1966.
3. Bendy, R., and Landman, M.: A survey of infections in a community hospital, J. M. Soc. New Jersey **61:** 454, 1964.

Spread of infection in hospitals

WILLIAM R. SANDUSKY, M.D.
CHARLOTTESVILLE, VA.

From the Department of Surgery, University of Virginia Medical Center

Microorganisms enter the hospital in or on people, in or on inanimate objects, in air currents, and occasionally in or on lower animals or insects. Here they are harbored in a variety of reservoirs which include the following: patients with infections, either overt or inapparent; healthy carriers; inanimate surfaces; particles capable of being airborne such as dust, lint, or shed epidermal squames; unsterile solutions; food; lower animals and insects. From these reservoirs pathogens may be disseminated by contact or by air.

The organisms most frequently responsible for hospital-acquired infections are the coagulase-positive hemolytic staphylococcus, to an increasing extent the gram-negative bacilli, and to a very limited extent the group A hemolytic streptococcus.

Some people harbor pathogenic staphylococci regularly, others rarely. The nose, the skin, and the intestine, in this order, are the usual sites of carriage. Nasal carriage is so common that it is generally regarded as a "normal" condition. Multiplication usually takes place on the lining of the vestibule of the nose. This is the area to be cultured when searching for nasal carriers, and this is the area from which transfer by fingers is apt to occur. Carriage and dissemination are not synonymous. It is doubtful that very many staphylococci are introduced into the air during ordinary breathing or even coughing. It takes vigorous respiratory activity such as sneezing or nose blowing to disperse these organisms. More likely they are removed from the nose by hands and transferred to other sites. In fact, skin carriage usually represents nothing more than simple transfer from the nose.

Serious infections that are due to gram-negative bacilli are being seen with increasing frequency. Given moisture and very little nourishment, these organisms multiply at room temperature. Hence, gram-negative bacilli may be found in solutions, anesthesia apparatus, respirators, tubing, water traps, or any other moist place. Moreover, because of their normal habitat, self-contamination is the origin of many wound and urinary tract infections.

Streptococci may be found in the throat of otherwise healthy individuals. Although carriers or persons with overt infection contaminate their environment, it is generally held that streptococci are distributed by contact.

The opportunities for a surgical patient to develop infection are almost countless. Instruments, materials, and solutions expected to have been sterilized before use almost invariably can be relied upon to be sterile; however, when they are not sterile they become unsuspected hazards in the transmission of bacteria.

During the course of a surgical operation,

the chances for dissemination of microorganisms include violations of aseptic technique, such as carelessness in degerming the hands of the surgical team and the skin of the operative area, failure to recognize and to change promptly gloves that become punctured during operation, inadequate exclusion of the patient's skin from the incision and ineffective masking. These lapses are abetted by improperly clothed surgical teams and visitors, uncontrolled traffic in and out of the operation room, the presence of personnel with overt infection, and faulty ventilation.

Outside the surgical suite disregard for aseptic protocol may find expression in the performance of venipuncture, catheterization, needle biopsy, lumbar puncture, or other procedures for diagnosis or treatment. The injudicious use of the indwelling intravenous catheter should be emphasized as a source of infection. Additional factors contribute to the origin of sepsis. These include failure to isolate patients and to exclude personnel with infection, laxity in the techniques of isolation and wound dressing, inappropriate disposal of dirty materials in such places as open bedside wastebaskets, or simply the neglect of people to wash their hands following contact with patients or after urination or defecation. Faulty air-conditioning equipment or improper ventilatory practices in the wards as well as in the operation room may be the distributing media for pathogens. Housekeeping, laundry methods, dietary facilities, and food preparation must not be overlooked as sources of sepsis.

The formidable list of sources for bacterial contamination suffers from the fact that precise, quantitative knowledge of the relative value of each pathway is not available; moreover, the ability to culture microorganisms from a given site does not necessarily signify clinical infection. Controversy envelops the subject relative to the importance of contact spread compared with airborne spread and of inanimate surfaces compared with man as the principal reservoir. These are old debates, and the answers are not readily apparent. The evidence is contradictory; yet, in weighing it one concludes that, in the setting of the modern hospital, contact is the most important means of dissemination and man the chief source of sepsis.

REFERENCES

1. Altemeier, W. A.: Some epidemiological considerations of surgical infections, *In* Proceedings of the National Conference on Institutionally Acquired Infections, Minneapolis, 1963, pp. 118-125.
2. Colbeck, J. C.: Control of infections in hospitals, American Hospital Association, Chicago, 1962.
3. Proceedings of the National Conference on Institutionally Acquired Infections, Minneapolis, 1963.
4. Walter, C. W.: Surfaces, their importance and control, *In* Proceedings of the National Conference on Institutionally Acquired Infections, Minneapolis, 1963, pp. 27-34.
5. Williams, R. E. O., Blowers, R., Garrod, L. P., and Shooter, R. A.: Hospital infections: Causes and prevention, ed. 2, Chicago, 1966, Year Book Medical Publishers, Inc.

Isolation techniques and their effectiveness

JOHN F. BURKE, M.D.
BOSTON, MASS.

From the Department of Surgery, Harvard Medical School

Until a fail-safe method is devised which prevents transfer of bacteria from patient to environment to patient, the necessity of concentrating patients with bacterial disease and individuals with inefficient host resistance in hospitals will ensure continued incidents of hospital-acquired infection. The general outlines of this problem have been understood since the work of Pasteur and Lister, but no effective and efficient solution has yet been devised. The attempts made to protect patients from cross infection have generally been called "isolation techniques," and it has always been recognized that the airborne and contact routes of bacterial spread are the major vehicles of bacterial transfer. In the hospital setting, airborne spread has classically been controlled by placing sufficient distance or barrier between each patient so that airborne bacteria were unlikely to be carried from one patient to another. Contact spread has classically been controlled by avoiding patient-to-patient contact and by providing a method which prevented clinical and nursing personnel from acquiring and carrying the patient bacteria. Over the years, although the basic philosophy of preventing airborne and contact bacterial spread had not changed, there have been countless technical changes and innovations in the actual methods used. The very fact that these isolation techniques have not been standardized but have been constantly changed and rearranged is adequate testimony to the fact that no effective and efficient system exists in modern hospital practice.

The primary responsibility for the failure to evolve a unified body of procedures which prevents cross infection in hospitals rests in the increasing complexity and cost of inpatient care. Today's patient is moved throughout the hospital for diagnostic and therapeutic reasons. His bed is placed close to his neighbor's in order to efficiently use the expensive and short hospital floor area. Patient care is administered by a large number of highly trained medical and paramedical personnel who may have responsibilities throughout the hospital rather than in a single unit. Diagnosis and treatment are likely to be carried out with the use of complicated electronic, mechanical, and chemical equipment which must be shared by the entire hospital population. These forces have added compromise after compromise to the originally uncomplicated philosophy of "isolation technique" until, today, it is hardly recognizable as an organized system.

It has become clear that any effective solution to the problem of bacterial spread must not only take into consideration the isolation of patients but must also protect the hospitalized patient whose host resistance is defective and who runs an extraordinary risk of bacterial infection. In order to accomplish these ends, a number of innovations in isolation techniques tending to revise the system completely have been made in the past few years. These include: (1) the use of an efficiently designed isolation ward, (2) the use of environmental ultraviolet radiation, (3) the use of plastic envelope and indirect patient access, (4) laminar airflow environments, and (5) combinations of one or more of these.

At this time no unified system has been developed which is practically applicable to the problem of preventing cross infection in the general hospital. However, considerable progress has been made, for instance, in the area of the patient whose host resistance is defective through the use of a combination of indirect patient access and laminar airflow systems. It also seems reasonable to anticipate an economic and efficient solution to the entire problem of hospital isolation techniques along lines which have already begun to be developed. In order to solve these problems in the general hospital, it appears that a method must be evolved which is highly adaptable and inexpensive, maintenance free, and simply operated. Although the system has not yet been devised, it appears it will incorporate many of the points of the various systems already under experimental study.

Survival or death from sepsis

GEORGE H. A. CLOWES, Jr., M.D.
BOSTON, MASS.
From the Department of Surgery, Harvard Medical School

Treatment of the patient suffering from life-endangering sepsis is at the opposite end of the scale from isolation and prophylaxis in the over-all problem of dealing with infection. Successful therapy is dependent upon an understanding of the demands placed upon the various organ systems and their physiologic responses essential for survival. Of equal importance are the metabolic and other causes rendering one or more of their responses insufficient which leads to death.

The course of fulminating invasive sepsis usually passes through three phases on the way to recovery: (1) shock, (2) isolation of the process by inflammation, reticuloendothelial function, and immunologic activity, and (3) a more or less prolonged period of resolution.

Products from invasive bacteria and necrosing tissue tend to cause shock by a variety of mechanisms for the great part related to alterations of metabolism and membrane permeability throughout the body as well as in the immediate area of infection. Hypovolemia is secondary to translocation of extracellular fluid into a "third space" (edema, gut water, ascites, etc.) and to some extent into the cellular compartment. Pulmonary vascular resistance and decreased myocardial contractility lead to right heart failure. Moderate hypoxemia ($pO_2 < 80$ mm. Hg) accompanies the development of pulmonary interstitial edema and capillary congestion which is in part due to microemboli and intravascular thrombosis. Focal alveolar collapse occurs as surfactant production diminishes. If cardiac output declines below a minimum of 2.5 L. per square meter per minute necessary to deliver oxygen to the tissues, anaerobic glycolysis and a progressive metabolic acidosis eventuate in death. The normal alarm responses (sympathoadrenal activity, corticoid and antidiuretic hormone secretion) lead to vasomotor venous and arteriolar constriction accompanied by water retention by the kidneys. Increased sensitivity of the respiratory center causes hyperpnea elevating respiratory work further adding to the circulatory demand for perfusion of the respiratory muscles.

Therapy at this stage must be designed to support vital functions primarily of the respiratory and cardiovascular systems until localization occurs. Of greatest value is restoration of the blood volume by intravenous administration of albumen or plasma with supplemental Ringer's solution to replace functional extracellular water. The amount of fluid given must be guided by measurements of central venous pressure supplemented when possible by blood volume measurements with radioactive-iodinated albumen. Digitalis, isoproterenol, and other ionotropic substances may restore myocardial contractility. Hydrocortisone in pharmacologic doses (500 mg. every 6 hours for 1 day) acts not only as a moderate vasodilator to improve perfusion but also may reduce pulmonary inflammation and restore membrane permeability toward normal. The use of a well-controlled respirator insufflating 50 percent oxygen not only increases the blood pO_2 but reduces the work of respiration. To hasten the localization of infection and to reduce the introduction of toxic products into the circulation, the appropriate antibiotic determined by smear and culture must be given in effective doses. Of course, effective exteriorization or isolation of a known focus by surgical means (drainage, excision, tourniquet, etc.) will produce rapid improvement.

When equilibrium is established between the body and the progress of the infection by its inflammatory localization, certain stresses remain. An elevated demand for circulation continues necessitating cardiac outputs up to 150 to 200 percent of the normal resting value. Pneumonitis may progress on to atelectasis and bronchopneumonia. Pulmonary insufficiency is responsible for 60 percent or more of the deaths within the first 10 days. Coronary occlusion and myocardial failure account for another 25 percent, probably as a result of the prolonged circulatory demand amounting to as much as 200 percent of the normal resting value. To satisfy this, cardiac indices of 5 to 6 L. per square meter per minute are commonly observed. Prevention of hyperthermia and respiratory support will go far to reduce the load on the pulmonary and cardiovascular systems.

The energy expenditure measured in calories seldom exceeds 3,000 kcal. per day, an elevation of 40 to 50 percent. However, in the presence of ileus and starvation, a problem not infrequently encountered in peri-

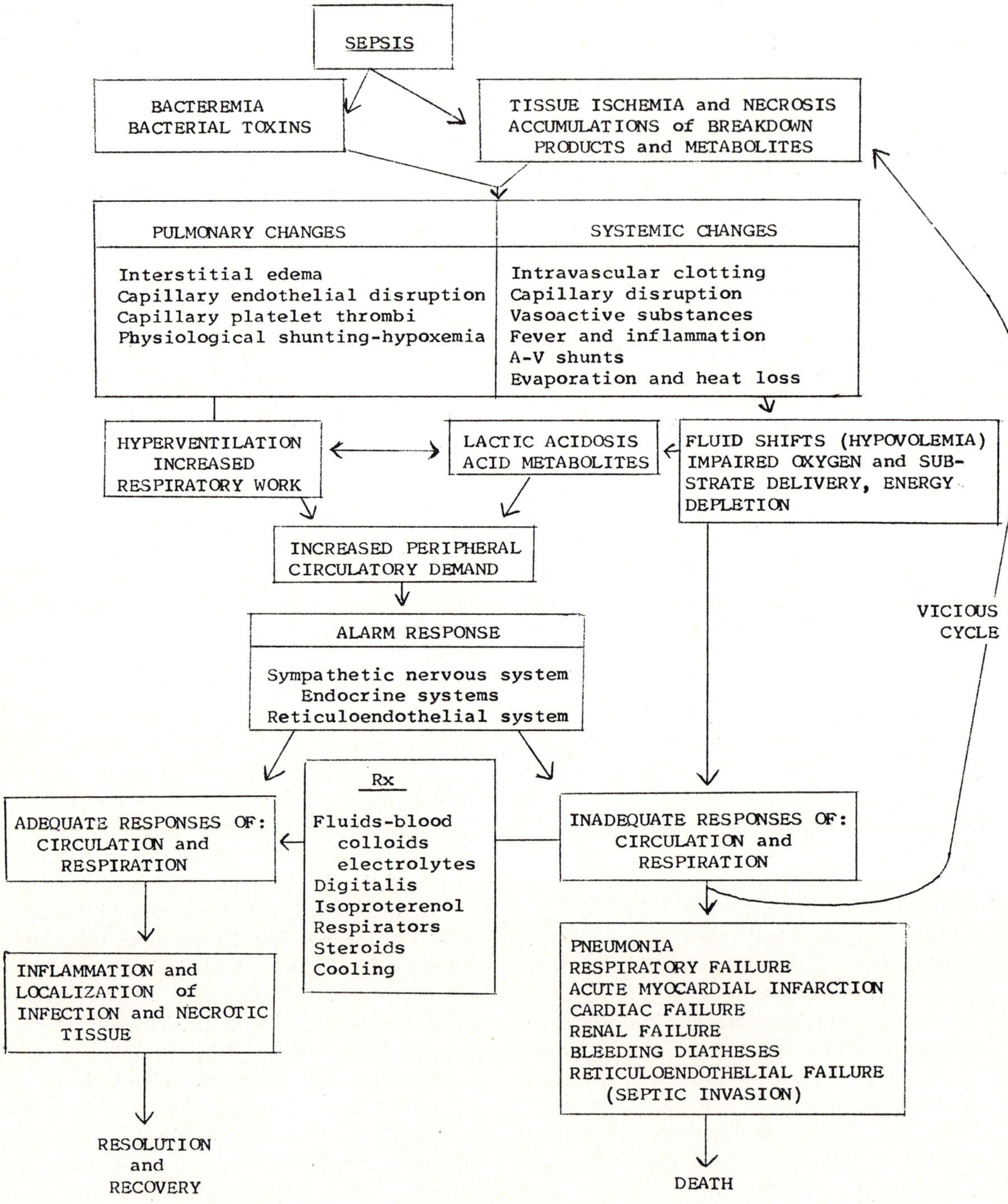
SEPSIS
BACTEREMIA
BACTERIAL TOXINS
TISSUE ISCHEMIA and NECROSIS
ACCUMULATIONS of BREAKDOWN
PRODUCTS and METABOLITES
PULMONARY CHANGES
Interstitial edema
Capillary endothelial disruption
Capillary platelet thrombi
Physiological shunting-hypoxemia
SYSTEMIC CHANGES
Intravascular clotting
Capillary disruption
Vasoactive substances
Fever and inflammation
A-V shunts
Evaporation and heat loss
HYPERVENTILATION
INCREASED
RESPIRATORY WORK
LACTIC ACIDOSIS
ACID METABOLITES
FLUID SHIFTS (HYPOVOLEMIA)
IMPAIRED OXYGEN and SUB-
STRATE DELIVERY, ENERGY
DEPLETION
INCREASED PERIPHERAL
CIRCULATORY DEMAND
ALARM RESPONSE
Sympathetic nervous system
Endocrine systems
Reticuloendothelial system
VICIOUS
CYCLE
Rx
Fluids-blood
colloids
electrolytes
Digitalis
Isoproterenol
Respirators
Steroids
Cooling
ADEQUATE RESPONSES OF:
CIRCULATION and
RESPIRATION
INADEQUATE RESPONSES OF:
CIRCULATION and
RESPIRATION
INFLAMMATION and
LOCALIZATION of
INFECTION and NECROTIC
TISSUE
PNEUMONIA
RESPIRATORY FAILURE
ACUTE MYOCARDIAL INFARCTION
CARDIAC FAILURE
RENAL FAILURE
BLEEDING DIATHESES
RETICULOENDOTHELIAL FAILURE
(SEPTIC INVASION)
RESOLUTION
and
RECOVERY
DEATH

Fig. 1.

tonitis, the catebolic wastage becomes severe. This is magnified by the fact that in the presence of sepsis far greater quantities of protein are broken down as indicated by urinary nitrogen. This in turn leads to protein depletion, reduced immunoglobulin production, and respiratory failure. Thus, every effort must be directed toward maintenance of caloric intake, if possible by the gastrointestinal tract, otherwise by continuous carbohydrate and amino acid infusion. In certain respects, which include excessive protein breakdown to form carbohydrate and incomplete metabolism of mobilized fat, the behavior of the septic patient resembles that of the diabetic patient. Observations by ourselves and others suggest that promising results in conserving protein may be obtained with very small doses of insulin during glucose infusion.

In summary, the general concepts expressed concerning the mechanisms of survival or death from extensive sepsis are presented in Fig. 1. From this it is apparent that all therapeutic efforts are directed toward supporting and shifting inadequate responses toward those which are adequate to support the vital processes necessary for survival while localization and ultimate recovery take place.

The question and answer period

Dr. Altemeier: For which bacterial infections do you insist upon isolation?

Dr. Burke: In the last few years this has become a more complicated problem than it used to be. Five or six or perhaps 10 years ago the bacteriologists would have given us a list of bacteria which they considered virulent, and we would have taken their word for it. It is now perfectly obvious that in some of the situations we face in clinical medicine, particularly when host resistance is very low, any bacteria can be a virulent one.

I think the question can be answered by saying that any infection, regardless of the type of bacteria, should be separated from the hospital at large, and in addition I would say that any patient who has a reduced host resistance should be in some way protected.

Dr. Altemeier: Dr. Sandusky, what is your attitude toward the question and the problem upon which it is based? In many instances a member of the hospital infections committee—he may be a bacteriologist—bases his diagnosis on a culture report. Specifically which types of infections should be isolated?

Dr. Sandusky: I agree with Dr. Burke. We base our decisions to isolate or not to isolate on whether or not there is clinical evidence of sepsis; the bacteriology may not be forthcoming right away. Other groups requiring isolation are those who are at risk because of others in the hospital—protective isolation, if you will.

Dr. Altemeier: Dr. Pulaski, what do you think?

Dr. Pulaski: I think the first priority should go to the individual who is a menace to others in the hospital whether they are patients or staff. These are the "heavy shedders" of organisms into the environment, whether the shedding is from a large draining abscess of soft tissue or peritoneal cavity or whether it is from lungs via sputum and exudate.

Dr. Altemeier: My own ideas are as follows. Staphylococcal infections should certainly be isolated and so should beta-hemolytic streptococcal infections, Clostridia infections, and Pseudomonas infections. And, in addition, any serious infection, particularly those in which the organisms are still unknown.

Dr. Altemeier: Dr. Pulaski, do high doses of the synthetic penicillins have the same effect on gram-negative infections that natural penicillins are reputed to have?

Dr. Pulaski: The penicillinase-resistant penicillins such as methicillin, oxacillin, and the like have a relatively low capability of action on the gram-negative organisms. This is not compensated for or enhanced by large doses, namely 6 to 12 Gm. a day. You will recall that Dr. Barnes recommended 10 million units of penicillin every 2 hours. This is 6 Gm. of penicillin G every 2 hours. To repeat the answer, they do not progressively effect gram-negative organisms with increasing doses.

DR. ALTEMEIER: Are you referring to antibacterial effects or are you including in this the effect of these penicillins on the cell wall and the production of L-forms by the gram-negative bacteria?

DR. PULASKI: Those are separate but not entirely unrelated questions. I was referring initially to the fact that biosynthetic penicillins generally do not have any activity on the cell wall; therefore and generally, they do not act like penicillin G and this tendency of penicillin G to be more and more effective with large doses is not shared by the biosynthetic penicillins.

DR. ALTEMEIER: We will come back to this point in just a moment. Dr. Pulaski, the use of Keflin for 1 week produced several blood cultures positive for Candida. Is this reported, and how can you manage it?

DR. PULASKI: This is a possibility with any broad-spectrum antibiotics and remember Keflin is one of those. The possibility is particularly real in an individual who for one reason or another is largely devoid of natural defenses. The treatment at the present time is supportive, and expectant antibiotic therapy has been extremely disappointing.

DR. ALTEMEIER: Any other thoughts from members of the panel on this subject? Dr. Clowes?

DR. CLOWES: I want to put in a word against prolonged preoperative use of antibiotics even if the anticipated operation carries an increased risk of infection. We have seen examples of superinfection associated with this prolonged use of these drugs.

DR. ALTEMEIER: We have a number of questions relating to the choice of penicillin and streptomycin as outlined by Dr. Barnes. The first of these: If the disc sensitivity shows resistance of the predominant organism to penicillin, do you change the antibiotic? Dr. Barnes?

DR. BARNES: I think that is a very important point. Prophylactic antibiosis should be directed to some particular organism that you believe will cause trouble in the postoperative period. When you find from cultures that you guessed the wrong organism or when you find that sensitivities are different from what you supposed, then the antibiotic therapy should be changed at once.

DR. ALTEMEIER: Where does the dosage of 10 million units of penicillin come from? Why not 2, 20, or 40 million, or 100 million units prophylactically, Dr. Barnes?

DR. BARNES: The reference to Campbell* in the course outline gives some of the background for this. This in turn is based on studies of the in vitro concentration necessary to produce bacteriostatic or bactericidal effects. Also consideration is given to the toxicity of the penicillin. Doses larger than that can, under certain circumstances, lead to toxic manifestations, but this in a series of over 100 patients reported that reference was a highly successful form of antibiosis. I would like to comment, if I may at this time, about the possibility of potassium intoxication. Penicillin G does have 1.7 mEq. of potassium per 1 million units, so if you are giving 10 million units of penicillin G you will be giving the patient 17 mEq. of potassium. This is an important consideration. When a patient has normal kidneys and good urinary output this will of course cause no difficulty at all. When you are dealing with a patient who has markedly impaired renal function, then, of course, this type of antibiotic therapy is not advisable.

DR. ALTEMEIER: Dr. Sandusky, do you use 10 million units of penicillin a day prophylactically?

DR. SANDUSKY: Not prophylactically. If one has an overwhelming infection, then I would go to large doses. But for prophylactic purposes, I have kept the daily dose of penicillin G at 600,000 to 1,200,000 units.

DR. ALTEMEIER: Suppose you are doing a low anterior resection for carcinoma of the rectosigmoid, what systemic antibiotic coverage would you use?

DR. SANDUSKY: Under such circum-

*Campbell, P. C.: Large doses of penicillin in the prevention of surgical wound infection, Lancet 2: 805, 1965.

stances, one does not know what organism may cause sepsis—streptococcus or hospital staphylococcus or enteric bacilli; therefore, I would give penicillin G, methicillin, and an agent that would be effective against the gram-negative enteric organism such as streptomycin or kanamycin or the newer antibiotic gentamicin.

Dr. Altemeier: Let me poll the panel. Under circumstances such as I have mentioned, resection of a carcinoma of the lower retrosigmoid area with anterior resection, how many would use prophylactic antibiotics? May I see a show of hands. One, two, three would; two would not.

Dr. Burke: I think this is a much more complicated thing than just showing of hands. There has to be a good reason for giving antibiotics, and if the operation goes well and you do not expect trouble, then you do not give antibiotics, but if things do not go well, then you give them at that time. The foot I would like to stand on is the one that says that in this kind of operation with everything being equal, you do not use any preventative antibiotics.

Dr. Altemeier: What is the incidence of postoperative wound infection after resection of the sigmoid or lower anterior resection?

Dr. Barnes: May I answer, because I am inclined to agree with Dr. Burke? The over-all rate would be between 10 and 15 percent, but I do not think this is a fair figure to use. A figure of this sort includes different conditions of the patients and different technical difficulties during the operation. When you put these together and use an over-all figure, it can be quite misleading. If you break these down into what you might regard as smooth, straightforward resections in a well-prepared bowel in a patient in reasonably good health, then the incidence of wound infection would probably drop down to 1 or 2 percent. It is in this latter group that there are specific indications for the use of prophylactic antibiotic therapy, and I feel these drugs should be used. In a situation in which the bowel is well prepared, the patient is in good shape, and things have gone smoothly technically, then I feel that the risk of infection is substantially less than the risk of prophylactic antibiotics.

Dr. Clowes: May I make a comment of a more general nature in this connection. Early administration of large doses of penicillin probably does make a considerable difference in the ultimate outcome of the traumatized patient. In a way, this is the same sort of thing, although the anterior resection is a controlled trauma with very little tissue necrosis. But the reason I raised my hand is that if I had to take a stand yea or nay, I would go yea. But I could not agree more with what these gentlemen say. I think that you have to use your brain on this thing in terms of the injuries that have been inflicted, remembering always that there is the race between the factors putting the patient into shock or rendering him incapable of responding with the defenses that are built up in inflammation, the reticuloendothelial system, and bacterial destruction by white cells. I think the seriously traumatized patient probably should be given a large dose of penicillin at the earliest possible moment.

Dr. Altemeier: Well, there you have it. Division of opinion on a very important and very common problem. I can tell you what the moderator does and what he has found to work best in his hands.

Under circumstances such as this, I give the patient 1 million units of penicillin G and 250 or 500 mg. of either tetracycline or chloramphenicol with 1,000 c.c. of IV, starting immediately preoperatively and continuously during the operation and for 2 or 3 days postoperatively. With this method in 113 elective colon resections, the incidence of infection has been 4 percent. This includes all blue-eyed patients, all fat patients, all patients on steroid therapy, in other words, everybody that I see without excluding any, because all these patients that you have, well not all but many of them, have predisposing factors or other associated diseases which contribute to infection.

Dr. Pulaski: Dr. Altemeier, may I come back to a point which was brought up earlier, namely 10 million units of penicillin at frequent intervals. Apparently Campbell did not have available penicillinase-resistant biosynthetic penicillins and for this reason she went on the principle, which is a valid one, that massive doses of penicillin G will suppress penicillinase producers if they are present in small numbers.

Dr. Altemeier: Dr. Burke, you describe techniques to protect the patients from organisms of others. How do you protect the patient from his own organisms?

Dr. Burke: This problem really comes into focus when one deals with transplantation problems and cancer chemotherapy problems and in areas like burns. I do not know that the problem has been completely solved. There are two areas that have to be dealt with. One is the respiratory system and the other is the gastrointestinal system. We have been able to control upper respiratory shedding reasonably well with bacitracin ointment in the nose, but this needs to be done only on those patients who have almost no host resistance left.

Dr. Altemeier: How would you advise setting up isolation techniques in a small understaffed community hospital (and I guess that would go for the large understaffed community hospital too) on the wards, in the intensive care unit, or in the recovery room?

Dr. Burke: Proper isolation techniques are not compatible with understaffing, you can not have your cake and eat it too. There is no way I know of to use the effective isolation procedures and not increase the number of people dealing with patients. The small hospital and the large hospital problem is, as Dr. Altemeier implies, exactly the same. Presently the only reasonable way to deal with the intensive care unit is to divide it into two areas—one where you have the physical facilities for isolating patients with sepsis and the undifferentiated part. This is very ineffective, but the best we can do at present.

Dr. Altemeier: Dr. Barnes, do you use local antibiotics to irrigate wounds?

Dr. Barnes: No, I think that careful debridement is the most important aspect in achieving nonseptic healing, and I feel that the systemic antibiotic therapy is the best means of getting the drug to the areas where it is required; it can be carried on for several days if indicated.

Dr. Altemeier: How about the rest of the members of the panel? How many of you irrigate operative wounds with antibiotic solutions for the prevention of infection? Could I see a show of hands. (The panel indicated agreement with Dr. Barnes.) The panel and moderator are in complete agreement.

Dr. Barnes, there are a lot of people concerned with your use of streptomycin. Some ask whether a broader-spectrum antibiotic should not be used. Should not an antibiotic be used which can be given intravenously? And some ask if you are concerned with nerve damage.

Dr. Barnes: Prophylactic antibiosis with penicillin and streptomycin is directed against two general catagories of organisms, those sensitive to penicillin G, a very large group indeed, and a group that might be insensitive to penicillin, principally the enteric organisms. Now what drugs should be used for those? I feel you should use a drug of very narrow sensitivity and not one of the very broad antibiotics because of the incidence of superinfection that will follow the use of a broad-spectrum antibiotic. If it is used in the usually recommended doses, streptomycin will not usually lead to eight nerve difficulties. In summary, the recommendation of penicillin and streptomycin is based on the fact that these two drugs will provide a sufficient coverage.

Dr. Altemeier: Dr. Pulaski, some one has directed the same question to you. What do you think about the combination of penicillin and streptomycin?

Dr. Pulaski: Penicillin and streptomycin continue to have one proved indication, and that is bacteremia and subacute bacterial endocarditis due to group D nonhemolytic streptococci. To the best of my knowledge, this is the one and the only proved indication.

DR. ALTEMEIER: Any other thoughts before we leave this question?

DR. CLOWES: Tuberculosis.

DR. ALTEMEIER: Correct. What are the best antibiotics for Pseudomonas infections in your opinion, Dr. Pulaski?

DR. PULASKI: The preferred antibiotic for Pseudomonas infections is polymixin B or its cousin polymixin E (Colistin). On the drawing board for tomorrow there are two extremely promising ones which probably are better than the polymixins. One is gentamicin; the other is one of the biosynthetic penicillins, carbenicillin, which is under study at the present time and can be used with about the same margin of safety as penicillins in general.

DR. ALTEMEIER: In my hands, gentamicin has proven as an experimental drug highly effective for Pseudomonas infections. There will be an international conference dealing with the various aspects of gentamicin at the University of Illinois on October 30 and 31 in Chicago. It is hopeful that this drug will be released for general use shortly thereafter. Dr. Pulaski, what precaution would you suggest should be taken by the surgeon with a long and thick mustache before doing any major surgical procedure? And along that line I might ask what about the junior or senior medical student who has a long beard? What prophylactic would you advise?

DR. PULASKI: I would think in terms of electrocautery! (Laughs.)

DR. BARNES: An example of the generation gap, I believe, Dr. Altemeier!

DR. ALTEMEIER: I believe so, too. It is interesting to see how many of the students shave their beards and mustaches before they come to the surgery service. I hope this is a matter of conscience rather than any other motivation.

There are many questions here related to methods the panel uses to decrease the incidence of thrombophlebitis caused by or associated with continuous intravenous therapy. Dr. Sandusky, what method do you use, or do you have this problem?

DR. SANDUSKY: We do have the problem. A survey made in our hospital showed that the incidence of thrombophlebitis was doubled when the indwelling intravenous catheter remains longer than 24 hours. By education and surveillance we have reduced the prolonged use of these catheters, and as a result the incidence of thrombophlebitis has fallen. When it is necessary to use the catheter longer than 24 hours we ask the house officer to write a note on the chart indicating the reason.

DR. ALTEMEIER: Dr. Barnes, you mentioned that abscesses require drainage not drugs. What about resections for lung abscesses? Do you use antibiotics here? And do you really mean that if you have a patient with an active abscess that you do not place that patient on antibiotic therapy?

DR. BARNES: This depends on the location of the abscess. The first point to be made is that someone who has an abscess should not be treated by antibiotics alone. This is primarily a surgical problem. Whether one adds antibiotics to surgical drainage depends on anatomic considerations. If the abscess is superficial and well localized and one has not cut across tissue planes at some distance from the abscess, I do not think a very strong argument can be made for adding antibiotics. On the other hand, when the abscess is deep and requires cutting across uncontaminated tissue planes, certainly antibiotic coverage is necessary.

DR. ALTEMEIER: I want to poll the panel on this. It is an important consideration in clinical practice. How many members of the panel would use penicillin and a broad-spectrum antibiotic in treating a lung abscess, or in the management of a patient with a lung abscess in which drainage was necessary?

DR. ALTEMEIER: Five. A little slow in coming up, but they all came up.

DR. CLOWES: I think this must be modified a little. Having grown up in thoracic surgery in the era when we really first had large quantities of effective drugs, we soon learned that the great majority of lung abscesses do not need draining provided you start the treatment with a drug to which the organism is sensitive, use it in adequate quantities, and use it for a long time. It has been demonstrated to me over and over again that the treatment of a lung abscess requires a minimum of 2 months of continuous antibiotic therapy and maybe 3. With that program the instance for drainage has been reduced to approximately 5 percent.

Dr. Altemeier: This is certainly true. Lung abscesses that require drainage must be less than 5 percent. I would like to give my own thoughts on whether or not you give an antibiotic to a patient with an abscess. I think that the determining factor in my way of thinking is whether or not there are systemic manifestations of invasiveness or activity of the infection. If there are, I prefer to use antibiotic therapy as an adjunctive measure starting it immediately before the abscess is drained and continuing it during the procedure. But if there is no sign of systemic involvement or effect, I would agree completely with the statement given by Dr. Clowes.

Dr. Altemeier: Dr. Sandusky, what is your definition of superinfection?

Dr. Sandusky: Superinfection defines the overgrowth on a wound or body cavity or surface of organisms initially present in small numbers after a predominant flora has been altered, that is, eliminated or suppressed by antimicrobial agents. The overgrowth of yeasts or staphylococci in the colon following "bowel prep" is a good example of this phenomenon. Superinfection is one of the classic risks associated with the use of antibiotics.

Dr. Altemeier: Almost everyone on the panel has received a question relative to how he tests the patient for sensitivity to penicillin. Dr. Pulaski, will you comment?

Dr. Pulaski: This is an area of extremely lively activity at the present time. It begins with what, to me as an old timer in this area, is a "shocker," namely the thesis that penicillin is not sensitizing at all. Yes, penicillin is not sensitizing at all. The sensitizer is a contaminant in the penicillin G product. This material I believe has been isolated and has been increasingly accurate in forecasting serious allergic reactivity of the patient to penicillin using a simple scratch test which is the eliminator of the very severely reacting and in those who are negative using intracutaneous innoculation.

Dr. Altemeier: May I express at this time my gratitude to the audience and to the members of the panel for your participation.

Amniocentesis: A new approach to some old problems in obstetrics

HENRY A. THIEDE, M.D.
JACKSON, MISS.
From the Department of Obstetrics-Gynecology, University of Mississippi Medical Center

The placenta has been the object of intensive biological study for several decades. Information about hormone synthesis, steroid metabolism, gas exchange, acid-base balance, and other homeostatic processes of the fetoplacental unit has gradually unfolded with the development of versatile and more sophisticated research tools. The full significance of many of these findings has not yet been appreciated, but one by-product of this research, the technique of amniocentesis, has already had a measurable effect on obstetrics.

Until recently, out of regard for the health and well-being of the fetus, the amniotic cavity was considered inviolable. It was animal experimentation which revealed that needle aspiration of amniotic fluid is not only simple but relatively safe for both mother and fetus. This opened many new avenues for human investigation. Equally important is the fact that the fetal milieu is now readily accessible to the clinical practitioner at any time throughout the second and third trimesters of pregnancy. The purpose of this article is to discuss some of the more significant recently developed clinical applications of amniocentesis which are beginning to find widespread acceptance in obstetrics-gynecology.

Samples of amniotic fluid can be readily obtained by percutaneous puncture as early as 16 weeks' gestation when the uterine fundus is midway between the umbilicus and the symphysis pubis. Before amniocentesis is attempted, the maternal bladder must be emptied. With the patient supine, the fetal position is ascertained by abdominal palpation and auscultation of the fetal heart tones. If the gestational age is less than 24 weeks, the patient is placed in moderate Trendelenburg to help displace the bowel from the lower abdomen. The abdominal skin is carefully prepared and draped. A small area of the anterior abdominal wall 2 to 3 cm. inferior to the umbilicus near the midline is infiltrated with local anesthetic. A 6 inch 20 gauge spinal needle with obturator in place is inserted through the area into the amniotic cavity on the side of the uterus containing the fetal small parts, but in a direction away from the fetus. Up to 50 ml. of fluid can be removed with impunity. After the needle is withdrawn, pressure is maintained over the aspiration site for 5 minutes. The patient is observed for 30 minutes and if the fetal heart rate is normal and there is no bleeding or pain, she is sent home. A dry tap occurs in about 5 percent of all attempts. This is more prevalent during late pregnancy when it is sometimes difficult to find a pocket of amniotic fluid (Fig. 1).

With meticulous sterile technique and careful attention to every detail, this procedure is relatively safe for both mother and fetus. Infection and the initiation of premature labor have not been a significant problem. However, 15 percent of amniotic fluid taps are bloody. The placenta is usually located high on the anterior or posterior uterine wall, but occasionally it implants in the lower uterine segment and is traversed at the time of amniocentesis. This presents the hazard of fetal hemorrhage from perforation of

Received for publication May 28, 1969.

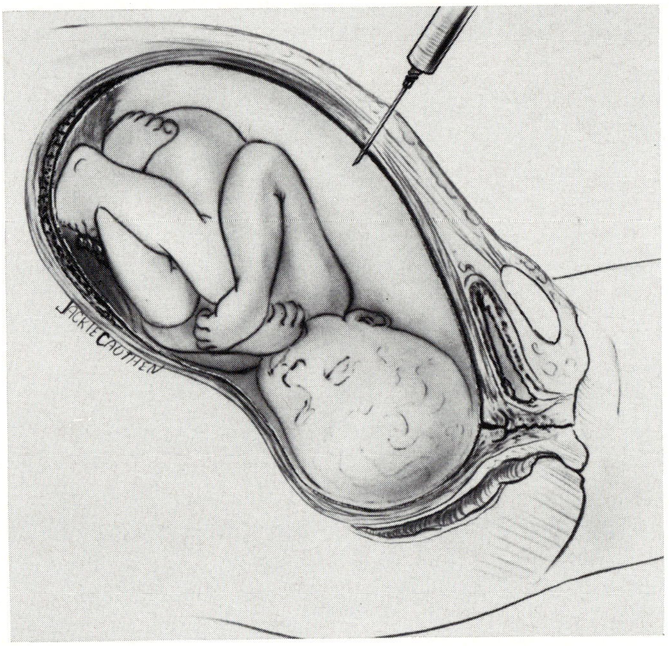

Fig. 1. This illustration of amniocentesis during the third trimester depicts the needle entering the abdomen in the midline below the umbilicus and above the empty urinary bladder. The needle must be directed away from the fetus as it enters the amnion.

a vessel on the fetal surface of the placenta. Although fetal erythrocytes can often be demonstrated in blood from the maternal antecubital vein following a bloody tap, reports of fetal distress from hemorrhage have been infrequent. Needle injury to the fetus or cord may also rarely occur. Because of these potential hazards, it is recommended that the pediatrician be routinely informed about every newborn infant in whom amniocentesis was performed or attempted, so that they will be alert for anemia or other unexpected trauma in the baby.

The list of indications for amniocentesis continues to grow. Some of these are more important than others either by virtue of their frequency of occurrence or by the usefulness of the information obtained. These indications can be categorized as fetal, placental, and maternal, as shown in the following outline:

Applications of amniocentesis

- A. Fetal
  1. Bilirubin determination
  2. Distress
  3. Pregnanetriol determination
  4. Enzyme analyses
  5. Developmental anomalies
  6. Hydrops
  7. Maturity studies
  8. ABO blood grouping
  9. Intrauterine transfusion
  10. Demise
- B. Placental
  1. Localization
  2. Suspected tumor
  3. Amniotic fluid volume
- C. Maternal
  1. Cytogenetic studies
  2. Polyhydramnios
  3. Therapeutic abortion

FETAL INDICATIONS

Rhesus incompatibility. Bevis,[1] Walker,[9] and Liley[3] were among the first to demonstrate a correlation between the level of unconjugated bilirubin in amniotic fluid and the degree of hemolytic disease in the fetus caused by rhesus incompatibility. There is little question that this observation was instrumental in popularizing amniocentesis in the United States. Obstetricians have been searching many years for a successful means of determining prenatally the severity of fetal involvement when erythroblastosis was suspected. It was partly in desperation, therefore, that many obstetricians overcame their ingrained regard for the sanctity of the fetal sac and began sampling amniotic fluid for quantitative bilirubin determinations.

The bilirubin analysis is very straightforward. Thirty milliliters of amniotic fluid is placed in a brown bottle (exposure to light may invalidate the results) and taken directly to the laboratory where it is centrifuged for 20 minutes at 2,000 r.p.m. A recording spectrophotometer is used to obtain an optical density curve from 300 to 650 mμ on an aliquot of the supernatant fluid. The optical density difference (Δ O.D.) between the peak at 450 mμ and a base line drawn on the curve from 365 to 550 mμ reflects the amount of bilirubin present in the sample. As in any laboratory determination this information must be correlated with the clinical history and physical findings. There are some pitfalls, but, in general, a rising or persistently elevated Δ O.D. is an indication of an affected fetus. Under these circumstances, if the gestational age approximates 35 to 36 weeks, induction of labor and neonatal exchange transfusion may be the treatment of choice. However, in women with a history of previous stillbirth caused by erythroblastosis, severe fetal involvement may be manifested as early as 24 weeks. It is in these cases that another use of amniocentesis may be effective, i.e., the technique of intrauterine transfusion. This is a very delicate procedure. Even in the hands of an experienced, highly skilled team, there is a fetal mortality rate of at least 10 percent per transfusion.[5] Fundamentally, the method consists first of instilling radiopaque medium into the amniotic cavity. Abdominal x-rays are taken 2 hours and 24 hours later. This accomplishes three things: (1) It clearly outlines the fetus. If generalized edema (hydrops fetalis) is already present, transfusion is probably contraindicated. (2) It establishes whether the fetus is swallowing amniotic fluid at a normal rate. If contrast medium is seen in the fetal small intestine at 2 hours, fetal distress is suspected because it is often associated with hyperperistaltic activity. If no contrast medium is found in the intestine after 24 hours, the fetus is either dead, too sick to swallow, or has a congenital deformity of the upper gastrointestinal tract. (3) The contrast medium usually found in the fetal intestine after 24 hours provides a target for the introduction of a Tuohy needle into one of the lower quadrants of the fetal abdomen under a fluoroscope with an image intensifier. About 10 ml., per 100 grams of estimated fetal weight, of packed, THAM–buffered, group O Rh-negative blood that is compatible with the mother's serum is slowly instilled into the fetal peritoneal cavity. This is repeated at intervals of 10 to 14 days until 35 to 36 weeks' gestation when delivery is effected by cesarean section.

Fetal maturity. There are occasions when it is essential to have a reasonably accurate estimate of the gestational age of the fetus. A good example is found in the management of the pregnant diabetic patient where to permit pregnancy to continue until term invites an unheralded intrauterine demise and where interruption of pregnancy too soon leads to death in the nursery from respiratory distress syndrome. The best results are obtained by delivery at 37 weeks. But a means for determining fetal age that is both reliable and entirely acceptable is lacking. Women frequently don't recall the exact date of their last menses or they misinterpret bleeding which may occur with nidation as being their last normal menses. Clinical estimation of fetal size, even in the hands of an experienced obstetrician-gynecologist, is frequently wide of the mark, especially in very small and very large babies. Furthermore, there are good data to show that the fetal size doesn't correlate well with fetal maturity. For example, large babies may be metabolically and functionally immature (as in cases of diabetes), and small babies may be the product of growth retardation in utero. Therefore, fetal skeletal measurements obtained by roentgenography or ultrasound are of limited usefulness. Roentgenographic demonstration of calcification in the distal femoral epiphyses of the fetus is usually consistent with a gestational age of 36 to 37 weeks, but unfortunately it is not seen in the fetograms of at least 15 percent of mature gestations. Moreover, growth-retarded infants have delayed epiphyseal ossification as well as small skeletal measurements. Absence of calcification, therefore, doesn't exclude the possibility of a mature fetus. Accordingly, obstetricians have been actively seeking a means for detecting maturity other than by fetal size. Emphasis has recently been placed on finding a means for determining the degree of fetal metabolic maturity. Amniotic fluid analysis may provide this answer.

Considerable data on the physicochemical composition of amniotic fluid have been available for many years. Only recently, however, has it been widely recognized that with increasing fetal age there is also an increase in amniotic fluid creatinine. The creatinine is presumed to be contributed by the fetal urine which is excreted into the amniotic fluid, but the reason for its gradual increase in concentration is not yet clear. The unconjugated bilirubin in amniotic fluid decreases with advancing pregnancy in the absence of rhesus incompatibility. This is probably a reflection of the increased capability of the fetal liver to conjugate bilirubin and excrete it via the biliary tract. Another parameter that can be measured relates to the types of exfoliated cells found in the amniotic fluid. When one drop of unspun fresh amniotic fluid is mixed with one drop of 1 percent Nile blue sulfate and examined microscopically, lipid-containing cells are seen as orange-colored anucleated squames. The other cell types stain blue. The percentage of orange-stained cells increases with advancing gestation. These are thought to originate from fetal sebaceous glands, and the increase in numbers is thought to be an indication of increasing functional maturity of the sebaceous glands.

Preliminary results suggest that if the creatinine level is 2 mg. percent or higher (Hare's[2] method), the bilirubin Δ O.D. at 0.00, and the orange cell count greater than 50 percent, the fetus is in all probability mature.[10] More studies are still necessary before these criteria can be used to form a basis for management of a specific clinical problem.

PLACENTAL INDICATIONS

Localization. Vaginal bleeding during the third trimester of pregnancy is often the result of partial separation of the placenta. The prognosis and subsequent management of this problem depend in large measure upon where the placenta is implanted. If the placenta covers the cervix or encroaches upon the lower uterine segment, further hemorrhage is likely at any time. Continuous hospitalization is necessary until the fetus approaches maturity whereupon pregnancy is promptly terminated, usually by cesarean section. The patient without a low implantation may be managed expectantly at home. Although a definitive diagnosis of placenta previa can be made by pelvic examination, this invariably precipitates uncontrollable hemorrhage and is, therefore, steadfastly avoided. Several indirect means for placental localization have been devised, but none of these has been entirely satisfactory. Soft tissue roentgenography tends to be inaccurate unless the problem holds special interest for the radiologist. Pelvic arteriography is accurate, but the procedure is too formidable. With isotopic scanning an unacceptably high incidence of false negatives is encountered in posterior implantations. The use of ultrasound scanning is quite satisfactory, but the equipment is expensive and considerable experience is required for reliable interpretation of the results. Amniography overcomes many of these objections. It requires no special equipment; it can be easily performed and interpreted by the obstetrician; it accurately localizes the placenta wherever the implantation site; and, as a bonus, the obstetrician has amniotic fluid to examine for evidence of intraovular bleeding, fetal well-being, and fetal maturity. To obtain an amniogram 50 ml. of amniotic fluid is removed and is replaced with 50 ml. of water soluble contrast medium. To avoid the unpleasant possibility of injecting this amount of contrast medium into the fetus or maternal soft tissue, it is suggested that the usual method of amniocentesis be altered slightly by threading a catheter through the needle and then withdrawing the needle. A free flow of amniotic fluid from the catheter should be demonstated before the contrast medium is injected. Three hours later standing anteroposterior and lateral films of the abdomen are obtained. If the mother is not allowed to void during that interval, both the maternal bladder and placenta are readily identified.

Trophoblastic neoplasm. Occasionally the clinician is confronted with the possibility that his patient has a placental tumor, such as a hydatidiform mole. Since this question often arises at 14 to 16 weeks, before a positive diagnosis of pregnancy can be made (18 to 20 weeks), the distinction between a normal intrauterine pregnancy and a trophoblastic tumor is difficult. Amniography can be useful here, also. Recovery of amniotic fluid by amniocentesis excludes the diagnosis of hydatidiform mole in most instances, but if no amniotic fluid is obtained, the question is unresolved. Under these circumstances 2 ml. of radiopaque medium is instilled under fluoroscopy. If the needle is in the uterine cavity and if the uterus contains a hydatidiform mole, the vesicles are clearly outlined by the contrast medium and the diagnosis is established. If the needle is in the uterine wall or in the fetus, this small amount of radiopaque medium is unlikely to cause any serious difficulties.

MATERNAL INDICATIONS

Genetic counseling. One of the most dramatic outgrowths of amniocentesis developed several years ago with the discovery that the fetal cells which are constantly found in the amniotic fluid are viable and can be readily propagated in tissue culture.[6, 7] After a short period of growth in vitro, these fetal cell cultures can be used for obtaining chromosome preparations. This not only provides a tool for diagnosing cytogenetic disorders prenatally, but it also permits the detection of heritable metabolic disorders in the fetus as early as 14 to 16 weeks of gestation.

To a pregnant woman, who has previously delivered a nondisjunction type of Mongoloid (Down's syndrome), it is a great relief to be assured at 4 months of gestation that her fetus is cytogenetically normal. The same information can be obtained for the pregnant woman who at age 40 or over stands a statistically greater risk of having conceived a Mongoloid. In the event that autosomal trisomy is encountered in the fetus, therapeutic abortion may be offered to the patient where it is legal to do so.[8]

There are at least 18 familial metabolic disorders which have been, or can be detected prenatally, early in the second trimester.[4] These include such defects as galactosemia, glucose-6-phosphate dehydrogenase deficiency, homocystinuria, orotic aciduria, etc. Successful management of these disorders is dependent upon early diagnosis in order that the missing precursors or metabolites can be supplied or that substances which tend to accumulate because of an enzyme deficiency can be avoided. Further, since the genetic sex of the fetus can be accurately determined by karyotypic analysis of the fetal cells, pregnancies in women heterozygous for certain other x-linked recessive disorders such as hemophilia and some types of muscular dystrophy can be managed in a more informed and confident manner than has previously been the case.

Termination of pregnancy. It is uncommon now to encounter a situation in which therapeutic evacuation of the pregnant uterus is essential to preserve the life of the mother. However, missed abortion and fetal death in utero, which may be associated with progressive maternal hypofibrinogenemia, constitute a clear-cut indication for emptying the uterus. Amniocentesis has proved to be useful here also. First, it helps to substantiate the clinical diagnosis of fetal death. The amniotic fluid is usually muddy in appearance and radiopaque medium instilled into the amniotic cavity fails to appear in the fetal intestine. Secondly, after removing from 125 ml. to a maximum 200 ml. of amniotic fluid, a like amount of sterile 20 percent saline is slowly instilled into the amniotic cavity. Labor and spontaneous evacuation of the uterus will result within 36 hours in the vast majority of patients. It is absolutely essential that the hypertonic saline be placed only in the amniotic cavity and not the maternal soft tissues, so replacement of the needle with a catheter is strongly advised. Although this procedure is not without some hazard to the mother, the morbidity is considerably less than that for a hysterotomy. Dilatation and curettage is contraindicated in a pregnant uterus any larger than a 12 to 14 weeks' gestation.

The concept of amniocentesis has already been expanded to include the development of methods and instruments with which to look into the amniotic cavity, such as the following: Give intrauterine fetal transfusions; perform intrauterine fetal surgery; monitor continuously during labor the fetal electrocardiogram, electroencephalogram, pH, and blood gases; and record the frequency and amplitude of uterine contractions. This continued emphasis on research in fetal medicine is stimulated by the growing realization that it is of primary importance to be wellborn.

SUMMARY

Amniocentesis, by definition, is the aspiration of fluid from the amniotic cavity. Whereas this was initially a procedure largely employed by those pursuing some form of clinical investigation, through a series of relatively unrelated events, it has become a valuable clinical tool—an office procedure—with which every practicing obstetrician ought to be thoroughly familiar. Amniocentesis serves two fundamental purposes. It provides a means of obtaining amniotic fluid in reasonably pure form for physicochemical analysis; it provides a means for the introduction of a variety of different materials into the amniotic cavity. These new diagnostic and therapeutic capabilities offer considerable promise of improved care for both mother and fetus.

REFERENCES

1. Bevis, D. C. A.: Blood pigments in haemolytic disease of the newborn, J. Obstet. Gynaec. Brit. Emp. **63:** 68, 1956.
2. Hare, R. S.: Endogenous creatinine in blood and urine, Proc. Soc. Exp. Biol. Med. **74:** 148, 1950.
3. Liley, A. W.: Liquor amnii analysis in the management of the pregnancy complicated by rhesus sensitization, Amer. J. Obstet. Gynec. **82:** 1359, 1961.
4. Nadler, H. L.: Prenatal detection of genetic defects, J. Pediat. **74:** 132, 1969.
5. Niswander, K. R., Westphal, M. C., and Seekree, S.: Amniocentesis in management of the Rh problem, Obstet. Gynec. **30:** 646, 1967.
6. Steele, M. W., and Breg, W. R.: Chromosome analysis of human amniotic fluid cells, Lancet **1:** 383, 1966.
7. Thiede, H. A., Creasman, W. T., and Metcalfe, S.: Antenatal analysis of human chromosomes, Amer. J. Obstet. Gynec. **94:** 589, 1966.
8. Valenti, C., Schutta, E. J., and Kehaty, T.: Prenatal diagnosis of Down's syndrome, Lancet **2:** 220, 1968.
9. Walker, A. H. C.: Liquor amnii studies in the prediction of haemolytic disease of the newborn, Brit. Med. J. **2:** 376, 1957.
10. Wiser, W. L., and Thiede, H. A.: Amniotic fluid and fetal maturity, South. M. J. **62:** 577, 1969.

Surgical techniques

Conducted by WILLIAM S. BLAKEMORE, M.D.

Ligation, stripping, and excision of varicose veins

W. ANDREW DALE, M.D.
NASHVILLE, TENN.
From the Vanderbilt Medical Center, St. Thomas Hospital, and Baptist Hospital

Operations for the removal of varicose veins of the legs are commonplace in any general hospital operating room in this country. The method described below has evolved from the trial of numerous variations of technique and is designed to be efficient, to minimize blood loss, to produce primary healing without infection, and to leave minimal scarring. The indications for surgery of varicose veins include those which are symptomatic in terms of pain and edema, or which cause cosmetic disfigurement.

Preoperative evaluation is done with the surgeon seated opposite the patient standing on a stool in front of a gooseneck lamp. This allows for direct eye-level inspection of the legs. Various tourniquet tests have been discarded as unimportant in the evaluation of legs from which varicosities are to be removed in their entirety.[1] Phlebography is reserved for patients whose histories suggest previous venous thrombosis or who have "unusual" varicose veins. The latter category consists of those patients whose varcosities are strictly unilateral, who are quite young, who have previously had a varicose vein operation, who have hemangiomata on the legs, or whose clinical syndrome is not representative of the usual primary varicose veins.

PREPARATION

Carbolfuchsin solution is applied to the skin with a swab stick to mark the veins preoperatively. Since the legs are scrubbed with pHisoHex for 5 minutes at bedtime and again in the morning prior to operation, the nursing service is requested to re-mark the area precisely with carbolfuchsin after each washing and also after the preoperative shaving. The red marks, then, are firmly in place when the patient reaches the operating room. During the preoperative period each patient is asked to wear pajamas rather than a gown to prevent one leg from cross-marking onto the other.

A slotted rack device* (Fig. 1) is attached to the foot of the operating table to hold the legs at a 30 degree elevation during the preoperative preparation and also during the operation. The multiple advantages of the elevated position include the release of technicians who would be required to elevate the legs during the circumferential preparation period, the avoidance of the necessity to place subcutaneous ligature material since very little bleeding occurs in the elevated position, the decrease in the total loss of blood, the general absence of subcutaneous hematoma formation, and the ready availability of the extremities for an incision at any point which may be required. The use of this rack usually eliminates the need for placing the patient in a prone position since the posterior aspect of the legs is readily available.

Preparation of the extremities is carried out with the feet placed on folded sterile towels supported by the rack (Fig. 2). A

Received for publication April 1, 1969.

*Zimmer Company, Warsaw, Ind.

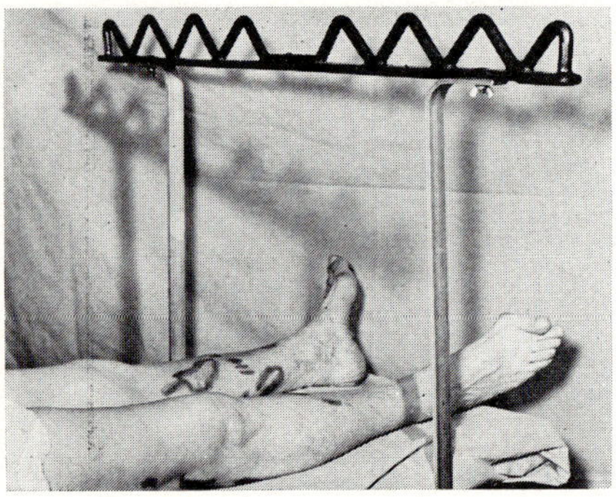

Fig. 1. The slotted rack attached to the foot of the operating table allows circumferential preparation and later operation without the necessity to hold the legs up.

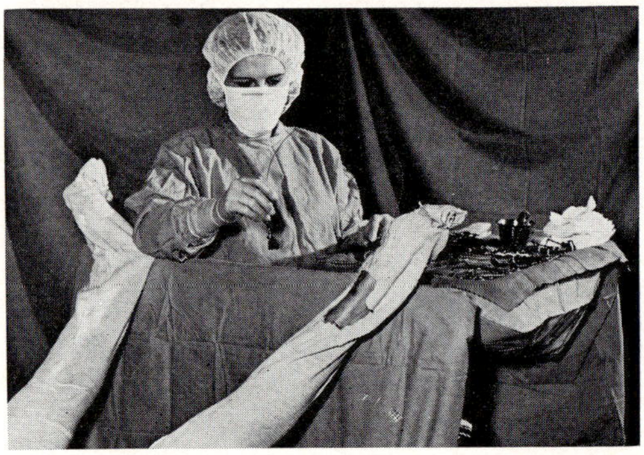

Fig. 3. The intraluminal vein stripper is passed from below upward within the greater saphenous vein.

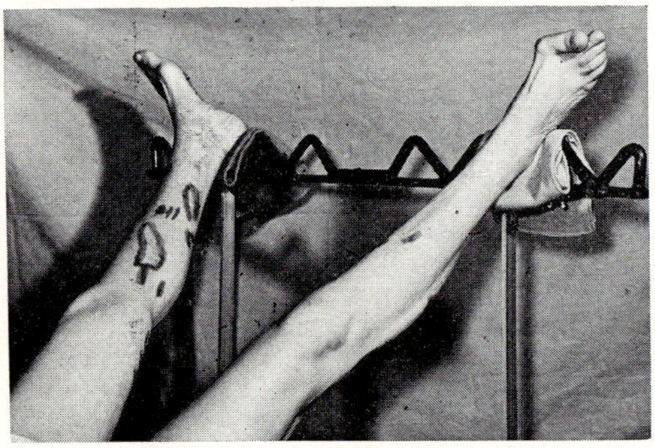

Fig. 2. The ankles are placed on sterile towels laid across the rack during the period of surgical preparation and draping.

double layer of orthopedic stockinette is then rolled over the feet and onto the upper thighs. The legs are temporarily elevated off the rack and sterile drapes are placed on the top of the operating table and across the supporting frame. The feet are then replaced on the rack.

SURGERY

Greater saphenous venous cannulation is initiated at the ankle by making a 2 cm. longitudinal incision just medial to the medial malleolus and by elevating the distal end of the greater saphenous vein out of the subcutaneous tissue. The distal end is tied with 3-0 plain gut, and an opening is made proximal to this to allow the vein stripper to be placed within the lumen (Fig. 3). A cable type of vein stripper is usually preferred, but any of a variety of intraluminal strippers may be used. The stripper is immediately threaded within the greater saphenous vein to the groin where its appearance can be seen and where it is easily palpated.

High ligation of the saphenous vein at its junction with the femoral vein in the groin is begun by cutting down upon the palpable end of the vein stripper as it lies buried in the groin. A short incision of 3 to 4 cm. is made directly over the metallic tip. This incision is made obliquely in the inguinal skin crease or higher, on the lower portion of the abdominal wall, if the patient is obese. In women particularly, the incision is placed above the pubic hairline so that it is later completely concealed.

Since the stripper tip is readily apparent, the femoral skin and fat tissues may be opened by cutting down onto the saphenous vein. Care is taken to insure that the stripper is actually within the saphenous vein and that it has not passed through some lower communicator into the femoral vein. An incision is made across the saphenous vein, and the proximal end is elevated to allow for the identification of tributary venous branches so that they may be divided. The saphenous vein itself is then doubly ligated with 3-0 silk flush at its entrance into the femoral vein. A small opening is made in the distal saphenous vein to allow the stripper to be drawn out of the

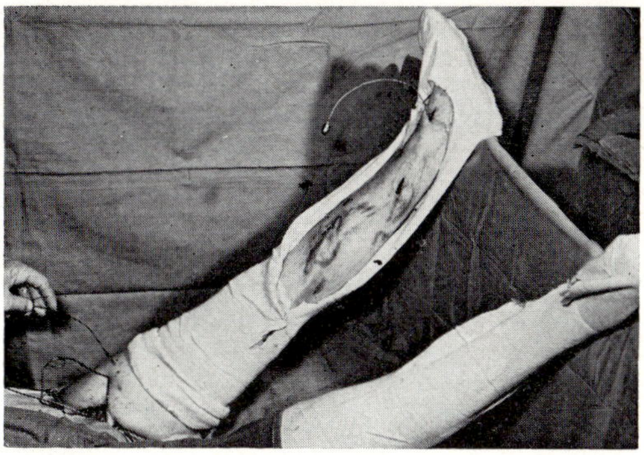

Fig. 4. The intraluminal vein stripper is left in place within the saphenous vein to identify its position while other marked varicosities are removed through other incisions.

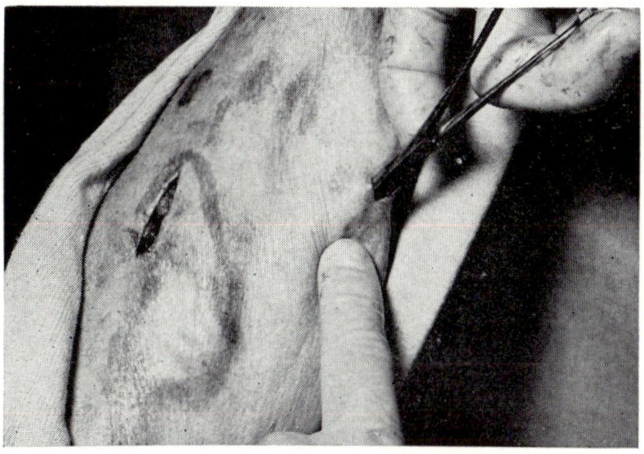

Fig. 5. A curved clamp is placed through a short longitudinal incision to seize the underlying vein and avulse it as radically as possible. Counterpressure from the finger aids seizure of the varicosity.

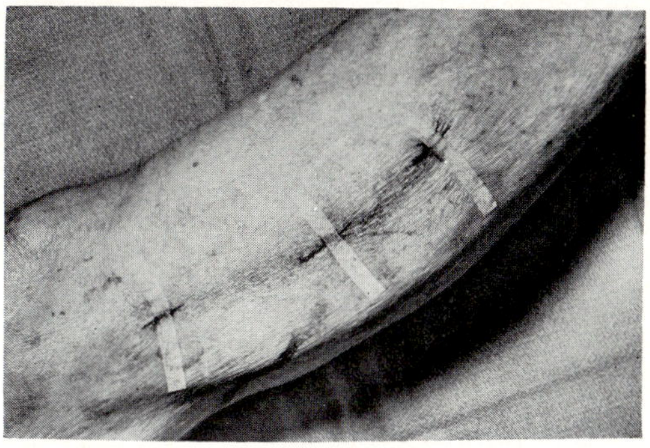

Fig. 6. The longitudinal incisions closed with Steri-strips.

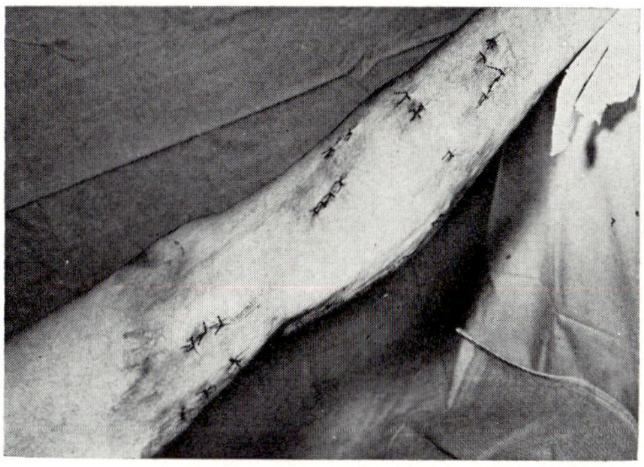

Fig. 7. The incisions closed with interrupted sutures.

vein. A ligature is placed about the vein and the indwelling stripper to prevent bleeding. The stripper is left in place to identify the position of the main saphenous vein throughout the remainder of the operation.

The excision of marked varicosities is done through the short longitudinal incisions where the varicosities are indicated by the dye marks. The scars from longitudinal incisions have a much better cosmetic end result than those from transverse incisions, and are therefore preferred (Fig. 4). An effort is made to make these incisions very short (less than 1 cm.) and to clamp the veins underneath the skin with the placement of a curved hemostat which is used to seize and avulse underlying and nearby varicosities. External counterpressure by the finger is often useful to push the varicosity into the jaws of the clamp (Fig. 5). Placing the legs in an elevated position minimizes bleeding and, therefore, also the need for buried ligatures. Excessive bleeding can be controlled by placing gauze packing in the wound for a few minutes.

Dissatisfaction with buried chromic or plain gut as materials for wound closure has occurred because these occasionally cause prolonged drainage and may lead to excessive skin pigmentation. The only buried suture materials used, therefore, consist of the 4-0 silk placed on the proximal end of the saphenous vein, of a single 3-0 plain gut suture placed in the fat of the groin incision, and of occasional subcuticular sutures of

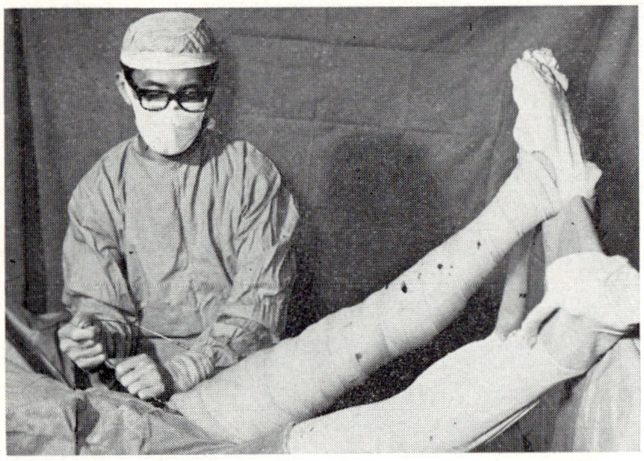

Fig. 8. Following closure of wounds and tight placement of an Ace bandage, the greater saphenous vein is stripped out through the groin incision.

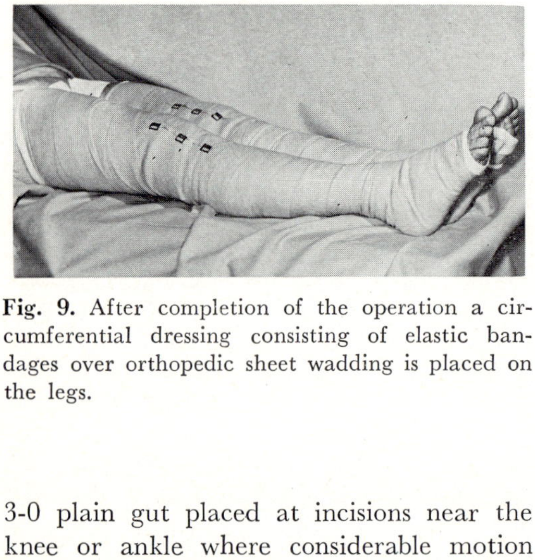

Fig. 9. After completion of the operation a circumferential dressing consisting of elastic bandages over orthopedic sheet wadding is placed on the legs.

3-0 plain gut placed at incisions near the knee or ankle where considerable motion may occur. The remainder of the incisions are closed with Steri-strips* (Fig. 6) or with 4-0 silk sutures (Fig. 7).

Vein stripping, with the use of the previously placed intraluminal stripper, is carried out only after all marked veins have been removed and the wounds have been closed (Fig. 8). A 6 inch elastic bandage is then very tightly wrapped about the entire extremity, and the stripping is performed. The groin portion of the wound is then held firmly for a period of 10 minutes. At the end of the 10 minute period the bandages are removed, and the groin wounds are closed with a single 3-0 plain gut suture in the fat and 4-0 skin silks.

Occasionally, when almost all of the marked veins are directly posterior, it is preferable to start with the patient prone, complete the posterior portion, cover the legs (with all incisions sutured) with a sterile sheet, roll the patient onto his back, and reprepare and drape the legs for the greater saphenous venous stripping.

Dressing is done at the end of the procedure while the extremities are still elevated on the frame. Orthopedic sheet wadding is wrapped about the legs from the toes to the proximal thighs. No other surgical dressings or sponges are necessary unless extra pressure is desired at a particular point. Elastic bandages are applied from the base of the toes to the thigh, and a small dressing is placed on each groin incision (Fig. 9).

This operation of ligation, stripping, and excision of varicose veins is a radical removal of all of the large varicosities from both legs at one time. The ordinary operating time of an experienced team is approximately 2 hours, with a range of 1 to 3½. Much of the efficiency of the procedure depends upon the scrub nurse who is called upon to manage a constantly shifting group of materials. If the varicose veins require more work than can be reasonably accomplished in one stage, it may be well to perform all the anterior work initially and defer the posterior veins to a later second stage with the patient in the prone position.

POSTOPERATIVE CARE

Postoperative care is aimed at simplicity. The patient is allowed out of bed the day of the operation, and thereafter is allowed to walk as much as desired, but is asked to refrain for 1 week from sitting with the legs in a dependent position. Very little pain is expected since the elevated position and the placement of firm wraps during the stripping prevent hematoma formation which is the cause of most of the postoperative pain. The dressings are allowed to remain without change for 7 days at which time all of the sutures are removed and replaced by strips

*3M, Box 3126, St. Paul, Minn. 55101.

of paper tape. After the first week, the elastic bandages are reapplied only from the toes to the knee and are maintained that way for approximately 2 more weeks or until all edema ceases.

Antibiotics are not used. Significant infection has occurred only once in the last 304 patients who underwent operation. Deep venous thrombosis of the calf or thigh veins has not been a particular problem although two pulmonary emboli have occurred in this group of patients. Both cleared successfully with intravenous heparin therapy being used for a period of 1 week and in neither patient has there been any evidence of postphlebitis damage.

The patient is asked to return to the office for re-examination at yearly intervals following the varicose vein operation. If recurrences appear, it is ordinarily better to place local anesthesia, open the skin, elevate the vein, tie it, and remove it rather than to use sclerosing agents. Such local excisions are easily carried out as an office procedure in 10 to 15 minutes, and their judicious use may prevent the necessity for a secondary formal operation several years later.

SUMMARY

This technique of operation for varicose veins not only allows easy access to all parts of the legs but also relies upon the elevation of the legs for hemostasis and thereby reduces blood loss and hematoma formation as well as limiting the size of skin incisions and the need for buried ligatures.

REFERENCES

1. Dale, W. A.: Peripheral venous disease, *in* Conn, H. F., and Conn, R. B., editors: Current diagnosis, Philadelphia, 1968, W. B. Saunders Company, vol. II, p. 291.
2. Meyers, T. T.: Surgical treatment of varicose veins with a note on sclerosing therapy, *in* Allen, E. V., Barker, U. W., and Hines, E. A., editors: Peripheral vascular diseases, Philadelphia, 1962, W. B. Saunders Company, p. 948.

A method of salvaging the bifurcated saphenous vein for use in femoral-to-popliteal bypass grafts

W. JASON McDANIEL, M.D.
GEORGE JOHNSON, Jr., M.D.
CHAPEL HILL, N. C.
From the Division of Vascular and Traumatic Surgery, Department of Surgery, University of North Carolina School of Medicine

In patients with occlusion of the superficial femoral artery, the only method currently in use that gives acceptable results is a bypass graft employing the greater saphenous vein.[2, 4] When arterial occlusion occurs below the inguinal ligament, bypass procedures employing the Dacron prosthesis or veins less than 5 mm. in diameter have proved unsatisfactory. For this reason, techniques that allow salvage of the variants of normal saphenous veins are greatly needed.

The technique described below has been employed in two cases of occlusion of the superficial femoral artery. In both of these patients the distal half of the saphenous vein consisted of two small branches, each less than 4 mm. in diameter. In one patient both branches were superficial; in the other, one branch was superficial and one was deep. The following technique made it possible in both cases to obtain a distal segment large enough to be used as a bypass.

TECHNIQUE

The greater saphenous vein was removed by the method of Darling, Linton, and Razzuk,[1] both distal branches being carefully preserved. The vein was dilated with heparin-saline solution; the adventitia was removed, and the small leaks were oversewed or ligated. The branches were then divided along the inner edges (Fig. 1, *A*), and a running Teflon-coated Dacron arterial suture was used to join the two posterior and the two anterior edges of both branches (Fig. 1, *B*). Thus one large vessel was formed, which was then used in the usual reversed fashion for a femoral-to-popliteal bypass graft.

Sutures used to anastomose the veins were tied to those used at the arteriovenous anastomosis, after the proper length had been determined. The heparin-saline solution leaked quite freely through the porous long anastomosis, but there was no leakage of blood after insertion of the graft into the arterial system. These grafts have functioned quite well in the two patients on whom this technique has been employed during the past 6 months.

DISCUSSION

It has been estimated that in 25 percent of the population the greater saphenous veins branch at midthigh. In such cases, Edwards[2] has obtained satisfactory results with a partial bypass graft using one of the branches as a prolonged patch graft over an endarterectomized segment of the proximal artery. The procedure described herein should give a smoother lumen than that obtained with Edwards'[2] procedure.

A method similar to the one we have described has been used by Hershey and Colman[3] in dealing with a short venous branch, and others are apparently using this technique.[5] Its use for a long-branched vein, however, has not previously been described in the literature.

The possibility of employing any tech-

Received for publication May 20, 1969.

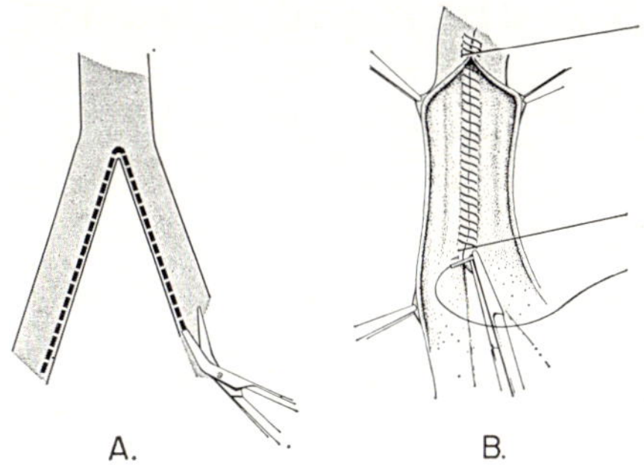

Fig. 1. *A,* The branches of the vein are opened medially. *B,* The anterior and posterior vessel walls are joined with a continuous suture.

nique for salvaging an inadequate saphenous vein makes it important to start dissection of the vein distally and not to divide any large distal branches until the entire vein has been exposed. Preoperative phlebograms may be of value in cases where the existence of a small or branched distal vein is a possibility.

CONCLUSION

A technique for salvaging a bifurcated saphenous vein and using it in a femoral-to-popliteal bypass graft is described, and the successful use of this procedure in two patients with occlusion of the superficial femoral artery is reported.

REFERENCES

1. Darling, R. C., Linton, R. R., and Razzuk, M. A.: Saphenous vein bypass grafts for femoropopliteal occlusive disease: A reappraisal, SURGERY **61:** 31, 1967.
2. Edwards, W. S.: The present status of femoral-popliteal arterial reconstruction, Ann. Surg. **168:** 1094, 1968.
3. Hershey, F. B., and Colman, C. H.: Atlas of vascular surgery, St. Louis, 1967, The C. V. Mosby Company, p. 104.
4. Linton, R. R., and Darling, R. C.: Autogenous saphenous vein bypass grafts in femoral popliteal arterial disease, SURGERY **51:** 62, 1962.
5. Morris, G. C.: Personal communication.

Editorial

Conducted by EDWIN H. ELLISON, M.D.

Cancer immunology and the surgeon

DONALD L. MORTON, M.D.
BETHESDA, MD.
From the Tumor Immunology Section, Surgery Branch, National Cancer Institute of the National Institutes of Health

The concept that immunity to cancer might be acquired in the same manner as immunity to infectious diseases is not new. This view was very popular during the early 1900's when remarkable immunity was induced against transplantable neoplasms of laboratory rodents. However, it soon became evident that this antitumor immunity was, in reality, homograft immunity directed against normal histocompatibility antigens in the tumor. Thereafter, interest in cancer immunology rapidly declined. During the long period of "Dark Ages" for cancer immunology that followed, most immunologists and experimental oncologists even doubted the existence of tumor-specific antigens.

However, interest in cancer immunology was reawakened by the work of Foley in 1953 and of Prehn and Main in 1957. These investigators conclusively demonstrated tumor-specific antigens in methylcholanthrene-induced sarcomas of mice. Their work was aided by the development of inbred strains of laboratory rodents which, through many years of inbreeding, had reached the genetic homogeneity of monozygotic twins. In these animals, grafts of normal tissues were permanently accepted when transplanted between members of the same inbred strain. However, tumor-specific transplantation resistance could be induced by presensitization with a transplant of tumor tissue which was allowed to grow for a time and then excised. These animals were then resistant to subsequent grafts of the same tumor. This immunity could be passively transferred to nonimmunized animals of the same inbred strain by sensitized lymphoid cells from immune donors but rarely by serum.

Submitted for publication Aug. 25, 1969; resubmitted Oct. 13, 1969.

During the past decade, there has been tremendous progress in cancer immunology. Cancer-specific antigens have now been demonstrated in almost every adequately studied viral or chemical carcinogen-induced neoplasm, as well as in certain spontaneous tumors of laboratory rodents. These tumor-specific antigens, initially demonstrated by tumor transplantation experiments, have now been demonstrated by a variety of classical immunologic techniques, including complement fixation, gel diffusion, and immunofluorescence reactions. Thus, cancer immunology has rapidly emerged as a new discipline, the conception of which resulted from the marriage of immunogenetics and tissue transplantation immunity and the development of which has been nurtured by knowledge and techniques borrowed from the fields of classical immunology and viral oncology.

Tumor-specific antigens can be divided into two large groups, depending upon whether the oncogenic agent is a virus or chemical carcinogen. Virus-induced tumors are characterized by common antigens. Any tumor induced by a certain virus will cross-react with all other tumors induced by the same virus, even though these tumors may be of different histological types. Therefore, specific transplantation immunity to virus-induced tumors can be elicited by immunization with the virus itself or any tumor induced by the same virus.

Neoplasms induced by chemical and physical carcinogens, in marked contrast to the viral-induced neoplasms, are antigenically diverse and contain antigens individually distinct for each tumor. Immunity induced against one chemically induced neoplasm usually will not cross-protect against another tumor of similar histological type and induced by the same carcinogen, even though both tumors may have originated simultaneously in the same animal.

Although it is logical to assume that human neoplasms contain cancer-specific antigens similar to those found in animal tumors, until recently there has been little evidence for the existence of such antigens. The tumor transplantation techniques successful in demonstrating the tumor-specific antigens of animal neoplasms have not been applicable to the study of human tumors. Therefore, early attempts to detect tumor-specific antigens in human neoplasms depended primarily upon serologic analysis of antisera against human tumor tissue produced in a foreign species, such as the rabbit. The great antigenic disparity between man and the rabbit results in the formation of many antibodies against normal tissue antigens contaminating the immunizing material. Thus, it is difficult or impossible to sort out antibodies against tumor-specific antigens which make up only a small part of these antigenically complex tissues and differentiate between qualitative and quantitative differences in the antigenic composition of normal and neoplastic tissues. For these reasons, most of the earlier reports suggesting the presence of tumor-specific antigens by these methods were not widely accepted.

Recently, however, sensitive immunological techniques have been used to detect antibodies, reactive with antigens of autologous tumor tissue, in the sera of patients with Burkitt lymphoma, malignant melanoma, neuroblastomas, osteogenic sarcomas, and other types of neoplasms. Thus, there is increasing evidence that human cancers, like animal neoplasms, contain tumor-specific antigens which are immunogenic in the autologous host. Therefore, tumor antigens can no longer be regarded as a laboratory curiosity and now must be seriously considered in relationship to human neoplastic disease.

In this respect, recent studies of particular interest to the surgeon demonstrate the importance of immunologic factors in human cancer. There is a remarkable correlation between the results of cancer surgery and cell-mediated immune reactions. Over 90 percent of patients with impaired immunologic reactivity to skin sensitization by dinitrochlorobenzene were found to be inoperable or developed early recurrence following definitive cancer surgery; whereas, patients with normal immunological competence had a good prognosis.

Additional evidence for the importance of immune mechanisms in host resistance against neoplasia is provided by recent reports of cancer developing in kidney transplant patients receiving immunosuppressive agents. This might have been expected since the immune mechanisms responsible for tumor specific immunity are similar to those causing rejection of genetically foreign grafts of normal tissues. Furthermore, during the evolutionary process, the homograft rejection response probably was developed to protect the host against neoplasia by the elimination of antigenically foreign clones of tumor cells.

Many empirical attempts at immunotherapy of human cancer have been made in the past, employing active and passive immunization. Although an occasional patient may have benefited from these attempts, the therapeutic potential of immunotherapy remains almost completely undeveloped at the present time. Obviously, the rational application of immunotherapy to human cancer must depend upon knowledge of the nature of tumor-specific antigens in human neoplasms, which, in turn, will depend upon the inducing agent. Since virus-induced tumors contain common antigens, immunization could be carried out with any neoplasm induced by the same virus. In contrast, it will be necessary to prepare a vaccine from each patient's own tumor when the inducing agent is a chemical carcinogen, since each neoplasm has individually distinct antigens. Therefore, effective immunotherapy will depend, to a large extent, upon a better knowledge of the nature of tumor-specific antigens in human neoplasms and methods for increasing the immune response against these antigens.

Since it has been difficult or impossible to cause regression of established tumors in animals by immunologic means, it is unlikely that immunotherapy *alone* will ever play the major role in the treatment of cancer. Furthermore, Southam's studies on the autotransplantability of cancer in man indicate that inoculation of 10^8 cells almost uniformly results in tumor growth at the inoculation site. A neoplasm, only one centimeter in diameter, contains approximately 10^9 tumor cells. Therefore, by the time most tumors are clinically detectable, they have already outgrown the patient's immune defenses, and it is unlikely that immunotherapy alone will ever bolster host defenses sufficiently to reverse this process in the patient with advanced disease.

However, immunotherapy is a logical adjunct to definitive cancer surgery for several reasons: (1) Patients who have only small foci of cancer cells remaining after surgical removal of the bulk of tumor are those most likely to benefit from immunotherapy because the tumor mass which must be destroyed by host immune responses is smallest at that time. (2) Surgical patients are most likely to respond from the immunologic standpoint to any immunotherapeutic maneuvers, since the cancer patient's immunological competence is greatest in the stage of localized cancer and progressively declines with advancing disease. (3) Immunotherapy would be expected to compliment rather than to interfere with other currently available methods of managing cancer recurrences following surgery, such as irradiation and chemotherapy.

For these reasons, the surgeon is ideally suited to utilize immunotherapy as a therapeutic tool and should welcome its development. One of the major obstacles to the clinical development of immunotherapy is the paucity of clinicians with adequate training in cancer immunology. Therefore, surgeons with a serious interest in cancer are invited to consider a period of special training in this rapidly advancing area of cancer research.

The crisis in surgical training

BASIL R. MEYEROWITZ, M.B., B.CH., M.D., F.R.C.S.

SAN MATEO COUNTY AND PALO ALTO, CALIF.

From the Surgical Service, San Mateo County General Hospital, and the Department of Surgery Stanford University School of Medicine

For many years, the better surgical training programs in the United States have been based at university-affiliated county or municipal hospitals or at private hospitals which had strong affiliations with hospitals of this type. This proved to be a beneficial arrangement for the local government agency because it provided a high level of comprehensive treatment at a relatively low cost for those citizens whose health was the government's responsibility; it was valuable from the teaching point of view because it provided a large volume and variety of patients. In recent years, there has been a move toward the setting up of contracts between local governments and medical schools to take over the function of the "charity" hospitals. This trend bespeaks the value of such a program for the local authority; and it indicates the willingness of the teaching hospital to continue and to strengthen these relationships.

The vast majority of the "charity" hospitals have labored under tremendous obstacles. They have had miniscule budgets; they have had antiquated and frequently condemned physical plants; and they have been understaffed and overloaded in terms of their physical facilities. Add to these obstacles a good dose of red tape and political interference, and one can see the typical county or municipal hospital so aptly described in the nation's newspapers and periodicals.

With the changing patterns of medical care that have evolved, especially in the large cities, an added burden has been placed on these hospitals deflecting them from their main course. One example is the abuse by the local community of the emergency room on nights and over weekends. Nonetheless, in general, they have provided good care, albeit somewhat austere, for the patients who have been obliged to seek their medical attention; and simultaneously they have provided good training grounds for prospective surgeons and continuing education for practicing surgeons. Not all the hospitals have been outstanding; however, the majority has been well above average on both these accounts.

To add to the woes of these hospitals and training programs, Medicare and Medicaid legislation have cut the very life from some of these institutions. They did this by channeling patients to private or community hospitals, thereby *diminishing the patient load* and leaving only a hard core of the "undesirables," the uninsurable patients, prisoners, social derelicts, alcoholics, and addicts. The "charity" hospitals are obviously unable to compete for patients, both structurally and organizationally with the local community hospitals which have sprung up in the past decade or two. These, in general, have been better financed and, because of their recent vintage, have far more attractive physical facilities. This has led to an impending crisis in surgical training which will soon become apparent. Surgeons who complete their training in the next ten to fifteen years are likely to have had a less intensive and more

Received for publication Oct. 20, 1969.

constricted training than is the case today; for example, surgeons returning from Vietnam will have acquired a certain expertise in multiple trauma, but if all local government hospitals disappear, with them will vanish many of the trauma units now being developed.

Of course, part of the blame must be placed on the local governments who have not kept themselves informed of developments; nor have they anticipated the rapid socioeconomic effects of the legislation introduced by the Federal Government. There are probably very few county or city hospitals the facilities of which could now comply with the federal regulations concerning Medicare; this is not a consideration with most of the community hospitals.

The solution to the problem appears difficult and almost unattainable. But solution is urgent. With the rapid rise in the cost of medical care, it is likely that alternative patterns of medical and surgical practice will evolve. More and more hospital-based physicians are likely to be appointed. For several reasons, this approach has been slow to be adopted by community hospitals. The large "charity" hospitals (including those not under the jurisdiction of medical schools) have had a greater experience of creating and filling such positions. One solution would be the rapid reconstruction of the "charity" hospitals to make them more acceptable to patients from all walks of life, thereby ensuring an adequate patient load. An alternative would be the subsidization of hospital-based physicians in community hospitals by the local government. The function of these physicians would then include the coordination of training programs with an affiliated teaching hospital.

It is curious that while the life and death struggle of "charity" hospitals is being enacted, several authorities are inflicting serious additional wounds to surgical programs in teaching institutions. The Federal Medicare program is considering the withholding of professional payment to physicians working with residents, unless the faculty staff man can be shown to have been in attendance from start to finish of the patient's hospitalization; this proposal would require that senior surgeons divert much of their activities into trivial matters. (A private man in the same setting may have his partner see his patients for him; not the faculty man.) Some private third party insurers already enforce nonpayment to staff men in teaching hospitals.

In California the Medi-Cal authority has forbidden payment to a physician receiving any remuneration from his county for work in the county hospital; this full-time or part-time surgeon must then forego a fee for service to involve the residents in his patients' care, should he bring the patients into the county institution. Alternatively, he could take the patients to a private hospital where payment would be made along the *usual and customary lines,* but the experience would be denied the residents based in the county hospital. Perhaps the final blow is the rumor now circulating that some malpractice insurance carriers are considering not covering teaching hospital surgeons, unless they personally do the operations on their patients.

All this bodes ill for surgical training; if major changes in the attitude of the Medicare and Medicaid administrators and the third party insurers do not occur, and if the trend of patients away from teaching facilities is not stopped, the American surgical trainee will be obliged to reverse the present trend and to spend a few years overseas in order to acquire the necessary skills essential for a competent well-trained surgeon.

"Letters to the Editors"

As part of the editorial section, the Editorial Board of SURGERY invites comments in the form of "Letters to the Editor" or further editorials which express differences or supporting views of prior editorials or recent papers published in SURGERY. The Editorial Board reserves the right to accept, reject, or excerpt letters without changing the views expressed. Letters must include name and address which shall be included if published. Letters and editorials may be submitted directly to the following:

Edwin H. Ellison, M.D. (or to)
Division of Surgery
Marquette School of Medicine, Inc.
7540 North Beach Drive
Milwaukee, Wis. 53217

Theodore Drapanas, M.D.
Department of Surgery
Tulane University School of Medicine
1430 Tulane Avenue
New Orleans, La. 70112

A LETTER TO THE EDITORS:

In the June, 1969, issue of SURGERY, Dr. Robert J. Touloukian[4] reported on an infant with renal vein thrombosis. He successfully removed the kidney but unfortunately concluded that nephrectomy is the treatment of choice.

First of all, the diagnosis of renal vein thrombosis can be made clinically. Prior to further studies, we must treat the infant's underlying shock and dehydration with plasma and intravenous fluids. Because of the characteristic clinical and roentgen findings, a nephrectomy should never be done because of a mistaken diagnosis of Wilm's tumor.[1] Furthermore, in Rickham and Johnston's 36 cases contralateral spread of the thrombus was not seen, and it has not been reported in the literature.[2] Rickham and Johnston prefer conservative management of renal vein thrombosis with heparin. They clearly state that "nonoperative management is indicated in the majority of cases of renal vein thrombosis." Stark[3] reported on 3 of his own cases and found 17 more in the literature which were treated conservatively.

Received August 25, 1969.

We are in the process of reporting a newborn infant who had bilateral flank masses, hematuria, and a swollen left testicle. Contrast material injected into the saphenous vein ascended through lumbar veins, completely bypassing the thrombosed inferior vena cava. Neither kidney visualized despite a drip pyelogram. We treated him with heparin and urokinase. He recovered and now, a year later, has good bilateral renal function.

If an infarcted kidney becomes infected or atrophies and causes hypertension, a nephrectomy is then indicated. Otherwise conservative therapy saves the kidney as well as the child.

REFERENCES

1. Raffensperger, J. G., and Abousleiman, A.: Abdominal masses in children under one year of age, SURGERY **63:** 514, 1968.

2. Rickham, P. P., and Johnston, J. H., editors: Neonatal surgery, New York, 1969, Appleton-Century-Crofts, Inc., p. 569.
3. Stark, H.: Renal vein thrombosis in infancy recovery without nephrectomy, Amer. J. Dis. Child. **108:** 430, 1964.
4. Touloukian, R. J.: Ideopathic vena cava thrombosis with renal infarction in the newborn infant: Survival following nephrectomy, SURGERY **65:** 978, 1969.

John G. Raffensperger, M.D.
Ruth Andrea Seeler, M.D.
700 S. Wood St.
Chicago, Ill. 60612

ERRATUM

In the December, 1969, issue of SURGERY, in the article, "Recurrent thromboembolism: Report of a case and inquiry into the nature of the fast antiplasmin," by Drs. H. Gans, J. R. Edson, B. H. Tan, and R. V. Ebert, there were two omissions on page 1018. Line 3 of the legend for Fig. 4 should have read: "0: Rabbit antihuman alpha$_2$-macroglobulin serum"; and lines 2 and 3 of the text should have read: . . . of the patient's plasma against rabbit antihuman alpha$_2$-macroglobulin were compared . . ."

Volume 67 *Number* 3

SURGERY

MARCH, 1970

Clinical surgery

A study of the danger of antibiotic preparation of the bowel for surgery

E. THURSTON THIEME, M.D.
GEORGE FINK, M.D.
ANN ARBOR, MICH.
From the Department of Surgery, St. Joseph Mercy Hospital

Preoperative oral antibiotic preparation of the bowel for surgery has been widely used in this country since antibiotics became available. This preparation shares with better anesthesia and better patient care the credit for the marked improvement in morbidity and mortality rates following colon surgery. Surgical technique as practiced by the relatively few surgeons of the preantibiotic period was undoubtedly as good as the technique now used by the many doing colon surgery. It is quite possible that less meticulous surgical technique is now successful because of the antibiotic preparation. Certainly, open anastomosis for colon surgery is widely accepted and the many special clamps for "aseptic anastomosis" are almost unknown.

However, dangers inherent to antibiotic preparation of the bowel previously recognized have recently been emphasized to the point that this preparation has been discontinued in certain institutions. Staphylococcal overgrowth, resulting in staphylococcal enterocolitis and wound infection, is the more dangerous complication of this preparation. This has been reported as a complication of 43 percent of patients by Altemeier and associates.[1] Polacek and Sanfelippo[5] have recently reported a 50 percent complication rate in patients who are given oral antibiotics, with diarrhea and wound infections being the greatest problem. The staphylococcus has frequently been cultured in the wound infections, but less frequently it has been cultured in the stools of those having postoperative diarrhea. The incidence of postoperative staphylococcal pseudomembranous enterocolitis varies greatly. However, staphylococcal overgrowth is considered by many authors to be the expected penalty paid for the use of oral antibiotics. The threat of contamination by pathogens of the colon at the time of operation is such that there must be strong reasons for giving up any method that might reduce this danger.

Inasmuch as antibiotic preparation has been routinely used before bowel surgery in this hospital, it was proposed to evaluate the dangers of this routine and to decide if a change of policy was warranted. Therefore, the primary purpose of this study was to evaluate the dangers of antibiotic preparation

Supported wholly by a grant from the Herrick Foundation.
Received for publication March 25, 1969.

and secondarily to observe the effect of the preparation on the intestinal flora. No attempt has been made to evaluate the benefits, as the use of antibiotic preparation is widespread in the country. This was a continuing study, not a retroactive chart study. One hundred twelve cases form the basis of this study.

The antibiotic preparation used followed three plans. Neomycin alone was used for 24 to 36 hours, never more than for 48 hours. Neomycin and a poorly absorbed sulpha (succinylsulfathiazole or phthalysulfathiazole) were combined for a short preparation, and, third, sulpha was given alone for more than 4 days, usually 7 to 10 days, before neomycin was added. Sulpha was used in doses of 8 to 12 Gm. per day and neomycin to a total dose of 10 to 12 Gm. Neomycin was never used for more than 48 hours, usually 24 hours. Tetracyclines were never used. Table I indicates the use of these three plans and the condition for which the operation was done. In considering bowel preparation, it is important to note that 36 percent of these patients presented with a clinically significant degree of obstruction. Preparation of such patients requires careful planning as castor oil and other purgatives may be dangerous, and mechanical preparation alone is not satisfactory. However, enemas and catharsis were used when possible; diet restriction was always used. The distribution of cases is considered typical of community practice with neoplasm predominating. All cases in which an antibiotic preparation of the bowel was used are included regardless of the type of operation performed.

Although no superiority could be shown statistically for any one of the three routines, there was a strong clinical impression that those patients with significant obstruction did much better with prolonged sulpha administration prior to the addition of neomycin. This was particularly true if diverticulitis was the cause of the obstruction.

This study to evaluate the dangers of antibiotic preparation of the bowel was planned to obtain a sterile rectal or colostomy culture before antibiotic preparation. If sulpha alone was used for more than 4 days, a culture was taken when neomycin was added. A third culture was taken just before operation after the preparation had been completed. A fourth culture of the bowel was taken at the time of operation. Cultures were taken after the first bowel movement and at the time of discharge. This series of 112 cases is not consecutive as an appreciable number of cases was discarded because of failure to obtain the necessary cultures. The fragmentary information available from the discarded cases is not included.

All cultures were taken from a sterile glove or by the sterile-tube technique. No specimen was taken from a bed pan or specimen carton. All specimens were inoculated and interpreted by the same medical technologist who had special training in this field. All cultures were inoculated on four differential plates: blood agar, phenol ethyl alcohol, eosin methylene blue, and Salmonella-Shigella agar. In addition, for greater sensitivity all specimens were inoculated into three broths for incubation and secondary agar plate culture. If the primary agar plate inoculation showed

Table I. *Use of antibiotic preparation*

Antibiotic	*Carcinoma*	*Diverticular disease*	*Ulcerative colitis*	*Closure colostomy*	*Others*	*Total*
Neomycin alone	11	2	2	5	9	29
Neomycin and sulpha, short preparation	18	10	2	2	4	36
Sulpha alone 4 days or more, then neomycin added	29	7	2	3	6	47
Total	58	19	6	10	19	112

no growth but growth was obtained from the secondary plating, this was considered to be an indication that the intestinal flora had been significantly reduced. Stool titration, as advocated by Cohn[4] and others, was not done. The broths used were heart-brain infusion, heart-brain infusion plus 10 percent saline, and selonite broth. The methodology of this study was formulated by the head of the department of bacteriology.

In the more than 620 stool cultures done for the 112 patients of this series there were 24 positive for staphylococcus in 17 patients. In this series, 7 of 112 patients had a positive culture before preparation. During the course of preparation an additional six had a positive culture, but five of the original were no longer positive. None of these 13 had a positive culture at operation. The one positive culture at operation was the only positive culture for that patient. During the postoperative period seven of 112 patients had a postive culture, four had had a positive culture preoperatively, and three were new patients. Three patients had a positive culture at discharge. This sporadic and nonpersistent occurrence of the staphylococcus is shown in Table II.

This is in marked contrast to Altemeier and co-workers'[1] report of staphylococcal overgrowth in over half of the patients receiving neomycin. Forty percent of the wound infections reported by Polacek and Sanfelippo[5] were atttributed to the staphylococcus. The sporadic and nonpersistent appearance of the staphylococcus in our series led to no case of postoperative overgrowth. In considering this lack of staphylococcus, we would emphasize that neomycin was never used for more than 48 hours and usually only 24 hours. Also, the tetracyclines were never used. Another factor that is harder to define is that of the hospital environment and patient population. Cohn[3] from New Orleans Charity Hospital reported a 50 percent occurrence of the staphylococcus in the stools of those patients. Altemeier and associates'[1] figures average about 15.8 percent. There is little information available concerning the occurrence of staphylococcus in stools before antibiotic preparation is started. The low incidence of 6.2 percent in this series may be an important factor in the lack of postoperative staphylococcal overgrowth. The socioeconomic status of the patient may produce a patient population already carrying the staphylococcus, and the hospital background may predispose to further infection. Azar and Drapanas[2] have considered the difference between ward and private patients to be important.

Because the occurrence of staphylococcus in this series was sporadic and nonpersistent,

Table II. *The distribution of cultures positive for staphylococcus as found in 17 of 112 patients studied by 620 stool cultures*

Patient No.	*Before preparation*	*After sulpha alone*	*Preparation completed*	*At operation*	*After first bowel movement*	*At discharge*
1	×					
2	×				×	×
3	×				×	
4				×		
5		×				
6						×
7		×				×
8	×		×		×	
9		×				
10		×				
11		×				
12					×	
13		×				
14					×	
15	×					
16	×					
17	×	×				

there could be no significant correlation between the type of preparation, the degree of obstruction, or the condition for which the operation was done and the occurrence of staphylococcus.

The explanation given for staphylococcal overgrowth has been that the preoperative preparation suppresses or eliminates normal flora allowing the unopposed staphylococcus to flourish. The implication of this is that the more successful the preparation, the more disastrous are the results. Our lack of staphylococcal overgrowth was not due to failure of our preparation if our results are compared with those of others. Forty-seven percent of the cultures of the bowel at operation grew no bacteria or only a species of Candida. The flora was significantly altered in an additional 27.5 percent inasmuch as *E. coli* was eliminated and growth of other bacteria obtained only on subcultures. In 25.5 percent of the cases the preparation was considered a failure because *E. coli* was demonstrated on culture with or without other bacteria at the time of operation.

All of the seven patients who had staphylococcus cultured from the postoperative stools had no growth of bacteria from bowel culture at operation. This is in accord with the theory that successful suppression of the normal flora leads to the growth of the staphylococcus. However, clinically, this was not staphylococcal overgrowth in this 6.2 percent of our patients, as these patients did not have staphylococcal enterocolitis or staphylococcal wound infection. The lack of clinical significance of these positive cultures may be explained by the growth of *E.* coli and other stool flora with the staphylococcus in all but one case. The one dominant culture of staphylococcus came from a normal-functioning colostomy following resection of the rectosigmoid colon. Undoubtedly, the rapid return of usual bowel flora postoperatively stopped any staphylococcal overgrowth. This occurred in 90.9 percent as shown by the cultures of the first bowel movement. The remaining 9 percent had either no growth or yeast at the time of their first bowel movement.

Pseudomembranous enterocolitis with or without staphylococcus in the stools has been reported for many years. This may or may not be associated with a surgical procedure. Altemeier and associates[1] have stated that changing the intestinal flora with antibiotics will predispose to staphylococcal enterocolitis.

Prohaska and associates[6] have very well reviewed the entire subject of postoperative diarrhea following antibiotic preparation of the bowel. Enterocolitis may be due to the enterotoxin of the staphylococcus without stool cultures showing the staphylococcus. The typical case is characterized by chills, fever, abdominal pain, and frequent mucoid watery stool. Azar and Drapanas[2] reported three deaths in their series of 445 cases and an over-all incidence of 10 percent. Polacek and Sanfelippo[5] reported a 27 percent incidence in 270 cases with two cases of fulminating enterocolitis. Cohn[3] reported only one in over 700 cases. Concomitant to the sporadic nonpersistent occurrence of staphylococcus during the postoperative course of the patients in this study, there was no case of fulminating or severe enterocolitis. Seventeen patients were considered to have diarrhea during their postoperative course. There was no constant or significant pattern to their stool cultures, and no staphylococcus was demonstrated on culture. We would point out that an anastomosis that functions poorly is a source of obstruction which can produce diarrhea.

Postoperative wound infection following colon surgery has been studied in many institutions. Altemeier and co-workers[1] have reported a 12.9 percent infection rate in surgical wounds and emphasized the role of the staphylococcus in colon surgery. Polacek and Sanfelippo[5] reported a 23 percent occurrence following antibiotic preparation with 40 percent attributed to the staphylococcus. Azar and Drapanas[2] emphasized the dangers of combining pre- and postoperative antibiotics. Their over-all wound infection rate was 19 percent. Twenty-four percent of the wounds had staphylococcus in the culture. One must consider the many variables, such as infection at the time of surgery, difficult bowel preparation, and the type of operation, when considering wound infections. Because the staphylococcus occurred only sporadically in the stool cultures of this series, it rarely joined in wound infection. Clinically, at the time of patient care, 14 wounds were considered infected but two wound cultures grew no bacteria. Of the 12 wound infections in 112 patients, four were expected from operative findings, two resulted from suture breakdown, and six were unexpected. Eight wound cultures grew stool flora, and in one additional case staphylococcus joined with stool flora. Half of these 12 patients had no growth from the bowel culture at operation and an additional 25 percent showed a significant reduction of stool flora with the elimination of *E. coli.* The figure of 10 percent wound infection despite a 75 percent successful bowel preparation agrees with other reports. The lack of staphylococcal wound infection in this series is unusual but not unexpected in view of its absence in the stools.

The routine use of postoperative antibiotics following colon surgery has been condemned by Azar and Drapanas[2] particularly if it was combined with preoperative preparation as this led to enterocolitis and wound infection.

Altemeier and co-workers,[2] who do not use antibiotics preoperatively, have recommended 3 days of postoperative parenteral antibiotics. Others have suggested the use of oral antibiotics specifically for the staphylococcus in the postoperative period. In this series 58 percent of the patients received postoperative antibiotics, usually penicillin and Chloromycetin. Eight of the 12 patients who developed a wound infection were given antibiotics immediately after operation, the other four only when the infection developed. Inasmuch as 42 percent of the patients in this series did not receive postoperative antibiotics, it is obvious that no routine was followed. We can conclude that in this experience the use of postoperative antibiotics did not lead to staphylococcal overgrowth and that their use did not prevent wound infection.

Because this study was done primarily to evaluate the dangers of staphylococcal overgrowth and because no staphylococcal overgrowth occurred, other postoperative complications are not reported in detail. Two deaths were due to myocardial infarction and pulmonary embolism, respectively. Two vaginal fistulas developed; one patient died after a prolonged septic course. Two suture lines broke down resulting in a septic course and a colostomy, but both patients survived. No incidence of "super infection" occurred.

In none of these usual complications did the staphylococcus play a dominant part.

CONCLUSIONS

Based on this active, not retroactive, study of 112 patients, it is demonstrated that the use of antibiotics to prepare the bowel for surgery can be done without danger from staphylococcal overgrowth. The preparation must be individualized if any degree of obstruction is present. No superiority could be shown for any one of the three methods used in this series except for the impression that prolonged sulpha aids the patient who has obstruction.

Cultures showed no bacterial growth from the bowel at surgery in 50 percent of the patients and a significant reduction of the flora with the elimination of *E. coli* in an additional 25 percent. This change in flora did not result in staphylococcal overgrowth nor did it protect from wound infection and the anticipated complications of colon surgery.

The low incidence of staphylococcus in this series before operation was continued in the postoperative course. It is suggested that the socioeconomic status of the patient population and the hospital environment may be important factors in the occurrence of the staphylococcus. Undoubtedly, the prompt return of the usual flora is a major factor in controlling staphylococcal overgrowth in the postoperative period. We feel that limiting neomycin to a maximum preparation of 36 hours with a dose of 10 to 12 Gm. is most important. The use of postoperative antibiotics did not eliminate wound infection nor did it produce staphylococcal overgrowth.

No attempt was made to prove the benefits of antibiotic preparation of the bowel but rather to reassure those who wish to use this preparation that it can be done safely.

SUMMARY

The dangers of antibiotic preparation of the bowel for surgery were studied in a series of 112 patients. The bowel was prepared by neomycin alone in 29 patients. For 36 patients neomycin and sulpha were used for a short preparation. Sulpha alone was used for more than 4 days (usually 7 to 10 days) with neomycin added for the final 36 hours in 47 patients. Catharsis, mechanical preparation, and diet restriction were used as indicated for each patient. Cultures were taken of the bowel before preparation. If sulpha was used more than 4 days, a second culture was taken before neomycin was added and a third when the preparation was complete. Cultures were taken at the time of surgery, immediately after surgery, and before discharge. The preparation used resulted in a bowel at surgery showing no growth or only yeast in 50 percent and a significant alteration in flora in an additional 25 percent. The change in flora did not result in staphylococcal overgrowth leading to staphylococcal enterocolitis or staphylococcal wound infection. It is concluded that antibiotic preparation of the bowel can be used safely.

REFERENCES

1. Altemeier, W. A., Hummel, R. P., and Hill, E. O.: Prevention of infection in colon surgery, Arch. Surg. **93:** 226, 1966.
2. Azar, H., and Drapanas, T.: Relationship of antibiotics to wound infection and enterocolitis in colon surgery, Am. J. Surg. **115:** 209, 1968.
3. Cohn, I., Jr.: Intestinal antisepsis, Am. Surgeon **25:** 498, 1959.
4. Cohn, I., Jr.: Intestinal antisepsis, Dis. Colon & Rectum **8:** 11, 1965.
5. Polacek, M. A., and Sanfelippo, P.: Oral antibiotic bowel preparation and complications in colon surgery, Arch. Surg. **97:** 412, 1968.
6. Prohaska, J. W., Farrell, M., Baker, W., and Collins, R.: Pseudomembranous (staphylococcal) enterocolitis, Internat. Abst. Surg. **112:** 103, 1961.

Transabdominal ligation-resection of the esophagus in cases of bleeding esophageal varices

I. BOEREMA, M.D., F.A.C.S. (Hon.)
P. J. KLOPPER, M.D.
A. A. HOLSCHER, M.D.
AMSTERDAM, THE NETHERLANDS

It is now clear from experience extending over the past 20 years that lowering of portal hypertension by means of various shunt operations does not influence the natural course of cirrhosis of the liver.

The portacaval shunt is followed by a large percentage of postoperative encephalopathy; furthermore, there is a disappointing operative mortality rate, largely because of hepatic insufficiency, ascites, jaundice, and coma.

The enthusiasm of many observers for shunt operations performed because of indications other than bleeding has waned markedly.

The direct attack upon the bleeding point by transthoracic transesophageal ligation of the varices[1, 2] has been tried in many clinics as a preliminary to the shunt operation which will follow when the patient is in better condition.

Another approach to acutely bleeding esophageal varices is an effort to decrease inflow of the portal blood into the varices. By lowering portal pressure the shunt operation lessens the risk of dangerous bleeding. However, the shunt operation does not completely stop venous inflow into the portal system, and therefore does not preclude recurrent bleeding. Weinberger[9] noted recurrent hemorrhage rather frequently; Hallenbeck and associates[5] did so in 25 percent of the cases. Furthermore, emergency portacaval shunt carries a high operative mortality rate. A reliable figure for the world literature probably lies between 50 and 66 percent. With careful selection of cases for operation, this high mortality rate obviously lessens. Laboratory tests of liver function do not give a reliable prognosis as to the outcome of the operation.

Of the different methods directed at blocking the inflow to the bleeding varices completely, ligation of the whole esophagus in the hiatus according to the method of Vossschulte[8] is most effective. However, this method is often followed by leakage of the esophagus when the ligature cuts through its walls; inflammation, abscesses, fistula, and death from peritonitis may ensue.

To obviate leakage (Fig. 1) the authors have employed their button-anastomosis technique which permits approximation of the esophageal wall above and below the ligature so that a leakproof resection of a 2 cm. length of the esophagus can be achieved, thus separating the portal blood bed completely from the esophageal varices. In all of our cases, the ominous bleeding ceased immediately (Fig. 2).

Recurrent bleeding having been observed in the postoperative phase from ulceration in the stomach in two instances attending this procedure, complete vagotomy in the hiatus has been added, with a concomitant anterior gastroenterostomy.

Having become convinced that all clinical and laboratory tests are inadequate for case selection, since January, 1967, we operated on all patients admitted to our wards with massive hemorrhage from varices. We soon discovered that there were losses in "good cases," and complete success in several apparently "lost cases" (Table I).

Submitted for publication April 15, 1969; resubmitted Aug. 4, 1969.

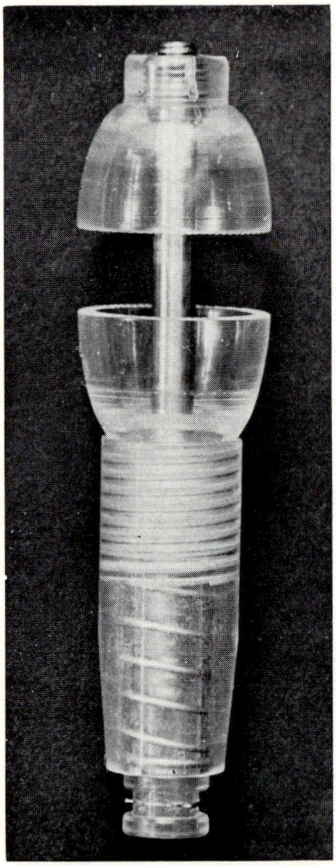

Fig. 1. Button used for sutureless transabdominal resection of the esophagus.

It has been our plan to operate on every patient who enters the hospital with severe bleeding or who has had severe hemorrhage a few days or weeks before. The technique is as follows (Fig. 3):

1. A median upper abdominal incision is made, with excision of xiphisternum, and a transverse incision of peritoneum overlying the esophagus in the hiatus.

2. The esophagus is mobilized. All veins on the esophageal wall and in the hiatus are ligated and transected. Both vagus nerves are divided. The esophageal wall is now clean all around, down to the muscular wall. A thick nylon thread is laid around the esophagus. A vertical incision, 7 cm. long, is made in the anterior wall of the stomach; all clots are removed from the stomach (these are often very voluminous). The upper half of the button is introduced into the esophagus by means of a gentle pull on the nasal thread by the anesthetist, carefully guided by the sur-

Table I

No. of patients	*Condition*	*Total hospital deaths*	*Survived*
Jaundiced	5	2	3
Comatose	4	1	3
Clinical ascites	12	7	5

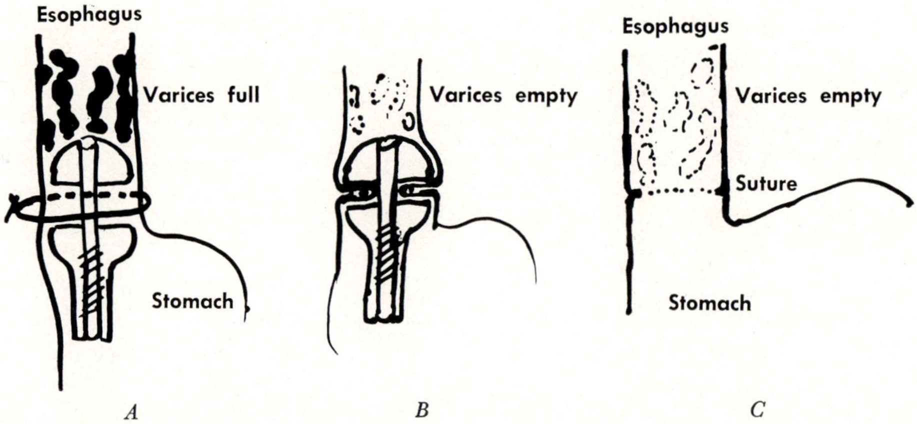

Fig. 2. *A,* Button in place, not closed; varices full of blood. *B,* Ligature tied, button closed; varices empty. *C,* Button and ligature sloughed loose and removed by traction upward through the mouth, or spontaneously through the rectum.

geon. The esophagus is ligated by the nylon thread on the tube of the upper half of the anastomosis button. The lower half of the button is pushed against the upper half; they are made to click together by the spring inside. The bleeding stops immediately after the ligation by the nylon thread; the inside of the stomach, now dry, is inspected for (very rare) bleeding gastric varices, which can be ligated by the Boerema-Crile technique.

3. An anterior antecolic gastrojejunostomy is made, with the gastrotomy opening being used. A Braun jejunojejunostomy is added.

4. A splenectomy is done only when no excessive blood has been lost, blood transfusions during operation have been few, the patient is in good condition, and the spleen is free from adhesions to the diaphragm or posterior abdominal wall.

5. In case of some oozing, a drain is left below the left diaphragm.

6. The esophagus is kept empty by continuous suction via a nasal tube halfway down the esophagus.

7. After about 3 days the nasal tube is removed and feeding with fluids by mouth is started.

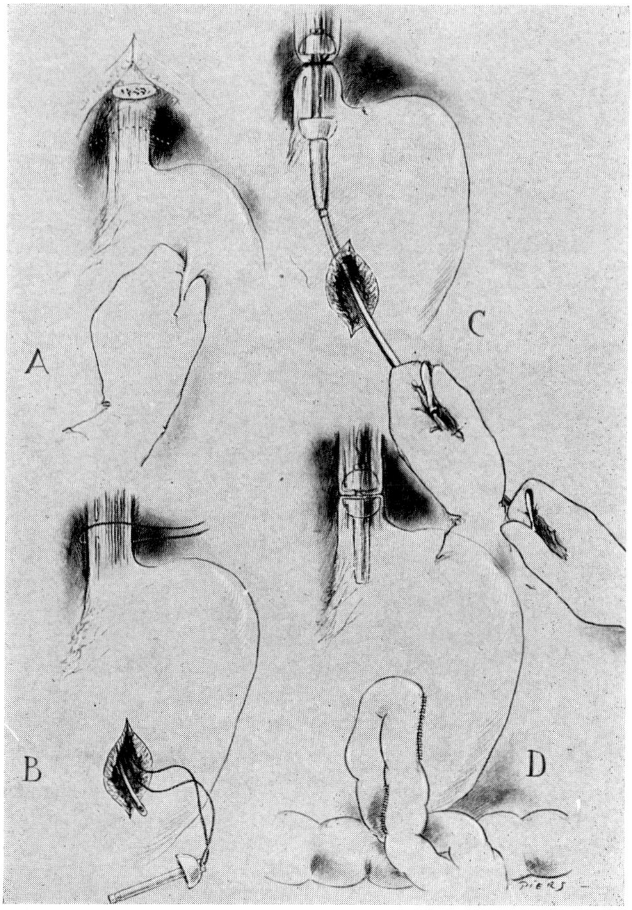

Fig. 3. *A,* Transverse incision through peritoneum on the esophagus in the hiatus. *B,* Vagotomy in the hiatus. Nylon string around the esophagus. Upper half of the button being pulled into the esophagus. *C,* Esophagus tied off on the button. Second half applied. *D,* Button closed. Segment of the esophagus caught between the two halves. Gastroenterostomy and anastomosis performed according to the method described by Braun.

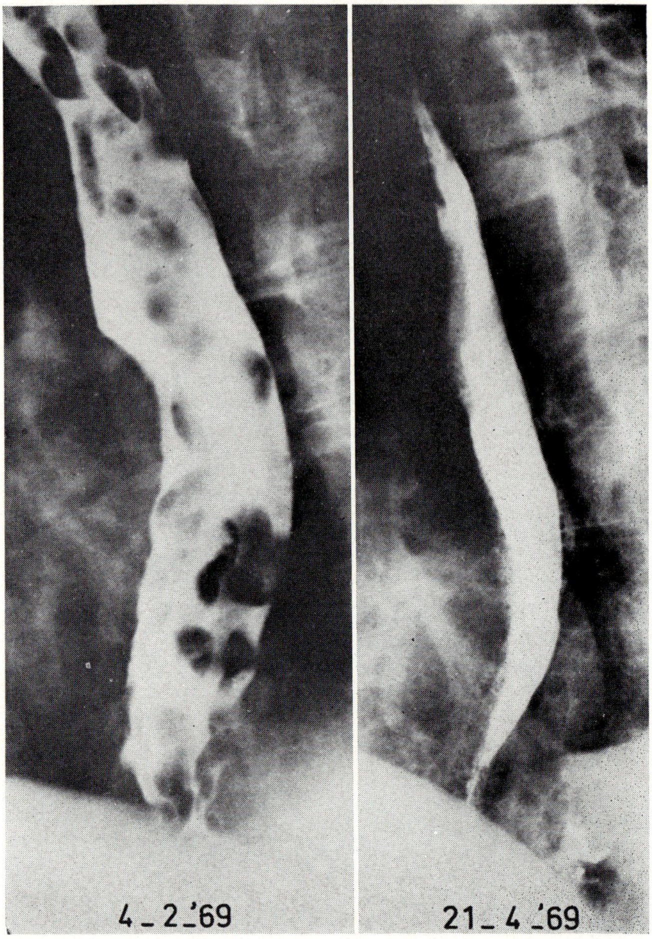

Fig. 4. X-ray of a 51-year-old man with cirrhosis. Varices full before operation; empty afterward.

8. On the twelfth day, with the patient under general anesthesia, the button is extracted through the mouth by the nasal thread. When the button, by earlier sloughing of the esophageal segment, has already descended into the stomach, the apparatus is allowed to pass through the gut and is recovered in the stool.

In all we have operated upon 34 patients, the youngest 9 years old, and the oldest 80. Twenty-four had cirrhosis, ten had portal hypertension from extrahepatic portal stenosis; one patient had never bled, but showed massive varices on the x-ray. Of our 34 patients, 12 (35 percent) died in the hospital within 2 months after operation. The surviving 22 patients, many of whom entered the hospital as "lost cases," went home in good condition; the bleeding had stopped completely and recurrent bleeding was not probable—not in the first years, and perhaps not even during the likely life expectancy of people with progressive Laennec's cirrhosis. In none of our surviving patients has recurrent bleeding been observed. However, our period of observations extends only to 2 years and 8 months. Ten patients have returned to normal work, to school, or to sport.

The mortality rate is obviously high, but certainly not much different from the risk of emergency shunt. Moreover, the shunt operation is done on a select group of patients. The more discriminating the selection, the lower the mortality rate, but also the smaller the group of patients. We have not excluded any patient, but have operated upon the entire group of those who presented with massive hemorrhage.

Certainly, evaluation of different methods is not to be based solely on the mortality rate of a favorable group of patients, but upon the survival rate of all patients admitted with massive hemorrhage from varices.

From our group only 12 patients would have been considered acceptable for an emergency shunt operation, adjudicated by the usual clinical observation and laboratory tests. From literature reports, it might be inferred that only six would have survived an emergency shunt operation. This would suggest that from our group of 34 patients only six (18 percent) would have been surgical successes. All the patients not operated upon would probably have died, from either persistent bleeding or recurrent bleeding, within a year.

Of our 34 patients, all of whom without exception underwent ligation and resection of the esophagus, 22 (65 percent) went home in good condition, the bleeding being arrested immediately and completely, and so far without recurrent bleeding (Fig. 4).

SUMMARY

All patients admitted to our hospital since Jan. 1, 1967, with bleeding esophageal varices have been operated upon. Those with massive bleeding were handled as emergency cases; those in whom bleeding ceased in the hospital were operated upon soon thereafter.

Sutureless ligation-resection of the lower esophagus was performed, complemented by vagotomy and gastrojejunostomy. Comatose, jaundiced, and ascitic patients were not excluded from the operative series.

REFERENCES

1. Boerema, I.: Bleeding varices of the esophagus in cirrhosis of the liver and Banti's syndrome, Arch. Chir. Neerl. **1:** 253, 1949.
2. Boerema, I.: Chirurgische hulp bij bloedingen uit varices van de oesophagus bij levercirrhose en bij het syndroom van Banti, Nederl. T. Geneesk. **93:** 4174, 1949.

2A. Boerema, I.: The resectability of gastric carcinoma, Ann. Surg. **142:** 228, 1955.

3. Boerema, I., Klopper, P. J., and Holscher, A. A.: Afbinding van de gehele slokdarm bij bloedende varices, Nederl. T. Geneesk. **111:** 1549, 1967.
4. Boerema, I., Klopper, P. J., and Holscher, A. A.: Traitement des varices oesophagiennes saignantes par ligature totale de l'oesophage, Presse Med. **75:** 1849, 1967.
5. Hallenbeck, G. A., Wallaeger, E. E., Adson, M. A., and Gage, R. P.: Results after portal systemic shunts in 120 patients with cirrhosis of the liver, Surg. Gynec. Obstet. **116:** 435, 1963.
6. Klopper, P. J.: Bloedende maagvarices bij portale hypertensie, Nederl. T. Geneesk. **105:** 521, 1961.
7. Klopper, P. J.: De chirurgische behandeling van oesophagusvarices, Geneesk. Bl. **49:** 31, 1959.
8. Vossschulte, K.: Dissektionsligatur des Oesophagus bei Varicen der Speiserröhre infolge Pfortaderhypertonie, Chirurg **28:** 186, 1957.
9. Weinberger, H. A.: Emergency portacaval shunt for esophagogastric hemorrhage, Arch. Surg. **91:** 333, 1965.

An intensive care bed for the initial diagnosis and treatment of severely ill patients

J. DONALD HILL, M.D.
ELMER E. JOHNSON
SAN FRANCISCO, CALIF.
From the Presbyterian Hospital and the Institute of Medical Sciences; Pacific Medical Center

Most surgeons have had the experience of being asked to see a patient who is in shock, or a preshock condition. On approaching the bed it is often difficult to examine the patient and appraise his condition because of the large number of tubes, intravenous lines, electrocardiographic lines, respirators, suction equipment, and monitors that surround him. The advances in treating severely ill patients have made all this diagnostic and therapeutic equipment necessary; however, the basic bed on which these patients are treated has become inadequate for the diagnostic procedures and therapeutic treatments that are available. Furthermore, not infrequently, useful information is not obtained, e.g., special x-rays and mixed venous pO_2, because the environmental situation makes it difficult or impossible.

The purpose of this report is to describe a bed that can be used in an intensive care ward during the initial diagnosis and treatment of severely ill patients. After the patient's condition has stabilized, the patient can be transferred to a bed in a conventional intensive care unit.

THE BASIC FRAME

Since it is very advantagous to be able to take x-rays through the bed, and to use an image intensifier, the basic frame is an x-ray table.*

Aided in part by United States Public Health Service Grants HE 06311 and FR 05566.

Received for publication March 28, 1969.

*Philips Electronic Instruments, Medical X-ray Division, Eindhoven, Netherlands.

The dimensions of the bed top are 77 inches by 28 inches. A polyurethan mattress 4 feet by 60 inches by 25 inches is put on the hard top surface. This mattress does not interfere with x-rays. Caster wheels are put on the four legs so that the bed can be moved easily in any direction (Fig. 1, *17*). One of these wheels has a lock that makes the bed stay in a fixed position when being used. The top of the bed of the bed is mobile so that it can be easily used for fluoroscopic work. The bed top will move 6 inches in both directions horizontally, and 3 feet in both directions longitudinally. This table motion is controlled by an electromagnetic switch (Fig. 1, *10*). If it is necessary to move the bed top only in the longitudinal direction, the horizontal direction can be fixed by locking the horizonal motion (Fig. 1, *14*). Underneath the bed top there is a mobile x-ray holder to take skull, chest, abdomen, or extremity x-rays. Along each side of the bed top there is a T-slot. This serves as a universal adaptor to which the accessory equipment can be added.

Accessory equipment.

Mobile lamp holder (Fig. 1, 1*).* A mobile lamp holder has been designed that can be attached at any point along the edge of the bed in the T-slot. This gives ample lighting for any minor surgical procedure.

Drape support (Fig. 1, 2*).* This can be used anywhere along the bed, but it is basically for the head and neck regions so that drapes can be kept off the patient's face and respiratory tubes and connections can be kept free during surgical procedures.

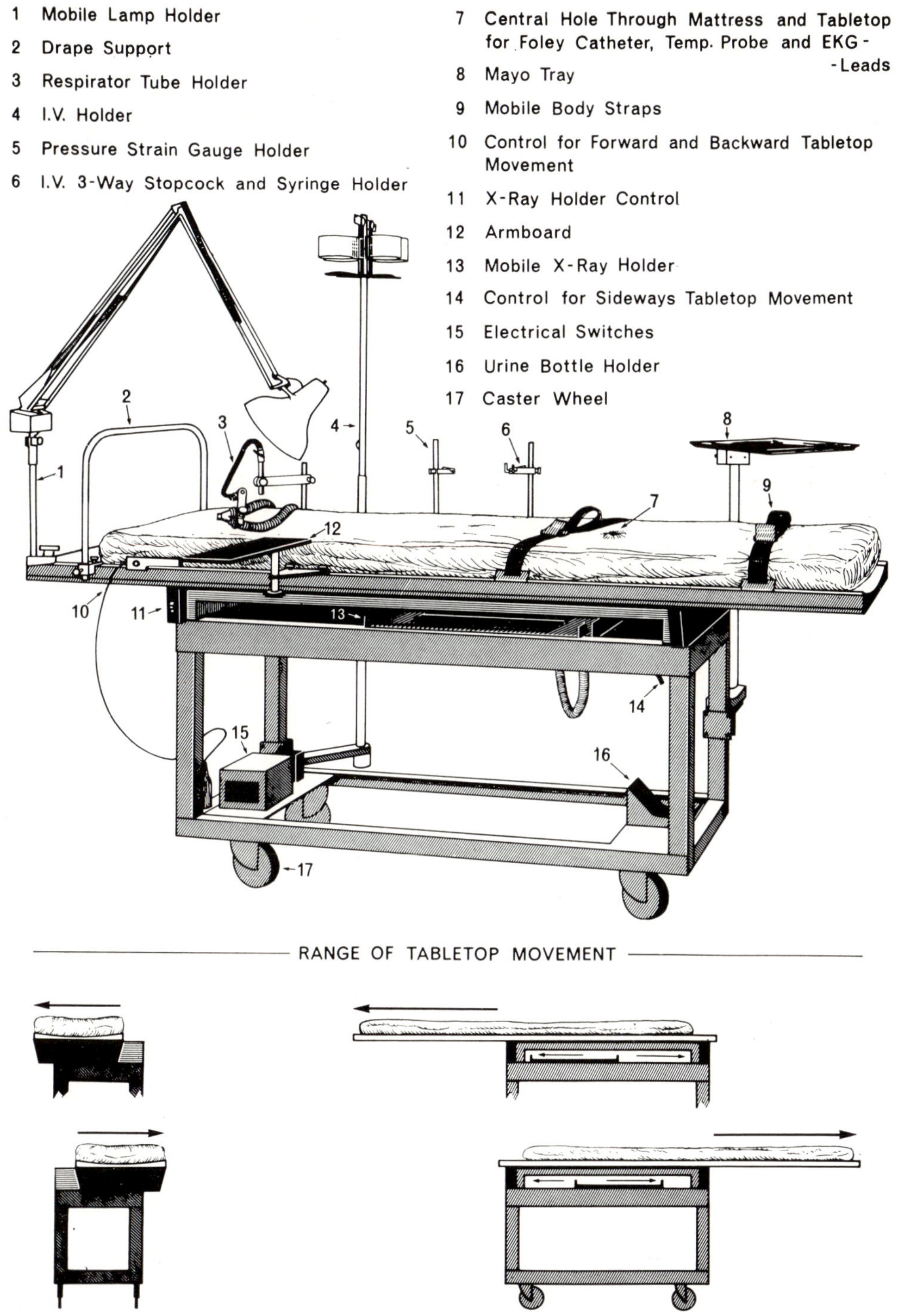

Fig. 1. Diagram of the table and accessory equipment. Also shown is the range of movement for the tabletop for radiologic use with an image intensifier.

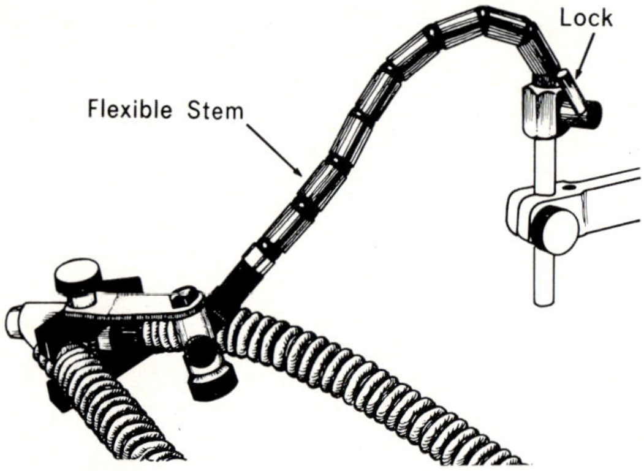

Fig. 2. Respiratory tube holder with a flexible stem. The flexible stem enables three-dimensional 360° positioning that can be held in the desired position by a single turn of the lock.

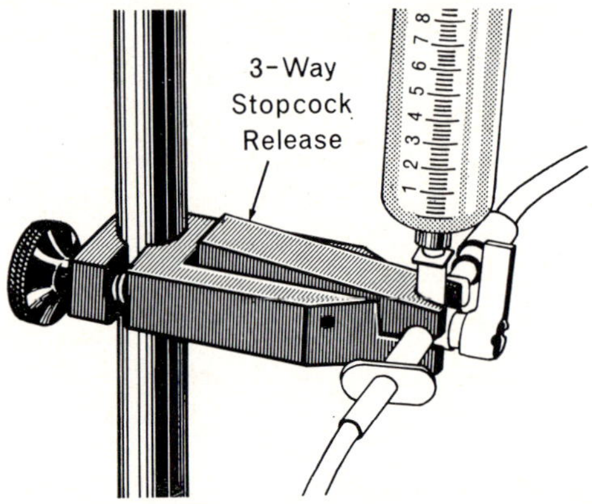

Fig. 3. The simple and single motion, three-way stopcock holder can be used with a syringe for drug injection or irrigation solutions, or for attachment of a venous manometer.

Respiratory tube holder (Fig. 1, 3, *and Fig. 2).* This respiratory tube holder can slide anywhere along the T-slot to a suitable position. The most advantageous feature, however, is the flexible connecting arm that can be made taut in any position that is desirable.

Intravenous holder (Fig. 1 4*).* The intravenous holder can swing forward or backward as desired. It also can be elevated. It holds four bottles that cannot be knocked off to the floor.

Pressure strain-gauge holder (Fig. 1, 5*).* This holder supports standard pressure strain gauges. It can be easily elevated or lowered to the correct level.

Three-way stopcock holder (Fig. 1, 6, *and Fig. 3).* This three-way stopcock holder and syringe is in a fixed solid position. It can be moved anywhere along the T-slot and elevated or depressed. Bolus intravenous injections can be easily added at the three-way stopcock. A central venous pressure manometer can be added at the stopcock if desired.

Central bed-top hole (Fig. 1, 7*).* In the middle of the bed at a position that would be between a patient's legs there is a hole 2 inches in diameter. This hole goes directly through the mattress and the bed. This hole carries the Foley catheter, electrocardiogram lines, and rectal temperature probes. This equipment ordinarily comes to the patient from the sides. They serve no purpose on the sides, and, furthermore, they get in the way. Therefore they have been brought through the middle of the bed out of the way.

Mayo tray (Fig. 1, 8*).* There is an attachable Mayo stand. This is used while doing surgical procedures. When not in use, it is removed.

Restraining strap (Fig. 1, 9*).* There are two mobile and removable restraining straps that slip into the T-slot. When not needed, they are removed.

Armboard (Fig. 1, 12*).* A mobile and detachable armboard fits anywhere into the T-slot.

Urine bottleholder (Fig. 1, 16*).* Via the Foley catheter that comes through the hole in the bed, the urine can be measured hourly and collected in a large urine bottle.

Not shown in the diagram, is a polyurethan foam wedge that can be inserted under the mattress at the head of the bed to elevate the head of the patient. Similarly, if the Trendelenburg position is desired, the wedge can be inserted at the foot of the bed.

DISCUSSION

This bed has a number of simple advantages. It enables one to diagnose effectively and efficiently and initially treat patients who are severely ill from any cause. Necessary x-rays can be taken easily, and catheters and pacemakers can be inserted and positioned. Tracheostomy, chest tube insertion, or any minor surgical procedure can be quickly performed. The patient can be treated for shock and simultaneously prepared for assisted circulation if necessary. The assisted circulation is then carried out while the patient is on this bed.

SUMMARY

A bed has been described that was designed and constructed for the initial diagnosis and treatment of severely ill patients. This type of bed is now necessary in an intensive care unit because of the advances in technology that are available and because of the aggressive approach now taken in the care of these patients.

Primary malignant tumors of the gallbladder: Report of 43 cases

MANIKCHAND RUKMANAPPA TANGA, M.B., B.S., M.S.
J. BURKE EWING, M.D., C.M., F.R.C.S.(C), F.R.C.S.(E), F.A.C.S., F.I.C.S.

OTTAWA, ONTARIO, CANADA

From the Department of Surgery, Ottawa General Hospital and University of Ottawa

A malignant tumor of the gallbladder was first described by Maximillian de Stoll[9] of Vienna in the year 1777. It was considered as a rare disease until Evarts Graham[18] showed that it constituted 8 to 10 percent of malignant tumors in female patients. About 6,000 lives were lost in the United States[1] because of this disease in 1963.[6] It occupies fifth place in gastrointestinal malignancy,[6] and it constitutes 3 to 4 percent of all malignancies. It is a highly lethal disease. Despite the great progress in medical sciences, the mortality rate from this disease has been steady for the past 50 years and cures few and far between. In his cumulative review, Strauch[30] reported a 1 percent 5 year survival.

The present study was undertaken in an attempt to discuss possible factors which might improve survival.

Forty-three patients with this disease were treated in Ottawa General Hospital between January, 1935, to June 30, 1967.

In the series reported by Gerst,[14] these cases constitute 0.018 percent of adult hospital admissions and 1.8 percent of biliary tract operations. In Arminski's[2] series, 1.12 percent of the patients undergoing biliary tract operations were found to have carcinoma of the gallbladder. Burdette[5] found this disease to constitute 0.01 percent of hospital admissions, and 1 percent of those with gallstones were found to have carcinoma. Thus, the incidence in those with gallstones is 100 times more than in those without. Thorbjarnarson and Glenn[33] reported that it constituted 1.86 percent of the benign biliary tract operations. In Strauch's[30] series, the incidence was 0.04 percent of hospital admissions. In our series, the incidence is 0.014 percent of hospital admissions and 0.81 percent of biliary tract operations.

Received for publication April 10, 1969.

The victims of this disease are predominantly female. Twenty-nine of our patients (67.44 percent) were female. The female-male ratio is approximately 2:1. In the series reported by Thorbjarnarson and Glenn,[33] the ratio between female and male was 3:1. Strauch[30] had the same ratio. Litwin[23] reported his female and male ratio to be 5:1. The increased incidence in female patients is probably caused by the increased frequency of gallstones and other biliary tract diseases in them.

Our youngest patient was 43 years old and the oldest was 90 years. The average age was 63.2 years. Thirty-nine or 90 percent of our patients were over 50 years of age. About half of the female patients were over 70 years of age, and only a quarter of the male patients were over 70 years. In Strauch's[30] series, 94.3 percent of his patients were over 50 years of age.

ETIOLOGY

Gallstones have been implicated in the development of carcinoma of gallbladder by

Vol. 67, No. 3, pp. 418-426

Table I

	Stones present	Stones not present	Not known
Male	9	2	3
Female	20	1	8
Total	29	3	11

Courvoisier,[8] Judd and Gray,[19] and Kehr.[20] In 32 of our patients, presence or absence of the gallstones was noted. Among these, 29 or 90.6 percent were known to have stones. The distribution of stones in male and female patients is shown in Table I.

Burdette,[5] Thorbjarnarson and Glenn,[33] Gerst,[14] Marcial-Rojas,[25] and Litwin[23] have reported similar percentages (83 to 90) of gallstones among those having carcinoma of the gallbladder. Thus, there is no controversy regarding this association. The real controversy lies between the relation of gallstones and carcinoma of the gallbladder.

Aschoff[3] and Lancereaux[21] advocated the theory that carcinoma was responsible for the formation of gallstones. This view is not widely accepted.

The stones are believed to cause carcinoma by mechanical irritation, autoirradiation, and associated inflammation. Petrov and Krotkina[28] produced carcinoma of the gallbladder in guinea pigs by intracholecystic implantation of glass tubes and radium. Fortner[11] produced the lesion in cats by similar implantation of methylcholanthrene. Because of this experimental work and because of the chemical similarity between the chemical carcinogens, bile salts and cholesterol, one wonders whether slight metabolic aberration would be responsible for the formation of gallbladder cancer.

Lazarus-Barlow[22] in 1914 asserted that carcinoma of the gallbladder is caused by autoirradiation of the gallbladder by stones. Fortner and Norris[12] could not confirm this hypothesis.

Comfort and associates[7] followed 112 patients with silent gallstones for a period of 10 to 25 years and none developed carcinoma. Burdette[5] states that 1 percent of patients having cholelithiasis would develop carcinoma of the gallbladder. Similar figures have been quoted by most authors. If gallstones are responsible for malignancy, this low percentage of carcinoma in those having gallstones cannot be explained. In a certain number of cases (10 percent), gallstones are absent. In these patients, some other factors may have been responsible for the development of carcinoma. It can, however, be argued theoretically that in these cases gallstones were present initially and these were passed later, after initiating the chain reaction which led to the formation of carcinoma.

Chronic infection, benign neoplasm of the gallbladder, and exogenous factors have been blamed but not with general acceptance.

All of our patients were of European extraction.

SYMPTOMS AND SIGNS

The exact duration of symptoms that are due to malignancy cannot be determined with certainty in the majority of cases. This is due to two facts. First, the carcinoma of the gallbladder is asymptomatic in its early course. It produces symptoms mainly by the spread of tumor beyond the gallbladder and involvement of the neighboring vital structures.

The second reason is, in the majority of cases, there is associated cholecystitis with cholelithiasis. The symptoms of malignancy may be superimposed upon chronic cholecystitis with the transition unnoticed by the patient, or the patient may not have any symptoms that are due to malignancy at all and present himself with symptoms of benign biliary tract disease.

The duration of symptoms in our patients varied between 1 day and 15 years. About 49 percent of our patients had symptoms for less than 3 months. The duration of symptoms in eight patients in whom the tumor was grossly localized to the gallbladder was between 2 days and 2 years. In seven of these eight patients, the duration was less than 1 year. Past history suggestive of biliary tract disease was present in nine of 43 (20.93 per-

Table II

Symptoms	*No. of patients*
Pain in the abdomen	37
Jaundice	18
Loss of weight	18
Nausea and/or vomiting	15
Loss of appetite	15
Fatty-food tolerance	11
Dark urine and/or clay-colored stools	7
Hematemesis and/or melena	3
Edema legs	2
Mass in abdomen	1

Table III

Clinical findings	*No. of patients*
Tenderness in upper abdomen	23
Jaundice	22
Palpable liver (metastatic in 10, tender in one)	21
Anemia	5
Palpable gallbladder	4
Rigidity in right hypochondrium	4
Cachexia	4
Ascites	3
Ill-defined abdominal mass	3
Intestinal obstruction	2
Thrombophlebitis of leg	1

cent) patients. The recent change in symptoms was persistent and severe pain, nausea, vomiting, jaundice, and loss of appetite. In Arminski's[2] series, past history of biliary tract disease was present in 52 percent of cases. It was 88 percent in Gardner's[13] patients.

Pain was the commonest symptom and was present in 37 of 43 (86 percent) of our patients. Jaundice and weight loss were the next common symptoms. The details of symptoms are given in Table II; the common findings on clinical examinations are depicted in Table III.

Jaundice was most commonly due to invasion of the biliary ducts and/or liver by malignancy. Only in three cases was the jaundice due to stones in the biliary tract. These findings are in variance with Thorbjarnarson and Glenn.[33]

Table IV

Investigative findings	*No. of patients*
Obstructive jaundice	11
Combined features of obstructive and parenchymatous jaundice	8
Liver function tests:	
Mild derangement	2
Moderate derangement	4
Severe derangement	2
Occult blood in stools	10
Anemia	6
Leukocytosis and increased neutrophil count	4
Raised blood urea nitrogen	4
Arteriosclerotic heart disease	6
Raised serum alkaline phosphatase	2
Severe hypokalemia	1

Table V

Radiologic studies	*No. of cases*
Plain film of abdomen	
Calcified gallbladder	1
Mass in right hypochondrium and elevation of right dome of diaphragm	1
Oral cholecystography	
Nonfunctionnig gallbladder	15
Stones in functioning gallbladder	4
Faint opacification of gallbladder	1
Barium swallow and upper gastrointestinal examination	
Pyloric obstruction	2
Swollen and congested duodenal mucosa	1
Duodenal ulcer with gastric retention	1
Extrinsic pressure on the duodenum	1
Duodenal diverticula	2
Barium enema	
Extrinsic mass pushing down	1
Hepatic flexure of colon	1
Liver scan	
Positive for metastasis	2

INVESTIGATIONS

The routine and special investigations were not of great help in diagnosis. The results are shown in Table IV.

The important findings are obstructive jaundice, anemia, occult blood in stools, leukocytosis, raised neutrophil count, deranged liver function tests. Increased serum alkaline phosphatase with very little increase in serum bilirubin is highly suggestive of hepatic metastases.

The radiologic studies were equally unrewarding (Table V).

In the majority of cases, a diagnosis of carcinoma of the gallbladder was not made clinically. In Litwin's[23] series, correct preoperative diagnosis was made in 19 percent of cases. This figure is a little higher than the generally reported figures. In only three (7 percent) of our cases was a correct preoperative diagnosis made. The commonest preoperative diagnosis was benign tract disease, the next common being carcinoma of the pancreas or bile ducts. In eight patients, the diagnosis was even missed at operation. In seven of these, the operative diagnosis was chronic cholecystitis with cholelithiasis. In the remaining one, diagnosis was acute cholecystitis with perforation of the gallbladder.

TREATMENT

In all but four patients, an abdominal exploration was carried out. Four patients died without having had surgical treatment, and in these patients, the diagnosis was made at autopsy. In only eight patients, six of whom were undiagnosed at operation, was the tumor removed completely. Our resection for cure rate was 18.6 percent. Glenn and Hays[15, 16] could resect the tumor in 32 percent of cases, and in Gerst's[14] series it was 16.66 percent. The operative procedures in these operable cases are shown in Table VI. The surgical procedures carried out in nonresectable tumors are shown in Table VII.

Table VI

Operative procedures	*No. of cases*
Cholecystectomy	5
Cholecystectomy, choledocholithotomy, T tube drainage	2
Cholecystectomy, common bile duct exploration, and T tube drainage	1

Table VII

Operative procedures	*No. of cases*
Laparotomy	4
Laparotomy and biopsy	17
Gastrointestinal short-circuiting	2
Partial gastrectomy	1
Cholecystostomy	2
Partial cholecystectomy	1
Cholecystectomy	3
Cholecystectomy and common bile duct exploration	2
Jejunostomy	1
Ileostomy	1

PATHOLOGY

In 39 cases, histologic proof of the disease was available. In the remaining four patients, the disease was identified at operation, but no biopsy was performed. Table VIII shows the details of the histologic findings.

Table VIII

Histologic findings	*No. of cases*
Adenocarcinoma	32*
Epidermoid carcinoma	3
Undifferentiated carcinoma	1
Carcinoma in situ	1
Mucoepidermoid ductular pattern of carcinoma	1
Angiosarcoma	1

*Of these cases of adenocarcinoma 3 were mucus producing, 2 duct cell, and 2 papillary.

In their paper, Fahim and co-workers[10] have described the mode of spread of carcinoma of the gallbladder. The modes of spread are: (a) pericholedochal and pancreaticoduodenal lymph nodes in 25 percent, (b) localized involvement of the vein and venules of the gallbladder in 12.1 percent, (c) invasion of nerves in 24 percent, and (d) localized involvement of the underlying liver in 25 percent.

Blood-borne metastases are uncommon. The distribution of metastases is shown in Table IX.

In addition to the above-mentioned metastases, there were some interesting findings. These were biliary cirrhosis in six cases, malignant ascites in six cases, perforation of gallbladder in five cases, biliary embolization to lungs in two cases. Pericholecystic abscess, in-

Table IX

Site	No. of cases
Liver	30
Omentum and peritoneum	11
Portal lymph nodes	9
Common bile duct	7
Duodenum	6
Colon	5
Cystic lymph nodes	3
Portal vein	3
Lung	3
Pancreas	3
Stomach	3
Celiac lymph nodes	2
Skin	2
Mediastinal lymph nodes	1
Vertebrae	1
Thyroid	1
Subpericardium	1
Spleen	1
Inferior vena cava	1
Brain	1
Ovary	1
Kidney	1
Small bowel	1

farction of liver, splenomegaly, cholemic nephrosis, cholecystoduodenal fistulas, thrombosis of portal and splenic veins with and without involvement by tumor were each observed in one patient.

In three patients, in addition to the gallbladder tumor, there were associated benign or malignant tumors. These were (1) an angiorhabdomyolipoma of the kidney in one patient, (2) a carcinoid of the appendix and a carcinoma in situ of the gallbladder in a second patient, and (3) a basal cell carcinoma of the face, a carcinoma in situ of the penis, and multiple tubular adenomata of the kidney in a third patient.

RESULTS AND FOLLOW-UP

Twenty-two patients, including the four who did not have an operation, died during the first hospital admission. This gave an operative mortality rate of 41.86 percent. Death during the first admission occurred in 51.16 percent of patients. Among the deaths during the first admission, only one was due to unrelated cause (myocardial infarction). In this case, carcinoma of the gallbladder was an incidental finding at autopsy. Even in this case there was metastasis to the cystic duct lymph node.

All the deaths occurring during the first admission were within 2 months after operation and were caused by the tumor or the usual postoperative complications. One patient, whose tumor was resected for cure, died the day of the operation because of cardiac arrest. He had severe preoperative hemorrhage and had cardiac arrest during operation.

Six more patients died during the second hospital admission and all died within 5 months after operation. Among these six patients, there was one patient who had a cholecystectomy for possible cure. She died because of malignant obstructive jaundice and hepatic coma.

One patient in whom the diagnosis was only established at histologic examination was readmitted 8 months after the first hospital discharge with metastasis to the incision. This was irradiated with little relief. She was readmitted for the third time with severe pain in the skin nodules. She died 1 year after operation.

The modes of death were jaundice and hepatic failure in 18 patients, intestinal obstruction in four cases, myocardial infarction in two patients, and cardiac arrest, bronchopneumonia, pulmonary edema, ascites, and postoperative shock in the remainder.

Thus, there were 14 patients who were discharged from the hospital after their treatment, palliative or curative. Of these, nine patients are known to have died of carcinomatosis. In seven patients, the duration of postoperative survival was less than 8 months; in one, 2 years; and in the other, 4 years. Three patients had widespread metastases and could not have possibly survived long. One patient is alive 5 months after operation with hepatic metastases. Our longest survival is 10 years and 9 months. She was alive at the time of last follow-up less than a year ago.

Strauch[30] had 1 percent 5 year survival in his patients. In Thorbjarnarson and Glenn's[33] series, three patients survived for more than 7 years out of his 90 patients. Chandler and Fletcher[6] had 3 percent 5 year survival, being 20 percent of those in whom the tumor was resected for cure. Appleman and his colleagues[1] from Mayo Clinic have reported 12.6 percent 5 year survival among those in whom the tumor was supposed to have been removed completely. Gerst[14] has had very good results. Seven (31.8 percent) of his 22 patients undergoing curative surgical treatment survived for more than 4 years. Eight of our patients underwent possible curative operation, and only one (2.5 percent) lived for more than 10 years. Among those who had only palliative surgical treatment, the longest survival was for 5 months.

DISCUSSION

It is evident from a review of the literature and from our cases that carcinoma of the gallbladder has an extremely poor prognosis. The results of treatment are very poor despite the rapid advances in the fields of anesthesia, surgery, and the allied sciences.

The mortality rate of such simple procedures as cholecystectomy, laparotomy, and biopsy is very high. In our hands, the operative mortality rate (60 days postoperatively) was 41.86 percent.

Carcinoma of the gallbladder does not have any typical symptoms in its early phase. The signs and symptoms are those of associated gallbladder disease, usually associated with gallstones. When the symptoms and signs that are due to malignancy, such as rapidly increasing jaundice, loss of weight, cachexia, loss of appetite, persistent severe pain, and distant metastases appear, the tumor is generally inoperable. Thus, there is a dilemma. Carcinoma of the gallbladder, when operable, is asymptomatic and when symptoms appear, it is inoperable. With the presently available resources, there is no way to diagnose a carcinoma of the gallbladder when it is operable for cure. Thus, it seems that the only way out of this problem is to screen all the patients with biliary tract disease and those with cholelithiasis.

The autopsy incidence of gallstones in persons aged 20 years or over is 10.2 percent according to Raul A. Marcial-Rojas.[25] The incidence of gallstones increases with age. One fruitful source would be to screen the general population with age 20 years or over for gallstones. Even though this is theoretically desirable, it is impractical because of the cost and lack of facilities for the entire population. Until a cheaper and simpler method is found, we cannot afford to screen the entire population for gallstones.

The next question is, if the gallstones and/or biliary tract disease are found during investigations or operation, what is to be done. Regarding the biliary tract disease, there is no dispute: These have to be treated. The controversy arises when the patients are found to have gallstones with little or no symptoms. The convincing answer to this problem has been given by Lund[24] in his paper. He followed 526 cases of cholelithiasis which were not operated upon initially, for a period of 5 to 20 years. Of these, 34 patients were absolutely asymptomatic; one third of these developed severe symptoms. Regardless of the severity of symptoms initially, 33.3 to 50 percent developed severe symptoms and/or complications.

Thus, all the so-called "silent gallstones" will not remain silent all the time. In his series, the mortality rate of cholelithiasis was 2.7 percent and in those over 60 years, it was 7.2 percent. Three patients (0.57 percent) developed carcinoma of the gallbladder. However, these figures could have been higher if 25 percent would not have had subsequent cholecystectomy.

The present mortality rate of elective cholecystectomy in good centers is less than 1 percent.[6] The risk of the development of carcinoma of the gallbladder in those with cholelithiasis is not higher than this. The risk of carcinoma per se, therefore, is not an indication for cholecystectomy. Glenn and Hays[17] have reported that 10 percent of patients over 65 years of age with gallbladder disease harbor carcinoma of the gallbladder. They also state that the mortality rate of elective cholecystectomy in patients under 50 years of age is 0.65 percent and in those over 65 years, it is 6.7 percent. The increased mortality rate is attributed to the development of acute cholecystitis, stones in the common bile duct, acute processes with minimal signs and symptoms, and carcinoma of the gallbladder.

McLaughlin[26] has reported that in persons over 70 years of age with biliary tract disease, 11 percent would be found to have carcinoma of the gallbladder. He advises elective cholecystectomy for cholelithiasis because of the risk of acute processes and carcinoma. Ross and Hickock[29] have reported a 7 percent incidence of gallbladder carcinoma in patients who had gallbladder operations beyond 70 years of age. In their hands, the mortality rate of elective gallbladder surgery was 2.8 percent and that of emergency surgery was 18.9 percent. Comfort and associates[7] followed 112 patients with cholelithiasis for a period of 10 to 25 years. Carcinoma did not develop in any. Ultimately, 21 percent of patients needed surgical treatment for nonmalignant complications.

Since 33.33 to 50 percent of patients with cholelithiasis develop severe symptoms and/or complications and since the mortality rate of emergency surgery is prohibitive, elective prophylactic cholecystectomy is justified. Risk of carcinoma further adds strength to the argument for elective prophylactic cholecystectomy.

In 1954, Glenn and Hays[15-17] wrote that whenever there is a suspicious lesion in the stomach or lung, they investigated and, if necessary, they operated to confirm or rule out a malignant lesion. They argue why should the biliary tract disease be ignored when 10 percent of patients over 65 years could have malignancy. Moreover, cholecystectomy is simpler than gastrectomy or thoracotomy. At present, the only effective measure against carcinoma is prevention.

Thus, it seems to us that prophylactic cholecystectomy is indicated for cholelithiasis in good-risk patients in centers which have acceptable mortality and morbidity rates. Both our long-term survivors were operated upon for gallstones, and carcinoma was diagnosed at histopathology.

In our series, there were at least four patients in whom the prognosis could have been improved. In one case, cholecystostomy was done for cholelithiasis because of poor general condition. The patient did not return for cholecystectomy when her general condition improved.

A year later, she returned with a mass in the right upper quadrant of the abdomen. Laparotomy revealed widespread metastases. Cholecystectomy as soon as possible and feasible could have prevented the carcinoma.

Another patient was admitted with complaints of weight loss, weakness, and lower abdominal pain. She was diagnosed as having hyperthyroidism and cystitis. A month later, an inoperable carcinoma of the gallbladder was found. In this case, the diagnosis was missed at the initial admission. Two other patients were diagnosed as having chronic cholecystitis with cholelithiasis and obstructive jaundice, 1 and 2 years previously. One patient was treated medically elsewhere. The other patient was advised to have an operation in this hospital, but he refused. Both the patients had inoperable carcinoma when they finally underwent surgical treatment.

Fahim and associates[10] have described in their classical paper the mode of spread of carcinoma of the gallbladder. It is evident that ideally in the treatment of carcinoma of the gallbladder, besides the gallbladder, the lymph nodes and lymphatics from the porta hepatis to duodenum, a contiguous wedge of the liver and the adjacent omentum should be removed. Thorek[34] in 1947 did a partial hepatectomy for local extension of carcinoma of gallbladder. Pack and co-workers[27] reported three cases of total right hepatic lobectomy for cancer of the gallbladder. In 1954, Glenn and Hays[15, 16] advocated radical cholecystectomy comprising the gallbladder, adjacent liver, omentum, lymphatics, and lymph nodes. In 23.5 percent of their cases, they did a radical cholecystectomy. Brasfield[4] in 1961 reported the first 5 year survival of carcinoma of the gallbladder treated by cholecystectomy and right hepatic lobectomy. In this case, the liver was invaded by contiguity. Thorbjarnarson and Glenn[33] have stated that if there is no contraindication, radical operation should be done. The contraindications are: (1) distant metastases, (2) involvement of both lobes of the liver, (3) hepatic artery and portal vein involvement, (4) intrahepatic extension along the bile ducts.

Appleman and his colleagues[1] from Mayo Clinic advocate extensive surgical treatment compatible with a low mortality rate as long as there is no contraindication.

In our series, no radical cholecystectomy or hepatic resections were done. However, in eight patients, radical cholecystectomy could have been done and four patients were candidates for total hepatic lobectomy.

In a fair number of cases, the duration of any symptoms is very short. In such cases, improvement in results can only be obtained whenever newer methods for early diagnosis become available.

In 1960, Thorbjarnarson[32] reported that 11 percent of his cases had superimposed acute cholecystitis. In none of these was the diagnosis of carcinoma suspected preoperatively. McLaughlin[26] reported that 36.4 percent of his cases of carcinoma of the gallbladder presented as acute cholecystitis.

We encountered superimposed acute or subacute cholecystitis in 18.6 percent. In these series, there were five cases (11.6 percent) of perforation of the gallbladder. To the best of our knowledge, this association has not been reported earlier. Since in some cases the diagnosis is not recognized at operation, thus negating the patient's chance of having radical cholecystectomy and (if needed) total hepatic lobectomy, it is wise to open all gallbladders in patients over 50 years to examine for the presence of cancer. If necessary, the suspicious lesions must be sent for frozen-section biopsy.

One patient had thrombophlebitis of the left leg 5 months prior to the diagnosis of the lesion. In another patient at autopsy, the portal and splenic veins were thrombosed without involvement by tumor. In certain intra-abdominal malignancies such as that of the pancreas, occurrence of thrombophlebitis of leg and intra-abdominal thrombosis is recognized.

There was another interesting problem. One patient had metastasis to the transverse colon and she was admitted with a history of vomiting. Electrolyte studies revealed severe hypokalemia. This hypokalemia could have been due to preoperative vomiting or profuse discharge from the diseased colon.

Since in the majority of cases the tumor is unresectable for cure, palliative methods will be indicated. Sullivan and associates[31] have reported effective palliation by prolonged chemotherapy through hepatic artery infusion.

SUMMARY AND CONCLUSIONS

1. Forty-three cases of primary malignant tumors of the gallbladder have been reviewed.

2. Carcinoma of the gallbladder is asymptomatic when curable. Occurrence of symptoms that are due to malignancy generally heralds incurability.

3. A plea to submit all cases of cholelithiasis including so-called "silent stones" and other forms of gallbladder disease to early cholecystectomy is made. This will reduce the occurrence of carcinoma, and carcinoma will be detected in an earlier stage.

4. More frequent use of radical cholecystectomy and total hepatic lobectomy when indicated would improve survival.

5. If for any reason cholecystectomy cannot be done during operation, the patient should be reoperated upon and the entire gallbladder should be removed as soon as feasible.

6. A continued search toward early diagnosis should be made.

7. Effective palliative treatment can be achieved in inoperable cases by prolonged intra-arterial chemotherapy.

REFERENCES

1. Appleman, R. M., Morlock, C. G., Dahlin, D. C., and Adson, M. A.: Long-term survival in carcinoma of the gallbladder, Surg. Gynec. & Obst. **117:** 459, 1963.
2. Arminski, T. C.: Primary carcinoma of the gallbladder, Cancer **2:** 379, 1949.
3. Aschoff, L.: Cited by Arminski.[2]
4. Brasfield, R. D.: Right hepatic lobectomy for

carcinoma of the gallbladder. A five year cure, Ann. Surg. **153:** 563, 1961.
5. Burdette, W. J.: Carcinoma of the gallbladder, Ann. Surg. **145:** 832, 1957.
6. Chandler, J. J., and Fletcher, W. S.: A clinical study of primary carcinoma of the gallbladder, Surg. Gynec. & Obst. **117:** 297, 1963.
7. Comfort, M. W., Gray, H. K., and Wilson, J. M.: Silent gallstones: A 10 to 25 year follow-up study of 112 cases, Ann. Surg. **128:** 931, 1948.
8. Courvoisier, L. O.: Casuistisch-Statistische Beitrage: Zur Pathologie und Chirurgie der Gallenwege, Leipzig, Germany, 1890, F. C. W. Vogel.
9. de Stoll, M.: Cited by Arminski.[2]
10. Fahim, R. B., McDonald, J. R., Richards, J. C., and Ferris, D. O.: Carcinoma of the gallbladder: A study of its modes of spread, Ann. Surg. **156:** 114, 1961.
11. Fortner, J. G.: Experimental induction of primary carcinoma of the gallbladder, Cancer **8:** 698, 1955.
12. Fortner, J. G., and Norris, W. P.: Determination of radioactivity of gallstones obtained from cases of gallbladder cancer, Cancer **8:** 687, 1955.
13. Gardner, L. W.: Primary carcinoma of the gallbladder, Harper Hosp. Bull. **14:** 186, 1956.
14. Gerst, P. H.: Primary carcinoma of the gallbladder: A thirty-year summary, Ann. Surg. **153:** 369, 1961.
15. Glenn, F., and Hays, D. M.: Carcinoma of the extrahepatic biliary tract, S. Clin. North America **33:** 479, 1953.
16. Glenn, F., and Hays, D. M.: The scope of radical surgery in the treatment of malignant tumors of the extrahepatic biliary tract, Surg. Gynec. & Obst. **99:** 529, 1954.
17. Glenn, F., and Hays, D. M.: The age factor in the mortality rate of patients undergoing surgery of the biliary tract, Surg. Gynec. & Obst. **100:** 11, 1955.
18. Graham, E. A.: The prevention of carcinoma of the gallbladder, Ann. Surg. **93:** 317, 1931.
19. Judd, E. S., and Gray, H. K.: Carcinoma of gallbladder and bile ducts, Surg. Gynec. & Obst. **55:** 308, 1932.
20. Kehr, H.: Introduction to the differential diagnosis of the separate forms of gallstone disease based upon his own experience gained in 433 laparotomies for gallstones, Philadelphia, 1901, P. Blackstone Son & Co.
21. Lancereaux, M.: Cited by Arminski.[2]
22. Lazarus-Barlow, W. S.: A lecture on the cause and cure of cancer viewed in the light of recent radio-biological research, Brit. M. J. **1:** 1001, 1914.
23. Litwin, M. S.: Primary carcinoma of the gallbladder. A review of 78 patients, Arch. Surg. **95:** 236, 1967.
24. Lund, J.: Surgical indications in cholelithiasis: Prophylactic cholecystectomy elucidated on the basis of long-term follow-up on 526 non-operated cases, Ann. Surg. **151:** 153, 1960.
25. Marcial-Rojas, R. A.: Unsuspected carcinoma of the gallbladder in acute and chronic cholecystitis, Ann. Surg. **153:** 289, 1961.
26. McLaughlin, C. W.: Carcinoma of the gallbladder, an added hazard in untreated calculous cholecystitis in older patients, SURGERY **56:** 757, 1964.
27. Pack, G. T., Miller, T. R., and Brasfield, R. D.: Total right hepatic lobectomy for cancer of the gallbladder; report of 3 cases, Ann. Surg. **142:** 6, 1955.
28. Petrov, N. N., and Krotkina, N. A.: Experimental carcinoma of the gallbladder, Ann. Surg. **125:** 241, 1947.
29. Ross, F. P., and Hickock, D. F.: Hernia and gallbladder surgery in patients over seventy, New England J. Med. **262:** 501, 1960.
30. Strauch, G. O.: Primary carcinoma of the gallbladder, SURGERY **47:** 368, 1960.
31. Sullivan, R. D., Norcross, J. W., and Watkins, E., Jr.: Chemotherapy of metastatic liver cancer by prolonged hepatic artery infusion, New England J. Med. **270:** 321, 1964.
32. Thorbjarnarson, B.: Carcinoma of the gallbladder and acute cholecystitis, Ann. Surg. **151:** 241, 1960.
33. Thorbjarnarson, B., and Glenn, F.: Carcinoma of the gallbladder, Cancer **12:** 1009, 1959.
34. Thorek, M.: Partial hepatectomy in carcinoma of the gallbladder, with case report, J. Internat. Coll. Surgeons **10:** 369, 1947.

Polyarteritis nodosa of the gallbladder

PATERNO REMIGIO, M.D.*
EDWARD ZAINO, M.D.
NEW YORK, N. Y.
From the Department of Pathology, Mary Immaculate Hospital Division, Catholic Medical Center of Brooklyn and Queens, and the Department of Pathology, Mercy Hospital

This is a report of two elderly patients with unsuspected polyarteritis nodosa in whom cholecystectomy showed characteristic vascular lesions. The mild joint and systemic manifestations had been considered to be of little significance because of their age.

CASE REPORTS

Case 1. A 71-year-old Caucasian woman was admitted to Mercy Hospital with anorexia, 5 pound weight loss, nausea, weakness, and pains in both ankles and knees of about 2 months' duration. She had received tranquilizers and sedatives. There was a past history of "tuberculosis for several years" with no history of chemotherapy.

On admission she was well developed, oriented, and pale; she had a blood pressure of 130/60, a pulse rate of 124 per minute, and a temperature of 102° F. She had definite tenderness of the right upper quadrant with no organomegaly. There was no swelling, heat, or redness of the joints. The ankle and knee joints had full motion although there was some pain on motion of both ankles. The remainder of the examination was negative.

Chest x-rays showed right pleural thickening and shift of the trachea to the right. The gall bladder series, gastrointestinal series, and barium enema were normal. The intravenous pyelogram showed a right renal calculus. The electrocardiogram was normal. The hemoglobin was 9.4 Gm. percent. White count was 6,780 per cubic millimeter with 81 percent polycytes, 15 percent lymphocytes, 2 percent monocytes, and 2 percent eosinophils. Sedimentation rate was 31 mm. per hour (Cutler). Serum amylase was 218 Somogyi units, and total protein was 5.7 Gm. with an albumin-globulin ratio of 2.9/2.8. She had a 2+ albuminuria with 8 to 10 leukocytes and 12 to 15 hyaline casts per high-power field. The platelets, serum calcium, phosphorous, alkaline phosphatase, and urea nitrogen were normal. The sputum and gastric aspirates were negative for acid-fast bacilli on smear and later on culture as well. The lupus erythematosus preparation was negative. The stools were negative for occult blood.

Hospital course. The patient had intermittent temperatures up to 105° with persistent right upper quadrant pain. A laparotomy was performed on the tenth hospital day at which time the gastrointestinal tract, the spleen, pancreas, and kidneys were grossly normal. A few fibrous adhesions were seen between the gallbladder and the liver. A cholecystectomy and wedge biopsy of the liver was done. No calculi were present; the microscopic sections of the gallbladder showed necrotizing angiitis in the wall (Fig. 1) and liver (Fig. 2) with fibrinoid necrosis. Most of the perivascular leukocytes were polymorphonuclear neutrophils with a few eosinophils, and a rare plasma cell and lymphocyte. She was given tetracycline, streptomycin, and isoniazid postoperatively. She became asymptomatic and afebrile and was discharged on the thirteenth postoperative day.

Case 2. A 69-year-old Caucasian man had three admissions to Mary Immaculate Hospital in 2 years.

His first admission was for obstructive jaundice with dark urine of 5 days' duration. The hematocrit was 37 percent; white count was 5,800 per cubic millimeter with 72 percent polycytes, 22 percent lymphocytes, 5 percent eosinophils, and 1 percent monocytes. The total bilirubin was 20.4 mg. percent, with 14 mg. percent as direct. The chest x-ray and telectrocardiogram were normal. A laparotomy was performed on the seventh hospital day at which time a cholecystectomy and choledochostomy were performed. The gallbladder showed chronic cholecystitis and

Received for publication April 3, 1969.

*Reprint requests: Mary Immaculate Hospital Division, Jamaica, N. Y. 11432.

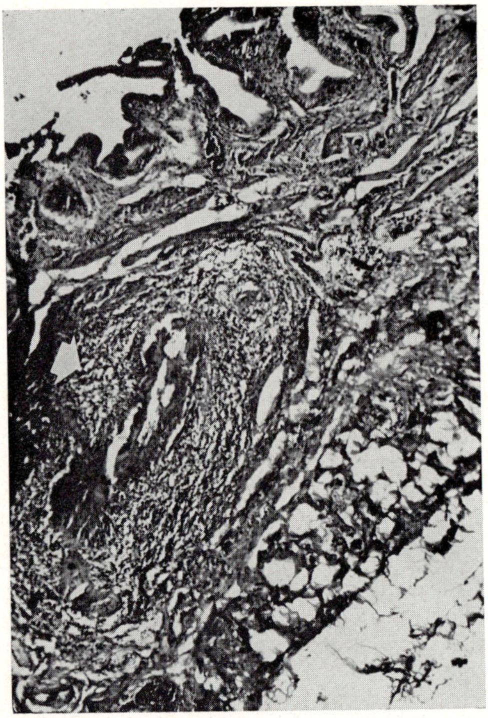

Fig. 1. Case 1: Section of the gallbladder with panarteritis (arrow). (Hematoxylin and eosin. Original magnification ×25.)

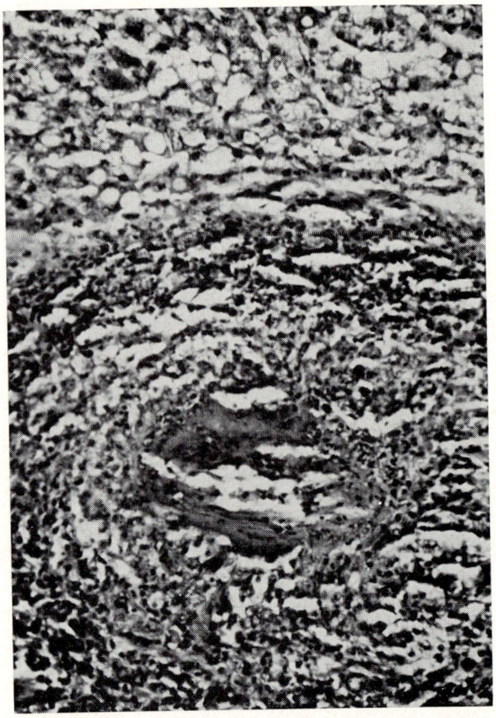

Fig. 2. Case 1: Section of wedge biopsy of the liver showing annular fibrinoid necrosis of the media and transmural exudation. The cells are mostly segmented neutrophils with a few eosinophils. (Hematoxylin and eosin. Original magnification ×250.)

cholelithiasis. The patient improved, became asymptomatic, and was discharged on the seventeenth postoperative day. The second admission was 8 months later with mild jaundice, epigastric pain, nausea, and vomiting. The bilirubin was 6.2 mg. percent, with 3.7 mg. percent direct. The blood urea nitrogen was 38 mg. percent, and total protein was 6.1 Gm. percent with an albumin-globulin ratio of 3.7 to 2.4. His symptoms and jaundice disappeared under conservative management, and he was discharged from the hospital on the fifth hospital day.

The third admission was 15 months later with frequency and difficulty in starting the urinary stream. There was now some substernal pain present on exertion; it was relieved by rest. A history was now obtained of recurring joint pains unassociated with redness or swelling. His vital signs were normal. The chest x-rays showed bilateral generalized fine nodular infiltrates. The intravenous pyelogram showed poor excretion and an enlarged prostate. The electrocardiogram was normal. His hemoglobin was 12 Gm. percent. White count was 19,000 per cubic millimeter with 1 percent bands, 90 percent polycytes, 4 percent lymphocytes, 3 percent monocytes, and 4 percent eosinophils. He had 4+ albuminuria with 25 to 30 erythrocytes and 5 to 10 leukocytes per high-power field. The initial blood urea nitrogen was 17 mg. percent and 236 mg. percent terminally. His creatinine rose to 13 mg. percent, the uric acid to 12 mg. percent, and the potassium to 7.1 mEq. per liter.

Hospital course. After admission he developed complete urinary retention. A suprapubic prostatectomy and bilateral vasectomy were performed. The prostate showed benign hypertrophy and a recent infarct. Thereafter he became progressively azotemic and despite peritoneal dialyses, intravenous fluids, and antibiotics, he died 44 days after operation.

Autopsy showed generalized polyarteritis nodosa in various stages with recent to organizing infarctions of the kidneys, pancreas, prostate, adrenals, heart, spleen, and lungs. The kidney (Fig. 3) and pancreas (Fig. 4) showed acute arteritis (Stage II) and healed lesions (Stage IV), respectively.

Review of the previously resected gallbladder (Figs. 5 and 6) revealed panarteritis in the third stage of organization. The urinary obstruction on

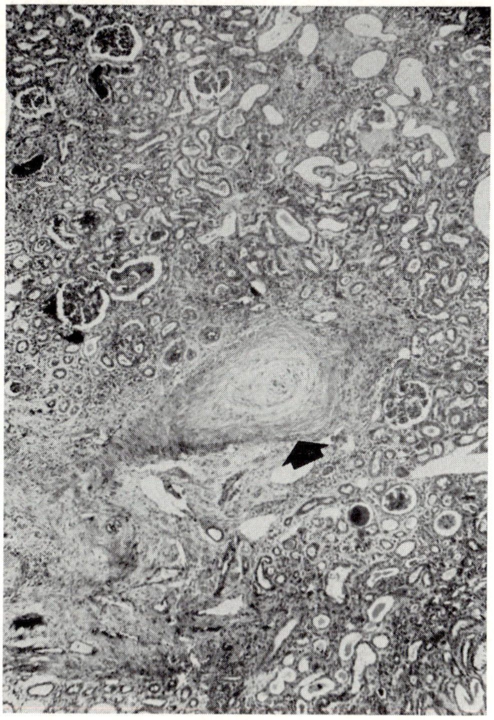

Fig. 3. Case 2: Section of the kidney showing healed-end arteritis, Stage IV (arrow). (Hematoxylin and eosin. Original magnification ×25.)

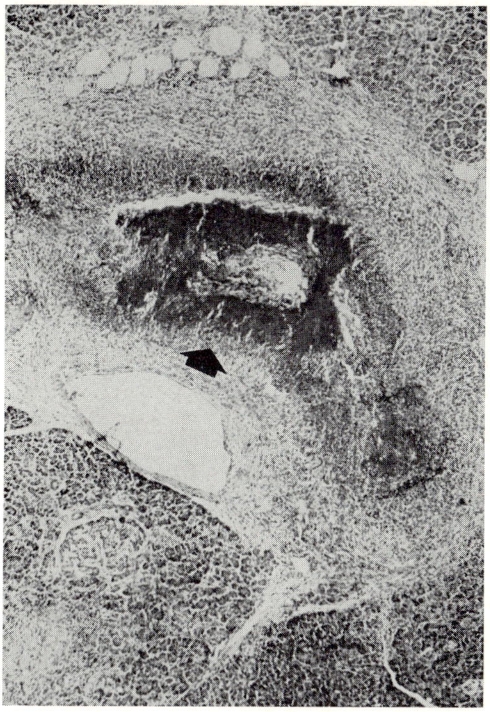

Fig. 4. Case 2: Section of the pancreas with panarteritis of medium size artery (arrow). (Hematoxylin and eosin. Original magnification ×10.)

the third hospitalization was due to polyarteritis of the prostate.

DISCUSSION

While the etiology of polyarteritis nodosa is still uncertain, there are findings favoring a hypersensitivity reaction: fibrinoid necrosis in the arteritis, frequent association with bronchial asthma, eosinophilia, and a response to steroid therapy. Eighteen percent of the patients have bronchial asthma and 94 percent of this group have eosinophilia.[3, 8] Patients without asthma, only 6 percent, had eosinophilia.[8] Mowrey and Lundberg[6] showed a general incidence of 18 percent eosinophilia. Muscle biopsy has been found to show diagnostic vascular lesions in up to 77 percent of the cases.[4]

The histologic changes in the arteries have been divided into four stages by Arkin[1]: alterative-degenerative stage, acute inflammatory stage, granulation tissue stage, and healed-end stage. The second stage is seen in the gallbladder and liver biopsy of Case 1, and the third stage is seen in the gallbladder of Case 2. At autopsy, the second case showed all stages of polyarteritis.

The organs often involved are listed in Table I. A presumptive clinical diagnosis can be made with a combination of the findings, especially when they refer to organs that are most frequently involved, such as kidneys, heart, liver, and gastrointestinal tract.[3] A detailed analysis of the clinical manifestations in 607 cases is rendered by Mowrey and Lundberg.[6] The diagnosis may be established by muscle and skin or testicular biopsy. Muscle biopsy should generally be performed in areas where there is myalgia or muscle tenderness. In its absence, Rose[7] suggests biopsy of the pectoralis muscle. Dahl and co-workers[2] examined the testes in 44 autopsy patients with this disease, and found polyarteritis in 86 percent of the cases. He estimated from numerous sections studied of autopsy material that a biopsy measuring

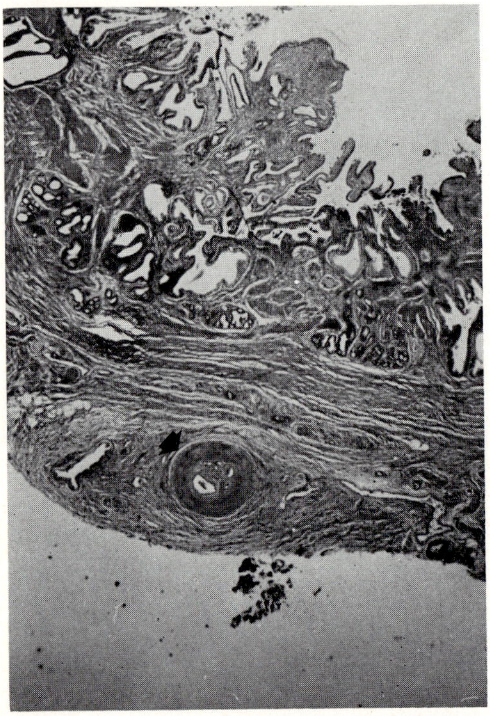

Fig. 5. Case 2: The gallbladder has Stage III arteritis at the serosa (arrow). (Hematoxylin and eosin. Original magnification ×10.)

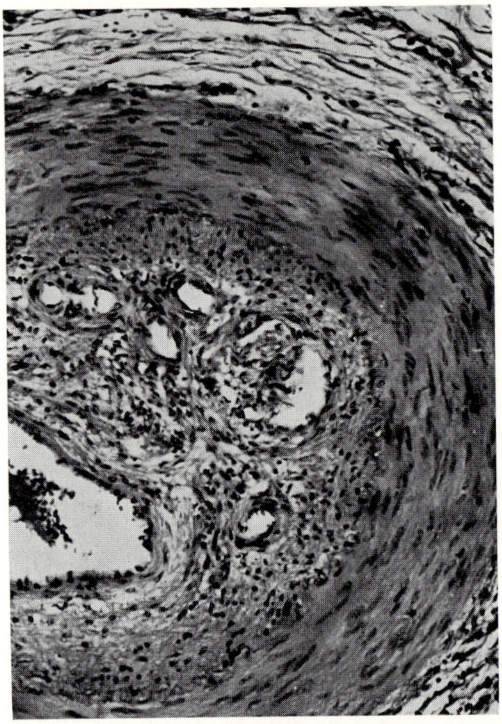

Fig. 6. Case 2: High-power magnification of the artery in Fig. 5, showing recanalization, mononuclear cells, and fibroblasts in a resolving arteritis. (Hematoxylin and eosin. Original magnification ×250.)

Table I. *Organs frequently involved in polyarteritis*

Organ	*Arkin*[1] (%)	*McCall and Pennock*[4] (%)	*Rose*[7] (%)
Kidney	80	100	79
Heart	70	78	32
Liver	65	78	—
Gastrointestinal tract	50	—	54
Pancreas	25	55	70
Mesenteric artery	30	—	—
Muscle	30	—	46
Peripheral nerve	20	—	36
Testes*	—	60	—
Adrenal	—	25	—

A dash indicates that no figure of frequency is given.

*Testes were involved in 86 percent of patients in Dahl and associates'[2] series.

6 by 4 mm. would give a 22 percent positive diagnosis of polyarteritis nodosa.

In retrospect, both of our cases had clinical features of polyarteritis nodosa, and the diagnosis may have been confirmed with extra-abdominal biopsy.

SUMMARY

Two patients are presented with clinical primary biliary disease. Both patients had cholecystectomy showing polyarteritis nodosa.

Elderly patients with vague, mild joint pains and right upper quadrant pain should be suspected for polyarteritis nodosa. The diagnosis may be confirmed by cutaneous muscle or testicular biopsy obviating the need for laparotomy.

REFERENCES

1. Arkin, A.: A clinical and pathological study of periarteritis nodosa. A report of five cases,

one histologically healed, Am. J. Path. **6:** 401, 1930.

2. Dahl, E. L., Baggenstoss, A. H., and DeWeered, J. H.: Testicular lesions of periarteritis nodosa with special reference to diagnosis, Am. J. Med. **28:** 222, 1960.
3. Griffith, G. C., and Vural, I. L.: Polyarteritis nodosa: Correlation of clinical and postmortem findings in seventeen cases, Circulation **3:** 481, 1951.
4. McCall, M., and Pennock, J. W.: Periarteritis nodosa, Ann. Int. Med. **21:** 628, 1944.
5. Maxeiner, S. R., Jr., McDonald, J. R., and Kirklin, J. W.: Muscle biopsy in the diagnosis of periarteritis nodosa; evaluation, S. Clin. North America **32:** 1225, 1952.
6. Mowrey, F. H., and Lundberg, E. A.: The clinical manifestations of periarteritis nodosa with emphasis on the hepatic manifestations, Ann. Int. Med. **40:** 1145, 1954.
7. Rose, G. A.: The natural history of polyarteritis, Brit. M. J. **2:** 1148, 1957.
8. Shulman, L. E., and McGehee, H.: Polyarteritis, *in* Hollander, J. L., editor: Arthritis and allied conditions; a textbook of rheumatology, Philadelphia, 1966, Lea & Febiger, Publishers, p. 802.

The clinical use of intraperitoneal cephalothin

MARTIN H. McMULLAN, M.D.
WILLIAM O. BARNETT, M.D.
JACKSON, MISS.
From the Department of Surgery, The University of Mississippi Medical Center

Our attention was first directed toward the possible superior efficacy of antibiotics administered intraperitoneally by experimental studies involving peritoneal contamination with toxic peritoneal fluid resulting from strangulation of small bowel segments.[3] Under standard conditions, penicillin and streptomycin were given intramuscularly in one group and intraperitoneally in another. There were more than twice as many survivors among the animals who received the antibiotic directly into the peritoneal cavity. Additional studies served to compare the efficacy of chloramphenicol and kanamycin when given intramuscularly, intravenously, and intraperitoneally. In the case of both antibiotics, the intraperitoneal route of administration gave superior results.

Upon the basis of these studies, we began the clinical utilization of intraperitoneal antibiotics. In a review of 105 cases of colon obstruction in our hospital, of which 16 cases were complicated by rupture, five patients received their antibiotics by the intraperitoneal route.[1] The mortality rate was 20 percent. Eleven patients were given antibiotics by the intravenous method, and the mortality rate was 54 percent. This experience is not sufficiently extensive at the present time to provide data of statistical significance; nevertheless, the results do suggest a trend which would support the conclusions gained from animal studies.

A later group of experiments was concerned with an evaluation of the possibility of eliminating the lethal properties of gangrenous bowel segments by the comparison of intravenous and intraperitoneal administration of cephalothin.[2] Survival was attained more than twice as often when the antibiotic was injected into the peritoneal cavity.

Comparative studies were carried out in which the efficacy of chloramphenicol, kanamycin, and cephalothin were evaluated following peritoneal contamination with gangrenous bowel segments. When kanamycin was used, the survival rate in experimental animals was 15 percent, while use of chloramphenicol was followed by a survival rate of 35 percent. Under similar conditions, cephalothin-treated animals survived at a rate of 80 percent.

We are convinced, as the result of experimental studies, that as the degree of peritoneal contamination increases, so must the dose of antibiotic be elevated in order to provide maximum chances for survival. Where cephalothin was used in a dose of 28 mg. per kilogram intraperitoneally to combat the lethal effects of a 10 cm. strangulated segment of bowel, the survival rate was 80 percent. Upon increasing the length of the gangrenous segment to 20 cm. and maintaining the same dose of cephalothin, the survival rate fell to 25 percent. With the subsequent increase of cephalothin to 56 mg. per kilogram, the survivors promptly increased to 69 percent.

TECHNIQUES

Most patients with peritonitis are rendered better operative risks if an intensive

Received for publication April 9, 1969.

preoperative period of treatment is carried out to include blood, fluid, electrolyte, etc., administration. Preoperative fluid and electrolyte correction is probably responsible, more than any other factor, for the improved survival rate in simple intestinal obstruction observed during this century. Yet, there is a considerable tendency to rush a patient with gangrenous bowel obstruction to surgery immediately without the benefit of such preparation despite the fact that he is suffering from all the derangements of the patient with simple obstruction and others in addition. Experimental evidence has shown conclusively that with the intraperitoneal administration of cephalothin, gangrenous bowel segments can be eliminated as sources of toxic materials. This approach could provide a reasonable preoperative period for correction of fluid and electrolyte deficiencies without undue progression of the deleterious effects of continuing peritoneal contamination.

Preoperative intraperitoneal antibiotics can be administered through a polyethylene tube which has been inserted only after the stomach and urinary bladder have been emptied. We have used a 14 gauge liver biopsy needle from which the sharp tips of both the needle and the obturator have been filed away in order to provide a blunt surface (Fig. 1). Under local anesthesia, a small transverse incision is made in the midline just above the umbilicus (Fig. 2). The fibrous tissue comprising the linea alba is also divided with the scalpel blade. The 14 gauge, blunt needle, with obturator in place, is then introduced and turned back and forth with gentle pressure in order to penetrate the preperitoneal tissues and the peritoneum. The needle should be angled at approximately 45 degrees with the surface of the abdomen and aimed away from any existing abdominal scars. The lack of resistance encountered after penetration of the peritoneum is readily apparent, and at this point the obturator is removed. A syringe can be attached to evaluate the characteristics of any free fluid that may be present within the peritoneum. The polyethylene tubing is then introduced through the needle after which it can be slipped gently over the tubing and removed. A few skin sutures around the tubing complete the procedure. We have found that polyethylene tubing with an internal diameter of 0.034 inch and an outside diameter of 0.05 inch passes through the needle with ease, and it also accepts the insertion of a 20 gauge needle. This needle is connected to a 1 L. solution of isotonic saline containing 5 Gm. of cephalothin. The solution is allowed to drip at a rapid rate consistent with the patient's comfort (Fig. 2).

In addition to the preoperative administration of intraperitoneal cephalothin for

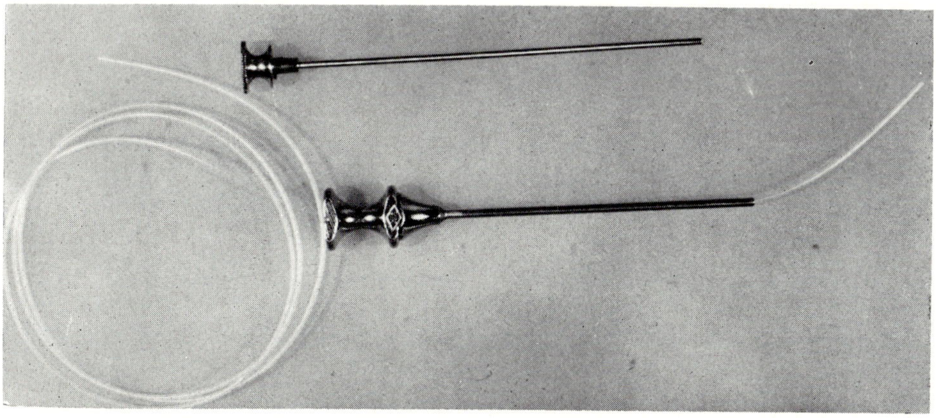

Fig. 1. Blunt needle and 14 gauge plastic tubing used for intraperitoneal placement.

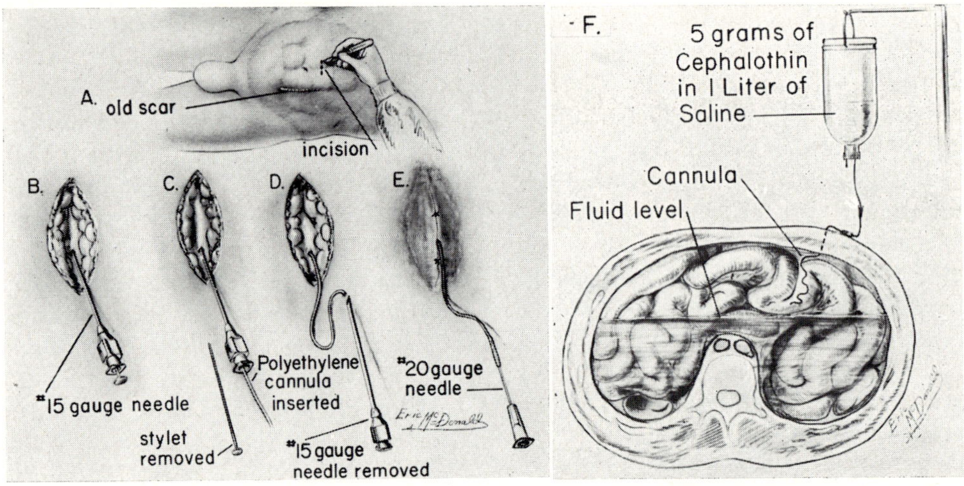

Fig. 2. Preoperative insertion of intraperitoneal polyethylene tubing. *A,* Small transverse incision above the umbilicus under local anesthesia. *B,* Needle introduced in lateral direction at angle of about 45 degrees. *C,* Tubing is introduced through needle after removal of stylet. *D,* Needle is slipped off over the plastic tubing. *E,* Small incision closed and 20 gauge needle connected to tubing. *F,* Antibiotic solution dripping into peritoneal cavity.

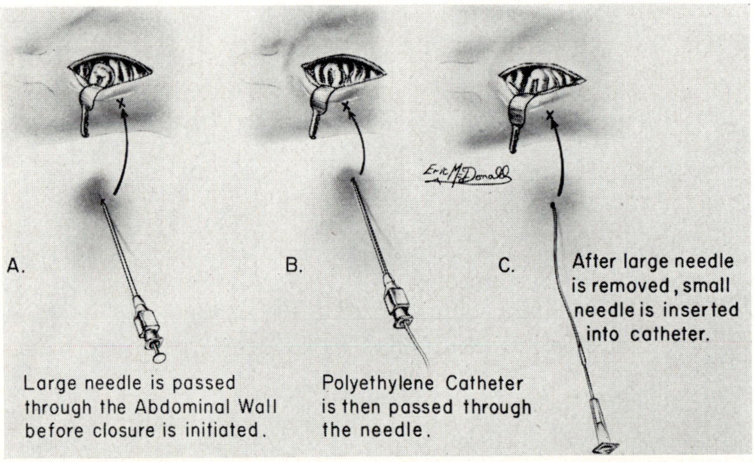

Fig. 3. Placement of intraperitoneal polyethylene tubing at time of operation.

suspected strangulation obstruction, we have now expanded this procedure into the intraoperative and postoperative periods as definitive therapy for purulent or potentially purulent peritonitis no matter what the etiology.

Where it is elected to insert a polyethylene tube at the time of operation, for the postoperative administration of the drug, a leakproof placement can be obtained by obliquely passing a large gauge needle through the abdominal wall under direct vision (Fig. 3). The tubing can then be passed through the needle after which the needle is removed (Fig. 3). Another acceptable method is the insertion of a No. 5 or 8 polyethylene pediatric feeding tube through a minute separate stab wound. Prior to closure of the abdomen, 2 Gm. of cephalothin in 20 c.c. of saline may be placed di-

Table I. *Cause of illness in 32 patients treated with intraperitoneal cephalothin*

Etiology	*No. of cases*
Penetrating wound of the abdomen	11
Small bowel obstruction	10
Appendicitis (perforated)	4
Acute cholecystitis	1
Sigmoid volvulus	1
Tube ovarian abscess	1
Perforated duodenal ulcer	1
Perforated colon (biopsy through proctoscope)	1
Rupture of duodenum from blunt trauma	1
Tuberculous enteritis with perforation	1

Table II. *Surgical procedures performed upon 32 patients treated with intraperitoneal cephalothin*

Surgical procedure	*No. of cases*
Small bowel resection	6
Closure of bowel perforations following trauma	5
Lysis of adhesions	4
Appendectomy	4
Hernia repair	4
Drainage of abscess	3
Colostomy and closure of colon perforations	3
Exteriorization of injured colon	3
Resection of unprepared right colon	2
Closure of perforated duodenal ulcer	1
Primary closure of sigmoid colon perforation	1
Cholecystectomy	1
Reduction of sigmoid volvulus and inversion of small gangrenous area	1
Bilateral salpingo-oophorectomy	1
Ileotransverse colostomy	1

rectly into the area of greatest contamination.

It is our practice to continue the intraperitoneal infusion of cephalothin for 3 to 4 days during the postoperative period.

CLINICAL EXPERIENCE

Intraperitoneal cephalothin has now been administered to 32 patients with abdominal complaints. The most common complaint among this group was penetrating wound of the abdomen with perforation of a hollow viscus (11 cases). Ten cases presented small bowel obstruction, while four cases of perforated appendicitis were included. The remainder included a wide variety of conditions as listed (Table I).

Surgical procedures carried out among these patients are listed in Table II. Five patients were given intraperitoneal cephalothin during the preoperative period, while administration of this antibiotic was initiated in six patients during the operation. In 21 instances, the intraperitoneal administration of cephalothin was started during the postoperative period. In the five patients in whom preoperative injection of the antibiotic was carried out, an opportunity to inspect the peritoneum during the subsequent operative procedure was afforded. There was no evidence of adverse reaction to direct peritoneal exposure to cephalothin in the diluted state as described above. It was possible to allow the antibiotic solution to drip into the peritoneal cavity at a relatively rapid rate without manifestation of discom-

Table III. *Clinical course in patients receiving intraperitoneal cephalothin*

	Postoperative day											
	1	*2*	*3*	*4*	*5*	*6*	*7*	*8*	*11*	*13*	*19*	*26*
Passage of flatus initiated (No. of patients)	0	4	8	10	3	4	0	0	0			
Bowel sounds present (No. of patients)	4	7	10	6	1	1						
Initiation of oral feedings (No. of patients)		1	4	8	8	2	6	1	1			
Patient became afebrile (No. of patients)		2	4	2	7	3	3	1	1	1	3	1

fort by the patients. Bowel sounds became present on the third postoperative day as a mean value among these patients (Table III). Passage of flatus was initiated on the fourth postoperative day (mean value) in most patients. In the average circumstance, oral feedings were initiated on the fifth postoperative day, while this figure was the eighth postoperative day in relation to the disappearance of fever. Superficial wound infections were observed in two patients, and a subphrenic abscess developed in one. Partial small bowel obstruction responded to nasogastric tube therapy on the eleventh postoperative day.

In this series of patients there were no deaths, nor were there ill effects from the intraperitoneal admission of the drug, such as respiratory depression, renal toxicity, bone marrow depression, eighth nerve toxicity, or hypersensitivity. In view of the fact that cephalothin is effective against the usual flora of gram-negative organisms and of the conclusion that it can be safely used in doses up to 12 Gm. per 24 hours, it may represent the antibacterial agent of choice for peritonitis.

SUMMARY

We report 32 patients who received intraperitoneal cephalothin management of various abdominal conditions. Five patients were given preoperative, intraperitoneal cephalothin, while six received the antibiotic during the operation. In 21 instances, intraperitoneal cephalothin was initiated during the postoperative period. There were no adverse reactions observed during this experience which could be attributed to the antibiotic. All patients recovered. The rationale for the superior efficacy of intraperitoneal antibiotics under certain circumstances is discussed, and the techniques involved are reviewed.

REFERENCES

1. Barnett, W. O., and Little, B. R.: Obstruction of the large bowel, South. M. J. **58:** 1493, 1965.
2. Barnett, W. O., Oliver, R. I., and Elliott, R. L.: Elimination of the lethal properties of gangrenous bowel segments, Ann. Surg. **167:** 912, 1968.
3. Dalton, M. L., Jr., and Barnett, W. O.: Investigations regarding the use of antibiotics in strangulation obstruction, Amer. Surgeon **27:** 721, 1961.

Mortality factors in major limb amputations for vascular disease: A study of 176 procedures

NORMAN ROSENBERG, M.D.
EDGARDO ADIARTE, M.D.
LESLIE J. BUJDOSO, M.D.
KLAUS D. BACKWINKEL, M.D.
NEW BRUNSWICK, N. J.
From the Vascular Surgical Services, Middlesex General Hospital and St. Peter's General Hospital

Amputation of the lower extremity is the oldest major surgical procedure, having been performed hundreds of years before the advent of anesthesia. It is a technically simple operation, which is often assigned to assistant surgical residents; yet the in-hospital mortality rate remains high,[1, 4, 7] and in most series is comparable to that resulting from open-heart surgery. Until 1942, the average death rate for midthigh amputation in the diabetic patient was 44 percent, with a range of 25 to 75 percent.[6] For combined groupings of diabetic and nondiabetic patients, a 42 percent mortality rate was not uncommon during this period[6] rising to as high as 51 to 66 percent when cellulitis and rapidly spreading gangrene were present.[2, 3, 5]

More recently, in the antibiotic era, the over-all mortality rate has ranged between 10 and 29 percent,[1, 4, 7] with most investigators reporting results nearer the lower figure. The death rate following this procedure still remains significantly high, prompting a re-examination of the factors, controllable and noncontrollable, which contribute not only to the loss of life but also to the high complication rate reported by most students of the problem.

CLINICAL MATERIAL

This study involves 176 major amputations performed over a 20 year period (1948-1967) (Table I). This series of cases represents, in the main, the personal experience of the senior author with most operations being performed by him or by surgical residents under his supervision. All were treated during the antibiotic era. All procedures were carried out for vascular insufficiency and its complications.

There were 105 amputations performed through the thigh. Seventy-one patients had below-knee amputations. The predominant indication for amputation was gangrene which was present in 159 limbs, and in almost all patients with diabetes. Other indications are listed in Table II. Operations that had been performed previous to the amputations and that are related to them are listed in Table III.

The series contains an almost equal number of diabetic and nondiabetic patients. Concurrent atherosclerotic heart disease was present in about 30 percent of the cases, and a similar number of patients had pulmonary emphysema.

Mortality rate. Thirty patients, or 17 percent, died following major amputation. The mortality rate in diabetic patients was 23.6 percent (21 of 89 cases), while only 10.3 percent of nondiabetic patients died after operation (9 of 87). Midthigh amputation proved more than twice as lethal as midleg amputation with a 21.9 percent versus a 9.9 percent mortality rate (see Table IV).

Age became a major factor only after the age of 60. However, 19 of the 30 patients who died, or 63 percent, were obese, and

Received for publication April 10, 1969.

Table I. *Statistical summary of 176 major lower extremity amputations performed during the 20 years from 1948 to 1967**

Data	No. of patients
Sex	
Male	101
Female	75
Age†	
Below 50 yr.	29
50 to 59	18
60 to 69	58
70 to 79	65
Above 80	6
Site of amputation	
Midthigh	105
Midleg	71
Diabetes	
Present	89‡
Not present	87

*Hospitals involved in the study were the Middlesex General Hospital with 112 cases and St. Peter's General Hospital with 64 cases.

†The age level ranged from 38 to 88 years.

‡Forty-four of the diabetic patients were male, and 45 female.

Table II. *Indications for amputation in the 176 cases being discussed*

Description	No. of cases
Precipitating vascular disease	
Peripheral atherosclerotic occlusion	156
Aortoiliac occlusion	1
Popliteal aneurysm	4
Arterial embolism (late cases)	12
Arterial injury	1
Phlegmasia cerulea dolens	2
Associated local pathology	
Gangrene	159
Necrosis at more distal amputation site	6
Extensive ulceration with infection	4
Intractable pain	5
Failure of prosthetic graft	2
Related major disease	
Heart disease	63
Arteriosclerotic	59
Rheumatic	4
Chronic bronchitis and emphysema	57
Diabetes-related states	
Diabetic neuropathy	51
Kimmelstiel-Wilson syndrome	30

Table III. *Previous related operations*

Description	No. of cases
Great toe amputation	19
Forefoot amputation	26
Midleg amputation	7
Midthigh amputation (opposite limb)	9
Lumbar sympathectomy	64
Arterial bypass graft	13
Embolectomy	6
Thromboendarterectomy	5
Exploration of artery	2
Excision of popliteal aneurysm	1
Peripheral nerve crushing	2

of the 30 deaths 27 or 90 percent had associated heart disease.

The causes of death are listed in Table IV. Despite the almost routine administration of antibiotics, sepsis played a major role, possibly reflecting the large number of diabetic patients in this series. Gas gangrene of the stump occurred twice. Cardiovascular deaths were prominent (myocardial infarction, cerebrovascular accidents, and pulmonary embolism).

Fig. 1 depicts our mortality experience on a year-by-year basis over the 20 years of this study. The markedly lower mortality rate over the last 5 year period is worthy of note.

Morbidity. Complications were numerous and are listed in Table V. Wound difficulties consisted of hematoma, skin necrosis, dehiscence, and an infection rate of 16 percent. Twenty-nine percent of patients developed evidence of coronary insufficiency or occlusion, and there was a 6.8 percent incidence of pulmonary embolism. Pneumonia occurred in 10 percent of patients. Forty percent developed or had urinary tract infection. Decubitus ulcer was experienced by almost 15 percent. Other problems are enumerated in Table V.

DISCUSSION

The very high mortality rate from major amputations in the lower limb prior to World War II has been emphasized. There was a marked improvement following the war, probably because of the widespread use of antibiotics. This seemed to be followed

Table IV. *Analysis of mortality statistics*

Data	*No. of patients*	*Mortality rate (%)*
Deaths	30 of 176	17
Males	19 of 101	18.7
Females	11 of 75	14.7
Autopsies (83%)	25 of 30	
Diabetic patients	21 of 89	23.6
Nondiabetic patients	9 of 87	10.3
Above-knee amputations	23 of 105	21.9
Below-knee amputations	7 of 71	9.9
Mortality age level		
Below 50	2 of 29	
50-59	2 of 18	
60-69	11 of 58	
70-79	13 of 65	
80 and over	2 of 6	
Causes of death		
Septicemia	9	
Myocardial infarction	6	
Cerebrovascular accident	3	
Gas gangrene	2	
Pulmonary embolism	2	
Dilaudid narcosis	1	
Incarcerated hernia	1	
Uremia	1	
Associated obesity	19 of 30	63
Associated heart disease	27 of 30	90

Table V

Complications	*No. of cases*
Wound difficulties	
Hematoma	37
Skin necrosis	26
Major infection	29 (16%)
Dehiscence	12
Cardiovascular and pulmonary	
Coronary insufficiency	34 } (29%)
Coronary occlusion	17 }
Arrhythmia	26
Thrombophlebitis	11
Pulmonary embolism	12 (6.8%)
Pneumonia	18 (10%)
Urinary tract problems	
Incontinence	45
Catheterization required	42
Cystitis	33 } (40%)
Pyelonephritis	37 }
Uremia	9
Neuropsychiatric	
Disorientation	43
Postoperative psychosis	8
Cerebrovascular accident	12
Coma due to Dilaudid narcosis	2
Decubitus ulcer	26 (14.7%)

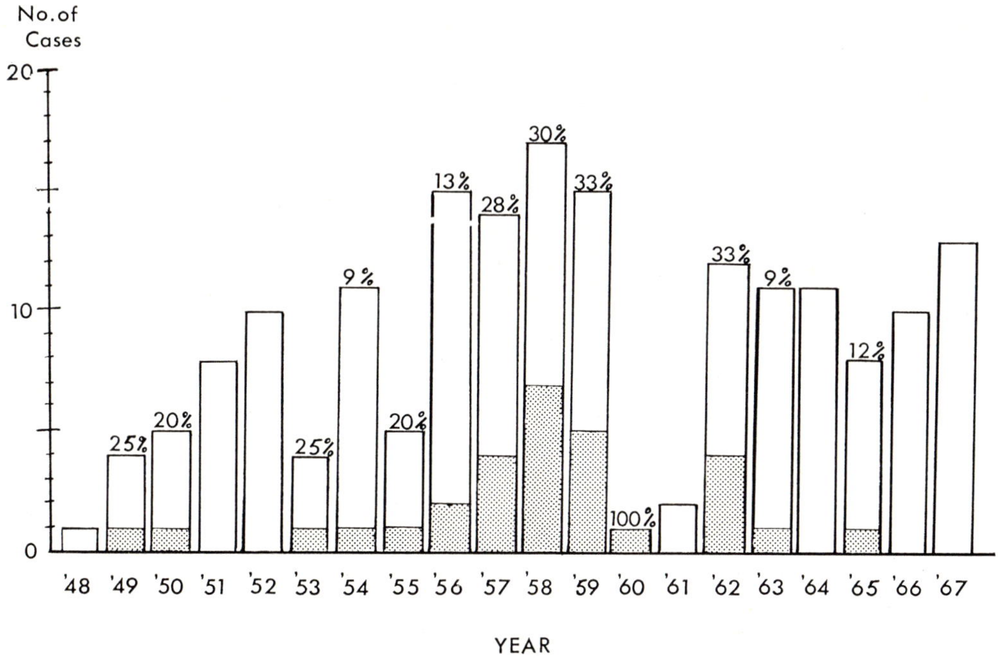

Fig. 1. Bar graph showing yearly mortality rate. The percent of deaths is indicated by the shaded areas.

in our series by a recurrence of higher mortality figures (see Fig. 1), which, however, were never as high as reported pre-war percentages. One might conjecture that, in recent years, the advent of arterial reconstruction procedures such as bypass grafting and endarterectomy had salvaged limbs in a considerable number of relatively younger, good-risk patients with segmental arterial disease who might otherwise have come to amputation, leaving a "scrap-basket," older, poorer-risk group of patients behind, with more extensive arterial disease and other medical complications to constitute our present amputation group. Disturbed by our high mortality rate in the 1955-1962 period, we began to consider all patients coming to major amputation as exceedingly "brittle" individuals who required the closest of observation and the most meticulous medical and nursing supervision.

Special attention was given to prevention of complications rather than solely to their treatment. The following regimen was adopted:

A. Prevention of wound (stump) difficulties
   1. Careful preoperative cleansing and preparation of skin
   2. Meticulous hemostasis, avoidance of tourniquets, limitation of the use of refrigeration technique
   3. Amputation at definitely viable levels
   4. Drainage of all stumps (at lateral wound angle)
   5. Open treatment of stump with delayed closure where infection seems likely to occur
   6. Leaving some sutures in for 14 days to avoid dehiscence
   7. Protection of stump from soiling by (a) use of indwelling catheter in the early postoperative period, (b) use of enema evacuation of the colon, and (c) protection of medial and posterior aspect of stump by plastic film
   8. The use of prophylactic antibiotics (Preoperative therapy is of additional value.)
   9. Adequate control of diabetes, when present

B. Prevention of decubiti
   1. Back care three times daily
   2. Frequent turning of patient
   3. Judicious use of "lamb-skin" robes and foam rubber
   4. Early mobilization from bed
   5. Maintaining nutrition of patient

C. Prevention of cardiovascular and pulmonary complications
   1. Bringing patient to operation in the best possible medical state (hydration, digitalis, etc.)
   2. Avoidance of insulin reactions in diabetic patients
   3. Prophylactic heparinization in all cases to prevent pulmonary embolism
   4. Encouraging coughing and deep breathing, intermittent positive-pressure breathing, and tracheal suction where indicated
   5. In-bed exercising of the stump and opposite limb and use of Balkan frame and trapeze bar for exercise of arms and shoulders

D. Prevention of urinary complications
   1. Routine indwelling catheter during early postoperative period covered by antibiotics or chemotherapeutic agents
   2. Maintenance of hydration to insure adequate urine flow

E. Prevention of neuropsychiatric complications
   1. Avoidance of large doses of opiates in elderly patients
   2. Avoidance of barbiturates, most tranquilizers, and antiemetics (Phenergan 12.5 to 25 mg. is commonly employed at night.)
   3. Side rails and loose restraints for protection of patient, where indicated
   4. Use of 3 to 5 mg. of Benzedrine occasionally in the morning in aged individuals to stimulate in the patients a greater interest in their food, their surroundings, and their moving about in bed
   5. Phlebotomy in patients with primary or secondary polycythemia to lower blood viscosity and improve flow char-

acteristics (This may help prevent cerebral and other thromboses.)

In addition, keeping unnecessary procrastination to a minimum is essential in the prevention of complications. Needless postponement of amputation will result in the following undesirable conditions: (1) It will prolong the period of ischemic pain and psychic stress; (2) it may permit the patient to become "toxic" and disoriented because of absorption of bacterial and tissue breakdown products, with adverse effects on vital organs; (3) nutrition and hydration will be affected by anorexia; (4) diabetes, if present, may become more difficult to control; (5) venous thrombosis may ascend to involve larger limb veins, increasing the chances for fatal postoperative pulmonary embolism.

Attention to the preventive regimen outlined above and avoidance of unnecessary delay have, we believe, led to a considerable improvement in survival statistics (see Fig. 1, 1963 through 1967).

CONCLUSIONS

1. A 20 year experience involving 176 major amputations through the lower limb is presented.

2. There was a 17 percent over-all mortality rate, 22 percent for midthigh and 10 percent for midleg procedures.

3. The presence of diabetes mellitus was associated with a 2.3-fold increase in the mortality rate.

4. The death rate was also higher in the aged, the obese, and in those with underlying heart disease.

5. A year-by-year analysis of our mortality figures discloses possible factors responsible for major fluctuations.

6. A program of management of these poor-risk patients is outlined, and its efficacy in lowering mortality and morbidity rates is suggested.

REFERENCES

1. Dale, W. A., and Jacobs, J. K.: Lower extremity amputations, Ann. Surg. **155:** 1011, 1962.
2. Herrmann, L. G., and Gibbs, E. W.: Phantom limb pain; its relation to treatment of large nerves at time of amputation, Am. J. Surg. **67:** 168, 1945.
3. Mandelberg, A., and Sheinfeld, W.: Diabetic amputations; analysis of 128 cases, Am. J. Surg. **71:** 70, 1946.
4. Otteman, M., and Stahlgren, L. H.: Evaluation of factors which influence mortality and morbidity following major lower extremity amputations for arteriosclerosis, Surg. Gynec. & Obst. **120:** 1217, 1965.
5. Perlow, S., and Roth, H. A.: Amputation for gangrene due to occlusive arterial disease, SURGERY **25:** 547, 1949.
6. Silbert, S.: Mid-leg amputations for gangrene in the diabetic, Ann. Surg. **127:** 503, 1948.
7. Thompson, R. C., Delblanco, T. L., and McAllister, F. F.: Complications following lower extremity amputation, Surg. Gynec. & Obst. **120:** 301, 1965.

Contralateral arterial grafts

LEÓN BIALOSTOZKY, M.D.
RAÚL LEGASPI, M.D.
LORENZO RISH F., M.D.
FEDERICO MORALES M., M.D.
MEXICO CITY, MEXICO
From the Department of Cardiovascular Surgery, Centro Hospitalario 20 de Noviembre (ISSSTE)

Since vascular grafts (plastic or homologous vein) have been implanted to bypass one or more obstructions, many lives and, especially, many limbs have been saved.

The majority of arterial obstructions are produced by atheromatous plaques. Proximally and distally to these obstructions there is a relatively normal artery. An anastomosis with grafts can be made in this place with satisfactory results, as long as there is no important obstruction distal to the anastomosis. The distal vascular bed plays the most important role in the etiology of arterial graft thrombosis.

Frequently, the general condition of an elderly patient with obstructive atherosclerotic disease is aggravated by the presence of diabetes mellitus or cardiac, pulmonary, or renal diseases. In these patients, a surgical procedure increases the already poor prognosis, not only for the extremity, but also for the patient's life.[7, 12, 13, 16]

The procedure here recommended, which implies less surgical aggression, is the revascularization of the ischemic extremity with a plastic or venous graft taken from the unobstructed common femoral or external iliac artery to the contralateral femoral or iliac, distal to the obstruction. This is done under superficial general anesthesia or peridural block; the technique is simple, with minimal trauma and maximum speed.[5, 9, 11, 17]

Submitted for publication April 19, 1969; resubmitted May 16, 1969.

MATERIAL AND METHOD

From December, 1965, to January, 1969, at the Centro Hospitalario 20 de Noviembre, 20 patients have been operated upon, 7 female and 13 male. Their ages ranged from 33 to 76 years, with an average of 61 years.

All patients had clinical and radiologic studies made: preoperative translumbar aortogram in 20 cases (100 percent) and postoperative studies in 10 patients (50 percent). The clinical picture was very similar in 19 of the 20 patients, with cardioangiosclerosis in 19 cases, high blood pressure in 4, auricular fibrillation in 5, pulmonary emphysema in 14, diabetes mellitus in 7, renal disease in 1, and obesity in 4. Intermittent claudication and signs of ischemia of the lower extremities were the causes for hospital admission of all patients.

Table I shows a summary of the diagnosis, operation, anesthesia, type of graft, postoperative x-rays, patency, and the postoperative condition of the patient.

The surgical procedure (Fig. 1) was performed under peridural anesthesia in six cases, and superficial general anesthesia in 14 cases. Bilateral supra- or infrainguinal incisions were made; the external iliac or common femoral arteries were dissected bilaterally and terminolateral anastomoses were performed. The graft was placed subcutaneously anterior to the pubic bone. When the external iliac arteries were used, they were

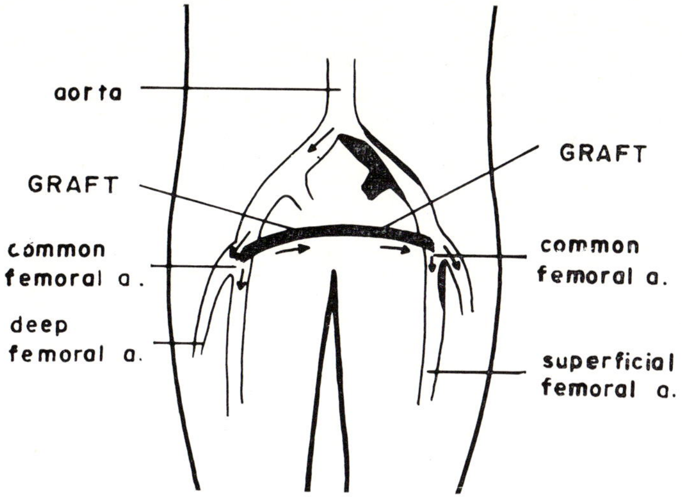

Fig. 1. Drawing of crossover graft from right to left femoral artery anterior to the pubic bone.

approached extraperitoneally. The anastomoses were done with 4-0 arterial silk.

RESULTS

The outcome was good, because the end result, namely the saving of the lower limb, was obtained with a minimum of surgical trauma. Of the 20 patients operated upon, 18 obtained immediate relief (Table I). The patency of the grafts was as follows: (1) less than 1 month in 5 patients (25 percent) and (2) over 1 month, up to 28 months in 14 patients (70 percent). One patient (5 percent) was lost to follow-up.

Two patients had homologous saphenous vein grafts and 18 had Dacron grafts (Fig. 2).

The patient with a graft patency of 28 months (Fig. 3) was a 33-year-old policeman with a gunshot wound in the right inguinal region and no arterial pathologic condition distally. A crossed saphenous vein graft was performed because of severe infection and massive hemorrhage of the right femoral artery.

Of the 20 patients, 13 are alive (65 percent) and 6 are dead (30 percent). In one the follow-up was lost. Five patients had auricular fibrillation, and three died of cerebral emboli (see Table I).

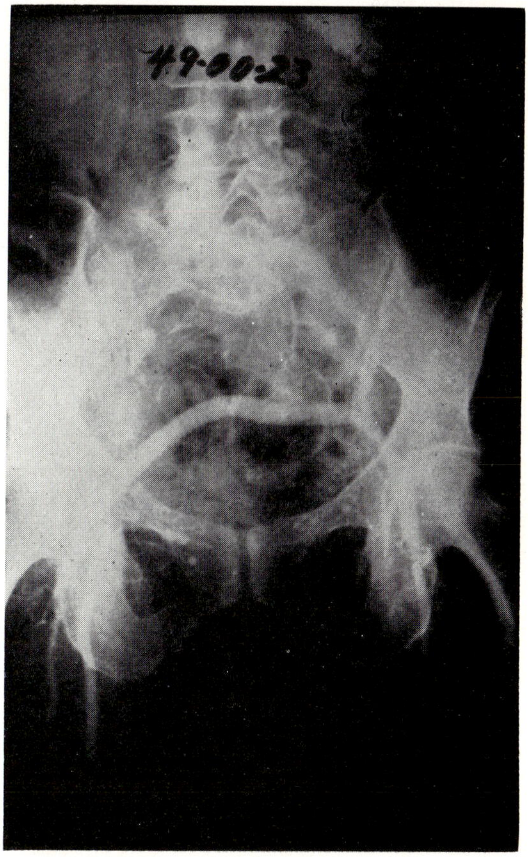

Fig. 2. Graft from left external iliac to right femoral artery.

Table I. *Contralateral arterial grafts*

	Name	*Age*	*Sex*	*Other diseases*	*Diagnosis*
1	G. S. J.	70	F	1. Cardioangiosclerosis 2. High blood pressure 3. Pulmonary emphysema 4. Auricular fibrillation 5. Arterial insufficiency of lower extremities	Right iliac artery obstruction (5/13/66)
2	M. M. F.	30	M	1. Gunshot wound infected right inguinal region	Inguinal and femoral skin infection, femoral artery infected and bleeding (9/19/66)
3	T. L. E.	60	F	1. Cardioangiosclerosis 2. Auricular fibrillation 3. Diabetes mellitus 4. Renal disease 5. Pulmonary emphysema 6. Arterial insufficiency of lower extremities	Right common iliac artery obstruction (8/21/66)
4	C. A. A.	56	M	1. Cardioangiosclerosis 2. High blood pressure 3. Pulmonary emphysema 4. Diabetes mellitus 5. Arterial insufficiency of lower extremities	Right common iliac artery obstruction (4/20/67)
5	L. G.	73	M	1. Cardioangiosclerosis 2. Pulmonary emphysema 3. Arterial insufficiency of lower extremities	Total right iliac and partial left iliac artery obstruction (4/13/67)
6	N. N. N.	70	F	1. Cardioangiosclerosis 2. Auricular fibrillation 3. Pulmonary emphysema 4. Obesity 5. Arterial insufficiency of lower extremities	Right iliac artery obstruction (12/24/67)
7	L. R. H.	66	F	1. Cardioangiosclerosis 2. Auricular fibrillation 3. Pulmonary emphysema 4. Diabetes mellitus 5. Obesity 6. Arterial insufficiency of lower extremities	Left iliac artery obstruction (11/4/66)
8	P. H. R.	65	M	1. Cardioangiosclerosis 2. Pulmonary emphysema 3. Obesity 4. Arterial insufficiency of lower extremities	Left iliac artery obstruction (2/25/67)
9	L. L. B.	76	M	1. Cardioangiosclerosis 2. High blood pressure 3. Pulmonary emphysema 4. Arterial insufficiency of lower extremities	Both iliac arteries obstructed (5/18/67)
10	G. L. M.	60	M	1. Cardioangiosclerosis 2. Pulmonary emphysema 3. Diabetes mellitus 4. Arterial insufficiency of lower extremities	Right iliac artery obstruction (10/11/67)

Surgery	Anes-thesia	Graft	Post-operative x-rays	Patency	Evolution
Left external iliac to right femoral (5/15/66)	Block	Dacron	5/23/66	6 mo. Nov., 1966	Death of cerebral embolus 6 months postoperatively
Left external iliac to middle third of superficial femoral artery, right common iliac artery ligation (9/22/66)	General	Vein	No	28 mo. Jan., 1969	Well
Left external iliac to right common femoral artery (8/23/66)	General	Dacron	9/5/66	28 mo. Jan., 1969	Well
Left external iliac artery to right femoral (4/25/67)	General	Dacron	4/29/67	Lost follow-up	
Laparotomy 4/15/67, right axillary to right femoral and crossed right femoral to left femoral artery (4/16/67)	General	Dacron	No	24 hr.	Death of acute renal insufficiency and probable myocardial infarction
Left iliac artery to right femoral (12/25/65)	Block	Dacron	No	2 weeks	Death of cerebral embolus 1/7/66
Right external iliac to left femoral (11/8/66)	General	Vein	11/24/66	17 days	Death 11/25/66 of myocardial infarction
Right iliac to left femoral (2/27/67)	Block	Dacron	3/7/67	23 mo. Jan., 1969	Well
Left axillary to left femoral and crossed graft left femoral to right femoral (5/22/67)	General	Dacron	6/15/67	20 mo. Jan., 1969	Well
Left iliac to right femoral (10/13/67)	General	Dacron	No	15 mo. Jan., 1969	Well, excellent right pedal pulse

Continued on following page.

Table I—*Cont'd*

	Name	*Age*	*Sex*	*Other diseases*	*Diagnosis*
11	P. V. J.	56	M	1. Two myocardial infarcts in 1962 2. Pulmonary emphysema 3. Arterial insufficiency of lower extremities	Left iliac and left superficial femoral obstruction down middle third (6/8/67)
12	L. R.	62	M	1. Cardioangiosclerosis 2. In 1962 aorto bilateral iliac graft	Obstruction of right limb of aortic graft and aneurysm of left iliac artery at the anastomosis (10/16/67)
13	B. L. E.	68	M	1. Cardioangiosclerosis 2. Pulmonary emphysema 3. Diabetes mellitus 4. Obesity 5. Arterial insufficiency of lower extremities	Obstruction of terminal aorta (8/15/67)
14	R. L. D.	62	M	1. Cardioangiosclerosis 2. High blood pressure 3. Diabetes mellitus 4. Arterial insufficiency of lower extremities	Right iliac artery obstruction (9/3/67)
15	M. A. I.	69	M	1. Cardioangiosclerosis 2. Diabetes mellitus 3. Arterial insufficiency of lower extremities	1. Right iliac artery obstruction 2. Gangrene of right fourth toe 3. Complete obstruction of right popliteal artery
16	S. S. L.	66	F	1. Myocardial infarct, August, 1967 2. Obesity 3. Arterial insufficiency of lower extremities	Terminal aorta obstruction (1/25/68)
17	M. C. F.	55	M	1. Cardioangiosclerosis 2. Arterial insufficiency of lower extremities	Left iliac artery obstruction (9/1/68)
18	O. G. G.	58	F	1. Rheumatic heart disease 2. Auricular fibrillation 3. Repeated emboli to lower extremities 4. Arterial insufficiency of lower extremities	Left iliac artery obstruction (9/1/68)
19	S. S. L.	60	M	1. Cardioangiosclerosis 2. Pulmonary emphysema 3. Arterial insufficiency of lower extremities	Left iliac artery obstruction, left superficial artery obstruction of middle third (9/15/68)
20	M. F. J. R.	59	M	1. Cardioangiosclerosis 2. Malnutrition 3. Arterial insufficiency of lower extremities	Total obstruction of right iliac artery, partial obstruction of left iliac artery (6/4/68)

Surgery	*Anes-thesia*	*Graft*	*Post-operative x-rays*	*Patency*	*Evolution*
Right external iliac to lower third of left superficial femoral artery (6/10/67)	Block	Dacron	8/1/67	19 mo. Jan., 1969	Well
Aneurysm resected, left external iliac to right femoral (10/21/67)	Block	Dacron	No	27 mo. Jan., 1969	Well
1. Right axillary to right femoral 2. Right femoral to left femoral	General	Dacron	No	Clotted after 12 hr.	Death 7 days postoperatively of gastrointestinal bleeding 8/25/67
Left iliac to right femoral (9/5/67)	Block	Dacron	No	16 mo. Jan., 1969	Well
1. Left external iliac to right femoral 2. Bilateral sympathectomy 3. Fourth right toe amputation (12/2/67) 4. Above-knee amputation (gangrene of right foot and leg) (12/23/67)	General	Dacron	No	13 mo. Jan., 1969	Stump healed well, graft pulsating
Right axillary femoral bypass and femoral to femoral crossover graft (2/5/68)	General	Dacron	2/27/68	13 mo. Jan., 1969	Well
Right femoral to left femoral artery (9/6/68)	General	Dacron	No	4 mo. Jan., 1969	Well
Right femoral to left femoral artery (9/2/68)	General	Dacron	No	Oct., 1968	Death of cerebral embolus 10/1/68, one month post-operatively
Right iliac to left femoral artery (9/20/68)	General	Dacron	9/24/68	3 mo. Jan., 1969	Graft pulsating well
Right axillary to femoral artery and crossed right femoral to left femoral artery (6/7/68)	General	Dacron	7/7/68	7 mo. Jan., 1969	Well

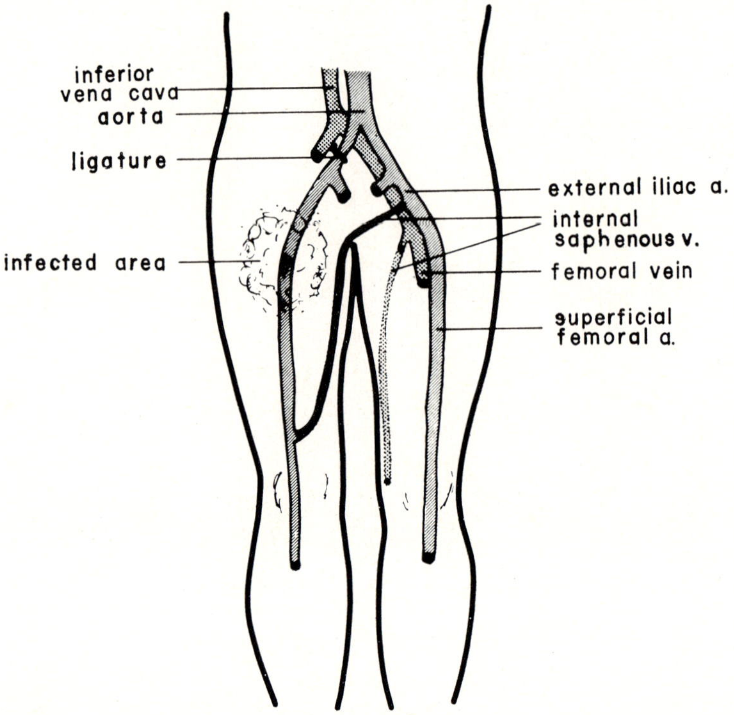

Fig. 3. Infected right femoral area. Crossed graft (vein), from left external iliac artery to lower one third of right superficial femoral artery.

In Patient 1 (Table I), the crossed graft was patent for 6 months until the day she had a cerebrovascular accident which caused her death. This accident was due to an embolus from the fibrillating heart. Although they were on anticoagulant therapy, Patients 6 and 18 in auricular fibrillation died as a result of cerebral emboli 2 weeks after operation.

Patient 5 died 24 hours postoperatively with acute renal insufficiency and probably with a myocardial infarction. This last patient underwent an important surgical stress that was due to two surgical interventions in less than 48 hours. In the first procedure a transperitoneal laparotomy was performed; nothing could be done because of severe atherosclerotic disease of the aortic and iliac arteries. In the second intervention 24 hours later, an "axillary-femoral" and a femoral-to-femoral bypass was placed, which worked well. The two operations, however, led to the patient's death (Fig. 4).

Patient 7, in auricular fibrillation, with two previous cerebrovascular accidents, died from a myocardial infarction 17 days later. The day before the patient died, an aortography was done, demonstrating the permeability of the crossed-vein graft.

Patient 13 died 7 days postoperatively of massive gastrointestinal bleeding.

In Patient 15, the crossover graft was patent 7 months postoperatively, but because of a poor arterial bed distal to the obstructed popliteal artery, an above-knee amputation had to be done 3 weeks later.

In Patients 2 and 11, the crossed grafts were placed from the external iliac artery to the lower third of the contralateral superficial femoral artery. In Patient 2, there was infection of the subcutaneous tissues as well as infection and bleeding of the femoral artery at the upper third of the right thigh (Fig. 3). In Patient 11, the obstruction of the superficial femoral artery was at its middle third, with fairly normal distal arteries. In both cases we obtained good distal pulses.

All these patients, with one exception (M.

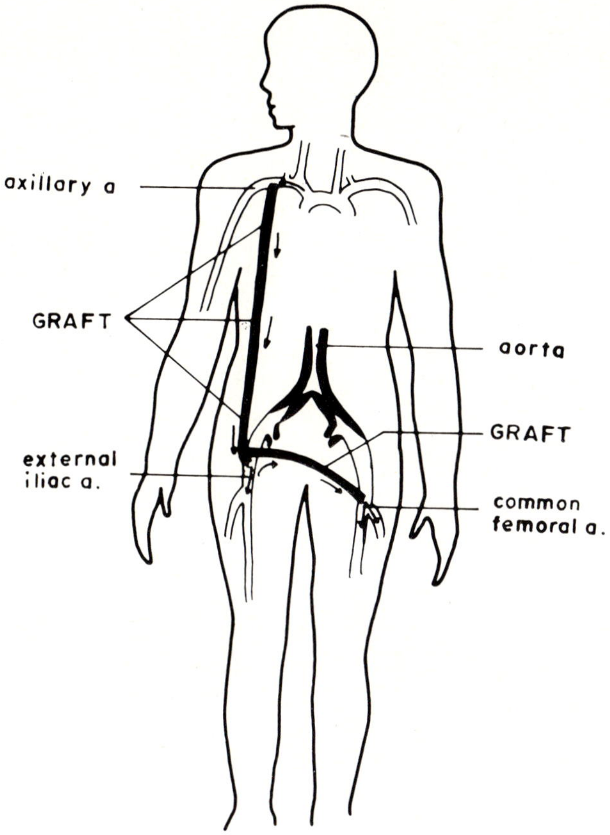

Fig. 4. Drawing which shows axillar-femoral graft and a crossover graft from the right femoral to the left femoral artery.

M. F., 33 years old), were more than 56 years of age, and five more than 70. This is important, because all of them had other illnesses: pulmonary emphysema, hypertensive and arteriosclerotic cardiac disease, renal disease, auricular fibrillation, diabetes mellitus. These added conditions increased even further the surgical risk in patients that required surgery, especially major surgery performed on the aorta and its branches.

The postoperative period was not stormy, as is usual in the patients operated transperitoneally, where the handling of abdominal viscera requires the use of postoperative nasogastric tube, intravenous fluids, laboratory tests, and bed rest for a minimum of 3 days.

With this procedure, the patient may get up from bed the same day of the operation and may have food by mouth. If his general condition improves, he may leave the hospital in a much shorter time than the patients operated upon transperitoneally.

After the crossed graft is placed, there is an increase of the blood flow through the deep femoral artery. Since in most of the cases the superficial femoral artery has a partial or a total obstruction, the deep femoral artery is almost always free of disease. This procedure improves the condition of the entire limb increasing the blood flow through the large and small collaterals.[10] At a later date and if the general condition of the patient has improved, a femoropopliteal graft may be placed.

CONCLUSIONS

Every elderly patient in poor general condition with obstruction of one iliac artery, in whom a laparotomy implies a greater risk,

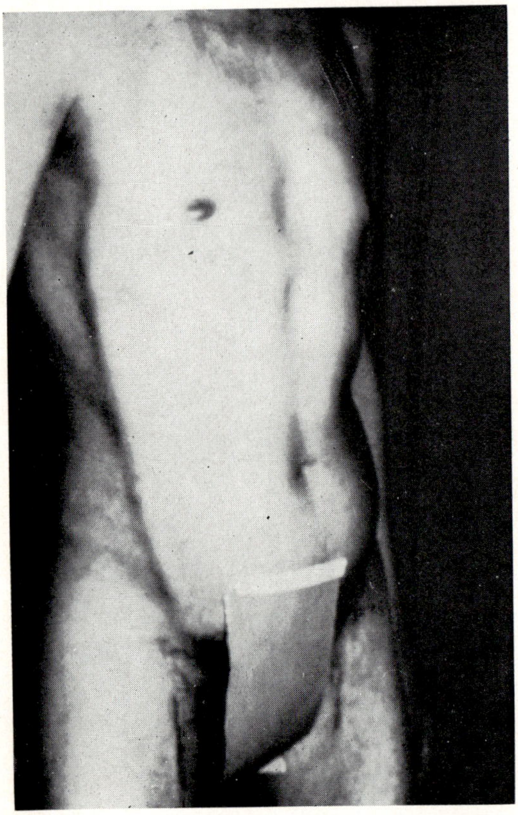

Fig. 5. Patient No. 20 with right axillary-femoral graft.

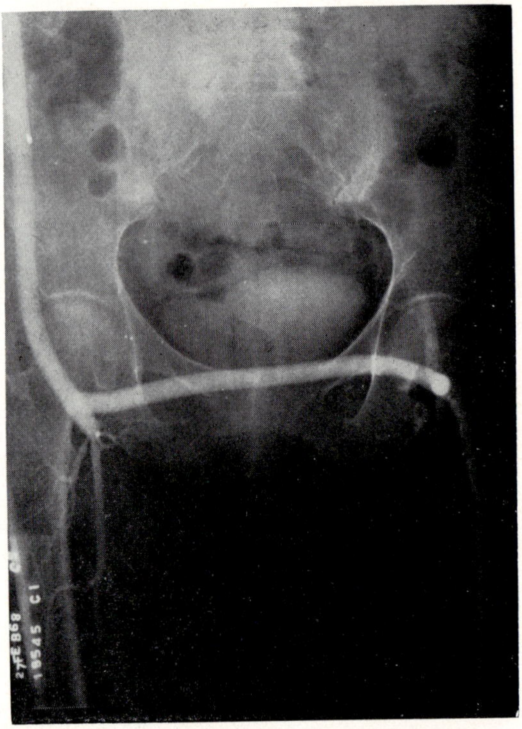

Fig. 6. Axillary-femoral and femorofemoral Dacron graft.

should have a crossed graft going from one unobstructed iliac artery or common femoral artery to the contralateral femoral artery. In case of complete obstruction of the terminal aorta[2, 4, 6-8, 12, 13, 15] or infected aortofemoral bypass,[3, 14] an "axillary-femoral" graft should be placed followed by contralateral femorofemoral graft (see Figs. 4 to 6).

In case of infection,[1] the crossed graft should be placed far away from the infected area (Fig. 3).

Even though this procedure is not new, it is certain that it has not been used frequently enough and for this reason we propose that this surgical method be kept in mind.

SUMMARY

In the Centro Hospitalario 20 de Noviembre, 20 patients have been operated upon, 7 of whom were female and 13 male. Their ages ranged between 33 and 76 years, with an average of 61 years.

All patients had clinical and angiographic studies (translumbar aortography) made. Only in 10 was a postoperative aortography done, demonstrating the correct functioning of the grafts.

This paper describes a procedure in which a graft is placed subcutaneously from the common femoral or external iliac artery on one side, crossing anterior to the pubic bone to the contralateral common femoral or external iliac artery without penetrating the peritoneal cavity.

Eighteen of the 20 patients operated upon obtained relief; 14 grafts were patent from 2 weeks to 28 months. Six patients died postoperatively, three of cerebral emboli. Most of these patients were old, with cerebral, cardiac, renal, or endocrine problems. These diseases must be considered a limiting factor in the operative procedure, which has to be performed under superficial general anesthesia, peridural block, or local anesthesia.

It is not necessary to open the abdominal cavity because these vessels are located in the retroperitoneum (external iliac artery) or subcutaneously in the femoral area (femoral artery). The postoperative period is not stormy; on the contrary, the patient may have his meals by mouth and get up the same day of the operation.

REFERENCES

1. Bialostozky, K. L., Blanco, C. M., Rodríguez, S. J., and Cedeño, M. A.: Injerto vascular femoral contralateral en arteritis aguda postraumática, Rev. Méd. ISSSTE, México **2:** 159, 1967.
2. Bialostozky, K. L., Blanco, C. M., and Cedeño, M. A.: Injerto "axilar-femoral," Arch. Inst. Cardiol Méx. **38:** 560, 1968.
3. Blaisdell, F. W., DeMattei, G. A., and Gauder, P. J.: Extraperitoneal thoracic aorta to femoral bypass graft as a replacement for infected aortic bifurcation prosthesis, Amer. J. Surg. **102:** 583, 1961.
4. Blaisdell, F. W., and Hall, A. D.: Axillary-femoral artery bypass for lower extremity ischemia, SURGERY **54:** 563, 1963.
5. Chavez, C. M., Hardy, J. D., and Tucker, F. H.: Cross-leg bypass, Arch. Surg. (Chicago) **94:** 357, 1967.
6. Lewis, C. D.: A subclavian artery as a means of blood supply to the lower half of the body, Brit. J. Surg. **48:** 574, 1961.
7. Louw, J. H.: Splenic-to-femoral and axillary-to-femoral bypass grafts in diffuse atherosclerotic occlusive disease, Lancet **2:** 1401, 1963.
8. Louw, J. H.: The treatment of combined aortoiliac and femoropopliteal occlusive disease by splenofemoral and axillofemoral bypass grafts, SURGERY **55:** 387, 1964.
9. McCaughan, J. J., Jr., and Kahn, S. F.: Crossover graft for unilateral occlusive disease of the iliofemoral arteries, Ann. Surg. **151:** 26, 1960.
10. Morris, G. C., Jr., Edwards, W., Cooley, D. A., Crawford, E. S., and De Bakey, M. E.: Surgical importance of profunda femoris artery, Arch. Surg. (Chicago) **82:** 32, 1961.
11. Papadopoules, C. D.: Cross-leg femorofemoral bypass, Amer. J. Surg. **111:** 216, 1966.
12. Pierangeli, A., and Guernelli, N.: The axillofemoral bypass as a treatment of the obstruction of the aorto-iliac junction in the poor-risk patients, J. Cardiov. Surg. **8:** 353, 1967.
13. Sauvage, L. R., and Wood, S. J.: Unilateral axillary bilateral femoral bifurcation graft: A procedure for the poor risk patient with aortoiliac disease, SURGERY **60:** 573, 1966.
14. Shaw, R. S., and Baue, A. E.: Management of sepsis complicating arterial reconstructive surgery, SURGERY **53:** 75, 1963.
15. Vetto, R. M.: The treatment of unilateral iliac artery obstruction with a transabdominal, subcutaneous, femorofemoral graft, SURGERY **52:** 342, 1962.
16. Warren, R.: Bypass arterial graft between splenic and iliofemoral arteries, Arch. Surg. (Chicago) **72:** 57, 1956.
17. Wertheimer, P.: Les derivation arterielles contralaterales, Lyon Chir. **59:** 350, 1963.

Arteriovenous vein graft for chronic hemodialysis: A preliminary report

MARK MOZES, M.D., F.A.C.S.
BARUCH J. HURWICH, M.D.
RAPHAEL ADAR, M.D.
HESKEL E. ELIAHOU, B.A., M.D.
HARRY BOGOKOWSKY, M.D.
TEL AVIV, ISRAEL
From the Department of General and Vascular Surgery and the Department of Nephrology, Tel-Hashomer Government Hospital and Tel Aviv University Medical School

The surgically created radial arteriovenous fistula introduced in 1966 by Brescia and associates[1] has been accepted over the Teflon-Silastic external arteriovenous shunt[5] in a large number of dialysis centers around the world.[2-4, 6] It has survived for longer periods of time with fewer complications and is preferred by patients and staff.

The arteriovenous fistula (AVF) has usually been created above the wrist without much difficulty, but some failures occur. These are due to absence of a vein of adequate caliber in the vicinity of the arteries in the wrist, or to thrombosis of the major forearm veins because of prior phlebitis or as a complication of multiple venipunctures. The female patient with small veins poses a special problem, for even if a fistula can be created the veins may be too small for successful dialysis by venipuncture and may eventually thrombose.

A new technique has been devised for AVF failures that are due to inadequate forearm veins. A saphenous vein autograft serves to bridge the gap between the radial or ulnar artery at the wrist and a large vein just below the antecubital skin crease.

Supported by the Jeanne Goetzel Foundation.
Received for publication April 7, 1969.

SURGICAL TECHNIQUE

The axilla, forearm, groin, and thigh are prepared for operation. Axillary nerve block is induced and, if necessary, the local tissues about the wrist are infiltrated with 1 percent Novocain. The radial (or ulnar) artery is exposed at the wrist in the usual manner. Assuming that there is no suitable vein available for creation of the simple AVF, the skin of the groin and thigh is also anesthetized. A 25 to 30 cm. segment of the long saphenous vein, from the saphenofemoral junction distally, is removed through two or three separate small incisions, in the same manner as the saphenous vein is procured for femoropopliteal grafting in the leg. A transverse incision in the upper forearm, just below the antecubital skin crease, exposes one of the large veins in this area, and a subcutaneous tunnel connecting the two forearm incisions is made by means of a long blunt instrument introduced from above and below. Aqueous heparin, 5,000 units, may be given intravenously at this point. The vein graft is interposed between the artery above the wrist and the antecubital vein by means of end-to-side anastomoses with 6-0 silk. On removing the clamps from the artery and the slings from the vein, a palpable pulsation is felt over the graft and a bruit is heard over the length of

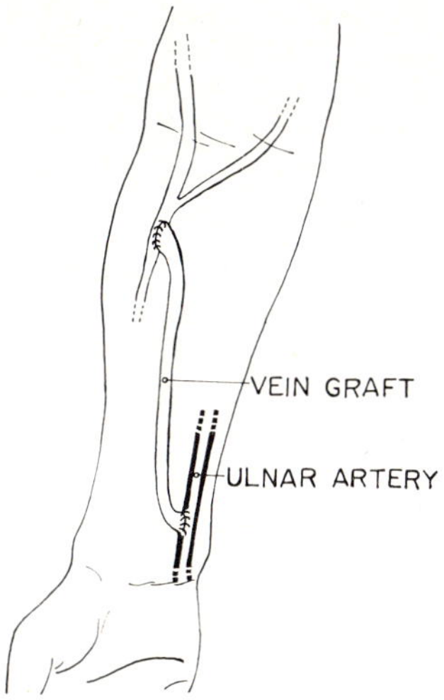

Fig. 1. The arteriovenous vein graft fistula (artist's drawing).

the graft and the anastomoses. The completed procedure is illustrated in Fig. 1, and brachial angiography is presented in Fig. 2.

PRELIMINARY RESULTS

We have created two arteriovenous vein graft fistulas in female patients in each of whom there had been two unsuccessful attempts to create a radial AVF. The graft fistulas are now a month old, and both are used for intermittent hemodialysis by venipuncture technique.

COMMENT

Despite a relatively short follow-up period, some advantages are already apparent. Technically, the anastomoses are easier to perform because of the better caliber and substance of the saphenous vein. So far we have not encountered any swelling of the hand or unsightly tortuosity of the veins of hand or forearm. Both of these phenomena were frequent sequelae of the regular AVF, and proved quite bothersome to the patient.

Final evaluation depends on a longer follow-up period. At present, we recommend this procedure for patients in whom the conventional AVF cannot be constructed or has failed.

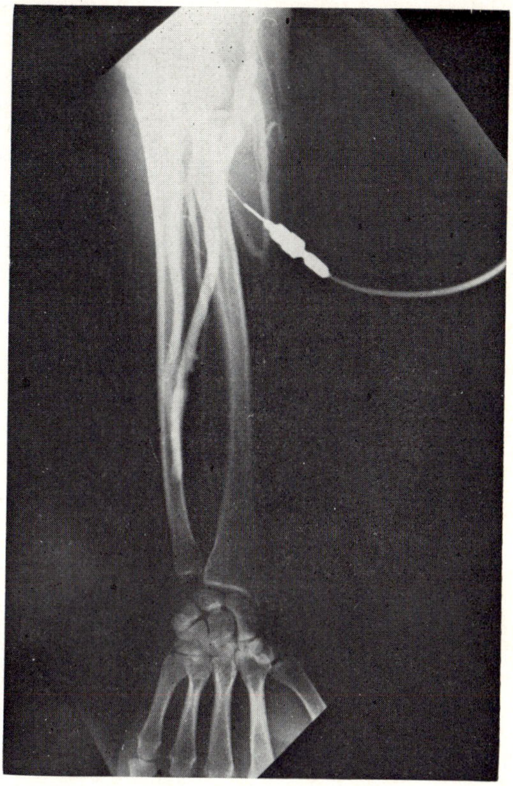

Fig. 2. Brachial angiography illustrating function of the AVF graft.

SUMMARY

A new method is described for creating an arteriovenous fistula for use in hemodialysis by venipuncture technique in patients who have proved unsuitable for creation of the usual AVF.

A segment of long saphenous vein is inserted as a bridge between an artery at the wrist and a vein below the antecubital skin crease. The 25 to 30 cm. vein graft may serve as a site for venipuncture in patients who have no other suitable veins for hemodialysis.

Two such graft arteriovenous fistulas have been created in female patients in whom previous attempts to create the standard AVF had failed.

REFERENCES

1. Brescia, M. J., Cimino, J. E., Appel, K., and Hurwich, B. J.: Chronic hemodialysis using venipuncture and a surgically created arterio-

venous fistula, New England J. Med. **275:** 1089, 1966.

2. Cohen, S., Lidsky, I., Kest, L., Kastagir, B., and Vertes, V.: Experiences with arteriovenous fistulas, Tr. Am. Soc. Artif. Int. Organs **14:** 421, 1968.
3. Hanson, J. S., Carmody, M., Keogh, B., and O'Dwyer, W. F.: Access to circulation by permanent arteriovenous fistula in regular dialysis treatment, Brit. M. J. **4:** 586, 1967.
4. Menno, A. D., Zizzi, J., Hodson, J., and McMahon, J.: An evaluation of the radial arteriovenous fistula as a substitute for the Quinton shunt in chronic hemodialysis, Tr. Am. Soc. Artif. Int. Organs **13:** 62, 1967.
5. Quinton, W. E., Dillard, D., and Scribner, B. H.: Cannulation of blood vessels for prolonged hemodialysis, Tr. Am. Soc. Artif. Int. Organs **6:** 104, 1960.
6. Salomon, J., Vidne, B., Robson, M., Rosenfeld, J., and Levy, M. J.: Our experiences with the use of arteriovenous fistula in chronic dialysis: Modified surgical technique, SURGERY **63:** 899, 1968.

Long-term arterial catheterization for repeated blood sampling

ROGER V. MOSELEY, M.D.
DONALD B. DOTY, M.D.
WASHINGTON, D. C.
From the Division of Surgery,
Walter Reed Army Institute of Research,
Walter Reed Army Medical Center

Important guides for the care of critically ill patients are found in the study of arterial blood. Physical examination and clinical judgment alone are unequal to the challenge of adapting modern technology to the resuscitation of the severely injured patient. Optimal adjustment of a respirator, for example, may require determination of gas tension and pH of arterial blood several times an hour during critical phases, and periodically for several weeks during a stormy convalescence. When measurement of cardiac output by dye-dilution technique is needed, continuous sampling of arterial blood is essential.

The techniques for obtaining arterial blood samples currently in use have several shortcomings. Repeated arterial punctures are uncomfortable to patients as well as potentially injurious to the artery. In addition, the possibility of arteriovenous puncture with admixture of venous blood may produce a significant, unrecognized source of error.[1] It is the usual experience that an indwelling catheter rarely remains open for more than 2 or 3 days, and catheter irrigation inevitably produces embolization of clot. A skin incision with attendant septic risk is often used to ensure accurate catheter placement. When used in measurement of cardiac output, a distally placed radial artery catheter may produce unreliable results that are due to uneven dye dilution in a vessel virtually occluded by the catheter.

In the care and study of battle casualties in Vietnam, a combination of familiar techniques was used to provide a convenient percutaneous catheterization method by which repeated arterial samples for both gas study and cardiac output measurement could be safely and painlessly obtained over periods of up to 2 weeks. The femoral artery was the preferred site because of its large diameter, superficial location, and relative proximity to the heart, which made the catheter suitable for cardiac output measurement as well as routine blood sampling. In patients with injury to a lower extremity, the brachial artery was used with good results.

METHOD

A Longdwel* Teflon catheter and obturator is placed in the femoral artery by percutaneous (Seldinger[2]) catheter technique. The skin is shaved and aseptically prepared. Local anesthesia is used to produce a small skin weal approximately one-half inch distal to the site of expected arterial puncture and to produce periarterial anesthesia, and then a 2 mm. skin incision is made with a No. 11 blade. An 18 gauge Cournand needle is inserted and the artery punctured at an angle of approximately 75 degrees to the skin, pointing toward the patient's head. When free flow of blood is obtained, a flexible tip guide wire, previously cut to a length of approximately 15 inches, is inserted through the needle. The needle is removed, and the

Received for publication March 24, 1969.

*Becton, Dickinson & Co., Rutherford, N. J.

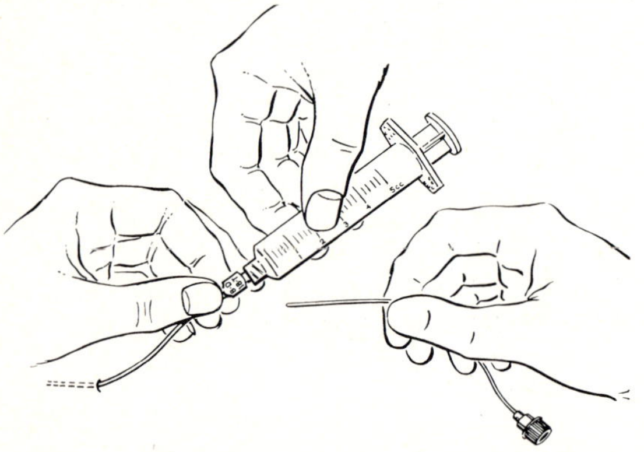

Fig. 1. The technique of obtaining repeated blood samples from an indwelling arterial catheter is shown. The operator steadies the catheter with his left hand and holds the obturator ready for reinsertion in his sterile-gloved right hand. The assistant withdraws the blood sample.

6 inch, 18 gauge Teflon catheter is advanced into the arterial lumen over the guide wire. Once in satisfactory position, the catheter tip will be located in the iliac artery approximately 3 inches distal to the aortic bifurcation. The guide wire is then removed and the Teflon obturator inserted to occlude the catheter. A small dressing is placed and the hub of the catheter securely taped to the skin. The obturator has a screw lock so there is no danger of it being extruded, and, since it protrudes slightly beyond the end of the catheter, blood cannot clot inside or at the tip of the catheter. Whenever blood samples are required, the obturator is removed and blood withdrawn. This is best done by two people, one of whom aseptically removes the obturator with a sterile-gloved hand and then easily slides it back in place after the assistant has drawn the sample (Fig. 1).

RESULTS

This method was successfully used in 70 combat casualties. Samples have been obtained and cardiac output measured through the same catheter for periods of up to 2 weeks. There were no significant technical difficulties or complications; local infection was not a problem, nor were there any changes in the distal arterial circulation. Patients were able to move freely and without discomfort both in and out of bed. Free flow of blood was nearly always seen when the obturator was removed, and only occasionally did the catheter have to be flushed with saline. Twice when shorter catheters were used, and once when the catheter was inadequately fixed to the skin, it was dislodged from the artery, but there was no resultant hemorrhage. One patient died of wounds after having a catheter in place for 10 days. At postmortem examination, there was a 1 by 2 mm. strand of soft fibrin near the tip of the obturator, but apart from this, there was no evidence of other thrombus around the catheter or of any reaction on the intima of the artery.

When an indwelling catheter was no longer needed, it was simply withdrawn and digital pressure applied to the puncture site for 10 minutes. Suture repair was never necessary as hemostasis was easily obtained when pressure was properly applied.

SUMMARY

A method of arterial catheterization is described which allows repeated sampling of arterial blood. It is well tolerated by patients and has the advantages of simplicity, reliability, and freedom from significant complications.

REFERENCES

1. Doty, D. B., and Moseley, R. V.: Reliable sampling of arterial blood, Surg. Gynec. & Obst. To be published.
2. Seldinger, S. I.: Catheter replacement of needle in percutaneous arteriography; new technique, Acta radiol. **39:** 368, 1953.

Catheter embolism

EMIL BLAIR, M.D.*
ROBERT HUNZIKER, M.D.
MARTIN E. FLANAGAN, M.D.
BURLINGTON, VT.
From the Departments of Surgery (Thoracic and Neurologic) and Radiology, The University of Vermont College of Medicine and the Medical Center Hospital

In recent years there has been an increasing number of reports of complications from intravascular plastic catheters.[2, 7, 8] Most of these have dealt with such problems as sepsis, but attention has been drawn more and more to embolization. The loss of a fragment of a plastic catheter evinces a great deal of anxiety because of the potential problem of thrombosis, perforation, or endocarditis. As a consequence, immediate removal is advised.[2] Recently a patient has been observed who, because of her condition, experienced a delay in removal of an embolized catheter. Daily x-rays of the chest permitted a sequential observation of the course of the catheter fragment which had extended through the superior vena cava, right atrium, right ventricle, and out the pulmonary artery.

CASE REPORT

F. L. B., a 17-year-old Caucasian girl, was involved in an automobile accident. Upon being brought to a local hospital, she appeared to be in shock and was deeply comatose with the left pupil dilated and fixed. In addition, she was found to have suffered a dislocation of the right elbow and was bleeding from a laceration of the face and from the vagina. There were multiple fractures of the pelvis. Following emergency resuscitation procedures including blood transfusion, the heart rate and blood pressure improved and became stabilized. It was apparent at this time that she had a left hemiplegia and that she had suffered intracerebral contusion and brainstem injury.

Four days after the accident the patient was transferred to the Neurosurgical Service of the Mary Fletcher Unit. At this time, the patient was semicomatose but responded to painful stimuli. Blood pressure was 130/90. A central venous pressure (CVP) catheter was inserted via an antecubital vein for monitoring. Neurologic examination at this time revealed continued left hemiparesis with withdrawal. There was a positive Babinski sign although she moved all extremities. She was started on Chloromycetin and Decadron, and also on hypothermia. A bilateral carotid angiogram revealed complete occlusion of the right internal carotid artery with excellent filling of the right middle cerebral artery from the left side. There was marked general swelling of the right cerebral hemisphere. It was confirmed that the patient was pregnant and threatening to abort. Orthopedic consultation resulted in the decision to wait until her condition improved before doing any reparative procedures on the dislocated right elbow.

A chest x-ray on the twentieth day revealed the CVP catheter lying in the superior vena cava. The catheter coiled through the right atrium into the right ventricle and out of the pulmonary artery so that the distal end was lying peripherally in the right lung field. Inquiry failed to reveal the cause of the catheter embolism. There was no evidence of parenchymal changes such as infarction. Successive films revealed changes in catheter position (Fig. 1). X-ray on the twenty-seventh day showed the catheter to be almost entirely in the pulmonary artery. Because of the patient's condition, attempts at removal of the catheter were delayed. The next day the catheter was found

Supported in part by United States Public Health Service Grant No. 11493.

Received for publication April 7, 1969.

*Present address: Department of Surgery, University of Colorado School of Medicine, 4200 East 9th Ave., Denver, Colo. 80220.

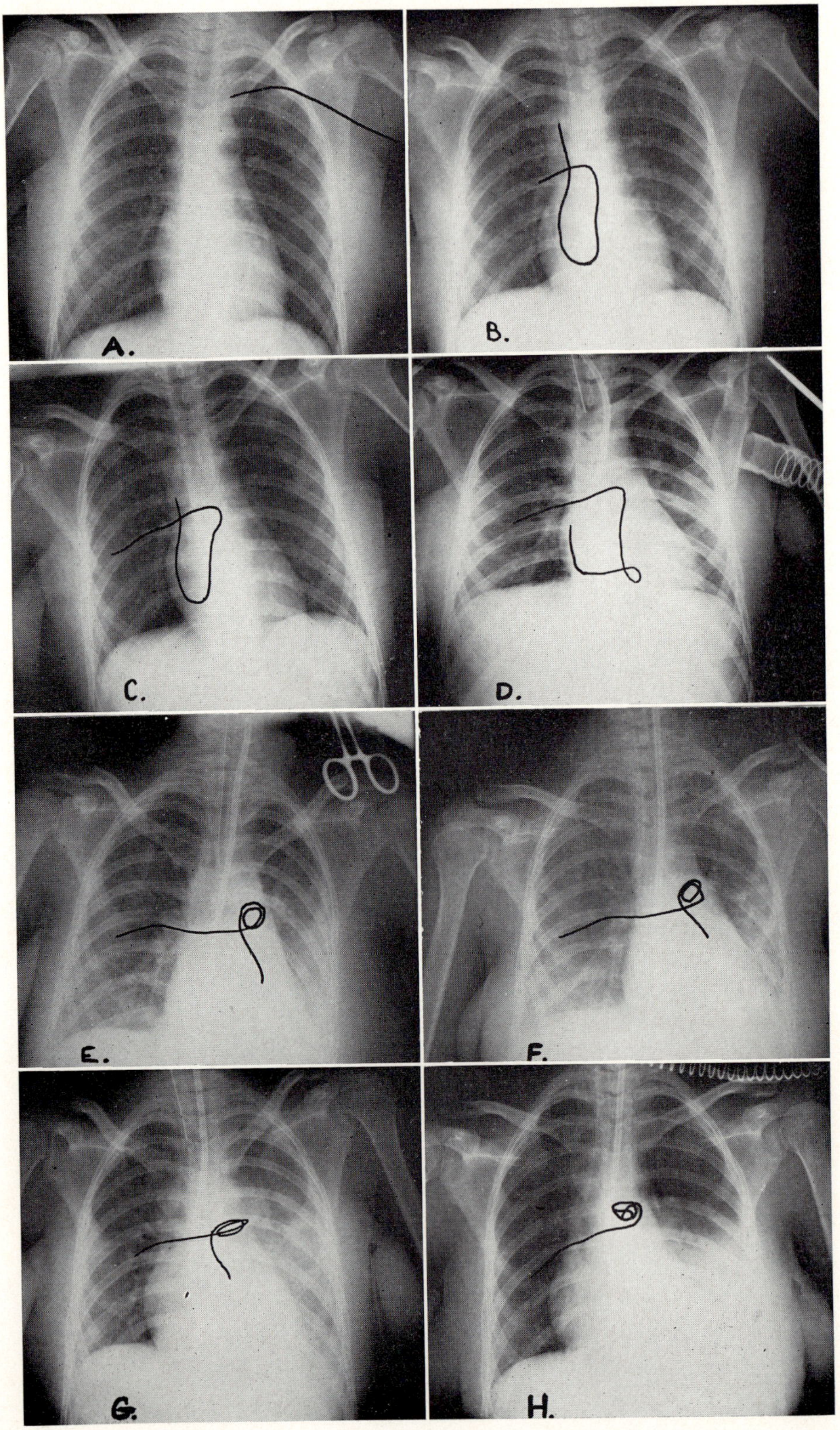

Fig. 1. *A,* CVP catheter inserted via antecubital vein. *B-H,* Catheter fragment positions 2 to 8 days.

coiled in the main pulmonary artery with the distal limb in the right branch. Fear of thrombus formation prompted the decision to operate. This was the eighth postembolus (twenty-eighth hospital) day. At operation, heart movements appeared vigorous and normal. Palpation of the pulmonary artery revealed several loops of the catheter in the main artery. The anterior surface of the artery was compressed between the forefinger and the thumb with the catheter between the fingers. The catheter was then pressed to the surface of the artery and grasped with a Babcock clamp. An incision 1 cm. in length was made directly over the palpated catheter. The catheter immediately popped into the incision, and was picked up and removed. The length of the catheter was approximately 37 cm. This was an Intracath commercial type. The patient withstood the thoracotomy satisfactorily. There was no evidence of thromboembolism from the catheter or other complications 1 year later.

DISCUSSION

While the apparent first report in the human of embolization of a fragment of intravenous polyethylene catheter was reported by Turner and Sommers[7] in 1954, Tuell and co-workers[6] noted such an incident in a dog in 1948. Most published reports deal with a single or several cases, with two recent reviews.[2, 8] In order to develop information relative to the problem, to its management, and to the outcome, these cases were reviewed again, as well as several others. Pertinent data were extracted and appear in Table I. The most common entry site was a vein in the arm, usually the antecubital (80 percent). The next most common was a leg vein (12 percent). The site of lodgment of the catheter fragment proved somewhat variable. As might be anticipated, in approximately 30 percent the fragment was in the superior vena cava, inferior vena cava, right ventricle, right atrium, or trailed through two of these chambers. The next most common site was an arm vein (26 percent), followed by pulmonary artery (18 percent). It is of interest that in at least 11 percent of the reported patients, the site of lodgment was never defined.

The mechanism for loss of the catheter was noted in only 33 of 61 cases, being unknown in a disconcerting 46 percent of this collected series of 61 patients. The most common was severance of the catheter by the needle through which the catheter had been passed (52 percent). The next most common was a spontaneous break in the catheter (27 percent) and finally detachment of the catheter fragment from the cannula or adapter (21 percent). Two predominant factors were noted with respect to the mechanism. One was undue or careless catheter manipulation by the nurse or the physician. The second was excessive movement of the patient. It is apparent from the collected data that a definitive correlation exists between the entry site and the mechanism involved. The antecubital vein proved notorious for being the worst possible place of intravascular cannulation because of excessive movement at the elbow.

Complications are noted in Table II. Information was available in 57 patients. In 44, or 77 percent, there was none. Atrial fibrillation occurred in one patient with death, thromboses in five with two deaths,

Table I. *Catheter emboli*

Entry site	*No.*	*%*	*Lodge site*	*No.*	*%*	*Mechanism*	*No.*	*%*
Arm vein	49	80	Arm vein	16	26	Needle cut	17	52
Leg vein	7	12	SVC, IVC, RA*	18	30	Spontaneous break	9	27
Neck vein	3	5	RA, RV*	6	10	Detachment	7	21
Miscellaneous	2	3	PA*	11	18	Total	33	100
Total	61	100	Miscellaneous†	3	5	"Disappeared"	28	46
			Unknown	7	11			
			Total	61	100			

*Single chamber or combined. SVC = superior vena cava; IVC = inferior vena cava; RA = right atrium; RV = right ventricle; PA = pulmonary artery.

†Subclavian vein; saphenous vein; iliac artery.

perforation in two with two deaths, and endocarditis in five with two deaths, and in two patients the problem was unspecified. Recovery or follow-up was recorded in 47 of 61 patients. The fragment of the catheter was retrieved in 31 patients or 52 percent and not recovered in 16. These patients survived and had been observed for periods extending up to 1 year with one as long as 6½ years.[4] There was a total of 14 deaths in the group of which seven were considered to have been due primarily to the catheter embolus or in which the embolus was a principal factor. The time interval was reported in 56 of 61 patients and evaluated (Table III). Catheter retrieval was accomplished in the majority within 24 hours. Of the 35 survivals without complications, 29 were free of the catheter or asymptomatic within 4 weeks. There were three patients with retained catheters in whom there were no symptoms after 1 year. The incidence of complications was spread rather evenly, appearing within 24 hours and extending through 3 months in 10 of 13 patients (Table III). The deaths were related to the approximate period of the complications. Lodgment in the heart proved of particular concern and was the site of most complications, as well as all of the deaths.

There was a great deal of concern on the part of the staff with regard to the delay in extraction of the catheter from the pulmonary artery of our patient. While her condition had not improved particularly at the time of the removal, the ultimate lodgment and curling of the entire fragment in the main pulmonary artery prompted the decision for surgical intervention. On the basis of the review of the literature, it would appear this was wise, since thrombi formed fairly frequently in the pulmonary arterial segment of lodgment of the embolus. At the time of removal, there was no evidence of thrombus, neither locally nor on the basis of pulmonary emboli.

The true incidence of embolization of indwelling plastic catheters is not known, since many probably are not reported.[2, 8] The oft-noted advantages of inert plastic catheters are borne out by the fact that the majority of patients apparently encountered no complications. Nevertheless, this review strikingly demonstrates that there is a sufficiently significant complication rate (23 percent) and, more important, a serious death rate (12 percent of series and over 50 percent of complications) that is due directly to the catheter. The need for critical care of indwelling intravenous catheters is obvious.

Since the principal problem relates to the site of entry at the antecubital vein, it would appear that this is the worst place for im-

Table II. *Catheter emboli—outcome*

Results	*No.*	*%*
Complication		
None	44	77
Atrial fibrillation	1 (1)*	2
Thrombosis	5 (2)	9
Perforation	2 (2)	3
Endocarditis	5 (2)	9
Total	57	100
Survived		
Operation	31	52
Not recovered	16	26
Died		
Primary	7	11
Unrelated	7	11
Total	61	100

*Numbers in parentheses indicate number of deaths.

Table III. *Catheter emboli—time interval*

	Days			*Weeks*	*Months*			
Data	*<1*	*1 - 3*	*5 - 7*	*2 - 4*	*1 - 3*	*4 - 6*	*7 - 12*	*12+*
Survivals	15	2	5	7	2	0	1	3
Complications	0	3	3	2	2	0	1	2
Deaths	0	1	1	1	2	0	0	2
Right heart	1	2	3	5	4	0	2	3

plantation of the indwelling catheter. If for some reason this appears to be necessary, then measures should be taken to fix the arm so that there would not be excessive movement at the elbow. Catheter manipulation and detachment can be avoided easily by the exercise of care in the preparation and in the handling of catheters. Agitation and excessive movement of patients have been noted to be two of the principal factors. It is quite obvious that a disturbed patient cannot be manacled to his bed. Rather a better selection of site of entry and proper fixation of the catheter as well as constant observation and inspection would reduce the incidence of embolic complications to a minimum.

There is uniform opinion that when a catheter fragment embolizes, it should be removed immediately. Most of them, since they occur in veins of the arm, can be removed once identified by local incision over the site with direct removal. Those in the right heart necessitate thoracotomy although recent reports indicate this can be done by a pervenous route.[5] The safest method for removal in a patient who does not present any serious risks is by thoracotomy. No particular devices for bypassing the heart are necessary since the catheter can be easily palpated. With a small incision over the site of the catheter, the fragment is removed with facility. Early removal is essential also because it is obviously less of a hazard and risk to make a small incision in the superior vena cava or the right atrium rather than the right ventricle or the pulmonary artery.

Localizing the catheter may at times be rather difficult and this may account for the reason that in a high proportion of patients the first evidence was noted simply that the catheter had "disappeared." Also the fact that in many of these patients neither the time interval nor the outcome was known demonstrates that embolism can occur relatively frequently and can easily be missed. Once a catheter is suspected of having been lost, then immediate films should be taken of the extremity involved and of the chest.[3] If the catheter cannot be visualized adequately, venography has been recommended as being of value.[8] If this fails, then cardiopulmonary angiography will demonstrate the catheter as a filling defect within the contrast media.

SUMMARY

A case of catheter embolism is reported. The mechanism for its loss was not determined, the catheter "disappearing." Delay in operation permitted tracing the course of the fragment. Within 1 week the fragment was coiled within the pulmonary artery. Removal was accomplished with ease by a small arteriotomy. The incidence of complications from embolized catheters was deduced to be about 23 percent with one half resulting in death.

REFERENCES

1. Coblentz, D. R.: Radiographic detection of plastic catheter embolus, California Med. **105:** 357, 1966.
2. Doering, R. B., Stemmer, E. H., and Connolly, J. E.: Complications of indwelling venous catheters with particular reference to catheter emboli, Am. J. Surg. **114:** 259, 1967.
3. Funke, J., Grove, J. H., and Lindenfield, F. H.: Plastic cathter embolus, radiographic localization, M. Radiog. & Photog. **37:** 56, 1961.
4. Lamprecht, W.: Zur Kasuistik iatrogener intrakardialer Fremdkörper, Chirurg. **36:** 182, 1965.
5. Massumi, R. A., and Ross, A. M.: Atraumatic nonsurgical technic for removal of broken catheters from cardiac chamber, New England J. Med. **277:** 195, 1967.
6. Tuell, S. W., Martin, W. B., and Laufman, H.: Complications from the use of plastic intravenous tubing, Quart. Bull. Northwestern Univ. M. School **22:** 353, 1948.
7. Turner, D. D., and Sommers, S. C.: Accidental passage of a polyethylene catheter from cubital vein to right atrium, New England J. Med. **251:** 744, 1954.
8. Wellman, K. F., Reinhard, A., and Salazar, E. P.: Polyethylene catheter embolism, Circulation **37:** 380, 1968.

Studies on the effect of 2-phenyl-2-(2-pyridyl)-thioacetamide (antigastrin) on canine gastric acid secretion

JAIME ISAZA, M.D.
KYOJI SUGAWARA, M.D.
RICHARD TIONGCO, M.D.
M. MICHAEL EISENBERG, M.D.*
GAINESVILLE, FLA., AND MINNEAPOLIS, MINN.
From the Departments of Surgery, College of Medicine, University of Florida, and Mount Sinai Hospital and University of Minnesota

A synthetic nonanticholinergic compound 2-phenyl-2-(2-pyridyl)-thioacetamide,† provisionally named "antigastrin" has been found to exert a strong inhibitory effect on gastric acid secretion stimulated by exogenous gastrin II, synthetic pentagastrin, or a meat meal.[3, 6]

Controversy directed at the specificity of suppression of gastrin-stimulated secretion[3, 6] or at the nonspecificity in the action of the compound against histamine or insulin-stimulated (vagal) gastric secretion[5, 8] has not been satisfactorily settled. The following series of experiments were undertaken to evaluate the effects of antigastrin on the gastric secretory response to a variety of stimuli, i.e., endogenously produced gastrin, vagal activation by 2-deoxy-D-glucose and histamine, and, if possible, to establish specificity of action.

METHODS

Four mongrel dogs (14 to 18 kilograms in weight) were prepared with denervated fundic pouches (Heidenhain) and isolated innervated antrums. Five additional dogs were prepared with both denervated fundic pouches and gastric fistulas placed just proximal to the antrum. All operative procedures were performed with aseptic technique and intravenous sodium pentobarbital anesthesia. Following a postoperative recovery period of at least 3 weeks, experiments were initiated by fasting the dogs for 18 hours. Only animals with 0.1 c.c. or less acid output during a 30 minute basal period were studied.

2-Phenyl-2-(2-pyridyl)-thioacetamide was dissolved in a vehicle consisting of 2.5 ml. of dimethylsulfoxide (DMSO).[9] Gastric secretion was collected every 15 minutes from the pouches and the gastric fistulas and titrated with 0.1N NaOH with Töpfer's reagent as pH indicator.

All data were submitted for statistical analysis, and the significance of the differences of the means was determined by the t test for unpaired values.

RESULTS

1. Endogenous gastrin. Release of endogenous gastrin was stimulated by perfusion of the antral pouch (in dogs with isolated innervated antrums and Heidenhain pouches) with acetylcholine (ACh) 0.1 percent in saline solution at a rate of 160 ml. per hour with a peristaltic pump (Harvard Apparatus Company). Following achievement of a steady plateau of gastric secretion

Supported in part by National Institutes of Health Grants No. AMO 2372-10 and No. AM 12921-01.

Submitted for publication Feb. 25, 1969; resubmitted May 1, 1969.

*Reprint requests: Department of Surgery, 2215 Park Avenue, Minneapolis, Minn. 55404.

†Compound SC-15396, G. D. Searle Company.

Vol. 67, No. 3, pp. 462-467

from the denervated fundic (Heidenhain) pouch, a single intravenous dose of test material was administered. Acetylcholine perfusion was maintained throughout the duration of the experiment. Control experiments were performed with acetylcholine background alone, acetylcholine infusion with 2.5 ml. DMSO injection, and with 10, 20, 40, 80, and 160 mg. of antigastrin in 2.5 ml. DMSO superimposed on acetylcholine-driven secretion.

A constant state of Heidenhain pouch acid output was usually achieved after 90 minutes of ACh perfusion; secretion was slightly but not significantly inhibited by the 2.5 ml. DMSO injection. Within 30 minutes following the injection of antigastrin dissolved in DMSO, however, significant suppression of fundic pouch secretion occurred. The degree and duration of effect was dose dependent (Table I, Fig. 1) Maximal inhibition ranged from 45.2 ± 11 percent with 10 mg. to 93.9 ± 1.9 percent for the 160 mg. of antigastrin. Duration of maximal inhibitory effect was less than 60 minutes with doses of 10 and 20 mg.; doses of 40 mg. or greater caused sustained inhibition lasting 120 to 180 minutes (duration of the experiment).

2. Vagus. In dogs with gastric fistulas and Heidenhain pouches, a series of control experiments was performed to determine response to strong vagal stimulation by administration of a single intravenous dose of 150 mg. per kilogram of 2-deoxy-D-glucose (2-DG) dissolved in 15 ml. of saline.[7] In subsequent experiments test material consisting of either 2.5 ml. of DMSO alone or a dose of antigastrin dissolved in DMSO was injected intravenously 15 minutes following the administration of 2-DG. Gastric secretory output was monitored for at least 180 minutes after injection of the test material.

Gastric fistula response to 2-deoxy-D-glucose with superimposed DMSO revealed a slight but not significant inhibition, by the vehicle, of vagally driven gastric secretion (Fig. 2). Twenty milligrams of antigastrin dissolved in DMSO did not produce an inhibitory effect significantly different from DMSO alone. Approximately 20 percent inhibition occurred with 40 mg. of antigastrin, but suppression also failed to meet statistical significance (p=0.1). Eighty milligrams of antigastrin clearly and significantly blunted the mean peak response to 2-DG by 40 percent (Fig. 3). Doses of 160 mg. of antigastrin

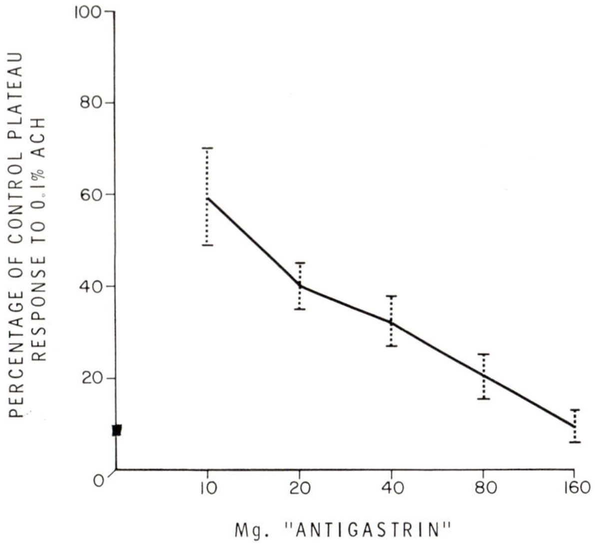

Fig. 1. Dose-response curve to antigastrin, based on the maximal 1 hour Heidenhain pouch output, presented in percentages of ACh control plateau secretion. Increasing antigastrin dose serially depresses secretion from control levels.

Table I. *Heidenhain pouch acid outputs—percentage of control plateau response*

Injection	No. of dogs	No. of experiments	Plateau response (mEq./15 min.)			
				1	2	3
DMSO alone	4	10	0.49 ± 0.089	96.7 ± 4.7	96.8 ± 6.5	83.9 ± 4.3
DMSO and "antigastrin"						
10 mg.	2	5	0.34 ± 0.026	75.0 ± 10.0	64.1 ± 2.4	61.2 ± 7.6
p =			> 0.2	< 0.05	< 0.01	< 0.02
20 mg.	4	10	0.58 ± 0.084	62.1 ± 4.5	33.9 ± 4.3	38.1 ± 4.7
p =			> 0.4	< 0.01	< 0.01	< 0.01
40 mg.	3	9	0.48 ± 0.098	68.0 ± 7.1	32.9 ± 4.9	32.2 ± 4.3
p =			> 0.4	< 0.01	< 0.01	< 0.01
80 mg.	4	10	0.44 ± 0.050	65.8 ± 6.3	23.3 ± 4.2	20.6 ± 4.3
p =			> 0.6	< 0.01	< 0.01	< 0.01
160 mg.	3	10	0.45 ± 0.063	64.7 ± 21.3	16.5 ± 6.1	8.1 ± 2.3
p =			> 0.7	< 0.01	< 0.01	< 0.01

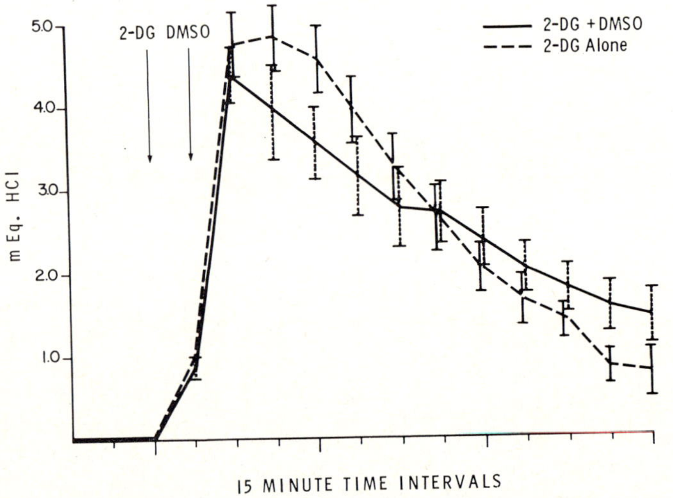

Fig. 2. Gastric fistula secretory output response to 2-deoxy-D-glucose alone (broken line) and 2-deoxy-D-glucose and DMSO (solid line). Mean of 22 experiments in five dogs. DMSO did not significantly retard acid stimulation by 2DG ($p > 0.1$).

provoked retching which made data interpretation difficult; those results have been discarded.

3. Histamine. A constant plateau of gastric acid secretion from dogs with gastric fistulas and denervated fundic pouches was obtained by continuous intravenous infusion of 0.5 mg. per hour of histamine base. After attainment of a steady state for at least four 15 minute samples, a single intravenous dose of either 2.5 ml. of DMSO or 40 or 160 mg. of antigastrin was administered.

Significant inhibition of histamine-driven gastric acid secretion from both the denervated fundic pouch and gastric fistula, to a degree of 46 percent and 43 percent, respectively, was produced by 40 mg. of antigastrin and lasted throughout the duration of the experiment (3 hours) (Figs. 4 and 5). Once again, however, the 160 mg. dose of

15 minute time intervals						
4	*5*	*6*	*7*	*8*	*9*	*10*
85.4 ± 6.1	83.2 ± 4.4	89.4 ± 6.1	82.6 ± 6.7	88.7 ± 6.6	91.0 ± 6.6	92.2 ± 8.3
56.7 ± 6.6 < 0.02	54.8 ± 11.0 < 0.02	63.6 ± 17.3 > 0.1	68.7 ± 19.2 > 0.04	71.9 ± 23.1 > 0.3		
43.2 ± 4.9 < 0.01	45.5 ± 6.6 < 0.01	51.7 ± 8.5 < 0.01	55.4 ± 10.4 < 0.01	52.2 ± 6.5 < 0.01		
32.5 ± 6.0 < 0.01	32.4 ± 6.7 < 0.01	33.1 ± 7.3 < 0.01	34.8 ± 6.9 < 0.01	33.9 ± 7.5 < 0.01	34.3 ± 9.1 < 0.01	44.2 ± 6.9 < 0.01
22.0 ± 6.6 < 0.01	18.1 ± 4.1 < 0.01	20.7 ± 4.5 < 0.01	24.5 ± 5.8 < 0.01	25.8 ± 5.9 < 0.01		
6.1 ± 1.9 < 0.01	8.8 ± 3.4 < 0.01	15.6 ± 6.5 < 0.01	13.4 ± 6.8 < 0.01	17.8 ± 7.8 < 0.01	18.6 ± 8.4 < 0.01	17.3 ± 7.9 < 0.01

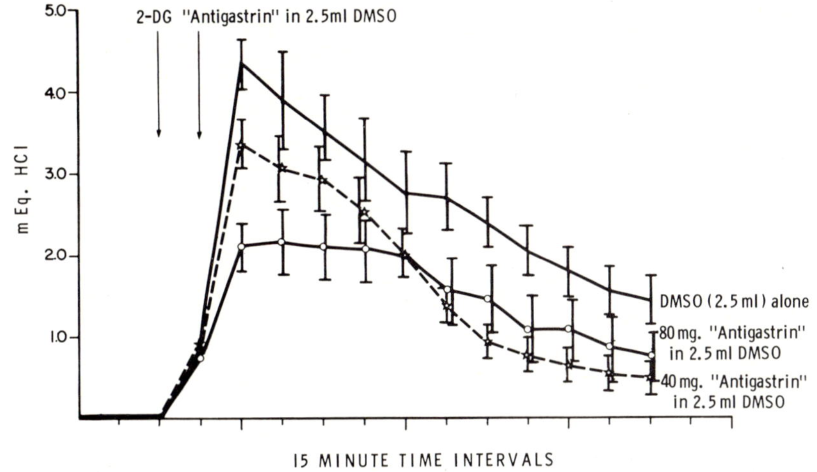

Fig. 3. Inhibition of 2-deoxy-D-glucose—stimulated gastric secretion with 40 and 80 mg. of antigastrin. Mean of nine control and 19 test experiments in five dogs. Suppression by 40 mg. of antigastrin is not statistically significant ($p = 0.1$). Suppression by 80 mg. of antigastrin is statistically significant ($p < 0.01$).

antigastrin invoked nausea and retching, in six out of eight experiments, and these data (with the high dose) were thereby considered invalidated and have been discarded.

DISCUSSION

These data show that intravenous 2-phenyl-2-(2-pyridyl)-thioacetamide is capable of acting as a powerful inhibitor of gastric secretion and that the inhibition is dose related. The studies examine the effect of antigastrin on vagal-, histamine-, and endogenous gastrin-stimulated gastric secretion and demonstrate that although suppression of gastrin is clearly more profound than blockage of histamine- or vagal-driven secretion, all three modalities are, in fact, retarded. The suggestion of lack of specificity of the inhibitory effect against gastrin stimulation is, therefore,

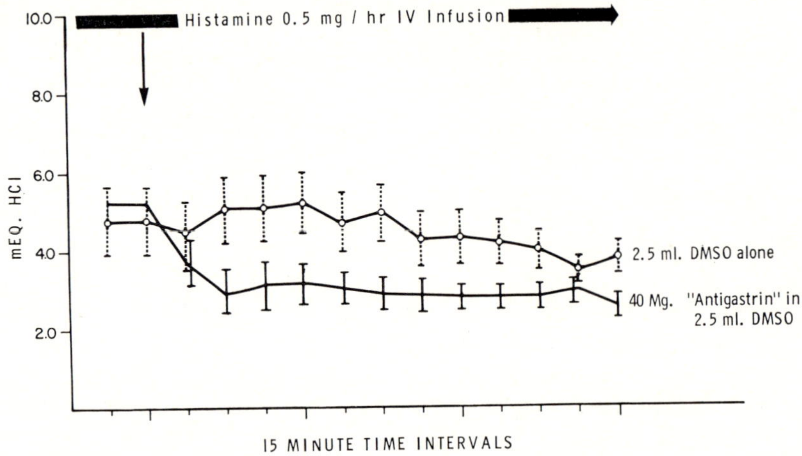

Fig. 4. Inhibitory response of histamine-stimulated gastric fistula output to 40 mg. of antigastrin. Mean of 17 control and eight test experiments in five dogs. Vertical arrow indicates time of antigastrin injection. A significant 46 per cent secretory depression is shown.

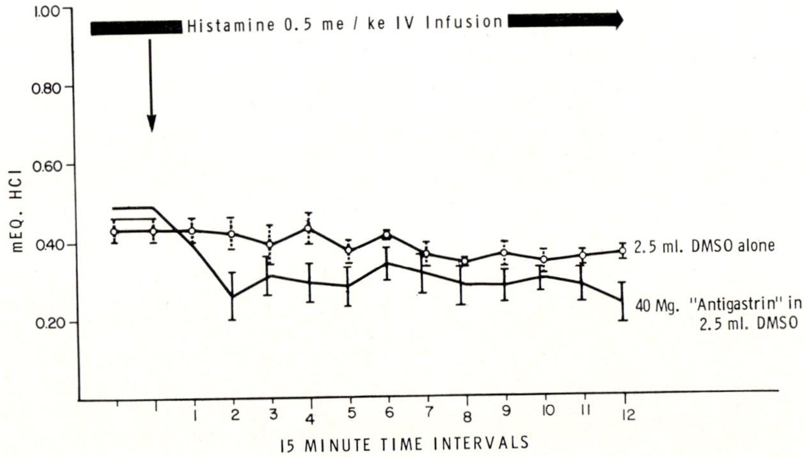

Fig. 5. Inhibitory response of histamine-stimulated, denervated (Heidenhain) fundic pouch secretion to 40 mg. of antigastrin. Mean of 17 control and eight test experiments in five dogs. Vertical arrow indicates time of antigastrin injection. A significant 43 per cent secretory depression is shown.

again raised. Bedi and associates,[3] using dogs with vagally innervated fundic pouches, could *not* obtain inhibition of histamine-stimulated gastric secretion with an intravenous dose of 20 mg. of antigastrin per 15 minutes, and Cook and Bianchi[6] could *not* demonstrate a significant inhibition of a test meal with oral doses of 10 to 15 mg. per kilogram. Subsequently, however, Connell and co-workers[5] and Gillespie and associates,[8] using higher intravenous, oral, or intrajejunal doses of antigastrin (10 mg. per kilogram), obtained significant inhibition of histamine-stimulated gastric secretion in vagally innervated or denervated pouches; they concluded that antigastrin is not a *specific* gastrin antagonist. Although we obtained similar results with smaller total intravenous doses of 40 or 80 mg., the use of a higher dose (160 mg.) in our experiments is considered to have given invalid data because of the emetic-like effect at this level. It seems possible, therefore, that the inhibition noted in Connell and associates[5] and Gillespie and co-workers'[8] studies may, in part at least, be artifactual on the same basis.

The mechanism by which low doses of antigastrin inhibit histamine- or vagally activated secretion in these experiments is not yet clear. The phenomenon of vagally stimulated gastrin release is established,[1, 2, 4, 11, 12] and it is also recognized that gastrin is an important potentiating agent for other gastric stimuli.[10] The specificity of antigastrin against gastrin-stimulated secretion cannot, therefore, be ruled out and interference with histamine and vagal stimulation in our experiments may merely represent the inhibition of potentiating background gastrin. Although 85 percent inhibition of insulin-stimulated secretion by compound SC-15396 in an *antrectomized* dog has been reported,[5] the possibility remains that such inhibition may have been based on the emetic effect of the large doses of inhibitor used rather than on direct interference with vagal effect. Finally, the possibility of other, nonantral, sources of endogenous gastrin have not been ruled out by antrectomy.

SUMMARY

The inhibitory properties of 2-phenyl-2-(2-pyridyl)-thioacetamide (antigastrin: compound SC-15396) have been studied against a background of endogenous gastrin-, vagal-, and histamine-stimulated gastric secretion in dogs. Under the conditions of these experiments antigastrin has been shown to be a potent inhibitor of gastric secretion, more powerful against gastrin-stimulated than against vagally or histamine-stimulated acid, but effective against all three modalities; suppression was dose related.

The precise role and specificity of antigastrin in inhibition of nervous- or histamine-stimulated juice is not clear; interference with histamine- and vagally stimulated gastric juice may merely represent inhibition of potentiating background gastrin. The enormous potential value of compounds of this type for both experimental and clinical investigative studies in gastrointestinal physiology is emphasized.

The authors wish to acknowledge the excellent technical assistance of Miss Cathy Holm and Mr. William Rush, Jr.

REFERENCES

1. Albe, L.: Significance of vagal release of gastrin during the nervous phase of gastric secretion in dogs, Gastroenterology **44:** 463, 1963.
2. Anderson, S., and Grossman, M. I.: Effect of denervation and subsequent resection of antral pouches on secretion from Heidenhain pouch in response to gastrin and histamine, Gastroenterology **51:** 4, 1966.
3. Bedi, B. S., Gillespie, G., and Gillespie, I. E.: Effects of a specific gastrin antagonist on gastric acid secretion in pouch dogs, Lancet **1:** 1240, 1967.
4. Burstall, P. A., and Schofield, B.: The effects of pyloric antrectomy on the secretory response of Heidenhain pouches in dogs to central vagal stimulation, J. Physiol. **123:** 168, 1954.
5. Connell, A. M., Sircus, W., Hill, R. A., Macleod, I. B., and Thomson, C. G.: A gastric secretion antagonist's effect, Lancet **2:** 720, 1967.
6. Cook, D. L., and Bianchi, R. G.: SC-15396, a new anti-ulcer compound possessing antigastrin activity, Life Sc. **6:** 1381, 1967.
7. Eisenberg, M. M., Emas, G. S., and Grossman, M. I.: Comparison of the effect of 2-deoxy-D-glucose and insulin on gastric acid secretion in dogs, Surgery **60:** 111, 1966.
8. Gillespie, G., McCusker, V. I., Bedi, B. S., Debas, H. T., and Gillespie, I. E.: Further experimental observations on the gastric acid secretion inhibitor, SC-15396, Gastroenterology **55:** 81, 1968.
9. Jacob, S. W., and Wood, D. C.: Dimethyl sulfoxide (DMSO), toxicology, pharmacology, and clinical experience, Am. J. Surg. **114:** 414, 1967.
10. Passaro, E. P., Gillespie, I. E., and Grossman, M. I.: Potentiation between gastrin and histamine in stimulation of gastric secretion, Proc. Soc. Exper. Biol. & Med. **114:** 50, 1963.
11. Pe Thein, M., and Schofield, B.: Release of gastrin from the pyloric antrum following vagal stimulation by sham feeding in dogs, J. Physiol. **148:** 291, 1959.
12. Woodward, E. R., Robertson, C. R., Fried, W., and Shapiro, H.: Further studies on the isolated gastric antrum, Gastroenterology **32:** 868, 1957.

Esophageal mucosal regeneration following experimental prosthetic replacement of the esophagus

BERNARD J. LEININGER, M.D.
HOWARD PEACOCK
WILLIAM E. NEVILLE, M.D.
HINES, ILL.
From the Veterans Administration Edward Hines, Jr., Hospital

Esophageal mucosal repair is seen in patients sustaining chemical burns of the esophagus. Foroozan and associates[3] reported regeneration of the entire esophageal mucosa following sloughing of the esophageal mucosa in a patient with pemphigoid. There remains considerable controversy over the manner and type of esophageal mucosal regeneration in man. Some authors[5, 7] have felt that esophageal repair is accomplished by gastric mucosal proliferation, particularly in the region of the cardioesophageal junction. Other authors[3] have suggested that esophageal mucosa regenerates from either deep mucous glands or from undifferentiated mesodermal elements of the submucosa. It is the purpose of this communication to report esophageal mucosal regeneration and the manner in which it takes place following prosthetic replacement of the esophagus in dogs.

MATERIAL

Eighteen mongrel dogs weighing between 10 to 20 kilograms, underwent right thoracotomies through the fifth or sixth intercostal space. The azygous vein was divided and 5 to 6 cm. of the middle third of the esophagus was excised. A Dacron-Silastic tube prosthesis, 7 to 9 cm. in length and 3 cm. in diameter, was sutured to the cut ends of the esophagus (Figs. 1*A* and 1*B*). The prosthesis* was constructed by covering a coarse Dacron mesh with Silastic. The wall was 1.5 mm. in thickness affording a certain amount of tubular rigidity. All anastomoses were made with one layer technique of running suture. The animals were divided into Groups A and B according to the type of suture material used. Group A consisted of 12 dogs in which nonabsorbable synthetic suture was employed. Group B consisted of six dogs in which chromic catgut suture was used. The prosthesis was telescoped into the lumen of both the proximal and distal esophagus for a distance of 1 cm. Care was taken to prevent devascularization of the esophagus through excessive mobilization of the resected ends of the esophagus. Tension on the suture line was lessened by purposely inserting a prosthesis that was longer than the resected esophagus. No attempt was made to cover the prosthesis with either mediastinal pleura or free fascial grafts. The chest was closed and the air was evacuated from the right pleural space by means of an intercostal catheter connected to an underwater sealed drainage bottle. Antibiotics were not administered. All animals were fed a mushy diet beginning on the third postoperative day and continuing until the time of death or killing.

RESULTS

Seven of the 12 dogs in Group A died within 8 days after operation. Leakage from one or both anastomoses with resultant empyema and mediastinitis was the apparent cause of death in all. The remaining five dogs were killed between 7 and 12 months after operation. These animals were main-

Received for publication March 19, 1968.

*Prostheses were constructed by the Dow Corning Center for Aid to Medical Research, Midland, Mich.

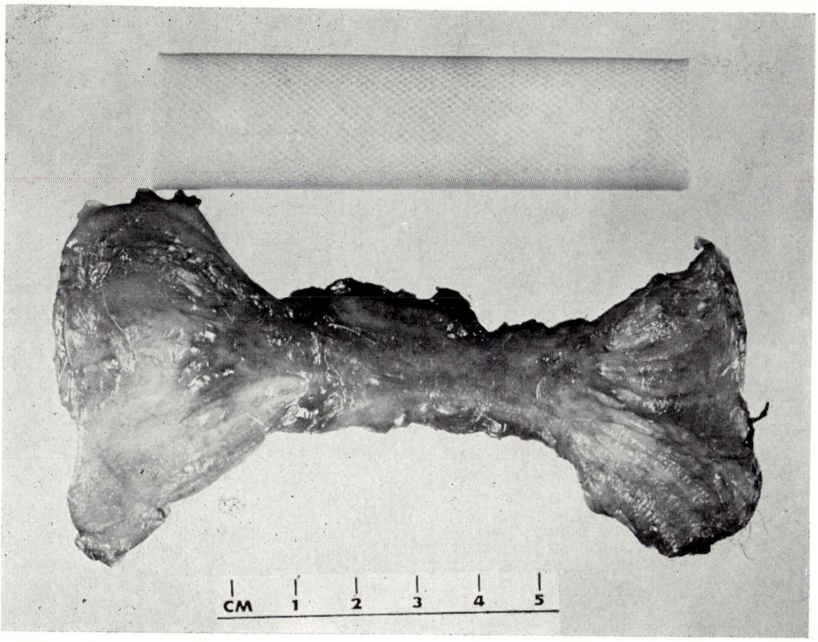

Fig. 1*A*. The tubular Dacron-Silastic prosthesis that was used is shown. The resected esophagus from an animal in Group B has been opened longitudinally showing the mucosal surface. Note the marked stenosis, shortening, and absence of mucosal lining in the neo-esophagus. The prosthesis in this animal sloughed at 3 weeks.

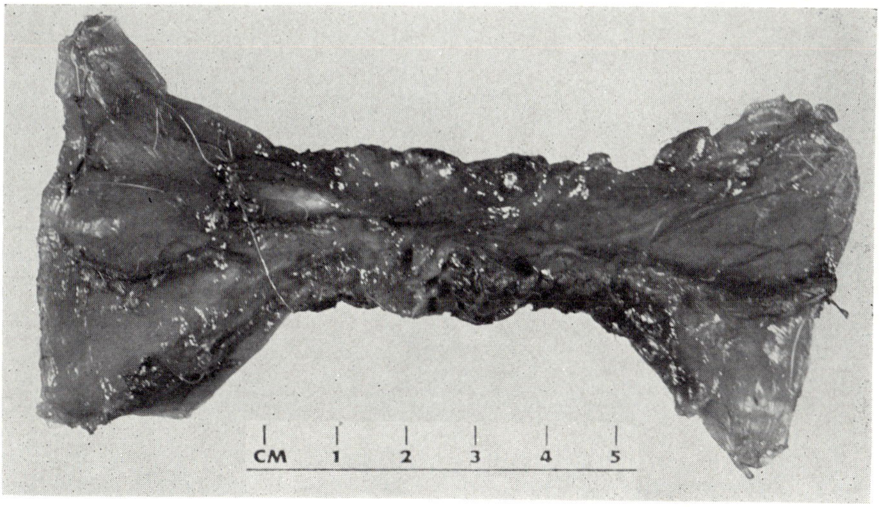

Fig. 1*B*. The external surface showing the fibrous reaction in the region of the neo-esophagus. The entire wall of the neo-esophagus consisted in fibrous connective tissue.

tained throughout on a mushy diet and at the time that they were killed had a mean weight loss of 11 percent of body weight as compared with their preoperative weight. Labored deglutition with occasional regurgitation was observed particularly in the first 4 weeks after operation. Esophagoscopy was performed postoperatively at the third, fifth, and seventh week. The esophageal prosthesis was visualized in all five dogs at 5 weeks, in three dogs at 7 weeks, and in none of the dogs at 9 weeks.

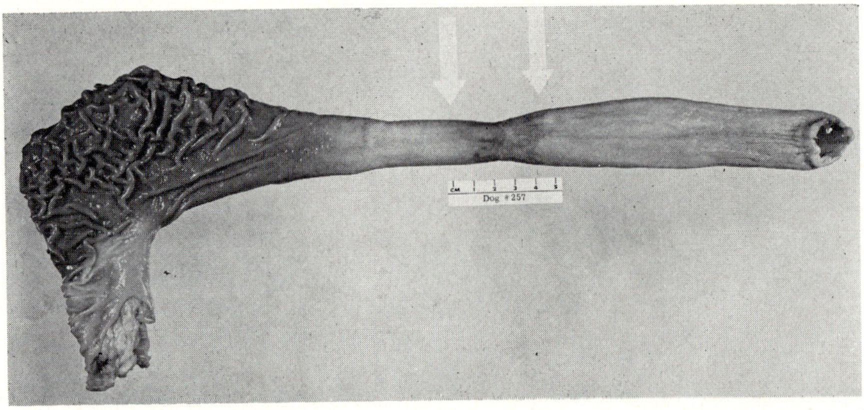

Fig. 2*A*. The esophagus and stomach turned inside out. This specimen is from a dog in Group A that was killed at 10 months. Note the minimal degree of narrowing of the neo-esophagus, also the dilatation of the proximal esophagus.

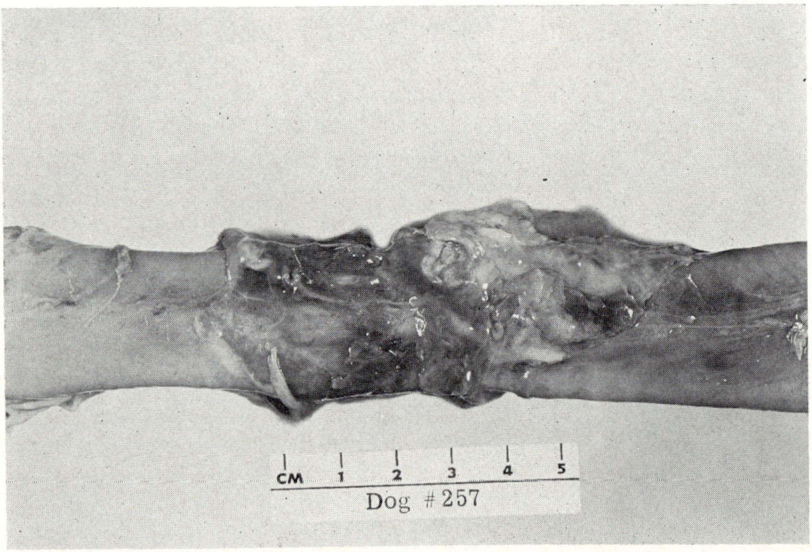

Fig. 2*B*. The external surface of the esophagus of the same animal. Note the adhesions and fibrotic tissue in the region of the neo-esophagus.

The autopsy findings of the five dogs killed in Group A showed the prosthesis to have been sloughed in all instances. Periodic antemortem endoscopic examinations indicated that the prostheses had been sloughed sometime between the fifth and ninth postoperative week in all of the animals. None of the prostheses were recovered in the gastrointestinal tract at autopsy. The neo-esophagus that formed in the area of the sloughed prosthesis was adherent to the lung and adjacent mediastinal structures. There were no findings to suggest recent or chronic infection in the mediastinum or pleural spaces.

Gross findings of the autopsies showed the following: (1) There was muscular hypertrophy and dilatation of the proximal esophagus, (2) the neo-esophagus was contracted in length, (3) the neo-esophagus showed some concentric narrowing internal diameters measuring from 2.5 to 3.0 cm.,

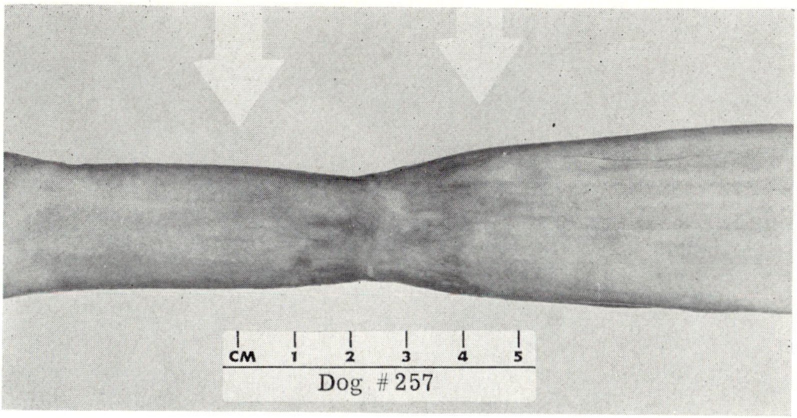

Fig. 2*C*. The esophagus turned inside out showing the smooth mucosal surface of the neo-esophagus.

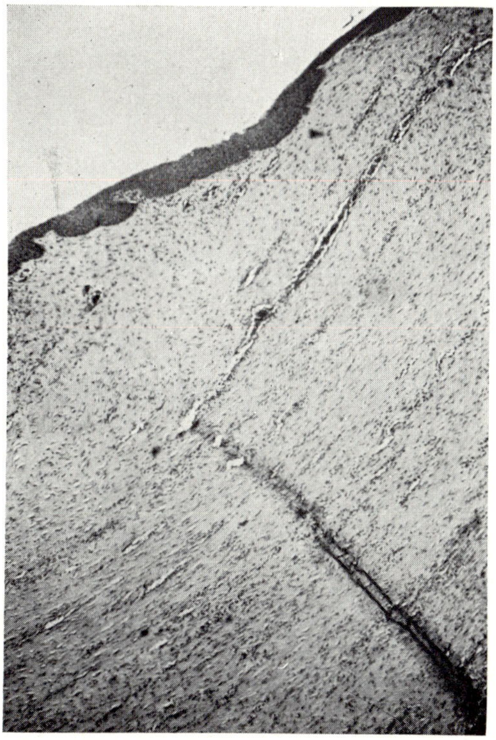

Fig. 2*D*. Section showing the thin layer of stratified squamous epithelium over a thick layer of fibrous connective tissue. Muscle layers were not present in the neo-esophagus.

(4) the neo-esophagus was firm and fixed to the surrounding structures (Figs. 2*A* to 2*D*).

Microscopically there was a complete squamous epithelialization of the entire length of the neo-esophagus in all five of the animals. This stratified squamous epithelium was thinner than the normal esophageal mucosa. The wall of the neo-esophagus consisted entirely of fibrous connective tissue. There were no muscle layers or mucous glands present.

Three of the six dogs in Group B died within 10 days after operation. The cause of death was again from empyema and mediastinitis secondary to leakage from the esophageal-prosthetic anastomosis. The three surviving dogs were killed after 3 to 4 weeks. All of the animals were having considerable difficulty in eating. At autopsy the prosthesis was found in the stomach in one, in the large bowel in another, and in the third animal the prosthesis was recovered ante mortem on the twentieth day in the stool. Pleural spaces and the mediastinum were free of fluid and/or infection in all. The neo-esophagi at the site of the prostheses were all structured to less than 1 cm. in diameter. In the region of the resected esophagus there were fibrotic segments varying from 5.5 to 6.5 cm. in length that formed a neo-esophagus. Lung and mediastinal structures were adherent to these segments. Microscopic examination of these segments showed an absence of muscular layers, mucous glands, and esophageal mucosa. The wall of the neo-esophagus was made up of fibrous connective tissue, and at each end there was an ingrowth of squamous epithelium.

The esophagus proximal to neo-esophagus showed dilatation and muscular hypertrophy.

DISCUSSION

The mechanism and type of esophageal mucosal regeneration is poorly understood in man. Hayward[5] states that columnar epithelium of the esophagus found below a stricture in man is a result of metaplasia. He states that this is secondary to the erosive effect of gastric secretion on the esophagus as a result of an incompetent cardioesophageal sphincter. Barrett[1] holds that a columnar-lined lower esophagus below a benign stricture is a congenital abnormality. Van de Kerckhof and Gahagan[9] stripped 2 cm. of the esophageal mucosa of dogs from just above the cardioesophageal junction. Fifty percent of the animals died from esophageal stricture; however, in the survivors the defect was covered with squamous epithelium, and there was no upward growth of gastric mucosa.

Caution is necessary in extrapolating experimental esophageal findings in the dog to humans. It is particularly true in this study. Absence of esophageal peristalsis first in the prosthesis and later in an aperistaltic neo-esophagus represents a greater liability in a horizontal than in an upright position. Perhaps because of this difference in posture the canine esophagus is naturally better developed and more durable than the esophagus of man.

The desirability of a satisfactory esophageal prosthesis is apparent to all dealing with esophageal problems. Patients with carcinoma of the middle or upper thirds of the esophagus are frequently in such a catabolic state as to make replacement of the esophagus with stomach or large or small bowel a formidable procedure. The functional aspect of the esophagus is rather simple, i.e., to transport food and oral secretion from the mouth to the stomach, notwithstanding the more sophisticated maneuvers of emesis and belching. It would appear then that a prosthesis functioning as a simple conduit would be a satisfactory substitute. Leakage from the esophageal-prosthetic anastomosis and the sequelae therefrom has been the major problem. Sloughing of the graft and stenosis have been later complications. One can reason that if one prostheses is successful then the cause of failure is technical and hence correctable. Invaginating the prosthesis into the esophagus, preventing devascularization by minimal mobilization of the ends of the esophagus, and eliminating tension on the suture lines are all technical lessons that have been learned; yet success has remained sufficiently unpredictable to warrant against clinical application.

Although the two groups in this study were relatively small, the findings were consistent. In Group B the prostheses were sutured with absorbable material and sloughed between the second to the fourth week. Squamous epithelialization did not have time to progress across the neo-esophagus resulting in stenosis. Microscopic sections of the ends of the neo-esophagus showed a thin layer of stratified squamous epithelium extending 0.5 to 1 cm. beyond the point where muscle layers and mucous glands were present, thus indicating that the process of epithelialization was, in fact progressing.

In Group A synthetic nonabsorbable suture material was used holding the prosthesis in place long enough to permit squamous epithelialization to advance around the outside of the graft. When the graft sloughed, epithelialization had progressed sufficiently to prevent stenosis. The neo-esophagus histologically consisted of fibrous connective tissue lined by a rather thin layer of stratified squamous epithelium. In our initial microscopic examinations of the neo-esophagus, mucous glands and muscle layers were thought to have regenerated; however, closer scrutiny showed these structures to be, in fact, part of the resected ends of the esophagus pulled into the neo-esophagus as a result of fibrosis. Muscular hypertrophy, dilatation, and elongation of the proximal esophagus and the shortening of the neo-esophagus prompted us to perform a successful resection of the neo-esophagus with a primary anastomosis in one animal. We are unable to think of a clinical situation to which this technique would be applicable.

The weight loss in these animals can be ascribed to several factors. Mobility studies were not performed on these animals although both endoscopic and pathologic examinations showed the neo-esophagus to be firm and nonexpansile. All had a moderate amount of dysphagia which was probably more a result of the adynamic segment than the relatively minor degree of stenosis. Also, diarrhea was a problem to some extent in all of the animals. This was thought to be due in part to the constant mushy diet.

SUMMARY

A neo-esophagus consisting of fibrous connective tissue resulted from bridging a resected portion of the middle third of the canine esophagus with a prosthesis. If the prosthesis was sutured with absorbable material, the graft sloughed at 2 to 4 weeks resulting in stenosis without mucosal epithelialization of the neo-esophagus. Esophageal prostheses held in place for 5 to 9 weeks with permanent synthetic sutures showed squamous epithelialization of the entire neo-esophagus. Epithelialization was demonstrated to have been a process of regeneration from the mucosal edges of the esophagus. Clinical and experimental implications of these findings are discussed.

REFERENCES

1. Barrett, N. R.: The lower esophagus lined by columnar epithelium, SURGERY **41.** 881, 1957.
2. Barrett, N. R.: Benign stricture in the lower esophagus, J. Thoracic & Cardiovas. Surg. **43:** 703, 1962.
3. Foroozan, P., Enta, T., Winship, D. H., and esophageal mucosa in pemphigoid, Gastroenterology **52:** 548, 1967.
4. Fryfogle, J. D., Cyrowski, E. A., Rothwell, D., Rheault, E., and Clark, T.: Replacement of middle third of the esophagus with a silicone rubber prosthesis, Dis. Chest **43:** 464, 1963.
5. Hayward, J.: The treatment of fibrous stricture of the esophagus associated with hiatal hernia, Thorax **16:** 45, 1961.
6. Lister, J., Altman, R. P., and Allison, W. A.: Prosthetic substitution of thoracic esophagus in puppies: Use of Marlex mesh with collagen or anterior rectus sheath, Ann. Surg. **162:** 812, 1965.
7. Mossberg, S. M.: The columnar-lined esophagus (Barrett syndrome)—an acquired condition? Gastroenterology **50:** 671, 1966.
8. Schuring, A. E., and Ray, J. W.: Experimental use of Dacron as an esophageal prosthesis, Ann. Otol. Rhin. & Laryng. **75:** 202, 1966.
9. Van de Kerckhof, J., and Gahagan, T.: Regeneration of the mucosal lining of the esophagus, Henry Ford Hosp. M. Bull. **11:** 129, 1963.

Cholesterol absorption following reversal of the upper and lower halves of the small intestine

ROGER L. GEBHARD, M.D.
HENRY BUCHWALD, M.D., PH.D.*
MINNEAPOLIS, MINN.
From the Department of Surgery, University of Minnesota Medical School

Cholesterol absorption has been shown to be affected by several factors, including bile acids,[5, 8, 9] pancreatic enzymes,[7] and association with fatty acids.[10] It has been stated that selective, or at least preferential, cholesterol absorption occurs in the ileum.[6] In an experiment published in 1964,[4] we demonstrated that the entire small intestine of the rabbit is capable of cholesterol absorption but that, with normal bowel continuity, there appeared to be preferential cholesterol uptake by the distal half of the small bowel. We next wished to consider whether this preferential distal absorption was the result of a site-specific intrinsic mechanism or the result of the relative location of ileum and jejunum.

METHODS

Ten white, New Zealand, 6 to 8 pound rabbits were prepared by surgically interchanging the distal and proximal halves of small intestine. Three side-to-side anastomoses were utilized between umbilical tape occlusions to direct intestinal flow. In this fashion, distal duodenum was anastomosed to proximal ileum, distal ileum to proximal jejunum, and distal jejunum to the intestinal side of the ileocecal valve. These animals thus had the ileum proximal to the jejunum with the duodenum and the pancreatic and biliary ducts left in situ.

The cholesterol "absorptive capacity" of the test animals was compared with that of ten weight- and sex-matched normal control animals (findings of these rabbits have previously been reported[4]). All animals were housed in identical cages and fed the same diet (standard Nutrena rabbit pellets). No analyses were performed on operated animals until they had regained their preoperative weights and were eating normally.

"Absorptive capacity" was defined as the average whole blood cholesterol radioactivity measured over 6 consecutive days subsequent to the forced feeding of a standard 10 mg. dose of cholesterol-4-^{14}C (0.4 μc per milligram) dissolved in corn oil. Extraction of whole blood cholesterol was performed by the method of Abell and associates[1] in all instances. One milliliter blood samples were utilized. Radioactivity was determined with a Packard Tricarb liquid-scintillation spectrometer with 0.3 percent 2,5-diphenyloxazole in toluene as the flour. A modified Liebermann-Burchard reaction, with color analysis in a Coleman Junior Spectrophotometer, was used for cholesterol quantitation.

RESULTS

As shown in Table I, the average absorptive capacity of the ten operated animals was 2,272 counts per minute per milliliter of whole blood with a standard error of the mean of 326 c.p.m. per milliliter. This was essentially identical to the average control animal value of 2,458 c.p.m. per milliliter with a standard error of the mean of 302

Supported by United States Public Health Service Grant No. HE-11901 and the American Heart Association Grant No. 67825.

Received for publication April 11, 1969.

*Established Investigator, American Heart Association.

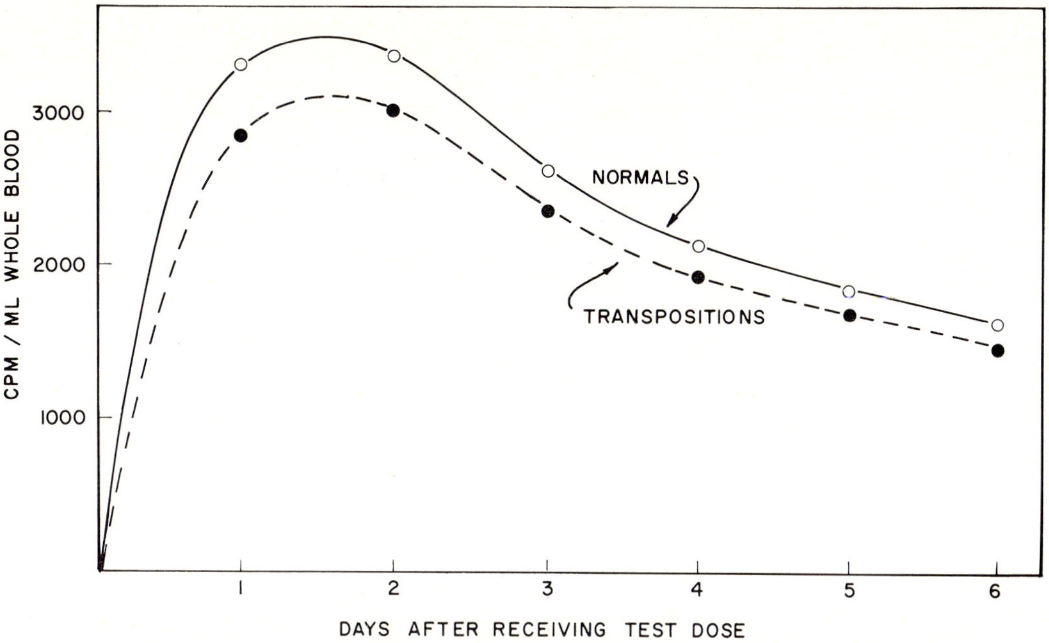

Fig. 1. Graphic comparison of average daily whole blood cholesterol radioactivity values for test and control animal groups.

c.p.m. per milliliter. The p value of the differences between the means of the two groups was not statistically significant ($0.7 > p > 0.6$). The absorption curves of the daily values are graphically demonstrated in Fig. 1. It can be seen that the curves have the same form, with peak values reached between 24 and 48 hours, followed by an exponential falloff.

Table I also compares the average whole blood cholesterol levels and specific activities of the two groups. The average cholesterol concentration of the animals with transposed small intestinal halves was 86.9 mg. percent while that of the control animals was 91.4 mg. percent. Specific activities averaged over the 6 day periods were 2,698 c.p.m. per milligram for the test group and 2,693 c.p.m. per milligram for the control animals. Again, no statistically significant difference between the test group and the control group could be found.

Table I. *Absorptive capacity, milligrams percent whole blood cholesterol, and specific activity of control and transposition test groups*

	Control	*Transposition*
Six day average whole blood radioactivity in in counts per minute per milliliter ± S.E.	2,458 ± 302	2,272 ± 326
Average whole blood cholesterol levels in milligrams per milliliter ± S.E.	91.4 ± 3.8	86.9 ± 5.2
Specific activity in counts per minute per milligram	2,693	2,698

DISCUSSION

In the previously reported experiment,[4] bypass of the rabbit's distal small intestine resulted in only 14 percent of normal absorption (see Table II). Bypass of the proximal small intestine yielded 19 percent of normal absorption. When the quantitative average absorption capacity of the two parts is summated, they yield less than one third of the control radioactivity value. These findings, combined with the demonstration of a statistically significant 21 percent de-

Table II. *Summary of cholesterol absorptive capacity data previously reported for control, ileal bypass, jejunal bypass with ileocecal valvuloplasty, and ileocecal valvuloplasty rabbits*

Group	*Average 6 day whole blood radioactivity in counts per minute per milliliter ± S.E.*	*Percentage of control value*
Control	2,458 ± 302	100
Ileal bypass	341 ± 48	14
Jejunal bypass with ileocecal valvuloplasty	468 ± 64	19
Ileocecal valvuloplasty	1,934 ± 225	79

crease in cholesterol absorption induced by rendering the rabbits' ileocecal valves incompetent, suggest that transit time through the small bowel significantly influences quantitative cholesterol absorption.

In the present experiment, control and operated groups of rabbits had comparable lengths of small intestine in continuity and both had functioning ileocecal valves. There was no reason, a priori, to assume that they did not also have similar transit times. In the animals with interchanged intestinal segments, the time in transit through the proximal small bowel (now ileum) should be equivalent to that of the bypassed animals having only ileum in continuity. Thus only about 19 percent of normal absorption should occur in the proximal segment. Since a normal total amount of cholesterol was absorbed by animals with transposed small bowel, the distal segment (now jejunum) can be assumed to be responsible for the remaining absorption. Similarly, it can be argued that in a rabbit with an intact small intestine, with a 10 mg. cholesterol dose, approximately 20 percent of absorption will occur proximally and 80 percent will occur distally. There appears to be no evidence, in the rabbit, for intrinsic specificity of cholesterol absorption in either half of the small intestine. Any relative difference in absorption between jejunal and ileal segments is probably due to the time necessary to prepare cholesterol for absorption, so that whichever segment is distal will be responsible for the major share of cholesterol absorption.

These results are analogous to Booth and co-workers'[2, 3] findings for fatty acid absorption. These authors demonstrated that the distal intestine becomes more important in the absorption of fatty acids as the ingested load increases. There is suggestive evidence that jejunal cholesterol absorption may also occur in man. Simmonds, Hofmann, and Theodor[11] have found a decreasing concentration of prepared labeled cholesterol micelles in passage through the human jejunum, representing significant absorption of this form of cholesterol. Micellar cholesterol may be the absorbable form of dietary cholesterol following the digestive processes of dispersion and emulsification.

SUMMARY

Reversal of the continuity of jejunal and ileal segments resulted in no change in total cholesterol absorption. Based on this finding and those of a previous study, it has been demonstrated that there does not appear to be an ileal or jejunal site in the small intestine of the rabbit which is specific or selective for cholesterol absorption. It is suggested that utilizing a moderately large oral feeding of crystalline cholesterol (10 mg.) in the rabbit will result in maximum absorption in the distal half of the small intestine regardless of the relative continuity of intestinal segments. Transit time in the small intestine seems to strongly influence quantitative cholesterol absorption.

REFERENCES

1. Abell, L. L., Levy, B. B., Brodie, B. B., and Kendall, F. E.: A simplified method for estimation of total cholesterol in serum and demonstration of its specificity, J. Biol. Chem. **195:** 357, 1952.
2. Booth, C. C., Read, A. E., and Jones, E.: Studies on the site of fat absorption. I. The sites of absorption of increasing doses of I^{131}-labeled triolein in the rat, Gut **2:** 23, 1961.
3. Booth, C. C., Alldis, D., and Read, A. E.: Studies on the site of fat absorption. 2. Fat

balance after resection of varying amounts of small intestine in man, Gut **2:** 168, 1961.

4. Buchwald, H., and Gebhard, R. L.: Effect of intestinal bypass on cholesterol absorption and blood levels in the rabbit, Am. J. Physiol. **207:** 567, 1964.
5. Buchwald, H., and Gebhard, R. L.: The essential role of bile in the intestinal absorption of cholesterol, SURGERY **61:** 791, 1966.
6. Byers, S. O., Friedman, M., and Gunning, B.: Observations concerning the production and excretion of cholesterol in mammals. XI. The intestinal site of absorption and excretion of cholesterol, Am. J. Physiol. **175:** 375, 1953.
7. Hernandez, H. H., Chaikoff, I. C., and Kiyosu, J. Y.: Role of pancreatic juice in cholesterol absorption, Am. J. Physiol. **181:** 523, 1955.
8. Ivy, A. C., Suzuki, R., and Prasod, C. R.: Obligatory function of a continuous flow of normal bile for cholesterol absorption, Am. J. Physiol. **193:** 521, 1958.
9. Mueller, J. H.: The assimilation of cholesterol and its esters, J. Biol. Chem. **21:** 1, 1915.
10. Pihl, A.: The effect of dietary fat on the intestinal cholesterol absorption and on the cholesterol metabolism in the liver of the rat, Acta. physiol. scandinav. **34:** 183, 1955.
11. Simmonds, W. J., Hofmann, A. F., and Theodor, E.: Absorption of cholesterol from a micellar solution: Intestinal perfusion studies in man, J. Clin. Invest. **46:** 874, 1967.

Intestinal strangulation in rats monocontaminated with *Sphaerophorus necrophorus*

C. E. YALE, M.D., D.Sc.*
V. R. DOWELL, Jr., Ph.D.**
CINCINNATI, OHIO
From the Cincinnati Veteran's Administration Hospital and the Department of Surgery, University of Cincinnati

Numerous animal experiments involving the suppression or elimination of the intestinal bacteria have emphasized their fundamental importance in intestinal strangulation.[1, 17] Although many different species have been implicated, the significance of the gram-negative, nonsporulating, anaerobic bacilli of the family Bacteroidaceae is unknown. The Bacteroidaceae are the predominant microorganisms of the normal stool of man and other mammals.[6, 12] They are associated with a variety of polymicrobic infections in man[10, 14] and are frequently isolated from pathologic materials, including the exudate from a segment of strangulated intestine[2, 3, 15] when proper anaerobic procedures are employed. Many of the Bacteroidaceae have not been adequately studied. Consequently, their classification is controversial and their role in pathogenesis is poorly understood.[5, 9, 13, 14] *Sphaerophorus necrophorus (Bacteroides funduliformis, Fusiformis necrophorus)* is one of the more than fifty species presently classified in this family.[5]

The use of germ-free animals provides a unique research method for investigations of host-parasite relations under well-defined conditions. This report summarizes a study of intestinal strangulation in rats monocontaminated with *S. necrophorus* by three separate methods.

Submitted for publication March 21, 1969.
Resubmitted May 14, 1969.

*Present address: Department of Surgery, University of Wisconsin Medical School, 1300 University Avenue, Madison, Wis. 53706.
**Present address: National Communicable Disease Center, Atlanta, Ga. 30333.

MATERIALS AND METHODS

Twenty-seven, 258 to 412 gram germ-free Sprague-Dawley rats of mixed sexes were individually caged, nine animals in each of three flexible film isolators. Each isolator constituted a separate experiment, but all of the experiments were done simultaneously.

Experiment 1, strangulation after direct intraintestinal contamination. Nine germ-free rats were anesthetized with intramuscular sodium pentobarbital (25 mg. per kilogram of body weight) and, through a midline abdominal incision, a 10 cm. segment of distal ileum (about 10 percent of the total length of the small intestine) was isolated by ligating each of its ends with 2-0 silk. The bowel was divided above and below the ligatures, and an inverted end-to-end anastomosis with interrupted 6-0 silk was done to restore the continuity of the bowel. The venous return from the test segment was ligated in one third of the animals, the arterial and venous supply in a second third, and the last 3 animals served as control studies. One cubic centimeter of the pure culture of *S. necrophorus* was injected through a No. 27 needle into the lumen of the test segment of each of the nine rats. The abdominal wall was closed in two layers with 5-0 chromic catgut.

Postoperatively, the animals were given feed and water as desired. Initially, at 1,

2, 4, and 7 days, and weekly thereafter until death or killing, the activity, weight, temperature, white blood cell count (WBC), and hematocrit of each animal were determined. At death or killing after 8 weeks, an autopsy was performed.

Experiment 2, strangulation after intraperitoneal contamination. Each of nine germ-free rats was given an intraperitoneal injection of 1 c.c. of the pure culture of *S. necrophorus.* Their activity, weight, temperature, WBC, and hematocrit were determined initially and at 1, 2, 4, 7, and 11 days after injection. At this time, the operations described in Experiment 1 were repeated, except no additional culture was placed into the isolated test segments. Postoperatively, the protocol of Experiment 1 was followed, and an autopsy was done at death or killing after 6 weeks.

Experiment 3, strangulation after oral contamination. All nine rats were denied food and water for 12 hours and then given 36 c.c. of water to drink containing 4 c.c. of the pure culture of *S. necrophorus.* Fresh water was not added to the water bottle until 12 hours later. The animals were monitored as in Experiment 2 for 18 days, when they were operated upon as in Experiment 1, except, once again, no culture was injected into the test segments. Postoperatively, the protocol of Experiment 1 was followed and an autopsy performed at death or killing after 5 weeks.

Bacteriology. The *Sphaerophorus necrophorus* culture was isolated from the blood of an infant in the nursery of the Cincinnati General Hospital. A stock culture was maintained in modified Brewer's thioglycollate broth (BBL). It was transferred to fresh medium at 2 to 4 week intervals, incubated at 37° C. for 24 hours, and then stored at 4° C. For these animal experiments the organism was grown in a continuous culture apparatus[7] using modified Brewer's thioglycollate broth containing 0.002M glucose at a dilution rate of 0.68 hour^{-1}. The culture at this dilution rate contained 4×10^9 viable organisms per cubic centimeter and appeared as small gram-negative bacilli with bipolar staining in Gram-stained smears. Samples of the culture were sealed in vials which were then sprayed with 2 percent peracetic acid solution and passed into the isolators on the day of the experiments.

Samples of the ileal stool at operation, stool from each rat and material from each isolator at weekly intervals, and the peritoneal cavities at death or killing were placed in freshly boiled and cooled modified Brewer's thioglycollate broth, tubed in 10 ml. quantities in 16 by 150 mm. screw-capped tubes. After 4 to 7 days' incubation at 37° C., aliquots of the broth cultures were streaked on blood agar plates (trypticase soy agar containing 5 percent sheep blood volume for volume) and incubated both aerobically and anaerobically[8] at 37° C. for 5 to 7 days. Gram-stained smears of the cultures, feces, and ileal contents were examined by direct microscopy.

RESULTS

Experiment 1, strangulation after direct intraintestinal contamination. The animals with hemorrhagic (venous) strangulation lived an average of 15 hours after operation, those with ischemic (arterial and venous) strangulation lived 143 hours, while two out of the three without strangulation lived to be killed after 8 weeks (Table I). The combination of necrotic bowel and *Sphaerophorus necrophorus* was lethal in this experiment.

Postoperatively, the three animals with ischemic strangulation lost about 100 grams by death. Those without strangulation lost 50 to 80 grams in 2 to 4 days, regained the loss by 4 weeks, and changed little thereafter. The animals with venous strangulation died so rapidly that their postoperative laboratory values were not obtained.

The temperatures of the survivors varied little in the postoperative period. The temperatures of those animals with ischemic bowel were 4 to 5° C. below normal for 2 to 3 days before death. The initial WBC rose to 20,000 during the first week in the control animals and remained near this level until they were killed. The WBC of

Table I. *Intestinal strangulation in rats monocontaminated with* Sphaerophorus necrophorus

Experiment No.	*Route of contamination*	*Type of strangulation*	*No. of animals for analysis*	*Survival time of individual animals (hours)*
1	Intraintestinal	None	3	275,* —,† —†
		Venous	3	8, 18, 19
		Arterial and venous	3	9, 116, 254
2	Intraperitoneal	None	2	8, —†
		Venous	3	27, —,† —†
		Arterial and venous	3	158,* —,† —†
3	Oral	None	2	—,† —†
		Venous	3	11, 25, —†
		Arterial and venous	3	—,† —,† —†

*Died of simple chronic intestinal obstruction.
†Killed 5 to 8 weeks after operation.

those with ischemic strangulation rose to 30,000 to 60,000 at 2 to 4 days and dropped to 16,000 to 27,000 at 1 week. The hematocrit of the control animals and those with ischemic strangulation dropped from 50 percent at operation to 35 percent at 1 to 2 days, and averaged 40 percent at 1 week.

At autopsy, the animals with venous strangulation had a very hemorrhagic, dark red, distended, thinned-out test segment which was usually leaking the intraluminal contents. There was 2 to 5 c.c. of dark red fluid in the peritoneal cavity. The segments with arterial and venous strangulation were white, thin, occasionally distended with gas, and necrotic. There was no peritoneal fluid. After 8 weeks, the test segments in the control animals were intact but markedly thinned, distended, and measured 1.5 cm. diameter by 8 to 10 cm. long. They were filled with thick, whitish-yellow mucus mixed with the small amount of retained stool. There were a few peritoneal adhesions about the test segments.

The initial stool cultures from all the animals and the culture of the isolator were sterile. By the end of the first postoperative week fecal smears of all the surviving animals showed large numbers of gram-negative bacilli. *Sphaerophorus necrophorus* was isolated in pure culture from the weekly samples of feces and materials from the isolator until after the fifth postoperative week. At that time the two survivors from this experiment were combined with the surviving animals from Experiments 2 and 3. Cultures at the termination of the experiments revealed *S. necrophorus* and *Staphylococcus epidermidis,* a secondary accidental contaminant.

Experiment 2, strangulation after intraperitoneal contamination. One animal died 12 hours after the intraperitoneal injection of *S. necrophorus.* At autopsy its cecum was distended with gas to twice the size of that of a germ-free animal. The eight remaining animals lost 10 to 30 grams during the first 2 days and gradually regained their preinjection weights. No significant change in the activity, temperature, WBC, or hematocrit was noted.

After 11 days, the animals were operated upon, and five of the eight lived until killing at 6 weeks (Table I). There was no significant difference in survival of any of the three groups. One control animal died after 8 hours and the autopsy was unremarkable. One animal with venous strangulation died after 27 hours, and the cecum was massively distended with gas similar to that found in the one animal that died after the intraperitoneal injections. One animal with ischemic strangulation died of simple chronic intestinal obstruction after 158 hours.

Postoperatively, each animal lost about 40 grams during the first four days and then began to gain. After 6 weeks, all weighed within 20 grams of their initial weights.

Very little change in temperature was observed in the survivors. The initial average hematocrit of 45 percent dropped to 35 percent at 1 day in the control and ischemic strangulation groups, while it fell to 30 percent in those animals with venous strangulation. All hematocrits were above 40 percent after 2 weeks. The WBC had dropped 2,000 to 5,000 in all groups at 24 hours. At 4 days in both groups with necrotic test segments, the WBC was about 20,000 and ranged from 15,000 to 40,000 over the next 4 weeks. After operation, the WBC never returned to normal in any of the groups.

At killing, the control animal had a dilated, intact test segment similar to that found in the control animals of Experiment 1. Each of the strangulated test segments was a 2 to 3 cm. diameter thick-walled "cyst" which was filled with small amounts of stool and thick yellow mucus. These "cysts" were adherent on all sides to loops of intestine or omentum through which they obtained their blood supplies. There was no peritoneal fluid.

Initially, the isolator and the stools from all the animals were sterile. At operation no organisms were observed in smears of the ileal contents, but large numbers of gram-negative bacilli were observed in the feces of all animals. *Sphaerophorus necrophorus* was isolated in pure culture from the ileal and fecal material at operation, and from all the postoperative stool and isolator samples for the next 4 weeks. At this time *S. epidermidis* was also detected, as previously mentioned.

Experiment 3, strangulation after oral contamination. All nine animals lived to be operated upon 18 days after the oral feeding of *S. necrophorus*. Each rat lost 15 to 30 grams within 48 hours after the feeding, but had regained this weight at 1 week. Although the weight loss may have been due to the dietary restrictions, it was our impression that the animals were somewhat less active after the feeding. However, the serial temperatures, WBC's, and hematocrits showed no change.

At operation, one animal died shortly after receiving the usual intramuscular dose of sodium pentobarbital. Six of the remaining eight lived until they were killed after 5 weeks (Table I). Two of the three animals with venous strangulation died 11 and 25 hours after operation. At autopsy, they had the typical findings of venous strangulation described in Experiment 1.

Postoperatively, the values of the weight, temperature, WBC, and hematocrit of the animals corresponded to those animals in the same groups described in Experiment 2.

At killing, the animals with ischemic strangulation had the same autopsy findings as described in Experiment 2, while the findings in the control group were similar to those in Experiments 1 and 2. The single animal with venous strangulation which lived until it was killed had a 2 cm. diameter cystic mass located between several loops of intestine. This mass represented either an interloop abscess or a very thin revascularized test segment filled with old fecal material, blood, and a little mucus.

Initially, the isolator and all stools from the animals were sterile, but *S. necrophorus* was detected in the feces of the animals 24 hours after oral feeding and in all subsequent cultures. Although no organisms were observed in Gram-stained smears of the ileal contents at operation, cultures of this material revealed *S. necrophorus*. *Staphylococcus epidermidis* was also detected in cultures of feces and various materials from the isolator during the latter part of the experiment.

DISCUSSION

A similar ischemic or hemorrhagic intestinal strangulation was uniformly fatal in rats with a conventional bacterial flora.[17] In contrast, up to 15 percent of the small intestine can be hemorrhagically strangulated and 75 percent ischemically strangulated in the germ-free rat without a death.[16] Although *S. necrophorus* had little effect on the germ-free rats after either oral or intraperitoneal injection, its combination with necrotic tissue was lethal.

Hemorrhagic strangulation appeared to be more toxic than ischemic strangulation in all three experiments. This may be due to the additive effect of a nonlethal blood loss or the bacterial potentiating action of the blood.[4, 11] Although the surgical procedures were identical in all experiments, there were fewer fatalities in Experiments 2 and 3. This could have been due to increased host resistance after the intraperitoneal or oral contaminations, or it may be possible that the number of organisms in the small intestine of these animals was not sufficient to initiate an infection of the test segment. In normal animals, the Bacteroidaceae are found in large numbers in the colon, in contrast to relatively small numbers in the small intestine,[12] and it is likely that there was a similar distribution preoperatively in the monocontaminated animals. The fact that no organisms were observed in direct smears of the ileal contents but large numbers of gram-negative bacilli were seen in smears of the feces at the time of operation tends to support this view.

Spaerophorus necrophorus is a gram-negative, nonspore-forming, strictly anaerobic, highly pleomorphic organism. It appears as cocci, bacilli, filaments 80 to 100 μ long and 0.75 to 1.5 μ thick, spherical bodies, and even L forms in appropriate media.[7] It is a normal inhabitant of the oral cavity and the intestinal and genitourinary tracts of man and animals. The organism is associated with a variety of infections in man, ranging from relatively benign lesions to fulminating processes complicated with septicemia, and is frequently isolated in pure culture. Numerous animal diseases (calf diphtheria, labial necrosis of rabbits, liver abscess in various animals, and foot rot in sheep) have also been attributed to this organism. Isolates from animal infections are usually more pathogenic for laboratory animals than those from human sources. Rats are usually resistant to infection by animal as well as human strains. Animal strains produce two types of toxin (beta and gamma) while the human strains produce only beta toxin.[13]

Although these experiments prove only that *S. necrophorus* can be lethal in intestinal strangulation in monocontaminated rats, it is possible that this organism or other Bacteroidaceae may be an important factor in death from intestinal strangulation in the human.

SUMMARY

Although vast numbers of gram-negative, nonspore-forming, anaerobic bacilli of the family Bacteroidaceae inhabit the intestinal tract of man, their significance in intestinal strangulation is unknown. Therefore, the natural course of intestinal strangulation was studied in a series of germ-free rats monocontaminated with a highly pleomorphic member of this family, *Sphaerophorus necrophorus*.

Contamination of a small intestinal test segment at the time of either ischemic or hemorrhagic strangulation was fatal. Neither oral nor intraperitoneal contamination, alone, was toxic. Although ischemic strangulation several days after oral contamination was not fatal, hemorrhagic strangulation resulted in several deaths. This result might be explained by the added stress of a nonlethal hemorrhage, or by the bacterial potentiating action of blood.

These experiments suggest that the intestinal Bacteroidaceae may be an important lethal bacterial factor in death from intestinal strangulation.

The authors wish to acknowledge the advice of Drs. W. A. Altemeier and E. O. Hill of the Department of Surgery, University of Cincinnati, Cincinnati, Ohio. We would also like to acknowledge the expert technical assistance of Mr. Mathew Maley.

REFERENCES

1. Barnett, W. O., Oliver, R. I., and Elliott, R. L.: Elimination of the lethal properties of gangrenous bowel segments, Ann. Surg. **167:** 912, 1968.
2. Bishop, R. F., and Allcock, E. A.: Bacterial flora of the small intestine in acute intestinal obstruction, Brit. M. J. **1:** 766, 1960.
3. Bornside, G. H., and Cohn, I., Jr.: Bacteriology, spectrophotometry and toxicity in strangulation intestinal obstruction, J. A. M. A. **179:** 526, 1962.
4. Bornside, G. H., and Cohn, I., Jr.: Hemoglobin as a bacterial virulence—enhancing factor in fluids produced in strangulation intestinal obstruction, Am. Surgeon **34:** 63, 1968.

5. Breed, R. S., Murray, E. G. D., and Smith, N. R.: Bergey's manual of determinative bacteriology, ed. 7, Baltimore, 1957, The Williams & Wilkins Company.
6. Donaldson, R. M., Jr.: Normal bacterial populations of the intestine and their relation to intestinal function, New England J. Med. **270:** 938, 1964.
7. Dowell, V. R., Jr., Loper, J. C., and Hill, E. O.: Constancy of deoxyribonucleic acid base composition in the transition of *Sphaerophorus necrophorus* from bacilli to large bodies, J. Bact. **88:** 1805, 1964.
8. Mueller, J. H., and Miller, P. A.: A modification of Rosenthal's chromium-sulfuric acid method for anaerobic cultures, J. Bact. **41:** 301, 1941.
9. Prevot, A. R.: Manual for the classification and determination of the anaerobic bacteria, first American ed., translated by Fredette, V., Philadelphia, 1966, Lea & Febiger, Publishers.
10. Saksena, D. S., Block, M. A., McHenry, M. C., and Truant, J. P.: Bacteroidaceae: Anaerobic organisms encountered in surgical infections, SURGERY **63:** 261, 1968.
11. Simmons, R. L., Diggs, J. W., and Sleeman, H. K.: Pathogenesis of peritonitis. III. Local adjuvant action of hemoglobin in experimental *E. coli* peritonitis, SURGERY **63:** 810, 1968.
12. Smith, H. W.: The development of the flora of the alimentary tract in young animals, J. Path. & Bact. **90:** 495, 1965.
13. Smith, L. DS., and Holdeman, L. V.: The pathogenic anaerobic bacteria, Springfield, Ill., 1968, Charles C Thomas, Publisher.
14. Wilson, G. S., and Miles, A. A.: Topley and Wilson's principles of bacteriology and immunity, ed. 5, London, 1964, Edward Arnold (Publishers) Ltd.
15. Yale, C. E.: Experimental strangulated intestinal obstruction, SURGERY **66:** 338, 1969.
16. Yale, C. E.: Ischemic intestinal strangulation in germfree rats, Arch. Surg. In press.
17. Yale, C. E., and Altemeier, W. A.: Intestinal obstruction in germfree rats, Arch. Surg. **91:** 241, 1965.

Lymphatic absorption of intraperitoneal endotoxin in the dog

RONALD DANIELE, M.D.
HIRA SINGH, M.D.
HUBERT E. APPERT, PH.D.
FREDERICK W. PAIRENT, PH.D.
JOHN M. HOWARD, M.D.
PHILADELPHIA, PA.
From the Departments of Surgery, Physiology, and Biological Chemistry, Hahnemann Medical College

It is generally accepted that substances with a large molecular weight are absorbed from extracellular fluid spaces via the lymphatic system. Bacterial endotoxin is believed to have a molecular weight in the range of 700,000. It might, therefore, be postulated that endotoxic substances produced during peritonitis are absorbed into the bloodstream predominantly by way of the lymphatic system. The purpose of the present study has been to evaluate this concept on the basis of the experimental intraperitoneal injection of endotoxin in the dog.

The lymphatic drainage of the dog's peritoneum has been studied by Higgins and Graham[6] who followed the passage of graphite particles from the peritoneal cavity. These particles became visible in sternal lymphatics leading to the right duct well before they could be identified in the lymph of the left thoracic duct. Similarly, Courtice and Steinbeck[4] studied the absorption of plasma labeled with Evans blue from the peritoneal cavity of cats. These investigators showed that about 10 percent of the labeled plasma could be recovered in the lymph collected from the intubated left thoracic duct during a period of 5 hours. Approximately twice that amount was recovered from the intubated right thoracic duct. At the end of the 5 hours, only about 2 percent of the injected plasma was present in the blood.

Blood levels, clearance from the blood, and tissue distribution of intravenously injected endotoxin have been studied in rats[1] with the use of ^{131}I, and in rabbits, mice, and dogs with the use of ^{51}Cr.[2, 8] The current experiments were designed to investigate the rate of absorption and the tissue distribution of ^{51}Cr-labeled *Escherichia coli* endotoxin in control and lymph duct cannulated dogs, following its intraperitoneal injection.

METHODS

Ten mongrel dogs of either sex, weighing between 15 and 20 kilograms, were studied. The first five served as control animals. Under sodium phenobarbital anesthesia, chromium-51–tagged endotoxin (Bacto-Lipopolysaccharide *E. coli* 026:B6, Difco Laboratories, Detroit, Mich.) was injected into the peritoneal cavity in doses of either 1 or 2 mg. per kilogram of body weight. Injection was made via a tiny incision in the abdominal wall to ensure that the solution entered the peritoneal cavity.

In the second group of five experiments, a similar injection was performed following cannulation of the right and left thoracic ducts at the base of the neck. The ducts were cannulated with a fine polyethylene catheter. Additional animals were excluded

Supported by Grants AI-04064, HE-04182, and HE-05553 from the National Institutes of Health.
Received for publication Feb. 4, 1969.

because cannulation of the right lymph duct could not be achieved.

A femoral artery and vein were cannulated for continuous measurement of arterial pressure and for serial blood sampling, respectively. Blood samples were collected hourly, and lymph from the right and left thoracic ducts was collected continuously in periods of 1 hour each for a total of 8 hours.

At the termination of the experiment, the animal was killed and the amount of endotoxin remaining in the peritoneal cavity was determined by infusion of 500 ml. of cold saline into the peritoneal cavity, manually mixing the fluid within the cavity and then aspirating the peritoneal contents for assay purposes. In addition, immediate autopsy permitted removal of the liver, kidney, spleen, lung, stomach, intestines, and abdominal lymph nodes. The organs were rinsed, weighed, and homogenized in cold saline solution according to the method of Braude and associates.[2] The amount of endotoxin recovered in each organ was calculated as a percentage of the dose initially injected after measurement of the specific activity of the homogenate of the respective organ.

The endotoxin was labeled with $^{51}CrCl_2$ after the method of Braude and co-workers.[2] The endotoxin was diluted in 0.9 percent sodium chloride solution to a concentration of 1 mg. per milliliter. The radioactivity of the resultant solution was measured with a well-type solid scintillation detector, and the specific activity of the sample was calculated and used to determine the amount of radioactive material injected.

In order to test the relationship between ^{51}Cr activity of the lymph and endotoxin activity, bioassay experiments were performed with mice. In these experiments, the radioactive lymph recovered from the dogs was injected into mice and the toxicity quantitated by $L.D._{50}$ measurements. Prior to the radioactive labeling procedure, an intraperitoneal dose of 0.22 mg. of endotoxin per kilogram of body weight was required to produce an $L.D._{50}$ in mice. Subsequent to labeling of the endotoxin with ^{51}Cr. and exhaustive dialysis of the preparation, an $L.D._{50}$ of 0.19 mg. per kilogram of body weight was determined for the endotoxin. The specific activity (ratio of c.p.m. to $L.D._{50}$ value) of the labeled preparation was calculated and was compared with the specific activity of the lymph recovered from the right thoracic duct of a dog treated with ^{51}Cr-endotoxin. The results indicated that the endotoxin recovered from the lymph in these experiments maintained its toxicity in passage from the peritoneal cavity. Therefore, the radioactivity of all samples was taken as an actual measure of endotoxin concentration.

Blood volume was estimated as 9 percent of body weight.

RESULTS

The recovery and distribution of the radioactivity expressed as the percentage of that injected is shown in Table I. Total blood levels shown in Table I were calculated from the concentration at the termination of the experiment and in every experiment this sample had the maximal radioactivity.

Table I. *Distribution of intraperitoneal ^{51}Cr-endotoxin* (E. coli) *in control dogs**

Experiment No.	*Duration (hr.)*	*Blood*	*Liver*	*Spleen*	*Lungs*	*Kidney*	*Lymph nodes*	*Peritoneal cavity washings*	*Total recovery*
1	6	6.4	9.0	1.8	4.5	2.3	—	—	—
2	8	11.2	7.2	2.1	2.8	4.0	—	—	—
3	10	7.9	11.9	3.0	7.9	4.4	2.0	23.0	60.1
4	8	10.3	8.1	1.4	6.4	6.0	3.0	30.0	65.2
5	8	7.3	6.4	1.9	7.8	3.8	—	38.0	65.2
Average		8.7	8.5	2.0	5.8	4.0	2.5	30.3	63.5

*Percent of injected radioactivity.

Table II. *Distribution of intralymphatic* ^{51}*Cr-endotoxin* (E. coli) *in cannulated dogs**

Experiment No.	*Duration (hr.)*	*Blood*	*Liver*	*Spleen*	*Lungs*	*Kidney*	*Heart*
1	10	4.1	1.6	2.2	1.3	2.0	—
2	9	2.8	2.5	1.8	2.0	2.1	—
3	8	1.6	1.0	0.9	1.1	3.0	—
4	8	3.8	2.6	2.0	5.3	5.9	0.3
5	8	2.2	1.3	1.0	2.1	0.02	0.06
Average		2.9	1.8	1.6	2.4	2.6	0.2

*Percent of injected radioactivity.

In the five uncannulated control dogs, the maximal radioactivity in the blood ranged between 6.4 to 11.7 percent of the injected dose, a mean of 8.7 percent. In the cannulated animals the blood level was significantly lower, ranging from 1.6 to 4.1 percent of the injected dose, with a mean of 2.8 percent.

The recovery of radioactivity in the right lymph duct ranged between 5 to 24 percent (mean 15.1 percent) of the injected dose, while the recovery from the left thoracic duct ranged from 6.5 to 9.6 percent (mean 5.7 percent).

The mean values for the amount of injected endotoxin recovered from the liver, spleen, lungs, and kidneys were approximately equal to each other (2 to 4 percent of the injected dose). About one third of the injected dose of endotoxin could be recovered from the peritoneal cavity 8 hours following its injection.

DISCUSSION

The tissue distribution of endotoxin in this series of experiments was similar to that found by other investigators.[1, 2, 7, 8] Starzecki and associates[8] found that in dogs the highest concentrations of labeled endotoxin after intravenous injection could be recovered from the liver and spleen (2 to 4 μg per gram of tissue). The concentration of endotoxin in the lymph nodes, lungs, adrenals, and kidneys was considerably lower. The investigators did not calculate total recoveries. It would appear from their data, however, that if organ weight was considered the endotoxin found in the liver, spleen, and lungs at the end of 24 hours could account for most of the endotoxin which had been injected.

Braude, Carey, and Zalesky[2] studied the tissue distribution of chromium-labeled endotoxin in rabbits. They found that about 17 percent of the intravenously injected endotoxin could be recovered in the liver within 2 hours after its injection into the bloodstream. About 1 to 2 percent of the injected endotoxin could be found in the lungs and another 1 to 2 percent in the intestines. The spleen contained less than 1 percent.

It appears that very little information is available concerning the fate of intraperitoneally injected endotoxin, a problem pertinent to peritonitis, for it is probable that many bacteria in peritonitis release their endotoxin into the inflamed peritoneal cavity.

Barnes, Lupfer, and Henry[1] found that in rats, only 10 percent of the intraperitoneally injected dose of ^{131}I-labeled Flexner dysentery antigen was absorbed into the bloodstream after 18 hours. The rest was retained by the visceral organs. Our observations also indicate that a large amount of endotoxin injected intraperitoneally is not immediately absorbed but remains in the peritoneal fluid. In two experiments in which the measurements were made 8 hours after injection (Table II), the stomach, intestine, and mesentery retained a large amount of the endotoxin (22 and 28 percent of the total recovered radioactivity). These observations emphasize the importance of local mechanisms within the peritoneal cavity in delaying or minimizing the absorption of the toxins.

The recovery of endotoxin from right and left thoracic ducts indicates that the lym-

Stomach and intestine	Lymph nodes	Urine	Right lymph duct	Thoracic duct	Peritoneal cavity washings	Total recovery
—	3.0	—	18.5	5.2	34.0	71.9
—	2.0	—	24.2	6.5	17.0	60.9
—	—	—	14.3	9.6	42.0	73.5
13.9	—	3.8	5.4	5.4	15.6	64.0
27.8	0.5	8.3	12.7	1.8	41.4	99.2
20.9	1.8	6.1	15.0	5.7	30.0	73.9

phatic drainage of the peritoneal cavity of the dog is similar to that of other species.[3, 4] The recovery of endotoxin from the right lymph duct greatly exceeded that recovered from the left thoracic duct in all but one experiment (Table II), although the volume of lymph collected from the left duct far exceeded that from the right side (59 versus 4.7 ml. per hour).

Little information is available about the drainage of the peritoneal cavity of the human. If the drainage of the human peritoneal cavity is similar to that of the dog, then it would appear that during peritonitis a substantial amount of endotoxin may bypass the left thoracic duct and enter the circulation through the right thoracic duct. Cannulation of the left thoracic duct is feasible in humans and has been performed by several investigators.[9] The simultaneous cannulation of both left and right thoracic ducts in humans has often been performed by Falor.[5] It is quite conceivable that long-term cannulation, particularly of the right lymph duct, might find an occasional clinical use in partially draining bacterial toxins from the peritoneal cavity, thereby decreasing the quantity absorbed into the system.

SUMMARY

During a period of 8 hours following the injection of ^{51}Cr-labeled endotoxin into the peritoneal cavity of dogs, 15 percent of the injected endotoxin could be recovered from the lymph of the right thoracic duct, 6 percent from the left thoracic duct. The amount of endotoxin recovered from the right (15 percent) and left (6 percent) ducts exceeded the total extraperitoneal recovery (14.2 percent) of endotoxin from the other organs studied.

REFERENCES

1. Barnes, F. W., Jr., Lupfer, H., and Henry, S. S.: The biochemical target of Flexner dysentery somatic antigen; studies on the rat using antigen labeled with I^{131}, Yale J. Biol. & Med. **24:** 384, 1952.
2. Braude, A. I., Carey, F. J., and Zalesky, M.: Studies with radioactive endotoxin; correlation of physiologic effects with distribution of radioactivity in rabbits injected with lethal doses of *E. coli* endotoxin labelled with radioactive sodium chromate, J. Clin. Invest. **34:** 858, 1955.
3. Courtice, F. C., Harding, J., and Steinbeck, A. W.: The removal of free red blood cells from the peritoneal cavity of animals, Australian J. Exper. Biol. & Med. Sc. **31:** 215, 1953.
4. Courtice, F. C., and Steinbeck, A. W.: The lymphatic drainage of plasma from the peritoneal cavity of the cat, Australian J. Exper. Biol. & Med. Sc. **28:** 161, 1950.
5. Falor, W. H.: Bilateral scalene lymph node excision: Bilateral thoracic duct cannulation, Pacific Med. Surg. **72:** 350, 1964.
6. Higgins, G. M., and Graham, A. S.: Lymphatic drainage from the peritoneal cavity in the dog, Arch. Surg. **19:** 453, 1929.
7. Rowley, D., Howard, J. G., and Jenkin, C. R.: The fate of p^{32}-labeled bacterial lipopolysaccharide in laboratory animals, Lancet **1:** 366, 1956.
8. Starzecki, B., Reddin, J. L., Gran, A., and Spink, W. W.: Distribution of endotoxin-^{51}Cr in normal and endotoxin-resistant dogs, Am. J. Physiol. **213:** 1065, 1967.
9. Werner, B.: Thoracic duct cannulation in man. I. Surgical technique and a clinical study on 79 patients, Acta. chir. Scandinav. **353:** 1, 1965. (Suppl.)

Studies on the functional and biochemical changes during kidney preservation

PAUL A. LOTKE, M.D.*
SORELL L. SCHWARTZ, PH.D.**
BETHESDA, MD.
From the Naval Medical Research Institute, National Naval Medical Center

The recent success with renal transplantation has emphasized related problems in this field, notably that of whole organ storage. Improvement in methods for organ preservation will depend on a better understanding of the biochemical and functional changes that occur in cells during storage and on the development of reliable determinations of the viability and transplantability of stored organs. As an approach to this goal, we have investigated some of the changes that occur in canine kidneys during hypothermic storage under normobaric and hyperbaric conditions, as well as after treatment with hydrocortisone and chloroquine.

Functional changes in the stored kidney were evaluated in vitro by determination of the para-aminohippurate (PAH) uptake and oxygen consumption. The concentration of PAH is a reflection of tubular transport events and evaluates, in part, the ability of the proximal tubular cells to perform an integrated cell function.

Enzymatic changes associated with the stability of lysosomal organelles were examined. de Duve and Wattiaux[3] suggested that the subcellular particles are important in the processes of intracellular digestion and autolysis. Under slightly acidic conditions these membrane-delimited small organelles contain several hydrolytic enzymes which can break down different types of macromolecules. The lytic potentialities of lysosomal enzymes and their release under certain conditions suggest that they are responsible for cell necrosis.[1]

In consideration of the role that lysosomes may have on the storage of kidneys, free and bound lysosomal enzyme activity was evaluated to determine if these parameters might predict the extent of the tissue injury occurring during storage. In addition, we studied the agents known to stabilize the lysosomal membrane, i.e., hydrocortisone and chloroquine,[15] to determine their ability to prolong kidney storage.

METHODS

Canine kidneys were perfused with a solution of equal parts of homologous serum and lactated Ringer's solution. To this mixture was added either hydrocortisone (0.001M) or chloroquine (0.005M). The whole kidney was stored in a thermoelectric cooler[7] at 2° C. under normobaric conditions or three atmospheres (gauge) of oxygen for up to 72 hours. At specific time intervals, cortical sections were removed from the kidneys for functional and enzymatic evaluation.

Functional studies. Cortical sections were

The assertions or opinions contained herein are the private ones of the authors and are not to be construed as official or reflecting the views of the Navy Department or the Naval Service at large. The experiments reported herein were conducted according to the principles enunciated in the "Guide for laboratory animal facilities and care" prepared by the Committee on the Guide for Laboratory Animals Resources, National Academy of Sciences–National Research Council.

Received for publication Feb. 25, 1969.

*Present address: Hospital for Special Surgery, 535 East 70th Street, New York, N. Y. 10021.

**Present address: Department of Pharmacology, Georgetown University Schools of Medicine and Dentistry, Washington, D.C.

studied by the simultaneous in vitro determination of PAH uptake and oxygen consumption with the use of previously described procedures.[6] All experiments were performed in the conventional Warburg apparatus. Cortical sections of 0.4 mm. thickness were sliced in a Stadie-Riggs microtome. Tissue slices weighing approximately 300 milligrams were placed in the main compartment of each vessel which contained 2.7 ml. of a solution containing NaCl, 115 mM.; KCl, 10 mM.; sodium acetate, 11 mM.; calcium chloride, 0.75 mM.; phosphate buffer (pH 7.4), 7.5 mM.; and sodium para-aminohippurate (PAH), 7.4 $\times 10^{-5}$ mM. The gas space was filled with oxygen. The vessels were shaken in a water bath at 25° C., and oxygen consumption was recorded during a 30 minute period. Oxygen uptake was expressed as QO_2 (c.c. of O_2 per gram of wet weight per hour).

After 1 hour in the bath, the vessels were removed and chilled immediately. The slices and solutions were assayed for PAH content. The extent of the accumulation within the cortical slice is estimated by measuring the slice to media (S/M) ratio for PAH.

Biochemical assays. The adjacent cortical tissue was sectioned and assayed for the lysosomal enzymes, acid phosphatase (AcPase) and acid ribonuclease (AcRNAase), in both the sediment and supernatant fractions.

Aliquots of renal cortex weighing approximately 1 gram were homogenized in ice-cold 0.9M sucrose (1:10 wet weight to volume) with the use of a glass homogenizer with a motor-driven Teflon pestle. Red cells, whole cells, connective tissue, and other debris were removed by centrifugation at 11 $\times$ g for 2 minutes. The sediment was discarded and the resultant supernatant considered as the whole homogenate. In order to separate the total sedimentable acid hydrolase activity, the homogenate was then centrifuged at 150,000 $\times$ g for 60 minutes. The sediment was resuspended and diluted according to the needs of the enzyme assay and adjusted to contain a final concentration of 0.1 percent Triton X-100 in 0.05M acetate buffer, pH 5. The supernatant was treated in a similar fashion.

Acid phosphatase (orthophosphoric monoester phosphohydrolase, E.C.3.1.3.2.) activity was determined according to a previously described procedure with p-nitrophenylphosphate being used as the substrate.[12] The activity is expressed as the number of millimicromoles of p-nitrophenol liberated per milligram of protein per minute.

Acid ribonuclease (polyribonucleotide l-oligonucleotidotransferase (cyclizing) E.C.2.7.-3.10.) activity was determined by previously described methods.[12] Activity is expressed as the change in optical density (O.D.) at 260 mμ per 30 minutes per milligram of protein under the conditions of the assay.

Protein was determined by the method of Lowry and associates,[8] utilizing bovine albumin as the reference standard.

All data is presented as the mean ± standard error of the mean. Paired comparisons were made by Student's t test.[14] Multiple comparisons were made by a multiple range test utilizing the Neuman-Keuls method.[16] Statistical significance is considered as $p = 0.05$ or less.

RESULTS

Functional studies. The effects of the duration of cold storage and lysosomal stabilizing agents on PAH uptake and oxygen consumption are shown in Figs. 1 to 4. At all points except the 12 hour measurement in Fig. 1 and the 36 hour measurement in Fig. 3, there was a significant difference between the treated groups and the control group. There was no significant difference between the hydrocortisone-treated group and the chloroquine-treated group.

These results indicate that storage with perfusate containing hydrocortisone or chloroquine significantly increases the ability of kidney slices to concentrate PAH and consume oxygen as compared with kidneys stored without these agents. Second, these functions are maintained at higher levels for longer periods of time when the kidneys are stored in hyperbaric oxygen rather than under normobaric conditions.

Analysis of "free" and "bound" lysosomal enzymes. The data presented in Tables I and

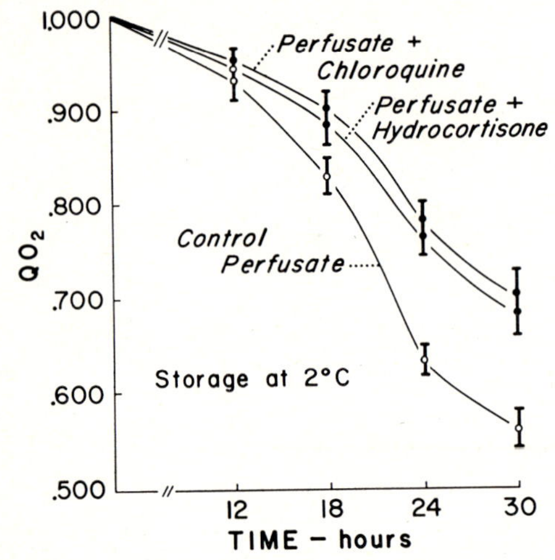

Fig. 1. Oxygen consumption of cortical slices after storage at 2° C. in normobaric environment. Mean ± S.E., N ≧ 24.

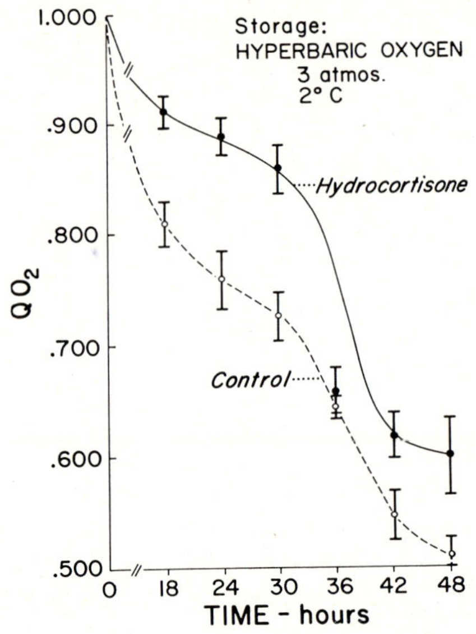

Fig. 3. Oxygen consumption of cortical slices after storage at 2° C. in 100 percent oxygen at 3 atmospheres of pressure. Mean ± S.E., N ≧ 16.

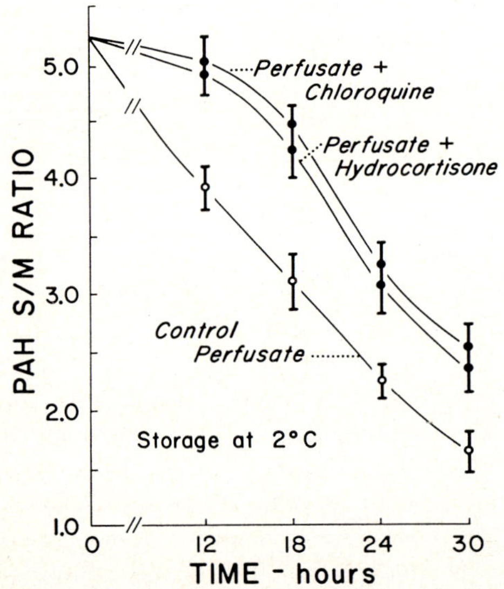

Fig. 2. PAH uptake of cortical slices after storage at 2° C. in normobaric environment. Mean ± S.E., N ≧ 16.

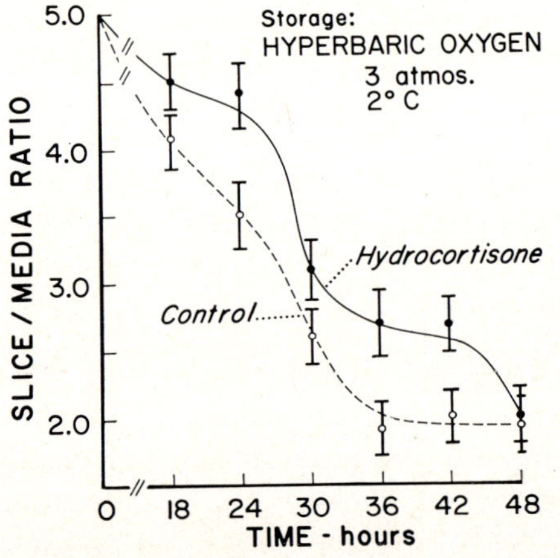

Fig. 4. PAH uptake of cortical slices after storage at 2° C. in 100 percent oxygen at 3 atmospheres of pressure. Mean ± S.E., N ≧ 16.

II represent the specific activities obtained from the untreated tissue under normobaric and hyperbaric conditions. With the Student's t test, it was concluded that no significant differences existed between the values shown for the untreated control tissue and the corresponding values obtained for tissues treated with hydrocortisone.

Table I shows the specific activities of enzymes in tissues stored at 2° C. under normal oxygen tension for periods up to 30 hours. With the multiple range test, it was found that for the supernatant AcPase activity ("free enzyme") the values at 0 and 3 hours are significantly lower than the value obtained at 30 hours, and that some

Table I. *Specific activities of lysosomal enzymes in untreated renal cortices stored at 2° C. under normal oxygen tension*

Storage time (hours)	Acid phosphatase (micromoles p-nitrophenol liberated/min./mg. protein)			Acid ribonuclease (change in O.D. 260 mμ/30 min./mg. protein)		
	Sediment	Supernatant	N	Sediment	Supernatant	N
0	20.14 ± 1.27	18.41 ± 1.50	6	1.09 ± 0.16	0.71 ± 0.14	6
3	21.29 ± 1.27	16.11 ± 1.96	5	1.19 ± 0.17	0.36 ± 0.13	5
6	25.89 ± 2.19	23.59 ± 3.34	5	1.41 ± 0.17	0.89 ± 0.22	5
12	23.59 ± 2.42	25.30 ± 1.32	9	1.29 ± 0.25	0.90 ± 0.22	5
18	20.14 ± 2.70	20.71 ± 1.04	5	1.51 ± 0.23	0.95 ± 0.08	5
24	20.71 ± 2.30	24.16 ± 1.96	9	1.58 ± 0.23	0.76 ± 0.14	7
30	30.49 ± 1.67	27.61 ± 1.50	5	1.67 ± 0.13	1.10 ± 0.30	5

but not all of the values between 6 and 24 hours are significantly different than the 0 and 3 hour activities. No significant differences were noted for the supernatant AcRNAase activity or from the sedimentable fractions ("bound enzyme").

Table II represents the sedimentable and supernatant activity of AcPase obtained in tissues stored in a hyperbaric oxygen atmosphere. For the supernatant activity, all values between 0 and 48 hours are significantly lower than 72 hour values. No differences were found to exist among the data between 0 and 48 hours. No significant differences were noted to exist within the sedimentable values.

Table II. *Specific activity of acid phosphatase in untreated renal cortices stored at 2° C. under hyperbaric oxygen tension*

Storage time (hours)	Acid phosphatase (micromoles p-nitrophenol liberated/min./mg. protein)		
	Sediment	Supernatant	N
0	20.14 ± 1.27	18.41 ± 1.50	5
12	19.91 ± 1.32	15.71 ± 2.19	8
24	24.80 ± 2.24	16.68 ± 1.04	6
36	20.42 ± 1.61	15.65 ± 0.86	5
42	25.14 ± 1.32	17.83 ± 1.44	5
48	16.51 ± 2.53	18.41 ± 1.78	5
72	19.33 ± 0.63	40.73 ± 0.75	5

DISCUSSION

These studies of PAH metabolism and oxygen consumption indicate the beneficial effects of the storage in hyperbaric oxygen. The level of in vitro function remains at higher levels for longer periods of time in the kidneys stored in hyperbaric oxygen than those stored under normobaric conditions. This corroborates the studies of others who have demonstrated in vivo the benefits of hyperbaric oxygen storage.[9] In addition, the results demonstrate that hydrocortisone and chloroquine have the ability to prolong function as measured in vitro in the stored kidneys. Whether this is due to their effect on the lysosomal membrane itself or other cell membranes and processes cannot be directly evaluated by this approach.

The enzymatic studies demonstrate several interesting points. The values for the supernatant activity of the acid phosphatase after normobaric storage begin to become significantly elevated above the control values after 3 to 6 hours of storage. This same rise in supernatant activity occurs between 48 and 72 hours in the hyperbaric oxygen–stored kidneys. These studies indicate that the release of enzymes into the supernatant fractions occurs as a function of time, and second, that the release of enzymes can be retarded by storage in hyperbaric oxygen. Similar phenomena have been documented by others under a variety of circumstances including liver stored at 37° C.,[2] and with in vivo high altitude ischemia.[11]

It is also of interest to note that the limit of transplantability of whole kidneys after normobaric hypothermic storage is 6 hours,[5] and in hyperbaric storage it is 48 hours.[10] The correlation of the rise in enzyme levels to transplantability has clear clinical implications and may apply to the assessment of functional viability of a potentially transplantable organ.

The results showed that there were no significant differences in the release of AcPase between kidneys treated with hydrocortisone and those left untreated. This is unexpected since hydrocortisone is a known lysosomal stabilizer. One possible explanation for this may be that the stabilization imparted by the low temperature may be significantly greater than that which can be imparted by the concentration of hydrocortisone used.

The observation that AcRNAase activities were unchanged while alterations in AcPase occurred is not necessarily inconsistent. Somewhat similar results were obtained in a study of the relationship of EDTA-induced renal vacuolization to renal lysosomal enzyme changes.[12] This may be related to the heterogeneity of content lysosomes and the existence of various species of these organelles.[4, 13]

SUMMARY

In summary, we have studied renal cortical sections after storage at 2° C. in normobaric and hyperbaric oxygen conditions by a lysosomal enzyme assay and an in vitro cellular function test. The results indicate that (1) By in vitro measurements, the drugs known to be lysosomal-stabilizing agents protect cell function from the deleterious effects of storage, (2) the release of lysosome enzymes into the supernatant fractions is delayed by hypothermia and hyperbaric conditions, and (3) the rise in enzyme levels may be used as an indication as to the extent of tissue injury occuring during storage.

REFERENCES

1. de Duve, C.: Lysosomes and cell injury, *in* Thomas, L., et al., editors: International symposium on injury, inflammation, and immunity, Baltimore, 1964, The Williams & Wilkins Company, pp. 283-312.
2. de Duve, C., and Beaufay, H.: Tissue fractionation studies. 10. Influence of ischemia on the state of some bound enzymes in rat liver, Biochem. J. **73:** 610, 1959.
3. de Duve, C., and Wattiaux, R.: Functions of lysosomes, Ann. Rev. Physiol. **28:** 435, 1966.
4. de Duve, C., Pressman, B., Gianetto, R., Wattiaux, R., and Appelmans, F.: Tissue fractionation studies. 6. Intracellular distribution patterns of enzymes in rat liver tissues, Biochem. J. **60:** 604, 1955.
5. Dempster, W. J., Kountz, S. L., and Jovanovic, M.: Simple kidney-storage technique, Brit. M. J. **5380:** 407, 1964.
6. Lotke, P. A.: Lysosome stabilizing agents for hypothermic kidney storage, Nature **212:** 512, 1966.
7. Lotke, P. A., and Dolan, M. F.: Thermoelectric cooler for whole organ freezing and thawing, Cryobiology **1:** 289, 1964.
8. Lowry, O. H., Roberts, N. R., Wu, M., Hixon, W. S., and Crawford, E. J.: The quantitative histochemistry of brain. II. Enzyme measurements, J. Biol. Chem. **207:** 19, 1954.
9. Manax, W. G., Block, J. H., Longerbeam, J. K., and Lillehei, R. C.: Successful 24-hour in vitro preservation of canine kidneys by combined use of hyperbaric oxygen and hypothermia, SURGERY **56:** 275, 1964.
10. Manax, W. G., Block, J. H., Eyal, Z., Lyons, G. W., and Lillehei, R. C.. Hypothermia and hyperbaria, J. A. M. A. **192:** 85, 1965.
11. Nelson, B. D.: Hepatic lysosome and serum enzyme alterations in rats exposed to high altitude, Am. J. Physiol. **211:** 651, 1966.
12. Schwartz, S. L., Hayes, J. R., Ide, R. S., Johnson, C. B., and Doolan, P. D.: Studies of the nephrotoxicity of ethylenediaminetetraacetic acid, Biochem. Pharmacol. **15:** 377, 1966.
13. Shibko, S., and Tappel, A. L.: Rat kidney lysosomes, isolation and properties, Biochem. J. **95:** 731, 1965.
14. Snedacor, G. W.: Statistical methods, Ames. 1946, Iowa State College Press.
15. Weissman, G.: Labilization and stabilization of lysosomes, Fed. Proc. **23:** 1038, 1964.
16. Winer, B. J.: Statistical principles in experimental design, New York, 1962, McGraw-Hill Book Company, Inc.

Use of saphenous vein homografts for arterial reconstruction: A preliminary report

DAVID A. TICE, M.D.
ERNESTO SANTONI, M.D.
NEW YORK, N. Y.
From the Departments of Surgery, New York University School of Medicine and the New York Veterans Administration Hospital

Occasionally, suitable autogenous saphenous vein is not available for arterial reconstruction. When this occurs, the only substitute is a synthetic graft. The experience with synthetic materials versus autologous vein for femoral-popliteal artery bypass procedures has shown autologous vein to be preferable with a higher long-term patency rate.[1] The following is a preliminary report on the clinical use of saphenous vein homografts for vascular reconstruction.

MATERIALS AND METHODS

Patients undergoing saphenous vein ligation and stripping are asked to sign separate permission to donate the veins to the tissue bank. Patients undergoing vascular reconstruction are informed and sign permission for the use of homograft veins, if it becomes necessary.

The upper one half of the greater saphenous vein from the groin to the knee is removed from the donor under direct vision through several small transverse incisions. All branches are individually ligated and divided. If the vein segment is greater than 10 mm. in diameter, aneurysmal, or otherwise diseased microscopically, it is not used (Fig. 1). Suitable veins are irrigated with a solution containing penicillin and streptomycin in normal saline. A small portion is sent for microscopic examination and culture. Veins that are not sterile are discarded. After preparation, the harvested vein is placed in a sterile sealed jar and stored at –50° C. until used. All veins in this series have been used within 60 days. On the morning of the operation a vein is thawed and small portions again removed for culture and microscopic examination. Femoral-popliteal artery bypass is performed in the usual manner, with a reversed segment of the homograft vein being used. If the vein segment is used for a patch, the unused portion is discarded. Angiography is performed in the operating room before the incisions are closed. All patients receive antibiotic therapy postoperatively.

Received for publication March 6, 1969.

RESULTS

Six patients have had femoral-popliteal artery bypass, with homograft vein. Two patients have had a vein patch with homograft; one had a right vertebral endarterectomy with a vein patch, and the other had a vein patch applied to superficial femoral artery for severe stenosis (Table I). Angiography was performed in all patients in the operating room. The angiograms were similar in appearance, following reconstruction, to angiograms obtained in patients having femoral-popliteal bypass, with autograft veins (Fig. 2).

Failure of the graft occurred in one patient who had a prior femoral-popliteal bypass with an 8 mm. Dacron graft. His distal runoff was fair, and when the Dacron graft closed, severe ischemic changes developed and a homograft vein bypass was performed. This did function well; however,

Table I. *Pertinent clinical details and current status of 8 patients having revascularization with saphenous vein homografts*

Patient	Age	Chief complaint on admission	Location of lesion	Date of procedure	Type of procedure	Current status
V. T.	55	Claudication for 4 months, gangrene of fourth right toe	Occlusion distal third right superficial femoral artery, runoff +++	2-5-1968	Femoral-popliteal bypass—Dacron 8 mm.	
		Failure of the Dacron bypass and localized wound infection		4-4-1968	Femoral-popliteal bypass vein, obtained March 26, 1968	Cellulitis progressed, right above-knee, March 15, 1968
K. N.	70	Bilateral claudication for 6 years, gangrene of right big toe	Bilateral superficial femoral occlusion, runoff ++	4-26-1968	Right femoral-popliteal bypass vein, obtained March 26, 1968	No palpable pulses, lesion healed, bypass patent by angiography
			Total occlusion of left superficial femoral artery	12-5-1968	Left femoral-popliteal bypass vein, obtained Sept. 9, 1968	Palpable pulses, no symptoms
J. L. H.	58	Claudication for 2 years, operation on right side at another hospital, on physical examination no pulses below femoral artery	Right superficial femoral occlusion, runoff +++	6-21-1968	Femoral-popliteal vein, obtained May 7, 1968	Palpable pulses, no symptoms, February, 1968
C. G.	46	Transient ischemic attacks, 1967, unsteady gait	Stenosis of vertebral arteries: right—80%, left—30%	6-24-1968	Patch right vertebral vein, obtained May 21, 1968	Palpable pulses, no symptoms
J. S.	67	Left leg pain and coldness, right bilateral claudication for 10 years, gas endarterectomy, 1967, right above-knee amputation, September, 1967	Narrowing of left superficial femoral artery just above anastomosis	7-16-1968	Arteriotomy and patch of superficial femoral vein, obtained May 21, 1968	Palpable pulses, no symptoms
P. I.	55	Left claudication for six weeks, burning left sole, diabetic	Superficial femoral occlusion, left, runoff ++	7-17-1968	Left femoral-popliteal vein bypass, obtained May 22, 1968	Palpable pulses, no symptoms
M. A.	40	Large ischemic ulcer,right foot	Superficial femoral occlusion, right, runoff 3+	12-13-1968	Right femoral-popliteal vein, obtained Dec. 3, 1968	Palpable pulses, ulcer healed, no symptoms

above the knee amputation was performed for ascending infection and gangrene.

To date, all other patients have patent grafts as indicated by palpable peripheral pulses and disappearance of ischemic symptoms.

DISCUSSION

It is unlikely that this method of preservation preserves the viability of all cellular components in the homograft. Microscopic examination of the vein segments before and after preservation shows little change in

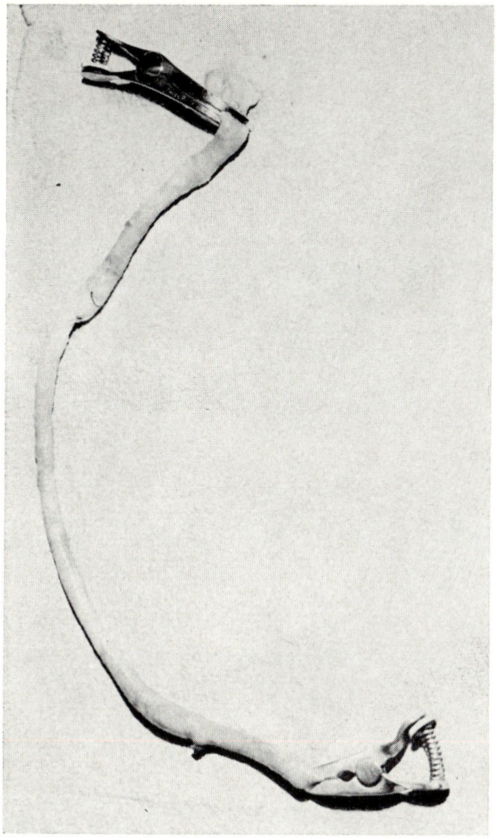

Fig. 1. A segment of saphenous vein averaging 8.5 mm. in diameter and stored for 44 days at –50° C. This photograph was taken just prior to a femoral-popliteal bypass.

architecture. The endothelial layer shows some fragmentation and some separation after preservation; the smooth muscle and connective tissue appear to be unchanged (Fig. 3, *A-D*). Prolonged patency of these homografts suggests that the endothelial layer is replaced by host endothelium. The ultimate fate of collagen and smooth muscle is not clear. Whether they remain undisturbed and serve as a conduit or whether invasion of the homograft by host cells occurs with replacement of connective tissue by the recipient's own collagen, is not clear.

Questions may be raised concerning the ultimate fate of vein homografts in view of the discouraging results with cadaver arterial homografts in the past decade. The early methods of preserving these cadaver grafts have been shown to contribute to accelerated degenerative changes when placed in a biologic system. The current experience with preservation of aortic valve homografts suggests that high-energy sterilization and storage of tissues at low temperature (–50° C.) is the method of choice.[2] Saphenous vein removed under sterile conditions in the operating room can be cultured, irrigated with an appropriate antibiotic solution, and stored immediately at

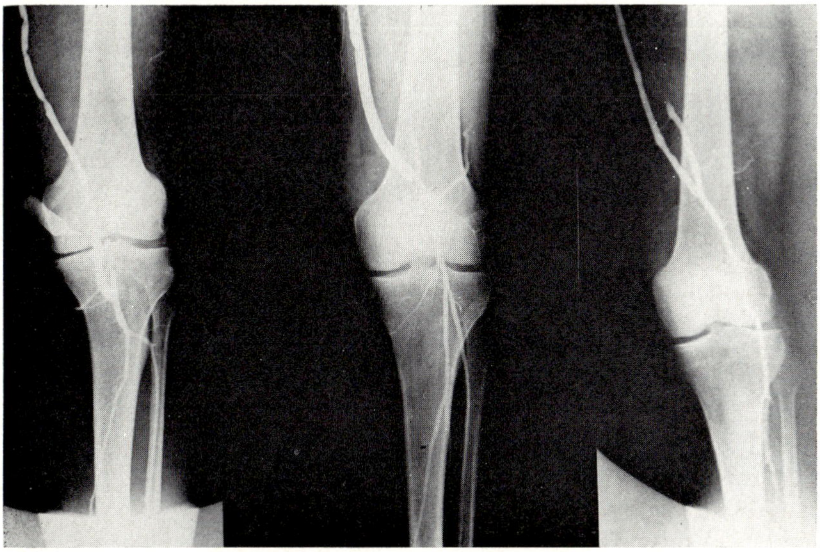

Fig. 2. Intraoperative arteriograms in three patients following femoral-popliteal bypass with a saphenous vein homograft.

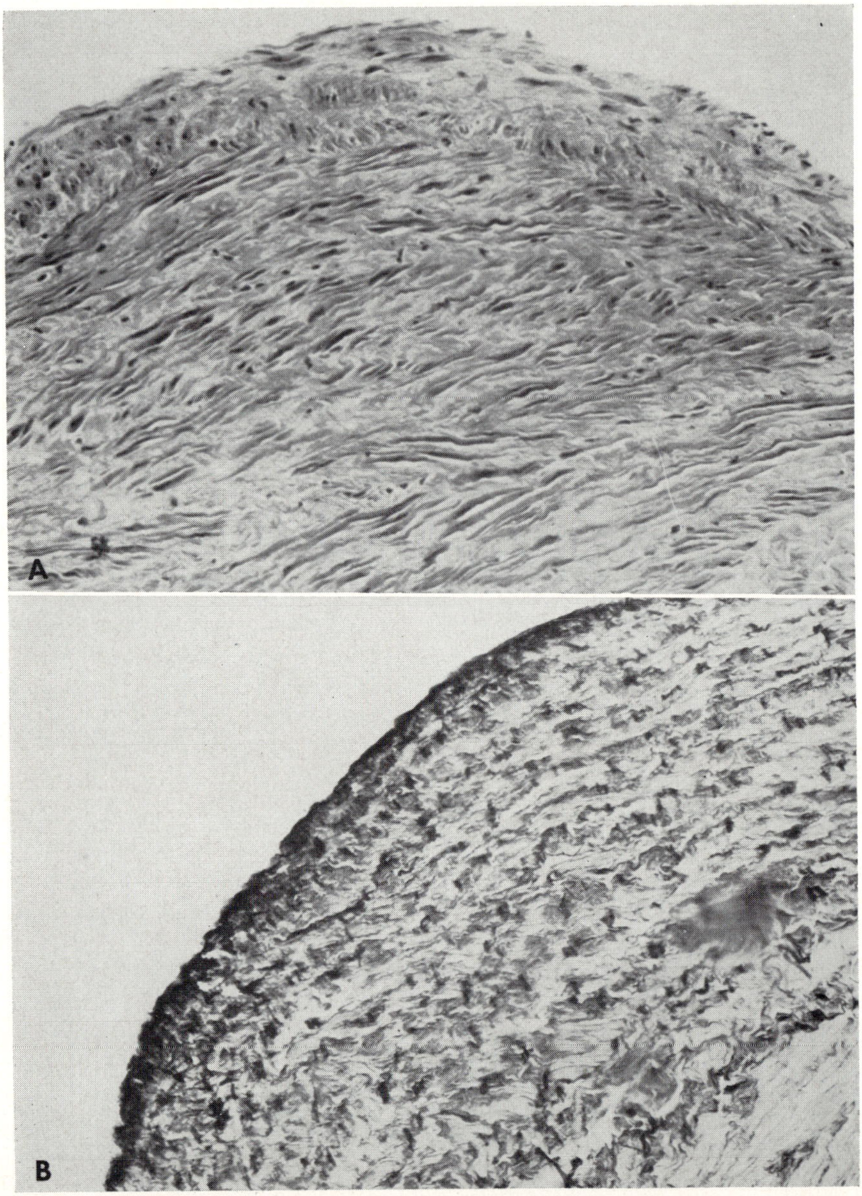

Fig. 3. *A,* Hematoxylin and eosin stain showing the histologic appearance of vein prior to preparation and storage. *B,* Elastica van Gieson's stain showing the connective tissue content and distribution in the same vein as shown in *A.*

–50° C. Additional high-energy sterilization is not necessary, as it seems to be when cadaver tissues are employed. To date, all patients have had primary healing of wounds without early or late infection.

Other factors contributing to the poor results with arterial homografts may have been related to differences in structure. Unlike veins, arteries require a plentiful blood supply through the vasa vasorum. Also, it is well recognized that arteries are one of the target organs for the atherosclerotic process, whereas veins are virtually never involved. The poor results with cadaver arterial homografts were probably due to all of the factors previously considered. In this initial

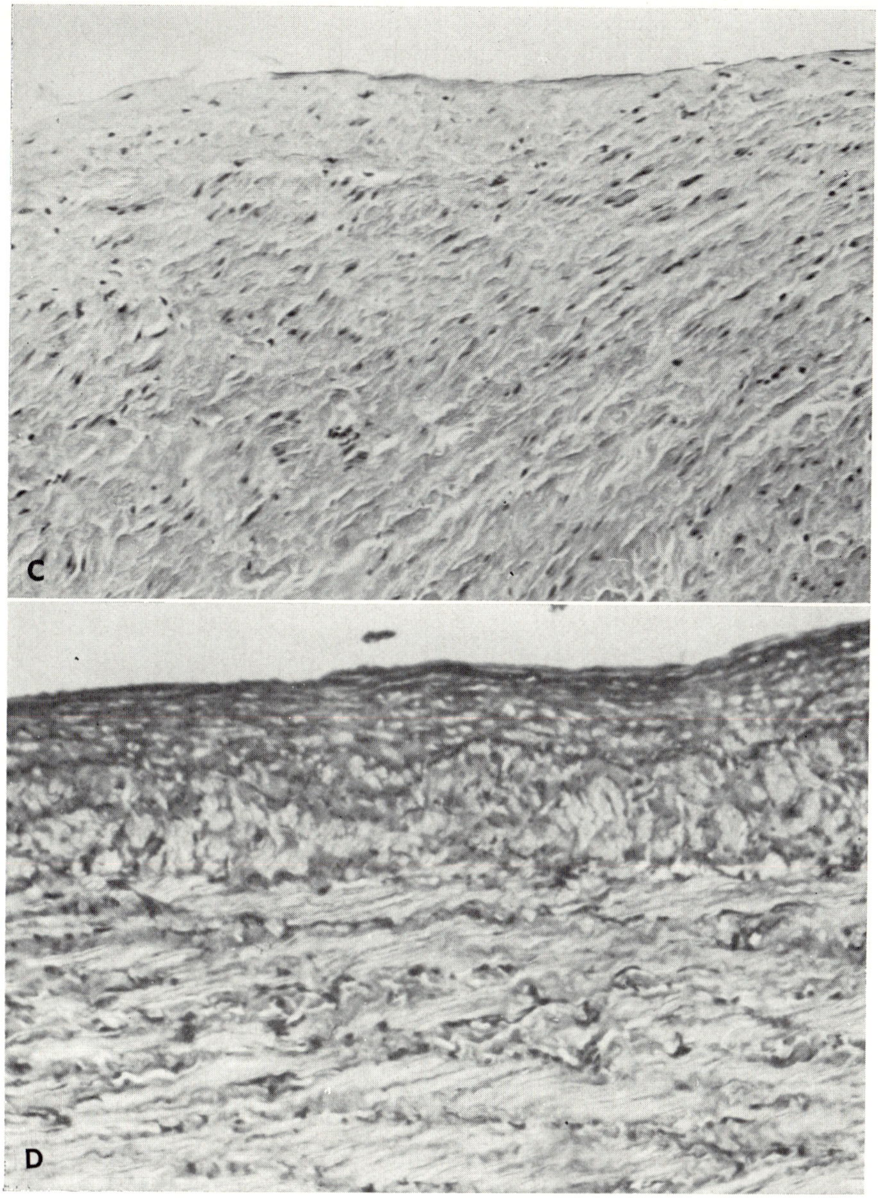

Fig. 3. *C,* Hematoxylin and eosin stain showing the histologic appearance of a vein stored for 44 days at –50° C. *D,* Elastica van Gieson's stain showing the connective tissue content and distribution in the same vein as shown in *C.*

experience, there appears to be no difference between vein homografts and vein autografts, when used for vascular reconstruction.

If this preliminary experience is confirmed by longer follow-up, then the possibilities of procuring vein segments from cadaver donors, as well as from live donors, would make available a larger source of homografts.

SUMMARY

To date, eight patients have had homologous saphenous veins used for revascularization procedures. Six of the seven patients with femoral-popliteal bypass have patent grafts (range, 4 to 14 months). Homograft vein patch was used in two patients: one with right vertebral endarterectomy, and a second with proximal superficial femoral artery stenosis. Preliminary results suggest that saphenous vein homografts, when removed, prepared, and stored in the manner described, can be used successfully for revascularization procedures. Continued follow-up will be necessary to determine the ultimate long-term fate of vein homografts.

REFERENCES

1. DeWeese, J. A., Terry, R., Barner, H. B., and Rob, C. R.: Autogenous venous femoropopliteal bypass grafts, SURGERY **59:** 28, 1966.
2. Harris, P. D., Kovalik, A. T. W., Marks, J. A., and Alm, J. R.: Factors modifying aortic homograft structure and function, SURGERY **63:** 45, 1968.

The progressive nature of pulmonary contusion

ROBERT L. FULTON, M.D.
EDWARD T. PETER, M.D., PH.D.
ALBUQUERQUE, N. MEX.
From the Department of Surgery, University of New Mexico School of Medicine

Because of an increasing number of high speed automobile accidents, contusion of the lung has become a more common clinical problem.[2] As has been described, pulmonary contusion is severe, often associated with other chest injuries, and frequently fatal.[1, 2] While it is not surprising that patients with pulmonary contusion have poor alveolar gas exchange, it has been noticed that the respiratory function appears to deteriorate during the several hours immediately after injury.[1, 4] This fact excited interest to explore the apparently increasing physiologic deficit which develops after direct lung injury or pulmonary contusion.

In this study, an estimate of the time course of oxygen transport and CO_2 elimination during the 24 hours immediately after injury was made. The effect of intermittent positive-pressure breathing on blood gas alterations was observed at various times after injury. Histologic examinations of contused lungs were made at various intervals during the first 24 hour period. Flow rates of blood through the injured lung were measured, and pulmonary vascular resistance was calculated over a period of 30 minutes after injury. It was observed that both the physiologic and histologic alterations increased with time.

METHODS

Blood gas studies. Six adult mongrel dogs were anesthetized with Nembutal (30 mg. per kilogram of body weight) and intubated with an endotracheal tube. Animals were placed on a Bird Mark 7 intermittent positive-pressure respirator. A right thoractomy was performed. Polyethylene catheters (18 gauge tubing) were inserted into the pulmonary artery through right ventriculotomies. Similar polyethylene catheters were inserted into the pulmonary venous drainage of the right middle and upper lobes. Venous catheters were placed in such a fashion that the pulmonary venous drainage from the experimental lobes was not impaired. The three catheters were then exteriorized and fashioned with stopcocks to allow withdrawal of blood samples. The upper lobe of the right lung was contused with an air-driven hammer constructed for this purpose. The hammer was driven a distance of 2 inches under 50 pounds per square inch pressure. After the entire upper lobe was contused, the lung was replaced into its anatomic position and the chest was closed with the use of chest tube drainage to evacuate air. The animals were then removed from the respirators. Blood samples were drawn at 30, 60, 90, and 120 minutes after contusion. Thirty seconds prior to measurements, the dogs were placed on intermittent positive-pressure breathing (IPPB) in order to decrease the possibility of atelectasis not caused by the injury. The blood samples were drawn 30 seconds after the dogs had again been taken off the IPPB. The PO_2, PCO_2, and pH of the pulmonary venous and arterial blood was immediately determined with a Radiometer pH meter and blood gas analyzer. At the end of 2 hours, the animals were again placed on the

Supported by the Albuquerque Veterans Administration Hospital Project Number 4-68.

Submitted for publication March 19, 1969; resubmitted June 20, 1969.

respirator for 30 minutes. The respirator delivered a 60 percent oxygen-air mixture (approximate) at a pressure of 20 to 25 cm. H_2O. After 30 minutes, blood gas determinations were again repeated.

In another group of six dogs, pulmonary contusion was produced in a similar manner. Thoracotomies were closed under sterile conditions, and the animals were kept alive for 24 hours without special precaution. After 24 hours, the thoracotomies were reopened and the pulmonary artery and veins of the right upper and middle lobes were cannulated. Thoracotomies were again closed. The animals were taken off the respirators, and blood gas determinations were made. Animals were then submitted to 30 minutes of IPPB as above and the blood gas determinations were repeated.

Histologic study. Microscopic sections of contused lungs were obtained from another group of animals in which pulmonary contusion was produced in the same manner as described above. Specimens were taken immediately after contusion, at 1 hour and 2 hours after injury. No special respiratory support was given these animals. All specimens of lung tissue were taken during inspiration. The tissue was fixed in either formalin or Bouin's solution and stained either with Mallory's trichrome method or with periodic acid–Schiff, hematoxylin and eosin, orange-green, and celistine blue stains. Photomicrographs were made with a Leitz light microscope.

Blood flow and vascular resistance study. Six dogs were anesthetized as before, placed on a Bird intermittent positive-pressure respirator with a cuffed endotracheal tube and a right thoracotomy was performed. The pulmonary artery was cannulated with a large bore polyethylene cannula (13 gauge) through a right ventriculotomy. Either a 12 or 14 F biliary T tube was placed into the main pulmonary vein of the middle lobe. One limb of the "T" extended into the left atrium, the other into the pulmonary vein and the long limb was attached to a 3-way stopcock. The P.A. cannula and the T tubes were then attached to Statham strain gauges (23d) for pressure measurements. An Electronics for Medicine multichannel recorder was used for recording pressures. Blood flow was measured by clamping the atrial limb of the T tube and opening the long limb of the tube into a graduated cylinder. Blood was collected for exactly 30 seconds. Four to six measurements of blood flow were obtained before the middle lobe was contused (control). Similar measurements were obtained at 5 minutes after contusion and at 30 minutes after injury. Pulmonary vascular resistance was calculated in peripheral resistance units (PRU) as

$$R = \frac{\text{pul. art. pressure} - \text{pul. vein pressure (mm. Hg)}}{\text{blood flow (c.c./min.)}}$$

RESULTS

Blood gas studies. Pulmonary venous blood from the contused right upper lobe was found to become progressively less saturated with O_2 from the time of injury up to (and perhaps beyond) 24 hours. The absolute difference in PO_2 as measured in millimeters of mercury between the control lobe and the contused lobe is shown in Fig. 1. The average experimental values of PO_2 in the control lobe minus the PO_2 in the contused lobe are shown with their standard error of the means. The average control pulmonary venous PO_2 over the 2 hour period was 82 mm. Hg (essentially a normal value at the altitude of this laboratory which is 5,500 feet above sea level). The differences between the PO_2 of the control observations and the experimental observations at 30, 60, 90, and 120 minutes were 21.6 ± 10.3, 37.1 ± 14.8, 38.7 ± 11.0, and 37.7 ± 11.6 mm. Hg, respectively. Interestingly, the probability that the control and experimental means differ increased with time: $p > 0.1$, $0.05 < p < 0.1$, $p = 0.05$, and $0.01 < p < 0.05$, respectively, at 30, 60, 90, and 120 minutes after injury (t test evaluation). At 24 hours, the difference between control and experimental PO_2 was 57.7 ± 24.0 mm. Hg ($p < 0.05$). The correlation between the increasing PO_2 deficit

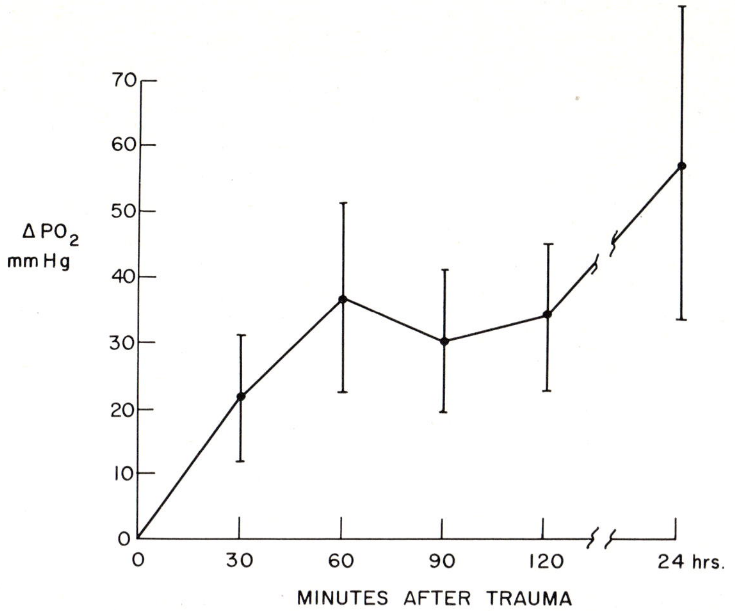

Fig. 1. PO_2 difference between control and contused lung versus time after injury.

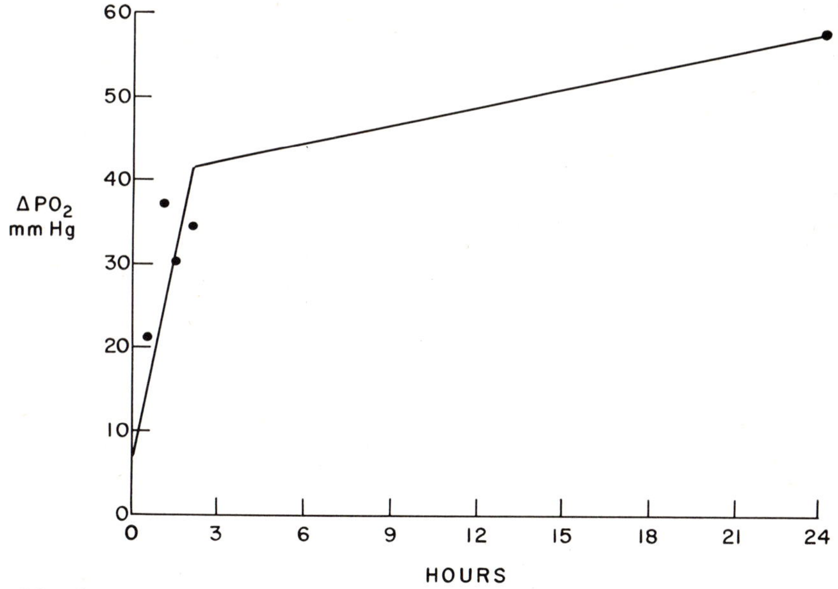

Fig. 2. PO_2 difference between control and contused lung versus time after injury.

and time for 2 hours was + 0.82 and for 24 hours, + 0.75 ($p \sim 0.05$). Fig. 2 depicts a regression line analysis of these data. The slope of the first line segment is 0.26 mm. Hg per minute and for the second segment approximately 0.03 mm. Hg per minute. These data confirm the hypothesis that a progressive oxygen diffusion barrier across the contused lung develops after a 24 hour period.

The response of pulmonary venous PO_2 to IPPB is shown in Fig. 3. At the end of

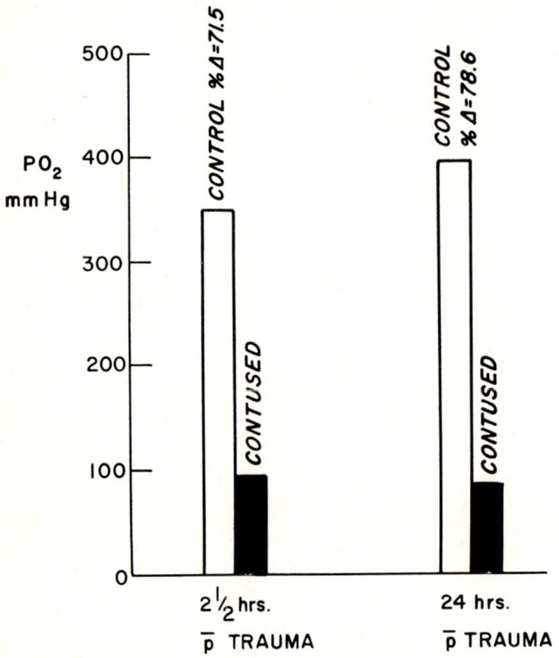

Fig. 3. Differences between control and contused lobes (PO_2) on respirators 2½ and 24 hours after trauma.

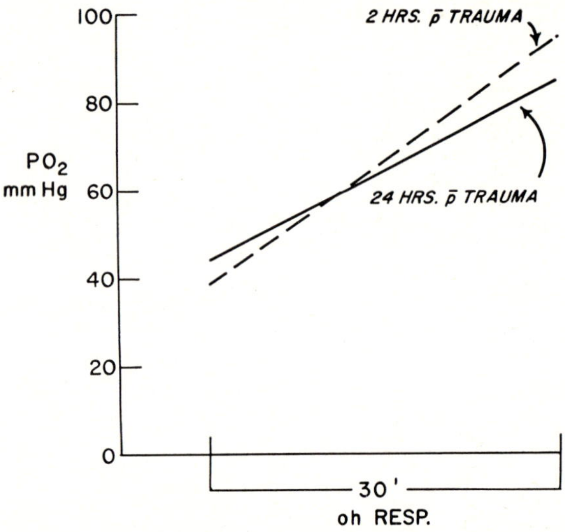

Fig. 4. Change in PO_2 on respirator 2 and 24 hours after contusion.

2 hours after trauma and after 30 minutes on the respirator, the mean control pulmonary venous PO_2 was 95 mm. Hg, a difference of 71.5 percent ($p < 0.01$). A difference of 78.6 percent was observed at 24 hours after trauma (297.5 and 85.1 mm. Hg, for control and experimental means, respectively, $p < 0.01$). There was no significant difference ($p > 0.1$) before or during positive-pressure ventilation of pulmonary venous PO_2 determinations of the contused lung at either 2 or 24 hours after injury. That is, IPPB did not produce a significant increase in the PO_2 of pulmonary venous blood of the contused lung. Fig. 4 depicts the slopes of the response curves of pulmonary venous PO_2 of the contused lobe to IPPB. There is a slight (but not statistically significant) indication that as the lesion progresses it becomes more difficult to produce normal oxygenation. The values in this graph depict the mean values of the PO_2 measurements.

PCO_2 retention across the injured lung was observed, but because of the experimental design, it was not shown to be either significant or progressive. Fig. 5 illustrates the difference between the mean pulmonary venous PCO_2 values of the traumatized and control pulmonary lobes. Except for the values at 24 hours ($p < 0.05$) there was no significant difference in the PCO_2 between control and traumatized lobes. The PCO_2 of the pulmonary venous blood of the contused lobe after IPPB was still higher than that of the control lobe. The differences are depicted in Fig. 6. At 2 hours after injury there was no significant difference between the control and after-injury values, but at 24 hours the difference is significant ($p < 0.05$). Again, IPPB did not produce a significant difference in the PCO_2 values of the contused-lobe venous blood at either 2 hours (8.6 mm. Hg) or at 24 hours (16 mm. Hg). There is some indication that a progressive CO_2 barrier develops, but this has not been proved.

It is likely that the PCO_2 values measured reflected the total CO_2 content of the animals. The pulmonary artery PCO_2 values were not elevated and more often than not demonstrated a low PCO_2. That some CO_2 retention did occur is indicated by the data, but because a small area of the total lung was involved in the injury it would not be

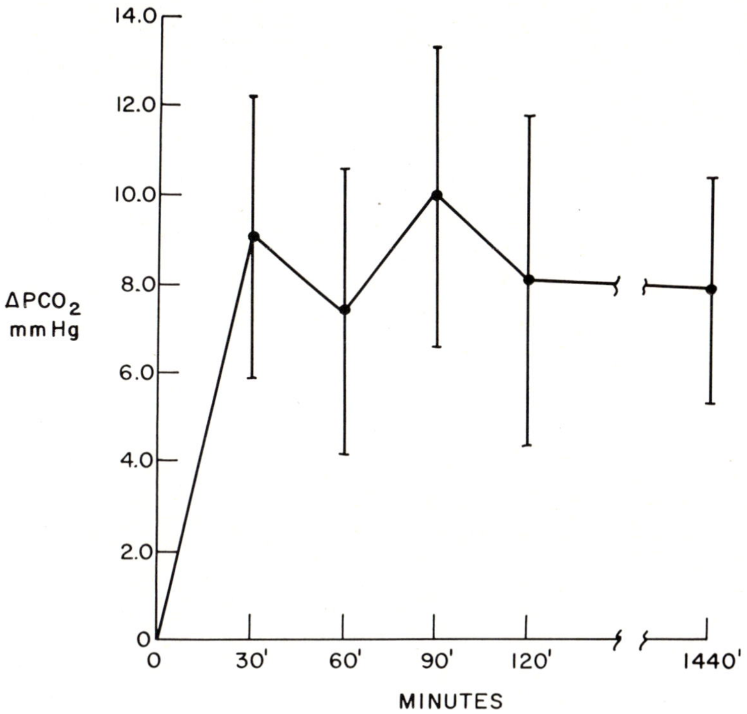

Fig. 5. Δ PCO_2 between contused and control lobes.

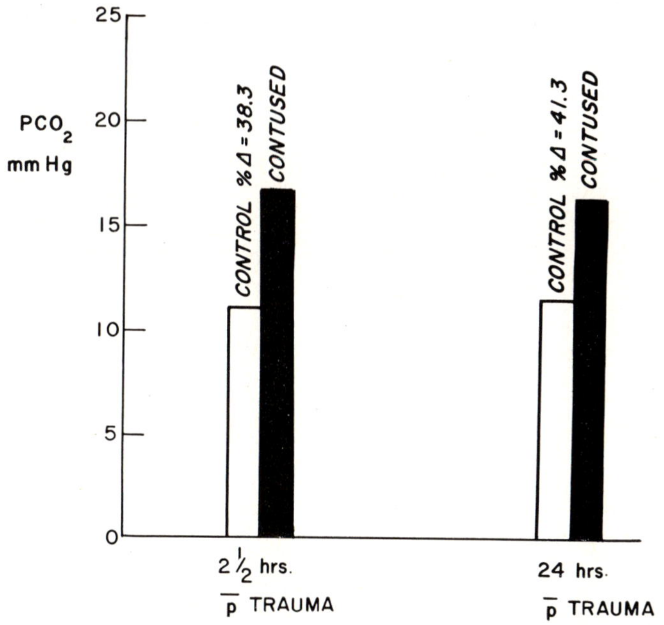

Fig. 6. PCO_2 after 30 minutes on respirator.

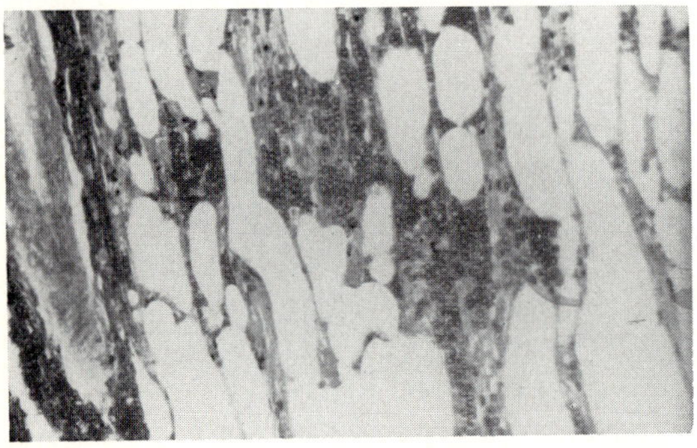

Fig. 7. Immediately after contusion interstitial hemorrhage is seen without significant atelectasis. There is very little edema present at this time.

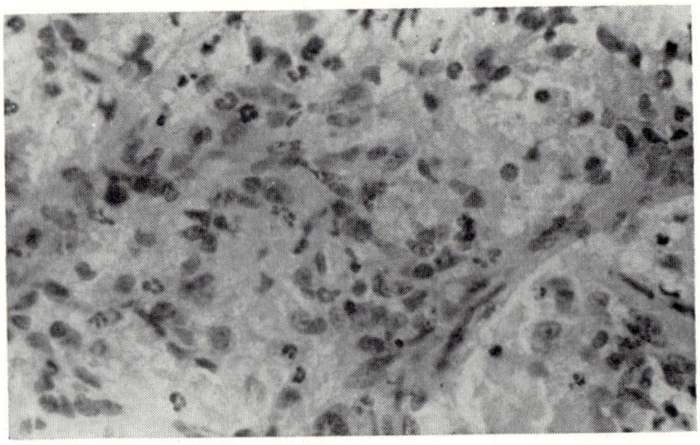

Fig. 9. Biopsy taken at 24 hours after contusion shows almost complete loss of architecture of the lung. There is rather massive interstitial edema and round cell infiltration at this time.

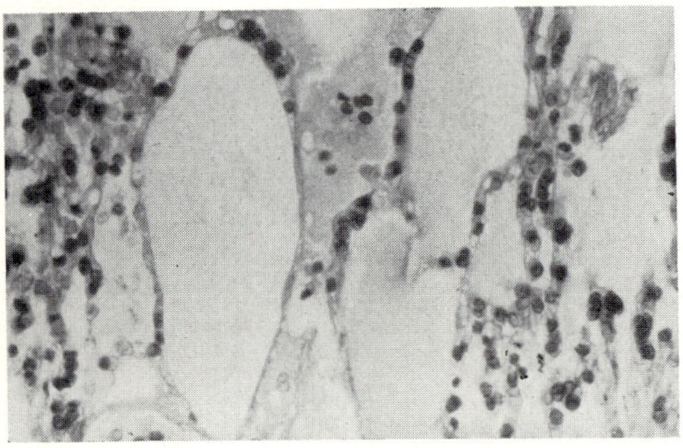

Fig. 8. Biopsy of the lung taken at 2 hours after contusion shows significant interstitial edema without appreciable cellular infiltration. Architecture is still preserved at this time.

expected that significant elevations of CO_2 would occur.

Microscopic pathology. Examination of biopsies of the dog's lung taken immediately after contusion and at 1, 2, and 24 hours after injury demonstrated the development of a progressive lesion. Initially (Fig. 7) there is destruction of alveoli with some hemorrhage into the interstitial space and the alveoli. There is little collapse of the alveolar structure, however. Within 1 to 2 hours (Fig. 8) the injured lung begins to show accumulation of edema. There is, in addition, a moderate infiltration of mononuclear and polymorphonuclear cells. The alveolar architecture can still be demonstrated. By 24 hours (Fig. 9) the architecture of the lung is almost obliterated by a massive accumulation of inflammatory cells, primarily mononuclear elements. Polymorphonuclear cells are also present in abundance and together with the monocytes tend to obscure the hemorrhage. Edema, i.e., protein-containing fluid, is also present. The lesion of pulmonary contusion, then, seems initially to be due to hemorrhage followed by an increasing infiltration of nucleated cells and edema until the pulmonary architecture is obliterated.

Pulmonary blood flow and resistance. Blood flow and pressure measurements taken as described indicate that an increase in resistance across the vascular bed of the injured lung occurred. Fig. 10 demonstrates the increase in resistance and decrease in flow as a function of time after injury. There is an initial stepwise increase in vascular resistance in 5 minutes, followed by a more gradual increase over the next 25 minutes. The average control resistance in six animals was 0.75 ± 0.27* PRU. The average control flow was 18.2 ± 5.6 c.c. per minute. At 5 minutes after injury the resistance had increased to 0.98 ± 0.29 PRU, and the flow had decreased to 13.07 ± 5.03 c.c. per minute. Thirty minutes after contusion, the resistance was 1.23 ± 0.31 PRU while the flow was 9.9 ± 3.6 c.c. per minute. Both the 5 and 30 minute values differed from the con-

*Standard deviation.

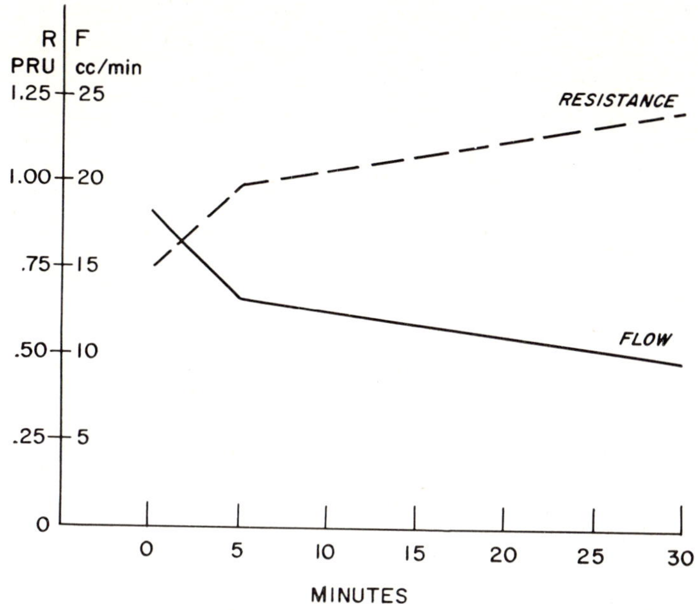

Fig. 10. Correlation of vascular resistance and flow of contused lung and time.

trol values significantly ($p < 0.05$). The difference between the 5 and 30 minute values, however, however, were not significant ($p \simeq 0.10$). There was a significant ($p \simeq 0.01$) negative correlation (–0.89) between flow and time and a significant ($p << 0.01$) positive (+0.94) correlation between resistance and time. It is, therefore, concluded that pulmonary contusion produces a progressive increase in pulmonary vascular resistance which leads to a decreased flow across the injured lung.

DISCUSSION

Pulmonary contusion appears to be a progressive lesion, at least during the first 24 hours. From examination of the biopsy specimen of contused dog lung, it is not difficult to surmise why a progressive gas diffusion barrier develops after contusion. The injury does not produce much more than hemorrhage initially. Edema is not particularly marked immediately after injury. Alveolar collapse or destruction of architecture does not seem to occur initially. Because of the injury, edema begins to accumulate in the interstices of the lung. This fluid enters the interstitium and the alveoli. It must, of course, be brought there by the pulmonary artery blood and probably develops as a time-related function of flow and injury. Following the influx of edema, the cellular response to injury occurs. While in other areas of the body this response is thought to be helpful, in the lung it tends to be harmful in that it places tissue between the alveolar air and capillary blood. This response must also be time dependent.

As the edema and cellular elements enter the lung the diffusion distance for O_2 and CO_2 increases, resulting in lowered pulmonary venous oxygen saturation and CO_2 retention. Other mechanisms which can lead to lowered respiratory exchange have also been reported following pulmonary contusion. Garzon and associates[3] showed that lung compliance was greatly decreased and that mean respiratory resistance increased following pulmonary injury in man. They did not, however, take serial measurements close to the time of injury but indicate that the lesion may become fatal after an initial satisfactory clinical course. Nichols and coworkers[5] showed that pulmonary surfactant assays from dogs with contused lungs became abnormally low in 24 to 48 hours after trauma. It is noted that the surfactant values were normal at 24 hours. Their data on blood gases and histologic examination corroborate this study. Various other investigators[1, 2] have noted that the clinical course of patients suffering from chest injuries often deteriorates with the passage of time and suggest that the lung injury is the cause.

The response of the injured lung to intermittent positive-pressure respiration was demonstrated in this study. Intermittent positive-pressure breathing does not appear to reverse the diffusion barrier which develops. It becomes increasingly more difficult to oxygenate and remove CO_2 with the passage of time after injury. The absence of a significant response to IPPB suggests that atelectasis is a minor and relatively unimportant part of the physiologic derangement. If major bronchi are crushed or obstructed with secretions, atelectasis may occur and become a major problem, but with the contusions produced in this study, major bronchial injury did not occur. It seems likely that the main component of injury is the accumulation of alveolar and interstitial edema and invasion of the lung with cellular elements. Certainly, changes occur in lung compliance and airway resistance. These effects could be related to injury of the minor bronchi or by compression of the alveoli by edema. It would be anticipated that respiratory mechanics could be improved with IPPB if some of the effect of contusion was at the bronchiolar level, since a diffiusion block that is due to edema and cellular infiltration would not be expected to respond markedly to low pressure IPPB and higher airway oxygen content. That is, if the distance between alveolar cavities and capillaries was markedly increased by edema or cellular elements, it would not be expected that the pressures and airway O_2 content used in this study would reverse the apparent diffusion barrier.

It would be further anticipated that if blood flow decreases through the injured lung then the total oxygen transport would be decreased. This study shows a progressive decrease in pulmonary blood flow caused by pulmonary contusion. It is demonstrated that the pulmonary vascular resistance increases with time following injury. The resistance increase is perhaps due to the accumulation of edema with increasing interstitial pressure and collapse of small capillaries, direct injury to capillaries, or to an increase in viscosity of the blood by loss of water as edema. This study does not indicate the nature of the vascular derangement. It does show, however, that hemodynamic changes occur which are progressive.

SUMMARY

A progressive diffusion barrier to oxygen and a progressive increase in vascular resistance were shown to occur following pulmonary contusion in the dog. The oxygen diffusion barrier was not decreased by IPPB. Histologic examination of the injured lung indicates that edema and cellular infiltration are partially responsible for the progressive nature of the injury.

REFERENCES

1. Alfano, G. S., and Hale, H. W.: Pulmonary contusion, J. Trauma **5:** 647, 1965.
2. DeMuth, W. E., and Smith, J. M.: Pulmonary contusion, Am. J. Surg. **109:** 819, 1965.
3. Garzon, A. A., Seltzer, B., and Karlson, K. E.: Physiopathology of crushed chest injuries, Ann. Surg. **168:** 128, 1968.
4. Hopkinson, B. R., Border, J. R., and Schenk, W. G., Jr.: Experimental closed chest trauma, J. Thoracic & Cardiovas. Surg. **55:** 580, 1968.
5. Nichols, R. T., Pearce, H. J., and Greenfield, L. J.: Effects of experimental pulmonary contusion of respiratory exchange and lung mechanics, Arch. Surg., **96:** 723, 1968.

Responses of skeletal muscle pH to injury: A new technique for determination of tissue viability

IRWIN R. BERMAN, M.D.*
MICHAEL D. LEMIEUX, M.D.
GENE V. AABY, Lieutenant Colonel, MC, USA
WASHINGTON, D. C., AND NEW YORK, N. Y.
From the Division of Surgery, Walter Reed Army Institute of Research, and the Department of Surgery, New York University Medical Center

Changes in hydrogen ion activity on the surface of organs and tissues are reliable experimental indicators of the degree to which metabolic activity in those tissues has shifted to the buildup of products of anaerobic metabolism.[1-4] Consequently, surface pH is logically assumed to be related to the adequacy of perfusion of the tissues being examined. In the intact kidney with occluded arterial inflow, surface hydrogen ion activity rises sharply and returns to normal after restoration of blood flow.[3] In hemorrhagic shock, fall in surface pH of skeletal muscle may actually precede a measurable fall in blood pH or rise of lactic acid in the blood.[4] Surface pH measurement may thus represent the most sensitive parameter by which adequacy of specific tissue perfusion may be assessed and closely monitored.

Since skeletal muscle accounts for a large portion of oxidative metabolism, it is reasonable that measurement of surface pH could have a valuable surgical application in assessment of limb viability following ischemia or trauma. A historic lesson of combat surgery is that the inexperienced surgeon often performs inadequate debridement because of the lack of objective evidence of nonviability of tissue. Furthermore, technically perfect arterial reconstructions have been performed in extremities with irreversible damage from ischemia. Over-enthusiastic, excessive debridement of viable tissue and limbs is likewise unacceptable.

Conventional criteria for estimation of viability of skeletal muscle include direct observation of color, consistency, contractility, bleeding, and the use of various staining methods. The latter techniques have definite limitations which render them impractical or imprecise for clinical application. The present study was designed to evaluate the technique of electrometric surface pH measurement in assessment of skeletal muscle viability following crush, thermal, and high velocity missile injury.

MATERIALS AND METHODS

The principles of laboratory animal care as promulgated by the National Society for Medical Research were observed. Twenty albino rabbits, weighing 2 to 3 kilograms, were anesthetized with intravenous sodium pentobarbital and methoxyflurane administered by the open-drop method. A 3 cm. incision was made through the skin and subcutaneous tissues of the lateral aspect of the thigh and deepened through the investing fascia, avoiding injury to muscle. Surface pH measurements were made on the underlying muscle with an Instrumentation Laboratories' Combination pH Glass Electrode Model 14043 held in light contact with the muscle surface and connected to an Instrumentation Laboratories Model 245 Delta-

Received for publication March 25, 1969.

*Department of Surgery, New York University Medical Center, 550 First Avenue, New York, N. Y. 10016.

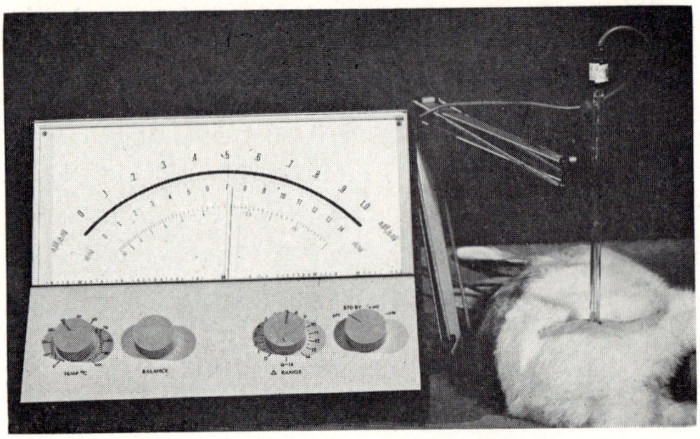

Fig. 1. Deltamatic pH/MV electrometer and electrode used for skeletal muscle surface pH measurements.

matic pH/MV Electrometer (Fig. 1). The instrument was calibrated with standard pH reference buffer solutions.

In 10 rabbits, crushing injury was created across the muscle of the lateral aspect of the thigh with a pair of Kocher clamps. The clamps were applied over a thin sheet of polyethylene to prevent contact of metal with muscle and left in place for 5 minutes. Serial pH determinations were made on the surface of normal and injured areas during a 2 hour period following injury. The injured area was then marked with metallic clips, the wound closed, and the animal returned to its cage. These wounds were reopened after 24 hours for a second measurement of surface pH. Then a correlation was made between this parameter and tissue staining after intravenous Patent Blue V dye.[5]

In 10 rabbits, a graded thermal injury was applied to the muscle by electrocautery with a Bovie Electrosurgical Unit, Model CSV. Three 1 cm. square areas of injury were created by varying the coagulation current in contact with muscle. Char injury was first produced with a current setting of 40 held in contact for 5 seconds. A lesser injury was then inflicted with a current setting of 25 to 30 for the same length of time. The setting was then reduced to 20 and held in contact with muscle for 10 seconds. These areas were arbitrarily designated as "severe," "moderate," and "mild" thermal injury, respectively. Serial pH measurements were performed on the surface of each of the burned areas and over normal muscle. Results were then correlated with the degree of hypoperfusion indicated by tissue staining following intravenous Patent Blue V dye. After 24 hours, wounds were reopened and examined for gross and pH changes as well as staining characteristics accompanying vital dye infusion.

The effects of high velocity missile injury were studied in two beagle dogs. These animals were anesthetized with intravenous sodium pentobarbital and subjected to soft tissue wounding of each proximal hind limb with a 0.25 inch steel sphere traveling in excess of 2,000 feet per second. Animals were studied 2 to 3 hours following wounding. The entrance and exit wounds were fully exposed by incision and fasciotomy. Repeated skeletal muscle surface pH measurements were then made on multiple areas of traumatized muscle to determine differences in pH between normal tissue and muscle that usually would be excised in a similar combat wound occurring in man. Muscle debridement was not performed. Intravenous Patent Blue V dye was infused 4 hours after injury and again 24 hours later to correlate results of this parameter with gross changes and surface pH measurements. Results of all pH determinations were subjected to statistical analysis, and probability was determined by Student's nonpaired t test.

Table I. *Skeletal muscle surface pH measurement accompanying crush, thermal, and high velocity injury*

Description	*Mean*	*Range*	*S.E.**	*Significance*
Crush injury				
Normal	7.479	7.358-7.610	0.025	$p < 0.001$
Crush	6.585	6.334-6.875	0.058	
Thermal injury				
Normal	7.557	7.340-7.722	0.046	N.S.
Mild	7.631	7.443-7.742	0.055	
Moderate				
Immediate	6.914	6.600-7.241	0.066	$p < 0.001$
30 minutes	7.449	7.165-7.584	0.050	$p < 0.001$
Severe	7.652	7.205-7.828	0.110	N.S.
High velocity				
Normal	7.786	7.568-8.065	0.025	$p < 0.001$
Injured	7.280	7.178-7.448	0.041	

*S.E. = standard error.

RESULTS

The results of surface pH measurement of skeletal muscle subjected to crush, thermal, and high velocity missile injury are expressed in Table I and Figs. 2 and 3. Immediately following crush injury, the muscle was white and obviously totally ischemic, and the surface pH varied minimally from normal. However, fall in pH was progressive during the 30 minutes following injury. During this time, traumatized muscle became more reddish in color, as blood flow to the injured area was restored. pH of injured skeletal muscle was stable by 1 hour after injury, with mean pH fall of 0.894 ± 0.065 pH units ($p < 0.001$). Surface pH of adjacent normal muscle remained stable during this period with transition from normal to acid pH values regularly occurring at the point of gross demarcation of the crush injury. On the day following injury, pH also changed sharply at the point of demarcation outlined by the metallic clips and by tissue staining after intravenous Patent Blue V dye (Fig. 4). At this time, however, pH change was in the opposite direction. Surface pH of crushed tissue was always higher than that of surrounding normal tissue, still with the sharp line of demarcation observed on the day of injury.

There was no detectable fall in surface pH of skeletal muscle subjected to "mild" thermal injury. However, surface pH of skeletal muscle that was burned more severely ("moderate") regularly demonstrated a transient significant pH fall, followed by restoration to normal levels within 30 minutes following injury (Fig. 2). Mean fall in pH in moderately burned areas was 0.655 ± 0.078 ($p < 0.001$). Restoration to normal values after 30 minutes was also statistically significant ($p < 0.001$). Intravenous administration of Patent Blue V dye after burning caused staining in minimally burned areas but initial failure of staining in areas subjected to moderate injury. However, the latter areas subsequently became bright blue, concomitant with rise in surface pH values toward normal. Areas of most severe injury (char) were not stained by the dye, and pH did not fall. Twenty-four hours later charred tissue was usually alkalotic.

High velocity missile injury with the symmetrical steel sphere seemed to cause less gross tissue destruction than that occurring after injury with an M-16 rifle, a high velocity weapon currently used in combat areas. The usual small wound of entrance and larger exit wound were nevertheless created, with areas of muscle appearing definitely devitalized by conventional clinical criteria. Surface pH of traumatized muscle was consistently lower than normal muscle. Average pH fall in apparently devitalized

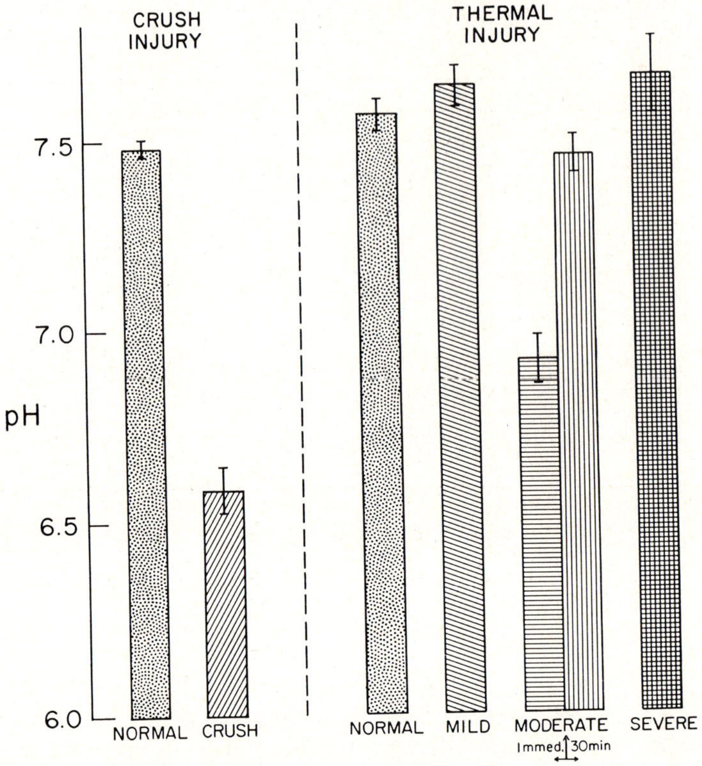

Fig. 2. Skeletal muscle surface pH following crush and thermal injury. Values expressed represent the mean of all determinations ± standard error.

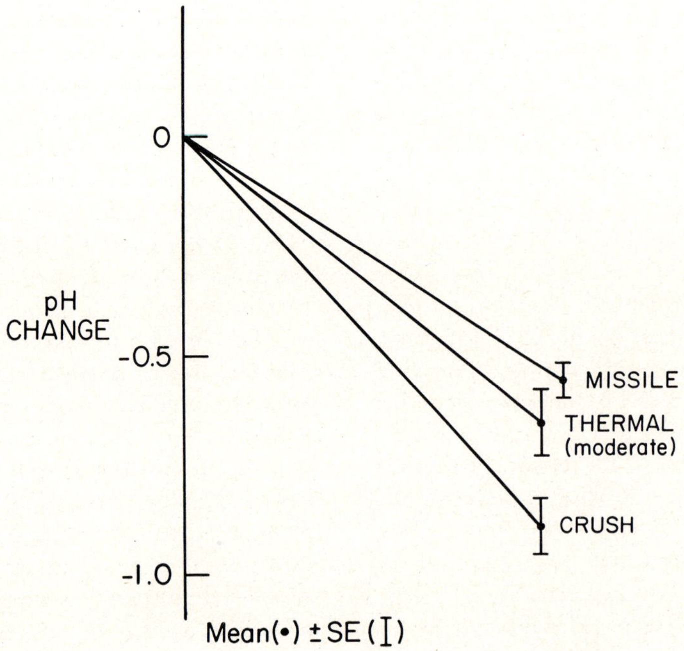

Fig. 3. Skeletal muscle surface pH changes following crush, burn, and missile injury. Values expressed represent the mean of all determinations ± standard error.

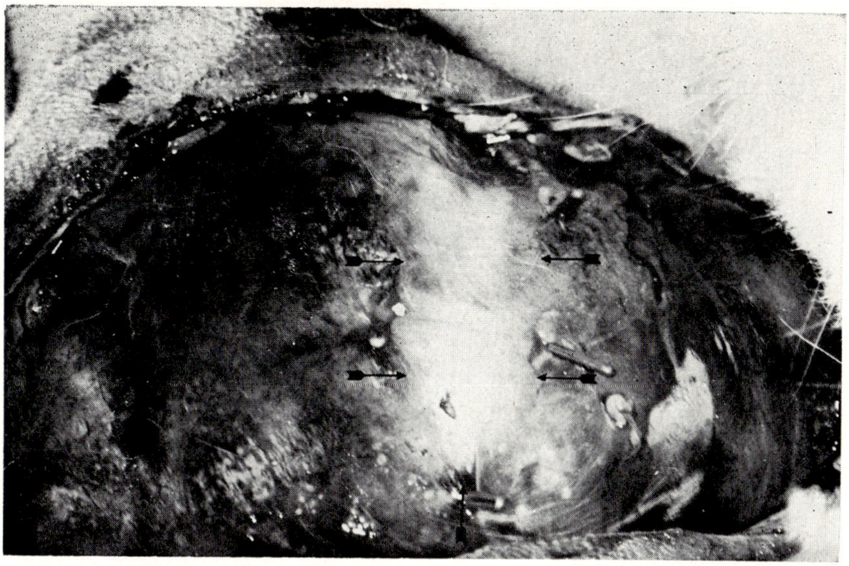

Fig. 4. Staining of tissues accompanying Patent Blue V dye administered intravenously after crush injury. The unstained area (arrows) corresponds to area of crush.

areas was 0.506 ± 0.037 pH units (Fig. 3). Muscle staining after infusion of Patent Blue V dye was poor on the day of injury, except in one wound in which correlation of staining with grossly devitalized muscle seemed reliable. Twenty-four hours later, however, demarcation by gross observation, vital dye infusion, and fall in muscle surface pH were all possible. The shift to alkaline pH of apparently devitalized muscle which was observed 24 hours after crush and severe burn injury had not occurred after missile injury.

DISCUSSION

Diminution of surface pH of skeletal muscle after wounding suggests that cellular metabolic activity in traumatized muscle readily shifts to the accumulation of products of anaerobic glycolysis. The extent of this transition in the acute period after injury would appear to be directly related to the extent of tissue devitalization and local accumulation of lactic acid and other acid metabolites.[1, 2]

Correlation of surface pH with intravenous infusion of vital dyes indicates that changes in surface hydrogen ion activity are directly related to alterations in tissue perfusion. The absolute fall in pH of muscle injured by crush or high velocity missile and the transient fall in pH in tissue subjected to moderate thermal injury reflect such alterations in perfusion. In moderately burned areas, correlation of the restoration of pH to normal values with the appearance of staining after vital dye infusion further indicates that tissue perfusion was restored toward normal by 30 minutes following injury. The slight rise in surface pH in tissue subjected to minimal burn may be the reflection of augmented tissue perfusion. Although consistent, this change is not statistically significant.

Failure of charred muscle to demonstrate a fall in pH is believed to reflect absolute tissue devitalization with cellular death and total metabolic failure. After 24 hours, charred areas, as well as those subjected to crush injury, regularly demonstrated an increase in surface pH values above those in normal muscle, with distinct lines of demarcation from normal muscle. However, this phenomenon was not observed 24 hours after high velocity missile injury. It is likely that the total devitalization that followed crush and char injury probably did not occur with the less uniform though equally severe injury inflicted by a high velocity missile. It would thus appear that tissues absolutely deprived of blood supply do not demonstrate the same capacity for maintaining surface acidosis as those in which some measure of perfusion is maintained. It is not clear from these studies whether this represents diminished capacity for anaerobic glycolysis[2] or loss of integrity of the cell membrane.

Demonstration of changes in surface hydrogen ion activity of injured muscle suggests that electrometric measurement of surface pH may be useful in assessing and monitoring tissue viability in cases of severe peripheral vascular insufficiency and direct trauma. Such a clinical adjunct could be of special value in the following instances: for wounds of critical areas in which extensive debridement might result in unnecessary alteration of appearance or function (e.g., face, hand), for areas in which viable muscle could better protect another surgical procedure (e.g., femoral vascular repair), and for difficult areas in which massive trauma is accompanied by a high incidence of redebridement and/or infection (e.g., pelvis, retroperitoneum). Since equilibration of electrode and muscle surface is not usually instantaneous, however, direct application to combat surgery may be somewhat cumbersome with currently available instrumentation.

The results of this study would suggest that significant devitalization has occurred after injury when repeated surface pH determinations demonstrate significant variation from obviously normal tissue. When this difference exists and when the tissue being studied is acidotic, it is likely that impairment of perfusion has been recent. When the tissue in question is significantly alkalotic relative to obviously normal muscle, absolute devascularization or death has probably occurred considerably earlier. Theoretically, these findings would render the techniques of surface electrometric measurement most applicable in the acute period following injury or vascular insult when precise definition of viability is most difficult. Additional studies are now in progress to correlate the extent of change in surface pH with ultimate tissue death or survival following high velocity missile injury and vascular occlusive disease.

SUMMARY AND CONCLUSIONS

Surface electrometric pH of skeletal muscle demonstrates significant changes after crush, thermal, and high velocity missile injury. The anatomic correlation of these changes with the distribution of vital dye indicates that surface hydrogen ion activity of skeletal muscle is readily altered by changes in tissue perfusion. Further studies will be directed toward definition of the extent of pH change which is consistently associated with tissue death.

REFERENCES

1. Couch, N. P., Maginn, R. R., Middleton, M. K., Appleton, D. R., and Dmochowski, J. R.: Effect of ischemic intervals and temperature on renal surface hydrogen ion concentration, Surg. Gynec. & Obst. **125:** 521, 1967.
2. Couch, N. P., and Middleton, M. K.: Effect of storage temperature on the electrometric surface hydrogen ion activity of ischemic liver and heart, Surgery **64:** 1099, 1968.
3. Dmochowski, J. R., Couch, N. P., Kempf, R. N., and Appleton, D. R.: Electrometric surface pH of the ischemic kidney and the effect of hypothermia, J. S. Res. **6:** 45, 1966.
4. Lemieux, M. D., Smith, R. N., and Couch, N. P.: Effect of hemorrhage and infusion on electrometric surface hydrogen ion activity and redox potential of skeletal muscle, S. Forum **19:** 1, 1968.
5. Randolph, J. G., Leape, L. L., and Gross, R. E.: The early surgical treatment of burns. I. Experimental studies utilizing intravenous vital dye for determining the degree of injury, Surgery **56:** 193, 1964.

Massive megacolon and megaileum in childhood due to tuberculous stenosis of the ascending colon

JAMES J. PATTON, M.D.
THOMAS C. MOORE, M.D.
TORRANCE AND LOS ANGELES, CALIF.
From the Pediatric Surgical Service, UCLA–Harbor General Hospital, Torrance, and the Department of Surgery, University of California School of Medicine, Los Angeles

It has been estimated that from 12 to 25 million cases of infectious tuberculosis exist in the world today.[3] The hazard in childhood has been reduced substantially in the United States[36] and Western Europe[25] but remains a problem in areas in which public health programs are less developed.[3, 20, 28, 29, 31] The same is true for tuberculous involvement of the gastrointestinal tract. It rarely is encountered in the United States but does appear more frequently in other areas in the Near and Middle East and India.[5, 6, 21, 23, 34, 37]

It has seemed desirable to report a case of acquired massive megacolon and megaileum in childhood as a rare complication of alimentary tract tuberculosis.

CASE REPORT

The patient, a 12-year-old Mexican boy, was admitted to the UCLA–Harbor General Hospital on October 1, 1968, because of intermittent, crampy abdominal pain which had been present during the previous 1½ years. The pain largely was generalized, but at times it was localized to the right lower quadrant. It frequently occurred about one-half hour after eating and generally was associated with loud borborygmi that were quite audible. Abdominal distension initially was noted approximately 9 months prior to admission to the hospital. It had increased gradually since that time. The patient had had several loose stools each day over the previous several months. No blood or mucus was noted in the stools, and they were not foul smelling. There was no vomiting. The child had become quite anorexic at the time of his admission to the hospital. His height and weight had not changed since his arrival from Tijuana, Mexico, two years earlier.

The patient's health while in Tijuana was reported to be good. There had been no serious repiratory infections, coughing, hemoptysis, night sweats, or exposure to tuberculosis. He had been skin tested yearly in Tijuana for tuberculosis. The results of these tests were not known. In addition, there was no history of dysuria, hematuria, fever, or chills.

On physical examination, the patient was found to be cachectic, pale, and chronically ill in appearance (Fig. 1, *A*). Even though 12 years of age, he was the average height, 48 inches, for a six-year-old, and he weighed 49 pounds, average for a seven-year-old. His weight did not reflect the true degree of his cachexia. A significant, but nonmeasurable, amount of his weight was due to factors which produced his abdominal distension, retained feces, and a greatly thickened ileocecal area. Temperature, pulse, respirations, and blood pressure were within normal limits. The lungs were clear to auscultation and percussion, and there was no evidence of abnormality.

The abdomen was markedly distended and diffusely tympanitic. It was nontender. Peristaltic sounds were quite active and loud. No masses were encountered on rectal examination and the stool was soft, pale brown, and guaiac positive. His extremities and face were quite cachectic in appearance. There was no evidence of significant lymphadenopathy.

The hemoglobin was 7.4 Gm. percent and the hematocrit was 26 percent. The leukocyte count was 4,600 per cubic millimeter. The blood urea nitrogen was 11 mg. percent, and the creatinine was 0.5 mg. percent. Multiple stool examinations revealed numerous white blood cells but were

Received for publication April 21, 1969.

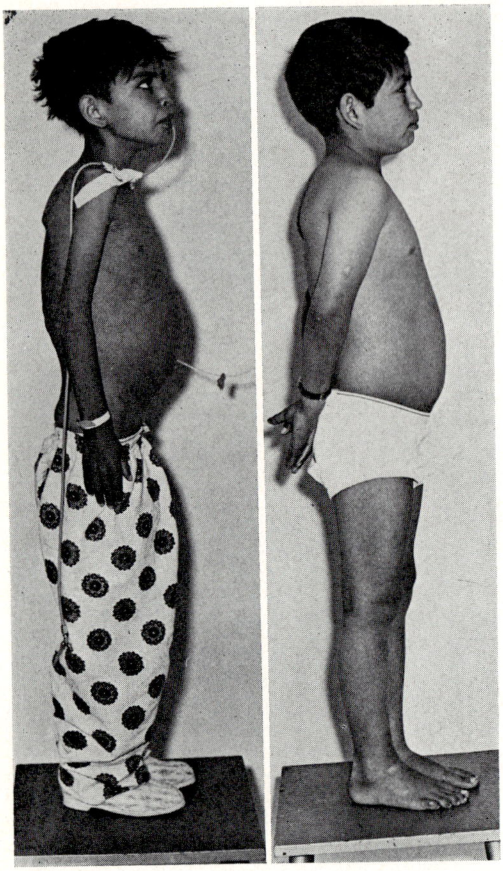

A *B*

Fig. 1. Photographs of the patient. *A,* Before and *B,* four months after resection of the massive megacolon and megaileum. The abdomen was greatly distended and the patient's arms and face showed evidence of marked cachexia prior to operation. The gain of weight and restoration to normal health are documented in the postoperative photograph.

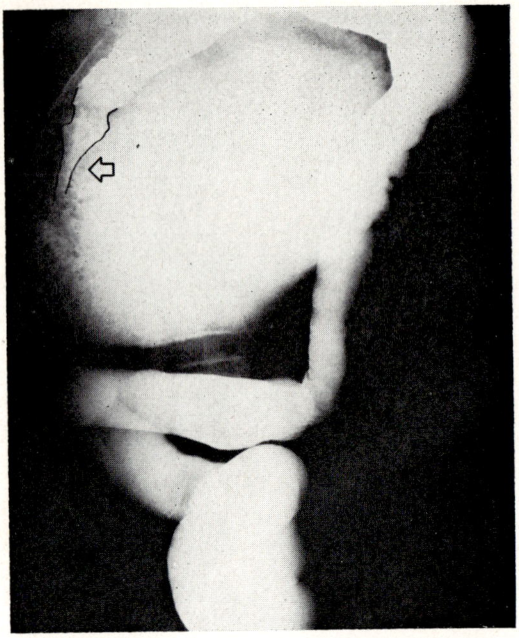

Fig. 2. Barium enema demonstration of a normal sigmoid descending and transverse colon with a stenotic area of ascending colon (arrow and retouched) leading into the greatly dilated area of megacolon and megaileum.

negative for ova, parasites, and pathogenic bacteria. Study of the sputum, gastric washings, urine, and stool were negative for mycobacterium tuberculosis. Adrenal stimulation with ACTH showed a normal cortisol increase. The findings on sigmoidoscopic examination were within normal limits. A skin test with intermediate purified protein derivative produced a 10 mm. area of induration.

Roentgen examination of the chest showed calcified hilar lymph nodes but no evidence of parenchymal disease. A bone age of 6 years was estimated from wrist films. Flat and upright films of the abdomen revealed dilated loops of bowel with air-fluid levels. A barium enema demonstrated a normal descending and transverse colon and a marked narrowing of the ascending colon which communicated with huge cavity (Fig. 2). Roentgen study of the upper gastrointestinal tract showed displacement of the small intestine to the left by a large space-occupying mass (Fig. 3). Subsequent films demonstrated marked dilatation of the distal ileum which appeared to form a part of the mass.

Cystoscopic examination and the cystogram were within normal limits. Some narrowing of the left ureteropelvic junction with a mild degree of hydronephrosis was found on intravenous pyelographic study.

The anemia was partially corrected by blood transfusions and treatment with isoniazid (INH) and para-aminosalicylic acid (PAS) was initiated prior to operation because a tentative diagnosis of intestinal tuberculosis had been made. Abdominal exploration was carried out on October 18, 1968. A massively dilated distal ileum and proximal ascending colon were found. The huge megacolon and megaileum were proximal to an area of marked colonic narrowing which was surrounded by an inflammatory mass composed of omentum, mesocolon, and enlarged mesocolic lymph nodes. Enlarged lymph nodes also were found in the mesentery of the cecum and ileum.

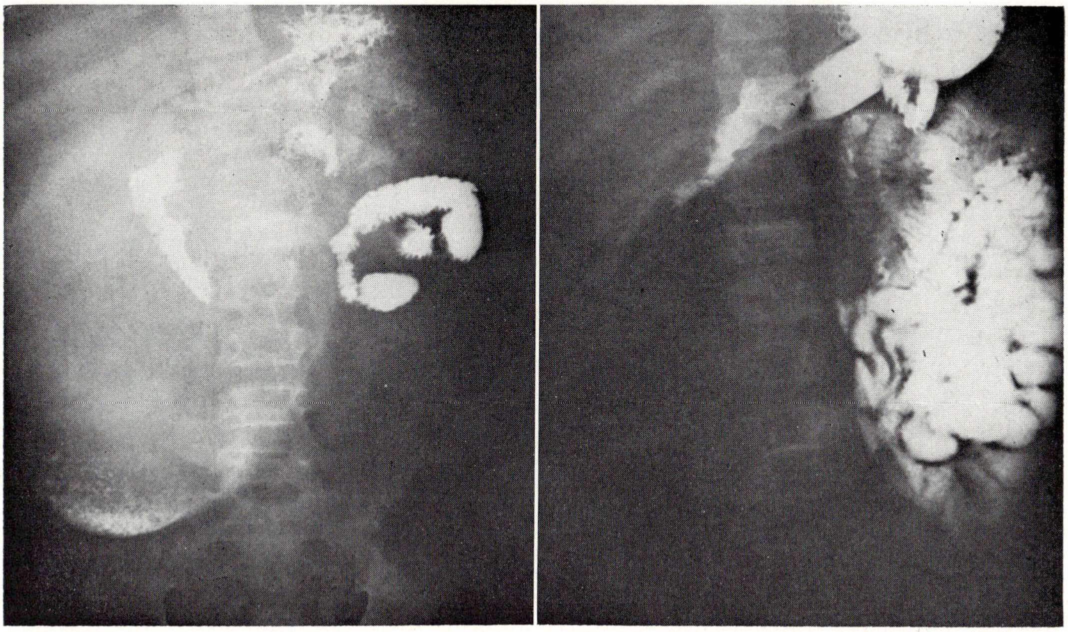

A B

Fig. 3. Roentgen study of the abdomen showing *A*, the large "mass" of dilated, feces-filled ileum and ascending colon faintly outlined with residual barium and *B*, the displacement of the barium-filled small intestine to the left by the "mass."

The right colon and distal ileum were resected and an end-to-end ileo–transverse colostomy was performed.

Examination of the resected specimen showed a markedly dilated and thickened distal ileum and proximal ascending colon which terminated abruptly in an area of marked stenosis (Fig. 4). The stenosis extended for approximately 2 cm. and had a circumference of 3 mm. The wall of the dilated ascending colon measured 0.5 cm. in thickness and the mucosa of this section of colon had a cobblestone appearance with areas of dark red mixed with areas of light gray and yellow. The distal ileum and the ileocecal valve also were dilated greatly. The mucosa of the distal ileum was normal in appearance.

Microscopic examination of the area of stenosis revealed extensive ulceration, scarring, and chronic inflammation (Fig. 5). Multiple zones of caseation necrosis were noted. In some areas, these zones of caseation necrosis extended through the muscularis and into the serosa. Many Langhan's giant cells were present. Other areas of the dilated ascending colon showed extensive mature scar tissue and chronic inflammation. Sections of mesenteric lymph nodes showed extensive caseation necrosis and many Langhan's giant cells. Acid-fast stains of the resected tissue showed organisms typical of *Mycobacterium tuberculosis* and cultures for *M. tuberculosis* (human) from this tissue were positive.

The postoperative course was uneventful. The patient did quite well and was discharged from the hospital on the eighth postoperative day. He was maintained on INH and PAS after operation. Four months following operation, his weight had increased by 20 pounds to 69 pounds and his height was 50½ inches (Fig. 1, *B*). Follow-up intravenous pyelography has demonstrated no change in the degree of ureteropelvic obstruction. This condition continues to be followed by our urologic colleagues who feel that no further surgical intervention is indicated at present.

DISCUSSION

Prior to the advent of antituberculous chemotherapy, involvement of the gastrointestinal tract in chronic pulmonary tuberculosis was so frequent an occurrence that it was considered by some authors to be part of the same disease and was almost uniformly fatal as late as 1910.[1] The reported incidence has varied in autopsy cases from 50 to 90 percent[9, 24] and in clinical cases from 6 to 28 percent.[26, 27] Biedent, in 1903, reported a 31.6 percent incidence in an autopsy study

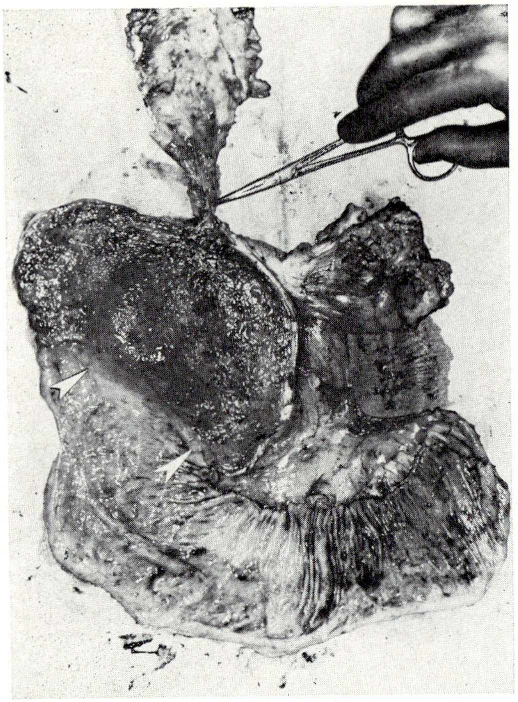

Fig. 4. Photograph of the surgical specimen portraying the area of stricture (hemostat) and the greatly dilated distal ileum and ascending colon. The massively dilated ileocecal valve is shown (arrows).

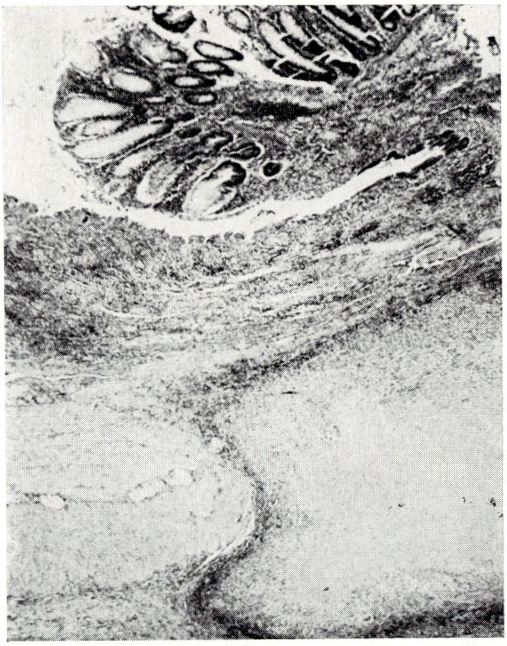

Fig. 5. Photomicrograph of one end of the area of stricture showing colonic ulceration, scarring, and caseous necrosis. Acid-fast stains identified tubercle bacilli in this area, as well as in regional lymph nodes.

of 1,346 children, and Cullen[19] in 1940, showed a 74 percent incidence in 125 children.

The use of antituberculous drugs has reduced, markedly, the incidence and mortality of tuberculous enteritis in the Western Hemisphere. Even in 1949, with only PAS and streptomycin available, Mitchell and Bristol[27] showed that the over-all incidence of tuberculous enteritis had decreased to 1.3 percent.

The majority of reported series of tuberculous enteritis have shown the occurrence to be highest in young adults in their third and fourth decades. Sixty percent of Cullen's[19] series of 734 cases were between 20 and 39 years of age, and the mean age in the 346 cases reported by Mitchell and Bristol[27] was 28.2 years. Only a small number, however, have been seen in children.[2, 5, 6] The youngest reported patient with tuberculous enteritis was two months old.[19] The youngest patient to have been operated upon for this disorder was ten years old.[6]

Tuberculosis of the intestine may be of the secondary type, occurring as a complication of pulmonary tuberculosis. Ukil,[37] in 1942, found pulmonary lesions in 95 percent of 1,000 patients with intestinal tuberculosis. Many cases of tuberculous enterities doubtless are due to swallowed bacilli.[4] In some areas of the world a higher incidence of intestinal tract tuberculosis due to causes other than pulmonary disease may be found. In a recent report from Iraq, Hamandi and Thamer[23] observed that only 10 percent of their 86 cases of intestinal tuberculosis had pulmonary disease.

The ileoceal region has been the site most frequently involved in gastrointestinal tuberculosis. The reported incidence of involvement has ranged from 50 to 90 percent.[7, 9,

[16, 18, 19, 30, 32, 37, 41, 42] The second most frequent site is the ascending colon, varying from 10 to 40 percent.

A variety of clinical presentations, hypertrophic, ulcerative, or both, have been encountered in the comparatively small number of cases which have been reported in the recent years.[8-14, 17, 22, 33, 39, 40, 48] Only in India have cases similar to ours been recorded.[5, 6, 15] None of these cases involved children.

The outcome in cases of intestinal tuberculosis is dependent on the ability to control the pulmonary infection and on the character of the intestinal involvement and its complications. Secondary complications, such as the anemia and cachexia encountered in our case, may pose additional problems. The massive megacolon and megaileum which resulted from the stenotic intestinal tuberculosis in our patient is a most unusual complication of this illness in childhood. The rapid restoration of our patient to health with a 20 pound weight gain in the initial four months after resection of the disordered intestine and the initiation of drug therapy was quite gratifying.

SUMMARY

An unusual case of massive megacolon and megaileum due to tuberculous stenosis of the ascending colon in childhood is reported. The patient was a twelve-year-old Mexican boy who had roentgen evidence suggesting previous pulmonary tuberculosis. He had marked abdominal distention and was severely cachectic and anemic. He was managed successfully by resection of the greatly enlarged ileum and ascending colon with the area of ulceration and stenosis, followed by primary end-to-end ileo–transverse colostomy. Treatment with INH and PAS was initiated prior to and continued after operation. A weight gain of 20 pounds was recorded in the first four months after operation. His tuberculous enteritis was documented by histologic finding of acid-fast bacilli in the area of ulceration and stenosis and by identification of the organism on culture.

Complications of gastrointestinal tuberculosis are considered and the hazard of this disorder in childhood is discussed. Massive dilatation of the ascending colon and ileum secondary to tuberculous stenosis in childhood has not been described.

The successful result in this case suggests the advisability of resection of the ulcerated and stenotic area with the greatly dilated proximal intestine, supplemented with antituberculous therapy in the management of this disorder.

REFERENCES

1. Abrams, J. S., and Holden, W. D.: Tuberculosis of the gastrointestinal tract, Arch. Surg. **89:** 282, 1964.
2. Adams, R., and Miller, W. H.: Surgical treatment of intestinal tuberculosis, Surg. Clin. N. Amer. **27:** 656, 1946.
3. Alvarez Pagan, M., and Sifontes, J. E.: Abdominal tuberculosis in children, Bol. Asoc. Med. P. Rico **57:** 118, 1965.
4. Amerson, J. R., and Martin, J. D., Jr.: Tuberculosis of the alimentary tract, Amer. J. Surg. **107:** 340, 1964.
5. Anand, S. S.: Hypertrophic ileo-cecal tuberculosis in India with a record of fifty hemicolectomies, Ann. Roy. Coll. Surg. **19:** 205, 1956.
6. Anand, S. S., and Pathak, I. C.: Surgical treatment of abdominal tuberculosis with special reference to ileocecal tuberculosis, J. Indian Med. Ass. **37:** 423, 1961.
7. Anscombe, A. R., Keddie, N. C., and Schofield, P. F.: Cecal tuberculosis, Gut **8:** 337, 1967.
8. Babrow, M. L., and Friedman, S.: Tuberculosis appendicitis, Amer. J. Surg. **91:** 389, 1956.
9. Bentley, G., and Webster, J. H. H.: Gastrointestinal tuberculosis, Brit. J. Surg. **54:** 90, 1967.
10. Bloch, C., and Peck, H. M.: Radiologic notes: Case 214, J. Mount Sinai Hosp. N. Y. **30:** 451, 1963.
11. Bloch, C., and Peck, H. M.: Radiologic notes: Case 227, J. Mount Sinai Hosp. N. Y. **31:** 75, 1964.
12. Castleman, B., and Kibbee, B. U., editors: Case Records of the Massachusetts General Hospital: Case 46181, New Eng. J. Med. **262:** 930, 1960.
13. Castleman, B., and Kibbee, B. U., editors: Case Records of the Massachusetts General Hospital: Case 20-1961, New Eng. J. Med. **264:** 562, 1961.
14. Castleman, B., and Kibbee, B. U., editors: Case Records of the Massachusetts General

Hospital: Case 76-1961, New Eng. J. Med. **265:** 801, 1961.
15. Chawla, S., Bery, K., and Indra, K. J.: Enterolithiasis complicating intestinal tuberculosis, Clin. Radiol. **17:** 274, 1966.
16. Cirolini, W.: Tuberculosi del cieco, Fracastoro **59:** 777, 1966.
17. Cole, B. K., Oddsen, G., Winkleman, E. I., and Van Orstrand, H. S.: Gastrointestinal tuberculosis, Cleveland Clin. Quart. **34:** 265, 1967.
18. Crawford, P. M., and Sawyer, H. P.: Intestinal tuberculosis in 1,400 autopsies, Amer. Rev. Tuberc. **30:** 568, 1934.
19. Cullen, J. H.: Intestinal tuberculosis, a clinical pathological study, Quart. Bull. Sea View Hosp. **51:** 143, 1940.
20. Debroise, A., Senghor, G., Dan, V., et al.: Incidence et formes cliniques de la tuberculose infantile dans le service pediatric du Centre Hospitalier Universitaire de Dakar, Bull. Soc. Med. Afr. Noire Lang. Franc. **12:** 416, 1967.
21. Dinner, M.: Tuberculosis of the gastrointestinal tract in the non-white population of the Transvaal, S. Afr. J. Surg. **3:** 97, 1965.
22. Eidex, M. F., and Rosenbaum, L. J.: Tuberculosis of the ascending colon mimicking carcinoma, Missouri Med. **62:** 32, 1965.
23. Hamandi, W. J., and Thamer, M. A.: Tuberculosis of the bowel in Iraq; a study of 86 cases, Dis. Colon Rectum **8:** 158, 1965.
24. Jordon, G. L., Jr., and De Bakey, M. E.: Complications of tuberculous enteritis occurring during antimicrobial therapy, Arch. Surg. **69:** 688, 1954.
25. Kleinschmidt, H.: Der Leutig Stand der Kindertuberculose in Deutschland, Munchen. Med. Wschr. **107:** 1919, 1965.
26. Kornblum, S. A., Zale, C., and Aronson, W.: Surgical complications of intestinal tuberculosis as seen at necropsy, Amer. J. Surg. **75:** 498, 1948.
27. Mitchell, R. E., and Bristol, L. J.: Intestinal tuberculosis. An analysis of 346 cases. Diagnosed by routine intestinal radiography on 5,529 admissions for pulmonary tuberculosis, 1924-1949, Amer. J. Med. Sci. **227:** 241, 1954.
28. Magol, P. M., and Alvarez Pagan, M.: Manejode la tuberculosis en la infancia, Bol. Asoc. Med. P. Rico **59:** 20, 1967.
29. Ramachandren, R. S., and Purnaggen, S.: Tuberculosis in children, Indian Pediat. **3:** 218, 1966.
30. Rankine, J. A.: Tuberculosis of the ileocecal area, J. Int. Coll. Surg. **18:** 202, 1952.
31. Rueda, D. R., Carrada, T., and Xelhuantzin, M.: Tuberculosis en niños y adolescentes, Rev. Med. Hosp. Gen. (Mexico) **28:** 829, 1965.
32. Schwatt, H., and Steinbach, M. M.: Tuberculosis of the intestines, Amer. Rev. Tuberc. **8:** 9, 1923-24.
33. Singer, A., and Supplice, J.: A case of ileocecal tuberculosis, J. Mount Sinai Hosp. **30:** 491, 1963.
34. Tandon, H. D., Prakash, A., Rao, V. B., Prakash, O., and Nair, S. K.: Ulceroconstrictive disorders of the intestine in northern India: A pathologic study, Indian J. Med. Res. **54:** 129, 1966.
35. Taneja, O. P., Taneja, S., and Lal, A.: Intestinal obstruction in infancy and childhood, Arch. Surg. **97:** 544, 1968.
36. Trauger, D. A.: Tuberculosis in children in the United States; trends and current status, Clin. Pediat. **5:** 685, 1966.
37. Ukil, A. C.: Early diagnosis and treatment of intestinal tuberculosis, Ind. Med. Gaz. **77:** 613, 1942.
38. Virmani, P.: Ulcerative tuberculosis of the colon, Brit. J. Surg. **50:** 550, 1963.
39. Waggener, H. U., Muldoon, J. P., and Heaton, J. R.: Asymptomatic tuberculous enteritis simulating carcinoma of the cecum, J. A. M. A. **171:** 1337, 1959.
40. Walton, T. T., Jr., Elmendorf, E. A., and Kowierschke, S. W.: Tuberculous enterocolitis, Texas J. Med. **61:** 830, 1965.
41. Weisberg, A., and Luongo, V.: Coexistent pulmonary and ileocecal tuberculosis, New York J. Med. **61:** 1765, 1961.
42. Winter, J., and Goldman, M.: Tuberculosis of the terminal ileum, Gut **7:** 478, 1966.

Intrauterine midgut strangulation in a gastroschisis defect

JAY L. GROSFELD, M.D.
H. WILLIAM CLATWORTHY, JR., M.D.
COLUMBUS, OHIO
From the Department of Surgery, Division of Pediatric Surgery, The Ohio State University College of Medicine and Children's Hospital

Gastroschisis is an uncommon developmental defect through the anterior abdominal wall through which evisceration of the majority of the midgut may take place during intrauterine existence. Since the eccentric musculofascial opening is small, the eviscerated gastrointestinal tract is usually quite edematous and may actually be incarcerated or rarely even strangulated. The embryogenesis of this defect, as described, is related to the early failure of the development of one of the lateral embryonic mesodermal folds that form the developing abdominal wall.[1, 2] Fortunately, associated major congenital malformations are infrequent with this isolated lesion, although the expected incomplete rotation and fixation of the midgut is an obvious accompaniment of the extra-abdominal position of the viscera.

In 1957, Kiesewetter[3] reported a patient with an infarction of the midgut secondary to incarceration of the bowel and its mesentery in a tight gastroschisis defect. The present report concerns an infant with what appears to have been an intrauterine strangulation of the midgut in a gastroschisis defect with resultant intrauterine infarction of the majority of the gastrointestinal tract and the subsequent development of an acquired jejunal atresia. This previously unreported complication of gastroschisis provides additional support for the theories and experimental observations of Louw and Barnard[4] relating mid–small bowel atresia to intrauterine vascular catastrophes.

Received for publication June 19, 1969.

CASE REPORT

B. B. was the product of a gravida 4, para 4, abortus 0, 29-year-old Caucasian woman. The prenatal course was complicated by excessive weight gain and ankle edema. Four weeks prior to the estimated date of confinement, a male infant with a birth weight of 6 pounds 4 ounces was delivered vaginally following a 3½ hour uncomplicated labor. At delivery the infant was noted to have eviscerated infarcted bowel through a small right paraumbilical defect. The umbilical cord was intact. The infant breathed spontaneously and received an Apgar score of nine at one and five minutes. The patient was transferred to the Columbus Children's Hospital at age three hours. On admission, physical examination revealed a temperature of 97° F., blood pressure 90/60 mm. Hg, pulse 140 beats per minute, respiratory rate 38 per minute. Loops of gangrenous infarcted bowel were seen in a small gastroschisis defect measuring 1 cm. in diameter, just to the right of the umbilicus, which was entirely intact (Fig. 1). The abdomen was quite distended and dull to percussion. Bowel sounds were hypoactive. The anus was patent but tight, and no meconium was noted on rectal examination. Erect and recumbent x-rays of the abdomen revealed three large air-containing portions of intestines, and no evidence of free air (Fig. 2). The chest x-ray revealed some elevation of the diaphragm incident to abdominal distention. A nasogastric tube was inserted into the stomach and 300 c.c. of bilious material was aspirated. The abdomen appeared to flatten significantly. Laboratory data showed a hemoglobin of 14.5 Gm. percent; hematocrit, 46 percent; pH, 7.4 units; P_{CO_2}, 28 mm. Hg; CO_2, 24 mEq. per liter; chloride, 104 mEq. per liter; sodium, 139 mEq. per liter; potassium, 5 mEq. per liter; calcium, 6.5 mg.; bilirubin, 9 mg. percent; Coombs' test, negative. The white blood cell count was 21,000 per cubic millimeter, with a slight increase in polymorphonuclear cells. The urinalysis was unremarkable. At operation the infarcted bowel was

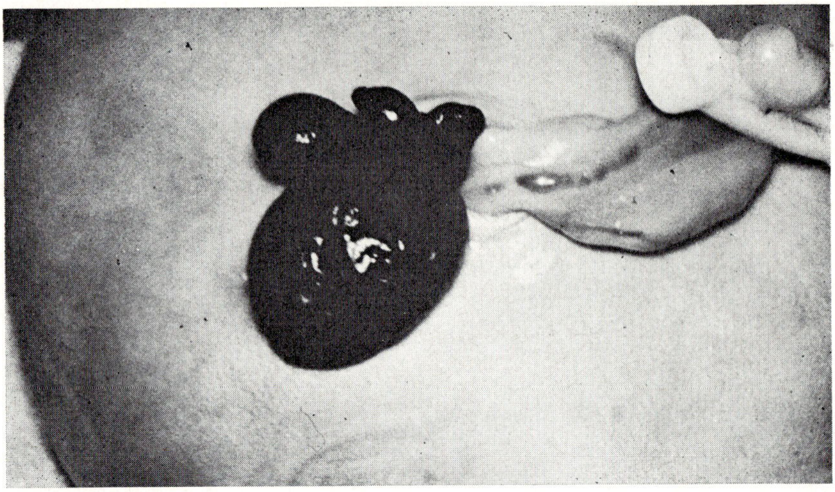

Fig. 1. A close-up photograph of the abdominal wall of the patient demonstrating the extremely small, eccentrically located paraumbilical gastroschisis defect. The umbilical cord is normal. There is no sac. The amorphous mass of shrunken gangrenous tissue extruding from the defect is all that is left of the majority of the midgut.

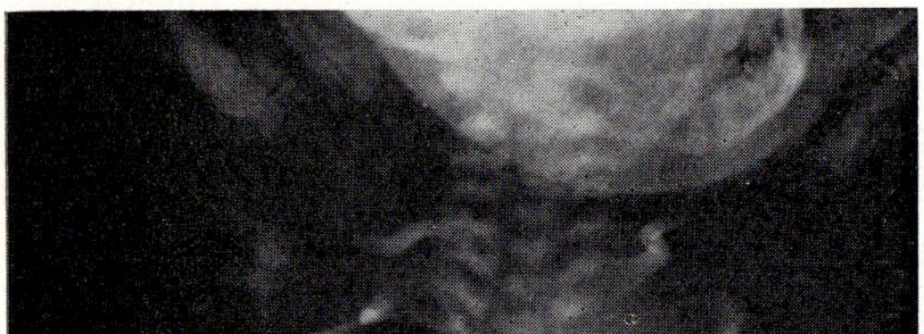

Fig. 2. Preoperative upright "babygram" showing evidence of high complete intestinal obstruction consistent with jejunal atresia in an infant with midgut infarcted in a gastroschisis defect.

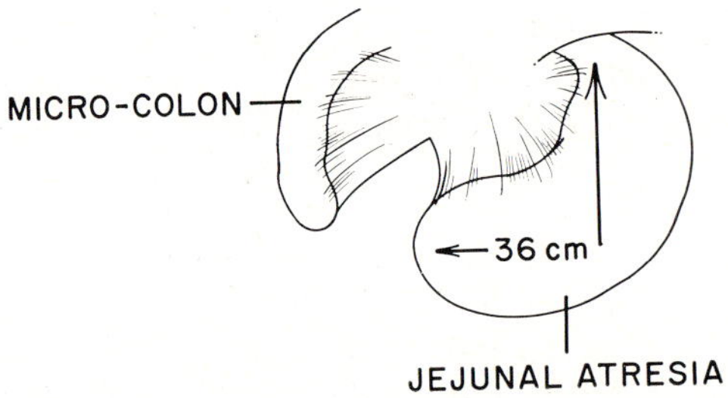

Fig. 3. Diagrammatic representation of intra-abdominal findings at time of operation: jejunal atresia, minimal length of small bowel, and a V-shaped mesenteric defect.

excised with the margins of the gastroschisis defect and the umbilicus. The infarcted bowel was shunken and represented most of the midgut. There was a jejunal atresia 36 cm. from the ligament of Treitz with a large V-shaped defect in the mesentery between the end of the atresia and a blind end of microcolon (Fig. 3). The appendix and cecum appeared to be within the infarcted mass. An end-to-side jejunocolostomy and a decompression Witzel-type jejunostomy were performed. Because of the small size of the defect and the lack of bowel to fill the abdominal cavity, a primary layered abdominal closure was possible in this particular instance of gastroschisis. Postoperatively, the patient was managed by intravenous hyperalimentation via a central venous silastic cannula. Persistent functional obstruction required reoperation on two separate occasions. Resection of the end-to-side anastomosis and a new end-to-end bowel anastomosis were performed at age one month. The previous anastomosis had been patent. This second anastomosis also failed to function, and an exteriorization procedure was done at age two months. Once again the anastomosis was patent. Ganglion cells were present in the bowel wall. The patient's nutrition was almost entirely supported by intravenous hyperalimentation; a 2 pound weight gain was observed, and yet the infant failed to thrive and died from gram-negative (pseudomonas) sepsis at the age of four months.

DISCUSSION

Strangulation of the intestine as the result of compression of its blood supply in a tight gastroschisis defect is a very rare occurrence, Kiesewetter's[3] case report in 1957 being the only previously such reported instance in the literature. There are some significant differences between his case and the present report. In the previously reported study, the bowel was intact, of uniform size, and recognizable in continuity, whereas an atresia was observed in the present instance and the infarcted bowel was greatly shrunken, suggesting that the catastrophic event occurred much earlier in intrauterine life. These findings also give further direct clinical evidence to support Louw and Barnard's[4] theory of the etiology of jejunoileal atresia, being directly related to an intrauterine vascular catastrophe involving the small bowel. The problems associated with the short bowel syndrome and alimentation in such an infant are beyond the scope of this report.

CONCLUSIONS

The second instance of intrauterine midgut strangulation in a tight gastroschisis defect is presented in a newborn infant in whom the process occurred early in intrauterine life and resulted in a vascular catastrophe and subsequent jejunal atresia.

REFERENCES

1. Duhamel, B.: Embryology of exomphalos and allied malformations, Arch. Dis. Child. **38:** 142, 1963.
2. Hutchin, P.: Somatic anomalies of the umbilicus and anterior abdominal wall, Surg. Gynec. Obstet. **120:** 1075, 1965.
3. Kiesewetter, W. B.: Gastroschisis, Arch. Surg. **75:** 28, 1957.
4. Louw, J. H., and Barnard, C. N.: Congenital intestinal atresia; observations on its origin, Lancet **2:** 1065, 1955.

Improved operative technique for gastric duplication

JOHN J. WHITE, M.D., C.M.
W. W. MORGAN, M.D.
BALTIMORE, MD.
From the Division of Pediatric Surgery of the Department of Surgery, The Johns Hopkins University School of Medicine.

Duplications of the gastrointestinal tract are interesting and uncommon lesions. Stomach duplications appear to be the rarest type; only 55 cases had been reported up to 1967.[1] Most have shared a common wall with the stomach along the greater curvature, and in these, some variety of gastric resection usually had been performed.

A huge duplication along the greater curvature of the stomach was diagnosed in a newborn infant admitted to the Childrens' Medical and Surgical Center of The Johns Hopkins Hospital. Inasmuch as the blood supply to the cyst and stomach was derived from the gastroepiploic arteries, which were in the sulcus along the common muscular wall shared by both, it was possible to excise the cyst walls and strip off all the cyst mucosa without entering the stomach or sacrificing its integrity. This technique appears to be applicable to most gastric duplications and, possibly, to duplications elsewhere in the gastrointestinal tract.

CASE REPORT

A one-day-old girl (JHH No. 128 41 95) was noted to have a tense, sausage-shaped mass in her abdomen running from the left upper quadrant across the midline to the right lateral portion of the abdomen (Fig. 2*A*). The mass was mobile and nontender and appeared to cause no distress. Chest roentgenogram showed hemivertebrae of T_3 and T_4. Abdominal films and intravenous pyelogram demonstrated a cystic mass occupying the left upper quadrant of the abdomen which passed over to the right lateral abdomen under the liver, displacing the stomach to the right and the remainder of the intestines to the left quadrant (Fig. 1). With a preoperative diagnosis of gastric duplication, laparotomy was performed on the second day of life. A complete duplication along the greater curvature from cardia to pylorus was found. Three hundred and fifty cubic centimeters of gray-green fluid were aspirated, and the cyst was managed by the technique described. Histologic examination confirmed a dupli-

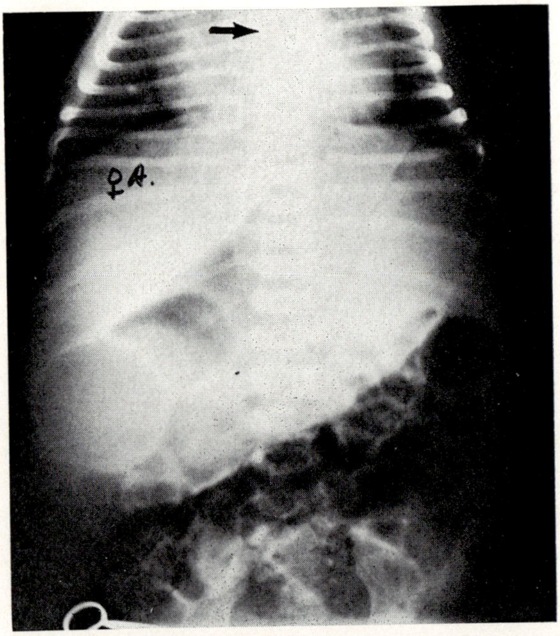

Fig. 1. Preoperative intravenous pyelogram. "Total body opacification" well outlines the walls of the cyst, which runs from the left upper quadrant to the right lateral portion of the abdomen. The gastric air is shifted toward the midline, and the intestines to the left lower quadrant. Thoracic hemivertebrae are indicated by the arrow.

Received for publication July 24, 1969.

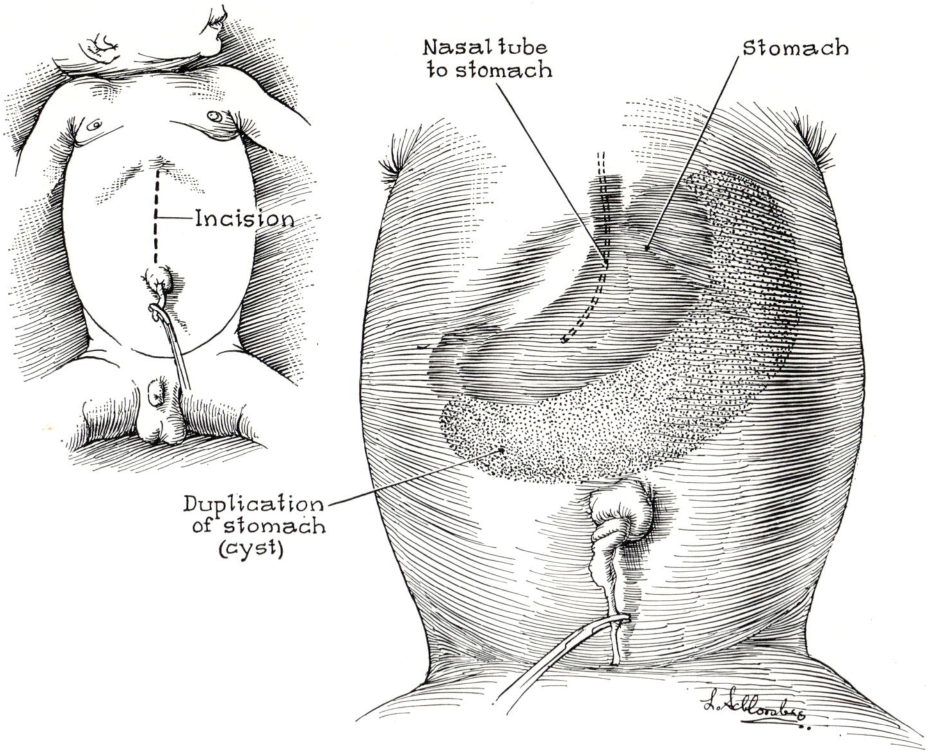

Fig. 2*A*. Operative technique. A midline epigastric incision provides excellent access to the cyst which runs along the greater curvature of the stomach from fundus to pylorus.

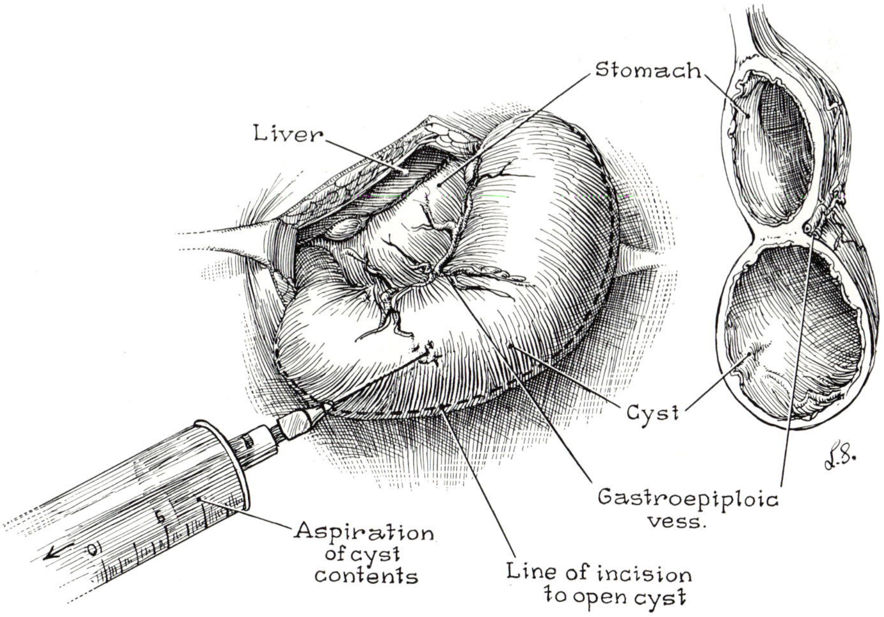

Fig. 2*B*. The cyst is aspirated of its contents for easy handling and to prevent peritoneal contamination. The gastroepiploic blood supply which is common to both cyst and stomach lies in the sulcus between the two.

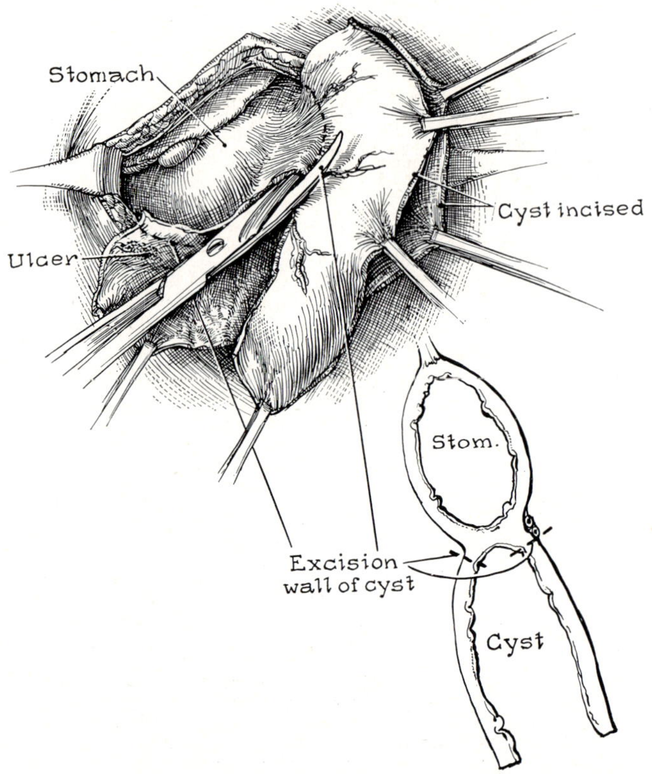

Fig. 2*C*. The cyst is first incised along its outer border and, then, each wall is excised down to the common wall with the stomach. The gastroepiploic vessels are preserved.

cation with gastric and intestinal epithelium; there was ulceration in the distal intestinal part. The stomach was never entered. Her postoperative course was entirely benign; feedings were started on the second day following operation. When last seen at age 1½ years, she was thriving.

TECHNIQUE

The operative steps are illustrated in Fig. 2. Through a midline epigastric incision, which allowed optimal exposure of the fundus, the preoperative diagnosis of duplication of the stomach was confirmed (Fig. 2*A*). The cyst along the greater curvature was first aspirated of fluid to prevent spillage into the peritoneal cavity (Fig. 2*B*). With realization that the common blood supply to the stomach and cyst arose from the gastroepiploic arteries which ran in the sulcus along the contiguous border of the duplication cyst and the stomach (Fig. 2*B*), the cyst was laid open along its outer wall. Each of the flaps so produced was resected back to the common wall between cyst and stomach, carefully preserving the gastroepiploic arteries (Fig. 2*C*). The small mucosal strip on the remaining cyst wall, lying along the greater curvature of the stomach, was then stripped from the muscularis (Fig. 2*D*). This 2 to 3 cm. area of mucosa, from cardia to pylorus, was easily removed. Finally, the transverse colon was sutured to the denuded greater curvature (Fig. 2*D*).

DISCUSSION

Duplications of the intestinal tract are either tubular or cystic. The former communicate with the bowel lumen proper through one or more openings, and generally present with symptoms of vague abdominal pain, bloating, or discomfort; less commonly, there may be intestinal bleeding resulting from ulceration of contiguous intestine by secretions from aberrant gastric mucosa. Cystic duplications tend to present with intestinal obstruction as the cyst enlarges as the result of retained secretions or

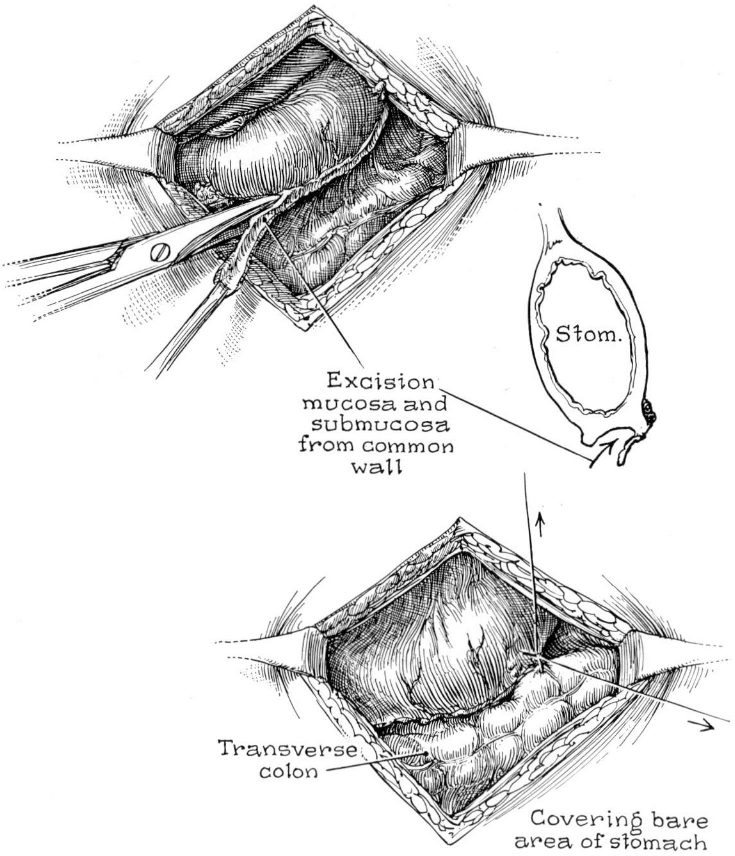

Fig. 2*D*. The mucosa of the cyst is stripped from the common muscular wall with the stomach, and the colon is sutured to the bare area as coverage.

with acute perforation of an ulcer. The infant presented had a cystic duplication, the common finding with stomach duplications. It was tensely filled with 350 c.c. of fluid and showed early ulceration of the intestinal mucosa at the distal aspect. Fortunately, it was diagnosed before obstruction or perforation.

The embryology of intestinal duplications remains uncertain. The older theory, proposed by Bremer,[5] of incomplete resolution of the solid stage of intestinal development, does not provide satisfactory explanation. Certain duplications, particularly the tubular, may result from double organization, i.e., the fusion of two embryos.[6, 11] Other duplications may represent dorsal enteric fistulas or the split notochord syndrome.[2] These neurenteric cysts generally occur in the foregut and are frequently associated with abnormalities of the thoracic spine.[10] Vertebral anomalies were noted in 5 out of the 8 esophageal duplications reported by Mellish and Koop[9] and hemivertebrae of T_3 and T_4 were present in our case.

The majority of duplications are found within the leaves of the dorsal mesentery of the contiguous bowel and participate in the same blood supply. Thus, their removal requires excision of the adjacent normal bowel as well. Probably related to its developmental rotation and its pouchlike enlargement, the main vessels to the stomach enter proximally and distally and travel along the greater and lesser curvatures. The blood supply to cyst and stomach runs between the two and does not envelop both together as elsewhere in the intestinal tract. This was the situation in this case, and in the photographs of the case presented by Kiesewetter.[7] It appears, then, that most gastric duplications can probably be excised without compromise of blood supply to the stomach proper.

The sequelae of duplications, cystic engorgement with retained secretions, and pain or bleeding from peptic ulceration, result from their mucosal activity. After excising all of the gastric duplication except the common wall with the stomach, it seemed rational to render the remaining strip of duplication impotent by stripping off the residual mucosa. This easily accomplished maneuver left only a small denuded muscular strip of duplication remaining. This area was covered with the transverse colon to reduce the danger of adhesions. There have been no sequelae to date, 1½ years later.

Rectal mucosal stripping has been advocated as therapy for several conditions in the gastrointestinal tract, including a few instances of duplications. It has been used in Hirschsprung's disease,[4, 14] and other rectal lesions,[13] and appears to be applicable in the management of long tubular duplications as well, where an excessive length of normal adjoining bowel might have to be sacrificed during resection. Wrenn[15] has reported successful management of such a duplication of the small intestine by completely stripping the mucosa through multiple transverse incisions. Ravitch and Scott[12] have successfully employed mucosal stripping in the treatment of duplication of the entire colon and rectum. Patient No. 1 of Ladd and Scott[8] apparently had such a procedure for a long esophageal duplication, with a satisfactory 16 year follow-up. Bishop and Koop[3] mention partial excision of a duplication of the stomach and duodenum, leaving the common wall intact and stripping away the mucosa. In all these instances, this approach has provided satisfactory management. It would appear to be applicable whenever preservation of intact bowel is desirable.

SUMMARY

A duplication cyst of the stomach, lying along the entire greater curvature, was removed from a newborn infant. Since the blood supply to cyst and stomach proper ran in the sulcus along the common muscular wall between them, it was possible to excise all of the cyst except the common wall without sacrificing stomach or compromising its blood supply. The mucosa was easily stripped from the remaining area, defunctioning the cyst. This operative technique appears to be applicable to most gastric duplications and probably to duplications elsewhere in the intestinal tract.

REFERENCES

1. Bartels, R. J.: Duplication of the stomach—case report and review of the literature, Amer. Surg. **3:** 747, 1967.
2. Bentley, J. F. R., and Smith, J. R.: Developmental posterior enteric remnants and spinal malformations, Arch. Dis. Child. **35:** 76, 1960.
3. Bishop, H. C., and Koop, C. E.: Surgical management of duplications of the alimentary tract, Amer. J. Surg. **107:** 434, 1964.
4. Boley, S. J., Lafer, D. J., Kleinhaus, S., Cohn, B. D., Mestel, A. L., and Kottmeier, P. K.: Endorectal pull-through procedure for Hirschsprung's disease with and without primary anastomosis, J. Pediat. Surg. **3:** 258, 1968.
5. Bremer, J. L.: Diverticula and duplication of the intestinal tract, Arch. Path. **38:** 132, 1944.
6. Duhamel, B.: Concerning the embryology of intestinal duplications, Ann. Chir. Inf. **8:** 55, 1967.
7. Kiesewetter, W. B.: Duplication of the stomach: A case report, Ann. Surg. **146:** 990, 1957.
8. Ladd, W. E., and Scott, H. W., Jr.: Esophageal duplications or mediastinal cysts of enteric origin, SURGERY **16:** 815, 1944.
9. Mellish, R. W., and Koop, C. E.: Clinical manifestations of duplication of the bowel, Pediatrics **27:** 397, 1961.
10. Neuhauser, E. B. D., Harris, G. B. C., and Berrett, A.: Roentgenographic features of neurenteric cysts, Amer. J. Roentgen. **79:** 235, 1958.
11. Ravitch, M. M.: Hind gut duplication—doubling of colon and genital urinary tracts, Ann. Surg. **137:** 588, 1953.
12. Ravitch, M. M., and Scott, W. W.: Duplication of the entire colon, bladder, and urethra, SURGERY **34:** 843, 1953.
13. Ravitch, M. M., and Sabiston, D. C.: Anal ileostomy with preservation of the sphincter, Surg. Gynec. Obstet. **84:** 1095, 1947.
14. Soave, F.: Hirschsprung's disease—technique and results of Soave's operation, Brit. J. Surg. **53:** 1023, 1966.
15. Wrenn, E. L., Jr.: Tubular duplication of the small intestine, SURGERY **52:** 494, 1962.

Surgery for duodenal and gastric ulcer in infancy and childhood

J. E. STRODE, M.D.
JOHN F. BALFOUR, M.D.
HONOLULU, HAWAII
From the Department of Surgery, Straub Clinic

Over the years, ulcers of the stomach and duodenum occurring in infancy and childhood have been given scant consideration in comparison with the voluminous literature, both clinical and experimental, that has accumulated relative to similar lesions in adults. This is easily understandable because of the discrepancy in frequency of occurrence of these conditions in these different age groups. However, in recent years, pediatricians and surgeons interested in the problems of childhood have become aware that these lesions are more common than were previously recognized. This has come about by more frequent x-ray investigation of symptoms such as vomiting, diarrhea, abdominal pain and discomfort, poor appetite, malnutrition, and other abdominal symptoms of a bizarre nature which were not previously thought indicative of an organic lesion of the upper digestive tract. Recent refinements in x-ray equipment and techniques enable recognition of gastric and duodenal deformities not apparent before. At the Straub Clinic since 1922, we have had occasion to operate upon children for only two duodenal ulcers and one gastric ulcer, and upon one individual of 18 years of age for a stomal ulcer resulting from a gastroenterostomy undergone for a duodenal ulcer at age 15. During this time more than 1,500 adults have been operated upon for similar lesions.

Gross,[11] in his book, *The surgery of infancy and childhood,* published in 1953, makes no mention of gastric ulcer and gives scant space to the subject of duodenal ulcer. He mentions that in two instances they had undertaken laparotomy for control of exsanguinating hemorrhage and on two occasions gastrojejunostomy had been performed for stenosis resulting from duodenal ulcer. He stated that mechanical obstruction is best treated by posterior gastroenterostomy and the surgeon should not be tempted to perform any type of resection.

Received for publication Sept. 2, 1969.

Ten years later Schuster and Gross[20] stated that the incidence of peptic ulcer disease in children is an unknown but suspiciously high figure and that the frequency with which the diagnosis is made unquestionably varies with the diligence with which the condition is searched for by both the radiologist and the pathologist.

Swenson's[22] book on pediatric surgery published in 1962 makes no mention of gastric ulcer or other lesions of the stomach. He said of duodenal ulcers, "This rare disease of childhood may result in severe hemorrhage in the newborn and there may be perforation in infancy. In older children there may be pain which is similar to the ulcer dyspepsia of adults." He further stated that "surgical treatment had not been used except in children with severe bleeding or pyloric obstruction. One reason for the conservative attitude of physicians and surgeons is the limited knowledge concerning the fate of a child following subtotal gastrectomy."

Lucas and Benson,[14] in 1967, stated that peptic ulcers in infancy and childhood are no longer considered a rare disease. In the vast majority of instances they can be managed satisfactorily by conservative measures. They reported a chronic duodenal ulcer with recurrent hemorrhage in a boy of ten treated by hemigastrectomy and vagotomy with a successful outcome.

Raffensperger and associates[19] noted, in 1966, that a surgeon called upon to treat an infant with a bleeding peptic ulcer has little data upon which to base his decision for therapy. They reported that at the Cook County Children's Hospital in Chicago, eighty patients, from newborn infants to 16 year olds, had a diagnosis of gastric or duodenal ulcer which had been made at autopsy, laparotomy, or roentgenographic examination covering the years 1937 to 1965. Twenty-three ulcers which complicated burns were not included. There were 21 babies in the newborn to 14 days of age group. All 13 gastric perforations occurred in this age group, and there were four perforated and four bleeding duodenal ulcers. The 32 infants from 15 days to one year old represented the largest single group, with 18 perforated and 16 bleeding duodenal ulcers. They noted that children between the ages of one and six years were remarkably free from the complications of peptic ulcer since there was only one perforation and two bleeding duodenal ulcers in this age grouping. The 21 children from seven to sixteen years of age commenced to have an ulcer pattern resembling that found in adults. They pointed out that is is possible that the diarrhea and malnutrition so frequently encountered in infancy may actually be manifestations of a chronic ulcer. Early and more frequent recourse to barium examination of the stomach and duodenum was recommended, since many such ulcers have deep indurated craters which should be easily recognizable, especially with recent improvement in x-ray equipment.

Gieske and Storey,[10] in 1966, reported the results of an analysis of duodenal ulcers in infancy at The Johns Hopkins Hospital between the years 1955 and 1963. There had been 15 primary ulcers and 27 secondary to either stress or medication. Of the latter 8 were diagnosed clinically and 19 at autopsy, a number indicating a need for increased awareness of ulcer disease in the ill child.

Three of the primary ulcers required surgery; two for perforation and one for intractability, a vagotomy and pyloroplasty being done. In 12 medically treated patients, two are known to have had recurrence of symptoms.

Moore,[16] in 1965, reported on a questionnaire on gastric resection in infancy and childhood gathered from members of the Surgical Section of the American Academy of Pediatrics and members of the Surgical Section of the British Association of Pediatric Surgery. Information concerning 113 gastric resections during the first 12 years of life was collected. Ninety-eight distal resections had been done with a 10 percent operative mortality rate and four late deaths, three the result of cancer. Forty-four percent were done in the first two years of life, and all the deaths occurred in patients six years of age or younger. Five were four months of age or younger. All deaths occurred in individuals with bleeding or perforation or both. Indications for opreation were most frequently due to complications of duodenal ulcer, representing 39 cases; two were for gastric ulcers and one for marginal ulcer. Thirteen were cases resulting from complications of ingestion of toxic material, eleven for duplication of the stomach, seven for benign neoplasms, and seven for malignant lesions. The most striking observation made was uniform growth and development following distal gastric resection, regardless of the amount of the stomach removed. Normal growth occurred in the few total gastrectomies reported. Billroth II type of reconstruction was carried out in 83 percent of the operations for peptic ulcer and no discernible difference was noted between Billroth I and Billroth II types of anastomosis. Fifteen cardioesophageal resections were done principally for stricture and esophageal varices: Thirteen patients survived and the striking observation was that only three developed in a normal manner. The original condition causing esophageal varices no doubt also contributed to lack of normal development.

Wilson and Ellison,[25] in 1965, reviewed the course of eight children with the Zollinger-

Ellison syndrome. Three children with less than total gastrectomy all died, while five with total gastrectomy were living and apparently doing well in spite of residual tumor. Their ages ranged between eight and fifteen years; those who lived were developing in a normal manner.

Tudor,[24] in 1967, reporting the experience at the Quain and Ramstead Clinic, said that 10 percent of the stomach x-rays of children revealed a peptic ulcer and that a similar experience had been reported by others interested in this problem. In their series, 24 peptic ulcers occurred during the first two years, 34 between age two and seven, 54 from seven to twelve, and three between twelve and sixteen years of life. There had been eight gastric ulcers, one associated with a duodenal ulcer.

In 1959, the Children's Peptic Ulcer Registry of the Bismark Medical Foundation of Bismark, North Dakota, was organized to collect unpublished cases of peptic ulcer in children and periodically to publish studies of their occurrence. It has also acquired copies of all medical articles involving peptic ulcer in children which have appeared in the world literature since the first article by Von Siebold in 1826. The report of this Registry as of January 1, 1967, showed the total number of cases collected to be 513, of which 242 were male. There had been 450 duodenal ulcers and 63 gastric ulcers. Ages ranged from birth to 17 years. The report of April 1, 1968, showed that 461 cases of gastric and duodenal ulcers had been subjected to surgery in this age group; the operation consisted of gastroenterostomy, gastric resection, pyloroplasty, or simple closure, some of which were combined with vagotomy.

In 1964, Barber and associates[1] at the Mayo Clinic made a study of 109 duodenal ulcers occurring in childhood and concluded that there is a 50 percent chance that a duodenal ulcer which begins in childhood will persist or recur in adolescence or adult life if medical treatment alone is employed. They pointed out that a carefully taken history of adult patients with a duodenal ulcer will often reveal the fact that the ulcer process had been present, although perhaps unrecognized, since childhood. Ten of the 109 patients did not respond to medical therapy and were operated upon. Five had posterior gastroenterostomy and five a gastric resection. Eight patients had been traced and each developed normally without recurrence of ulcer.

CASE REPORTS AND COMMENTS

The first four cases to be reported deal with the duodenal ulcer problem occurring in infancy and childhood. Two elective gastroenterostomies resulted in the development of stomal ulcers and two patients underwent emergency surgical treatment for exsanguinating hemorrhage.

Case 1. A Chinese boy of ten developed a bleeding stomal ulcer seven months following gastroenterostomy for pyloric obstruction. He was first seen on February 18, 1931, complaining of severe epigastric pain, nausea, vomiting, and loss of weight. The pain had been intermittent with remissions of two to four months' duration but with increasing severity and longer duration. Two years prior to being seen, he had been x-rayed and was told he had considerable 24 hour gastric retention. He had been placed on Sippy treatment with marked relief for a few months; then symptoms had recurred. At the time of our examination, the only positive physical finding was marked emaciation. The red blood cell count was 4,900,000 per cubic millimeter with hemoglobin 56 Gm. percent. X-ray examination showed a duodenal cap deformity with marked gastric retention.

After due preparation, including gastric lavage, intravenous fluids, and blood transfusion, the patient was operated upon on February 21, 1931. Exploration revealed a duodenal ulcer on the anterior wall apparently near perforation. The stomach was markedly dilated. The ulcer was covered over with omentum and a posterior short loop gastroenterostomy was performed. The patient left the hospital at the end of one week and three months later was feeling well and weighed 57 pounds, a gain of five pounds in weight. He was seen again at seven months after operation, at which time he was complaining of epigastric pain and vomiting. Blood examination showed 3,300,000 red blood cells per cubic millimeter, hemoglobin 30 Gm. percent, and there was blood in the stools. It was urged that the patient enter the hospital for further study and treatment. This was not done for another two months; meanwhile the epigastric pain had become more severe and the patient more anemic and emaciated. There was tenderness to the left of the umbilicus on palpation. The red blood cell count was now 1,800,000 per cubic millimeter, hemoglobin 40 Gm. percent, and blood was still present in the stools. On fluoroscopic and x-ray examination, there was no evidence of barium passing through the pylorus. The gastroenterostomy opening was small and irregular with a collection of barium to the left of the stoma, suggesting a large stomal ulcer crater (Fig. 1). The patient was given three blood transfusions, each of 300 to 400 c.c., with marked clinical improvement. At operation on December 17, 1931, a large ulcer was found in the jejunum, just to the left of the stoma penetrating into and prevented from perforating by the transverse mesocolon. The site of the previous duodenal ulcer seemed to be healed or was at least quiescent. A subtotal gastric resection was done to include the limbs of the anastomosis with a Billroth II reconstruction (Fig. 2). This patient was last seen on February 20, 1942, at 20 years of age. He was 6 feet 2 inches tall and normally developed; and he stated that he had had no further epigastric distress.

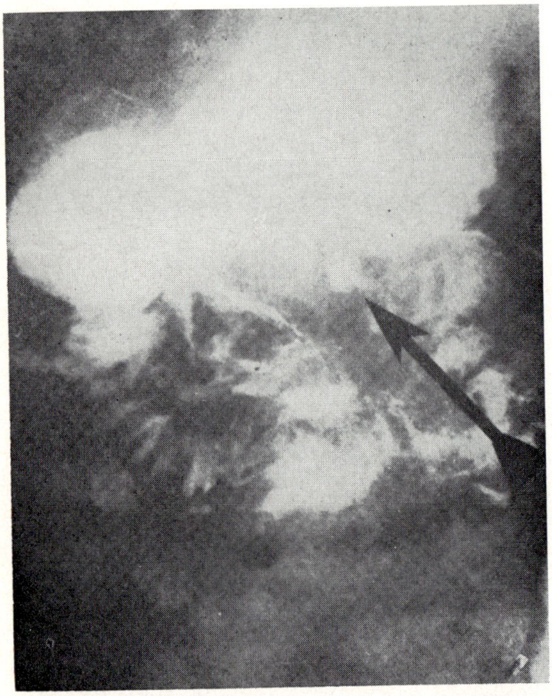

Fig. 1. Stomal ulcer crater at site of gastroenterostomy is shown (Case 1).

Case 2. A gastric resection was performed for a bleeding duodenal ulcer upon a boy of nine months. On October 21, 1949, one of us (J. E. S.) was called to assist Dr. Herbert Rothwell of Kahuku Plantation Hospital on Oahu with an operation upon this nine-month-old male infant with the following history.

At birth on January 9, 1949, the baby after normal delivery weighed 7 pounds 3 ounces and was of normal development; his progress was uneventful until October 7, 1949. At this time the baby became irritable, began to vomit, and had loose stools and weight loss. Stool examination showed a trace of occult blood. One week later gross blood was passed per rectum. Over the next 14 days, the patient vomited coffee-ground material and passed large quantities of bright red blood. Gastric and colon x-rays were interpreted to be negative. During the time of observation,

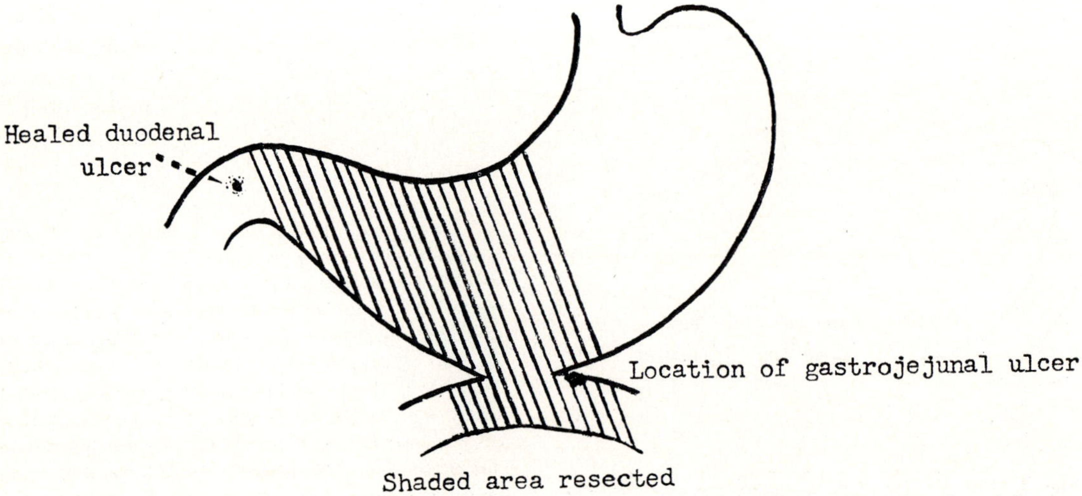

Fig. 2. Area resected in the treatment of the stomal ulcer is shown (Case 1). (Figs. 1 and 2 courtesy of *The American Journal of Surgery* **21:** 240, 1933.)

the infant received 8,000 c.c. of blood. On October 21, 1949, the abdomen was explored through a right rectus paramedian incision under drop ether anesthesia. The preoperative impression was that the bleeding came from a duodenal ulcer. A longitudinal incision was made across the pylorus and duodenum, and a duodenal ulcer on the posterior wall with a spurting artery in the center was found and closed with sutures of chromic catgut. It was thought advisable to resect the stomach rather than attempt closure of the long gastroduodenal incision and conversion into a pyloroplasty. About 50 per cent of the stomach was removed and reconstruction was by Billroth II anastomosis. The patient made a good recovery and four years later a gastrointestinal study did not reveal any unexpected abnormality. The patient is now 19 years of age, 6 feet 4 inches tall, weighs 190 pounds, and is in the Marine Corps in Vietnam. This is one of the first recorded cases of successful gastric resection in an infant of this age group.

Case 3. A young man of 18 years of age was first seen in July, 1935, with a history of having been operated upon for an intractable duodenal ulcer at the age of 13, at which time a posterior gastroenterostomy had been done. For the past several months, he had been suffering from epigastric pain and nausea. Physical examination and x-ray study indicated that he had developed a stomal ulcer. At exploratory laparotomy on July 18, 1935, a stomal ulcer was found. The distal three fourths of the stomach along with the stomal ulcer was excluded by a Devine type of operation, as shown in Fig. 3. The patient made a good recovery, and 19 years later he was living in California and wrote that he was feeling fine and had no further trouble with his stomach.

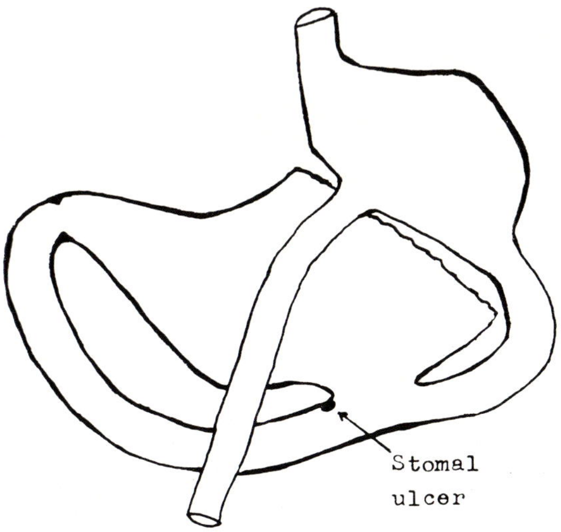

Fig. 3. The Devine type of gastric exclusion used in the treatment of the stomal ulcer is illustrated (Case 3).

Comment. This exclusion operation was advocated by Devine of Melbourne, Australia, in the late 1920's.[7, 8] He stated that the higher the exclusion, the greater the reduction in gastric acidity. However, the operation soon fell into disrepute because of the high incidence of recurrent ulcers. The senior author used this procedure in twelve instances before it was discontinued because one patient soon after operation died from peritonitis, the result of rupture of a stomal ulcer. Devine reported three cases of stomal ulcer treated by this procedure with satisfactorty results at the end of three years. No doubt the successful outcome in the case being reported resulted from excluding the antrum and a large part of the body of the stomach allowing sufficient acid to come in contact with the antrum so that release of gastrin was prevented.

At a recent meeting of the American Surgical Association (April 30 to May 2, 1969), a report was made from the University of Iowa relative to gastric bypass in the treatment of obesity and in seven cases of duodenal ulcer.[15] Seventy percent gastric exclusion had been used in the treatment of the duodenal ulcers, and while the period of observation had been short, results to date had been satisfactory. They too had observed that the higher the gastric exclusion, the greater the resulting anacidity. Much more extensive use of this procedure followed by a number of years of observation will be necessary to determine its merits in the treatment of duodenal ulcer.

Case 4. This patient was operated on at Barnes Hospital, St. Louis, Missouri, by Dr. Balfour, then a surgical resident. The patient was a 14-year-old Negro girl who underwent a subtotal gastric resection for control of a massively bleeding duodenal ulcer. Preoperative localization of the bleeding point was demonstrated by angiography, after a negative gastrointestinal series had been performed.

The patient was admitted to the hospital on December 7, 1965, because of melena and weakness. She gave a history of irregular eating habits for three months prior to admission and had complained of epigastric burning in the early morning

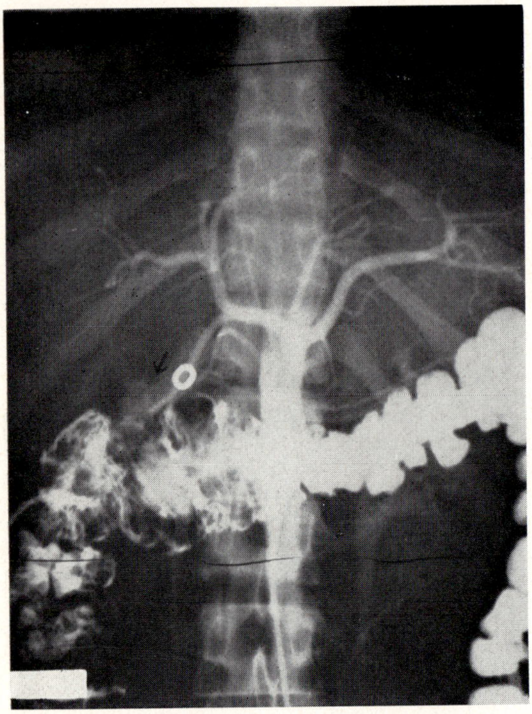

Fig. 4. Contrast material demonstrating the celiac artery and its branches is shown (Case 4). Arrow points to pooling of contrast material in area corresponding with the duodenal bulb from previous upper gastrointestinal series. This area was free of contrast material on the plain film taken before injection.

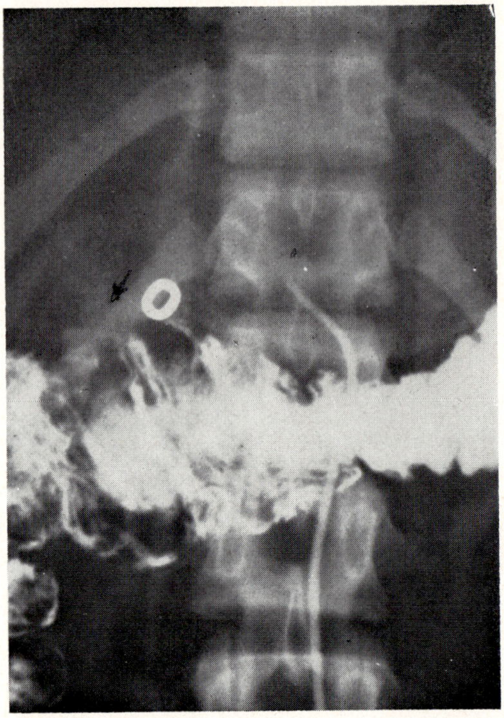

Fig. 5. Contrast material remaining in this area after all vascular structures are cleared of blood (Case 4). Fortunately, in this case, arteriographic findings were not obscured by the barium residual in the colon from upper gastrointestinal series taken the day before.

for several weeks. She noted melena for three days and became dizzy and fainted on the day of admission. Her pulse was 110 beats per minute, hemoglobin 7.4 Gm. percent, and hematocrit 26 per cent. A nasogastric tube was passed, yielding coffee-ground material and some streaks of red blood. Whole blood was transfused, and the following morning an upper gastrointestinal series was obtained, with no abnormality seen. By the following morning, December 9, 1965, she had received seven units of whole blood, continued to run a tachycardia, and passed bright red blood through her nasogastric tube. At this point, selective celiac arteriography was performed, showing pooling of contrast material in the area of the duodenal bulb (Figs. 4 and 5). This area conformed to the configuration of the duodenal bulb as seen on the upper gastrointestinal series taken the previous day. She was taken immediately to the operating room. A duodenal ulcer, 1.25 cm. in diameter, which was actively bleeding, was found. A 65 percent subtotal gastrectomy was performed. The patient had an uneventful convalescence and has done well since discharge. When last seen a year and a half after surgery, she was free of nutritional or recurrent ulcer problems.

Comment. The frequent inability to localize a bleeding point with conventional x-ray studies in patients suffering from gastrointestinal hemorrhage has been well documented.[2-4] Case No. 4 represents such a problem. This, together with a small percentage of patients who remain undiagnosed after a laparotomy and continue to bleed despite a blind subtotal gastrectomy or pyloroplasty with vagotomy, makes this a serious problem. Selective arteriograms have been useful in localizing bleeding points in a high percentage of cases as long as the active bleeding was present at the time of the study.[2, 3] It has been estimated that active bleeding of 0.5 ml. per minute must be present at the time of the study for adequate visualization.[29]

Baum and associates[3] reported one death in over 600 celiac and superior mesenteric arteriograms, and this was in a critically ill patient with advanced intra-abdominal malignancy. It was questionable as to whether her death could be attributed to the procedure. The only complications were local hematomas at the puncture site in 12 patients. They state that the only major contraindication to the examination is severe arterial disease that involves the femoral vessels. Although the indications would be infrequent, this method can certainly be well adapted to the pediatric age group. Recently, refinements in this tecnique with the use of direct magnification arteriography have improved the success rate in localizing bleeding points.

The next case was that of a gastric ulcer with characteristics similar to those occurring in adults.

Case 5. A 14-year-old boy was seen on December 29, 1957, complaining of epigastric pain of two months' duration. On examination he was acutely tender in the epigastrium and x-ray study showed a large penetrating ulcer of the lesser curvature (Fig. 6). The boy had undergone much psychic trauma as the result of family troubles and was being cared for by the Salvation Army. The size of the ulcer associated with acute epigastric tenderness made its rupture seem a definite possibility, and this associated with the difficulty of adequate medical therapy made the decision to resect the lesion seem justifiable. Approximately 50 per cent of the stomach, including the ulcer, was removed; reconstruction was performed by a retrocolic isoperistaltic Polya-Hofmeister anastomosis. The patient made a good recovery and three months later had gained three pounds in weight. He has been lost to further followup.

Comment. Gastric ulcer occurring in infancy and childhood is much less frequent than duodenal ulcers. The few that have been recognized by our Department of Pediatrics have responded well to medical therapy. We have had no occasion to operate on gastric ulcers in this age group to control hemorrhage or to close a perforation.

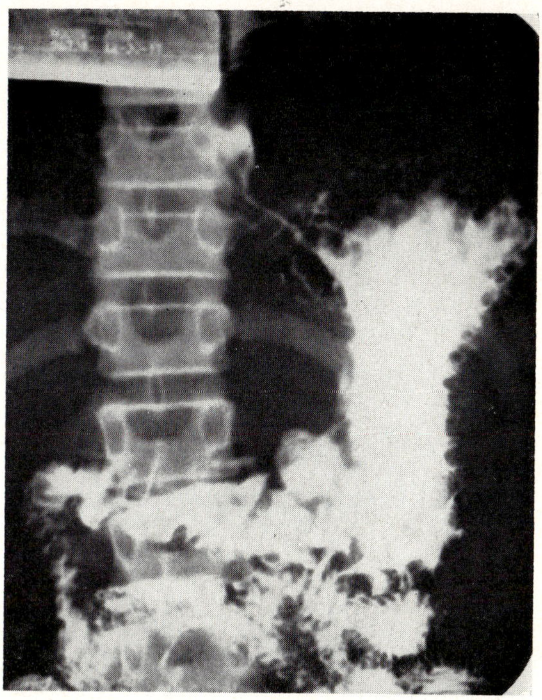

Fig. 6. The gastric ulcer of the lesser curvature is seen (Case 5).

DISCUSSION

From our own experience over the years at the Straub Clinic and from perusal of current literature, it is evident that surgery for gastric and duodenal ulcers in infancy and childhood occurs relatively infrequently in comparison with similar lesions in adults. However, with wider interest being taken in attempting to explain some of the more common and frequently unusual symptoms occurring in this age group by more frequent resort to barium studies of the upper gastrointestinal tract, more organic lesions are being found. This is particularly true in respect to duodenal ulcers, which in everyone's experience occur much more frequently than do gastric ulcers. It appears to be the unanimous conclusions of those experienced in such problems that in the very young most of these lesions heal following medical treatment or, probably in the vast majority of instances, no treatment at all. Only in those instances where hemorrhage becomes alarming or when such ulcers perforate, surgery is indicated and then the most conservative measures should be used to take care of the emergency. As children grow older, they begin to fall into the ulcerogenic pattern as it occurs in adults. No one has had sufficient experience to determine at what age this takes place. In our own experience we have had two stomal ulcers develop following gastroenterostomy for duodenal ulcers; one, a boy whose symptoms began at age seven, was operated upon at ten and developed a recurrent ulcer seven months later. The other developed this complication at 18 years of age, having had his original surgery at age 13. Others have reported similar experiences; it would thus seem to us that when the surgeon is called upon to correct an intractable duodenal ulcer as an elective procedure in this age group, a definitive operation is indicated, either an antrectomy, hemigastrectomy and vagotomy, or vagotomy and a drainage procedure. In our experience gastric ulcers in adults with few exceptions should be resected, one reason being that they respond poorly to medical treatment. The mortality and morbidity associated with conservative treatment is higher than with surgical removal, and the results of surgery for such conditions with few exceptions are most gratifying. Gastric ulcers in an adult always harbor the possibility of being malignant in spite of all efforts to prove their benignancy. This is rarely, if ever, a factor for consideration in infancy and childhood. Thus, it is our conclusion that if the surgeon is called upon to treat an intractable gastric ulcer in childhood, the same procedure should be used as in adults, namely, resection of the ulcer with the antrum. Most of these ulcers lie in the distal part of the stomach and their removal can almost always be accomplished without removing more than 50 to 60 percent of this organ. We have never found it necessary or advisable to do a vagotomy for gastric ulcer because the recurrence rate is negligible. Vagotomy is not an innocuous procedure and apparently has little to offer in the treatment of gastric ulcers in comparison with the treatment of duodenal ulcers.

CONCLUSIONS

Surgical lesions of the stomach and duodenum occur in infancy and childhood with relative infrequency in comparison with adults. More careful investigation with x-ray study in this age group suffering from abdominal symptoms reveals a higher incidence of organic lesions than has been suspected in the past. Angiography may be of benefit in cases where more conventional x-ray studies fail to demonstrate bleeding points. Duodenal ulcers are of more common occurrence than gastric ulcers in the young. In the very young, hemorrhage and perforation are the only complications needing consideration in the treatment of peptic ulcers. Control of the hemorrhage and closure of the perforation only need be done. As children grow older, a more definitive type of operation should be borne in mind, and the older the child becomes, the more closely he approaches the ulcerogenic diathesis common to the adult. Enough experience has now been gained to eliminate the fear of subsequent lack of development of the growing child following gastric resection, regardless of the age of the individual.

REFERENCES

1. Barber, K. W., Jr., Lynn, H. B., Dushane, J. W., and Priestly, J. T.: Surgical treatment of complicated duodenal ulcer in childhood, Postgrad. Med. **35:** 175, 1964.
2. Baum, S., Nusbaum, M., Blakemore, W. S., and Finkelstein, A.: The preoperative radiographic demonstration of intra-abdominal bleeding from undetermined sites by percutaneous selective celiac and superior mesenteric arteriography, SURGERY **58:** 797, 1965.
3. Baum, S., Nusbaum, M., Clearfield, H., Kuroda, K., and Tumen, H.: Angiography and the diagnosis of gastrointestinal bleeding, Arch. Intern. Med. **119:** 16, 1967.
4. Baum, S., Nusbaum, M., Kuroda, K., and Blakemore, W.: Direct serial magnification arteriography—as an adjunct in the diagnosis of surgical lesions of the alimentary tract, Amer. J. Surg. **117:** 170, 1969.
5. Berkowitz, D.: Fatal gastrointestinal hemorrhage diagnostic implications from a study of 200 cases, Amer. J. Gastroent. **40:** 372, 1963.
6. Birke, G., and Engstedt, L.: Melena and hematemesis: A follow-up investigation with

special reference to bleeding of unknown origin, Gastroenterologia **85:** 97, 1956.

7. Devine, H. B.: Basic principles and supreme difficulties in gastric surgery, Surg. Gynec. Obstet. **40:** 1, 1925.
8. Devine, H. B.: Gastric exclusion, Surg. Gynec. Obstet. **47:** 239, 1928.
9. Frazer, J. W., Jr.: Malignant lymphomas of the gastrointestinal tract, Surg. Gynec. Obstet. **108:** 182, 1959.
10. Gieske, J. P., and Storey, B.: Duodenal ulcer in infants, Bull. Hopkins Hosp. **18:** 499, 1966.
11. Gross, R.: The surgery of infancy and childhood, Philadelphia, 1953, W. B. Saunders Company.
12. Jones, F. A., Read, A. E., and Stubbe, J. L.: Alimentary bleeding of obscure origin: A follow-up study and commentary, Brit. Med. J. **1:** 1138, 1959.
13. Leger, J. L., Ricard, P. M., Leonard, C., and Piette, J.: Ulcère gastrique perforé chez un nouveau-né avec Survie, Un. Med. Canada **79:** 1277, 1950.
14. Lucas, C. E., and Benson, C. D.: Chronic bleeding duodenal ulcer in childhood managed by hemigastrectomy and vagotomy, SURGERY **61:** 478, 1967.
15. Mason, E. E., and Chikashi, T. O.: Gastric bypass. Meeting of the American Surgical Association, April 30-May 2, 1969.
16. Moore, T. C.: Gastrectomy in infancy and childhood. The results of an international survey, Ann. Surg. **162:** 91, 1965.
17. Nusbaum, M., and Baum, S.: Radiographic demonstration of unknown site of gastrointestinal bleeding, Surg. Forum **14:** 374, 1963.
18. Nusbaum, M., Baum, S., and Blakemore, W.: Clinical experience with the diagnoses and management of gastrointestinal hemorrhage by selective mesenteric catheterization. Meeting of the American Surgical Association, May 1, 1969.
19. Raffensperger, J. G., Condon, J. B., and Greengard, J.: Complications of gastric and duodenal ulcers in infancy and childhood, Surg. Gynec. Obstet. **123:** 1269, 1966.
20. Schuster, S. R., and Gross, R. E.: Peptic ulcer disease in childhood, Amer. J. Surg. **105:** 324, 1963.
21. Stern, M. A., Perkins, E. L., and Nessa, N. J.: Perforated gastric ulcer in a two-day old infant, Lancet **49:** 492, 1929.
22. Swenson, O.: Pediatric surgery, ed. 2, Des Moines, 1962, Meredith Publishing Company.
23. Ternberg, J. L., and Koehler, P. R.: The use of arteriography in the diagnosis of the origin of acute gastrointestinal hemorrhage in children, SURGERY **63:** 686, 1968.
24. Tudor, R. B.: Peptic ulcerations in childhood, Pediat. Clin. N. Amer. **14:** 109, 1967.
25. Wilson, S. D., and Ellison, E. H.: Total gastric resection in children with the Zollinger-Ellison syndrome, Arch. Surg. **91:** 165, 1965.

Repair of intracardiac defects after previous constriction (banding) of the pulmonary artery

JAROSLAV STARK, M.U.Dr., C.Sc.
MICHAEL TYNAN, M.B., B.S.
EOIN ABERDEEN, F.R.C.S., D.C.H.
DAVID J. WATERSTON, M.B.E., F.R.C.S.
RICHARD E. BONHAM-CARTER, M.A., F.R.C.P.
GERALD R. GRAHAM, B.A., M.D.
JANE SOMERVILLE, M.R.C.P.
LONDON, ENGLAND
From the Thoracic Unit and the Department of Clinical Physiology, The Hospital for Sick Children

Pulmonary artery constriction (banding) is well-established as a palliative treatment for infants with a large left-to-right shunt at ventricular level. It can be performed with a low mortality rate.[1, 2, 21, 26, 29, 31] The object of pulmonary artery constriction is to improve severe heart failure by decreasing pulmonary blood flow and pulmonary artery pressure. This allows the patient to survive to an age when corrective surgery can be done more safely and reduces the risk of pulmonary vascular disease.

We present here the results of corrective surgery in 28 children who had pulmonary artery constriction in infancy.

CASE MATERIAL AND METHODS

From March, 1966, to April, 1969, 28 patients (aged 3½ to 12 years) had corrective operations for cardiac lesions which had required pulmonary artery constriction in infancy (Table I). The lesions necessitating the palliative procedure were defects of the ventricular septum (V.S.D.) in 25 cases. Three other patients had a V.S.D. as part of a more complex lesion: endocardial cushion defect in one, transposition of the great arteries in one, and double-outlet right ventricle in one case. Twenty-six patients were under one year of age at the time of pulmonary artery constriction. Persistent heart failure despite full medical therapy was the indication in all these cases.

The technique of pulmonary artery constriction with the use of a plaited silk ligature has been described previously.[29] A patent ductus arteriosus was ligated at the same operation in 8 patients and at a previous operation in one. One patient had a coarctation of the aorta resected, patent ductus divided, and pulmonary artery constricted at the same operation. The patient with transposition of the great arteries had a Blalock-Hanlon operation 3 weeks after the pulmonary artery constriction.

After the palliative operation, patients were seen at least yearly. They were reinvestigated from 3 to 9 years after pulmonary artery constriction.

Physical examination. Eleven patients were cyanosed at rest, 3 only on effort. Eight had clubbed fingers. Cardiac catheterization and angiocardiography were performed in all patients prior to the corrective operation.

Cardiac catheterization. The pulmonary artery was entered and pressures recorded distal to the constriction in 22 cases. The

Supported in part by the British Heart Foundation.
Received for publication June 30, 1969.

Table I. *Diagnosis at operation*

Diagnosis	*No. of patients*
V.S.D. (25 cases)	
Single	16
Multiple	8
Spontaneous closure	1
V.S.D. (3 cases) associated with:	
Endocardial cushion defect	1
Transposition of the great arteries	1
Double-outlet right ventricle	1
Total	28

Table II. *Pulmonary artery pressure distal to the band at cardiac catheterization*

Pressure (mm. Hg.)	*No. of patients*
< 30	20*
30 - 40	3
40 - 50	2
> 50	1
Not measured	2

*In 4 patients the distal pulmonary artery pressure could be recorded only at operation.

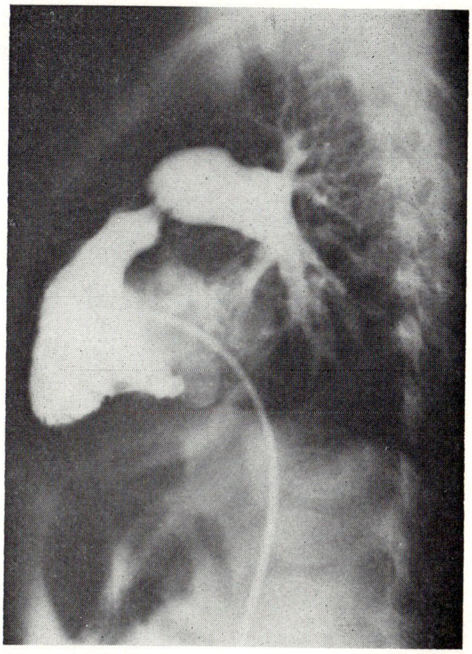

Fig. 1. Lateral projection of the right ventricular angiocardiogram of patient No. 24. The pulmonary artery constriction is close to the pulmonary valve.

stenosis of the pulmonary artery above the valve was confirmed by withdrawal traces from the pulmonary artery to right ventricle in 21 cases. In one patient, no evidence of constriction was found, the pulmonary artery pressure being at systemic level. The distal pulmonary artery pressure was elevated above normal (35 to 50 mm. Hg) in another 5 of these patients (Table II).

Subvalvar pulmonary obstruction was found in addition to the pulmonary artery constriction in one case.

Thirteen patients with V.S.D. also had a patent atrial septum which proved at operation to be a secundum atrial septal defect (A.S.D.) in 4 and a small patent foramen ovale in 9.

A left-to-right shunt at ventricular level was found in 12 patients, and in 2 of these the shunt was larger than 2.5:1. Seven patients had a bidirectional shunt, and in 4 the shunt was only right to left. No shunt could be demonstrated by oximetry in 5 patients.

Angiocardiography. All patients were studied by Elema biplane angiocardiography. With the realization that multiple V.S.D. were common in this series, left ventricular cineangiography in the left anterior oblique projection was performed in addition in 6 of the later patients.

The defect or defects were demonstrated in all patients but one, in whom the defect was proved at operation to have closed spontaneously.

In one patient, no evidence of pulmonary artery constriction was found at angiocardiogram, at cardiac catheterization, or at operation. The position of the pulmonary artery constriction, when present, was always identified. This was quite variable, being at any point along the pulmonary artery from the valve (Fig. 1) to the bifurcation (Figs. 2 and 3).

In 3 patients the right ventricular angiocardiogram (Fig. 4) revealed additional subvalvar pulmonary stenosis. In only one of these was it possible to identify a separate subvalvar pressure gradient.

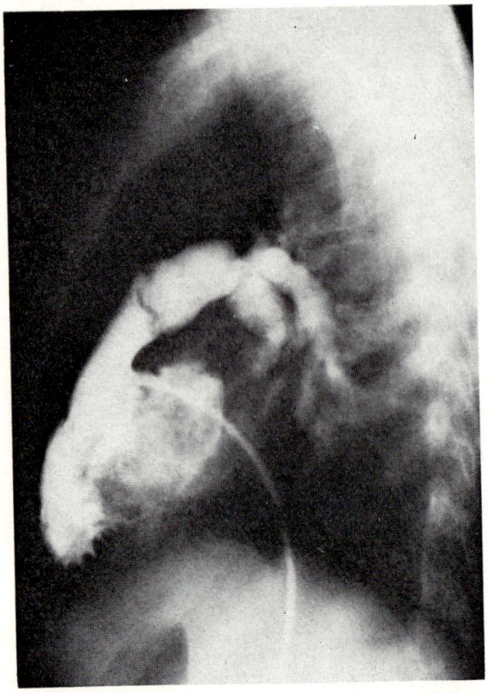

Fig. 2. Lateral projection of the right ventricular angiocardiogram of patient No. 18. The constriction is at the bifurcation.

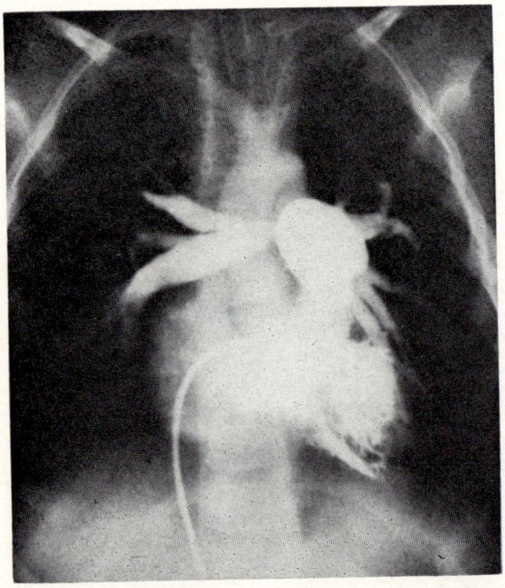

Fig. 3. Anteroposterior projection of the right ventricular angiocardiogram of patient No. 18. This is later in the series than Fig. 2 and demonstrates narrowing of the right pulmonary artery resulting from the constricting ligature. Aorta opacifies via the ventricular septal defect.

A

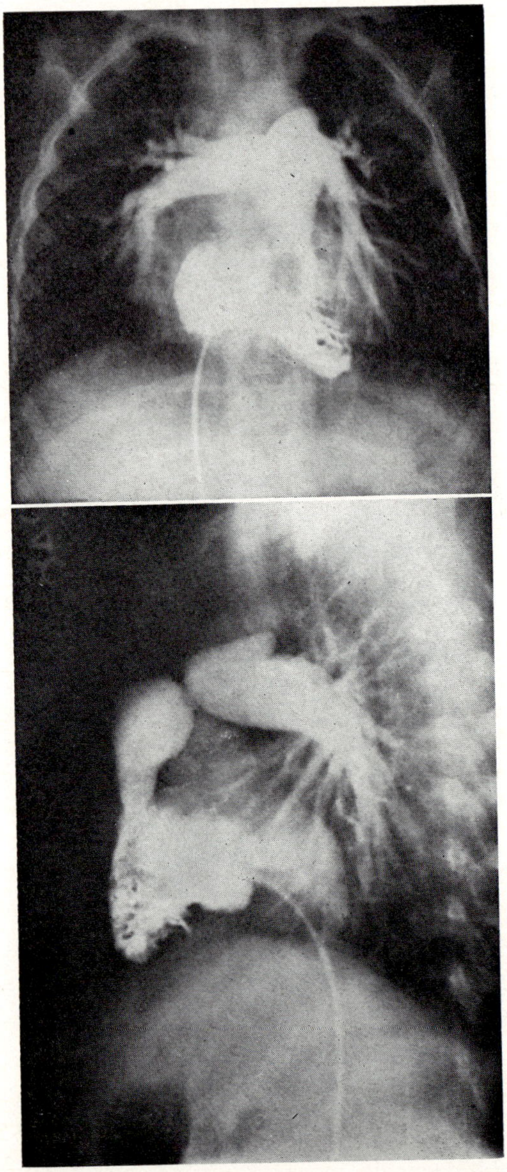

B

Fig. 4, *A and B.* Anteroposterior and lateral projection of the right ventricular angiocardiogram of patient No. 17. Infundibular stenosis is present. The narrowing resulting from the constricting ligature is demonstrated.

CORRECTIVE OPERATION

The corrective procedure was performed 3 to 10 years after the pulmonary artery constriction. The age of patients at the time of operation was 3½ to 12 years (mean, 6 years 4 months) and weight 25 to 54 pounds (mean, 38 pounds 4 ounces). The diagnosis at corrective operation is shown in Table I.

Roller pumps and a Kay-Cross type disc oxygenator were used in all but one patient in whom a membrane oxygenator was used. The ascending aorta was cannulated in 21; the femoral artery was cannulated in 7. The right ventricle was opened by a transverse or oblique incision.

Findings (Table III). The defect was single in 16 patients. Fifteen of these involved the membranous septum and one the muscular. Twelve defects measured more than 10 × 15 mm. at operation; 2 of these were larger than 30 × 40 mm., there being only a rim of septal tissue, i.e., there was nearly a common ventricle.

Eight patients had multiple V.S.D. Six of them had a defect of the membranous septum with additional muscular defects, while 2 had multiple muscular defects with intact membranous septum.

Spontaneous closure of the V.S.D. had occurred in one patient.[30]

The patient with an endocardial cushion defect had a large V.S.D. and an ostium primum type of A.S.D. with completely cleft mitral and tricuspid valves. The patient with transposition of the great arteries had an A.S.D. created operatively 4 years previously; his V.S.D. measured 12 × 17 mm. The patient with a double-outlet right ventricle had a ventricular defect which measured 20 × 18 mm.

OPERATIVE TECHNIQUE

Pulmonary artery. In all cases, the constricting ligature was embedded in fibrous tissue and removal was not possible. The pulmonary artery was incised longitudinally across the constriction and reconstructed either by a transverse closure of the incision (4 patients) or by inserting a patch of pericardium (23 patients). In one instance, the pulmonary artery required no reconstruction because there was no constriction (Table III).

The constriction was close to the bifurcation in 8 patients. In 3 of these, the left or right pulmonary artery was involved, and it was necessary to extend the patch into the affected main branch.

Ventricular septal defect. The defect in the membranous septum was small enough to be closed by direct suture in 3 cases. All other membranous septal defects were closed with a Dacron patch.

In some cases, it was found difficult to close the multiple muscular defects by the usual method. Closure was achieved by passing No. 3-0 silk deep mattress sutures through the muscular septum. The sutures were passed from outside the heart to the opposite side of the defect and tied on the epicardial surface of the heart over Dacron buttresses.

Infundibular resection. Resection of infundibular muscle to relieve the obstruction was performed in 3 cases with subvalvar pulmonary stenosis.

A.S.D. In addition to the V.S.D. a secundum A.S.D. was closed by direct suture in 3 and by a Dacron patch in one patient. A patent foramen ovale was closed in one patient.

Complex lesions. The endocardial cushion defect was repaired with a Dacron patch in the V.S.D. and the A.S.D. The clefts in the mitral and tricuspid valves were repaired by suture.

The transposition of the great arteries was corrected by Mustard's[20] operation, the V.S.D. being closed by direct suture through the tricuspid valve.

In the patient with the double-outlet right ventricle, the V.S.D. was closed with a Dacron patch with the use of Kirklin's technique.[16]

POSTOPERATIVE CARE

In the immediate postoperative period, special attention was paid to respiratory management. Artificial ventilation via face mask, nasotracheal tube, or tracheostomy was used in 18 patients, 4 of them requiring ventilation for longer than 5 days (maximum was 26 days). The management of postoperative arrhythmias is dealt with below.

RESULTS

Twenty patients survived the operation and were discharged from hospital; 19 of

Table III

No.	Age at Banding (mo.)	Age at Correction (yr.)	Catheterization data before correction: Systolic pressure mm. Hg R.V.	P.A.	Systemic	V.S.D. shunt	Data on: Type and size of the defect (mm.)
1	8	3 6/12	100	30	100	L → R	Membranous, 14 × 15
2	2	3 9/12	140	25	100	None	Four muscular
3	7	4 6/12	90	30	100	L → R	Membranous, 35 × 25
4	3½	4 3/12	75	25	80	L → R	Membranous, 10 × 17
5	2½	7 3/12	87	22*	87	Bidirectional	Membranous, large
6	4	5	80	18	88	None	Membranous, moderate
7	1¾	6 6/12	110	20*	110	L → R	Membranous, 16 × 9; muscular, 6 × 10
8	2	7 3/12	88	30*	100	L → R	Membranous, 25 × 25
9	4	9	80	—	80	Bidirectional	Membranous, 20 × 20
10	2½	9	100	15	125	Bidirectional	Membranous, 25 × 20; 3 muscular
11	2¾	4 9/12	80	24	85	R → L	Membranous, 25 × 35; 1 muscular
12	4	7 3/12	80	20	86	R → L	Membranous, 25 × 10; 4 muscular
13	5	5 3/12	80	22	88	None	Muscular, 10 × 10
14	21	12	90	—	93	L → R	Membranous, 10 × 14
15	7	9	90	35	110	None	Spontaneous closure
16	12	6	80	24	90	L → R	Membranous, 25 × 20
17	4	4 6/12	90	20*	88	Bidirectional	Membranous, 25 × 15
18	5	6 6/12	115	14	125	R → L	Membranous, very large
19	10	7	85	20	100	L → R	Four muscular
20	¾	4 6/12	115	10	100	L → R	Membranous, 40 × 20

R.V. = right ventricle; L.V. = left ventricle; A.S.D. = atrial septal defect; V.S.D. = ventricular septal defect; P.F.O. =

*Pressure taken during operation prior to correction.

†Pulmonary artery constriction in another hospital.

operation		*Systolic pressure after operation mm. Hg*					
Method of closure of V.S.D.	*Method of P.A. reconstruction*	*R.V.*	*P.A.*	*Systemic*	*Result*	*Follow-up*	*Comment*
Patch	Patch	40	30	100	Hospital death	—	Partial A-V block
Direct suture	Patch	40	35	125	Alive	Well at 3 yr.	P.F.O. closed, murmur of residual V.S.D.
Patch	Patch	30	25	80	Alive	Well at 3 yr.	Transient advanced A-V block
Patch	Arterioplasty	30	25	90	Hospital death	—	Complete A-V block
Patch	Patch	65	20	85	Hospital death	—	A.S.D. closed
Patch	Patch	60	25	100	Alive	Well at 3 yr.	Transient complete A-V block
Patch, direct suture	Patch	50	30	80	Alive	Well at 3 yr.	A.S.D. closed, complete A-V block, murmur of residual V.S.D.
Patch	Arterioplasty	60	30	110	Alive	Well at 2½ yr.	Murmur of residual V.S.D.
Patch	Patch	65	60	100	Alive	Well at 2½ yr.	Transient complete A-V block
Patch, direct suture	Patch	70	50	85	Hospital death	—	Complete A-V block
Patch, direct suture	Patch	65	60	70	Hospital death	—	A.S.D. closed, complete A-V block, infundibular resection
Patch, direct suture	Patch	40	40	75	Hospital death	—	Tracheostomy dislodged 6th postoperative day
Direct suture	Patch	60	30	100	Alive	Well at 2½ yr.	
Direct suture	Arterioplasty	35	30	110	Alive	Well at 2 yr.	Murmur of residual V.S.D.
—	Patch	40	38	105	Alive	Well at 1½ yr.	
Patch	Patch	60	30	125	Alive	Well at 1½ yr.	Murmur of residual V.S.D.
Patch	Arterioplasty	50	30	110	Alive	Well at 1½ yr.	Infundibular resection
Patch	Patch	60	30	90	Alive	Well at 1¼ yr.	Complete A-V block
Direct suture	Patch	50	30	85	Alive	Well at 1¼ yr.	Partial A-V block, residual V.S.D. despite second operation
Patch	Patch	95	30	100	Alive	Well at 1 yr.	Infundibular resection

patent foramen ovale; P.A. = pulmonary artey; mo. = month(s); yr. = year(s); wk. = week(s).

Continued on following page.

Table III—*Cont'd*

	Age at		*Catheterization data before correction*				*Data on*
			Systolic pressure mm. Hg				
No.	*Banding (mo.)*	*Correction (yr.)*	*R.V.*	*P.A.*	*Systemic*	*V.S.D. shunt*	*Type and size of the defect (mm.)*
21	7	7 9/12	100	20	110	Bidirectional	Membranous, 25 × 15; 3 muscular
22	3	5 9/12	100	40	85	None	Membranous, moderate
23	14	7 9/12	86	84	90	L → R	Membranous, 10 × 15; 1 muscular
24	10	5 6/12	85	16	85	R → L	Membranous, 25 × 15
25	3†	6	100	50	110	Bidirectional	Membranous, 15 × 12
Double outlet R.V. and V.S.D.							
26	3/4	7	100	50	100	L → R	Membranous, 20 × 8
Endocardial cushion defect							
27	4	7	120	40	120	Bidirectional atrial shunt	1° A.S.D.; large V.S.D.
Transposition of the great arteries and V.S.D.							
28	3	4 6/12	*L.V.* 100	10	100	Bidirectional atrial and ventricular	Membranous, 17 × 12

R.V. = right ventricle; L.V. = left ventricle; A.S.D. = atrial septal defect; V.S.D. = ventricular septal defect; P.F.O. =

*Pressure taken during operation prior to correction.

†Pulmonary artery construction in another hospital.

them are well and fully active. The patient who is limited in activity had a complete atrioventricular canal repaired but still has significant mitral regurgitation.

Pulmonary artery reconstruction. This was not necessary in the one patient in whom no evidence of pulmonary artery constriction could be found. In the remaining 27, reconstruction was satisfactorily achieved. After the repair, there was no pressure gradient across the reconstructed area in any of them. In 17 patients, a residual systolic pressure gradient of more than 5 mm. Hg from the right ventricle to the pulmonary artery was noted at infundibular level. In 8 of these, the systolic pressure difference was more than 20 mm. Hg (Table IV) and one of these died.

Closure of V.S.D. Seven of the 24 patients with V.S.D. died (Table V).

Table IV. *Right ventricle–pulmonary artery pressure gradient at infundibular level after correction*

Systolic gradient (mm. Hg)	*No. of patients*
0 - 10	14
10 - 20	6
20 - 40	5
> 40	3

Four of 12 patients with a single large or very large V.S.D. died. Three of 6 patients with a large V.S.D. in the membranous septum and additional muscular defects died.

No deaths occurred in the 7 patients with a moderately large V.S.D. (single in 4, multiple in 2).

operation		*Systolic pressure after operation mm. Hg*					
Method of closure of V.S.D.	*Method of P.A. reconstruction*	*R.V.*	*P.A.*	*Systemic*	*Result*	*Follow-up*	*Comment*
Patch, direct suture	Patch	30	25	100	Alive	Well at 9 mo.	Murmur of residual V.S.D.
Direct suture	Patch	75	40	95	Alive	Well at 5 mo.	—
Patch, direct suture	—	35	35	100	Alive	Well at 4 mo.	—
Patch	Patch	50	30	110	Hospital death	—	A.S.D. closed
Patch	Patch	30	30	100	Alive	Well at 6 wk.	—
Patch	Patch	40	30	95	Alive	Well at 1¼ yr.	Transient partial A-V block
Patch, 1° A.S.D.; Patch, V.S.D.	Patch	40	30	100	Alive	Limited activity at 1¼ yr.	Transient atrial flutter, mitral incompetence
Direct suture	Patch	*L.V.* 35	20	85	Hospital death	—	Complete A-V block

patent foramen ovale; P.A. = pulmonary artery; mo. = month(s); yr. = year(s); wk. = week(s).

Table V. *Operative mortality*

	Total	*Dead*
Type of V.S.D.		
Large single membranous defect	12	4
Large membranous defect and additional muscular defect(s)	6	3
Moderately large single membranous or muscular defect	4	0
Multiple muscular defects	2	0
Defect closed spontaneously	1	0
Endocardial cushion defect and large ventricular defect	1	0
Double-outlet right ventricle and large ventricular defect	1	0
Transposition of the great arteries and large ventricular defect	1	1
Total	28	8

Three of 4 patients with a large V.S.D. and an additional A.S.D. died.

Seven patients still have auscultatory findings of residual V.S.D. Four of these had multiple muscular V.S.D. One patient with persistent heart failure has had a second operation, but there is still clinical and angiocardiographic evidence of a V.S.D. All these patients are well, asymptomatic, and with a heart of normal size.

Endocardial cushion defect. The patient's general condition is improved, but there is still a pansystolic murmur suggesting significant mitral incompetence (Table V).

Double-outlet right ventricle and V.S.D. There is no clinical evidence of residual cardiac disease in this patient (Table V).

Transposition of the great arteries and V.S.D. This patient died 24 hours after operation (Table V).

Table VI. *Arrhythmias*

Rhythm before operation	*Rhythm after operation*	*No. of patients*	*Deaths*	*Pacemaker used (days)*
	No arrhythmia			
Sinus	Sinus	13	2	—
Sinus and nodal	Sinus and nodal	1	—	—
Partial (1°) A-V block	Partial (1°) A-V block	1	1	—
	Permanent arrhythmia			
Sinus	Partial (2°) A-V block	2	1	0, 0
Sinus	Complete A-V block	5	3	½, 3, 33, 1, 0
Partial (1°) A-V block	Complete A-V block	1	1	0
	Transient arrhythmia			
Sinus	Complete A-V block → sinus rhythm	2	—	12
Sinus	Advanced A-V block → sinus rhythm	1	—	20
Sinus	Partial (2°) A-V block → partial (1°) A-V block	1	—	0
Partial (1°) A-V block	Atrial flutter → partial (1°) A-V block	1	—	12

POSTOPERATIVE ARRHYTHMIAS (TABLE VI)

Fifteen patients showed no change in heart rhythm following operation. Three deaths occurred in this group. The remaining 13 patients can be divided into two main groups:

First, permanent arrhythmias occurred in 8 patients (i.e., throughout the follow-up period or until death).

Second, transient arrhythmias developed in 5 patients. Disturbances of atrioventricular conduction are classified according to Miller and Rodriguez-Coronel.[17]

I. Partial block: This is first degree (1°) and second degree (2°) atrioventricular block;

II. Advanced block: This is basically atrioventricular dissociation with occasional atrial or ventricular captures;

III. Complete block: There is no evidence of atrioventricular conduction.

Permanent arrhythmias. In all these patients, the abnormality of conduction was first observed in the operating room.

Five deaths occurred in this group; 4 were patients with complete atrioventricular block. In all 4 patients, epicardial pacemakers were used until death. The fifth death was in a patient with partial atrioventricular block who died 18 hours after operation.

Three survived with permanent arrhythmias; 2 are in complete and one in partial atrioventricular block. One survivor in complete atrioventricular block needed epicardial pacing for 33 days after operation but now, 9 months later, maintains a spontaneous ventricular rate of 60 per minute. Neither of the other 2 survivors has needed an artificial pacemaker, because their pulse rates have never been below 60 beats per minute.

Transient arrhythmias. There were no deaths in this group. Two patients with complete atrioventricular block reverted to sinus rhythm 3 and 12 days after the operation.

One patient developed partial (2°) atrioventricular block 2 days after the operation. Twenty-one days later she changed spontaneously to regular sinus rhythm with a prolonged P-R interval. This has persisted for the past 14 months.

The other patient developed advanced atrioventricular block with ventricular arrests giving rise to Stokes-Adams attacks 14 days after the operation. A transvenous pacemaker was inserted and she was paced for 20 days. She reverted spontaneously to sinus rhythm and has now remained in this rhythm for 2½ years.

Atrial flutter occurred in one patient following repair of an endocardial cushion defect. This was converted to sinus rhythm with prolonged P-R interval by D.C. countershock, without change to the present.

DISCUSSION

Reconstruction of the pulmonary artery. Pulmonary artery reconstruction was satisfactorily achieved in all cases and no death was attributable to this part of the operation.

The ligature of plaited silk had provoked a fibrous reaction and become incorporated in fibrous tissue.[3] The constriction was relieved by a longitudinal incision and the use of a pericardial patch or arterioplasty. In 6 patients, the ligature had cut almost through a part of the wall of the pulmonary artery, but was still incorporated in fibrous tissue and covered with endothelium. In one patient, part of the ligature was lying free in the lumen of the pulmonary artery, but there was still an adequate constriction.

Ideally, the pulmonary artery should be constricted by material which can be removed easily and does not require reconstruction of the pulmonary artery. Teflon tape has been described as such a material in some cases.[8, 11, 12, 24] We hesitated to use it because of reports of Teflon tape cutting through the pulmonary artery wall.[23, 25] Death from hemorrhage as the result of acute erosion of the pulmonary artery had not occurred in our first 209 cases. Subsequently we experienced this complication in Cases Nos. 210 and 218, i.e., 2 instances in a total of 235 bandings. Both these patients died. We continue to use a plaited silk ligature, but with further experience, we may change our technique.

Type and size of V.S.D. The type and size of V.S.D. dealt with at debanding was very often different from the V.S.D. we have closed without previous banding. Many V.S.D. in the presented series were very large, and the incidence of multiple V.S.D. was high. In 897 collected cases of closure of V.S.D. reported in adequate detail,[5, 13, 14, 22] only 35 (3.9 percent) had multiple defects—whereas 33 percent were multiple in the present series.

Multiple V.S.D. are often associated with pulmonary hypertension and the reported surgical mortality rate has been high in the past.[9, 14] Surprisingly few results have been reported recently.

In our experience, closure of multiple V.S.D. was difficult, as was the closure of very large V.S.D. Of 7 patients with auscultatory evidence of residual V.S.D., in 4 multiple V.S.D. had been present.

MORBIDITY AND MORTALITY RATES

Several series of V.S.D. (single or complex) with pulmonary artery constriction followed later by correction have been reported.[7, 8, 11, 12, 32] There have also been several case reports.[5, 6, 10, 18, 21, 23, 28] The overall mortality rate for all these cases was 21 percent (15 deaths of 71 cases).

One-stage repair of the V.S.D. can be done in infants. In those without severe pulmonary hypertension, excellent results have been achieved by the Ann Arbor group. They closed the V.S.D. in 10 infants under one year of age without a death. Pulmonary hypertension increased the operative risk considerably. Of 18 infants whose pulmonary artery pressure was 75 percent of systemic pressure or more, 5 (28 percent) died following V.S.D. closure.[27] The Mayo Clinic Group repaired V.S.D. in 21 infants of 6 months to one year of age with one death.[4]

We prefer pulmonary artery constriction (and later total correction) in infants with V.S.D. under 6 months of age. Over the age of 6 months, closure of an isolated V.S.D. is preferred. Patients with V.S.D. and previous pulmonary artery constriction are clearly a selected series; the size and multiplicity of their V.S.D. contrasts with other reported experiences. Selection is thus made from the difficult end of the V.S.D. spectrum, because without palliative operation, survival would have been unlikely.

The most important complication was an abnormality of atrioventricular conduction. Thirteen patients had a transient or permanent arrhythmia following the operation; 11 of these had large defects of the membranous septum either alone (8 cases) or associated with other defects (e.g., transposition of the great arteries, double-outlet right ventricle, A.S.D., or additional muscular septal defects). Four of the patients with complete heart block died (Table III). None of the survivors has needed a permanent pacemaker, although temporary pacing was necessary in 6 for up to 33 days. Heart block proved a special problem of the very large V.S.D., presumably because the atrioventricular bundle runs a long course in the exposed margin of the defect. However, surgical heart block has not been a problem in our cases of V.S.D. treated by closure without previous pulmonary artery constriction. For instance, heart block occurred once in 140 V.S.D. closures.

Four patients had an A.S.D. additional to the ventricular one. Three of these died, but this association may be no more than coincidence.

The morbidity and mortality rates in the presented series were closely related to the size of the defect. With one exception, only those patients died who had a large membranous V.S.D., alone or in association with additional muscular defects. In other words, the operative risk was determined by the type of V.S.D. and not by the pulmonary artery constriction.

SUMMARY

The results of corrective operation for lesions requiring earlier pulmonary artery constriction (banding) in 28 children are presented. Twenty-five patients had V.S.D. In 3 others, the defects were part of a more complex malformation. The data from cardiac catheterization and angiocardiography are presented. Reconstruction of the pulmonary artery was accomplished by pericardial patch or arterioplasty. No morbidity or mortality could be attributed to this part of the operation. One third of this series had multiple muscular V.S.D. Temporary or permanent heart block was the major postoperative complication. Eight patients died after operation. Death occurred only in patients with very large V.S.D. There have been no late deaths. Long-term results are good.

REFERENCES

1. Albert, H. M., Fowler, R. M., Craighead, C. C., and Atik, M.: A treatment for infants with intractable cardiac failure due to interventricular septal defect, Circulation **23:** 16, 1961.
2. Bernhard, W. F., and Filler, R. M.: Hyperbaric oxygenation: Current concepts, Amer. J. Surg. **115:** 661, 1968.
3. Berry, C. L.: Changes in the wall of the pulmonary artery following banding, J. Path. Accepted for publication, 1969.
4. Cartmill, T. B., DuShane, J. W., McGoon, D. C., and Kirklin, J. W.: Results of repair of ventricular septal defect, J. Thorac. Cardiov. Surg. **52:** 486, 1966.
5. Coleman, E. N., Reid, J. M., Inall, J. A., and Stevenson, J. G.: Ventricular septal defect repair in childhood, Brit. Heart J. **30:** 845, 1968.
6. Craig, T. V., and Sirak, H. D.: Pulmonary artery banding, J. Thorac. Cardiov. Surg. **45:** 599, 1963.
7. Dammann, J. F., Jr., McEachen, J. A., Thompson, W. M., Jr., Smith, R., and Muller, W. H., Jr.: The regression of pulmonary vascular disease after the creation of pulmonary stenosis, J. Thorac. Cardiov. Surg. **42:** 722, 1961.
8. Dobell, A. R. C., Murphy, D. R., and Gibbons, J. E.: Pulmonary artery debanding, Ann. Thor. Surg. **5:** 435, 1968.
9. Friedman, W. F., Mehrizi, A., and Pusch, A. L.: Multiple muscular ventricular septal defects, Circulation **33:** 35, 1965.
10. Grainger, R. G., Nagle, R. E., Pawidapha, C., Robertson, D. S., Taylor, D. G., Thornton, J. A., Verel, D., and Zachary, R. B.: Pulmonary artery banding for ventricular septal defect, Brit. Heart J. **29:** 289, 1967.
11. Hallman, G. L., Cooley, D. A., and Bloodwell, R. D.: Two-stage surgical treatment of ventricular septal defect: Results of pulmonary artery banding in infants and subsequent open-heart repair, J. Thor. Cardiov. Surg. **52:** 476, 1966.
12. Hallman, G. L.: Discussion of Dobell, A. R. C., Murphy, D. R. and Gibbons, J. E.: Pulmonary artery debanding, Ann. Thor. Surg. **5:** 441, 1968.
13. Kahn, D. R., Vathayanon, S., Stern, A. M., Fergusson, P. W., and Sloan, H.: Location of ventricular septal defect, Circulation **35-36:** Suppl. 2, 153, 1967.
14. Kirklin, J. W., McGoon, D. C., and DuShane, J. W.: Surgical treatment of ventricu-

lar septal defect, J. Thorac. Surg. **40:** 763, 1960.

15. Lynfield, J., Yao, A. C., Vichitbandhe, P., Rodriguez-Torres, R., and Karlson, K. E.: Complications following banding of the pulmonary artery for treatment of heart failure in infants with ventricular septal defect, Circulation **32:** Suppl. 2, 140, 1965.
16. McGoon, D. C.: Origin of both great vessels from the right ventricle, Surg. Clin. N. Amer. **41:** 1113, 1961.
17. Miller, R. A., Rodriguez-Coronel, A.: Congenital atrioventricular block in heart disease in infants, children and adolescents, in Moss, A. J., and Adams, F. H., editors: Heart disease in infants, children and adolescents, Baltimore, 1968, The Williams & Wilkins Company.
18. Mills, H., Kay, J. H., Magidson, O., Anderson, R. M., and Schniff, A.: Correction of congenital ventricular septal defect in a patient with previous surgically produced pulmonary artery stenosis, Amer. J. Cardiol. **6:** 976, 1960.
19. Murthy, K., Arcilla, R. A., Moulder, P. V., and Cassels, D. E.: Functional closure of the ventricular septal defect after pulmonary artery banding. An unusual late complication, J. A. M. A. **205:** 592, 1968.
20. Mustard, W. T.: Successful two-stage correction of transposition of the great vessels, SURGERY **55:** 469, 1964.
21. Reid, J. M., Barclay, R. S., Coleman, E. N., Stevenson, J. G., Welsh, T. M., and McSwan, N.: Pulmonary artery banding in congenital heart disease associated with pulmonary hypertension, Thorax **23:** 385, 1968.
22. Ritter, D. G., Feldt, R. H., Weidman, W. H., and DuShane, J. W.: Ventricular septal defect, Circulation **32-33:** Suppl. 3, 42, 1965.
23. Rohmer, J., Brom, A. G., Nauta, J.: Bands inside the pulmonary artery. A complication of the Muller-Dammann procedure, Ann. Thorac. Surg. **3:** 449, 1967.
24. Roe, B. B.: Discussion of Dobell, A. R. C., Murphy, D. R., and Gibbons, J. E.: Pulmonary artery debanding, Ann. Thorac. Surg. **5:** 442, 1968.
25. Schmidt-Habelmann, P., Sebening, F.: Erfahrungen mit der bandelung der pulmonalarterie, Thoraxchirurgie **14:** 541, 1966.
26. Senning, A.: Herzchirurgie beim Neugeborenen, Deutch. Med. Wschr. **93:** 1087, 1968.
27. Sigmann, J. M., Stern, A. M., Sloan, H. E.: Early surgical correction of large ventricular septal defects, Pediatrics **39:** 4, 1967.
28. Sirak, H. D., Hossier, D. M., and Clatworthy, H. W., Jr.: Defects of the interventricular septum in infancy. A two-stage approach to their surgical correction, New Eng. J. Med. **260:** 147, 1959.
29. Stark, J., Aberdeen, E., Waterston, D. J., Bonham-Carter, R. E., and Tynan, M.: Pulmonary artery constriction (banding): A report of 146 cases, SURGERY **65:** 808, 1969.
30. Stark, J., Tynan, M., and Aberdeen, E.: Spontaneous closure of ventricular septal defect following pulmonary artery constriction (banding), Amer. Heart J. In press.
31. Takahashi, M., Lurie, P. R., Petry, E. L., and King, H.: Clinical and hemodynamic effects of pulmonary artery banding, Amer. J. Cardiol. **21:** 174, 1968.
32. Vince, D. J.: Banding of the pulmonary artery in infancy: Selection of patients and results of main pulmonary artery banding in the treatment of congenital heart disease, Canad. Med. Ass. J. **97:** 1, 1967.

Localization of gastrointestinal hemorrhage by selective angiography

CHARLES F. FREY, M.D.
STEWART R. REUTER, M.D.
JOSEPH J. BOOKSTEIN, M.D.
ANN ARBOR, MICH.
From the Departments of General Surgery and Radiology of the University of Michigan Medical Center and Wayne County General Hospital

Percutaneous selective visceral angiography was first used to determine the location of active gastrointestinal bleeding by Baum and associates[2] in 1965. Since their report, angiography has proved to be a useful and reliable adjunct in the evaluation of otherwise unexplained gastrointestinal hemorrhage. Experimental work in dogs performed first by Nusbaum and Baum[11] later confirmed in our own laboratory[9] indicated that bleeding rates of 0.5 to 0.6 ml. per minute were demonstrable through the use of selective celiac or superior mesenteric angiography.

The site of gastrointestinal hemorrhage may be localized by selective angiography in two ways. If the patient is actively bleeding, contrast medium may extravasate into thc bowel lumen. Or, angiography may permit identification of the lesion responsible for intermittent or chronic bleeding, such as arteriovenous malformation, without actually demonstrating the bleeding per se.

Our experience with arteriography at the University of Michigan Medical Center is reviewed and correlated with that from other institutions in order to better define the role of arteriography in the localization of gastrointestinal hemorrhage.

METHODS

Angiographic technique. A radiopaque polyethylene catheter with an appropriate distal curve is inserted into the celiac, superior mesenteric, or inferior mesenteric arteries by a percutaneous femoral approach. If upper gastrointestinal bleeding is being investigated, celiac and superior mesenteric angiograms are performed; for lower gastrointestinal bleeding, the superior and inferior mesenteric arteries are injected. If the site is not known, then all three are injected. Approximately 35 ml. of 76 percent Renografin is injected at 12 ml. per second into the celiac and superior mesenteric arteries, and 15 ml. at 7.5 ml. per second into the inferior mesenteric artery. Serial films are exposed at the rate of 2 per second for 4 seconds, and 1 every 2 seconds for an additional 12 seconds.

MATERIAL

Between 1964 and 1969, we have studied 45 patients with active bleeding and 50 with inactive or chronic bleeding at the University of Michigan Medical Center and Wayne County General Hospital.

Most patients considered to have bleeding were passing bright red blood through mouth or anus or had obviously melanotic stools or continuing drop in hematocrit, although 3 patients had only 4+ guaiac stools. Inactive (intermittent) or chronic bleeders included patients without any current evidence of hemorrhage, or patients whose stools were 3+ guaiac or less.

These patients had angiography because of uncertainty as to the source of massive hemor-

Received for publication Sept. 4, 1969.

rhage or because of repeated episodes of gastrointestinal bleeding, the origin of which remained obscure after hematologic, endoscopic, and radiographic examinations, and even after operation.

RESULTS

Angiographically, active bleeding appears as an intraluminal accumulation of contrast medium which develops during the arterial phase and may persist through or beyond the venous phase.

The site of bleeding was visualized in 25 of the 45 patients with active bleeding (Table I). A lesion believed responsible for bleeding was found in 31 of 50 patients with chronic or intermittent bleeding (Table II).

DISCUSSION

Active gastrointestinal hemorrhage. In active bleeding, the extravasated contrast material will usually outline normal mucosal folds, but rarely, the pattern of accumulation will offer some clue as to the cause of bleeding. For example, in 2 patients a discrete round collection of contrast medium was recognized as being within an ulcer crater, and a similar, round collection occurred in a patient with a bleeding colonic diverticulum.

Uremic bleeding is often thought to occur as a diffuse ooze from long segments of small or large bowel. However, in 2 of 3 patients with uremia that we have studied by angiography, specific single bleeding arteries were identified in the bowel. These 2 patients had the densest collection of contrast medium of all the active bleeders.

The mucosa of the entire colon is often diseased in ulcerative or granulomatous colitis or typhoid fever. One patient each with these diseases was studied by angiography during active bleeding. The sites of bleeding appeared to be multifocal but were confined to a short segment of bowel.

Arterial bleeding was demonstrated at the esophagogastric junction in 3 patients. In each the bleeding was caused by a Mallory-Weiss tear.[14]

We have been unable to visualize extravasated contrast material related to bleeding

Table I. *Etiology of active hemorrhage visualized by arteriography in 25 patients*

Etiology	*No. of patients*
Upper gastrointestinal	
Duodenal ulcer	4
Gastric ulcer	1
Superficial gastric ulcer	3
Marginal ulcer	1
Carcinoma—stomach	2
Pancreaticojejunal anastomosis	1
Mallory-Weiss tear	1
Small bowel	
Chorionic adenoma destruens	1
Chorionic carcinoma	1
Jejunal ulcer associated with uremia	1
Ileocolic anastomosis	1
Colon	
Diverticulosis	4
Ulcerative colitis	1
Typhoid ulcer	1
Granulomatous colitis	1
Ulcerative colitis	1

Table II. *Lesions thought responsible for chronic or intermittent hemorrhage in 31 patients*

Etiology	*No. of patients*
Upper gastrointestinal	
Esophageal varices	5
A-V malformation—stomach	2
A-V malformation—duodenum	1
Hemangioma liver plus stomach	1
Mallory-Weiss tear	1
Leiomyosarcoma—duodenum	1
Aneurysm gastroduodenal artery	1
Aneurysm of marginal artery of colon	1
Small bowel	
Telangiectasis	1
Arteriosclerosis—vasa recta	5
A-V malformation	1
Regional enteritis	1
Hypervascularity—jejunum	1
Ileocolic anastomosis	1
Colon	
A-V malformation	5
Benign polyp sigmoid	1
Malignant polyp ascending colon	1
Carcinoma ascending colon	1

A-V = arteriovenous.

A 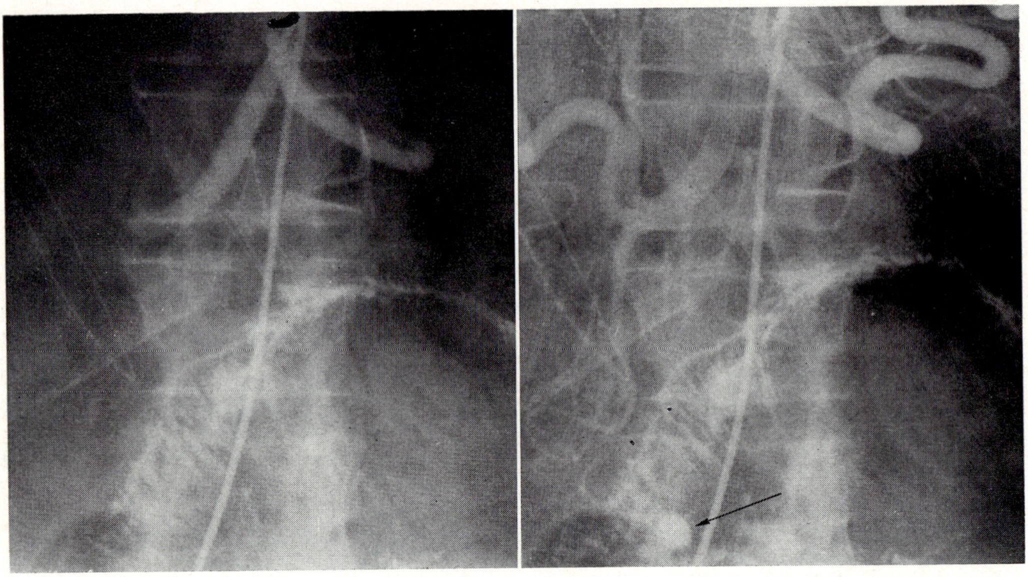 B

Fig. 1. Active gastrointestinal bleeding at rate of 1,500 c.c. per hour into a distal duodenal ulcer. *A,* Early arterial phase after celiac injection. Residual barium is noted within the bowel. *B,* Late arterial phase. Additional contrast medium (arrow) accumulates at the bleeding site. The smooth round configuration without evident mucosal pattern suggests bleeding within an ulcer.

varices, because of the dilution that occurs within the capillary bed. However, angiography is of aid to the surgeon in patients suspected of having variceal hemorrhage by ruling out arterial bleeding from duodenal or gastric ulcerations. Dilation of the hepatic artery and its branches and increased tortousity of intrahepatic arteries may help confirm the impression of cirrhosis. During the venous phase, visualization of esophageal varices or of other associated portal-systemic collaterals or demonstration of an enlarged spleen help confirm the presence of portal hypertension.[3, 4]

Extravasation of contrast material can be visualized by angiography when rates of bleeding are 0.5 to 0.6 ml. per minute in the dog. The extract rate demonstrable in man is unknown but is probably of the same order of magnitude. We have demonstrated bleeding on arteriograms in two patients who had apparently ceased to hemorrhage at the time of angiography, as judged by vital signs and follow-up. Of the 20 patients in whom active bleeding was not localized by angiography, slowing or cessation of hemorrhage was the explanation in most cases. Other failures of angiography included: (a) an obese patient in whom an actively bleeding right colonic diverticulum was not included on the film, and (b) an uremic patient with multiple coagulation defects who was probably bleeding diffusely.

The value of arteriography in the localization of active bleeding is exemplified by the following case reports.

Case 1. A 33-year-old alcoholic man with ankylosing spondylitis, treated with aspirin and cortisone, underwent a partial gastrectomy and gastrojejunostomy as the result of massive hematemesis and melena. Over the next month, he bled massively twice and each time an exploratory operation was performed, but the source of hemorrhage remained unknown. His course was complicated by a massive pulmonary embolus and renal failure. He arrived at the University of Michigan Medical Center with a Sengstaken-Blakemore tube in place. Two days later he again bled, requiring 4 L. of blood replacement in 90 minutes. He was thought to be bleeding from a diffuse gastritis. Arteriography was performed en route to the operating room. Bleeding was demonstrated at the junction of the third and fourth portion of the duodenum and the smooth round margins of accumulated

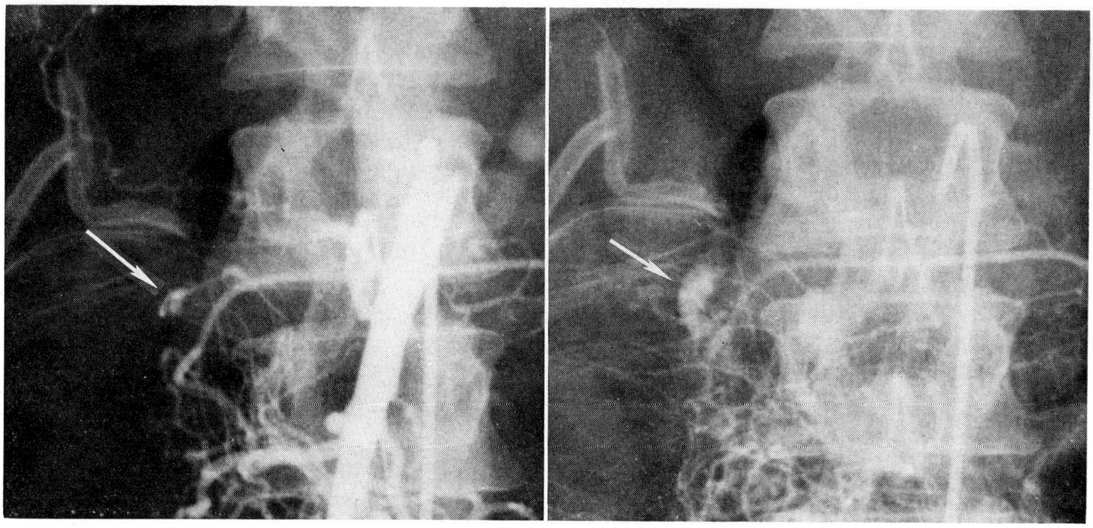

Fig. 2. Active bleeding at a pancreaticojejunostomy site. Clinically estimated rate 250 c.c. per hour. *A,* Early arterial phase after injection of superior mesenteric artery. Beginning intraluminal extravasation of contrast medium is recognized (arrow). *B,* Late arterial phase. Fully developed extravasation creates a pattern suggestive of duodenal mucosa.

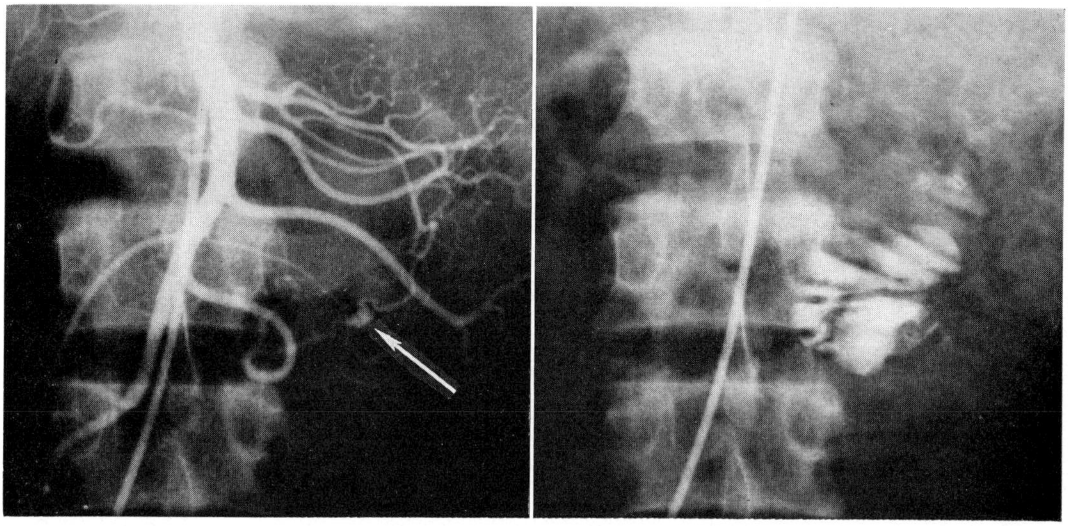

Fig. 3. Active jejunal bleeding in uremia. Clinically estimated rate 1,500 c.c. per hour. *A,* Early arterial phase demonstrates beginning extravasation (arrow). *B,* Fully developed extravasation densely opacifies a large area of jejunum with clearly demonstrated mucosal pattern.

contrast medium suggested an ulcer crater (Fig. 1). This was confirmed at operation.

Case 2. A 62-year-old man bled through his nasogastric tube 2 days after pancreaticoduodenectomy. The operation had been performed because of injury to the pancreas and duodenum incurred in an automobile accident. Two days later, after replacement of 12 units of whole blood, arteriography was performed. Bleeding was demonstrated in the jejunum and was correctly diagnosed as coming from the pancreaticojejunostomy site (Fig. 2). At operation, a single bleeding artery was found and ligated at the pancreaticojejunostomy anastomosis. The patient had no further hemorrhage and was discharged 3 weeks later.

Case 3. A 49-year-old man was admitted to the

University of Michigan Medical Center because of allergic vasculitis. The vasculitis was thought to have an infectious basis and was treated with cephalothin, kanamycin, and colistin. The patient became progressively oliguric. When the serum creatine was 10 mg. percent, he passed dark red clotted blood through the rectum and became hypotensive. Five liters of blood replacement were required over the ensuing week. Suddenly, hemorrhage became massive, and 7 L. of blood were administered in less than 18 hours. Arteriography was performed and a single bleeding point was identified in the proximal jejunum (Fig. 3). At operation, a single incision was made in the jejunum 3 feet from the ligament of Trietz and an arterial bleeder in the base of a shallow ulcer was identified and ligated. Subsequently, the patient was discharged after resolution of his vasculitis and renal failure.

CHRONIC OR INTERMITTENT GASTROINTESTINAL HEMORRHAGE

Intermittent or chronic hemorrhage from the gastrointestinal tract was believed to have been caused by a variety of lesions, including tumors, arteriovenous malformations, telangiectasias, aneurysms, and infarcts.

Tumors may be identified by the presence of "tumor vessels" which appear as irregular, short, serpiginous vessels with irregular branches. Previously existing arteries may be displaced, encased, or occluded. Some tumors, such as small bowel leiomyoma, are typically hypervascular.[5]

Aneurysms may appear as saccular dilatations of any intestinal artery and occur following trauma, operation, or as a result of congenital or arteriosclerotic defects. They may or may not be associated with intestinal bleeding.[15]

Telangiectasias or arteriovenous malformations were noted in the stomach, small bowel, and colon, and were most frequent in the colon. The early, dense opacification of veins draining the lesion helps in its identification.[10, 14] Active bleeding was not identified from arteriovenous malformations but, when excised, no further episodes of gastrointestinal hemorrhage occurred.

In patients with severe atherosclerosis of the mesenteric vessels, it has been postulated that occlusion of the vasa recta may infarct the underlying mucosa and lead to bleeding.[1, 7] Supposed sites of infarcts were identified at angiography by the premature termination of the vasa recta branches in 5 cases.

The value of angiography in the localization of the cause of chronic or intermittent bleeding is exemplified by the following case report.

Case 4. Over a period of 2 years, a 56-year-old woman had undergone numerous conventional barium studies because of anemia and guaiac-positive stools. An operation was performed because malignancy was suspected, but no source of bleeding was found. Thirty centimeters of terminal ileum was empirically resected. She continued to have chronic blood loss. One year after the resection, angiography was performed. An arteriovenous fistula was demonstrated in the proximal ascending colon (Fig. 4). At operation, no abnormality was noted, but the cecum and ascending colon were resected. When the specimen was carefully examined a small, reddish, punctate, mucosal discoloration was seen in the cecum, and a tangle of dilated submucosal veins was found under this at microscopic examination. Subsequently, the patient was found to have a conjunctival telangiectasis. On follow-up, she has had no further blood loss.

INDICATIONS FOR THE USE OF ARTERIOGRAPHY IN GASTROINTESTINAL HEMORRHAGE

Arteriography is indicated in the localization of massive gastrointestinal bleeding whenever the source of bleeding is not known, provided that vital signs can be stabilized. In experienced hands, the procedure requires one-half hour, and the diagnosis can be made while the operating room is prepared.

In performing arteriography on patients with massive gastrointestinal hemorrhage, it is essential that clinicians and arteriographers function as a team. A clinician should accompany the patient to the Radiology Department in order to monitor vital signs and to administer intravenous fluids or blood. The around-the-clock availability of a skilled angiographer is essential if angiography is to be employed in these emergency situations.

Exploration of the abdomen without pre-

A

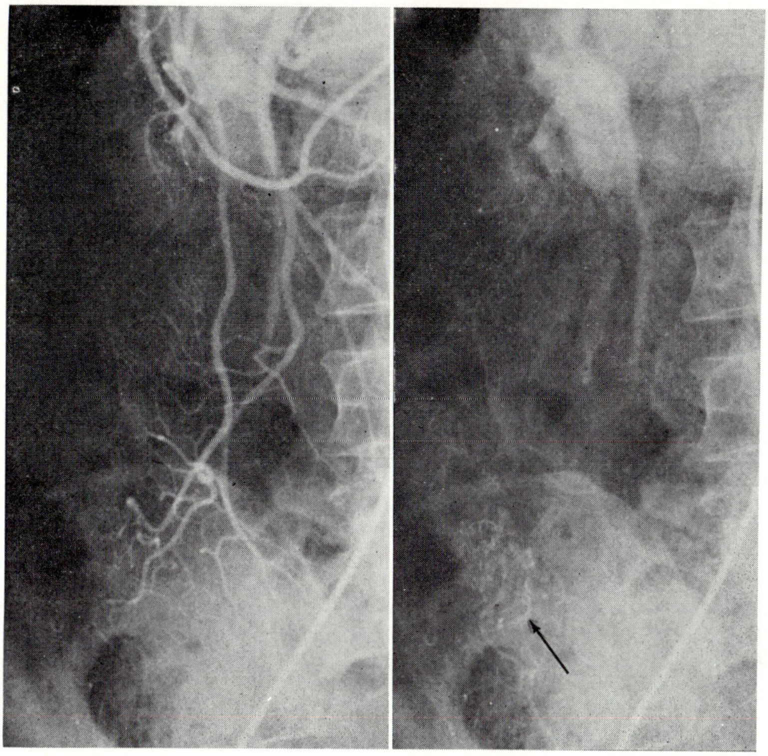

B

Fig. 4. Chronic active bleeder due to an arteriovenous fistula. *A*, Early arterial phase demonstrates no abnormality. *B*, Late arterial phase—early opacification of a small vein (arrow) is recognized. This vessel is distinguishable from the adjacent artery by slight difference in caliber and position and on later films (not shown) was seen to be contiguous with other veins. Bleeding is not demonstrated.

cise preoperative localization of the bleeding site may be a frustrating experience. Frequently the bleeding stops during the induction of anesthesia. Also the bowel may be filled with blood and lesions may not be recognized even on direct inspection of the mucosa. This is particularly true of the shallow ulcerations that are associated with uremia.

The incidence of unexplained bleeding in the upper gastrointestinal tract is reported by Foster and associates[8] to be approximately 6 percent. In the past, when the source of bleeding was known to come from the upper gastrointestinal tract but could not be further localized by conventional roentgen techniques or at operation, blind total gastrectomy was often performed. While vagotomy and pyloroplasty avoid some of the nutritional sequelae of gastrectomy, it does not decrease the incidence of rebleeding from a persistent source.

Unexplained bleeding from the small intestine may lead to repeated small bowel resections, and these in turn may cause a short bowel syndrome. Patients with diffuse vascular malformations can be particularly difficult to manage since the bleeding could potentially come from a number of different sites.[13]

When the bleeding is from the colon, accurate localization of the hemorrhage without the use of angiography is often impossible. The surgeon may be forced to perform multiple colotomies in the hope of finding a bleeding source[16] or to empirically resect the colon creating an ileocolostomy. The former procedure is hazardous and usually futile in the unprepared bowel[12]; the latter may result in troublesome diarrhea. In diverticulosis, localization of the bleeding diverticulum by angiography permits resection of a short appropriate segment of bowel. In patients with active bleeding from previously demonstrated granulomatous or ulcerative colitis, it is not essential to locate the precise site of bleeding since the entire diseased segment of bowel will be removed at operation.

Thus, in patients bleeding actively from the gastrointestinal tract, when the cause is not known with reasonable certainty from prior history or barium studies, angiography should be performed before operation. This is especially true of patients with intermittent bleeding who have often undergone multiple barium studies and frequently one or more operations without the source of hemorrhage being identified. When such an individual is admitted to the hospital actively bleeding, the initial procedure should be angiography. Arteriography is the most accurate procedure in localizing the source of bleeding, and the more active the hemorrhage, the better the chances of visualizing bleeding.

The patient with chronic or inactive intermittent bleeding should be evaluated initially by conventional methods, including barium studies and endoscopy. If these provide no information regarding the source or cause of bleeding, angiography should be performed before operation is considered. Some lesions, such as arteriovenous fistulas and superficial ulcers of the colon, can be identified only by angiography. Even under direct inspection of the mucosa small arteriovenous fistulas often cannot be recognized until the specimen is meticulously examined by the pathologist.[6, 14] Occasionally, lesions usually apparent on barium examinations, such as carcinoma polyps or regional ileitis, have been apparent only on angiograms.

COMPLICATIONS

Serious complications of selective visceral arteriography are infrequent and represent no risk different from other arteriographic procedures which utilize the percutaneous femoral approach.

In the last 3,000 cases of retrograde percutaneous femoral catheterizations, we have had 5 femoral artery thromboses, 3 severe hematomas, and 3 false aneurysms. All 11 complications were corrected surgically without further sequelae. In order to reduce the incidence of thromboses, the femoral pulse is monitored below the site of catheterization during the procedure. If the pulse is weak or absent, papavarine is injected into the femoral artery and the procedure is continued. If the pulse remains unpalpable in patients who are not bleeding, a full dose of intra-arterial heparin is also given, but obviously this cannot be used in patients with gastrointestinal hemorrhage.

SUMMARY

Selective visceral arteriography has proved useful in evaluating gastrointestinal hemorrhage and has detected the site of active bleeding in 25 of 45 patients (56 percent) with active bleeding, and 31 of 50 patients (62 percent) with intermittent or chronic bleeding.

Selective visceral arteriography is advocated as the primary procedure in patients with massive unexplained gastrointestinal hemorrhage, and in instances when previous operative procedures or conventional methods of diagnosis have failed to identify the site of hemorrhage.

REFERENCES

1. Aakhus, T.: The value of angiography in superior mesenteric artery embolism, Brit. J. Radiol. **39:** 928, 1966.
2. Baum, S., Nusbaum, M., Blakemore, W. S., and Finkelstein, A. K.: The preoperative radiographic demonstration of intra-abdominal bleeding from undetermined site by percutaneous selective celiac and superior mesenteric arteriography, SURGERY **58:** 797, 1965.
3. Baum, S., Stein, G. N., Nusbaum, M., and Chait, A.: Selective arteriography in the diagnosis of hemorrhage in the gastrointestinal tract, Radiol. Clin. N. Amer. **7:** 131, 1969.
4. Boijsen, E.: Selective angiography of the celiac axis and superior mesenteric artery in cirrhosis of the liver, Rev. Int. Hepat. **15:** 323, 1965.
5. Boijsen, E., and Reuter, S. R.: Angiography in the evaluation of inflammatory and neoplastic disease of the intestine, Radiology **87:** 1028, 1966.

6. Butsch, J. L., Dockerty, M. B., McGill, D. B., and Judd, E. S.: "Solitary" nonspecific ulcers of the colon, Arch. Surg. **98:** 171, 1969.
7. Corry, R. J., Bartlett, M. K., and Cohen, R. B.: Superficial erosions of the cecum. A cause of massive hemorrhage, presented at 10th Annual Meeting of Society for Surgery of the Alimentary Tract, New York, July 12-13, 1969.
8. Foster, J. H., Hickok, D. F., and Dunphy, J. E.: Changing concepts in surgical treatment of massive gastroduodenal hemorrhage, Ann. Surg. **161:** 968, 1965.
9. Frey, C. F., Ernst, C. B., Lindenauer, S. M., Bartlett, J. B., and Bookstein, J.: Use of arteriography in the diagnosis of occult gastrointestinal and traumatic intra-abdominal hemorrhage, Amer. J. Surg. **113:** 137, 1966.
10. Halpern, M., Turner, A. F., and Citron, P.: An angiographic study of abdominal visceral angiodysplasias associated with gastrointestinal hemorrhage: Hereditary hemorrhagic telangiectasia, Radiology **90:** 1143, 1968.
11. Nusbaum, M., and Baum, S.: Radiographic demonstrations of unknown sites of gastrointestinal bleeding, Surg. Forum **14:** 374, 1963.
12. Olsen, W.: Hemorrhage from diverticular disease of the colon: The role of emergency subtotal colectomy, Amer. J. Surg. **115:** 247, 1968.
13. Pierce, W. S., and Davis, A. N.: Massive bleeding from a diffuse vascular malformation of the small intestine, Arch. Surg. **98:** 336, 1969.
14. Reuter, S. R., and Bookstein, J. J.: Angiographic localization of gastrointestinal bleeding, Gastroenterology **54:** 876, 1968.
15. Reuter, S. R., Fry, W. J., and Bookstein, J. J.: Mesenteric artery branch aneurysms, Arch. Surg. **97:** 497, 1968.
16. Taylor, F. W., and Epstein, L. I.: Treatment of massive diverticular hemorrhage, Arch. Surg. **98:** 505, 1969.

Surgical techniques

Conducted by WILLIAM S. BLAKEMORE, M.D.

Hemostasis during liver resections

WILLIAM R. CLARK, JR., M.D.*
ROBERT P. LEATHER, M.D.
ALBANY, N. Y.
From the Department of Surgery of the Albany Medical College of Union University

Partial resections of the liver remain hazardous operations in spite of an enormous regenerative capacity. The principal reasons for this are the extreme vascularity of the liver, the softness of its parenchyma which in the normal organ does not hold sutures well, and its intolerance of ischemia for more than short periods.

Securing hemostasis of the parenchymal hepatic vessels is a most important feature of this operation and one of the most time-consuming elements. Done by the conventional clamp and tie method, it requires

Received for publication July 21, 1969.
*Present address: Moyer Clinic, Baraga, Mich. 49908.

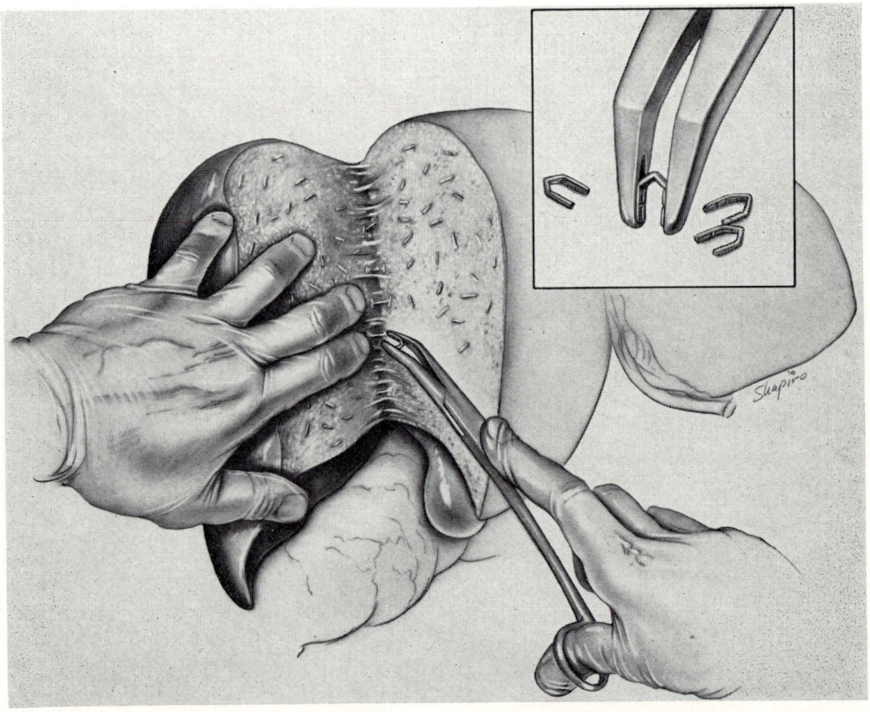

Fig. 1. A short segment of intrahepatic vessel is exposed and clipped prior to division. The insert shows the narrow jaws of the clip holder; the angle at the tip facilitates placing the clip flush with the hepatic parenchyma.

frequent halts, the utilization of hands often needed for exposure, and repetition because of low efficiency. When the method of dividing the hepatic parenchyma with the scalpel handle is coupled with the use of Hemoclips (Edward Weck & Company, Inc., New York, N. Y.), most of these difficulties are avoided, time is saved, and blood loss is reduced.

The appropriate hepatic artery and portal vein are temporarily occluded during the hepatic parenchymal dissection. The illustration shows most of the details (Fig. 1). The narrowness of the Hemoclip necessitates only minimal exposure of the vessel prior to accurate placement of the clip. This can be provided by the scalpel handle which does not cut the vessel. Securing the vessel in a Hemoclip requires only one free hand and can be done without pulling on the vessel or tearing the attached parenchyma in an effort to provide more exposure. Assistants remain free to maintain exposure. Three sizes of clip are available, and even the larger vessels can be occluded in a single clip. Hemostasis is secure, and necrosis of the vessel wall does not occur so that delayed hemorrhage is not a problem. Mattress sutures are rarely needed; unnecessary necrosis along the line of resection is thus avoided. And thus, a method for providing rapid hepatic parenchymal hemostasis by the use of Hemoclips has been described.

Editorial

Conducted by THEODORE DRAPANAS, M.D., *and* EDWIN H. ELLISON, M.D.

A Pacific-wide view of surgery

SIR DOUGLAS ROBB
AUCKLAND, NEW ZEALAND

It is relatively easy these days for the Westerner to catch glimpses of most of the territories of the world that have formerly been out of easy reach or have been thought to be of little interest. He can speed in, spend a few hours or days looking around, and speed back to his workhouse at home. He will have noted the obvious differences in his field of activity from that which he is used to. He may quickly lose everything save a hazy impression of cocoanut palms, tropical flowers, the balmy evenings, and the amiable inhabitants. He may—in moods more generous, more conscientious, more egotistical, more guilty, who knows which?—feel he should do something about it. He may want to send some equipment, or seek to persuade a junior colleague to go out and work for a while, or do some other tangible thing. Or he may take time to ponder the situation more deeply, should his largeness of soul still seek an outlet.

In the last of these moods, a panel discussion on surgical and medical education was held in Honolulu in October, 1969, at the Eleventh Congress of the Pan-Pacific Surgical Association, with some of the less developed Island territories in the West and South Pacific particularly in mind. Micronesia, the Solomons, Papua–New Guinea, Fiji, and Samoa were referred to, all the panelists and chief speakers—surgeons, internists, and administrators in education and health—having had first-hand experience in the field. Herein lay the chief lesson. It takes personal experience of the whole situation—and the more of it the better—to generate useful reactions. It is not enough to slam down a lot of new equipment, or build a fine hospital such as we would like to have at home, or even to supply teams of Western-trained workers. The particular climate, the food, the economy of the country, its importance (or the reverse) to major powers for strategic purposes, the services available to maintain electrical, mechanical, and other equipment, and the means of transport and communication between villages and islands are all important. But most important of all are the people themselves. Often they have had only a brief period of contact with Europeans, and the real effect of the teaching of missionaries and schoolmasters can only be guessed at. They may lose, are losing, or have lost, their evolved order of society, and the system of customs and sanctions that it had built up. We may not ourselves like the look of this, but we are obliged to study it. It is even more important that we turn around, look at ourselves and our own systems, and ask how much better off we are than they. We must decide what elements of ours can help them in their seemingly unwilling and inevitable clash with the West. We must seek to gain their confidence and their desire for our presence and help. We must not feel frustration, or show it, at the many disappointments we will inevitably meet. One of the panelists reminded us of Diderot's address to the Tahitians, with reference to the coming of the Europeans in the eighteenth century. "They will come with the crucifix in one hand, and a dagger in the other, to cut your throats, or force you to their customs and opinions. Under their rule, you will eventually be as unhappy as they are."

Received for publication October 30, 1969.

 Vol. 67, No. 3, pp. 558-560

Other points that emerged from the discussion underlined individual consideration of each situation. In Okinawa, for example, any assistance must be frankly transitory, in anticipation of the return to Japanese association and control. In American Samoa, a more durable relation between the Samoans and the Americans was likely to be needed. The same could be said of most of the territories under discussion, Western Samoa being an example of independence already achieved, but where continued professional assistance would be needed for a considerable period. In some, if not most, areas the greatest needs of all were for elementary hygiene, sanitation, and good nutrition. The humdrum work of malaria eradication and health education promises, even today, far more benefit than the introduction of the men and equipment for the practice of modern biochemical and electronic medicine. Many territories have no medical pathologist or radiologist but also need the elementary medical and surgical services which can be provided without them. It is galling to a Westerner to see defects left untouched that his colleagues at home could easily rectify. It must be a matter of sensible priorities, however, not only within the field of medical endeavor, but also as between medical and other important fields, such as education, public works, transport, and communications. We must keep our heads. If we put in modern cardiology today, we will have to go back and fully computerize the hospital in five years' time—and so on.

The impossibility, apart from the undesirability, therefore, of imposing Western standards and methods in any degree of completeness, was accepted. When this is applied to nursing and medical personnel recruited from the local inhabitants and trained in their schools and hospitals, further problems arise. All agree that the object should be indigenous self-sufficiency as soon as reasonably possible. Progress toward this varies from area to area and is assisted by postdiploma training which is available in the larger hospitals, for example, in Suva, Fiji, and in countries like Australia and New Zealand, where the selected Suva diplomate is given temporary registration and is trained and treated in all respects as the local doctors are. He returns to his own territory on completion, since his diploma does not allow practice in Western countries.

Several speakers referred to the Suva School of Medicine—which dates from 1882 and has a great record of training and service to many Pacific Islands—and also to the newer Medical School in Port Moresby in Papua. The Suva School is run by the Department of Medical Services and has a course lasting five to seven years, according to the attainments of the entering student. The clinical training is carried out largely at the Colonial War Memorial Hospital in Suva. Students have come from all Pacific countries. Essentially practical, they have gone out to outer villages and islands where no other help except nursing could have been provided. A few Fijians have taken University medical courses in Australia or New Zealand, but the bulk of them are limited to practice in their own countries. Selected men and women have had postdiploma training in Australia, New Zealand, and elsewhere, and have become admirable doctors in such fields as obstetrics, anesthesia, surgery, public health, and cardiology.

The professional recognition of these people remains a problem. If they attain Western qualifications, they are likely to be lost to their countries. The higher diplomas currently offered in Australia and New Zealand are designed for sophisticated Western practice, and not for the type of medicine and surgery that is so important in their own countries. Perhaps special diplomas could be set up by colleges or universities to meet the just needs of this very able and worthy section of the profession in the Pacific.

Both the Papuan and Suva Schools have new universities growing up alongside them —the University of Papua–New Guinea and the University of the South Pacific, respectively. Problems here are again difficult. There are relatively few medical students with sufficient prior schooling to sustain a normal Western course in these universities, apart from the considerable demands that would be required for staff and equipment. If, in fact, such a course were set up, there would be a strong tendency to fit the graduates for work in a Western environment and not one where they are needed. Compromise arrangements will need to prevail for five to ten years, at least. Development could prove to be more rapid than we can guess now. A great deal depends on the general educational and social progress in the various territories.

A great impression was made on those present by maps showing the vast areas involved—Micronesia alone covers an area equal to that of U.S.A.—and illustrations and accounts of actual incidents experienced. Examples were a 48 hour trip in a small boat in open ocean to assist in two obstetrical emergencies and the transport of patients by canoe across open waters.

Both the challenge and the difficulties were presented, and interest was aroused. Who can tell what fresh knowledge and new values may be established through mutual understanding and contacts betweeen East and West across the Pacific?

Volume 67 Number 4 SURGERY

APRIL, 1970

Clinical surgery

"Fiberduodenoscopy"—early diagnosis of cancer of the papilla of Vater

ITARU OI, M.D.
TADAYOSHI TAKEMOTO, M.D.
KOMEI NAKAYAMA, M.D.
TOKYO, JAPAN
From the Institute of Gastroenterology, Tokyo Women's Medical College

Direct observation of the duodenum has always been a dream of endoscopists. Until now, most endoscopists have had little success in visualizing even the duodenal bulb, though many endoscopists have tried to inspect the duodenum under direct vision with their instruments, described as duodenoscopes.

Recently, with our Fiberduodenoscope, made by Machida Company under our direction, the papilla of Vater could be directly observed in approximately half of the cases examined. Duodenal ulcer, duodenal diverticulum, and duodenal polyp could be diagnosed endoscopically without much difficulty. Moreover, a small cancer of the papilla of Vater could be diagnosed before operation by direct observation and aiming biopsy with our Fiberduodenoscope, even though its early diagnosis has been fairly difficult with available diagnostic procedures. We also succeeded in cannulating the papilla of Vater for the purpose of examining the pancreas by injecting the radiocontrast material to opacify the ducts.

Received for publication Aug. 28, 1969.

INSTRUMENT

Our Fiberduodenoscope (Fig. 1) is 105 cm. in length and 11 mm. in diameter. Its short tip, including side-viewing lens and air and biopsy channels, can be flexed 127 degrees, extended 82 degrees, and rotated 90 degrees. This instrument necessarily uses the cold light system. The "small-bite" biopsy forceps is controlled by the examiner while viewing the suspicious area.

RESULTS OF OBSERVATION OF THE DUODENUM

"Fiberduodenoscopy" can be performed under local pharyngeal anesthesia (as can "fibergastroscopy") and takes less than 30 minutes. The Fiberduodenoscope is inserted into the duodenal bulb, and the first portion of the duodenum is visualized in every case. The papilla of Vater could be seen in about half of the 105 cases examined. Fig. 2 shows how this instrument may be passed to the ligament of Treitz.

Diagnosis of duodenal ulcer is not difficult with the use of this instrument. It is especially valuable in determining the stage of healing of ulcer by direct visualization. Duo-

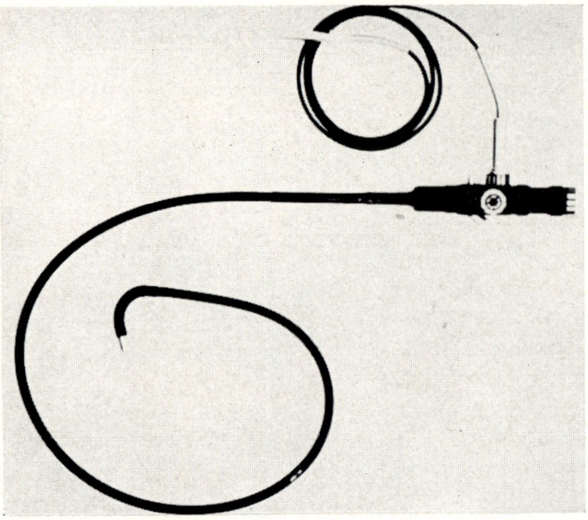

Fig. 1. Fiberduodenoscope (FDS-Lb, made by Machida Company).

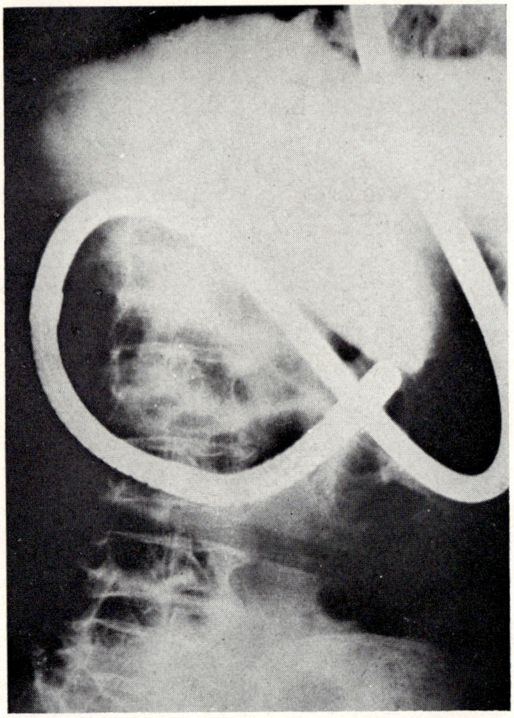

Fig. 2. The Fiberduodenoscope may be passed to the ligament of Treitz.

denal polyps and diverticula can be observed, just as those of the stomach. Endoscopically, the papilla of Vater is a whitish-colored hemispherical protrusion with concentric ditches and is confirmed by intermittent excretion of bile. Following stimulation by pancreozymin, the B bile is seen coming out from the orifice which is usually located at the tip of the papilla of Vater (Fig. 3).

CANCER OF THE PAPILLA OF VATER

Although patients with cancer of the papilla of Vater develop symptoms earlier than those with cancer of the pancreas and can be diagnosed relatively easily, nevertheless, there are not many cases in which the diagnosis had been made consistently.

We have diagnosed cancer of the papilla of Vater in two cases with our Fiberduodenoscope. One was a 69-year-old man who had suffered from jaundice which had worsened over a two-week period. X-ray examination of the upper gastrointestinal tract was negative. At fiberduodenoscopy, we could observe a small crater just under the papilla of Vater surrounded by granular elevation of the mucosa with blood clot (Fig. 4). Biopsy specimen was positive and operation was performed. The lesion was a plate-like tumor with protrusion of the papilla restricted to the papillary area without suggestions of infiltration. The tumor resected by transduodenal papillectomy measured less than 3 cm. (Fig. 5) and was diagnosed microscopically as adenocarcinoma (Fig. 6). In the other patient, a tumor lying length-

Fig. 3. Normal papilla of Vater; B bile coming out from the orifice of the papilla as the result of stimulation of pancreozymin.
Fig. 4. Cancer of the papilla of Vater; small crater surrounded by granular elevation of the mucosa with blood clot.
Fig. 5. Resected specimen of cancer of the papilla of Vater.
Fig. 6. Microscopic picture of cancer of the papilla of Vater.

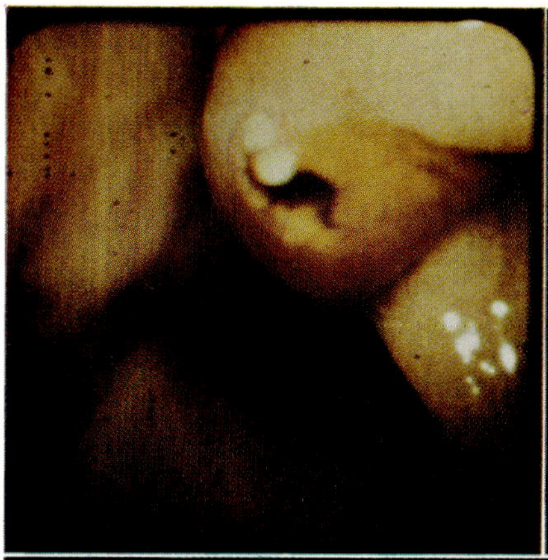

Fig. 3

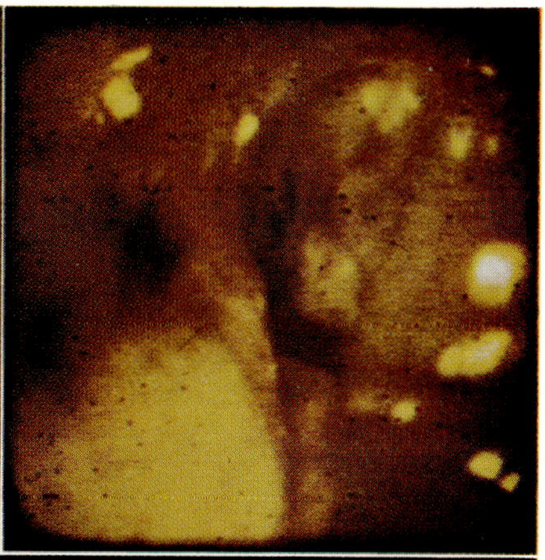

Fig. 4

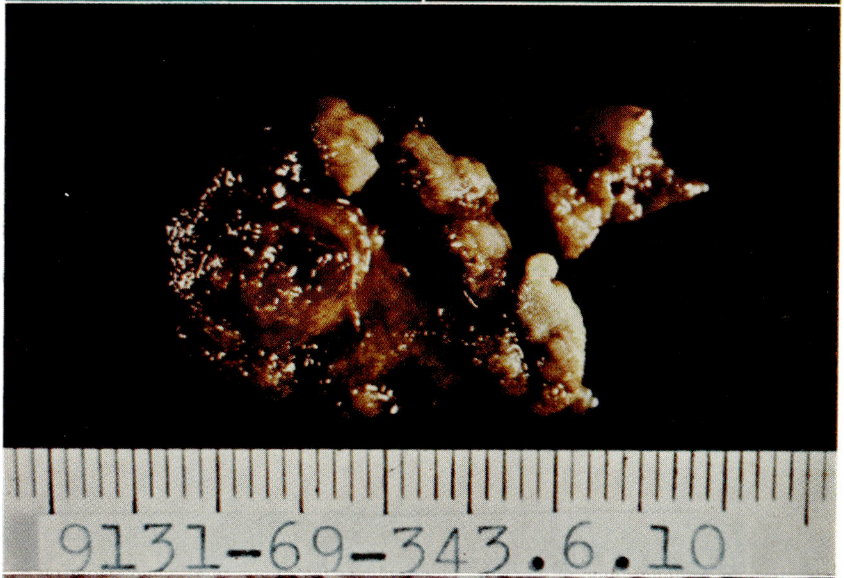

Fig. 5

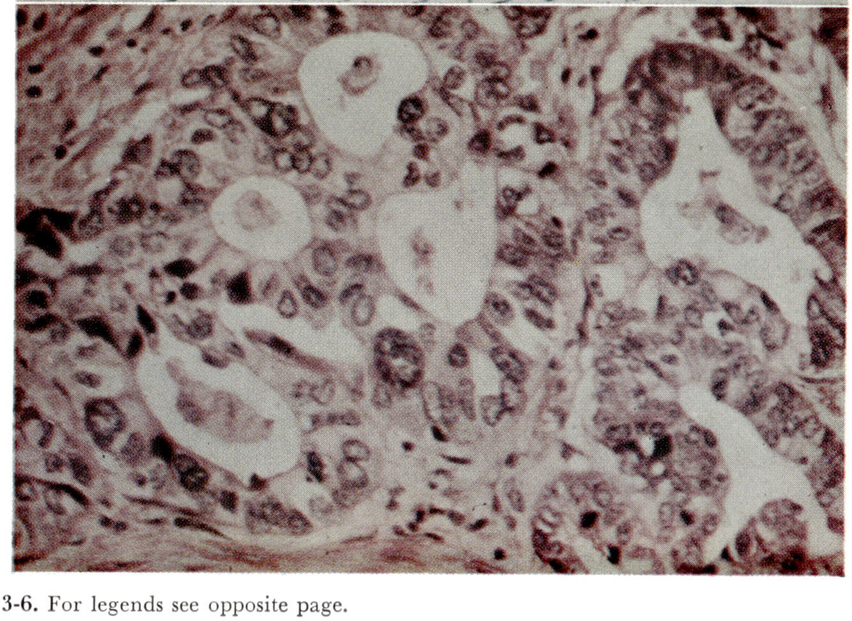

Fig. 6

Figs. 3-6. For legends see opposite page.

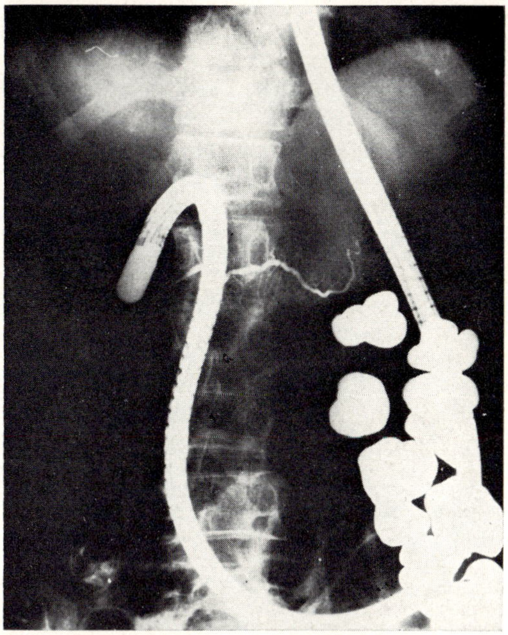

Fig. 7. Endoscopic pancreatography.

wise in the second portion of the duodenum was seen and at first was believed to be the dilated common bile duct. Beneath the lower end of this tumor, we observed an enlarged papilla of Vater with a red granular orifice. The same operation was performed and the excised cancer measured less than 2 cm.

Fiberduodenoscopy makes it possible to recognize cancer of the papilla of Vater at an early stage, which enhances the possibilities for cure.

CONCLUSION

Although many endoscopists have tried to observe the duodenum under direct vision, most have had little success. Our Fiberduodenoscope permits visualization of the papilla of Vater in about half the cases. Duodenal ulcer, duodenal diverticulum, and duodenal polyp can be diagnosed without much difficulty.

We have diagnosed cancer of the papilla in an early stage in two patients by direct observation and biopsy with the Fiberduodenoscope. In addition, we have cannulated the papilla of Vater and succeeded in opacifying the pancreatic duct with radiocontrast material with the Fiberduodenoscope (Fig. 7). "Fiberduodenoscopy" should become an important procedure in the diagnosis of the lesions of the duodenum and pancreas, especially in the detection of cancer of the papilla of Vater.

Removal of residual biliary tract calculi without reoperation

R. MAZZARIELLO, M.D.
BUENOS AIRES, ARGENTINA
From the Liver and Biliary Tract Department of the Center of Investigations and Medicochirurgical Teaching, Ward XV, Rivadavia Hospital

Despite the technical, radiographic, and prophylactic advances of modern times, postoperative cholangiographies through Kehr tubes occasionally reveal the presence of "immediate" residual calculi in the biliary tract, thus giving rise to a vexing situation vis-à-vis the patient.

In a logical desire to avoid reoperation, various methods, such as clamping of drainage tubes, choledochoclysis, hyperpressure in association with antispasmodics, or the dissolution of stones within the common bile duct, have been employed in an endeavor to eliminate them. However, none has gained general acceptance because of the uncertain results obtained and the numerous sessions required with the consequent annoyance to the patient and discouragement of the surgeon.

Although there are isolated publications on the instrumental extraction of residual calculi, it was Mondet[5] who first reported great success with a specially designed forceps. My personal experience with this method commenced in 1964 and has been the object of successive publications.[1-4] I feel that my series of patients is now sufficiently large to allow more definite conclusions concerning its efficacy.

MATERIAL AND METHODS

Thin patients, short and straight-drainage outlets, T tubes of suitable size, and not too large calculi contribute toward a successful extraction through the fistulous tract, the patency of which is indispensable. Contrariwise, obese patients, long and angulated fistulous tracts, and narrow T tubes may be regarded as unfavorable factors though they are capable of correction. For obvious reasons large calculi (over 15 mm.) and biliary ducts of narrow diameter constitute formal contraindications to the employment of the method under consideration.

The foregoing facts should be carefully evaluated during postoperative cholangiographies. The same applies to the functional condition of the duodenal papilla because if there is no inflammatory reaction it may be possible to eliminate calculi by pushing them into the duodenum.

In patients with residual calculi the following circumstances should be borne in mind in order to determine the opportune moment for our method to be employed, viz., (1) the formation of perifistular fibrous tissue, and (2) the approximation which always takes place between the common bile duct and the skin. Therefore, the longer one waits the better the chances of extracting the calculi without complications, and in the meantime clinical treatment may suffice to eliminate them. Originally a period of 60 days was allowed to lapse before attempting instrumental removal, but we gradually shortened it to 20 to 30 days in some patients.

The majority of cases can be treated without hospitalization. However, it is mandatory when the patient is in a bad state of health, when he lives far away, or when the

Received for publication June 16, 1969.

Reprint address: Republiquetas 6320, Buenos Aires, Argentina.

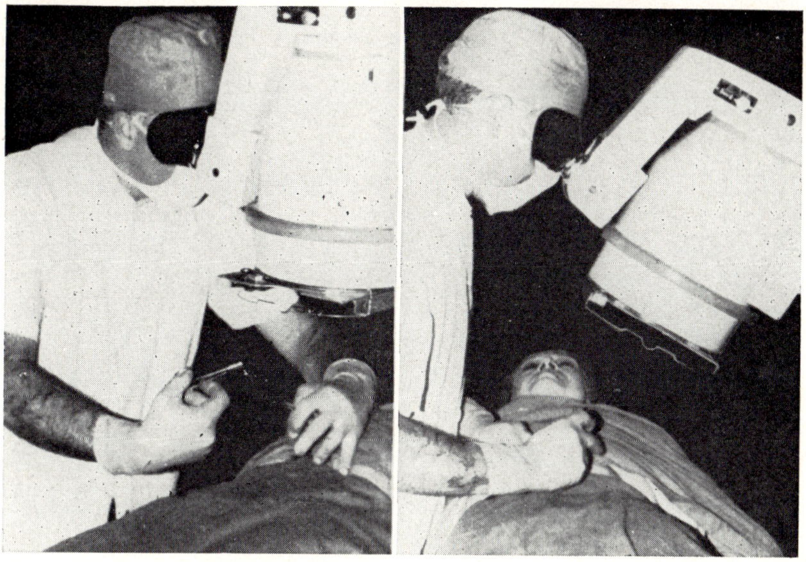

Fig. 1. Extraction of residual calculi through fistulous tract after removal of T tube. Fluoroscopic intensifier enables every step of the procedure to be followed closely without interference with the operator's hands.

nature of his problem requires constant and strict supervision. The patient should always be told the objective aimed at in order to assure his cooperation. The prior preparation of the patient depends upon his temperament and his reaction to local stimuli. Although in many cases we have not administered analgesics, it may be advisable to do so. In a very few instances we have used Pentothal.

A good and uninterrupted fluoroscopic vision and a fistulous tract of reasonable diameter are essential for the success of the procedure. In order to assure a good image, an intensifier either with direct vision or coupled to a television screen should always be used. This setup enables every step of the extraction to be followed comfortably and without any risk (Fig. 1).

The extraction having been decided upon, the main biliary passage is filled with contrast medium and the T tube is then removed. If a clear image is not obtained of the biliary passage as well as of the tract from the skin wound down to the site of the choledochotomy, contrast medium should be injected again by means of a sound until total filling of the fistulous tract has been accomplished.

Next, the extraction forceps should be carefully threaded through the fistulous tract and passed into the common bile duct until it is possible to grasp the stone or stones in the biliary ducts. The forceps should be withdrawn with very gentle movements (Fig. 2).

The Mondet[5] forceps has been found ideal for this procedure (Fig. 3). It is sufficiently thin and flexible to adapt itself to the curves of the different fistulous tracts. Different types of instruments, like the Randall and Leger forceps, were used before finally adopting almost entirely the last named and that devised by Mondet[5] (Fig. 4). We even had a special flexible forceps constructed which was provided with a plastic cover and a device for the continuous injection of contrast medium (Fig. 5). Another instrument which we tried was a specially constructed sound resembling the catheter used for the extraction of urethral stones. The point to be made clear is that rather than obtaining an ideal instrument it is essential to have an easy-to-thread fistulous tract. When such is

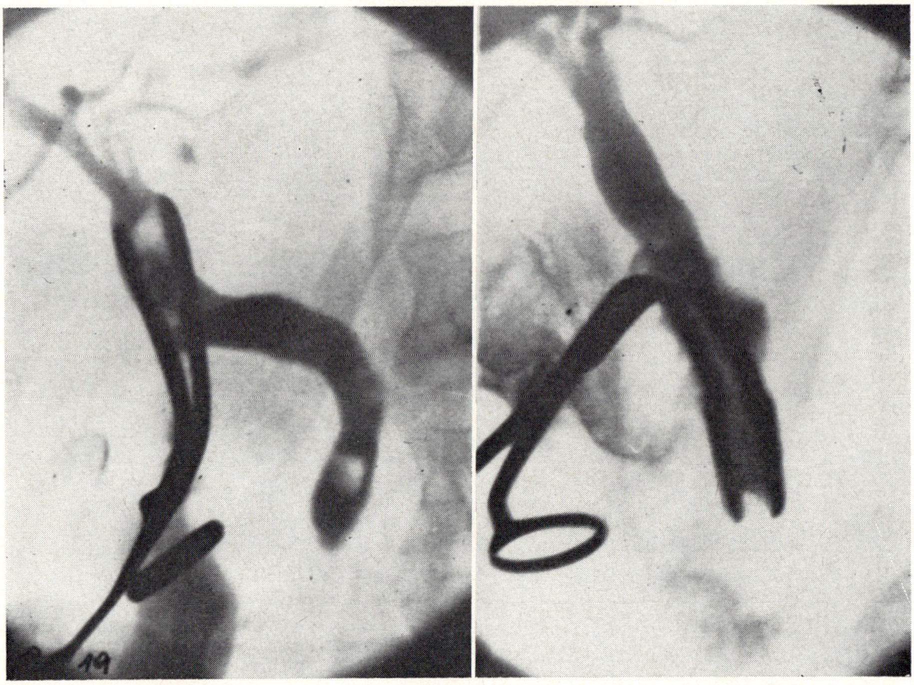

Fig. 2. Removal of residual calculi in the hepatic duct and in the terminal portion of the choledochus. Note difference in the curves of the forceps used in these two extractions.

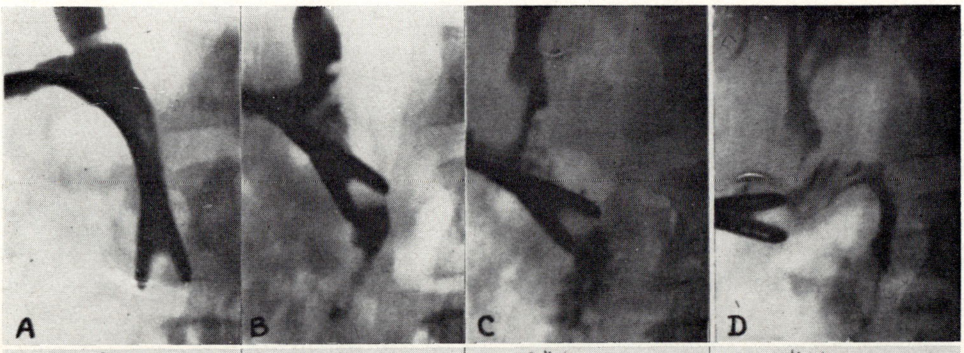

Fig. 3. Radiographic sequence showing use of Mondet forceps in the extraction of residual calculus in the terminal portion of the common bile duct.

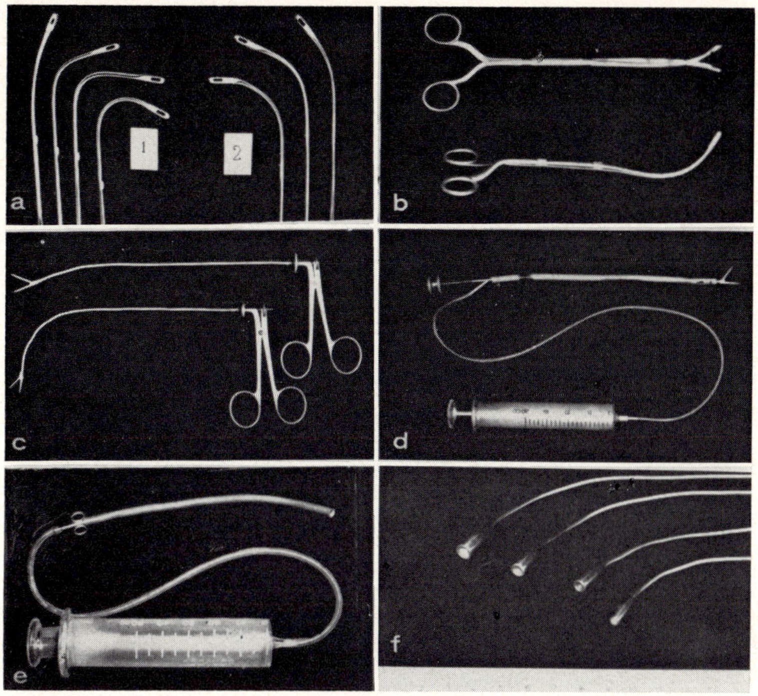

Fig. 4. Most commonly used instruments in the 74 cases reported. *a,* Modified Randall forceps *(2);* its curves are less pronounced and it is longer and thinner. *b,* Leger forceps, with longer curves. The thinner extremities enable easier penetration of the intrahepatic ducts and terminal portion of the common bile duct. This type of forceps opens widely at the extremity without appreciable increase in the width of the body. *c,* Mondet forceps. Its flexibility enables adaptation to the curves of fistulous tracts. *d,* Forceps designed by the author. It is provided with a device for continuous injection of contrast medium and is flexible enough to adapt itself to the most difficult tracts. *e,* Aspirating concave-tipped rubber sound. *f,* Concave-tipped bougies. They are especially useful for impelling small calculi into the duodenum.

not the case, it is necessary to increase its diameter by dilating procedures and eventually some degree of correction in direction may also be necessary so as to enable an easier introduction of the forceps and larger calculi to be removed.

Dilation may be accomplished in a single session by means of Béniqué's sounds, Hegar bougies of progressively greater diameter, or with Nélaton-type plastic sounds provided with a stylet. These procedures should be carried out with great care and always only if no obstacle whatever is found in introducing the instrument used to obtain dilation. The correct course followed by the instrument should be kept under permanent fluoroscopic control.

Should it be considered that the dilation obtained is not sufficient to enable the stone to be extracted, the last bougie passed through the fistulous tract should be left in situ for 24 hours. It should then be changed for a larger size until obtaining the desired dilation. This delay will in no way disturb the patient; on the contrary, it will contribute toward the success in removing the calculi.

It is astonishing how the diameter of a fistulous tract can be enlarged with the method referred to and how the forceps can thus be introduced into places which seem unreachable. Plastic sounds, being flexible but having a certain degree of rigidity, enable an easy passage to be created. They are introduced up to the entrance to the common bile duct and are then fixed to the

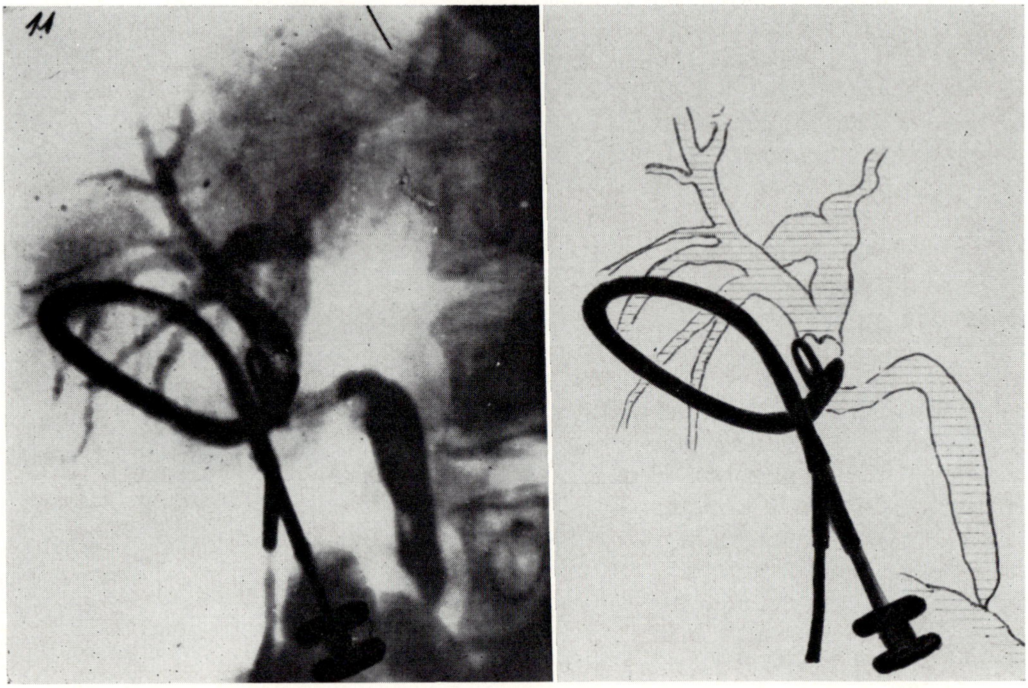

Fig. 5. Use of forceps designed by the author in the extraction of a common bile duct calculus. Removal was successfully accomplished despite pronounced curves of fistulous tract.

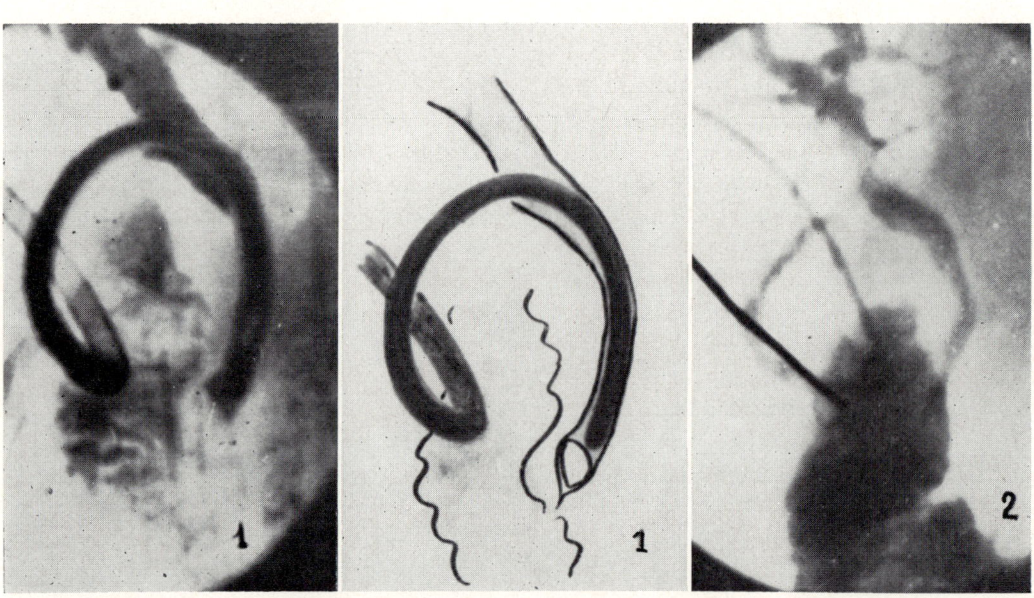

Fig. 6. Continuous action of plastic sound enabled calculus to pass into duodenum. The sound had been left in situ to dilate the fistulous tract *(1)*, and it brought about spontaneous expulsion of the calculus 24 hours later.

skin by means of adhesive tape, leaving them unclamped to avoid biliary retention (Fig. 6).

In some cases in which we aimed at correcting the course of a fistulous tract, the stones were pushed deeper into the biliary ducts and in more than one occasion calculi in a terminal position were driven into the duodenum within 24 to 48 hours. This passage through the sphincter became another means of eliminating residual calculi but in order to be successful it is indispensable that the area in question be free from inflammatory or spasmodic strictures.

Continuous fluoroscopic control constitutes the best way of determining whether a free passage can be obtained through the duodenal papilla. We prefer extracting the stones but if the terminal portion cannot be reached with the forceps then there is no recourse but to endeavor to push them into the duodenum with other instruments. Elimination in this manner can only be achieved if the calculi are sufficiently small (up to 5 mm.).

Manipulation of the instruments must be very gentle and if a sound is left in situ for continuous impulsion its diameter should not be excessive so as to avoid compression of Wirsung's duct. If the patient experiences pain, he will require antispasmodics and analgesic agents. The sound should be provided with perforations to assure an adequate bile discharge.

In some patients we have speeded the propulsion of residual calculi into the duodenum by means of a specially constructed concave-tipped metal bougie. We have also had patients in whom olive-tipped bougies were used to obtain sufficient dilation of the duodenal papilla to enable elimination of small-sized fragments of calculi with the aid of abundant lavage of the biliary passages.

In the case of a patient in whom other procedures had failed we used aspiration with a sound into whose concave tip the stone fitted comfortably. This sound contained a hollow stylet connected to a 50 c.c. syringe with which a sudden vacuum was created upon contacting the calculus.

In the event of failure of all attempts to remove residual calculi and before contemplating reoperation, enlargement of the fistulous tract may be resorted to by means of a small incision through the superficial layers of the abdominal wall without reaching the peritoneum. In this manner it is sometimes possible to correct complicated sinous tracts and thus facilitate access to the common bile duct. Should this last attempt fail, then a regular choledochotomy can be performed immediately, simply by inducing a deeper anesthesia.

RESULTS

Our series comprises 74 patients in 64 of whom (86 percent) residual calculi were successfully removed without reoperation during the period 1964 to 1968 (Table I).

The interval between original choledochotomy and calculi extraction in keeping with the procedure we have described averaged 34 days (limits ranging between 18 and 120 days).

Localizations of the residual calculi are listed in Table II.

Table I. *Results of instrumental extraction of residual calculi*

Year	No. of cases	Successes	Failures	Sessions required for calculi extraction				
				1	2	3	4	Total
1964	4	2	2	1	1	2	–	9
1965	10	8	2	4	2	3	1	21
1966	12	10	2	5	6	–	1	21
1967	21	18	3	14	5	2	–	30
1968	27	26	1	18	6	1	1	37
Total	74	64 (86%)	10 (14%)	42	20	8	3	118

Table II. *Localization of the residual calculi*

Site	*No. of cases*
Terminal portion of common bile duct	36
Other portions of the common bile duct	24
Left hepatic duct	5
Left hepatic duct and common bile duct	5
Terminal portion and other portions of the common bile duct	3
Both hepatic ducts	1
Total	74

Table III. *List of complications*

Complications	*No. of cases*
Pain, colic, and vomiting	10
Cholangitis, transient fever	7
Cholangitis, transient icterus	2
Accidental creation of false passage in the fistulous tract	1

Extraction was the most commonly used method. Impulsion into the duodenum was resorted to on 14 occasions either as the only procedure or as a complement to extraction. Aspiration was employed only once.

Previous dilation of the fistulous tract became necessary in 34 of the successfully treated patients. Most of these dilations were motivated by far-removed drainage openings. Generally speaking more sessions were also needed to treat these patients.

Four of the patients were first seen with a T tube introduced into a dilated cystic duct, and residual calculi were extracted in two of these patients. In another two the T tube had been eliminated or become displaced within 10 and 15 days, respectively, of the original operation. Recanalization of the fistulous tract with gradual dilation was feasible because of its having been kept patent by biliary hypertension. However, the tract closed rapidly as soon as such hypertension ceased. As a matter of fact this complication was also observed in cases of displacement of indwelling dilating bougies, thus making recanalization impossible.

Other failures were due to tracts with extreme angulation, strictures, or other causes which prevented the calculi from being reached.

No lesions attributable to the method herein described were found in patients who had to be submitted to a new operation for the extraction of residual calculi which could not be otherwise removed.

In Table III are listed the complications that were met. As will be observed, their nature is insignificant and as they were mostly observed in our first patients they should be attributed more to our lack of experience than to the method itself. It should be noted, however, that all of these complications were easily overcome.

There was one instance of accidental creation of a false passage in the fistulous tract. Fluoroscopic control enabled its immediate discovery and insertion of a fine probe into the fistulous tract, after which dilation was continued without further trouble.

Excellent recuperation took place in all the patients submitted to calculi extraction without reoperation, the immediate effects being manifested by disappearance of the inflammatory and spasmodic reactions produced the calculi in the region of the sphincter of Oddi.

Long-term control of our patients has afforded ample proof as to the excellence of the method under consideration.

SUMMARY

The extraction of residual calculi through the biliary passages, without reoperation and with hardly any complications, is reported by the author.

This procedure was applied successfully in 64 out of a total of 74 cases, and is particularly recommended in patients whose general condition renders further surgery inadvisable.

REFERENCES

1. Mazzariello, R. M.: La extracción instrumental de los cálculos biliares residuales, Bol. Soc. Arg. Cir. **27:** 640 & 709, 1966.
2. Mazzariello, R. M.: (Relato I. Goñi Moreno) Tratamiento de la litiasis residual de las vías

biliares con la extracción instrumental. Análisis sobre 37 casos, Bol. Soc. Cir. B.Air. **51:** 516, 1967.

3. Mazzariello, R. M.: La extracción incruenta de cálculos biliares residuales, Buenos Aires, 1968, Editor H. F. Martínez de Murguía.
4. Mazzariello, R. M.: Nuevos aportes a la extracción instrumental de cálculos biliares residuales, Bol. Soc. Arg. Cir. **29:** 404, 1968.
5. Mondet, A.: Técnica de la extracción incruenta de los cálculos en la litiasis residual del colédoco, Bol. Soc. Cir. B.Air **46:** 278, 1962.

Local gastric hypothermia in gastroduodenal hemorrhage

BORIS A. PETROV
NICOLAY N. KORENEV
MOSCOW, UNION OF SOVIET SOCIALIST REPUBLICS
From Sklifosovsky Emergency Surgery Institute

Our experience of many years has shown that in 70 percent of all cases massive hemorrhage occurs in patients with gastric or duodenal ulcer. The remaining 30 percent may be attributed to gastric cancer, esophageal varices, accompanying portal hypertension, gastric erosions, heart diseases, hiatus hernia, and a few other bizarre conditions. It is difficult sometimes to secure a correct diagnosis; in these cases urgent x-ray examination in the supine position is of great help. It is carried out after a hemostatic blood transfusion (150 ml.) and not before the shock condition of the patient is properly managed.

In the case of bleeding gastric or duodenal ulcer, we have two ways of treatment. If the hemorrhage is not massive, the blood pressure being not lower than 120 mm. Hg and the hemoglobin concentration, 60 to 70 percent, we prescribe bed rest, blood transfusion, and a dietary regimen. Three to 4 weeks later a stomach resection is usually performed. In cases of massive hemorrhage with the blood pressure below 100 mm. and the hemoglobin concentration less than 50 percent an urgent operation is performed only when the hemorrhage has lasted not more than 24 to 48 hours.

It has been noted that after 3 to 5 to 10 days after onset of hemorrhage the risk of operation increases considerably, particularly in the group of elderly and old patients suffering from arteriosclerosis, diabetes, and respiratory insufficiency.

For these patients local gastric hypothermia is indicated. Based on experimental data, it was shown at Wangensteen's surgical clinic at the University of Minnesota that gastric hypothermia causes (a) diminution of pepsin and HCl secretion, (b) lowered gastric motility, (c) reduction of gastric blood flow owing to arterial spasm. These effects contribute to establishing conditions favorable for the arrest of gastrointestinal hemorrhage: The blood clot is not digested by the inactivated gastric juice, and the reduced arterial inflow secures a better fixation of the clot in the lumen of the vessel.

This method of local hypothermia has also been applied is some European countries.[1-3]

In the Sklifosovsky Emergency Surgery Institute (1965) together with the engineer, G. D. Svidersky, we created a special apparatus for local gastric hypothermia (Fig. 1). With the aid of two devices the temperature of the inflow circulating fluid (alcohol 50 percent with water) is lowered down to –5° C.; the outflow temperature measures usually 1 to 2° C. The apparatus safely prevents the overfilling of the stomach, and the strength of the rubber balloon (wall thickness, 0.5-0.75 mm.) assures against rupture. Accurate monitoring of the gastric temperature and regulation of the quantity of fluid in the balloon are constantly carried out during the whole procedure. In experimental investigations on dogs, it was established that a lowering of the gastric temperature down to 10 to 12° C. was achieved only after an hour's cooling. In order to maintain the gastric mucosal temperature at this level, the gastric hypothermia needs to be continued for 2, 3, and occasionally 4 hours.

Received for publication June 3, 1969.

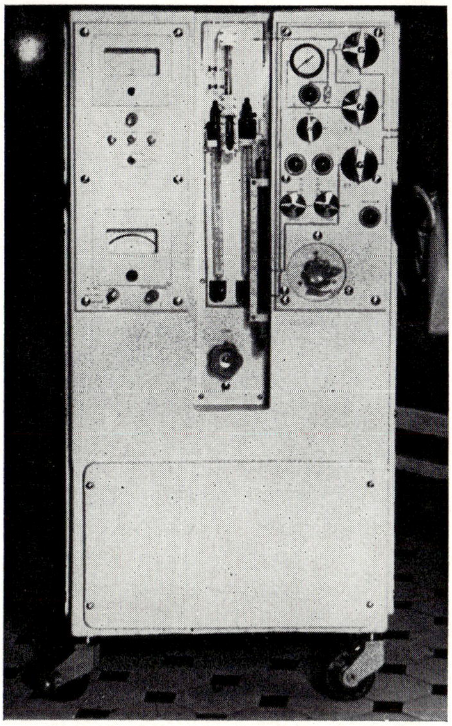

Fig. 1. Apparatus for local gastric hypothermia.

Local gastric hypothermia actually reduces the secretory response to histamine, inhibiting the function of parietal and chief cells thus prolonging considerably the latent period of gastric secretion. The proteolytic activity of the gastric juice was not always reduced, its potential digestive power hovering near the lower limits of normal. Histologic studies of the cooled stomach of dogs have shown that moderate cooling does not cause morphologic destructive changes in the gastric mucosa and musculature. In all cases only a mild edema of the mucosa and submucous layers was noted.

METHOD OF HYPOTHERMIA

The patient's stomach is properly washed out in order to remove accumulated blood and blood clots, after which the gastric balloon is introduced per os under local anesthesia and filled to 600 to 1,000 ml. of fluid previously cooled to –5° C. The system of circulation is put into action. The hypothermia lasts 4 to 5 hours. The patient is warmed by means of an electric blanket to maintain the rectal temperature in the normal range. The patient is given up to 1,000 ml. of blood, and vitamins and cardiac stimulants are given. At the end of the hypothermic period, the balloon is emptied by suction and is slowly withdrawn from the stomach.

In the period of 1965 to 1968 local hypothermia has been employed in 58 patients out of a total of 390 patients with gastric bleeding (in 252 of these patients the bleeding was from ulcer). There were 44 men and 14 women. All patients were in a very grave condition. In 49, the bleeding started 3 to 12 days before admission. The arterial pressure was 100 mm. Hg or less; three patients suffered from arterial hypertension. The hemoglobin concentration was 45 to 50 percent. In 37 patients the observed arterial pressure was 80 to 90 mm. Hg, and the hemoglobin concentration was 25 to 32 percent; in eight patients the arterial pressure was 60 mm. Hg and the hemoglobin concentration was 20 to 25 percent; in three patients the arterial pressure was zero and the hemoglobin concentration was 20 to 24 percent. In order to locate precisely the source of bleeding, urgent x-ray examination was made in 31 patients. In eight cases, this examination could not be made because of the extremely poor condition of the patients. We failed to establish the correct diagnosis in 16 patients before hypothermia. Six patients suffered from concomitant diseases: Two had diabetes, two had hemophilia and thrombocytopenia, one had active lung tuberculosis, two patients suffered from recent attacks of myocardial infarction.

Thus, local hypothermia was applied in those patients in whom an urgent operation was contraindicated because of prolonged hemorrhage, in some patients because of an obscure diagnosis, and in all the patients in this series because of their extremely grave condition.

Table I shows that the arrest of bleeding was achieved by means of hypothermia in all 58 patients (in 45 definitely, and in 13 bleeding was renewed). In 42 out of 58 patients the hemodynamic conditions were restored rapidly during hypothermia, the well-being of the patients improving dra-

Table I

Causes of bleeding	*No. of patients*	*Arrest of bleeding*		*Died from repeated bleeding*	*Urgent operation*	*Died after operation*
		Temporarily	*Definitely*			
Duodenal ulcer	25	1	24	—	2	1
Gastric erosion	4	—	4	—	—	—
Portal hypertension	5	4	1	2	3	1
Gastric ulcer	14	7	7	3	4	1
Peptic ulcer of anastomosis	3	—	3	—	—	—
Gastric cancer	3	1	2	—	—	—
Other sources (burns of stomach and other)	4	—	4	—	—	—
Total	58	13	45	5	9	3

matically. In some patients, restoration of hemodynamic conditions occurred rather slowly. Complete arrest of hemorrhage was achieved in 24 out of 25 patients with bleeding duodenal ulcer; in one patient bleeding resumed again.

In cases of bleeding gastric ulcer we managed to stop the hemorrhage completely in only 7 out of 14 patients. The bleeding recurred in seven patients; four of them required urgent operation, and one patient died.

Only in one out of four patients with bleeding esophageal varices, the hemorrhage was stopped definitely. A month later an operation of portacaval shunt was successfully performed and the patient left the hospital in good condition. Three other patients died from recurrent bleeding.

In four patients severe bleeding was caused by gastric erosions. Such hemorrhages are particularly dangerous since their source cannot be identified either by anamnesis or by x-ray examination. A single application of gastric hypothermia was sufficient to achieve arrest of bleeding. A subsequent gastroscopy confirmed the diagnosis of erosions.

Instances of bleeding from other sources (chemical burns of stomach, peptic ulcer of anastomosis) were also successfully treated by local gastric hypothermia.

CONCLUSIONS

1. Local gastric hypothermia is an efficient method of arrest of bleeding in duodenal ulcer. Operating upon the patient is quite good.

2. In order to prevent recurrent bleeding in ulcer after hypothermia, an immediate operation should be performed as soon as gastric improvement is achieved with the use of hypothermia.

3. If the etiology of massive bleeding remains obscure, local hypothermia should be employed with studies directed at determining the source of bleeding when hemorrhage has been controlled.

REFERENCES

1. Dollinger, M. R., and Morgan, L. R.: Local cooling in the management of acute upper Gastrointestinal bleeding, Amer. J. Surg. **3:** 651, 1966.
2. Gibbons, W. D.: Gastric hypothermia (Wangensteen): A preliminary report on cooling and "freezing" with the use of a new machine, Med. J. Aust. **30:** 220, 1966.
3. Grampton, R. S., Coli, J. R., Yerys, P., Buetow, G. W., and Glaubitz, J. P.: Experience with gastric hypothermia for active upper gastrointestinal tract hemorrhage, SURGERY 55: 607, 1964.
4. Petrov, B. A., and Korenev, N. N.: Local hypothermia of stomach in gastroduodenal hemorrhage, Chirurgiya (Rush.) **6:** 10, 1966.
5. Wangensteen, O. H., Root, H. D., Jensen, C. B., Imamoglu, K., and Salmon, P. A.: Depression of gastric secretion and digestion by gastric hypothermia: Its clinical use in massive hematemesis, SURGERY **44:** 265, 1958.
6. Wangensteen, O. H., Salmon, P. A., Griffen, W. O., Paterson, J., and Fattah, F.: Studies of local gastric cooling as related to peptic ulcer, Ann. Surg. **150:** 346, 1959.

Hemodynamic alterations and results of treatment in patients with gram-negative septic shock

GEORGE J. MOTSAY, M.D.*
RONALD H. DIETZMAN, M.D.**
ROBERT A. ERSEK, M.D.***
RICHARD C. LILLEHEI, M.D., PH.D.
MINNEAPOLIS, MINN.
From the Department of Surgery, University of Minnesota Medical School

In the past decade, gram-negative bacteria have replaced the gram-positive as the leading cause of death from septicemia. Only hemorrhage and myocardial infarction exceed gram-negative sepsis as a cause of shock.[9] Despite the increasing interest in gram-negative shock, the mortality rate remains at 60 to 80 percent in most large series when a positive blood culture accompanies the shock. Most investigators now agree that it is the endotoxin contained within the cell wall of all gram-negative bacteria which is responsible for the shock picture.

Studies describing the hemodynamics of this syndrome have been inconsistent. This investigation provides data on fifteen patients with gram-negative sepsis, treated by the clinical shock unit at the University of Minnesota Hospitals. A form of therapy is presented which has been uniquely successful in our hands.

MATERIALS AND METHODS

Hemodynamic studies. Over the past three years, our shock team has studied 150 patients with various problems causing shock. From this group we have obtained fifteen patients who suffered shock as a result of gram-negative bacterial sepsis (Table I). These patients were referred from various hospital departments and treated and investigated in their own ward with the aid of a mobile shock cart previously described.[5] Most patients were studied within two hours of the onset of shock, and base-line hemodynamic measurements were obtained on all prior to treatment (Table II).

An arterial cannula was inserted into the radial artery via a small cutdown or percutaneous puncture, and the arterial pressure recorded continuously from a No. P23AA Statham transducer. Intraluminal position of the arterial cannula was confirmed by the quality of the pulsatile flow.

Central venous pressure was measured on a No. 23AA Statham transducer attached to a polyvinyl catheter threaded into the superior vena cava or right atrium via the brachial, cephalic, or subclavian vein. Its position was established roentgenographically.

The cardiac output was measured by the indicator-dilution technique which uses indocyanine green dye in a concentration of 5 mg. per milliters and an MD4 densitometer module. The cardiac index and total peripheral resistance were calculated from the cardiac output, mean arterial and right atrial pressures, and body surface area by using standard formulas.[2] Urine volumes were recorded half-hourly or hourly by catheter drainage.

Supported by United States Public Health Service Grant No. HEO2941, United States Army Contract, The Commonwealth Electric Fund, and the Minnesota Heart Association.

Received for publication July 2, 1969.

*Medical Fellow in Surgery.

**Sterling-Winthrop Cardiovascular Research Fellow.

***Medical Fellow in Surgery.

Table I. Clinical data

Patient No.	Sex	Age	History	Source	Blood culture
1	71	M	Perforated sigmoid cancer	Peritonitis	*E. coli*
2	53	F	Foley catheter drainage	Urinary infection	Klebsiella
3	54	F	Rectovaginal fistula	Urinary infection	Klebsiella
4	62	F	Biliary cutaneous fistula	Cholangitis	Klebsiella
5	40	F	Foley catheter	Urinary infection	Klebsiella
6	37	F	Septic abortion	Infected uterus	*E. coli*
7	18	F	Septic abortion	Infected uterus	*E. coli*
8	60	M	Foley catheter	Urinary infection	Klebsiella
9	41	F	Subtotal urinary diversion	Pelvic abcess	Klebsiella
10	35	F	Septic abortion	Infected uterus	*E. coli*
11	25	M	Foley catheter	Urinary infection	Klebsiella
12	67	M	Enterocutaneous fistula	Abdominal abcess	*E. coli*
13	51	F	Pancreatitis and mass	Pancreatic abcess	Klebsiella
14	43	M	Postoperative central venous catheter	Infected intravenous site	Pseudomonas
15	57	M	Entercutaneous fistula	Abdominal abcess	*E. coli*

TREATMENT

Although each patient was treated individually, certain guidelines have emerged as experience is gained in treating these high risk patients (Table III).

A brief but thorough physical examination is made with emphasis on observation of skin temperature, pulse pressure, and mental status. If there is doubt about the airway, an endotracheal or nasotracheal tube is passed. The additional problem of gram-negative infections in tracheostomies can be lessened by using endotracheal or nasotracheal tubes whenever possible. Tracheostomy is done only if respiratory assistance beyond 48 hours is required.

If the central venous pressure is 10 cm. H_2O or less, intravenous fluids are started, and the choice depends on the needs. If the hematocrit is below 30 percent, blood is given if available. Otherwise, plasma or balanced salt solutions are used. We also use molecular weight dextran (40,000 molecular weight) frequently, but keep the volume used in any 24 hour period under 600 ml. Some patients respond favorably to fluid administration with an increasing urine output, a rising blood pressure, warming extremities, and clearing of the sensorium.

If the response to fluids is only temporary or does not occur and the central venous pressure reaches its upper limits of normal, 10 to 15 cm. H_2O, we use steroids or, less often, phenoxybenzamine to correct the pooling in the viscerocutaneous microcirculation which is responsible, in part, for the hypotension of gram-negative infection. Our choice is methyprednisolone as an intravenous bolus in a dose of 30 mg. per kilogram given over a five-minute period.

After a period of two to four hours, this same dose of steroids may be repeated if the

Table II. Hemodynamic data

Patient No.	Blood culture	BP before shock (mm. Hg)	Base-line hemodynamic data in shock BP (mm. Hg)	CVP (mm. Hg)	CI (L./min./M.^{2})	TPR (dynes/sec./cm.$^{-5}$)	Urine (c.c./hr.)
1	*E. coli*	130/70	80/40	6	6.43	613	10
2	Klebsiella	120/80	70/50	4	2.29	445	5
3	Klebsiella	110/50	85/20	9	2.76	391	6
4	Klebsiella	125/80	90/30	4	3.48	600	0
5	Klebsiella	110/80	90/40	5	4.10	835	322
6	*E. coli*	120/70	50/30	18	2.04	535	10
7	*E. coli*	120/80	90/40	3	4.29	943	5
8	Klebsiella	110/70	85/40	9	5.42	378	15
9	Klebsiella	130/84	70/40	12	3.45	584	25
10	*E. coli*	120/80	85/40	8	4.79	440	60
11	Klebsiella	120/80	100/40	3	5.90	486	25
12	*E. coli*	130/85	45/20	5	2.50	334	5
13	Klebsiella	120/80	70/38	11	5.40	448	15
14	Pseudomonas	130/80	68/32	3	3.67	438	2
15	*E. coli*	120/80	80/42	3	3.94	530	5
Mean values		121/	77/	5.8	4.08	533	9.8

BP = blood pressure; CVP = central venous pressure; CI = cardiac index; TPR = total peripheral resistance.

desired effects on the circulation are not achieved. If a beneficial response to corticosteroids is initially obtained, warming skin, rising urine output, elevation in blood pressure, etc., then no further methyprednisolone is given.

The use of digitalis is considered if there is a history of heart disease or signs of cardiac failure. Positive inotropic agents, such as isoproterenol or levoterenol, are also occasionally used for cardiac stimulation but only after vasodilation has been accomplished with methyprednisolone or phenoxybenzamine. When phenoxybenzamine is used, then it is given intravenously in a dose of 1 mg. per kilogram. This dose is diluted in 100 to 200 ml. of 5 percent dextrose in water and dripped in over a one- to two-hour period.

Antibiotics are immediately given in all patients, even though the offending bacteria are not immediately known, but cultures of sputum, blood, urine, and wounds, etc., are taken before the antibiotics are started. Bactericidal drugs such as synthetic penicillins and kanamycin are preferred and initial doses are always given intravenously. Subsequently, the urine output, results of cultures, or sensitivity reactions may make it necessary to change antibiotics after dosage or even stop them completely.

RESULTS

Hemodynamic studies.

Arterial pressure. In each patient, there was a drop in arterial pressure from the preshock level to 90 mm. Hg or less, except in one patient (No. 11) whose pressure fell late. The mean systolic preshock level was 121 mm. Hg and the mean systolic pretreatment shock value was 77 mm. Hg (Table II).

Central venous pressure. The central venous pressure was elevated in only one patient. The mean value for all twelve patients in shock was 5.8 mm. Hg (8 cm. H_2O) (Table II).

Cardiac index. In all fifteen patients, the cardiac index was greater than 2.0 L. per minute per square meter and in eleven of the fifteen patients, the cardiac index was greater than 3.45 L. per minute per square meter. The mean value for all fifteen patients prior to therapy was 4.08 L. per minute per square meter (Table II).

Peripheral arterial resistance. The total peripheral resistance of the patients in shock varied from 334 to 835 dynes/sec./$cm.^{-5}$ with a mean value of 533 dynes/sec./$cm.^{-5}$ (Table II).

Clinical studies.

Urine flow. There was a marked reduction in the urine flow of all but two patients (Nos. 5 and 10) and these had received osmotic diuretics. Excluding these two patients, the mean value was 9.8 c.c. per hour before therapy (Table II).

Skin blood flow. All patients except No. 8

Table III. Treatment data

Patient No.	*Source*	*Treatment*				*Outcome*
		Antibiotics	*Volume*	*Vasodilator*	*Inotropic agent*	
1	Peritonitis	Kantrex, ampicillin	LMWD* plasma	POB† SC‡	Lanoxin	Survived
2	Urinary infection	Kanamycin, tetracycline	LMWD plasma	Decandron	Lanoxin	Survived
3	Urinary infection	Kanamycin, penicillin	Blood plasma	SC	Isuprel, lanoxin	Survived
4	Cholangitis	Kanamycin, penicillin	LMWD plasma	POB SM§	Isuprel, lanoxin	Died
5	Urinary infection	Kanamycin, ampicillin	Blood plasma	SM		Survived
6	Infected uterus	Chloromycetin, penicillin	Blood plasma	SM	Isuprel, lanoxin	Survived
7	Infected uterus	Ampicillin, kanamycin	LMWD plasma	SM		Survived
8	Urinary infection	Kanamycin, ampicillin	Plasma	SC		Survived
9	Pelvic abcess	Kanamycin, ampicillin	Blood plasma	SM	Isuprel	Survived
10	Infected uterus	Kanamycin, ampicillin	Blood plasma	SM		Survived
11	Urinary infection	Kanamycin, ampicillin	Blood plasma	SM		Died
12	Abdominal abcess	Kanamycin, ampicillin	Blood plasma	SM		Survived
13	Pancreatic abcess	Ampicillin, kanamycin	Blood plasma	SM		Survived
14	Infected intravenous site	Ampicillin, kanamycin	Plasma	SM		Survived
15	Abdominal abcess	Keflin, polymyxin	Plasma	SM		Survived

*LMWD = low molecular weight dextran.
†POB = phenoxybenzamine.
‡SC = Solu-Cortef.
§SM = Solu-Medrol.

demonstrated decreased cutaneous blood flow as was evidenced by the cold and pale fingers and toes.

Sensorial level. All patients but Nos. 10 and 14 were obtunded and out of contact with their surroundings. Analysis of the nursing notes indicates most of the patients became disoriented prior to any change in blood pressure, an extremely accurate premonitory sign of impending septic shock.

Survival. Two patients could not be resuscitated from shock and died. The ten other patients were all resuscitated and either left the hospital or subsequently were returned to their respective surgical or medical services.

Follow-up. Analysis of the hemodynamic data after successful therapy reveals a normalization of all measurements. There is a decrease of the elevated cardiac indices to the normal range and an elevation of the low total peripheral resistances. The blood pressure rises to its preshock value. The skin of the fingers and toes becomes warm and the urine flow is increased.

CONCLUSIONS

Hypotension occurs in about twenty-five percent of patients developing gram-negative septicemia.[7] This is a result of stagnation in the microcirculation of the skin and viscera and also a result of shunting around the microcirculation which further decreases nutritional blood flow. An almost constant finding is a narrowed arteriovenous oxygen difference which cannot be changed initially by the use of 100 percent O_2. Patients in gram-negative shock usually have an increased blood-lactate concentration which will fall toward normal if reversal of the

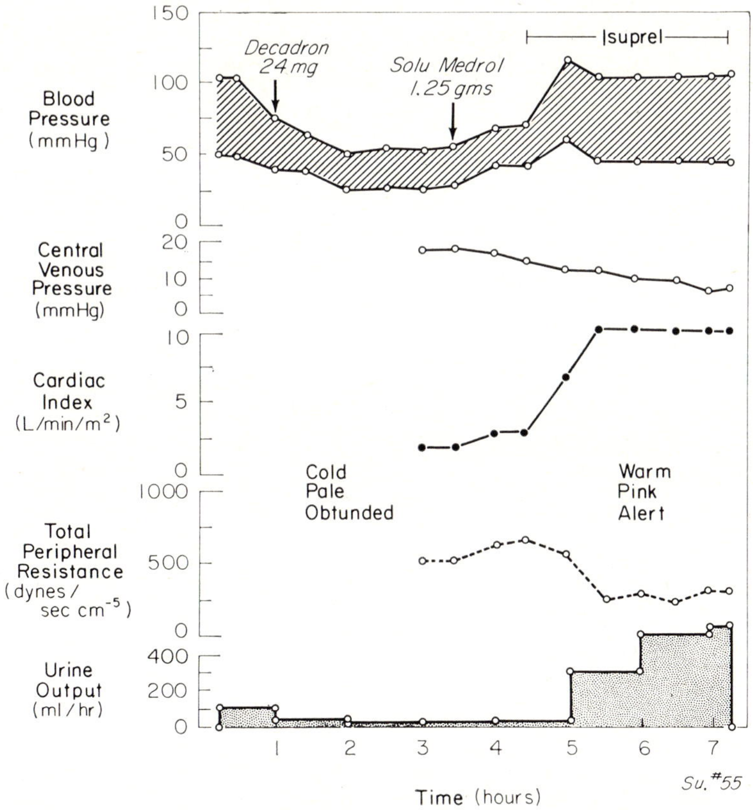

Fig. 1. Patient G. H., 37-year-old female, weight 45 kilograms. Graphic illustration of hemodynamic data from patient with gram-negative septic shock. Prior to being evaluated by our shock unit at three hours, she had been treated with a small dose of steroids at a community hospital.

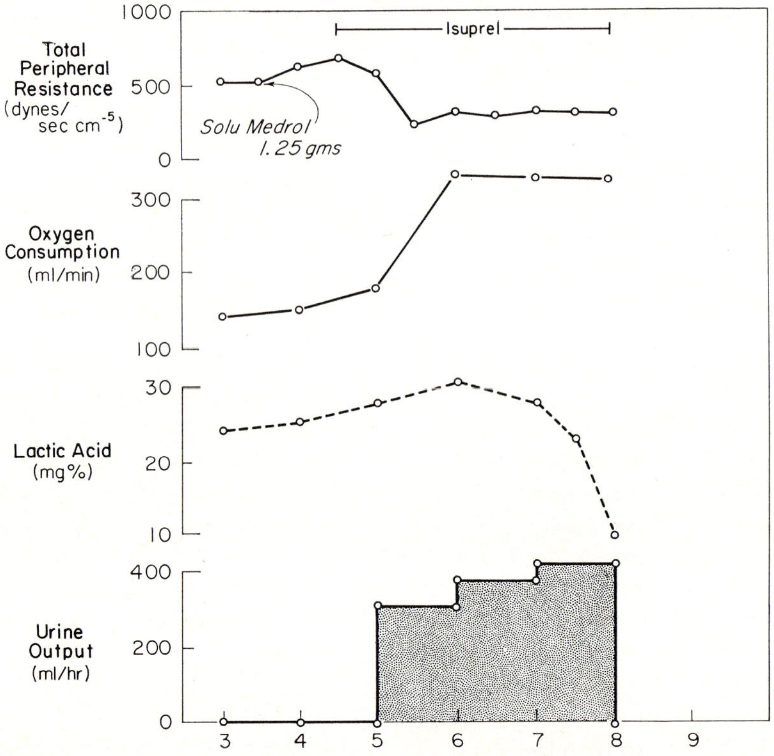

Fig. 2. Graphic illustration of metabolic data from patient in Fig. 1. Note the washout phenomenon of lactate associated with the rise in oxygen consumption.

hemodynamic alteration occurs and the stagnant, bypassed microcirculation is once again perfused (Figs. 1 and 2).

This series of patients demonstrates another indication for the existence of arteriovenous anastomosis, with the predominant alteration being one of normal or increased cardiac output associated with a low total peripheral resistance, as seen with an arteriovenous fistula. Furthermore, this hyperdynamic circulatory state is reversed with therapy. The elevated cardiac index and low total peripheral resistance approach normal values.

These findings differ markedly from those reported in gram-negative shock by Kwaan and Weil.[4] These investigators found a decreased cardiac index (mean value, 1.85 L. per minute per square meter) and an elevated total peripheral resistance (mean value, 1,649 dynes/sec./cm.$^{-5}$), while our patients had a normal or elevated index (mean value, 4.08 L. per minute per square meter) with a low total peripheral resistance (mean value, 533 dynes/sec./cm.$^{-5}$). One explanation for this marked discrepancy may be that Kwaan and Weil's patients were studied only after shock had existed for many hours. This is suggested by the fact that the mean systolic blood pressure of their patients was 59.8 mm. Hg compared with 77 mm. Hg for ours. Their survival rate of 12.5 percent (1/8) compared with our 87 percent (13/15) may also indicate differences in the stage of shock or differences in treatment (although their method of therapy is not indicated).

In this series, volume replacement was the keystone of therapy. The fluid given is usually a form of colloid and depends on the patient's hemoglobin level. The amount given is governed by the central venous pressure which is preferred in place of blood volume determinations, since the central venous pressure is easier to obtain and less subject to error. It also gives a dynamic picture of the right heart's ability to pump the blood presented to it. Strictly speaking, this does not represent the left ventricle's ability, but in most cases, the discrepancy is small. Although, patients in gram-negative septic shock may have a measured increased blood volume when Risa or tagged red cells are used, because the stagnation in the peripheral microcirculation immobilizes a good share of this volume, even though it is measured by the tag.

The use of volume is followed within minutes by the injection of methylprednisolone. The massive doses of methylprednisolone, 30 mg. per kilogram, have been shown in our laboratory to increase the survival of dogs given a predicably lethal dose of Difco endotoxin.[5] The results of this clinical study would also indicate these drugs have a salutary effect, although their specific mode of producting vasodilatation is not yet clear. They have been shown to stabilize cellular membranes and lysosomal membranes,[3] decrease sympathetic nerve activity,[1] and have a positive inotropic action on the heart.[8] These and other unknown effects may be significant. As we have gained experience with the steroids, we now administer the methylprednisolone almost simultaneously with the fluids. This has resulted in more prompt resuscitation and fewer late complications, especially pneumonias.

The choice of antibiotic coverage will vary from hospital to hospital and depend on the predominant organism and its sensitivities. In our environment, kanamycin is quite effective with 80 percent of the gram-negative organisms responsing at the dose range of 15 mg. per kilogram. A synthetic penicillin is also utilized intravenously at 2 to 4 Gm. every four to six hours. If renal shutdown is apparent after a few hours, the kanamycin must be reduced or stopped and the penicillin decreased. Recent reports by Martin and associates[6] indicate cephaloridine and gentamycin to be an effective combination in gram-negative infections.

When the results of the smears and cultures obtained prior to antibiotics coverage are known, the antibiotic program must be reassessed. Finally, we must emphasize the importance of finding the source of the sepsis and eliminating it by drainage, bypass, resection, etc., whenever possible. When we have failed to salvage patients from septic shock, it is usually due to failure to recognize and to eliminate the source of infection and/or a delay in the start of treatment.

SUMMARY

Fifteen patients with gram-negative septic shock have been presented. The hemodynamic data showed a normal or high cardiac index with a low total peripheral resistance. With a program of therapy based on volume supported by massive doses of steroids and appropriate antibiotics, a survival of 87 percent has been achieved.

REFERENCES

1. Dietzman, R.: Personal communication.
2. Hamilton, W. F., et al.: Comparison of the Fick and dye injection methods of measuring the cardiac output in man, Amer. J. Physiol. **153:** 309, 1948.
3. Janoff, A., Weissmann, G., Zweifach, B. W., and Thomas L.: Pathogenesis of experimental shock. IV. Studies on lysosomes in normal and tolerant animals subjected to lethal trauma and endotoxemia, J. Exp. Med. **16:** 451, 1962.
4. Kwaan, H. M., and Weil, M. H.: Difference in the mechanism of shock caused by bacterial infections, Surg. Gynec. Obstet. **169:** 371, 1969.
5. Lillehei, R. C., et al.: Treatment of septic shock, Mod. Treatm. **4:** 31, 1965.
6. Martin, C. H., et al.: Initial presumptive therapy for serious acute gram-negative rod infections, Abstracts of Eighth Interscience Conference on Antimicrobial Agents and Chemotherapy. Oct., 1968, p. 31.
7. Shubin, A. H., and Weil, M. H.: Bacterial shock—a serious complication in urologic practice, J. A. M. A. **185:** 850, 1963.
8. Tanz, R. D.: *In* Martin, L., and Pecile, A., editors: Inotropic actions of certain steroids upon cardiac tissue, hormonal steroids, biochemistry, pharmacology, and therapeutics, ed. 1, New York, 1964, Academic Press Inc.
9. Weil, M. H., Shubin, H., and Rosoff, L.: Fluid repletion in circulatory shock, J. A. M. A. **192:** 668, 1965.

Use of heparinized priming blood after whole-body perfusion

SAIT TARHAN, M.D.
EMERSON A. MOFFITT, M.D.
RICHARD O. LUNDBORG, M.D.
ROBERT B. WALLACE, M.D.
ROCHESTER, MINN.
From the Mayo Clinic and Mayo Foundation, Section of Anesthesiology and of Surgery

The needs for blood have been greatly increased with the development of more radical surgery. This demand frequently exceeds the available reserve of donors in most communities.[26] This is especially true in centers where cardiovascular surgery is done. Blood is frequently used for priming the pump-oxygenator, and additional blood also must be available to replace that lost during and after operation. Various methods have been described for saving and re-using blood, such as autotransfusion,[7, 26] utilization of the blood in the oxygenator for a second patient,[18] or use of a bubble oxygenator primed with a solution other than blood.

In most instances it is difficult to transfuse all the blood left in the oxygenator at the end of whole-body perfusion without overloading the patient. Feasibility of infusion of this blood to the same patient later during and after operation has been considered. Objections to this procedure have been (1) the possibility of contamination because of lack of a safe and practical method to recover the blood, (2) damage to erythrocytes in a prolonged perfusion, caused by mechanical trauma, (3) acidosis of this blood,[15] and (4) excessive bleeding in the patient because of heparin in the priming blood.

The purpose of this study was to evaluate a simple method of collecting heparinized blood from the pump-oxygenator at the end of whole-body perfusion and to determine the safety of transfusing this blood (instead of stored acid-citrate-dextrose blood) during the postoperative period after clotting has been re-established.

Supported in part by Research Grant GM-14919 from the National Institutes of Health, Public Health Service.
Received for publication May 1, 1969.

MATERIALS AND METHOD

One hundred patients were studied after whole-body perfusion was performed with the vertical-sheet oxygenator (Mayo-Gibbon). The mean perfusion time was 71 minutes (range 24 to 155 minutes). The prime contained acid-citrate-dextrose (ACD) blood up to 48 hours old. The diluents per 500 ml. of blood were 150 ml. of 5 percent dextrose in 0.45 percent NaCl, 65 ml. of 0.3M tris(hydroxymethyl)aminomethane (THAM), 4 mEq. of potassium chloride, 500 mg. of calcium chloride, and 3,000 units of heparin. The patients were heparinized with 9,000 units per square meter of body surface. Neutralization of heparin was with protamine sulfate, 1.3 times the total dose of heparin given to the patient, as previously described.[14]

At the conclusion of bypass, blood remaining in the extracorporeal circuit was collected via a stopcock in the line between the oxygenator and arterial pump (Fig. 1). Blood bags of 600 ml. capacity (Fenwal Laboratories, Division of Travenol Laboratories, Inc., Morton Grove, Ill.) were used.

 Vol. 67, No. 4, pp. 584-589

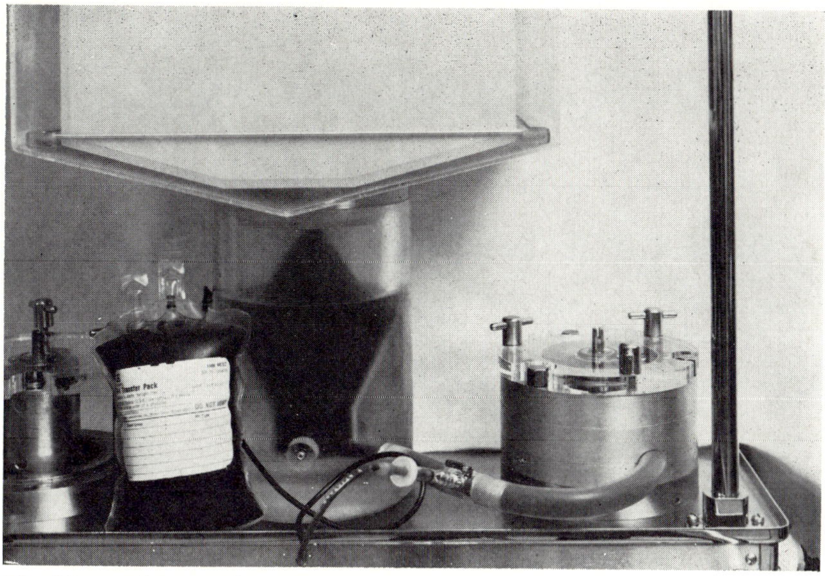

Fig. 1. Blood bag and connection to pump-oxygenator.

The inlet tubing was connected to a plastic extension of the stopcock for filling, and the blood was pumped into the bag.

A blood sample was drawn from the same site, for P_{O_2}, P_{CO_2}, and pH determination by electrodes (Instrumentation Laboratories, Inc., Boston) maintained at 37° C. Hematocrit value was determined by centrifugation for 20 minutes at 3,800 rpm. The value for standard bicarbonate was read from a Severinghaus slide rule.[22] Serum sodium and potassium values were obtained by flame photometry. The value for free plasma hemoglobin was determined by the method described by Lindberg and associates.[10]

The amount of postoperative blood loss, as measured by drainage from the chest tubes (per square meter of body surface), was recorded. This loss was compared with the blood loss of a group of 100 patients who had similar surgical procedures and who had received ACD blood during the same time interval after perfusion. Observations were made 8 and 24 hours after operation. Blood loss data of the two groups were compared by the Student's t test, with $p = 0.05$ accepted as the level of significance.

A heparin-protamine assay test as described by Woods[27] was done at the end of infusion of the heparinized blood in 41 patients to determine the presence of circulating free heparin.

Table I. *Comparison of priming blood with ACD blood*

Factor	*Priming blood (at end of perfusion)*	*ACD blood*[6] *(14 days old)*
pH	7.56	6.80
P_{CO_2} (mm. Hg)	24	150
P_{O_2} (mm. Hg)	328	40
Na^+ (mEq./L.)	127	150
K^+ (mEq./L.)	4.8	25
Ca^{++} (mEq./L.)	6[13]	<0.5
Standard HCO_3^- (mEq./L.)	24.5	7-10
Plasma hemoglobin (mg./100 ml.)	<40*	50
Hematocrit (%)	33.5	41.6[2]
Temperature (C.)	35	4

*Only 14 patients of the total had >40 mg. per 100 ml. of free hemoglobin.

RESULTS

Mean values of oxygen tension, the acid-base profile, and serum sodium and potassium levels are shown in Table I, compared with values for nonfresh ACD blood. Free plasma hemoglobin levels of more than

Table II. *Chest tube drainage (milliliter per square meter of body surface)*

Lesion	Infusion of heparinized priming blood: No. of patients	Postoperative blood loss: 8 hr.	Postoperative blood loss: 24 hr.	Infusion of ACD blood: No. of patients	Postoperative blood loss: 8 hr.	Postoperative blood loss: 24 hr.
Aortic valve replacement	23	361 ± 52*	492 ± 63	31	456 ± 67*	572 ± 73
Mitral valve replacement	30	334 ± 39	442 ± 53	14	350 ± 81	544 ± 109
Multiple valve replacement	17	501 ± 73	638 ± 81	14	390 ± 51	540 ± 75
Previous cardiac surgery	7	449 ± 102	590 ± 113	10	309 ± 42	423 ± 59
Atrial septal defect	3	315 ± 128	406 ± 129	4	227 ± 56	299 ± 45
Ventricular septal defect	5	946 ± 250	1,061 ± 259	8	389 ± 118	500 ± 137
Tetralogy of Fallot	3	528 ± 165	590 ± 188	3	779 ± 310	942 ± 387
Other cyanotic conditions	3	775 ± 229	862 ± 283	5	886 ± 205	1,247 ± 383
Miscellaneous congenital noncyanotic conditions	2	1,645 ± 10	1,954 ± 46	4	301 ± 51	391 ± 56
Reoperation for bleeding	7	—	—	7	—	—
Total	100			100		

*Mean ± S.E. There was no statistically significant difference between the means of the comparable subgroups.

Table III. *Details of Re-exploration of 14 patients*

Source of bleeding	Patients received heparinized blood	Patients received ACD blood
Aortotomy	3	2
Ventriculotomy (LV apex and LV wall)	1	1
Pericardium	1	0
Pericardial patch on pulmonary stenosis	0	1
Sternum	1	0
No surgical reason found	1	3
Total	7	7

40 mg. per 100 ml. of blood were found in 14 patients; 13 patients had between 100 and 150 mg., and one had 230 mg. Urine output of the 14 patients ranged from 1,500 to 2,400 ml. during the first 24 hours after operation.

Mean values for postoperative bleeding with standard errors are shown in Table II for the two groups who received heparinized or ACD blood. Re-exploration had to be done in seven patients in each group because of excessive bleeding. Causes of bleeding are shown in Table III; blood loss of these 14 patients was not included in Table II. Among the 41 patients who had a heparin-protamine assay, eight patients had free heparin in their blood; the appropriate amount of a second dose of protamine was given to neutralize this excess heparin, as described by Woods.[27] The chest drainage of these eight patients had not been excessive, prior to the injection of this second dose of protamine. All the patients whose chest drainage was more than average had a negative result of the heparin-protamine assay test.

No infection or septicemia was noted among the patients in this study. A total of 192 units of heparinized priming blood (range 200 to 1,800 ml. per patient) was recovered and reinfused. This represents the average saving of 1.9 units of ACD blood per patient.

DISCUSSION

The usual practice after whole-body perfusion is to replace blood loss with ACD blood (which may be as old as 3 weeks). The unphysiologic state of this ACD blood is well known[1, 20] (Table I). The adverse effects of low pH, hypocalcemia, hyperkalemia,[11] and excess citrate on cardiac function have been studied by Baue and associates[1] and others.[5] Various attempts have been made to correct these abnormalities, such as the addition of THAM for low pH,[1, 16] the addition of calcium,[1] and the use of ion exchange resins[12, 20] to remove the citrate and excess potassium.

Patients with cardiac disease who have had intensive treatment with digitalis and diuretics often have reduced total-body potassium even with the presence of normal levels of serum potassium.[14] It is unlikely that those patients with good renal function would have adverse effects from hyperkalemia of banked ACD blood. However, recalcification of ACD blood used in the oxygenator causes an elevated level of serum calcium, which is still present after operation.[14] This may be a level with significant inotropic effects unless the level of the ionized portion is not elevated. The decrease of total calcium concentration correlates with a decrease in cardiac output, which is sometimes seen on the evening of operation.[14] In these instances, the infusion of hypercalcemic blood should have a beneficial effect.

Diluted and appropriately treated ACD blood has been shown to be satisfactory for cardiopulmonary bypass in patients of all ages and regardless of the type of lesion.[21] In our study, blood gases, acid-base balance, and electrolytes remained at more normal physiologic levels in blood from the pump-oxygenator than in ACD blood, even after perfusions up to 155 minutes (Table I). The mean P_{CO_2} of 25 mm. Hg. (range 14.6 to 42.5) was responsible for the increased mean pH of 7.56 (range 7.39 to 7.70), and the basic factor responsible for the normal bicarbonate concentration (24.5 mEq. per liter) undoubtedly was the incorporation of THAM into the mixture.

Valtis and Kennedy[25] have pointed out that the oxygen dissociation curve of stored ACD blood shifts to the left, indicating that such blood after transfusion is at least temporarily incapable of releasing as large a volume of oxygen to the tissues as is normal blood. They found that this shift was still evident in some recipients' blood even after 24 hours and that changes were maximal in blood stored for a week. This work has been confirmed by others.[24] The abnormality in oxygen release, even if it lasts only a few hours, may be more important in the critically ill patient after cardiac surgery. It is reasonable to assume that priming blood, being relatively fresh (up to 48 hours old) and containing some of the patient's own blood, would have less an adverse effect than older ACD blood.

Since ACD blood is stored at 4° C., its rapid transfusion causes hypothermia in the recipient, unless it is warmed completely. It has been reported that transfusing 500 ml. of blood may lower the esophageal temperature as much as 1.5° C.[6] The relative viscosity of banked ACD blood is increased 15 percent after 15 to 21 days of storage,[24] which makes it more difficult to give rapidly. Cold blood can cause vasoconstriction and increased viscosity, which have deleterious effects on the microcirculation. This is important, especially in the presence of a low cardiac output, with vasoconstriction already present as a compensatory response.[14]

Hematocrit values averaged 33.5 percent in our study as compared with the 41.6 percent of the ACD blood.[2] Case and coauthors[3] reported that depression of the ventricular function curve did not occur until the hematocrit level was reduced to between 24 and 31 percent. The hematocrit level of diluted blood from the oxygenator does not seem to be low enough to jeopardize ventricular function.

The amount of free hemoglobin in the plasma is an indication of red cell destruction, although the patient's reticuloendothelial system removes some free hemoglobin. Free plasma hemoglobin of more than 40 mg. per 100 ml. in 14 patients was related to the duration of perfusion and the use of the intracardiac suction. This compares favorably with the levels of free plasma hemoglobin of 15-day-old ACD blood (Table I). This level of free hemoglobin is not expected to have any clinical significance.[23]

In open-heart surgery, numerous factors contribute to postoperative bleeding.[28] Circulating free heparin has been suggested as one of them,[19] yet reports of the need for complete heparin neutralization have been controversial.[4, 8] We attempted to determine the effects of infusion of heparinized blood on postoperative blood loss by comparing the chest tube drainage in the two groups of patients, as shown in Table II. There was no significant difference between the means of the matched subgroups. One should note that only a few patients had congenital lesions. Most of the latter patients were children who had less than 1 square meter of body surface. Between some of these subgroups, there were great differences in the mean blood loss, but there was no definite trend.

Re-exploration was necessary in seven patients in each group (Table III), and in most of these patients, a major bleeding point was identified. Inadequate surgical hemostasis has been the most important single factor for postoperative blood loss.[9, 14] Free heparin was not detected in the seven patients who received infusion of heparinized blood from the oxygenator by the heparin-protamine assay test.

Our practice is to over-neutralize rather than to under-neutralize the heparin. This is accomplished by giving a dose of protamine 1.3 times the total heparin dose by weight.[27] This amount of protamine and the short half-life[17] of heparin probably are sufficient for neutralizing the heparin in the blood infused after protamine is given, resulting in the small number of positive results to the heparin-protamine assay test, when this test is done at the end of infusion of heparinized blood.

SUMMARY AND CONCLUSIONS

Heparinized priming blood can be collected and infused to the patient safely for several hours after the whole-body perfusion, especially to a patient who has more than 1 square meter of body surface. This did not increase postoperative bleeding, as compared with the bleeding that occurred when nonfresh ACD blood was used. The saving of blood is substantial, which is particularly valuable for the patient with a rare blood group. Heparinized priming blood may have several therapeutic advantages over nonfresh ACD blood.

REFERENCES

1. Baue, A. E., Hermann, G., and Shaw, R. S.: A study of bank blood toxicity, Surg. Gynec. Obstet. **113:** 40, 1961.
2. Boyan, C. P.: Measurement and replacement of blood loss during surgery, American Society of Anesthesiologists Refresher Course Lectures, Las Vegas, Nev., Sept. 29, 1967.
3. Case, R. B., Berglund, E., and Sarnoff, S. J.: Ventricular function. VII. Changes in coronary resistance and ventricular function resulting from acutely induced anemia and the effect thereon of coronary stenosis, Amer. J. Med. **18:** 397, 1955.
4. Castaneda, A. R., and Varco, R. L.: Must heparin be neutralized following open-heart operations? J. Thorac. Cardiov. Surg. **52:** 716, 1966.
5. Corbascio, A. N., and Smith, N. T.: Hemodynamic effects of experimental hypercitremia, Anesthesiology **28:** 510, 1967.
6. Crocker, M. C.: Blood transfusion: A review, Anaesthesia **23:** 372, 1968.
7. Cuello, L., Vazquez, E., Rios, R., and Raffucci, F. L.: Autologous blood transfusion in thoracic and cardiovascular surgery, SURGERY **62:** 814, 1967.
8. Gans, H., Castaneda, A. R., Subramanian, V., John S., and Lillehei, C. W.: Problems in hemostasis during open heart surgery. IX. Changes observed in the plasminogen-plasmin system and their significance for therapy, Ann. Surg. **166:** 980, 1967.
9. Gilbert, J. W., Bronson, W. R., and Brecher, G.: Incidence of bleeding in cardiac surgery with extracorporeal circulation, Ann. N. Y. Acad. Sci. **115:** 302, 1964.
10. Lindberg, E. F., Berghuis, J., Theye, R. A., and Kirklin, J. W.: Plasma hemoglobin levels associated with use of a vertical-sheet pump-oxygenator (Mayo-Gibbon type), SURGERY **55:** 665, 1964.
11. Marshall, M.: Potassium intoxication from blood and plasma transfusions, Anaesthesia **17:** 145, 1962.
12. McLaughlin, E. D., Nealon, T. F., Jr., and Gibbon, J. H., Jr.: Treatment of bank blood by resins, J. Thorac. Cardiov. Surg. **40:** 602, 1960.
13. Moffitt, E. A., Rosevear, J. W., and McGoon, D. C.: Myocardial metabolism in open-heart surgery: Arterial levels of metabolites, electrolytes, oxygenation, and acid-base balance, Anesth. & Analg. **48:** 633, 1969.

14. Moffitt, E. A., Tarhan, S., and Lundborg, R. O.: Anesthesia for cardiac surgery: Principles and practice, Anesthesiology **29:** 1181, 1968.

15. Nahas, G. G., Malm, J. R., Manger, W. M., Verosky, M., and Sullivan, S. F.: Control of acidosis and the use of titrated ACD blood in open-heart surgery, Ann. Surg. **160:** 1019, 1964.

16. Nahas, G. G., Manger, W. M., and Ultmann, J. E.: Transfusion acidosis, Bibl. Haemat. **19:** 610, 1964.

17. Olsson, P., Lagergren, H., and Ek, S.: The elimination from plasma of intravenous heparin: An experimental study on dogs and humans, Acta Med. Scand. **173:** 619, 1963.

18. Replogle, R. L., Kevy, S. V., and Gross, R. E.: Some hematologic aspects of prolonged blood pumping: Observations from a series of paired perfusions, J. Thorac. Cardiov. Surg. **54:** 688, 1967.

19. Rothnie, N. G., and Kinmonth, J. B.: Bleeding after perfusion for open heart surgery: Importance of unneutralized heparin and its proper correction, Brit. Med. J. **1:** 73, 1960.

20. Sandler, J. L., Nealon, T. F., Jr., and Gibbon, J. H., Jr.: Restoration of stored bank blood to biochemical normalcy, J. A. M. A. **179:** 201, 1962.

21. Sessler, A. D., Taswell, H. F., Moffitt, E. A., and Kirklin, J. W.: Heparinized versus acid-citrate–dextrose blood for cardiopulmonary bypass, Mayo Clin. Proc. **40:** 859, 1965.

22. Severinghaus, J. W.: Blood gas calculator, J. Appl. Physiol. **21:** 1108, 1966.

23. Strumia, M. M., Crosby, W. H., Greenwalt, T. J., Gibson, J. G., 2nd, and Krevans, J. R.: General principles of blood transfusion. Section I. General considerations, Transfusion **3:** 307, 1963.

24. Strumia, M. M., and Strumia, P. V.: Alterations in banked blood, with special reference to hemostasis, Ann. N. Y. Acad. Sci. **115:** 443, 1964.

25. Valtis, D. J., and Kennedy, A. C.: Defective gas-transport function of stored red blood-cells, Lancet **1:** 119, 1954.

26. Wilson, J. D., and Taswell, H. F.: Autotransfusion: Historical review and preliminary report on a new method, Mayo Clin. Proc. **43:** 26, 1968.

27. Woods, J. E.: Studies on coagulation changes during and after extracorporeal circulation: With special reference to the effects of heparin and protamine, Thesis, Mayo Graduate School of Medicine (University of Minnesota), Rochester, 1965.

28. Woods, J. E., Taswell, H. F., Kirklin, J. W., and Owen, C. A., Jr.: The transfusion of platelet concentrates in patients undergoing heart surgery, Mayo Clin. Proc. **42:** 318, 1967.

Intensive care unit flow sheet

SCOTT G. KRAMER, CAPTAIN, MC, USN
CHARLES S. LIPSON, COMMANDER, MC, USNR
CHELSEA, MASS.
From the Department of Surgical Service and the Intensive Care Unit, Naval Hospital

Fig. 1. Twenty-four hour flow sheet.

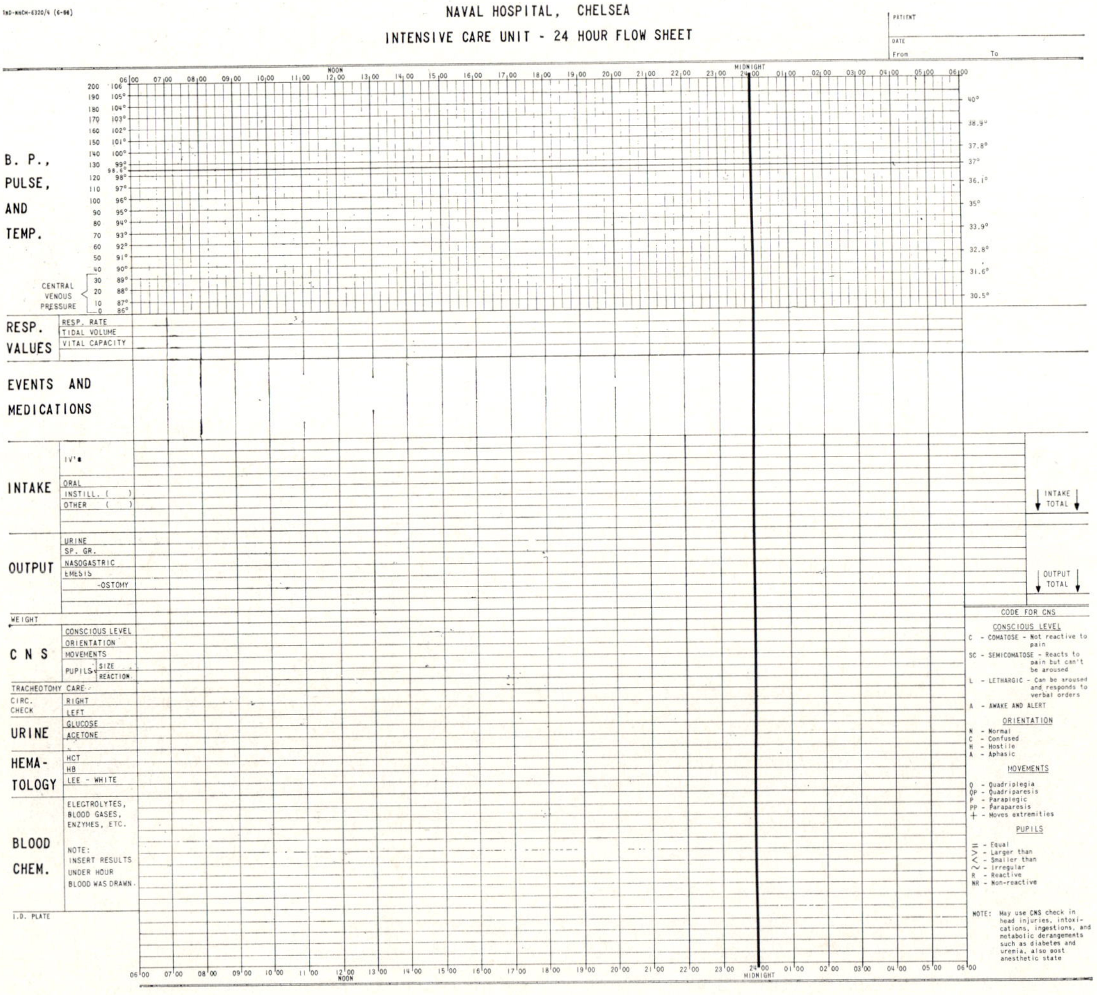

The opinions or assertions contained herein are those of the authors and are not to be construed as official or reflecting the views of the Navy Department or the Naval Service at large.

Received for publication May 20, 1969.

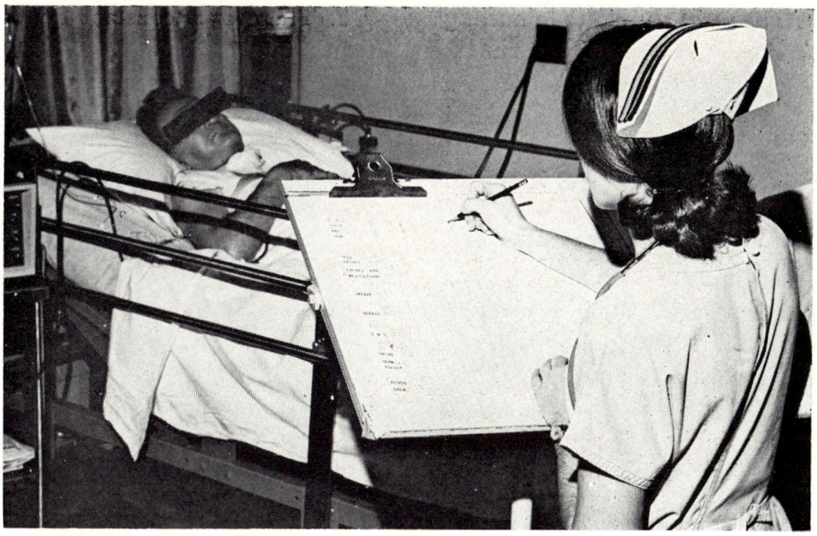

Fig. 2. Nurse records data at bedside as soon as they are taken.

There is a need for more concentrated record keeping in intensive care units. The intensive care unit has become a more complex area of patient care, and the variety of patients has greatly increased. Each case has its own peculiar needs in data recording so that, for instance, the diabetic patient needs one type of record, the head injury patient another, the respiratory distress patient another, and the postoperative patient still another, to mention a few. This has resulted in a proliferation of special record sheets for all types of cases.

In addition, current nursing notes, laboratory results, current medications, weight charts, intake and output sheets are also required—but too frequently not together in the same place. Consequently, collecting current data may involve several searches at rounds each morning. It is a task to leaf through many sheets in many places to find the information required. Also most data sheets will not accept a full day's data so that several sheets are necessary for each day's recording. Time intervals on sheets may vary in the same record.

We have developed a 24 hour flow sheet which overcomes many of the above difficulties (Fig. 1). It provides for all types of cases and allows complete data recording. It is kept at the patient's bedside, each new day's sheet being placed over the previous

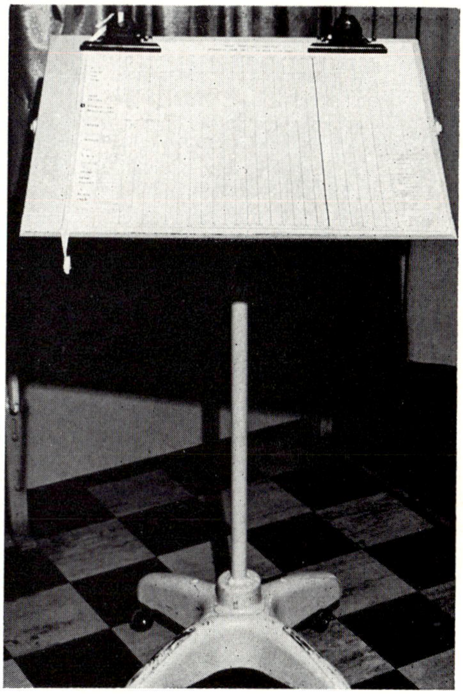

Fig. 3. Mobile lectern holds flow sheets which measure 22 by 24 inches.

day's (Fig. 2). The sheet correlates to nursing activities beginning at 6:00 A.M. and runs a full 24 hour period. Data are commenced at the hour at which the patient is admitted to the Intensive Care Unit. The sheet is kept on a mobile lectern that was fabricated in the hospital shop (Fig. 3).

We have found the chart to be quite useful. Its obvious advantages are:

1. It provides ready accessibility to complete current data, e.g., laboratory results are recorded under the time column that shows when the specimen was taken, and currently running fluids are indicated, as well as all vital signs and special checks.

2. There is a constant check on the patient's nursing care. Medications, tracheostomy care, and pulse checks among other items can readily be confirmed.

3. Nurses find this method of recording helpful in understanding the patient's changing condition and needs.

4. A change in the patient's condition is promptly noticed by attending personnel.

5. This record sheet provides for data keeping on all types of cases.

It is suggested that the 24 hour flow sheet is an improved method for keeping a record of the seriously ill patient.

Improved surgical technique for arteriovenous shunt implantation: Experiences with an all-Silastic shunt

LUIS A. ARAVENA
LEO KAPLAN, M.D.
ARTHUR GOLDING, M.D.
ARTHUR GORDON, M.D.
MORTON H. MAXWELL, M.D.
LOS ANGELES, CALIF.

From the Departments of Medicine, Pathology, and Surgery, Cedars-Sinai Medical Center, Mt. Sinai Hospital Division and from the Departments of Medicine and Surgery, UCLA Medical Center

Chronic hemodialysis became a reality only after the development of suitable techniques for the long-term maintenance of peripheral arteriovenous (A-V) shunts. In 1960 Quinton, Dillard, and Scribner[13] described a Teflon arteriovenous shunt. Later modifications resulted in the present Teflon-Silastic shunt currently used by most dialysis centers.[12]

Shunt survival for more than 1 year is rare and most centers continue to report an average shunt function of approximately 7-9 months.[2, 3, 6, 10, 11] The major causes of shunt failure are presumed to be stenosis of the proximal vessels, infection (resulting in thrombosis), bleeding, and false aneurysm formation. The present studies were undertaken in an attempt to devise techniques for insertion of an all-Silastic shunt which would overcome these problems.

MATERIAL AND EXPERIMENTAL SUBJECTS

Cannulas. Straight silicone tubes (Silastic),* measuring 0.3 cm. internal and 0.1 cm. external diameter, without tapered tips were used. A knitted Dacron skirt or Dacron velour was bonded to the Silastic cannula.

Design I. A Dacron skirt measuring 3.5 by 2.0 cm. was bonded to the Silastic cannula 1.5 cm. from the tip with Silastic medical adhesive silicone Type A (Fig. 1, *Design I*).

Design II. A 1.0 cm. length of tubular knitted Dacron with a 0.5 cm. internal diameter was similarly bonded to a Silastic cannula 1.5 cm. from the distal tip (Fig. 1, *Design II*).

Design III (control). A modified Quinton-Scribner cannula was fashioned, consisting of a straight Silastic tube with a tapered Teflon tip, measuring 1.5 cm. in length with 0.3 cm. internal and 0.05 cm. external diameter, inserted within it.

Experimental animals. Normal and bilaterally nephrectomized male and female mongrel dogs weighing 15 to 25 kilograms that were undergoing experimental hemodialysis were used.

METHODS

Anesthesia and presurgical preparation. Animals were anesthetized with intravenous sodium pentobarbital (25 to 30 mg. per kilogram).

Surgical technique. Under sterile conditions either the right or left common carotid artery and adjacent external jugular vein were approached in the ventral neck

Supported by General Research Support Grant No. 5-SO1FR 05468-07, National Institutes of Health Contract No. 69-82, and the University Medical Research Center.

Submitted for publication May 26, 1969; resubmitted July 28, 1969.

Reprint requests: Cedars-Sinai Medical Center, Mt. Sinai Hospital Division, 8720 Beverly Blvd., Los Angeles, Calif. 90048.

*Ultraflow Silastic rubber tubes manufactured by Travenol Laboratories, Morton Grove, Ill.

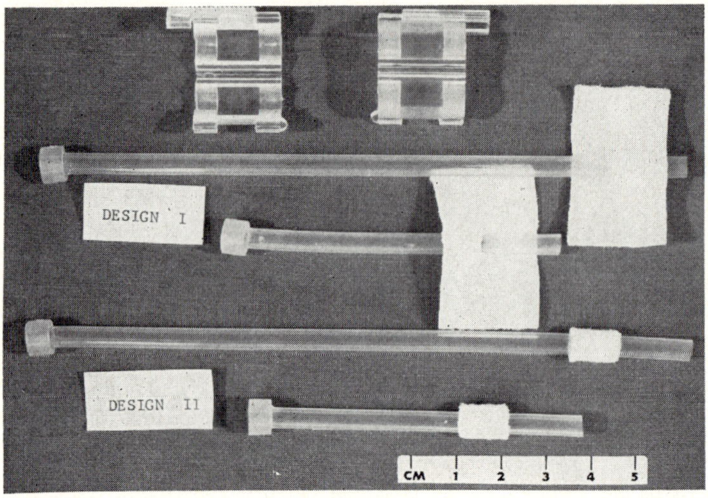

Fig. 1. Shows the two designs of Silastic cannulas with attached skirt and tubular Dacron with connector-split coupling device used for joining the arteriovenous cannulas.

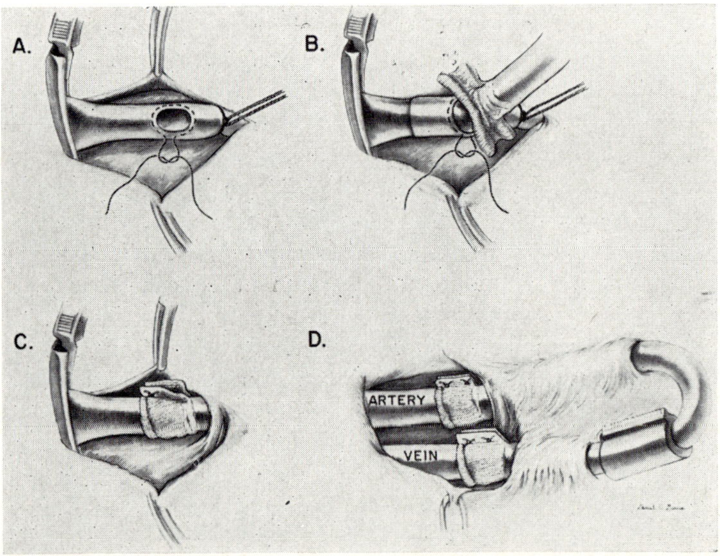

Fig. 2. *A* to *D,* Shows the surgical technique for implantation of Design I–type shunt.

through a 6 to 8 cm. longitudinal incision. The artery and vein were ligated distal to the cannula site and gently occluded proximally.

For implantation of Design I shunts a 6-0 silk purse-string suture was placed in the adventitia of the vessel. The latter was opened (Fig. 2, *A*) and without dilating the vessel the Silastic catheter was then gently introduced into the vessel lumen (Fig. 2, *B*) until the Dacron patch was adjacent to the vessel opening. The purse-string suture was then tied. Both halves of the Dacron patch were brought around the vessel and joined at the external wall of the vessel (Fig. 2, *C*) with two interrupted single sutures and one central double suture. The remaining Dacron skirt was trimmed external to the sutures (Fig. 2, *D*).

For implantation of Design II shunts, the vessels were partially transected and four 6-0

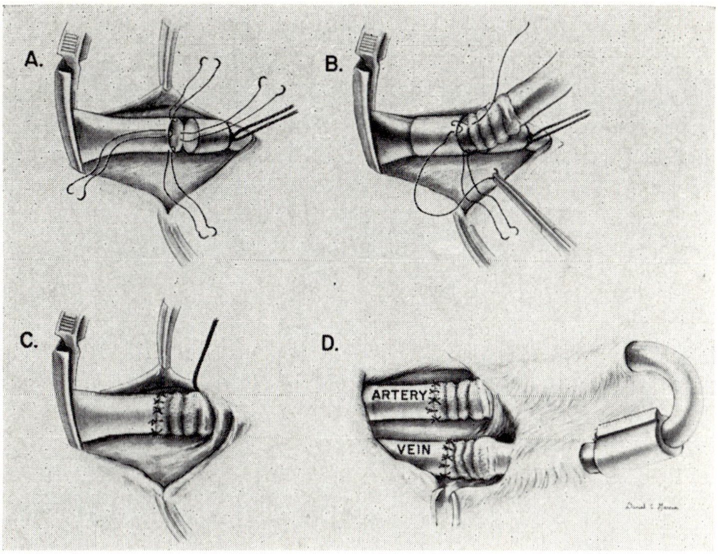

Fig. 3. *A* to *D*, Shows the surgical technique for implantation of Design II–type shunt.

silk horizontal mattress sutures were placed, prior to insertion of the cannula (Fig. 3, *A*). The catheter was gently inserted into the vessel lumen and the Dacron graft was then sutured to the vessel wall (Fig. 3, *C*).

For implantation of Design III shunts (Quinton-Scribner type) the standard surgical technique, as described by McDonald and Waterhouse,[9] was used.

Following implantation, these cannulas were flushed with 100 ml. of normal saline containing 2.5 mg. of heparin. No other anticoagulants were used for any study animal. The arterial and venous catheters were brought to the skin surface through individual subcutaneous tunnels and connected with a Travenol connector-split coupling. The vessel clamps were then removed and the surgical wound was closed, rinsed, and dried; neomycin sulfate ointment was applied and the wound was covered by dressings, which were supported with either a 4 or 6 inch elastic bandage placed around the neck.

Postshunt implantation follow-up. The animals were placed on intramuscular procaine penicillin (6,000,000 units) daily for 1 week and were observed closely for shunt function and local infection.

Blood flow. Blood flow through the shunt was measured at the completion of the operative procedure with a clinical flowmeter.*

Angiography. Arterial and venous angiograms were performed at various intervals in most of the animals. Under general anesthesia the arterial and venous cannulas were injected with 3 to 5 ml. of a 25 percent sodium Hypaque solution.

Pathology. At the termination of the study, the cannulated arteries and veins were carefully dissected and fixed in 10 percent neutral formalin.

Vessel samplings were prepared in paraffin blocks with cannulas in place. Sections were stained with hematoxylin and eosin, Gomori's trichrome, and Verhoeff's elastic tissue.

RESULTS

A-V shunt survival in normal animals. Table I summarizes our results with cannula Design I. Of ten normal dogs that underwent implantation of Design I, only one dog (I-2) had to be killed for purposes other than this study on the nineteenth day after

*Clinical flowmeter 1504, marketed by Allan L. Wolf Company, San Marino, Calif.

Table I. *A-V shunt survival in normal dogs (Design I)*

Dog No.	*Initial A-V shunt blood flow (ml./min.)*	*Functional A-V shunt (days)*	*Infection*	*Cause of A-V shunt termination*	*Remarks*
I-1	—	17	0*	Removed by animal	Removed entire shunt leaving Dacron patch over vessel—bleeding minimal
I-2	320	19	–	Terminated	Killed after acute experiment
I-3	328	55	–	Discontinued	Heparin given
I-4	285	44	–	Removed by animal	Removed arterial limb—bleeding minimal
I-5	310	29	–	Removed by animal	Removed arterial limb—bleeding minimal
I-6	345	53	–	Removed by animal	Removed arterial limb—bleeding minimal
I-7	320	118	–	Died	Pneumonia (autopsy finding)
I-8	410	16	+	Removed by animal	Removed arterial limb—bleeding minimal
I-9	340	15	+	Removed by animal	Removed entire shunt leaving Dacron patch over vessel—bleeding minimal
I-10	380	31	–	Removed by animal	Removed arterial limb—bleeding minimal

*None recorded.

Table II. *A-V shunt in normal dogs (Design II)*

Dog No.	*Initial A-V shunt blood flow (ml./min.)*	*Functional A-V shunt (days)*	*Infection*	*Cause of A-V shunt termination*	*Remarks*
II-1	—	17	0*	Terminated	Killed after acute experiment
II-2	350	16	0*	Removed by animal	Broke A-V shunt connector-split coupling device, bled to death
II-3	—	20	0*	Connector-splint coupling device failure	Uneven junction of A-V cannula clotted
II-4	310	47	–	Died	Died during an experiment
II-5	—	38	0*	Removed by animal	Broke Silastic A-V body, bled to death
II-6	310	33	–	Discontinued	Heparin given

*None recorded.

implant, with a functioning shunt. Dog I-3 was withdrawn from the study after a dose of heparin was administered for purposes of another experiment. Dog I-7 died of bilateral pneumonia, 118 days after implantation—but the shunt was functioning. For each of the remaining seven dogs shunt termination was due to extraction of the shunt by the animals. The average shunt survival for this group was 40 days with a range of 15 to 118 days. The average blood flow through the shunt was 337 ml. per minute with a range of 285 to 410 ml. per minute at the time of implantation. There were only two significant postoperative infections (Dogs I-8 and I-9). These responded promptly to local and systemic antibiotic therapy.

Table II summarizes the results obtained in six dogs in which Design II shunts were implanted. Dog II-1 was killed following an acute experiment. In Dog II-6, the experiment was terminated after the administration of heparin for purposes of another study. One dog (II-4) died in shock during an acute experiment. Dog II-3 broke the coupling device and bled to death. One dog (II-5) bit through the Silastic tubing and bled to death. Only one cannula clotted in this group (Dog II-3), and this was due to the improper junction of the A-V Silastic

Table III. *A-V shunt survival in bilaterally nephrectomized dogs undergoing hemodialysis*

Dog No.	*Design*	*Initial A-V shunt blood flow (ml./min.)*	*Functional A-V shunt (days)*	*Infection*	*Cause of A-V shunt termination*	*Remarks*
U.D.-1	I	—	7	−	Died	Uremia
U.D.-2	I	285	4	−	Died	Uremia
U.D.-3	I	—	5	+	Clotted	Venous limb, clotted during clamping
U.D.-4	I	310	9	++	Died	Uremia
U.D.-5	I	340	10	+	Died	Uremia
U.D.-6	I	360	22	+	Died	Uremia

Table IV. *A-V shunt with Teflon tip (Quinton-Scribner type) in normal dogs*

Dog No.	*Functional A-V shunt (days)*	*Infection*	*Cause of A-V shunt termination*	*Remarks*
1	3	−	Clotted	Venous side clotted (Dogs 1–5)
2	6	−	Clotted	
3	1	−	Clotted	
4	5	−	Clotted	
5	3	−	Clotted	
6	7	−	Removed by animal	Removed arterial limb—large hematoma prevented excessive bleeding
7	1	−	Clotted	Venous side clotted (Dogs 7–9)
8	6	−	Clotted	
9	9	−	Clotted	

cannulas within the connector-split coupling device.

Table III summarizes the shunt results in nephrectomized animals undergoing experimental hemodialysis. Shunt life was limited in these animals because all but one died of uremia within a short period of time. Shunt survival in this group, therefore, varied from 4 to 22 days. In no instance was survival altered by any problems with the shunt. All five shunts were patent and functioning at the time of death. There was one clotting episode in this group (U.D.-3). This occurred on the second day after implantation of the shunt, following prolonged clamping of the Silastic cannula, during a difficult hemodialysis. Declotting was readily accomplished and the shunt functioned well thereafter. This dog died of uremia on the fifth day. Four skin infections occurred in this group. In one of these animals the infection extended through the subcutaneous tissue down to the Dacron vessel juncture, but not into the vascular channels. All responded to antibiotic therapy.

Table IV summarizes the results obtained in nine normal dogs which underwent implantation of the Quinton-Scribner–type shunt as controls. Shunt termination in eight dogs was due to clotting originating in the venous limb, with propagation into the arterial cannula. One dog (No. 6) removed the arterial limb of the cannula. The average shunt life in this group of animals was 4 days with a range of 1 to 9 days.

Angiography. Angiographic studies of the arterial and venous limbs done at 1, 7, 14, 21, 30, 45, and 96 days after shunt implantation revealed no alterations of the blood vessel lumen proximal to the Silastic cannula

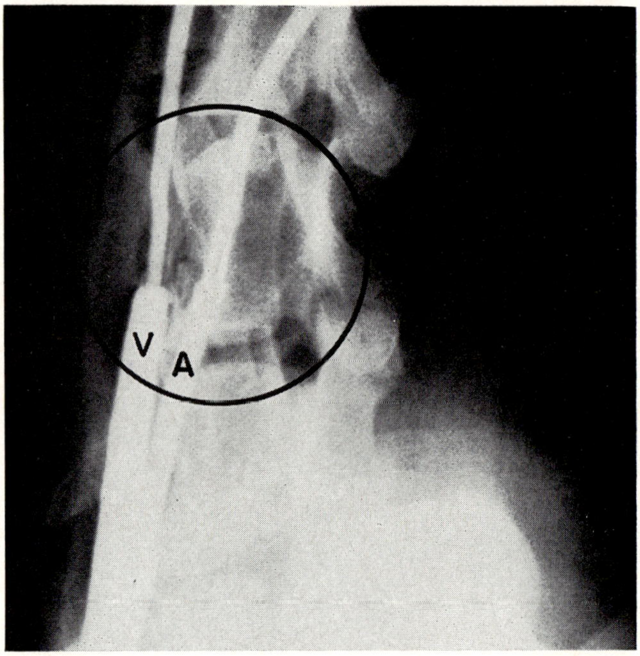

Fig. 4. Shows a patent arterial *(A)* and venous *(V)* angiogram taken at 96 days after shunt insertion (Dog I-7).

tip. Fig. 4 is a representative set of angiograms taken at 96 days in a dog with Design I–type A-V shunt cannulas.

Blood flows. Blood flow measured through the connected shunt immediately after implantation was 300 ml. per minute or greater in the majority of the animals. The blood flow rate was adequate for repeated dialysis for the duration of shunt survival in all animals.

Pathology. Microscopic alterations of cannulated segments of vessels up to the one hundred eighteenth day after implantation are progressive. Cannulated arteries showed enlarging internal and external diameters and increasing wall thickness. The inner linings generally showed surface necrosis and organizing fibrin with underlying lymphocytes in a dense matrix of collagen alternating with foci of fibrotic intima surfaced by endothelial cells. The internal elastic fibers were thinned and fragmented. The media was generally thickened by hypertrophied muscle. Fibrosis occurred at breaks in the internal elastic membrane. Fibrosis of the outer media blended with dense thick adventitia. Mold ridges on the external surface of the Silastic tubings produced vascular outpouchings with mural overlying necrosis.

Up to 118 days cannulated vein segments also showed progressively enlarging internal and external diameters and wall thickness. Areas of eroded intimal surface showed thin strips of fibrin, and endothelialized areas covered thick, transmural, laminated, and nodular connective tissue. The external mold ridges on the Silastic tubings again produced outpouchings of the wall where compression necrosis overlies dense mural fibrosis. The adventitial fibrohyaline scarring was uniform and quite thick.

DISCUSSION

To the best of our knowledge, the results obtained with these two designs represent the first published data on prolonged function of all-Silastic A-V shunts in dogs utilizing techniques and materials which could have applicability in man. Frasher[4] reported a technique for placing A-V shunts in dogs which required the use of stainless steel vessel inserts and complicated restraining harnesses to prevent excessive movement of the animals. With those techniques he achieved prolonged shunt survival of more than 60 days. In our experience successful maintenance of Teflon-Silastic shunts in dogs for more than 1 week was rarely achieved.

McDonald[7] indicated his inability to maintain patency of shunts in dogs for longer than 1 week when using the standard Teflon-tip Silastic cannula.

The causes of shunt malfunction are undoubtedly multiple. Increasing stenosis of the proximal cannulated vessel with subsequent decreasing flow and resultant thrombosis is the most common situation encountered. The stenosis can be due to: (1) continued trauma to the vessel wall by a rigid Teflon cannula tip; (2) necrosis of the vessel wall due to the circumferential ligatures used to secure the cannula; (3) the jet of arterial blood and turbulence of the endothelium of the cannulated vein; (4) chronic infection.

Our present shunt designs were directed toward elimination of certain of these factors. The absence of a Teflon tip reduces mechanical trauma to the vessel, and the elimination of circumferential ligatures about the vessel containing the Teflon tip reduces strangulation and subsequent injury to the vessel wall. The use of Dacron allows for tissue ingrowth decreasing mobility of the cannula, in addition to serving as a bacterial seal. Dacron cloths have been reported to inhibit soft tissue infection from reaching or involving the cannulated blood vessels. In the event of accidental shunt removal, the Dacron appears to serve a hemostatic function, preventing excessive bleeding. The larger-bore nontapered Silastic cannula possibly decreases turbulence and the jet effect on the venous side.

Our pathologic studies indicate less damage than those reported by Glashan and Walker[5] for the standard shunt, but nonetheless, significant progressive changes, attributable to external mold ridges of the Silastic cannulas, sutures, and exposure of the vein to arterial pressure, etc., were observed. The functional survival of these two new shunt designs is encouraging, particularly, since intravascular prostheses are more susceptible to thrombosis in dogs than man and long shunt survival was achieved in normal nonuremic dogs, not receiving anticoagulants.

The persistence and progression of morphologic changes occurring in the cannulated arteries and veins, even in the presence of soft nonreactive material, such as Silastic, suggest that these improvements in cannulation technique and design can decrease lesions and prolong cannula survival but do not eliminate these changes. Therefore, further new cannula designs and techniques of insertion are required if we are to eventually hemodialyze uremic patients without shunt complications.

REFERENCES

1. DePalma, J. R., Golding, A., and Maxwell, M. H.: Evaluation of A-V cannula malfunction and clotting using shunt angiography, Trans. Amer. Soc. Artif. Intern. Organs **15:** 278, 1969.
2. Dillard, D. H., and Pendras, J. P.: Cannula problems, Proc. Working Conf. on Chronic Dialysis, Seattle, Dec. 3-5, 1964, p. 10.
3. Foran, R. F., Golding, A. L., Treiman, R. L., and DePalma, J. R.: Quinton-Scribner cannulas for hemodialysis. Review of four years' experience, Presented at the annual meeting of the Southern California Chapter, Amer. Coll. Surgeons, Santa Barbara, Jan. 19, 1969.
4. Frasher, W. G., Jr.: Blood sampling by a chronic artificial external arteriovenous shunt in dogs, J. Appl. Physiol. **22:** 348, 1967.
5. Glashan, R. W., and Walker, F.: A histological examination of veins used in artificial arteriovenous ("Quinton-Scribner") shunts, Brit. J. Surg. **55:** 189, 1968.
6. Gombos, E. A., Hendler, E. D., and Hendler, R. G.: Arteriovenous shunt. Survival and pressure-flow relationships in the extracorporeal circuit of patients undergoing chronic hemodialysis, Proc. Europ. Dial. Transpl. Ass. **4:** 43, 1967.
7. McDonald, H. P., Jr.: Personal communications.
8. McDonald, H. P., Jr., Gerber, N., Michra, D., Wolin, L., Peng, B., and Waterhouse, K.: Subcutaneous Dacron and Teflon cloth adjuncts for Silastic arteriovenous shunts and peritoneal dialysis catheters, Trans. Amer. Soc. Artif. Intern. Organs **14:** 176, 1968.
9. McDonald, H., Jr., and Waterhouse, K.: Surgical technique of insertion of arterio-

venous shunts for regular dialysis therapy, Proc. Europ. Dial. Transpl. Ass. **3:** 337, 1966.
10. Pendras, J. D., and Smith, M. P.: The Silastic-Teflon arteriovenous cannula, Trans. Amer. Soc. Artif. Intern. Organs **12:** 222, 1966.
11. Quinton, W. E., Dillard, D. H., Cole, J. J., and Scribner, B. H.: Possible improvements in the technique of long-term cannulation of blood vessels, Trans. Amer. Soc. Artif. Intern. Organs **7:** 60, 1961.
12. Quinton, W. E., Dillard, D. H., Cole, J. J., and Scribner, B. H.: Eight months' experience with Silastic-Teflon bypass cannulas, Trans. Amer. Soc. Artif. Intern. Organs **7:** 237, 1962.
13. Quinton, W. E., Dillard, D. H., and Scribner, B. H.: Cannulation of blood vessels for prolonged hemodialysis, Trans. Amer. Soc. Artif. Intern. Organs **6:** 104, 1960.
14. Tenckhoff, H., and Schechter, H.: A bacteriologically safe peritoneal access device, Trans. Amer. Soc. Artif. Intern. Organs **14:** 181, 1968.

Scapulectomy: Indications and technique

TAPAS K. DAS GUPTA, M.D., PH.D.
CHICAGO, ILL.
From the Department of Surgery, Division of Surgical Oncology, University of Illinois College of Medicine

Scapulectomy for removal of tumors in the scapular region was orginally described by Syme[4] in 1864. In his monograph he described three patients on whom he had performed this operation. Although he did not clearly define the indications for scapulectomy, he showed the procedure to be feasible and practical. de Nancrede,[1] in his presidential address to the American Surgical Association Meeting in 1909, categorically stated that scapulectomy was an inferior operation. It thus fell into disrepute in this country, and the results of this operation were reported only occasionally thereafter. Pack and Ariel,[2] in 1958, mentioned this procedure but did not elaborate either in favor of or against it. It is thus apparent that the indications for scapulectomy have never been clearly defined, and consequently the end results have been unsatisfactory. It should be emphasized that scapulectomy has a limited role in surgery for neoplastic disease, and strict criteria must be set up for its performance, or a perfectly suitable operative procedure will not be utilized. *It should not, however, be considered as an alternative to interscapulothoracic amputation or the Tikhor-Lindberg operation.*

A scapulectomy is indicated in the following types of tumor:

A. Soft tissue tumors
   1. Low-grade fibrosarcoma invading the scapular muscles
   2. Desmoid-type tumor infiltrating the scapular muscles
   3. Liposarcoma arising from the adipose tissue in the scapular region where an adequate soft tissue excision necessitates excision of part or whole of the scapula
   4. Deeply invasive carcinoma of the skin for which there again must be wide excision including the scapula

B. Bone tumors
   1. Primary malignant bone tumor arising in the scapula (This is rare; however, scapulectomy may be useful in unusual cases of low-grade chondrosarcoma or of giant cell tumor of the scapula.)
   2. Solitary metastatic lesion, a very rare tumor (Although scapulectomy for this lesion was reported by Ryerson,[3] this procedure is rarely, if ever, indicated for metastatic scapular lesions.)

Scapulectomies in carefully selected patients have been performed with long-term cure and excellent functional results. The majority of these patients were able to resume normal activity with reasonable use of the arm shortly after the operation. The technique is described as follows.

OPERATIVE PROCEDURE

The patient is placed in the prone position with the arm resting in 90 degree abduction on an arm board. The arm should be draped so that an assistant can move the arm as required during the operation (Fig. 1, *A*).

An elliptical skin incision is then made, encompassing the tumor and extending from the tip of the acromion superolaterally to the paravertebral region inferomedially (Fig. 1, *A* and *B*). The lower end of the incision can

Partially supported by grants from the Carol Thomas Brigham Memorial Endowment Fund.
Received for publication May 7, 1969.

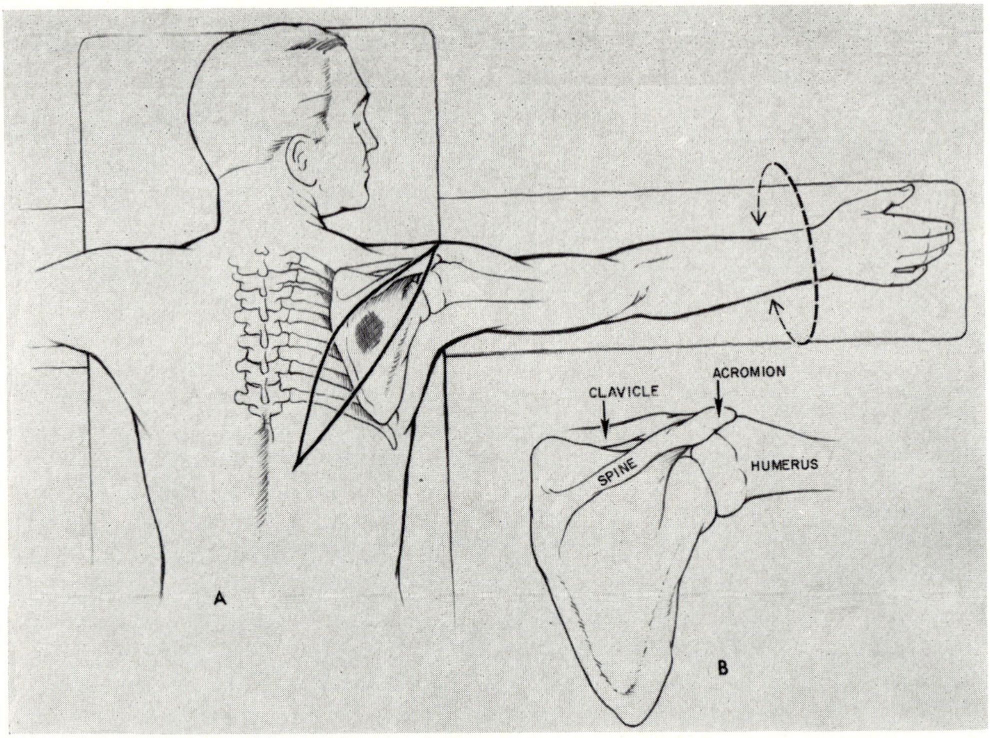

Fig. 1. *A,* The position of the patient and the incision for a tumor located in the center of the scapular region. The arm should be draped in such a way that an assistant can freely move the arm in order to facilitate the excision of muscular attachments. *B,* The scapula and its skeletal connections.

be extended to cross the midline if the tumor is so large as to make this necessary.

The medial and lateral skin flaps are raised as in a standard radical mastectomy. The superficial dorsal muscular attachment to the scapula is identified (Fig. 2). The attachment of the trapezius muscle to the scapular spine is completely resected and retracted superomedially, exposing the supraspinous muscle (Fig. 2). The attachment of the deltoid muscle to the lateral tip of the scapular spine is similarly resected and reflected laterally (Fig. 2). At this stage the rhomboid major muscle at the vertebral border, the latissimus dorsi inferiorly, the teres major and minor muscles laterally, and the infraspinous muscle can be easily identified.

The insertion of the latissimus dorsi muscle at the tip of the scapula is then excised and the muscle is retracted downward, exposing the tip (Fig. 3). The tip is then held by an assistant with a straight towel clip and pulled inferolaterally (Fig. 3). This provides traction to the muscles at the vertebral border, and excision of their scapular attachment is made simple.

The muscular attachments in the superior angle of the scapula are then resected along the vertebral border of the scapula. The levator scapulas, and the rhomboids, easily delineated, are then cut (Fig. 3). This maneuver can be quite simple if the assistant maintains constant traction at the tip of the scapula (Fig. 3). The inferior tip of the scapula is then rotated and a medial pull is applied while the arm is abducted (Fig. 4, *A*). This permits easy access and identification of the axillary contents. The contents are then retracted out of the operating field and the lateral muscles, teres major and minor, and the long head of the triceps, are cut (Fig. 4, *B*). Next, the supraspinous and

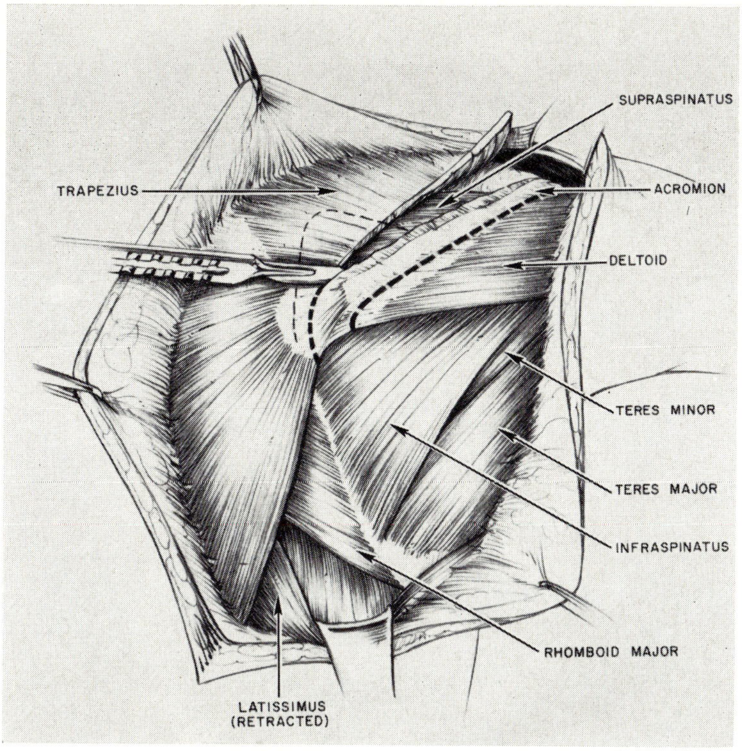

Fig. 2. The scapular muscles are exposed after raising the skin flaps. The trapezius muscle is then resected at the scapular spine. The dotted line shows the site of excision of the deltoid attachment. Reflection of trapezius exposes the supraspinous muscle.

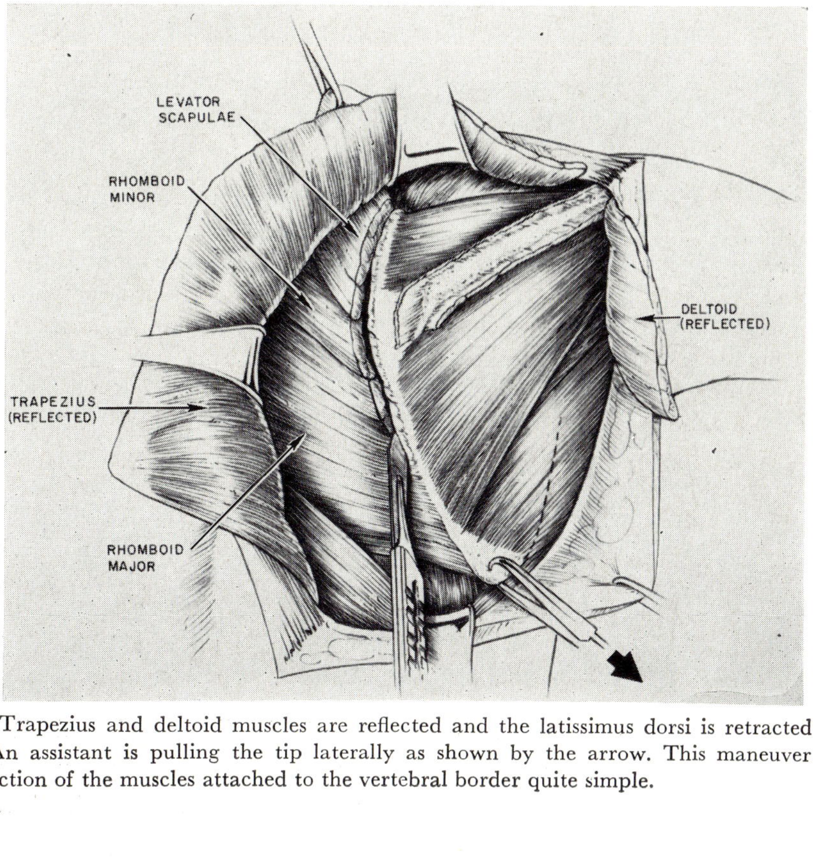

Fig. 3. Trapezius and deltoid muscles are reflected and the latissimus dorsi is retracted downward. An assistant is pulling the tip laterally as shown by the arrow. This maneuver makes the resection of the muscles attached to the vertebral border quite simple.

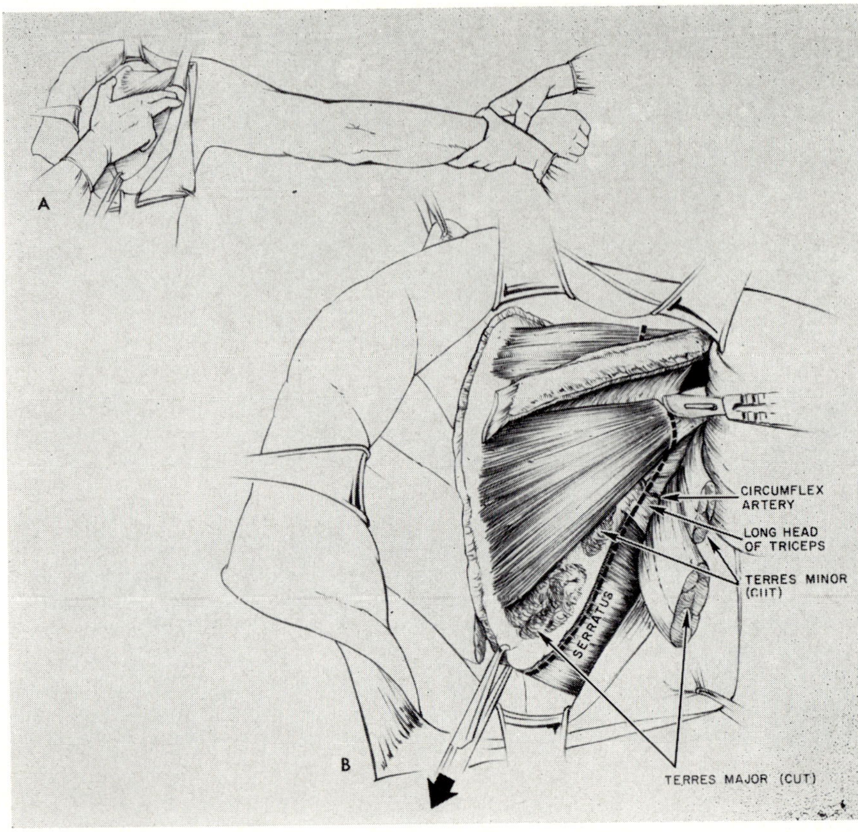

Fig. 4. *A,* Palpation of axillary contents. The axillary contents need to be retracted out of the operating field. *B,* The tip of the scapula is now pulled inferomedially and the muscles are cut. The dotted line shows the line of resection of supraspinous, intraspinous, and serratus anterior muscles.

intraspinous tendons and the attachment of serratus anterior muscles are cut, as shown in Fig. 4, *B*. The shoulder joint is then exposed and identified, and the spine cut near the acromion process by use of an osteotome (Fig. 5, *A*). Thus the acromioclavicular joint is kept intact. The only muscle remaining attached to the scapula, humerus, and shoulder joint is the subscapular, which is resected under the guidance of the operator's finger (Fig. 5, *B*).

A Gigli saw is then passed around the neck of the scapula, avoiding the glenohumeral joint. The scapula is resected and the specimen removed, care being taken to avoid injury to the glenohumeral joint (Fig. 5, *B* and *C*).

After proper hemostasis is achieved, the cut edge of the trapezius muscle is sutured to the deltoid muscle at the line of the previous position of the spine of the scapula (Fig. 6). The lateral margins of these muscular stitches incorporate the remnant of the acromion process (Fig. 6). The teres major and minor muscles are sutured to the chest wall (Fig. 6).

The suction catheter beneath each skin flap is then brought out through normal skin, the wound is closed by interrupted subcutaneous 3-0 chromic catgut sutures, and the skin margins are apposed by interrupted 3-0 Dermalon stitches. The suction catheters are then attached to a continuous suction device. A firm pressure dressing is applied and the arm is placed in a Velpeau dressing.

POSTOPERATIVE CARE

The patient should be allowed to ambulate early. The Velpeau dressing is removed after

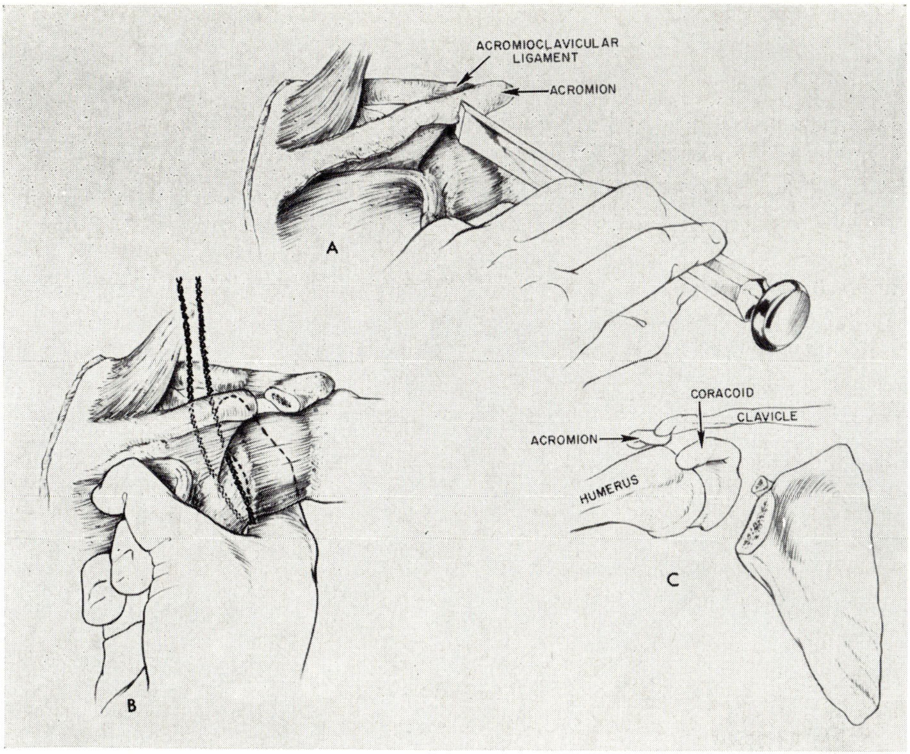

Fig. 5. *A,* The scapular spine is being cut with an osteotome. *B,* The subscapular muscle is cut under the guidance of the operator's finger. After this, a Gigli saw is passed around the neck of the scapula. *C,* The excised scapula with an intact shoulder joint.

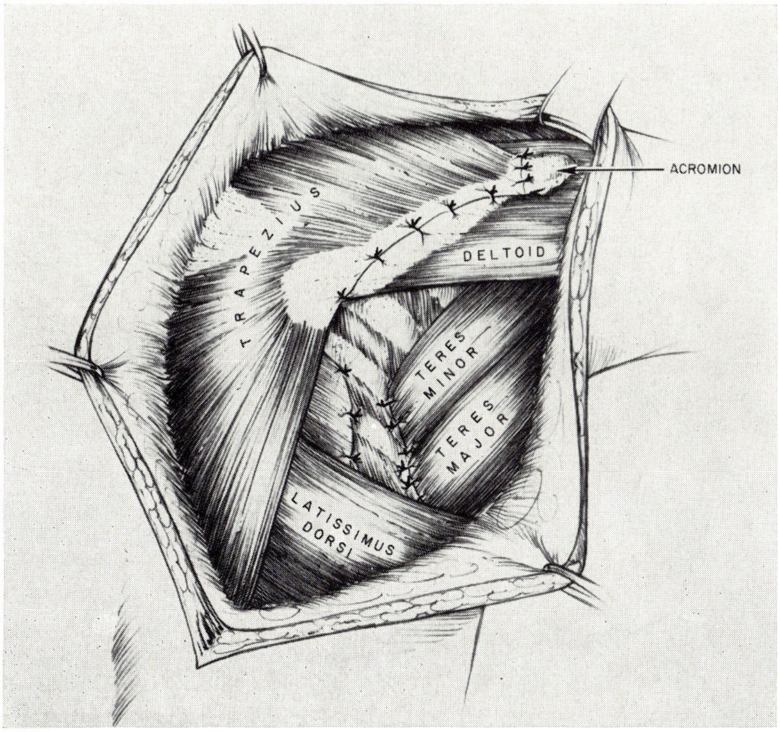

Fig. 6. The suture line between deltoid and trapezius muscles. The acromion process is shown at the top. The teres major and minor muscles are attached to the rib cage.

48 hours and replaced by an ordinary collar and cuff sling with the patient instructed to keep the arm in this sling during the day and supported on a pillow at night. By the end of the seventh day, active exercise, such as attempts at abduction, should be encouraged.

The patient should be seen by a physical therapist at this time for instruction in active and passive exercises. The suction catheters are removed by the eighth or ninth days and the skin stitches removed by the tenth to twelfth days.

A carefully organized physiotherapy program begun early after operation ensures maximum use of the extremity. In most instances the patient can return to normal work within 8 to 12 weeks after the operation.

REFERENCES

1. de Nancrede, C. B. G.: The end results after total excision of the scapula for sarcoma, Ann. Surg. **50:** 1, 1909.
2. Pack, G. T., and Ariel, I. R.: Tumors of the soft somatic tissues, New York, 1958, Paul B. Hoeber, Inc., Medical Book Division of Harper & Row, Publishers.
3. Ryerson, E. W.: Excision of scapula, J. A. M. A.: **113:** 1958, 1939.
4. Syme, J.: Excision of the scapula (monograph), Edinburgh, 1864, Edmonston and Douglas.

Spontaneous rupture of the esophagus

SAUL F. SALINAS IZAGUIRRE, M.D.*
JAMES T. HAGGERTY, M.D.
GERALD ECKERT, M.D.
ROCHESTER, N. Y.
From the Department of Surgery, Radiology and Medicine, St. Mary's Hospital

Perhaps one of the most commonly missed clinical diagnoses is spontaneous rupture of the esophagus. Although a compatible history and signs and symptoms are usually present, physicians rarely consider this entity because of its relatively infrequent occurrence. The tragedy of missed diagnosis lies in the fact that any delay in treatment greatly increases the mortality and morbidity rates. Fortunately, spontaneous rupture of the esophagus can be diagnosed easily by means of a chest x-ray and/or radiopaque swallow.

A clear differentiation must first be made between perforation and rupture because treatment and prognosis are quite dissimilar in each case. Perforation often involves a diseased esophageal wall and is more likely to result from instrumentation, such as the taking of a specimen for biopsy. The perforation defect nearly always is small and round and it may occur in any part of the organ.

Esophageal rupture, on the other hand, is an abrupt tear in an apparently normal and undiseased esophageal wall, precipitated by a sudden increase in intraluminal pressure. The laceration shows a predilection for site of occurrence and for direction of the rent. The cardinal factor in the pathogenesis of esophageal rupture appears to be the abruptness with which the rise in intraluminal pressure takes place rather than the level of the pressure attained.

The greatest incidence of rupture is in the lower portion of the esophagus. This area is composed entirely of smooth muscle fibers which spread out and constitute a comparatively thinner and weaker wall structure. In nearly all cases of rupture, the area of greatest susceptibility is the left posterolateral aspect of this region.[11] A longitudinally directed scar is the most commonly seen, although in the first case described in the literature[3] a transverse scar is reported.

The work of numerous investigators demonstrates that the muscle tissue is torn first and that the mucosa then herniates through it as the intraluminal pressure continues to rise. The mucosa possesses more than 50 percent of the holding power of the esophageal wall. In nearly all experimental cases, the mucosal defect is smaller than the muscularis one.

Derbes and Mitchell[9] showed that almost all experimentally produced ruptures are similar to those encountered clinically. Mackler[15] produced experimental rupture of the esophagus with an average pressure of 5 p.s.i. Derrick and co-workers[10] demonstrated that intraluminal pressures of 3 to 7.5 p.s.i. produced rupture of the intact human esophagus, whereas, if the esophageal mucosa is weakened by ulceration, esophagitis, or other causes, the detrimental level

Submitted for publication Feb. 22, 1969; resubmitted Sept. 23, 1969.

*Dr. Salinas Izaguirre is presently at the Department of Thoracic and Cardiovascular Surgery of St. Barnabas Hospital, New York, N. Y.

may be as low as 1 to 2.25 p.s.i. Any proximal or distal obstruction, such as esophageal stricture or the presence of a neoplasm, will evoke rupture at lower levels of intraluminal pressure.

SIGNS AND SYMPTOMS

Although the sudden increase in intraluminal pressure generally is associated with vomiting,[4, 5, 8, 25, 26] esophageal rupture may occur unaccompanied by vomiting[7] or other immediately notable stress (case 313328). It has been reported following labor, suprapubic prostatectomy, and diseases of the central nervous system. A history of dyspepsia is present in approximately 40 percent of cases, but many patients report no previous gastrointestinal disorders.

Clinically, the typical victim is a man of approximately 50 to 60 years of age who habitually consumes food and alcoholic beverages to excess. The catastrophe usually follows the ingestion of a heavy meal together with alcohol. Review of cases reported in the literature suggests that the high incidence of esophageal rupture among alcoholics is related to the correspondingly higher incidence of chronic esophagitis in this group.

Early symptoms of imminent esophageal rupture include the sudden onset of excruciating, epigastric, retrosternal pain described variously as burning,[14] crushing,[16] or knifelike tearing apart or bursting.[3] The pain is located in, or radiates to, the left lower chest and is markedly exacerbated by coughing and by deep breathing, indicative of its pleuritic origin. Shortness of breath is very pronounced. Surprisingly, dysphagia is not a frequent finding; some patients may even request something to drink for relief of epigastric pain. Fluid intake does not increase the retrosternal pain but aggravates the chest pain.

Probably the earliest and most significant sign of spontaneous rupture of the esophagus is mediastinal emphysema, with or without suprasternal involvement. Before actual perforation into the pleural cavity occurs, mediastinal and suprasternal emphysema are the most prominent and significant clinical findings.[29]

The extent of pleural involvement is determined to a great extent by the resistance of the mediastinal pleura to gastric content which is spilled into the mediastinum. The presence of hydropneumothorax and the lapse of time following perforation are indications of the severity of infection. An acid pH of the aspirated pleural fluid will certainly reveal contamination by gastric content. Involvement of the pleural cavity will decrease the chances of survival and diminish the likelihood of an uneventful recovery in these cases.

As the effects of the injury progress, a pleuritic type of pain appears, with definite impairment of respirations caused by hydropneumothorax and/or chemical and septic mediastinitis with or without emphysema. In an effort to reduce pain, the patient may splint his lower chest, which will precipitate a bilateral basilar atelectasis with superimposed pneumonia and increase the already present respiratory embarrassment. Cyanosis with rapid respirations and orthopnea may eventually lead to shock. Without definite treatment, shock or prostration coma can progress to irreversible stages.

DIAGNOSIS

The single most important diagnostic measure is the chest x-ray. It will reveal the presence of mediastinal or cervical emphysema,[14, 19, 20] pleural effusion, or hydropneumothorax. Radiological visualization of mediastinal emphysema prior to perforation of the mediastinal pleura was perhaps best described by Naclerio[18] as a "V"-shaped configuration. This sign represents a localized mediastinal, retrocardiac emphysema, the "V" shape corresponding to air in the mediastinal and diaphragmatic pleural space in the area of the lower esophagus.

The absence of prompt radiological evidence should not be misinterpreted. The appearance of air is not infrequently delayed. When the history and clinical findings are very suggestive of ruptured esophagus, the x-ray should be repeated in one hour and a radiopaque swallow should be performed at once. Again, a negative result of the swallow does not entirely rule out the possibility of esophageal rupture, since the afflicted area may be walled off or the thickness of the radiopaque substance may not allow the contrast medium to leak out. Massive edema can also be responsible for delay or prevention of the escape of contrast material through the perforation opening. Esophagoscopy has been suggested as a diagnostic measure[6] but edema and inflammation limit the feasibility of this procedure.

It is evident that early and accurate detection, prior to actual pleural involvement, requires considerable acumen on the part of the diagnostician. However, a timely diagnosis is particularly rewarding in these cases wherein so much depends upon prompt initiation of appropriate therapy.

When pleural complications have already arisen, a definite diagnosis can be made by radiopaque swallow[1] or by ingestion of a small amount of methylene blue, followed by performance of thoracentesis. In the presence of pleural effusion, the fluid obtained by thoracentesis is characteristically foul smelling, cloudy, brown in color, and often mixed with particles of food.

DIFFERENTIAL DIAGNOSIS

Most commonly rupture of the esophagus is misdiagnosed as perforated peptic ulcer. The pain associated with both conditions is almost identical in character and in location at the early stage. Chest x-ray and upright abdominal x-ray should provide a sufficient basis for differential diagnosis. The presence of air beneath the diaphragm usually rules out esophageal rupture, although Strauch and Lynch[27] have reported one instance of subdiaphragmatic rupture of the esophagus.

Other conditions need to be ruled out as well. The possibility of acute pancreatitis[12] should be considered. Enzyme studies will be of assistance here. Pulmonary embolism can readily be differentiated because it never causes mediastinal emphysema. Spontaneous pneumothorax rarely produces early pleural effusion, and pain is generally less severe. Myocardial infarction can be distinguished by means of an electrocardiogram.

PROGNOSIS AND TREATMENT

Time is an essential factor in the prognosis of this malady. The longer the time lapse between occurrence of rupture and initiation of treatment, the lower the expectancy of survival. Twenty-five percent of patients die during the first 12 hours.[28]

Although success has occasionally followed conservative management,[13, 22, 24] there has been no doubt since the first case of survival following surgical management was reported[2] that immediate open thoracotomy with repair of the laceration and pleural drainage,[17, 21, 23] including thorough irrigation and cleaning of the involved areas, is the treatment of choice.

Effective antibiotic therapy is of utmost importance. Infection must be promptly controlled. If it is allowed to progress, complications such as empyema, wound infection, disruption of the suture line, and mediastinal abscess must be anticipated. In cases of advanced infection, a residual esophagopleurocutaneous fistula will usually persist even after the infection has been effectively treated.

As soon as the diagnosis is suspected, a nasogastric tube should be inserted. This measure will markedly decrease the reflux of gastric content into the mediastinum and pleural cavity, thus reducing the severity of chemical or septic mediastinitis which is the main cause of shock and respiratory distress. Nasogastric suction of secretions should be carried out as needed and oxygen therapy and blood transfusion administered as indicated.

If surgical treatment is instituted within the first six to twelve hours, the postoperative course should be uncomplicated. Under no circumstances should the patient be denied the benefit of surgery. In a paper published in 1952, Ware and associates[30] made the interesting observation that "any maneuver which is performed to drain either the mediastinum or the pleural cavity will increase or prolong the life of the patient. The number of patients whose survival period was increased or prolonged may not be statistically significant, but such statistics do indicate that duration of life is increased by as simple a procedure as thoracentesis."

Death following surgical repair is usually a consequence of prolonged conservative management with late drainage of the mediastinitis and pyopneumohydrothorax. Without some form of treatment, the patients usually die within 48 to 72 hours. Massive and overwhelming sepsis is the main cause of death.

CLINICAL MATERIAL

Our experience is composed of 12 cases which occurred over a period of 27 years, from July 1, 1940, to June 30, 1967, in the city of Rochester, N. Y. The records of five hospitals were reviewed, although in two institutions no case of spontaneous rupture of the esophagus had been recorded during this period.

Table I. *Admitting diagnosis and time relationship*

Hospital and chart No.	Age, sex	Diagnosis on admission	*Time intervals* Symptoms to admission	Admission to diagnosis	Symptoms to treatment	Admission to discharge	Treatment	Survival and remarks
St. Mary's, 75764-66	40, F	Acute pancreatitis; pneumonia	7 days	9 days	16 days	28 days	Surgery	Alive
St. Mary's, 74049-66	45, M	Acute pancreatitis; right lower lobe pneumonia	8 hr.	7 days	8 days	9 days	Surgery	Died
St. Mary's, 84750-66	84, M	Acute sigmoid diverticulum	—	12 hr.	12 hr.	18 days	Surgery	Alive
St. Mary's, 28608-62	47, M	Spontaneous rupture of esophagus	8 hr. ?	—	12 hr.	21 days	Surgery	Alive
Genesee, 287246-62	68, M	Mallory-Weiss? Aspiration pneumonia?	3 hr.	3 days	3 days	13 days	Surgery	Died
Genesee, 308529-64	26, F	Pulmonary emboli; acute pulmonary edema	7 days	14 hr.	—	14 hr.	None	Died; diagnosis on autopsy
Strong Memorial, 210191-64	65, F	Sigmoid diverticulum? Hiatus hernia with peptic esophagitis?	4 hr. ?	6 hr.	10 hr.	27 days	Surgery	Alive
Strong Memorial, 313228-52	75, M	Gastric perforation? Dissecting aortic aneurysm?	5 hr.	—	—	8 hr.	None	Died; diagnosis on autopsy
Strong Memorial, 536902-64	52, M	Left hydropneumothorax	1–2 hr. ?	14 hr.	—	14 hr.	None	Died; diagnosis on autopsy
Strong Memorial, 575369-64	93, M	Mesenteric thrombosis? Acute pancreatitis? Acute cholecystitis?	17 hr.	4 days	—	4 days	None	Died; diagnosis on autopsy
Strong Memorial, 624755-66	41, M	Perforated duodenal ulcer? Spontaneous rupture of esophagus?	14 hr.	2½ hr.	17 hr.	21 days	Surgery	Alive
Strong Memorial, 11069-40	76, M	Coronary occlusion?	2 days	—	—	24 hr.	None	Died; diagnosis on autopsy

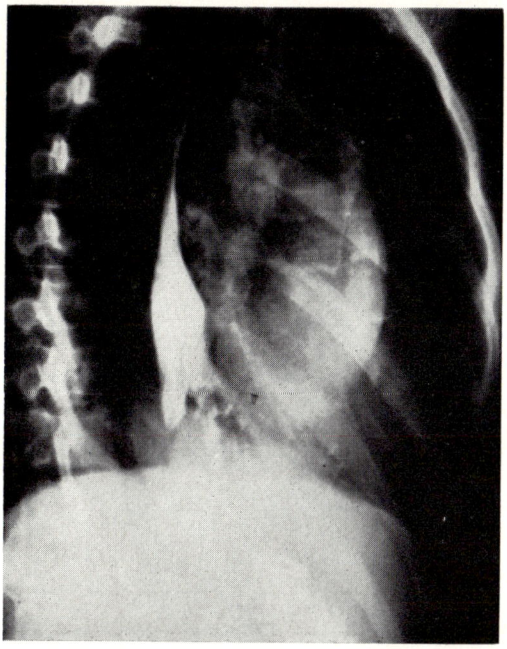

Fig. 1. This patient (case 75764) was operated on 9 days after admission to the hospital. His prolonged survival was probably attributable to noninvolvement of the pleural cavity coupled with early administration of large doses of antibiotics.

The ages of the patients ranged from 26 to 93 years, with an average age of 59.3. There were nine men and three women. The salient facts concerning each case are contained in Table I.

RESULTS

There were seven deaths in the total series of 12 patients. Five occurred in patients who had been treated conservatively and in whom the diagnosis was not made until autopsy. The mortality rate was 58.33 percent, including both the conservatively managed and the surgically managed patients. Among the surgical patients, the mortality rate was as low as 28.57 percent, whereas 100 percent of the patients who received conservative treatment alone died. Survival among the surgically treated patients might have been increased had the two patients who died received the indicated surgical intervention sooner.

Four of those who died did so within a period of 8 to 24 hours; one patient (case

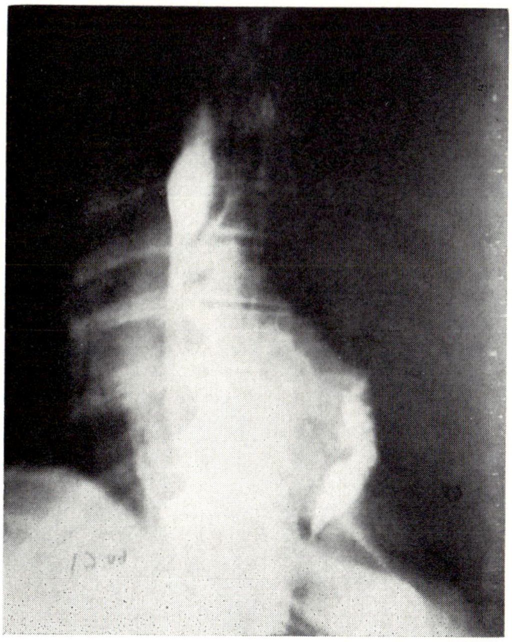

Fig. 2. In this patient (case 84750-66), barium swallow revealed the point of perforation to be in the lower third, left posterior aspect of the esophagus.

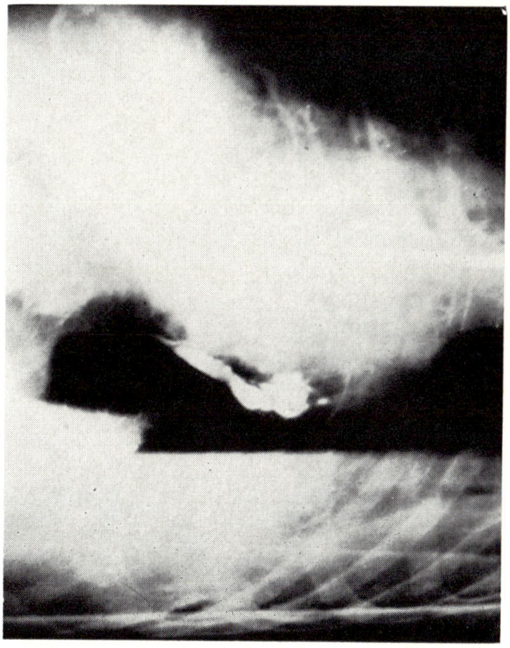

Fig. 3. Chest x-ray showed a left hydropneumothorax with an air fluid level of 5 cm. below the left rib cage in the same patient shown in Fig. 2.

575369) survived for four days following rupture. This extended survival can perhaps be explained by the frequency with which thoracenteses were performed. In the two patients who died following surgery, diagnosis was made seven days after admission to the hospital in the first patient and three days after admission in the second.

All of the five survivors underwent emergency surgical repair of the esophageal rent with drainage of the mediastinum and pleural cavity except one (case 75764) who was operated on nine days following admission (Fig. 1). This patient's survival was probably attributable to noninvolvement of the pleural cavity, coupled with administration of large doses of antibiotics early during hospitalization.

In only two patients was the correct diagnosis made at the time of admission to the hospital. Both received surgical treatment in a matter of hours. In the remaining patients the diagnosis was made during surgical procedures aimed at correction of other conditions such as acute pancreatitis.

Three patients had demonstrable suprasternal and/or supraclavicular subcutaneous emphysema on admission or shortly thereafter (cases 84750, 28608-62, and 313228-52). Only one of them was not surgically treated and he died eight hours later. The other two were discharged from the hospital 18 and 21 days later. Mediastinal and/or subcutaneous emphysema was radiologically demonstrable in three other patients (cases 84750-66, 536902-64, and 624755-66), but diagnosis was missed in the second patient, and this caused his death 14 hours after admission (Figs. 2 and 3).

SUMMARY AND CONCLUSION

Twelve cases of spontaneous rupture of the esophagus are presented with a total mortality rate of 58.33 percent. Early diagnosis followed by immediate surgical intervention reduced the mortality rate from 100 percent, as experienced with conservative treatment, to 28.57 percent.

A sudden and abrupt increase in intraluminal pressure is submitted as the precipitating cause of esophageal rupture. Definite predilection for site of occurrence and a characteristically longitudinally directed scar distinguish rupture from a perforation injury. Men of approximately 50 to 60 years of age, who habitually indulge in excessive quantities of food and alcoholic beverages, appear to be the individuals most prone to suffer spontaneous esophageal rupture. Diagnostic signs and symptoms are stressed, with emphasis on vomiting, epigastric pain, and mediastinal and/or suprasternal emphysema.

The clinical results obtained in this series once more emphasize the importance of performing open drainage of the mediastinum and pleural cavity with repair of the esophageal rent as soon as the diagnosis is established.

If the likelihood of spontaneous rupture of the esophagus is kept in mind, correct diagnosis can easily be made with the aid of a reliable history and the indicated radiological studies.

REFERENCES

1. Anderson, R. L.: Spontaneous rupture of the esophagus, Amer. J. Surg. **93:** 282, 1957.
2. Barrett, N. R.: Report of a case of spontaneous perforation of the esophagus successfully treated by operation, Brit. J. Surg. **35:** 216, 1947.
3. Boerhaave, H.: Atrocis, nec descripti pruis, morbi historia. Secundum medicae artis leges conscripta, Lugd. Bat. Boutesteniana, 1724. Translated in Bull. Med. Libr. Ass. **43:** 217, 1955.
4. Bowers, C. R., and Ferguson, D. H.: Rupture of the esophagus. Emetic dehiscence of the normal esophagus: Three new cases, Amer. J. Surg. **111:** 175, 1966.
5. Bruno, M. S., Grier, W. R. N., and Ober, W. B.: Spontaneous laceration and rupture of the esophagus and stomach, Arch. Intern. Med. **112:** 574, 1963.
6. Carter, R., and Hinshaw, D. B.: Use of the esophagoscope in the diagnosis of rupture of the esophagus, Surg. Gynec. Obstet. **120:** 1304, 1965.
7. Conte, B. A.: Esophageal rupture in absence of vomiting, J. Thorac. Cardiovasc. Surg. **51:** 137, 1966.
8. De Jode, L. R.: Spontaneous rupture of the esophagus with recovery following repair, Proc. Roy. Soc. Med. **58:** 431, 1965.

9. Derbes, V. J., and Mitchell, R. E.: Rupture of the esophagus, SURGERY **39:** 688, 1956.
10. Derrick, J. R., Harrison, W. H., and Howard, J. M.: Factors predisposing to spontaneous perforation of the esophagus, SURGERY **43:** 486, 1958.
11. Hochberg, L. A., and Parlamis, N.: Spontaneous perforation and rupture of the esophagus with a report of five cases, Amer. J. Surg. **102:** 428, 1961.
12. Hugh, T. B.: Spontaneous rupture of the esophagus, Brit. J. Surg. **52:** 73, 1965.
13. J. A. M. A. Editorial: Conservative management of esophageal perforation, J. A. M. A. **193:** 199, 1965.
14. Kyser, F. A.: Spontaneous perforation of the esophagus, Med. Clin. N. Amer. **43:** 3, 1964.
15. Mackler, S. A.: Spontaneous rupture of the esophagus: An experimental and clinical study, Surg. Gynec. Obstet. **95:** 345, 1952.
16. Marston, E. L., and Valk, H. L.: Spontaneous perforation of the esophagus: Review of the literature and report of a case, Ann. Intern. Med. **51:** 590, 1959.
17. Mathewson, C., Jr., Dozier, W., Hamill, J. P., and Smith, M.: Clinical experiences with perforation of the esophagus, Amer. J. Surg. **104:** 257, 1962.
18. Naclerio, E. A.: The "V" sign in the diagnosis of spontaneous rupture of the esophagus (an early roentgen clue), Amer. J. Surg. **93:** 291, 1957.
19. O'Connel, N. D.: Spontaneous rupture of the esophagus, Amer. J. Roentgen. **99:** 186, 1967.
20. Panaro, V. A., and Leslie, E. S.: Spontaneous rupture of the esophagus, Radiology **84:** 252, 1965.
21. Rossi, G., and Dreiling, D. A.: Spontaneous perforation of the esophagus: A report of four consecutive successfully treated cases, J. Mount Sinai Hosp. N. Y. **33:** 107, 1966.
22. Samson, P. C.: Postemetic rupture of the esophagus, Surg. Gynec. Obstet. **93:** 221, 1951.
23. Sanderson, R. G.: Spontaneous rupture of the esophagus. Report of survival without surgical management, Amer. J. Surg. **109:** 506, 1965.
24. Sealy, W. C.: Rupture of the esophagus, Amer. J. Surg. **105:** 505, 1963.
25. Smead, L. F.: Spontaneous rupture of the esophagus following vomiting, Amer. J. Surg. **13:** 497, 1931.
26. Sokolnicki, J.: Spontaneous rupture of the esophagus, Pol. Przegl. Chir. **38:** 132, 1966.
27. Strauch, G. O., and Lynch, R. E.: Subphrenic extrathoracic rupture of the esophagus: First reported case, Ann. Surg. **161:** 213, 1965.
28. Tesler, M. A., and Eisenberg, M. S.: Spontaneous esophageal rupture, Surg. Gynec. Obstet. **117:** 1, 1963.
29. Vanderlaan, W. P., and Maresh, G.: The significance of mediastinal emphysema, New Eng. J. Med. **235:** 617, 1946.
30. Ware, G. W., Schnider, B. L., and Davis, E. W.: Spontaneous rupture of the esophagus, Arch. Surg. **65:** 723, 1952.

Thymoma arising from undescended cervical thymus

C. E. RIDENHOUR, M.D.
J. H. HENZEL, M.D.
M. S. DeWEESE, M.D.
S. EARL KERR, M.D.
COLUMBIA, MO.
From the Departments of Surgery and Pathology, University of Missouri School of Medicine

Embryologic differentiation, descent, and resolution of the thymus gland provide many possibilities for abnormal findings in the fully developed neck. Lewis[7] summarized the findings in 34 cases of persistent cervical thymus, of which four were cysts. Seventeen cases of cervical thymic cysts have been documented,[5, 14, 16] and no neoplasm or malignant degeneration has been found. Thymoma developing from undescended thymus gland is an unusual occurrence, reported in only four previous cases.[1, 10, 12, 15] Two cases[1, 15] contained histologically malignant cells; however, neither had metastasized. We recently encountered in a middle-aged man a right submandibular neoplasm which proved to be a thymoma. Unusual clinicopathological features form the basis for this report.

CASE REPORT

T. T., a 47-year-old Negro man, was first admitted to the University of Missouri Medical Center in February, 1967, in a comatose state after a car-train accident. He had a subdural hematoma, left femoral shaft fracture, collateral ligament, and meniscus tears. After tracheostomy, bilateral temporal burr holes, and repair of the leg trauma, his condition stabilized and gradually improved over the ensuing three weeks. At admission a 3 cm., mobile, nontender, firm, right submandibular mass was detected deep to the cephalad portion of the sternocleidomastoid muscle. The mass was not attached to the carotid artery and did not displace adjacent structures significantly. No external skin sinuses or communication with the oropharynx was apparent. The patient stated that the mass had painlessly appeared in November, 1966, and had increased in size over the next four months. No history of congenital abnormality, chronic infectious disease, chest problems, or weight loss suggested metastatic malignancy.

Results of hemogram, urinalysis, uric acid, and liver function studies were normal. There was a slightly decreased albumin reading and slightly increased gamma globulin. Protein-bound iodine was normal with a low thyroid and red blood cell triiodothyronine uptake. The thyroid scan showed a mass displacing laterally the superior lobe of the thyroid. There was a poorly defined density in the right submandibular region. Barium swallow, chest x-ray, and upper gastrointestinal series yielded normal results. Submandibular gland neoplasm or lymphoma was considered the most likely diagnosis. The most likely organs for metastatic cancer from an occult primary site—oropharynx, parotid, thyroid, and larynx—were studied and no cancer was found.

On April 4, 1967, a right submandibular incision disclosed a 4 by 5 cm., nodular, solid mass deep to the sternocleidomastoid, adjacent to the submandibular gland, with no apparent connection to the oropharynx. Excisional biopsy was completed without difficulty. Neither additional masses nor lymphadenopathy was found. Definitive diagnosis was not possible with frozen section. Subsequent consultations confirmed the diagnosis of benign thymoma.

Gross pathology. The gray-white, well-encapsulated, smooth-surfaced mass measured 4.5 by 4.0 by 3.5 cm. It was moderately firm to rubbery.

Supported in part by grants from the American Cancer Society (CF Nos. 1958A and 2235A).

Submitted for publication May 9, 1969; resubmitted Sept. 15, 1969.

Address for reprints: C. E. Ridenhour, M.D., Clinical Instructor, Dept. of Surgery, University of Missouri School of Medicine, Columbia, Mo. 65201.

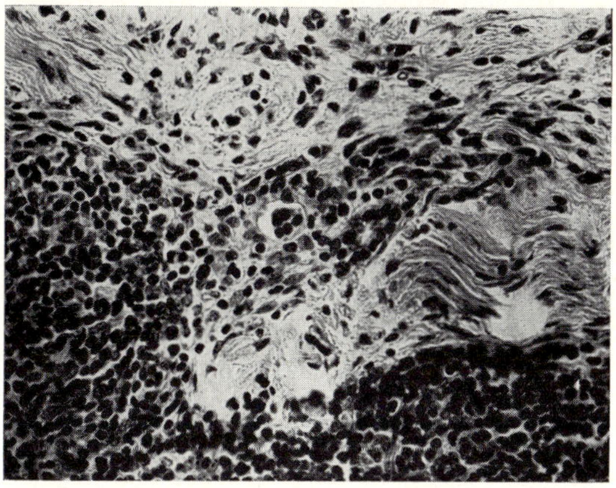

Fig. 1. Atypical lymphocytes are seen in the lower and left margins. The upper and right margins show spindle-shaped epitheloid elements. (Hematoxylin and eosin; ×400.)

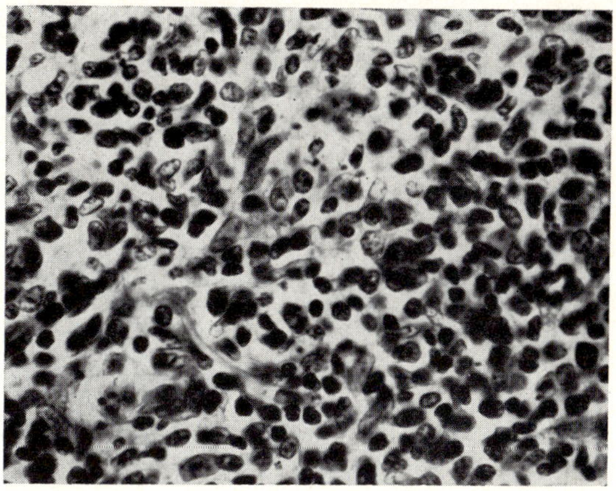

Fig. 2. Most of the thymoma disclosed a lymphocytic component with occasional areas of intermingling epithelial-like cells. (Hematoxylin and eosin; ×800.)

Cut surfaces showed pale brown homogeneous regions associated with prominent fibrous lacework areas. No gross hemorrhage, necrosis, or calcification is recognized.

Microscopic pathology. Numerous diverse sections revealed two cellular elements: lymphocytoid and epitheloid or spindle-shaped cells (Fig. 1). In some areas each is represented in a "pure" pattern, while others show varied intermingling (Fig. 2). There are frequent mitotic figures among the lymphocytic collections and occasional atypical forms (Fig. 3). The arrangement of the spindle-shaped cells gives the appearance of fibrous bands, but closer examination leads to doubt that these are connective tissue. Reticulum stains substantiate this impression. There is no evidence of Hassall's corpuscles or a definite lobular pattern. Within the capsule, several glandlike spaces lined by low cuboidal cells suggest epithelial cells blending with the epithelial component (Fig. 4).

The patient was discharged doing well. No evidence of myasthenia gravis, erythrocytic agenesis, acquired agammaglobulinemia, or Cushing's syndrome developed. Repeat barium swallow and chest x-rays have demonstrated no mediastinal involvement. Follow-up on an outpatient basis for the past two years shows no recurrence or further difficulty.

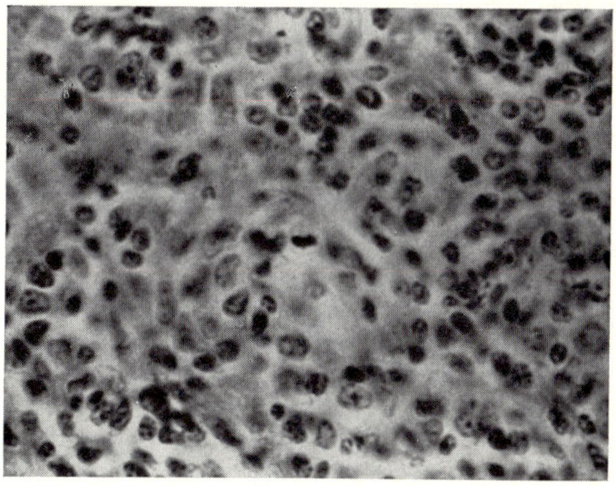

Fig. 3. Atypical forms and mitotic activity seen in areas where lymphocytoid cells predominate. (Hematoxylin and eosin; ×800.)

DIFFERENTIAL DIAGNOSIS

A single, solid, asymptomatic, submandibular neck mass in a middle-aged man presents a diagnostic challenge. Most of these prove to be metastatic neoplastic lymph nodes, with nasopharynx, thyroid, tonsil, tongue, and larynx the most likely primary sources.[11] Careful studies are necessary to evaluate these areas and, occasionally, tongue palpation under anesthesia with blind biopsy and open nasopharyngeal tissue biopsy will prove helpful. Other possibilities are lymphoma, salivary gland neoplasm, brachial cleft remnant, carotid body tumor, granuloma, or lymph node hyperplasia. Our case, as has been true in all previously reported cervical thymic masses, required excisional biopsy

A

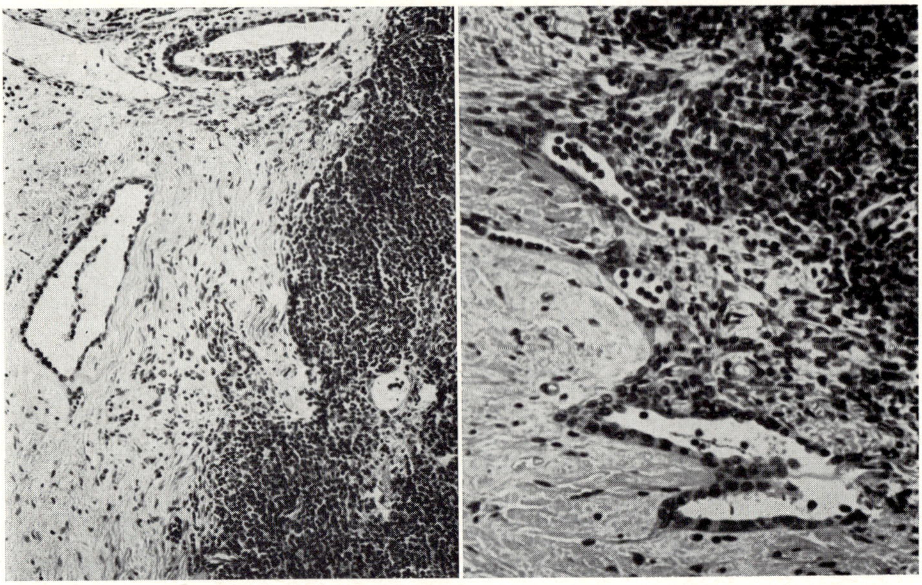

B

Fig. 4. *A,* Capsular region shows epithelial-lined sinuses adjacent to abundant lymphoid elements. No Hassall's corpuscles were seen in any of the sections. (Hematoxylin and eosin; ×160.) *B,* Higher magnification of one sinus discloses a low cuboidal cell lining merging with the lymphocytic element.

(or autopsy) for histological diagnosis. Although operating through a field for proposed cancer resection is undesirable, careful technique and proper placement of the incision reduce the chances for implantation and spread.

Widely diverse histological patterns in thymomas make precise diagnosis difficult. A lobular character separated by a loose fibrous connective tissue lacework identifies neoplastic change of the gland. Lymphocytes and syncytially arranged epithelial cells are found in the lobules, often with an overabundance of one type. Cell pleomorphism and undifferentiated embryonic cells make classification hazardous. When small cell lymphocytes predominate, differentiation from a lymphoma or metastatic oat cell carcinoma is difficult. Large epitheloid cells associated with epithelial-lined capsule sinuses identify the thymic origin. Microscopically, teratoma or germinoma may resemble thymoma; however, the presence of teratoid elements rules out any doubt. Mitosis in lymphocytes is usually seen only in rapidly growing tumors. Frequent mitotic figures (Figs. 2 and 3) and occasional atypical lymphocyte forms are recognized in our case.

Germinal centers have not been considered a feature of thymoma, which may be confused with Hassall's corpuscle, thymic lymph follicle,[9] or lymphoid hamartoma.[2] A case record (Fig. 5) shows diagnosis (at the Ellis Fischel State Cancer Hospital in 1953) of what was believed to be a benign cervical thymoma, while retrospective analysis supports the diagnosis of lymphoid hamartoma. An encapsulated 8 by 6 by 3.5 cm. tumor on cut section showed nodularity and a central mass of laminated cells surrounded by a broad zone of small lymphocytes resembling phagocytosis and lymphocytic cuffing as described by Castleman[2] (Fig. 5). Other than excisional biopsy no treatment was provided and the patient is living and well 15 years later.

DISCUSSION

Human thymic primordia appear toward the end of the sixth embryonic week as ventral outgrowths of the third pharyngeal pouches which migrate into the mediastinum

A

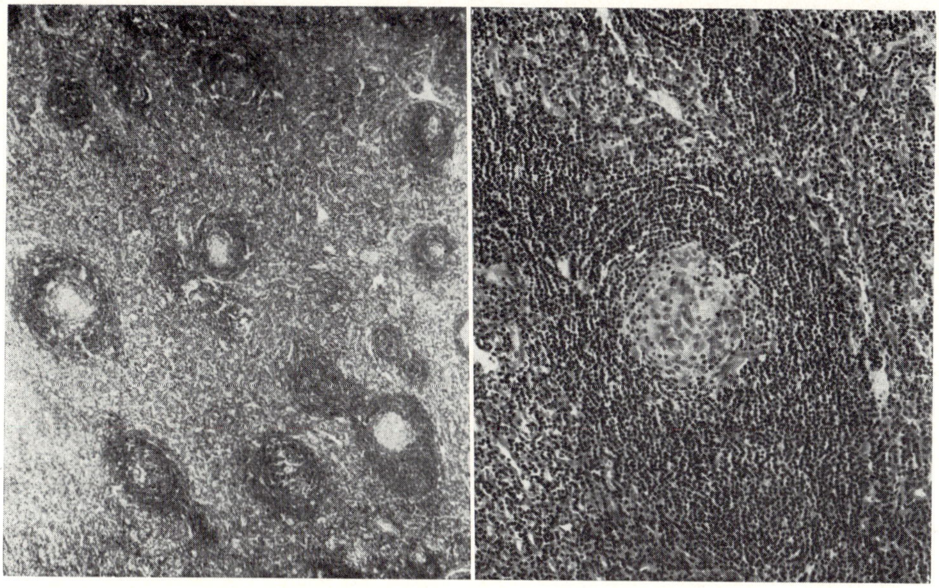

B

Fig. 5. *A,* Low magnification of lymphoid hamartoma (EFSCH 53-17,699) indicating lymphoid tissue with many germinal centers containing central degenerative, eosinophilic, whorl-like collections. (Hematoxylin and eosin; ×40.) *B,* Higher magnification shows broad zone of lymphocytic cuffing.

Table I. *Review of five cases of cervical thymoma*

Author, year	*Sex/age*	*Location*	*Source of study*	*Associated disease*	*Follow-up*
Wadon, 1934[15]	F/58	Upper trachea	Autopsy	Myasthenia gravis	Died of respiratory embarrassment
Boman, 1941[1]	F/71	Left neck	Autopsy	Atelectasis	Died
Pirkey, 1954[10]	F/11	Left neck	Excisional biopsy	None	Living and well, 5 mo.
Sease, 1956[12]	F/35	Suprasternal	Excisional biopsy	Questionable myasthenia gravis	Living and well, 17 yr.
Ridenhour, 1969 (the present report)	M/47	Right submandibular	Excisional biopsy	Acute trauma	Living and well, 24 mo.

by the middle of the eighth week. Ordinarily the thymus resides within the chest, enlarges to maximum size in puberty, then involutes after the period of greatest procreativity. Aberrant development may result in residual implants in the cervical path of descent, many of which have been treated by thymectomy.[7] In a patient of ours, a persistent thymic cord was found near a brachial cleft cyst. Thymic cysts without malignant degeneration have been documented in 17 cases.[5, 7, 14] Modes of pathogenesis of the cyst have been the subject of many reports, including failure of the thymopharyngeal duct to obliterate, as signified by a cuboidal or columnar epithelial lining,[5] cystic alteration of epithelial inclusion within lymphoid tissue,[4] infection,[7] and degenerative Hassall's corpuscles in ectopic cervical thymus.[14]

A summary of cervical thymoma cases is presented in Table I. Persistent thymic tissue is found predominantly in children,[7] whereas thymomas are generally discovered in middle-aged patients. No location predominates and all occur along the route of developmental descent. Two patients had associated myasthenia gravis, one quite mild. Except for one patient with respiratory embarrassment, most were asymptomatic and benign. This, of course, does not contraindicate extirpation to eliminate later complications.

Since cervical and mediastinal thymomas have a common derivation, it may be assumed that they behave similarly. Unfortunately, little is known of the natural history and degree of immunological function of thymomas. Reports have associated thymomas with myasthenia gravis, Cushing's syndrome, red cell agenesis, hypogammaglobulinemia, dermatomyositis, disseminated lupus erythematosus, and polymyositis.[6, 13, 17] Only myasthenia gravis has been noted with cervical thymomas.

The significance of histological interpretation of the degree of malignancy has been questioned.[5, 13, 17] A small proportion display microscopic signs of malignancy such as cellular pleomorphism and mitoses. The gross morphology and operative findings of the degree of invasiveness must often be used in predicting malignancy potential. Gross encapsulation of tumor and the absence of myasthenia gravis may be the best guides to a favorable prognosis.[17] Although most[6, 17] emphasize the predominant intrathoracic spread of thymomas, the question of embolic metastasis or permeation through the lymph stream has been discussed.[2, 8, 13] Cervical thymomas without mediastinal involvement demand careful study in each case of reported lymph node metastases which may represent heterotopic foci concomitantly responding to the same stimulus as the main thymus. Total local excision has provided adequate treatment, but removal of contiguous structures may become necessary if tumor invasion develops. Lymphatic metastasis of thymomas is very rare. Unless additional metastatic foci can be palpated, radical neck dissection is not indicated.

Thymomas have a variable response to irradiation without correlation with the histological pattern. Although we are not aware of reported irradiation in cervical thymomas, if total surgical extirpation is impracticable, a trial of irradiation might be considered rational in view of our current knowledge.

SUMMARY

A 47-year-old man had an isolated submandibular mass which excisional biopsy prove to be a thymoma in aberrant thymic tissue. A survey of world literature disclosed only four reported cervical thymomas. A lymphoepithelial cell variant and mitotic activity among the predominant atypical lymphocyte pattern were found. Lymphocytic cuffing, as seen in a lymphoid hamartoma case, is included to illustrate the difficulty in differentiating tumors resembling thymoma. The patient had none of the diseases occasionally associated with mediastinal thymomas and is well two years following surgical extirpation.

The authors thank Drs. J. M. Blumberg of the Armed Forces Institute of Pathology, J. B. Hazard of Cleveland Clinic, H. Rappoport for review of the pathological material, and John S. Spratt, Jr. for providing review material from the Ellis Fischel State Cancer Hospital.

REFERENCES

1. Boman, K.: Om thymusfoeraendringar vid myasternier, Nord. Med. **10:** 1625, 1941.
2. Castleman, B.: Tumors of the thymus gland, *in* Atlas of tumor pathology, Washington, D. C., 1955, Armed Forces Institute of Pathology, sec. V, fasc. 19.
3. Gaeckle, D. J., and Gerber, M. L.: Thymic cyst in the neck, Am. J. Surg. **103:** 755, 1962.
4. Henzel, J. H., Pories, W. J., and DeWeese, M. S.: Etiology of lateral cervical cysts, Surg. Gynec. Obstet. **125:** 86, 1967.
5. Indeglia, R. A., Shea, M. A., and Grage, T. B.: Congenital cysts of the thymus gland, Arch. Surg. **94:** 149, 1967.
6. Legg, M. A., and Brady, W. J.: Pathology and clinical behavior of thymomas: A survey of 51 cases, Cancer **18:** 1131, 1965.
7. Lewis, M. R.: Persistence of the thymus in the cervical area, J. Pediat. **61:** 887, 1962.
8. Lowenhaupt, E.: Tumors of the thymus in relation to the thymic epithelial anlage, Cancer **1:** 547, 1948.

9. O'Kabe, H.: Thymic lymph follicles. A histopathological study of 1,356 autopsy cases, Acta Path. Jap. **16(1)**: 109, 1966.
10. Pirkey, W. P.: Epithelioma of undescended thymus in a child, Arch. Otolaryng. **59**: 237, 1954.
11. Ridenhour, C. E., Yuen, P. F., and Spratt, J. S., Jr.: Metastatic carcinoma in cervical lymph nodes from occult primary sites, Missouri Med. **64**: 988, 1967.
12. Sease, C. I.: Cervical thymoma. A case report, Virginia Med. Monthly **83**: 345, 1956.
13. Shields, T. W., Fox, R. T., and Lees, W. M.: Thymic tumors, classification and treatment, Arch. Surg. **92**: 617, 1966.
14. Simons, J. N., Robinson, D. W., and Masters, F. W.: Cervical thymic cyst, Am. J. Surg. **108**: 578, 1964.
15. Wadon, A.: Thymoma intratracheale, Zbl. Allg. Path. **60**: 308, 1934.
16. Weller, R. W., Pearce, A. E., and Rapoport, M.: Thymic cyst of the neck, Arch. Path. **52**: 569, 1951.
17. Wilkins, E. W., Jr., Edmunds, L. H., Jr., and Castleman, B.: Cases of thymoma at the Massachusetts General Hospital, J. Thorac. Cardiovasc. Surg. **52**: 322, 1966.

A new operation for varicocele: Use of microvascular anastomosis

KOICHI ISHIGAMI, M.D.,
YOSHIYUKI YOSHIDA, M.D.
MASAO HIROOKA, M.D.
KIKUO MOHRI, M.D.
KYOTO, JAPAN
From the Second Surgical Division, Kyoto University Medical School (Director: Prof. Dr. Chuji Kimura)

There are two kinds of varicoceles: (1) the idiopathic, the most common type, and (2) the symptomatic, those that are due to kidney tumor, giant hydronephrosis, hepatic congestion, chronic constipation, etc. The pampiniform plexus is formed by three groups of veins: the cremasteric (posterior) group, the deferential (middle) group, and the spermatic (anterior) group, this last being usually the seat of varicocele. As the internal spermatic vein is thin, despite its long course, poor in muscle layer in its vascular wall, and lacking in effective valves except for the inflow points into the inferior vena cava or the renal vein, the blood flow in this vein tends to stagnate. In addition, the left testicle hangs down at a lower level as compared with the right one. The right internal spermatic vein opens obliquely into the inferior vena cava, while the left one enters the renal vein at a right angle. Therefore, the valvular insufficiency caused by congenital or acquired lesions easily induces the reflux into the internal spermatic vein and causes varicocele by exerting an elevated hydrostatic pressure on the pampiniform plexus. Ninety-seven percent of varicoceles occur on the left side only, while in 3 percent of cases the condition is bilateral. Recently, it is noticed that diseases, such as varicocele and orthostatic albuminuria or hypertension, may be caused by strangulation or compression of the renal or internal spermatic veins because of the arched renal or gonadal arteries,[5, 6] aortic superior mesenteric arterial pincers. Campbell[1] had paid attention to the anomalous lower polar renal vessel as a potential cause of varicocele, and an instance of its occurrence in a 13-year-old boy had been reported.

Many excellent treatments for varicocele have been reported as follows: (1) injection of sclerosing materials into varicocele; (2) resection of varicocele; (3) ligation of the internal spermatic vessels at a high level, ligation of the internal spermatic vein,[7] ligation and excision of the internal spermatic artery with the spermatic group of the pampiniform plexus[9]; (4) resection of the redundant scrotum; (5) elevation of the testicle; and (6) formation of tunnel, reduction of inguinal canal, and operation for inguinal hernia.[10]

Excision of the pampiniform plexus cannot remove the reflux in the internal spermatic vein and block the venous return at the level where the deep and superficial venous systems communicate with each other. Therefore, if the removal of the plexus is incomplete, it may possibly result in recurrence of varicocele or thrombus formation in the remaining plexus. And, if the removal of the plexus is complete, it may sometimes result in stagnation or marked swelling of the spermatic cord, testicular atrophy or hydrocele, epididymitis, etc., because of the damage of the internal spermatic artery or external spermatic nerve.[2, 4, 7, 11] On the other hand, ligation of the in-

Submitted for publication May 26, 1969; resubmitted June 27, 1969.

ternal spermatic vein cannot cure the varicocele in the cremasteric and deferential groups, and sometimes gives rise to the local phlebothrombosis.[2, 4, 7, 11]

These operations cannot accomplish two requisites for the ideal treatment of varicocele, that is, the removal of the reflux in the internal spermatic vein and the preservation of the venous return from the testicle, epididymis, etc. The ideal treatment for varicocele should remove all of the subjective and objective symptoms and prevent a patient from recurrence and testicular atrophy or hydrocele, etc.

In 1960, Palma and Esperòn[8] reported on the surgical treatment of the postphlebitic syndrome of lower limb in which the great saphenous vein on the opposite side was dissected free, brought into the diseased limb through the subcutaneous tissue adjacent to the pubic symphysis, and anastomosed to the femoral vein on the diseased side in end-to-side fashion. Inokuchi and co-workers[3] also presented the modified technique in which both veins were attached end-to-end by the blood vessel suturing apparatus. Impressed by these operations, we have recently performed a new operation to treat three men with varicocele. This relatively simple procedure could remove the varicocele and preserve normal venous return from the testicle.

METHOD

A skin incision, about 8 cm. in length, extending from below and medial to the anterior superior iliac spine to the pubic spine, is made 2 to 3 cm. above and parallel to Poupart's ligament and carried down to the aponeurosis of the external oblique muscle, under intratracheal intubations, or spinal anesthesia. An incision is made in the direction of the fibers of the external oblique and extended to the lateral side of the external inguinal ring. The lower flap of the aponeurosis is freed by blunt dissection down to include Poupart's ligament. Subsequently, venography of the left internal spermatic vein is performed by infusing 30 to 40 ml. of 76 percent Urografin into the pampiniform plexus. The findings on a venogram are useful in selecting the method of operation (Fig. 1). By digital palpation the internal inguinal ring is identified as a landmark. The fibers of the internal oblique and transverse muscles are separated 2 cm. above the internal inguinal ring. As soon as the last muscle fibers are separated, the varicosed veins are seen. These vessels run, at this point, between the peritoneum and the muscle wall. Then, the internal spermatic vein is dissected free preserving the internal spermatic artery and the nerves. The internal spermatic vein is not always single in number. Prior to the dissection of this vein, local anesthetics should be injected into its neighborhood to prevent it from contraction. When the varicocele is a mild case in which only the spermatic group of the pampiniform plexus is affected, the microvascular anastomosis is performed between the distal cut end of the internal spermatic vein and the mobilized great saphenous vein on the same side. However, in a severe case, the cremasteric and deferential groups are affected, and sometimes, valvular insufficiency of the external spermatic or deferential veins may occur in succession.[2] In such cases, the remaining plexus may be the cause of the postoperative complication.

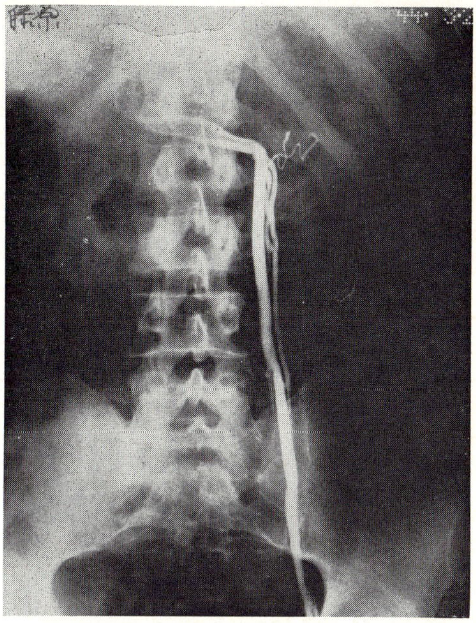

Fig. 1. Venogram of the left internal spermatic vein in Case 3.

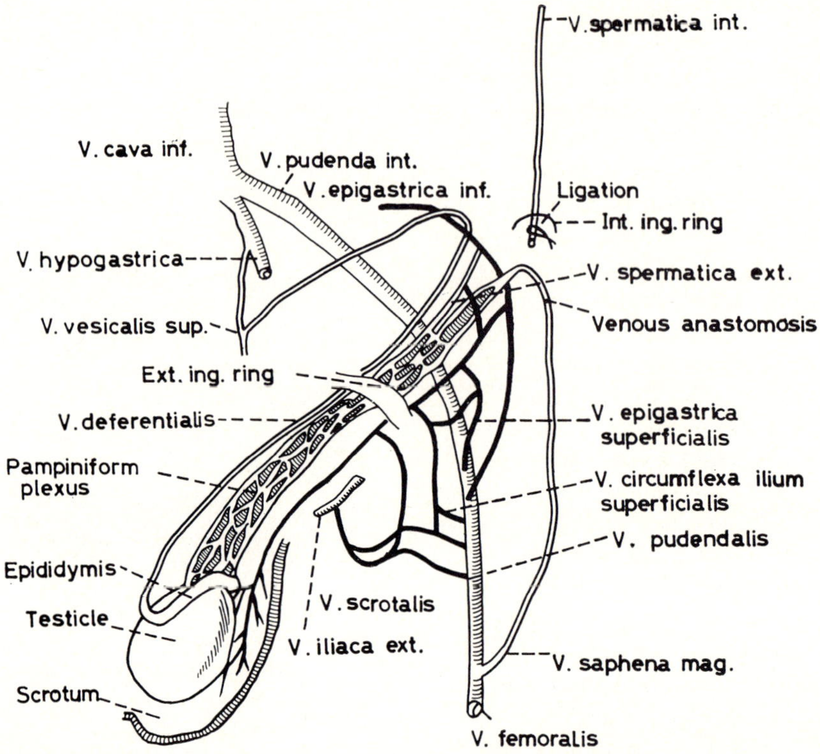

Fig. 2. Diagrammatic representation showing the use of microvascular anastomosis in the treatment of varicocele.

Sometimes, the venous anastomosis is impossible to perform because of the ramifications of the internal spermatic vein into several small branches. On such occasions, the sheath of the spermatic cord is incised, and the pampiniform plexus and the internal spermatic vein are dissected, preserving the deferent duct, the internal spermatic and deferential arteries, the external spermatic nerve, etc. Then, almost all of the plexus is excised, except for a distal healthy vein, about 2 cm. in length and of as large a diameter as possible.

As a second step of operation, the longitudinal skin incision, about 10 cm. in length, extending from 1 to 2 cm. cranial to Poupart's ligament in the caudal direction and running medial to the pulsation of the left femoral artery is made. The left great saphenous vein is dissected free about 7 cm. in length from its origin from the femoral vein. In order to prevent the mobilized vein segment from the spasm, the saline solution, with 1 ml. of 1 percent procaine and 10 mg.

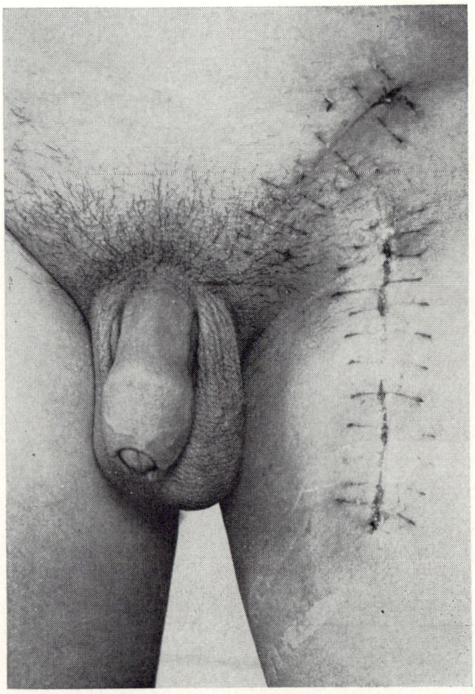

Fig. 3. Postoperative finding in Case 3.

of heparin per 100 ml. added, is infused into the vein through the vinyl tube. This solution is also injected from the base of the mobilized vein segment in the direction to its cut end to verify the effect of valve function. Then, the mobilized vein segment is brought into the left inguinal region through the subcutaneous tissue and the hole that was made in the lower flap of the aponeurosis from the left femoral region, paying attention to avoid its bending and twisting. After the testicle, epididymis, and spermatic cord are put back to the normal position, the end-to-end anastomosis is carried out between the mobilized great saphenous vein and the distal cut end of the internal spermatic vein (Method 1) or the preserved distal vein in the pampiniform plexus (Method 2), by using Inokuchi's blood vessel suturing apparatus (2.5 to 3.5 mm. in outside diameter). Fig. 2 shows diagrammatically the use of microvascular anastomosis in the treatment of varicocele. In Fig. 2, the veins, the lumina of which are shaded in black, play only an auxiliary role in the occurrence of varicocele. The anastomosis is quite easy to perform, as the internal spermatic vein is usually dilated remarkably. Both wounds of operation are drained to provide against hematoma formation because of the postoperative administration of anticoagulants. Early release from lying in bed and the intensive chemotherapy are necessary to prevent the patient from developing thrombus formation or infection.

Case 1, a 37-year-old man, was operated upon according to Method 2. Case 2, a 34-year-old man, and Case 3, a 24-year-old man were operated upon according to Method 1. Fifty milligrams of heparin and 26 to 56 mg. of Sintrom were administered for 6 to 8 days after operation. These patients were cured of their varicoceles with excellent results. Swelling in the left scrotum in Case 3 had disappeared completely on the fourteenth postoperative day, as shown in Fig. 3.

SUMMARY

Hitherto, many excellent operative treatments for idiopathic varicocele have been reported. However, none of them can accomplish two requisites for the ideal treatment, that is, the removal of the reflux into the internal spermatic vein and the preservation of the venous return from the testicle, epididymis, etc. Recently, we have invented a new operation for varicocele. We performed the microvascular anastomosis between the mobilized great saphenous vein and the distal cut end of the internal spermatic vein (Method 1) or a preserved distal vein in the pampiniform plexus (Method 2) with Inokuchi's blood vessel suturing apparatus, and could fulfill these two requisites. Three patients were cured of their varicoceles with excellent results.

REFERENCES

1. Campbell, M. F.: Varicocele due to anomalous renal vessel; an instance in a 13-year-old boy, J. Urol. **52:** 502, 1944.
2. Gösfay, S.: Untersuchungen der Vena spermatica interna durch retrograde Phlebographie bei Kranken mit Varikozele, Z. Urol. **52:** 105, 1959.
3. Inokuchi, K., Yagi, H., and Kusaba, A.: Reconstruction of blood vessels in the treatment for edema of lower limbs in phlebothrombosis, Shujutsu **17:** 92, 1963.
4. Kishimoto, T.: Operation for idiopathic varicocele, Shujutsu **15:** 273, 1961.
5. Nathan, H.: Observations on aberrant renal arteries curving around and compressing the renal vein; possible relationship to orthostatic proteinuria and to orthostatic hypertension, Circulation **18:** 1131, 1958.
6. Notkovich, H.: Variations of the testicular and ovarian arteries in relation to the renal pedicle, Surg. Gynec. Obstet. **103:** 487, 1956.
7. Olson, R. O., and Stone, E. P.: Varicocele; symptomatologic and surgical concepts, New Eng. J. Med. **240:** 877, 1949.
8. Palma, E. C., and Esperón, R. J.: Vein transplants and grafts in the surgical treatment of the postphlebitic syndrome, J. Cardiov. Surg. **1:** 94, 1960.
9. Palomo, A.: Radical cure of varicocele by a new technique; preliminary report, J. Urol. **61:** 604, 1949.
10. Sakabe, T.: Dancygier's operation for varicocele, Gekka Chiryo **8:** 587, 1963.
11. Shida, K., Saito, K., and Yanagida, O.: Operation for varicocele by ligating the spermatic vessels at a high level, Shujutsu **6:** 348, 1952.
12. Tseng, L.: Experiments of venography of the left spermatic veins in the patients suffering from varicosities, Arch. Jap. Chir. **33:** 973, 1964.

High systemic origin of the sole artery to the basal segments of the left lung: Findings, surgical treatment, and embryologic interpretation

EUGENE A. HESSEL, II, M.D.
EDWARD A. BOYDEN, PH.D.
STANLEY J. STAMM, M.D.
LESTER R. SAUVAGE, M.D.
SEATTLE, WASH.
From the Departments of Surgery, Biological Structure, and Pediatrics, University of Washington and Children's Orthopedic Hospital and Medical Center

This anomaly, occurring in an otherwise healthy boy, seems to have been unique in the following respects: First, the four basal segments of the left lower lobe were supplied solely by a large systemic artery, while both the superior segment and the left upper lobe were supplied by their usual pulmonary arterial branches; second, the systemic artery originated at one of the sites of a left lower bronchial artery and entered the lobe through the root of the left lung; third, the surgeon's attention had been attracted to this region by a continuous systolic-diastolic, machinery-like murmur heard all over the chest; fourth, this artery was utilized surgically in the hope of restoring normal pulmonary circulation by anastomosing it to the pulmonary artery of the left upper lobe; fifth, this maneuver did result in complete functional restoration of the lobe.

The only comparable instance of this particular anomaly, found in a search of the literature (and brought to our attention by McCotter's[23] article) is that reported in 1839 by the famous Viennese anatomist and scholar, Joseph Hyrtl,[17] then in Prague. It was fourth in a series of 15 autopsy reports recording venous anomalies. In one of these newborn infants, having absence of the integument over the anterior fontanelle and a left renal vein that emptied into the coronary sinus via a left cardinal vein, Hyrtl[17] notes that "the thoracic aorta gives rise to a pulmonary artery for the left lower lobe of the lung while the true left pulmonary artery supplies only the left upper lobe." This brief account suggests that perhaps in our case, also, the absence of the pulmonary artery to the left lower lobe might have been associated with other minor congenital anomalies, not visible in the living.*

CASE REPORT

L. R. (COH No. 09-58-20), aged 5½ years, was referred to the Children's Orthopedic Hospital and Medical Center in October, 1966, for evaluation of a heart murmur. There was a history of slight fatigue and slow growth, but no pulmonary complaints. His family history was unremarkable. On physical examination he appeared to be healthy, without cyanosis or clubbing. He was in the tenth percentile for height and twenty-fifth percentile for weight. His blood pressure was 115/45 with bounding pulses. There was fullness of the left precordium associated with a Grade 5/6 continuous systolic-diastolic, machinery-like murmur heard all over the upper precordium but most noticeable in the interscapular region and over the lower left posterior thorax. Chest x-rays revealed increased size of heart, prominent

Supported in part by Research Grant No. HD-00656-13, National Institutes of Health, United States Public Health Service.

Submitted for publication June 2, 1969; resubmitted June 20, 1969.

*At this time we wish to acknowledge assistance in "tracking down" cases supplied by the comprehensive articles of Findlay and Maier[13] and Sherrick and associates.[24]

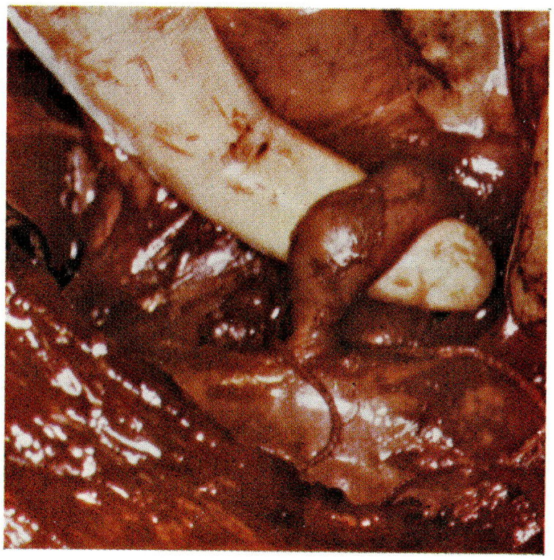

Fig. 1

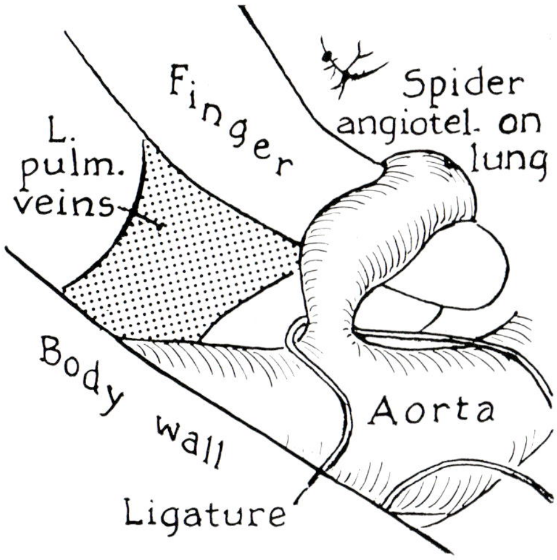

Fig. 2

Fig. 1. Kodachrome of anomalous artery taken at surgery.

Fig. 2. Explanation of Fig. 1. Head of patient is to the right. The left lung has been elevated, after left posterolateral approach to expose aorta and systemic artery (on finger). Note one of many angiotelectatic makings on lateral surface of pleura.

pulmonary artery, and increased flow to the left lung. Electrocardiogram showed left ventricular hypertrophy. The patient then underwent a left thoracotomy for closure of a suspected patent ductus arteriosus, but none could be found, and so the procedure was terminated and the patient made an uneventful recovery.

In June, 1967, he underwent a right heart catheterization, which revealed normal pressures and no oxygen step-up. Pulmonary arterial and right ventricular cineangiograms revealed no flow to the basal segments of the left lower lobe during the pulmonary phase, but during the systemic arterial phase, there was opacification of the left lower lobe. An aortogram established the presence of a large vessel arising from the descending thoracic aorta and supplying the left lower lobe. Bronchoscopy was normal. Bronchograms showed that branches of the left lower lobe bronchi were more slender, spread out, and with fewer branches than usual.

On September 25, 1967, he underwent a left posterolateral thoracotomy through the sixth intercostal space. An anomalous vessel was found arising from the descending thoracic aorta at about the level of the sixth vertebral body. The vessel entered the hilum of the left lung and thence into the left lower lobe. There was a vibrant thrill in the vessel through all phases of the cardiac cycle. At its origin, the vessel was 7 to 8 mm. in diameter, but just beyond this site, it dilated to about 15 mm. The left pulmonary artery was 10 to 12 mm. in diameter and appeared to supply only the left upper lobe. There were no other arteries to the left lung.

The left inferior pulmonary vein was very large. The left lower lobe felt heavy but contained no masses. It ventilated well. The visceral pleura of the left lower lobe was covered with many spider telangiectases.

The anomalous vessel was transected at its origin and the proximal end oversewed. It was then possible to bring the free end of the vessel up through a cleft in the hilum, to the anteroinferior surface of the left pulmonary artery, to which it was anastomosed, end to side. The patient made an uncomplicated recovery.

The patient was re-evaluated in January, 1968, at which time he was asymptomatic. There was no cyanosis and no murmurs could be heard. The chest x-ray and electrocardiogram were now normal. Again, right heart catheterization revealed normal pressures with no oxygen step-up. A pulmonary cinearteriogram now revealed normal flow into the left lower lobe. The arterial blood was 95 percent saturated on room air. Bronchograms were now normal.

ANATOMIC RELATIONS

The most striking feature was the balloon-like expansion of the artery to the left lower lobe as it arose from the anterior surface of the aorta about the level of the sixth thoracic vertebra. Fig. 1 is a colored print of the photograph made at the operating table after the left lung had been elevated to expose the aorta. Fig. 2 identifies the structures shown in the photograph. Fig. 3 indi-

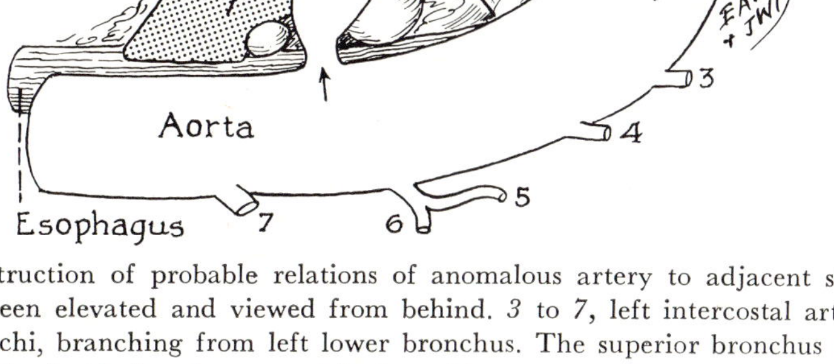

Fig. 3. Reconstruction of probable relations of anomalous artery to adjacent structures after left lung has been elevated and viewed from behind. *3* to *7*, left intercostal arteries; *7* to *10*, segmental bronchi, branching from left lower bronchus. The superior bronchus (No. 6) is not numbered, but lies just below the upper lobe bronchi.

cates the probable relation of this artery to adjacent structures and to other parts of the left lung when that organ was elevated to expose the aorta (compare Boyden[3] Fig. 102 and Plate 7). In 19.3 percent of 150 specimens, according to Cauldwell and associates,[8] a left bronchial artery can arise at as low a level as the seventh thoracic vertebra (see also Liebow's[19] Fig. 1). In our patient the systemic artery that supplied the left lower lobe arose somewhat higher and had no esophageal branches. It entered the lung within the territory of the left hilum (Fig. 3) and was superior in level to the inferior pulmonary vein. Just its position, therefore, and the fact that no other systemic artery was observed in this region raises the question as to whether this was not an enlarged bronchial artery. The solution is not a simple one. Perhaps the answer is to be found in the case history of a young woman of Breslau who was born without pulmonary arteries, who died of a cerebral hemorrhage at the age of 18, and whose lungs were meticulously dissected 50 years ago by a conscientious "Assistant" in pathology[14] (see Embryological interpretation).

SURGICAL TREATMENT

The operative procedure, as carried out by one of us (L. R. S.), was as follows: The "anomalous" artery was transected at its origin and the defect in the aorta closed. Its proximal end was then brought up through the hilum from the aorta (X^1, Fig. 4) and sutured to the inferior side of the left pulmonary artery (X^2, Fig. 4). Fig. 5 is a tracing of a Kodachrome taken at the end of the operation, showing where this anomalous artery was sutured to the left pulmonary artery—namely, at a level just deep to the retracted left superior pulmonary vein. Thus, the normal relations of pulmonary arteries to the left upper and lower lobes were completely restored.

Within four months or less, the patient had made a satisfactory recovery. As revealed by a pulmonary cinearteriogram, the flow into the left lower lobe was normal. The patient's arterial blood was shown to be 95 percent saturated in room air. Bronchograms made before the operation showed that at that time the left lower lobe bronchi were more widely spread and slenderer than normal, possibly as a result of contact with the high pressure arteries paralleling them.

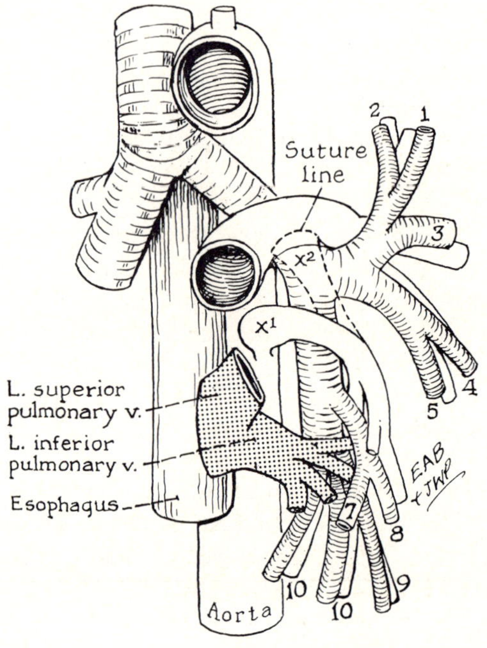

Fig. 4. Reconstruction of mediastinal view of root of left lung showing position of anomalous artery (X^1) before it was pulled up through the hilum and anastomosed (X^2) to the base of the left upper lobe pulmonary artery just before it arched over the left bronchus.

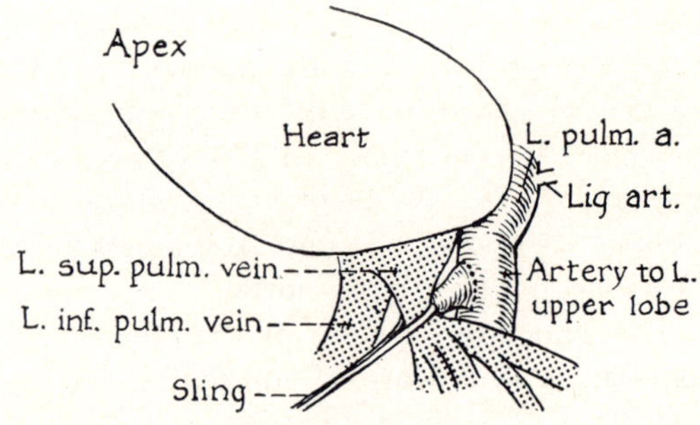

Fig. 5. Tracing of a Kodachrome, taken at end of operation, showing site of anastomosis from above. Note that the anomalous artery lies immediately deep to the left superior pulmonary vein.

Postoperatively, more of the lower lobe bronchi were visible and these showed an increase in diameter.

EMBRYOLOGICAL INTERPRETATION

The anomalous artery in this patient presents a rare example of a systemic artery arising high on the aorta, at the site of a bronchial artery, which in a period of 6½ years or less—and in the absence of the usual pulmonary artery—had induced a left ventricular hypertrophy but had failed to damage irreversibly, if at all, the respiratory tissue supplied by it.

Little is known about the origin of bronchial arteries beyond the fact that about 28 to 30 days after ovulation, in human embryos 4 to 5 mm. long, the common visceral plexus around the rudimentary lung buds is fed both by right and left "pulmonary" channels from the sixth aortic arches and by minute "systemic" channels descending around the esophagus into this plexus from the right and left dorsal aortae (compare Tobin,[25] Fig. 1). Supposedly, some of these minute systemic vessels become the stems of the future bronchial arteries; but the subsequent development of such vessels or their relation to the pulmonary arteries in successive stages has never been charted.* In microscopic sections of the lungs of 41, 118 and 140 mm. fetuses in our possession, the *bronchial* arterial system, if it exists at all as such, consists only of a minute capillary network closely investing the bronchi. Also, since this is connected to the more eccentrically placed pulmonary arteries by minute branches, it is even possible that much of the bronchial arterial system itself may develop in situ as offshoots of the pulmonary arterial plexus and later re-establish its connection with the aorta.

The *pulmonary* plexus of the embryo, by contrast, is a network of substantial arteries which, at first, forms a loose plexus about the growing bronchi. By the fortieth day after ovulation, this plexus has differentiated into definitive segmental arteries and their branches (see Wells and Boyden,[29] Plate 4). At this time, the bronchial system of vessels in the lung is almost invisible.

One way in which a portion of the pulmonary circulation may be taken over by a systemic artery was demonstrated by a 41 mm. human embryo in the Carnegie Collection which was "caught in the act."[4] An artery arose from the aorta just below the diaphragm, then passed up through the pulmonary ligament into the lung, and dropped down along the bronchi of the posterior basal segment to their terminations. (A similar case, in an adult, is shown in Boyden's[3] Fig. 120). Because this artery originated just above the celiac artery—and the latter had recently descended from a position high up in the "neck" region of the embryo—it was evident that the systemic artery, also, must have arisen in the neck. (For an account of this normal migration of visceral arteries, which takes place between the 5 and 19 mm. stages, see Evans,[11] p. 646 and Fig. 648). Significantly, the branches of this systemic artery differed in no way from the branches of the pulmonary arteries that supplied the rest of that lung.[4]

In the present case, the systemic artery to the left basal segments—if it were of the sort just described—did not descend but remained high up in the thorax. Therefore, it must have arisen from a left aortic arch above the zone from which arteries descend. Instances in which a systemic artery flows directly into a true pulmonary artery are not rare. Fraentzel's[14] case (Fig. 6) is one of the earliest. Here the dropping out of the proximal portion of a right pulmonary artery—together with the persistence of a right aortic arch, a right ductus arteriosus, and the distal portion of the right pulmonary artery—resulted in the transfer of aortic blood *directly* into the original pulmonary artery of the right lung. This flow continued from birth until the death of the patient from a cerebral abscess, at the age

*Wagenvoort and Wagenvoort[28] found 12 cases of anastomotic connections between bronchial and pulmonary arteries—some of large caliber—in 24 normal human fetuses and infants; but since these were found in sectioned blocks of tissue, information about their topographic relations is minimal.

Fig. 6

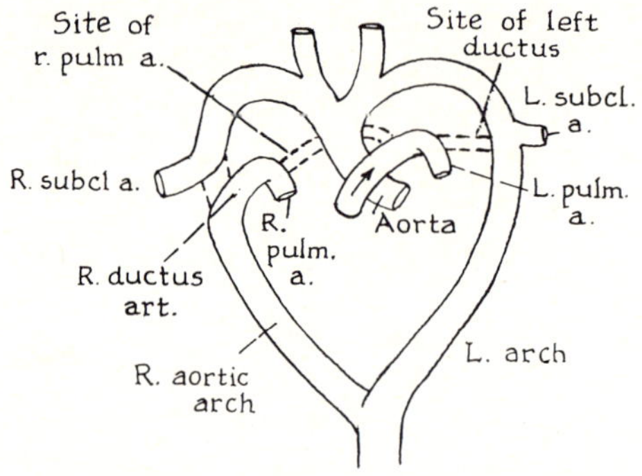

Fig. 7

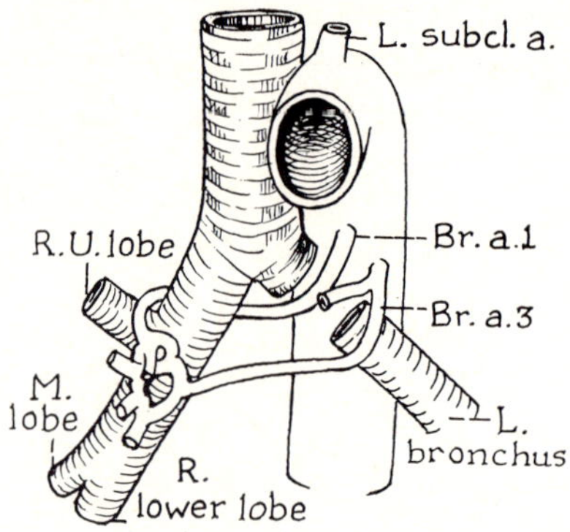

Fig. 6. Fraentzel's[14] case, in a 25-year-old servant maid who died of a cerebral abscess. The figure is after a diagram of Brenner's.[5] It illustrates the persistence of the right ductus arteriosus and the dropping out of the proximal portion of the right pulmonary artery—as a result of which pulmonary arteries of the right lung were perfused with oxygenated blood through a persisting right aortic arch, right ductus arteriosus, and distal stem of the right pulmonary artery.

Fig. 7. The bronchial arteries in Hülse's[16] case stuudy of an 18-year-old girl with persistent truncus arteriosus. This has been reconstructed by the writer from Hülse's precise account of his dissection of the lungs at autopsy. *Br.a.1,* bronchial artery to upper hilum of right lung; *Br.a.3,* bronchial artery to lower hilum of right lung. Note plexus between them. The branch between *1* and *3* is the bronchial artery to the left lung.

of 25. (Under such circumstances the artery may have become muscular.[26])

A second way in which a lobar pulmonary artery could have been taken over by a systemic artery is for it to have been tapped by a bronchial artery. An example of this is provided by Hülse's[16] case of a persistent truncus arteriosus in an 18-year-old girl. The patient had died of a cerebral hemorrhage. The pathologist had very carefully dissected the lungs. With the help of his sketch of the heart and his description, a reconstruction of the bronchial arteries has been made (Fig. 7).* The case is much like that of Edwards' Type 4 truncus (Fig. 1d, p. 112[10]). The definitive pulmonary arteries were entirely absent, the two ventricles communicated, and there was no conus arteriosus. Consequently, the lungs were supplied exclusively by two branches of the descending aorta. The most significant feature was a hilar arterial plexus interposed between the two aortic arteries to the right lung and the segmental arteries that followed the bronchi into the parenchyma. Because of this interposed barrier, it is suggested that the aortic branches entering the plexus were true bronchial arteries.

Indirect evidence for this is supplied by the experiments of Liebow and his colleagues[2, 20, 21] in ligating the pulmonary artery in newborn puppies and then letting them live for some 12 to 20 weeks. These authors noted that such lungs can maintain respiratory function while gradually increasing in size over a period of months. In summarizing his later work with rats, Liebow[18] shows how function was restored, namely, through penetration of the thick walls of the ligated pulmonary artery by the solid growing ends of the bronchial arteries.

That this was not the explanation in our case is suggested by the arteriograms. In the postoperative arteriogram, there is no suggestion of a network intervening between the sutured lower lobe artery and the segmental branches to the left lower lobe. The preoperative machine-like murmur can be explained, not by the obstruction of an intervening network, but by the narrow origin

*Feller's[12] diagram of this case, interpreting the truncus as continuing into a right aortic arch, is questionable. The present writer has redrawn it as a left arch (Fig. 7) in accordance with the author's description.

of this artery from the aorta and the resulting turbulence in the succeeding segment.

Therefore, it would seem that the anomalous artery in our patient is not a bronchial artery that had tapped the lower lobe arterial plexus but a high systemic artery that had retained its original embryonic connection with both the aorta and the pulmonary plexus. If so, it may be the first to have been shown to have arisen *above* the level from which celiac arteries descend into the lower thorax. Why didn't it become a bronchial artery? This leaves unanswered the question as to when and how bronchial arteries arise. (See Addendum.)

SURGICAL CONCLUSION

When surgical intervention is indicated, what is done should depend on the pulmonary findings. If the pulmonary tissue is severely diseased, it should be excised. If the pulmonary tissue is normal and has a normal pulmonary artery supply, the situation can be handled by merely ligating the anomalous systemic vessel, as one would do for a patent ductus arteriosus.[6, 9, 22] When one is dealing with what appears to be normal pulmonary tissue with a systemic origin of its pulmonary artery (i.e., no normal pulmonary arterial supply), the situation might be returned to normal by transferring the origin of the anomalous vessel to the side of the normal pulmonary artery that supplies the other lung or lobes. This approach was first suggested by Maier[22] in 1954, first successfully applied by Armer and associates[1] in 1961, and since that time reported by a number of other groups.[7] To our knowledge, our case is the first one in which such a transfer of a *lobar* artery of systemic origin was performed. This approach demands that the procedure be technically feasible, that the lung involved is relatively normal, and that the anomalous artery will function physiologically as a pulmonary artery (i.e., will distribute the blood near alveoli to permit gas exchange). That the latter assumption was valid in our case was supported by the fact that the postoperative pulmonary arteriogram showed perfusion of the left lower lobe, and yet there was no evidence of right-to-left shunting. The definitive evaluation of this fact awaits lobar bronchospirometry which cannot be accomplished yet because of the patient's size.

ADDENDUM

See article in press by E. A. Boyden, Anatomical Record, 1970, entitled "The time lag in the development of bronchial arteries."

REFERENCES

1. Armer, R. M., Schumacker, H. B., and Klatte, E. C.: Origin of the right pulmonary artery from the ascending aorta, Circulation **24:** 662, 1961.
2. Bloomer, W. E., Harrison, W., Lindskog, G. E., and Liebow, A. A.: Respiratory function and blood flow in the bronchial artery after ligation of the pulmonary artery, Amer. J. Physiol. **157:** 317, 1949.
3. Boyden, E. A.: Segmental anatomy of the lungs, New York, 1955, McGraw-Hill Book Company, Inc.
4. Boyden, E. A.: Bronchogenic cysts and the theory of intralobar sequestration: New embryologic data, J. Thorac. Surg. **35:** 604, 1958.
5. Brenner, F.: Ueber Defekte der rechten Lungenschlagader, Virchow Arch. Path. Anat. **298:** 394, 1936.
6. Campbell, D. C., Murney, J. A., and Dominy, D. E.: Systemic arterial blood supply to a normal lung, J. A. M. A. **182:** 497, 1962.
7. Caudill, D. R., Helmsworth, J. A., Daoud, G., and Kaplan, S.: Anomalous origin of left pulmonary artery from ascending aorta, J. Thorac. Cardiov. Surg. **57:** 493, 1969.
8. Cauldwell, E. W., Siekert, R. G., Lininger, R. E., and Anson, B. J.: The bronchial arteries. An anatomic study of 150 human cadavers, Surg. Gynec. Obstet. **86:** 395, 1948.
9. Cole, F. H., Alley, F. H., and Jones, R. S.: Aberrant systemic arteries to the lower lung, Surg. Gynec. Obstet. **93:** 589, 1951.
10. Edwards, J. E., Dry, T. J., Parker, R. L., Burchell, H. B., Wood, E. H., and Bulbanian, A. H.: An atlas of congenital anomalies of the heart and great vessels, Springfield, Ill., 1954, Charles C Thomas, Publisher.
11. Evans, H. M.: The development of the vascular system, II, *in* Keibel and Mall: Manual of human embryology, Philadelphia, 1912. J. B. Lippincott Company, pp. 570-709, Plate 48.
12. Feller, A.: Zur Kenntnis der angeborenen Herzkrankheiten. I. Mitteilung. Truncus ar-

teriosus communis persistens und seiner formale Enstehung, Virchow Arch. Path. Anat. **279:** 869, 1931.
13. Findlay, C. W., and Maier, H. C.: Anomalies of pulmonary vessels and their surgical significance, SURGERY **29:** 604, 1951.
14. Fraentzel, O.: Ein Fall von abnormer Communication der Aorta mit der Arteria pulmonalis, Virchow Arch. Path. Anat. **48:** 420, 1868.
15. Hayek, H. v.: Ueber ein Kurzschlusskreislauf (arterio-venöse Anastomosen) in der menschlichen Lunge, Z. Anat. Entwicklungsgesch. **110:** 412, 1940.
16. Hülse, W.: Beitrag zur Kenntnis der totalen Persistenz des Truncus arteriosus communis, Virchow Arch. Path. Anat. **225:** 16, 1918.
17. Hyrtl, J.: Venen-Varietäten, Med. Jahrb. Österr. St., N.F. **18:** 3, 1839.
18. Liebow, A. A.: Recent observations on pulmonary collateral circulation, Med. Thorac. **19:** 609, 1962.
19. Liebow, A. A.: Patterns of origin and distribution of the major bronchial arteries in man, Amer. J. Anat. **117:** 19, 1965.
20. Liebow, A. A., Hales, M. R., and Lindskog, G. E.: Enlargement of the bronchial arteries and their anastomoses with the pulmonary arteries in bronchiectasis, Amer. J. Path. **25:** 211, 1949.
21. Liebow, A. A., Harrison, W., and Hales, M. R.: Experimental pulmonic stenosis, Bull. Int. Ass. Med. Museums **31:** 1, 1950.
22. Maier, H. C.: Absence or hypoplasia of a pulmonary artery with anomalous systemic arteries to the lung, J. Thorac. Surg. **28:** 145, 1954.
23. McCotter, R. E.: On the occurrence of pulmonary arteries arising from the thoracic aorta, Anat. Rec. **4:** 291, 1910.
24. Sherrick, D. W., Kincaid, O. W., and Dushane, J. W.: Agenesis of a main branch of the pulmonary artery, Amer. J. Roentgen. **87:** 917, 1962.
25. Tobin, C. E.: The bronchial arteries and their connections with other vessels in the human lung, Surg. Gynec. Obstet. **95:** 741, 1952.
26. Valenzuela, C. T., Toriello, J., and Thomas, W. A.: Structural changes in intrapulmonary arteries exposed to systemic pressures from birth, Arch. Path. **57:** 51, 1954.
27. Verloop, M. C.: The arteriae bronchioles and their anastomoses with the arteriae pulmonales, Acta Anat. **5:** 171, 1948.
28. Wagenvoort, C. A., and Wagenvoort, N.: Arterial anastomoses, bronchopulmonary arteries, and pulmobronchial arteries in perinatal lungs, Lab. Invest. **16:** 13, 1967.
29. Wells, L. J., and Boyden, E. A.: The development of the bronchopulmonary segments in human embryos of horizons XVII to XIX, Amer. J. Anat. **95:** 163, 1954.

Pulmonary resection for massive hemoptysis

ANTONIO A. GARZON, M.D.
MARCIAL CERRUTI, M.D.
ANATOLE GOURIN, M.D.
KARL E. KARLSON, M.D.
BROOKLYN, N. Y.
From the Department of Surgery, Downstate Medical Center and Kings County Hospital

Massive hemoptysis is a life-threatening complication of several cardiopulmonary diseases. Hemoptysis has usually been treated nonoperatively, and surgical intervention has been reserved for those who fail to stop bleeding.[1, 11] It is difficult to evaluate published results of therapy because many reports make no clear distinction between massive and small amounts of blood loss. Massive hemoptysis has been defined previously as pulmonary bleeding of more than 600 ml. in a period of 48 hours.[2, 3, 7] The mortality rate for massive hemoptysis treated nonoperatively has been more than 50 percent in our institution.[2] However, when the mortality rate for nonoperative treatment was correlated with the rate of bleeding, it was found to be 78 percent in those patients bleeding 600 ml. or more in 16 hours. On the contrary, the mortality rate among those patients who required more than 16 hours to accumulate 600 ml. of blood loss was negligible. Therefore, we have redefined massive hemoptysis as 600 ml. within a period of 24 hours. Four years ago, we started to perform emergency pulmonary resection for hemoptysis of 600 ml. or more in 24 hours. This report deals with our experience.

MATERIALS AND METHODS

This series includes 35 patients, five women and 30 men, ages 20 to 64 years. Twenty-nine were bleeding actively at the time of operation. The other six had stopped bleeding at the time of pulmonary resection. Twenty-seven were bleeding from tuberculous lesions. Of these, 19 had acid-fast bacilli in the sputum cultures or in the resected specimens. Three patients were bleeding from bronchiectasis, three from lung abscesses, one from actinomycosis, and one from a bronchogenic carcinoma (Table I).

The designation of hemoptysis as massive was made by two attending physicians. Chest roentgenograms and pulmonary function tests, including vital capacity, forced expiratory volume, and maximum voluntary ventilation, were performed at the bedside in many cases. Surgeons were called in consultation, and emergency bronchoscopy was performed under topical anesthesia during bleeding to determine precisely the source of the hemorrhage.

All patients with massive hemoptysis were evaluated and classified into inoperable and operable groups. The criteria for inoperability were (1) bilateral far-advanced pulmonary disease with inability to localize the site of bleeding by bronchoscopy, (2) inoperable bronchogenic carcinoma with distant metastases, (3) vital capacity of less than 40 percent of predicted and/or a forced expiratory volume of less than 40 percent in the first second. A few patients in the operable group did not undergo operation because either the patient or his attending physician refused surgical intervention. However, the

Received for publication June 4, 1969.

majority of the patients with massive hemoptysis who were considered operable were resected.

Seven patients with acid-fast bacilli in the sputum had no effective antituberculosis therapy before resection. The remainder of the patients with acid-fast bacilli in sputum or resected specimens had received at least 2 weeks of adequate antimicrobial therapy.

Early in our experience, anesthesia was carried out with a bronchospirometric Carlens tube in place. However, in view of difficulties keeping the small lumina of Carlens tubes free of blood, a standard single lumen endotracheal tube was utilized in our later experience. To avoid airway obstruction by the blood, the bleeding bronchus was occluded frequently with an intraluminal blocker or the endotracheal tube was introduced into the contralateral bronchus.

Twenty-four lobectomies and 11 pneumonectomies were performed (Table II). Thirteen lobectomies were performed in patients with active tuberculosis. All of them were bleeding at the time of the emergency operation. Another six lobectomies were performed in patients with previous histories of tuberculosis and obvious tuberculous lesions in whom tubercle bacilli could not be demonstrated; all but one of these patients had emergency resections while bleeding. Five emergency lobectomies were performed for bronchiectasis and lung abscess.

Six pneumonectomies were performed in the face of active tuberculosis, four during bleeding. Two pneumonectomies were in patients with inactive tuberculosis, one while the patient was bleeding. One pneumonectomy was performed for lung abscess (actively bleeding), actinomyocosis, and bronchogenic carcinoma.

Table I. *Pulmonary resections for massive hemoptysis*

Diagnosis	*No. of patients*	
Tuberculosis		
Active	19	(17)*
Inactive	8	(6)
Bronchiectasis	3	(3)
Lung abscess	3	(3)
Actinomycosis	1	
Bronchogenic carcinoma	1	
	35	(29)

*The numbers in parentheses indicate the number of patients who were bleeding at the time of resection.

RESULTS

Lobectomy for active tuberculosis (Tables III and IV). In the 15 patients with active tuberculosis, four patients required tracheostomy for bleeding before the resection. There were three cases of aspiration pneumonitis. Two patients developed postoperative apical spaces which resolved without thoracoplasty.

Table II. *Pulmonary resections for massive hemoptysis: Type of operation and number of deaths (35 patients)*

	Lobectomy			*Pneumonectomy*		
		No. of deaths			*No. of deaths*	
Diagnosis	*No. of resections*	*Operative*	*Late*	*No. of resections*	*Operative*	*Late*
Tuberculosis						
Active	13 (13)*			6 (4)	1 (1)	1 (1)
Inactive	6 (5)		2 (2)	2 (1)	1 (1)	
Bronchiectasis	3 (3)	1 (1)				
Lung abscess	2 (2)			1 (1)	1 (1)	
Actinomycosis				1		
Bronchogenic carcinoma				1		
Totals	24 (23)	1 (1)	2 (2)	11 (6)	3 (3)	1 (1)

*The numbers in parentheses indicate the number of patients who had emergency resection during a massive bleeding episode.

Bronchopleural fistulas with localized empyema occurred in three patients. To close the fistulas, tailoring thoracoplasties were performed. There were no deaths in this group. All of the patients have been discharged from the hospital with their tuberculosis arrested.

Lobectomy for inactive tuberculosis. Four lobectomies were performed in patients with a history of tuberculosis but in whom no acid-fast bacilli could be demonstrated at the time of resection. One required tracheostomy before the resection to maintain the airway. Two patients had a postoperative apical space which closed spontaneously. Two developed bronchopleural fistulas; one of these patients required thoracoplasty. Two patients died in the postoperative period. One patient died 18 days after lobectomy. Postmortem examination showed small patchy areas of pneumonitis and severe fatty liver; the cause of the death was considered to be liver failure. The other patient died 4 months after operation with a bronchopleural fistula, localized empyema, and respiratory failure.

Lobectomy for bronchiectasis or lung abscess. In five patients with bronchiectasis or lung abscess, two required tracheostomies before operation; two developed aspiration pneumonitis; one had an apical space that closed spontaneously. One patient with bronchiectasis died within 24 hours of an emergency lobectomy for massive bleeding.

Table III. *Pumonary resections for massive hemoptysis: Cause of death (7 patients)*

Diagnosis	*Emergency operation*	*Cause of death*
1. Active tuberculosis	Pneumonectomy	Operative bleeding and aspiration
2. Active tuberculosis	Pneumonectomy	Bronchopleural fistula and empyema (postoperative day 38)
3. Inactive tuberculosis	Pneumonectomy	Operative aspiration and asphyxia
4. Inactive tuberculosis	Lobectomy (left upper lobe)	Delirium tremens, liver failure (postoperative day 18)
5. Lung abscess	Pneumonectomy	Operative bleeding and aspiration
6. Inactive tuberculosis	Lobectomy (right upper and middle)	Bronchopleural fistula, empyema, respiratory failure (fourth month after operation)
7. Bronchiectasis	Lobectomy (right lower lobe)	Respiratory failure (postoperative day 1)

Table IV. *Pulmonary resections for massive hemoptysis: Complications following lobectomy*

Diagnosis	*No. of patients*	*No. of patients with complications*	*Aspiration*	*Tracheostomy*	*Apical space*	*Bronchopleural fistula*	*Thoracoplasty*
Tuberculosis							
Active	13 (13)*	7 (7)	3 (3)	4 (4)	2 (2)	3 (3)	3 (3)
Inactive	6 (5)	3 (2)	2 (1)	1 (1)	1 (1)	2 (2)	1 (1)
Bronchiectasis	3 (3)	3 (3)	2 (2)	2 (2)	1 (1)		
Lung abscess	2 (2)	1 (1)			1 (1)		
Totals	24 (23)	14 (13)	7 (6)	7 (7)	5 (5)	5 (5)	4 (4)

*The numbers in parentheses indicate the number of patients who had emergency resection during a massive bleeding episode.

Table V. *Pulmonary resections for massive hemoptysis: Complications following pneumonectomy*

Diagnosis	*No. of patients*	*No. of patients with complications*	*Aspiration*	*Tracheostomy*	*Broncho-pleural fistula and empyema*	*Thoraco-plasty*
Tuberculosis						
Active	6 (4)*	2 (2)		2 (1)	1 (1)	(1)
Inactive	2 (1)	1	1	1		
Lung abscess	1 (1)					
Actinomycosis	1					
Bronchogenic carcinoma	1					
Totals	11 (6)	3 (2)	1	3 (1)	1 (1)	(1)

*The numbers in parentheses indicate the number of patients who had emergency resection during a massive bleeding episode.

The apparent cause of the death was respiratory failure. No pulmonary function tests had been performed preoperatively.

Pneumonectomy group (Tables III and V). Three patients required tracheostomy preoperatively to clear the tracheobronchial tree of blood. One patient with inactive tuberculosis developed a contralateral aspiration pneumonitis. There were three early operative deaths and one late death. One patient with tuberculosis and a destroyed lung suffered cardiac arrest during the induction of anesthesia. He was resuscitated and a pneumonectomy was performed, but he died on the operating table. Another patient with active tuberculosis had massive bronchial aspiration on the operating table and died before the operation could be finished. A patient with a lung abscess died during the operation, apparently from massive blood loss. One patient with a destroyed lung and sputum positive for tubercle bacilli had an emergency pneumonectomy. He developed a bronchopleural fistula, and a thoracoplasty was performed 20 days following the pneumonectomy. On the thirty-sixth postoperative day, he exsanguinated through the pleural drainage tube, bleeding from erosion of the pulmonary artery stump.

DISCUSSION

A number of reports have been published on the surgical treatment of massive hemoptysis,[5, 6, 8, 9] most concerned with single cases. More recently, reports involving series of patients have appeared. Some papers do not mention the amount of bleeding or the relationship of bleeding to the operative procedure.[4, 10]

Yeoh and associates[11] reported recently their surgical experience with massive hemoptysis in patients with pulmonary tuberculosis. They defined massive hemoptysis as loss of more than 200 ml. a day at least once during hospitalization. Surgical resection was performed when nonoperative treatment failed to control the bleeding. There were 11 lobectomies and two pneumonectomies. Postoperatively, three patients had roentgenologic evidence of bronchogenic spread of tuberculosis or aspiration pneumonia. One patient developed respiratory insufficiency. Two patients died. Amirana and associates[1] defined significant hemoptysis as 100 ml. or more per day in the hospital. In a selected group of these patients, they performed 15 resections without a death.

Because these operations are performed to arrest hemorrhage and prevent asphyxiation, details of technique in localizing the site of bleeding and assuring an airway are important. Localizing the bleeding was always done by bronchoscopy. When massive bleeding persisted during bronchoscopy, it was occasionally difficult to determine the exact source of bleeding. An inflatable rubber balloon at the end of the bronchoscope was used to isolate portions of the bronchial tree and to help locate the bleeding. This technique may also have saved the life of some patients by maintaining a dry airway to one lung during the massive bleeding episode. Usually, the bleeding during bronchoscopy subsided sufficiently to prepare the operating room for pulmonary resection. In a few instances, when the bleeding did not decrease, emergency bronchial blockage was utilized, the patient was transferred to the operating room, and the resection was performed with the airway to the site of bleeding blocked. A Fogarty catheter has been found to be an effective bronchial blocker because it can be introduced easily through the bronchoscope and inflated when in position. Tracheostomy had to be performed in several instances during bronchoscopy to maintain the airway clear of blood.

At the present time, we favor the blockage of the bleeding bronchus during bronchoscopy when massive bleeding occurs, introduction of an endotracheal tube, and immediate pulmonary resection. All of our resections were performed in a standard lateral position. Early in our experience we used Carlens tubes during anesthesia to protect the nonbleeding lung from aspiration, but these tubes did not work well in our hands. The lumina are too small to allow rapid aspiration of blood; this blood frequently accumulated on the bleeding side and leaked over to the contralateral side, creating a difficult aspiration problem. If bronchial blockage was not done, it was more satisfactory to introduce a regular single lumen endotracheal tube into the main bronchus of the nonbleeding lung and ventilate this lung alone until the bleeding bronchus was surgically occluded with a clamp.

The etiology of the lesion producing the bleeding or the activity of the tuberculosis at the time of resection did not influence the mortality rate. The incidence of aspiration pneumonia or the need of tracheostomy for bleeding was not related, either, to the etiology of tuberculosis. However, no bronchopleural fistulas were observed in patients requiring resection for nontuberculous lesions. The main factors which seem to influence the mortality rate were the extent of the pathologic process and the magnitude of the resection. In 24 lobectomies, 23 of them performed during active bleeding, there were only three deaths, and two of them were due to late complications. In 11 pneumonectomies, six of them performed while the patient was bleeding, three deaths occurred at the time of resection.

SUMMARY AND CONCLUSIONS

1. Thirty-five patients (24 lobectomies and 11 pneumonectomies) had pulmonary resection for massive hemoptysis. Twenty-nine resections were performed during the period of active bleeding and the remainder within 72 hours.

2. There were three deaths in the lobectomy group (13 percent) and four in the pneumonectomy group (36 percent). The combined mortality rate was 17 percent. This may be compared to a mortality rate of more than 50 percent in similar patients treated nonoperatively.

3. Our experience indicates that when the site of the massive bleeding can be resected by lobectomy, pulmonary resection is the treatment of choice for massive hemoptysis. Lesions requiring pneumonectomy should be treated nonoperatively until the risk of surgical intervention is clearly indicated to be lower than the risk of continuing hemorrhage.

REFERENCES

1. Amirana, M., Frater, R., Tirschwell, P., Janis, M., Bloomberg, A., and State, D.: An aggressive surgical approach to significant hemoptysis in patients with pulmonary tuberculosis, Amer. Rev. Resp. Dis. **197:** 187, 1968.
2. Crocco, J. A., Rooney, J. J., Fankushen, D. S., DiBenedetto, R. J., and Lyons, H. A.: Massive hemoptysis, Arch. Intern. Med. **121:** 495, 1968.
3. Ehrenhaft, J. L., and Taber, R. E.: Management of massive hemoptysis not due to pulmonary tuberculosis or neoplasm, J. Thorac. Surg. **30:** 275, 1955.
4. Epshtein, T. V.: Surgical methods in treat-

ing tuberculous patients with pulmonary hemorrhage and recurrent hemoptysis, Grudn. Khir. **5:** 60, 1965.

5. Ford, J. M., Clauss, R. H., Askari, S. A., and Wylie, R. H.: The surgical treatment of pulmonary hemorrhage in tuberculosis, J. Thorac. Surg. **35:** 341, 1958.
6. Linberg, E. J.: Emergency operation in patients with massive hemoptysis, Amer. Surg. **30:** 158, 1964.
7. Pursel, S. E., and Lindskog, G. E.: Hemoptysis: A clinical evaluation of 103 patients examined consecutively on a thoracic surgical service, Amer. Rev. Resp. Dis. **84:** 329, 1961.
8. Ross, C. A.: Emergency resection for massive hemoptysis in tuberculosis, J. Thorac. Surg. **26:** 435, 1953.
9. Ryan, T. C., and Lineberry, W. T., Jr.: Pneumonectomy for pulmonary hemorrhage in tuberculosis, Amer. Rev. Tuberc. **61:** 426, 1950.
10. Rzepecki, W., and Badmajew, P.: Hemorrhage in tuberculosis as an urgent indication for resection of pulmonary tissue, Dis. Chest **41:** 372, 1962.
11. Yeoh, C. B., Hubaytar, R. T., Ford, J. M., and Wylie, R. H.: Treatment of massive hemorrhage in pulmonary tuberculosis, J. Thorac. Cardiov. Surg. **54:** 503, 1967.

Recurrent pulmonary emboli following inferior vena caval plication

G. A. E. COUPLAND, M.B., F.R.A.C.S.
T. S. REEVE, M.B., F.A.C.S., F.R.A.C.S.
SYDNEY, AUSTRALIA
From the Department of Surgery, The University of Sydney at The Royal North Shore Hospital of Sydney

Recurrent pulmonary embolism may occur following ligation of the inferior vena cava, via collateral circulation in the gonadal and ileolumbar veins.[1, 2] Similar pathways may conduct emboli after inferior vena caval plication when thrombosis occurs at the site of caval plication. Patients with a patent inferior vena caval plication may complain of symptoms consistent with recurrent pulmonary emboli; the interpretation of these symtoms is difficult, but it is possible that emboli may pass through the site of caval plication.

The problem of recurrent pulmonary emboli after inferior vena caval plication has been studied in sheep and is the subject of this report. The aim of the study was (1) to determine if thrombosis at the site of inferior vena caval plication occurred regularly, and (2) to determine the efficiency of inferior vena caval plication in preventing an embolus from reaching the lungs.

METHOD

Nine sheep, weighing between 27 and 45 kilograms, were used. After intravenous anesthesia with Sodium Pentothal, an endotracheal tube was inserted and artificial respiration was maintained with a mechanical respirator. Anesthesia was maintained with repeated small doses of Sodium Pentothal. The right femoral vein was cannulated with a 1 mm. polythene catheter and passed into the lower inferior vena cava. Pressures were measured with a water manometer zero adjusted to the level of the inferior vena cava.

Through a right transverse muscle-splitting incision the inferior vena cava was exposed by extraperitoneal dissection. The vena cava was plicated with 4-0 Mersilene sutures placed 4 to 5 mm. apart so that each compartment would be approximately 3 mm. in diameter.

Pressure measurements were taken before clamping, after clamping, above and below the site of plication.

Immediately after the abdominal incision was closed a transfemoral inferior vena cavagram was made to demonstrate the patency of the plication. Twenty milliliters of 50 percent Hypaque was injected through the femoral vein cannula, and anteroposterior and lateral radiographs were taken. Further phlebograms were performed via femoral vein cannulation under a general anesthetic 10 days and 3 months after caval plication.

The first sheep was killed at the end of the first experiment to demonstrate that the operative technique resulted in 3 mm. compartments at the site of caval plication. The remaining eight sheep were killed 3 months after inferior vena caval plication and the

This work has been carried out under Grant 67-746 of the Postgraduate Medical Foundation of The University of Sydney and Surgical Research Funds of The Royal North Shore Hospital of Sydney, New South Wales, Australia.
Received for publication June 2, 1969.

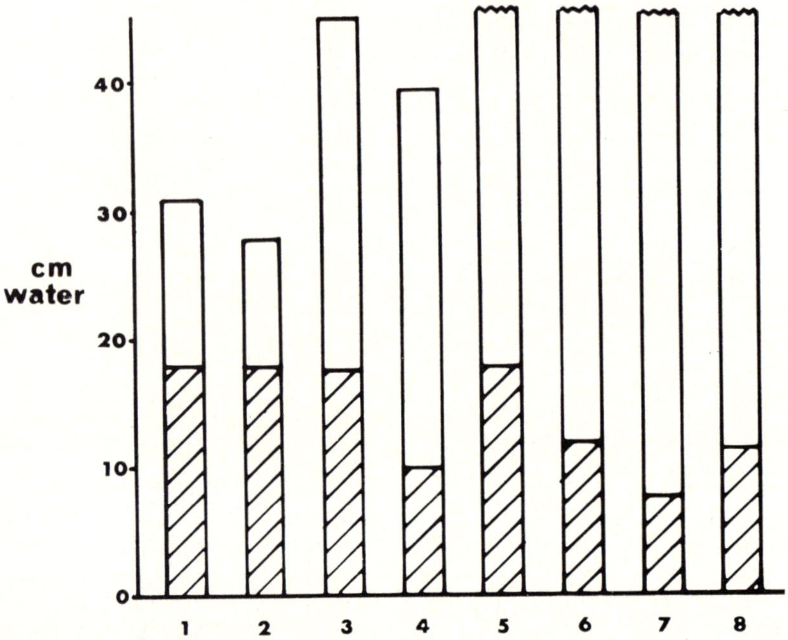

Fig. 1. Basal pressure levels in the inferior vena cava. Before clamping (cross-hatched area) and after clamping (clear area).

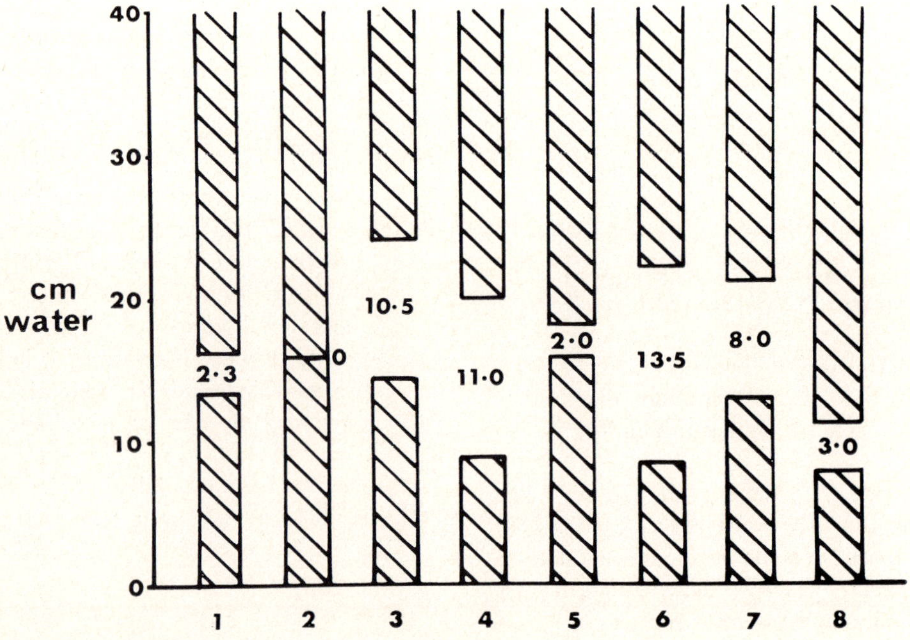

Fig. 2. Pressure gradients across vena caval plication.

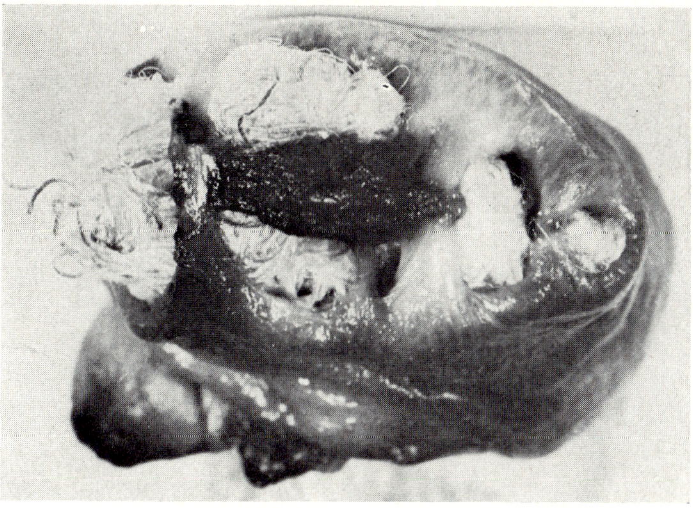

Fig. 3. Blood clot attached to the sutures in the center of the inferior vena cava.

inferior vena cava were excised and tested for patency.

RESULTS

The basal pressure levels in the inferior vena cava are shown in Fig. 1; a marked rise occurred after cross-clamping of the inferior vena cava in all cases. Pressures returned to the original level after the clamp was removed. The pressures above and below the plication were recorded and the gradient measured. The gradient was greater than 8 cm. of water in four animals (Fig. 2).

The inferior vena cava and common iliac veins were obtained when the sheep were killed. The plication from Sheep No. 1 allowed an embolus 1 cm. in diameter to pass through, but an embolus of greater diameter would not pass through. It was found that the sutures had pulled through into the center of the lumen of the vena cava thus enlarging the compartments created by the caval plication. A small amount of clot was found attached to the sutures in the center of the vena cava (Fig. 3).

In all other specimens the sutures had pulled through, enlarging the compartments. The compartments at the edge tended to become occluded while those in the center enlarged. Compartment size varied from complete occlusion to 10 mm. in diameter;

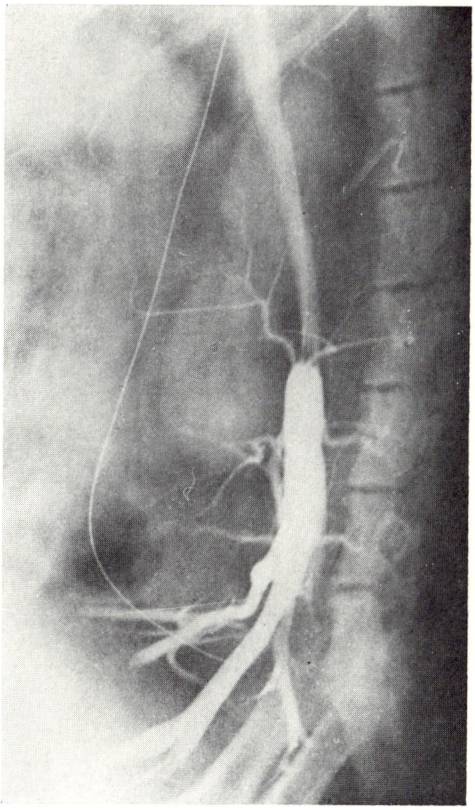

Fig. 4. Sheep No. 4, phlebogram demonstrating patency at the site of inferior vena caval plication.

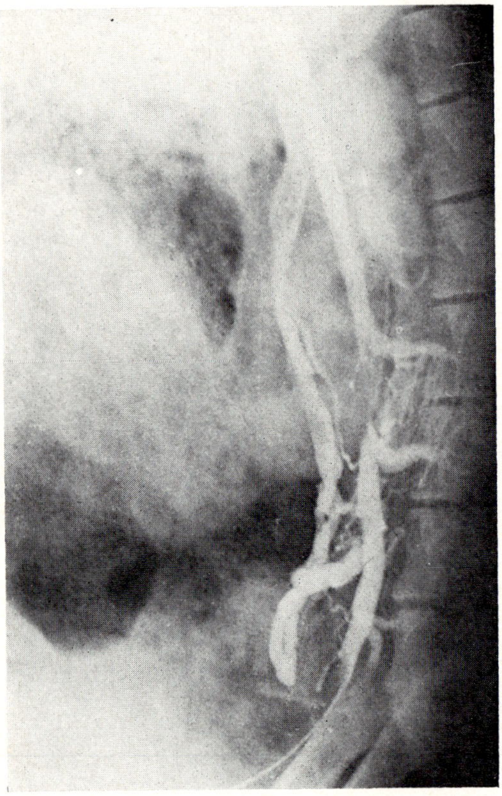

Fig. 5. Sheep No. 4, phlebogram demonstrating occlusion at the site of plication with extensive collateral circulation.

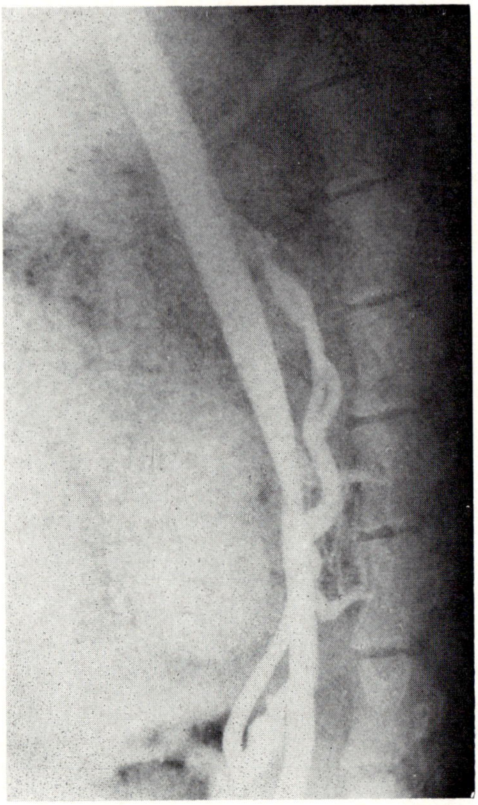

Fig. 6. Sheep No. 4, phlebogram demonstrating patency at the site of inferior vena caval plication after 3 months.

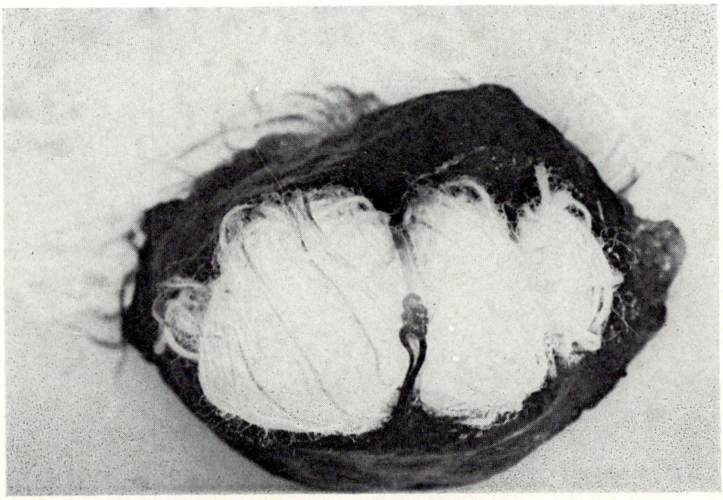

Fig. 7. Enlargement of the compartments created by inferior vena caval plication. Sutures in the center of the inferior vena cava.

in no specimen was the largest patent compartment smaller than 5 mm. in diameter.

All knots were identified and showed no evidence of unraveling. Phlebography demonstrated patency of all inferior vena caval plications immediately following operation (Fig. 4). Phlebography performed 10 days after inferior vena caval plication demonstrated that the site of plication was not patent in Sheep Nos. 4 and 8. Extensive collateral circulation was seen (Fig. 5).

Phlebography performed 3 months after inferior vena caval plication demonstrated that the site of plication was patent in all cases (Fig. 6).

Pressure recordings below the level of plication were not significantly different from those taken at the time of operation. The values for the Student's t test being: $0.1 > 2p > 0.05$ at 10 days and $0.4 > 2p > 0.3$ at 3 months.

DISCUSSION

In this study experimental animals were utilized to determine the adequacy of the suture method of plication in preventing distal emboli from reaching the lungs.

Thrombosis occurred in two sheep at 10 days as demonstrated by phlebography. Recanalization occurred in both cases and the cavae were shown to be patent. No clot was found at the plication site in these cases. The animals were not suffering from thrombotic disease as would be expected to exist in a clinical situation but the situation could be applied clinically when prophylactic inferior vena caval plication may be recommended.[3]

It has been demonstrated that the plications performed were not adequate to prevent significant embolization 3 months after plication. The process of enlargement of the compartments between the sutures occurs by the sutures pulling through into the lumen of the vena cava. A strand of endothelium accompanies the suture which is freely mobile; this allows a clot of greater diameter than the compartment to pass through (Fig. 7).

Recurrence of pulmonary emboli following inferior vena cava plication could be explained by the mechanism which has been demonstrated.

The studies also revealed that inferior vena caval plication should provide adequate protection against pulmonary embolization at the time of operation and for a limited time thereafter. Permanent protection in a clinical sense is unlikely to be provided.

SUMMARY

Nine sheep were subjected to inferior vena caval plication. In the eight sheep studied, it was demonstrated that the compartments created by the inferior vena caval plication enlarged allowing emboli of significant size to pass the plication.

The authors wish to thank Mr. R. Kearns, Wellcome Laboratories, The Royal North Shore Hospital of Sydney, for his technical assistance.

REFERENCES

1. Case Records of the Massachusetts General Hospital, Case 34, New Eng. J. Med. **227:** 360, 1967.
2. Gurewich, V., Thomas, D. P., and Rabinov, K. R.: Pulmonary embolism after ligation of the inferior vena cava, New Eng. J. Med. **274:** 1350, 1966.
3. Reeve, T. S., and Coupland, G. A. E.: Unpublished data, 1968.

Silver sulfadiazine and Sulfamylon Cream in the burned rat model: A comparative evaluation

DONALD P. DRESSLER, M.D.
WILLIAM A. SKORNIK, M.S.
CAMBRIDGE, MASS.
From the Department of Surgery, Harvard Medical School, The Cambridge Hospital, and The Holy Ghost Hospital

In 1963, Rittenbury and associates,[15] Pruitt and associates,[14] and others[13] revealed that, whereas the incidence of deaths resulting from burns had not changed appreciably over the years, the primary cause of death had shifted. The subsequent work of Teplitz,[18] describing the pathogenesis of Pseudomonas burn wound sepsis, resulted in a renewed interest in topical therapy by Moyer and co-workers,[12] Lindberg and co-workers,[10, 11] and others.[3, 4] Teplitz, using the standard Walker burned rat model,[19] demonstrated that the invasion of *Pseudomonas aeruginosa* proceeds at a known, prescribed rate, reaching 1×10^7 organisms per gram of skin within 72 hours following injury and seeding. Deaths resulting from Pseudomonas burn wound sepsis are directly related to the size of the wound and the number of bacteria in the subeschar tissue, and a topical agent must suppress the *Pseudomonas aeruginosa* bacterial count to less than 1×10^5 per gram, if deaths are to be prevented. Clinical data currently being reported show that topical therapy has resulted in a significant decrease in mortality rates. However, disadvantages of varying importance have been noted. Silver nitrate[1, 2, 12] therapy has resulted in severe electrolyte disturbances, occurrences of clostridial myositis, and increased cost of personnel and materials. In the patients treated with Sulfamylon Cream,* [3, 10, 11, 16, 20, 21] delayed eschar separation, increased insensible water loss, pain on application, and cutaneous reactions have occurred. Iatrogenic respiratory complications may also result from the use of these agents.[9]

Recently, a silver sulfadiazine ointment has been described as effective in the control of burn wound sepsis.[5-7, 17] The reported data, describing a mouse that had been burned over 30 percent of its body surface area and seeded with Pseudomonas, showed a significant discrepancy in results with Sulfamylon Cream from those being reported by other investigators using the Walker burned rat model.[19]

It was the objective of this study to compare the therapeutic effectiveness of topical silver sulfadiazine in Neobase to that of Sulfamylon Cream in the control of *Pseudomonas aeruginosa* wound sepsis in laboratory rats.

METHOD

A total of 356 female Sprague-Dawley rats were bred and raised in our facilities until the weight of each was 180 grams. They were fed Purina Rat Chow containing no antibiotics. The rats were anesthetized with an intraperitoneal injection of sodium pentobarbital (40 mg. per kilogram). The back was shaved with a No. 40 blade electric clipper and depilated. The depilatory (Nair)* was thoroughly washed off with warm water after two minutes. The animal was placed in a container designed to expose 50 cm.^{2} of the back, an area representing

Supported by National Institutes of Health Grant No. GM16210-02.
Submitted for publication June 23, 1969; resubmitted Sept. 2, 1969.

*Sulfamylon Cream (brand of mafenide) as acetate, Winthrop Laboratories, New York, N. Y.

*Carter Products, New York, N. Y.

Table I. *Experimental design of the mortality study showing the number of animals in each group*

	No treatment	*Neobase*	*Sulfamylon Cream*	*Silver sulfadiazine*	*CF 100*
Nonseeded	30	—	20	20	—
Seeded	55	45	55	50	30

Table II. *Experimental design of the bacteriology study showing the number of determinations in each group*

	No treatment	*Neobase*	*Sulfamylon Cream*	*Silver sulfadiazine*	*CF 100*
Nonseeded	5	—	5	5	—
Seeded	10	6	10	10	10

approximately 20 percent of the body surface of an 180 gram rat. The exposed back of each rat was immersed for exactly ten seconds in water maintained at 98° C. This resulted in a uniform, full-thickness burn.

Rats that were to be infected were seeded, ten minutes after scalding, by the application on the burn wound of 1 ml. of an 18 hour trypticase soy broth containing 1×10^8 organisms of *Pseudomonas aeruginosa.* All rats were weighed and placed in individual cages in an unsegregated room and given food and water ad libitum. The room was kept at constant temperature and humidity.

Topical therapy was started two hours after burning, or burning and seeding. Four agents were evaluated: (1) Neobase,* containing water, polyhydric alcohol esters, propylene glycol, liquid petrolatum, wetting agents (Aracel), and preservatives (methyl carbin); (2) Sulfamylon Cream 11.2 percent in a hydrophilic cream base; (3) silver sulfadiazine in Neobase; (4) CF 100.† The silver sulfadiazine was prepared as described by Fox and associates[5, 7] so that the final concentration was 30 millimoles per kilogram of Neobase ointment. Three grams of the agent being tested were applied daily with sterile tongue depressors. No attempt was made to wash off the previously applied agent or remove the eschar. Control animals received no topical agent. The experimental design for the mortality study is shown in Table I and for the bacteriology study in Table II. Animals were selected at random, but at least four of the experimental groups were represented at each immersion.

*Burroughs-Wellcome & Co., Tuckahoe, N. Y.
†Supplied by Dr. Charles Fox.

EVALUATION

Mortality study. Animals which lived for 21 days post burn were considered survivors; they were then put to death. Previous studies had revealed that all septic deaths occurred within this postburn period. All animals were weighed at the time of death. All results were analyzed statistically utilizing a 95 percent confidence coefficient as the criterion of significance.

Bacteriology study. Separate groups of rats were assigned to the bacteriology study. These animals were selected at random to be killed at three-day intervals post burn. Two seeded groups (untreated or treated with Neobase) survived long enough to permit representation on the first 12 days only. Animals were killed and bacteriology studies were performed 24 hours following the last treatment.

To eliminate postmortem changes which occur in the bacterial flora, blood and tissue samples were obtained while the animals were still alive. The animals were anesthetized with an intraperitoneal injection of sodium pentobarbital (40 mg. per kilogram). A 1 ml. sample of heart blood was aseptically drawn and immediately plated on blood agar. The eschar from the burned animals was excised with a sterile blade and discarded. One gram of tissue, including muscle, fat, and fascia, immediately underlying the burn wound, was removed for study. One gram of lung, kidney, and liver was also removed. Each tissue was immediately placed in a high-speed tissue grinder with 1 ml. of trypticase soy broth and ground for four minutes at 2,000 r.p.m. while immersed in ice. Each ground specimen was diluted serially and 1 ml. of each dilution poured onto agar plates. Colony counts were performed at 24 and 48 hours. The final count was determined from a plate containing from 30 to 300 colonies. Standard quantitative procedures were followed. The results are reported as the average logarithm of the bacterial count, since this more accurately reflects the logarithmic growth of the organisms.

Blood pH. Daily pH determinations were made on animals utilized for the mortality and bacteriology studies. Animals which received no treatment or were treated with Sulfamylon Cream or with silver sulfadiazine in Neobase were selected. The unanesthetized animal was placed in an open chamber and its tail washed with ethyl alcohol. The tip of the tail was amputated and 50 lambda of mixed blood was drawn into a heparinized capillary tube. The pH value of each sample was determined by the ultramicroelectrode technique (Radiometer). Digital readout permits full-scale reproducibility of ±0.001 pH units. Samples were obtained on five consecutive days from each of 20 normal animals to determine normal values. Thirty-eight, 49, and 36 determinations were made of the untreated rats, the rats treated with Sulfamylon Cream, and the rats treated with silver sulfadiazine in Neobase, respectively. The average pH value for each group was calculated. The results were subjected to standard statistical analysis.

Histology. Blocks of burn wound, lung, liver, and kidney were fixed in a 10 percent buffered formalin. The blocks were sectioned at a thickness of 6μ and stained with hematoxylin and eosin.

RESULTS

Mortality and bacteriology. Table III shows the mortality and bacteriology results among the burned, nonseeded animals. There was a three percent mortality rate among the untreated animals; no deaths occurred in the other groups. No positive blood cultures were seen in any group. Subeschar cultures of the untreated group and the group treated with silver sulfadiazine in Neobase showed an average of $10^{3.4}$ and $10^{1.2}$ bacteria per gram, respectively, compared to an insignificant number in the group treated with Sulfamylon Cream. The animals treated with silver sulfadiazine in Neobase had an average of $10^{1.2}$ bacteria per gram in the liver compared to no growth for the Sulfa-

Table III. *Results among burned, nonseeded animals*

	No treatment	*Neobase*	*Sulfamylon Cream*	*Silver sulfadiazine*
Mortality	3%	—	0%	0%
Incidence of positive blood cultures	0%	—	0%	0%
*Quantitative bacteriology**				
Skin	3.4 (2-9)†	—	0.4 (0-2)	4.2 (2-7)
Liver	0 (0)	—	0 (0)	1.2 (0-4)
Lung	0 (0)	—	0.4 (0-2)	0.8 (0-4)

*This figure represents the average logarithm (1 × 10^n) of the bacterial count per gram of tissue.
†Range

mylon Cream and an insignificant number in the lungs.

Table IV shows the results of mortality and bacteriology studies in seeded animals. Both no-treatment and Neobase groups had a mortality rate of 91 percent compared to 14.5 and 20 percent in the Sulfamylon Cream and silver sulfadiazine in Neobase groups, respectively. There was no significant difference between the Sulfamylon Cream and the silver sulfadiazine in Neobase groups. Average survival time was slightly higher in the latter group compared to the no-treatment and Neobase groups, but this was not significant. The mortality rate was 83.5 percent among seeded animals treated with CF 100. The average survival time for this group was 13.8 days.

In the seeded animals, no positive blood cultures were found among those treated with Sulfamylon Cream. This contrasts sharply with a 17 percent incidence of positive blood cultures in the silver sulfadiazine in Neobase group, 40 percent in the CF 100 group, and 83 and 100 percent in the control groups. Application of Sulfamylon Cream maintained the subeschar bacterial counts at 10^2 per gram. Among animals treated with silver sulfadiazine in Neobase, Neobase alone, or CF 100, no bacterial counts below 10^7 per gram were noted; the minimal count among animals which received no treatment was 10^5 per gram. Bacterial counts in liver and lung were somewhat higher in the silver sulfadiazine in Neobase and CF 100 groups than in the Sulfamylon Cream group.

Blood pH. The average normal determination was 7.378. There was no significant difference between this figure and those obtained from the Sulfamylon Cream group (pH 7.356 [$0.9 > P > 0.8$]), the silver sulfadiazine in Neobase group (pH 7.376 [$0.9 > P > 0.8$]), and the no-treatment group (pH 7.392 [$0.2 > P > 0.1$]).

Studies of the kidneys revealed no crystalluria. However, multiple renal abscesses were found in three animals which died in the silver sulfadiazine in Neobase group.

DISCUSSION

Topical silver sulfadiazine in Neobase and Sulfamylon Cream have been shown to be equally effective in reducing the number of deaths resulting from Pseudomonas burn wound sepsis in rats; CF 100 was not effective.

The ineffectiveness of the Neobase and the results of previous studies with the vehicle for the Sulfamylon Cream demonstrate that the base exhibits no antibacterial effect. The minimal mortality rate noted in the nonseeded animals treated with Sulfamylon Cream or silver sulfadiazine in Neobase, as well as those receiving no treatment, demonstrates the low toxicity of these agents.

All three agents (Sulfamylon Cream, silver sulfadiazine in Neobase, and CF 100) controlled bacterial invasion of liver and lung in experimental burn wound sepsis. Higher

Table IV. *Results among burned, seeded animals*

	No treatment	*Neobase*	*Sulfamylon Cream*	*Silver sulfadiazine*	*CF 100*
Mortality	91%	91%	14.5%	20%	83.5%
Average survival time (days)	7.7	6.2	8.4	8.3	13.8
Incidence of postive blood cultures	83%	100%	0%	17%	40.0%
*Quantitative bacteriology**					
Skin	7.3 (5-9)†	7.7 (4-9)	2.1 (0-7)	7.7 (7-9)	7.8 (4-9)
Liver	1.8 (0-4)	3.7 (0-8)	0.2 (0-2)	1.0 (0-7)	0.5 (0-3)
Lung	2.0 (0-5)	3.8 (0-7)	0.1 (0-1)	0.7 (0-4)	1.3 (0-6)

*This figure represents the average logarithm (1×10^n) of the bacterial count per gram of tissue.

†Range

subeschar bacterial colony counts among the rats treated with silver sulfadiazine in Neobase and those treated with CF 100 appear to parallel a significant incidence of positive blood cultures in these groups. The presence of renal abscesses among nonsurvivors in the silver sulfadiazine in Neobase group is disturbing.

Harrison and colleagues[8] have reported that C^{14}-labeled Sulfamylon is absorbed only during the first two hours following application, while there is yet a water interface between the wound and the cream. In spite of this, the subeschar bacterial count is suppressed below the critical level until the next application, 24 hours later. The inability of silver sulfadiazine in Neobase and CF 100 to effect equivalent suppression and the significant incidence of positive blood cultures suggest that the effectiveness of each application does not persist until the next, 24 hours later.

Neither the Sulfamylon Cream nor the silver sulfadiazine in Neobase significantly alters blood pH.

As found in clinical studies with other agents, it is often difficult to relate laboratory findings to clinical efficacy. Each effective mode of therapy has its advantages and disadvantages. The elevated subeschar counts and the presence of renal sepsis suggest that, to be effective, silver sulfadiazine in Neobase and CF 100 should be applied more frequently than Sulfamylon Cream.

CONCLUSIONS AND SUMMARY

Topical Sulfamylon Cream and silver sulfadiazine in Neobase have been shown to significantly reduce the number of deaths in rats resulting from Pseudomonas burn wound sepsis. Both agents have been shown to be equally nontoxic and do not influence acid-base balance beyond the alteration caused by the burn itself. CF 100 did not effectively prevent deaths in burned seeded rats. Sulfamylon Cream suppressed the subeschar bacterial colony counts and positive blood cultures significantly more than the silver sulfadiazine in Neobase. Renal sepsis was noted in three of the animals treated with silver sulfadiazine in Neobase.

ADDENDUM

Subsequent to completion of these studies, a new silver sulfadiazine preparation has been provided by Marion Laboratories, Kansas City, Missouri. When applied daily to the seeded, burned rats, the results were similar to that noted with CF 100 (85 percent mortality rate). In light of this and the high skin bacterial counts, a series of animals were treated with a topical application of silver sulfadiazine every eight hours for 21 days. In the seeded group, one death (4 percent) occurred at 17 days. The average subeschar bacterial count was 2×10^7 per gram and only one animal had a positive liver or lung culture. No deaths occurred in the nonseeded group. The subeschar bacterial count averaged 4×10^5 per gram and there was no growth in the liver or lung tissue. These results confirm the conclusion that with the use of silver sulfadiazine the suppressive effect is of shorter duration than with Sulfamylon Cream.

REFERENCES

1. Brentano, L., Moyer, C. A., Gravens, D. L., and Monafo, W. W., Jr.: Bacteriology of large human burns treated with silver nitrate, Arch. Surg. **93:** 456, 1966.
2. Burke, J. F., Bondoc, C. C., and Morris, P. J.: Metabolic effects of topical silver nitrate therapy in burns covering more than fifteen percent of the body surface, Ann. N. Y. Acad. Sci. **150:** 674, 1968.
3. Dressler, D. P., Rozin, R. R., Skornik, W. A., Bellas, A. E., and Soroff, H. S.: An evaluation of mafenide acetate in experimental burn wound sepsis, Arch. Surg. **95:** 1000, 1967.
4. Dressler, D. P., and Skornik, W. A.: Combined systemic and topical therapy of experimental burn wound sepsis, Arch. Surg. **95:** 1009, 1967.
5. Fox, C. L., Jr.: Silver sulfadiazine—a new topical therapy for pseudomonas in burns, Arch. Surg. **96:** 184, 1968.
6. Fox, C. L., Jr.: Comments subsequent to conference, Ann. N. Y. Acad. Sci. **150:** 978, 1968.
7. Fox, C. L., Jr., Rappole, B. W., and Stanfrod, W.: Control of pseudomonas infection in burns by silver sulfadiazine, Surg. Gynec. Obstet. **128:** 1021, 1969.
8. Harrison, H. N., Blackmore, W. P., Dressler, D. P., and Brown, D.: Absorption and metabolism of C^{14}-labeled Sulfamylon acetate, presented at the International Symposium of Pharmacological Treatment in Burns, Milan, 1968.

9. Ilahi, M. A., Billote, J. B., Aaki, A., Koumans, J. K., and Burke, J. F.: Occurrence of pulmonary hyaline membrane disease in burned guinea pigs treated with topical Sulfamylon, Surg. Forum **19:** 64, 1968.
10. Lindberg, R. B., Moncrief, J. A., Switzer, W. E., Order, S. E., and Mills, W.: The successful control of burn wound sepsis, J. Trauma **5:** 601, 1965.
11. Lindberg, R. B., et al.: Prevention of invasive *Pseudomonas aeruginosa* infection in seeded burned rats by the use of topical Sulfamylon Cream, Fed. Proc. **23:** 1725, 1964.
12. Moyer, C. A., Brentano, L., Gravens, D. L., et al.: Treatment of large human burns with 0.5% silver nitrate, Arch. Surg. **90:** 812, 1965.
13. Phillips, A. W., and Cope, O.: Burn therapy. II. The revelation of respiratory tract damage as a principal killer of the burn patient, Ann. Surg. **155:** 1, 1962.
14. Pruitt, B. A., Tumbusch, W. T., Mason, A. D., and Pearson, E.: Mortality in 1100 consecutive burns treated at a burn unit, Ann. Surg. **159:** 396, 1964.
15. Rittenbury, M. S., Maddox, R. W., Schmidt, F. H., Ham, W. T., and Haynes, B. W., Jr.: Probit analysis of burn mortality in 1831 patients: Comparison with other large series, Ann. Surg. **164:** 123, 1966.
16. Rozin, R. R., Skornik, W. A., Dressler, D. P., Ramirez, A. T., and Soroff, H. S.: Studies of insensible water loss from burns treated with para-aminomethyl benzene sulfonamide (Sulfamylon), Ann. N. Y. Acad. Sci. **150:** 778, 1966.
17. Stanford, W., Rappole, B. W., and Fox, C. L., Jr.: Clinical experience with silver sulfadiazine, a new topical agent for control of Pseudomonas infection in burns, J. Trauma **9:** 377, 1969.
18. Teplitz, C.: Pathogenesis of Pseudomonas vasculitis and septic lesions, Arch. Path. **80:** 297, 1965.
19. Walker, H. L., Mason, A. D., Jr., and Raulston, C. L.: Surface infection with *Pseudomonas aeruginosa,* Ann. Surg. **160:** 297, 1964.
20. Yaffee, H., and Dressler, D. P.: Topical application of mafenide: Its association with erythema multiforme and cutaneous reactions, Arch. Derm. In press.
21. Zawacki, B. E., Divincenti, F. C., and Moncrief, J. A.: The effect of topical Sulfamylon on the insensible weight loss of burned patients, Ann. Surg. **169:** 249, 1969.

Vasodepressor factor in declamp shock production

BOLEK BRANT, M.D.*
RICHARD P. ARMSTRONG, M.D.*
R. MARK VETTO, M.D., D.Sc.
PORTLAND, ORE.
From the Department of Surgery, University of Oregon Medical School and Veterans Administration Hospital

It is well known that varying degrees of hypotension, or declamping shock, frequently occur after loosening the proximal aortic vascular clamp during the course of abdominal aneurysm resection.

The three major known factors involved in the production of the declamping shock are: (1) profound metabolic acidosis resulting from washout of pooled anoxic blood, (2) large expansion of the vascular capacity of the legs caused by hypoxic vasodilation, and (3) the sudden loss of blood through the interstices of the prosthesis.[3] We have succeeded in controlling these factors in our abdominal aneurysmectomies by the administration of 40 mEq. of sodium bicarbonate and 80 μg of levarterenol into the body of the woven Teflon prosthesis prior to gradual declamping. Administered in this way, sodium bicarbonate works to correct the "washout" metabolic acidosis, while levarterenol acting directly on the myoneural receptors in the dilated arterioles constricts them, thus preventing the "bleeding out" into the expanded vascular compartment of the lower extremities. Woven Teflon prostheses are used, since they have been found to be more "blood tight" than other types of prostheses. The reported problems related to the use of Teflon have not occurred in our experience with more than 100 patients.

Received for publication April 18, 1969.
*Research Fellow, Department of Surgery, University of Oregon Medical School, Portland, Ore.

Concomitant with developing knowledge of the above mechanisms, we have been investigating a systemic vasoactive circulating factor, the existence of which has long been suspected.[2] In our laboratory, we have demonstrated the presence of a vasodepressor substance in the effluent blood from dogs' lower extremities following a resection of a segment of their aorta and placement of a Teflon sleeve graft.

METHODS AND RESULTS

General procedure: The study was performed on 38 dogs. Under Nembutal anesthesia the aorta between the renal arteries and the trifurcation was resected and replaced with a Teflon sleeve prosthesis. Both iliac veins were cannulated with large bore plastic cannulas for collection of hindlimb blood (Fig. 1). After 1½ to 2 hours of aortic cross-clamping, the clamps were released and 200 c.c. of effluent blood was collected in sterile precooled beakers. This blood was defibrinated and centrifuged at 2,500 r.p.m. at 4° C. for 20 minutes, and serum was separated. When introduced into anesthetized control dogs, via a cannula in the superior vena cava, this serum consistently produced a transient, but marked, drop in blood pressure.

Gel column separation. The active serum was passed through a series of cold Bio-Gel polyacrylamide columns and fractionated according to molecular weight. The gels were hydrated with distilled deionized water.

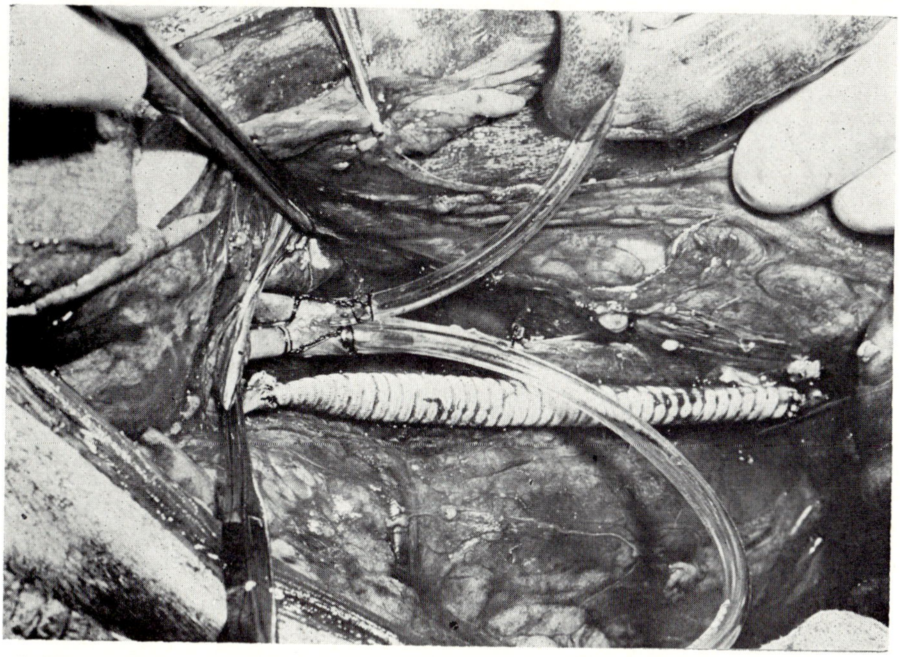

Fig. 1. The segment of the aorta between the renal arteries and the aortic trifurcation has been resected and replaced with a Teflon sleeve prosthesis. The iliac veins have been cannulated with large bore plastic cannulas for collection of hindlimb blood following aortic declamping.

With a Bio-Gel P-10 polyacrylamide column, fractions in the following molecular weight ranges were obtained: (1) greater than 17,000, (2) 17,000 to 10,000, (3) 10,000 to 4,500, and (4) less than 4,500. Of these only the fraction characterized by a molecular weight greater than 17,000 produced hypotension.

With a Bio-Gel P-200 which has a much higher molecular weight exclusion limit, fractions obtained were: (1) greater than 200,000, (2) 200,000 to 100,000, (3) 100,000 to 60,000, (4) 60,000 to 10,000, and (5) less than 10,000 (Table I). Of these, only the fraction of molecular weight 100,000 to 60,000 consistently produced hypotension (Fig. 2).

Controls. Several control fluids were injected into a control anesthetized dog. They included: (1) cold eluent used in gel fractionation (distilled deionized water), (2) cold serum obtained from normal dogs, and (3) cold serum obtained from dogs whose aortas were not clamped but who were anesthetized, operated upon, and kept asleep for 1½ to 2 hours. None of these control injections produced hypotension.

Table I. *Polyacrylamide gel column separation (4° C.)*

*Gel**	*Serum fractions (molecular weight)*
P-10	>17,000†
	17,000-10,000
	10,000-4,500
	<4,500
P-200	>200,000
	200,000-100,000
	100,000-60,000†
	60,000-10,000
	<10,000

*Gels were hydrated with distilled deionized water.
†Vasoactive fraction.

PHYSICAL CHARACTERISTICS

Injection of as little as 10 c.c. of active serum caused a detectable hypotension. The activity of the serum sample deteriorated in room temperature and became undetectable in 6 to 8 hours. Storing the serum at 4° C

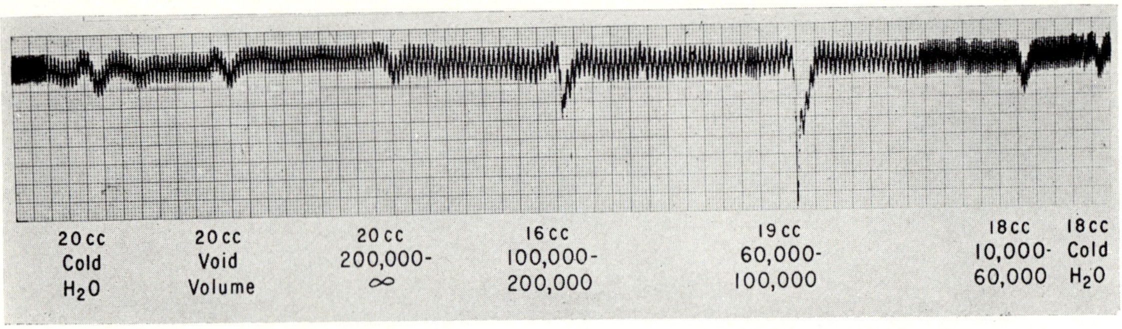

Fig. 2. This is a representative tracing of the intra-arterially monitored systemic blood pressure and its changes evoked by intravenous administration of different molecular weight fractions obtained with Bio-Gel P-200 column. The fraction of 60,000 to 100,000 produced a sudden short duration 35 mm. Hg drop in this animal's systemic blood pressure. Minimal activity of the immediately adjacent fractions was caused most probably by overlap in separation.

retarded, but did not eliminate, the deactivation process. There was no detectable activity in previously active serum following a 24 hour storage at 4° C.

Active serum samples, when placed in a water bath at 56° C. for 1 hour, lost all activity. However, freezing and thawing of the active serum did not seem to affect its vasodepressive activity. Furthermore, we observed that the active serum could be snap frozen at –90° C. and maintained at that temperature for at least 2 weeks without any deterioration of its activity.

COMMENTS

The molecular weight determinations and the above observations suggest that the vasodepressor factor may be a protein, or at least that the active factor may be attached to a protein. For this reason, the material may be subject to enzymatic deactivation. On the other hand, the described substance could be a precursor of one of the known vasodepressors; or it could be one of the catalyzing or activating enzymes involved in the production of such vasodepressors, not unlike some of the enzymes involved in the kallikrein-kallidin 9 (bradykinin) system. Bradykinin itself is a nonapeptide with molecular weight of 856.76, but some of the precursor proteins and catalyzing enzymes have molecular weights ranging from 50,000 to 150,000. In addition, the kallikrein-kallidin 9 system exhibits most of its vasodepressive activity in vitro at low pH (6.0 to 7.1), the upper limits of which correspond to pH levels encountered clinically after aortic declamping.

We have demonstrated that the described agent can indeed significantly lower the systemic blood pressure, and, even though it may not be of major importance in the production of the clinical syndrome of the declamping shock, it nevertheless represents one contributing factor. Although, multiple factors act in the production of declamping shock, the syndrome in clinical patients can now be adequately controlled with the regimen referred to above.[3]

Of more importance, in our opinion, is that this vasodepressive factor can be recovered from extremities that have been poorly perfused for these relatively short periods of time. While in this study the factor has been produced by cross-clamping the aorta during aortic resection, it would seem that generalized low perfusion states could result in production of greater amounts of this material from all poorly perfused vascular beds. The vasodepressive substance may then be a major factor contributing to increase in the severity of shock states from all causes. If this should be the case, new biochemical methods for treating shock suggest themselves. This approach would require the recovery of the vasodepressive substance from shock states, precise identification of its chemical structure, and the development of chemical means which would deactivate it without being toxic to the patient.

SUMMARY

A heat labile vasodepressor substance with a molecular weight of 60,000 to 100,000 exists in venous blood returning from the lower extremities of animals undergoing aortic declamping. Along with metabolic acidosis, vascular pooling, and prosthetic leakage, this substance contributes to the production of the syndrome of "declamping shock." It has been suggested that this material may be important in prolonging shock states of all types.

Technical assistance of Mr. Ronald A. Evenson is gratefully acknowledged.

REFERENCES

1. Barcroft, H., Darnhorst, A. C., McClatchez, H. M., and Tanner, G. M.: On the blood flow through rhythmically contracting muscle before and during release of sympathetic vasoconstrictor tone, J. Physiol. **117:** 391, 1952.
2. Malette, W. G., Armstrong, R. G., and Cricsuolo, D.: A second mechanism in hypotension following release of abdominal aortic clamps, S. Forum **14:** 292, 1963.
3. Vetto, R. M., and Brant, B.: Control of declamping shock, Am. J. Surg. **116:** 273, 1968.

The permanence of adequate incomplete vagotomy: A preliminary study in dogs

GUY LEGROS, M.D.*
CHARLES A. GRIFFITH, M.D.
SEATTLE, WASH.
From the Department of Surgery, University of Washington School of Medicine

In a previous study[12] we established a correlation between the adequacy of an incomplete vagotomy and its anatomic type. For example, after an incomplete vagotomy of one intact vagal trunk and consequent residual innervation of the entire ipsilateral mucosal surface of the stomach, acid secretion remained high with inadequate protection against ulcer. In contrast, if only a small branch from a trunk or gastric truncal division to the fundus of the stomach was left intact, only a small area of fundic mucosa remained innervated; this type of incomplete vagotomy had a low secretory potential and afforded adequate protection against ulcer. However, the permanence of the adequacy of this latter type of adequate incomplete vagotomy was questioned by the possibility of vagal reinnervation. The type of reinnervation of particular concern was that caused by sprouting as described by Murray[15] and Clark.[4] With the phenomenon of sprouting, by which microscopic collateral branches (or sprouts) may arise from intact vagal axons within the wall of the stomach and reinnervate the adjacent denervated mucosal cells, the small area of residually innervated mucosa of an adequate incomplete vagotomy might increase in size and become an inadequate vagotomy. The present study was, therefore, undertaken to determine whether the area of residually innervated mucosa remained the same or increased in size over a long-term period.

Aided by funds accruing from National Institutes of Health Grant No. AM08094.

Submitted for publication April 17, 1969; resubmitted June 16, 1969.

*Visiting Scientist. R. Samuel McLaughlin Research Fellow.

PRELIMINARY STUDIES

Because Clark[4] used cats in his investigations of vagal reinnervation of the stomach and we used dogs and rats in our studies, the anatomic distribution of the gastric vagi in cats was compared with that previously described in dogs[17] and rats.[13] Gross dissections of the vagal system from the neck to the abdomen in six cats showed a constant anatomic system that is the same as in dogs and rats. In six other cats the method of electric vagal stimulation in the presence of circulating neutral red[17] demonstrated that the vagi are distributed to the feline gastric mucosa in a pattern identical to the canine and rodent pattern: The anterior and posterior trunks innervate the anterior and posterior mucosal surfaces, respectively; each of the four branches of the esophageal plexus innervates two thirds to three fourths of the ipsilateral mucosal surface innervated by the trunk to which it contributes; and each terminal branch of the gastric truncal divisions innervates its own small segment of gastric mucosa. Thus, in all respects, the anatomic distribution of the gastric vagi was found to be the same in cats as in dogs and rats. We, therefore, concluded that the use of dogs in the present study would afford a valid comparison with Clark's[4] study in cats.

MATERIALS AND METHODS

Six adult mongrel dogs, weighing from 12 to 14 kilograms, were used. Three underwent the incomplete vagotomy studied by Clark,[4] namely, transection of the right cervical vagus nerve plus transection of the anterior abdominal vagal trunk, which leaves intact those fibers from the left cervical vagus nerve that form the left posterior branch of the esophageal plexus and contribute to the posterior vagal trunk. These dogs were designated as having "an intact branch of the esophageal plexus." The other three dogs underwent transection of the posterior vagal trunk plus transection of the anterior gastric truncal division just below the origin of its most proximal branch to the fundus of the stomach, taking care to preserve this proximal fundic branch. These dogs were designated as having "an intact fundic branch."

The area of residually innervated gastric mucosa was determined by electric vagal stimulation in the presence of circulating neutral red. The left cervical vagus nerve was stimulated in the dogs with an intact branch of the esophageal plexus, and the anterior abdominal vagal trunk was stimulated in the dogs with an intact fundic branch. The size of the area of mucosa that secreted the neutral red was recorded on gauze patterns placed on the mucosal surface as previously described.[12]

The dogs recovered uneventfully and were observed for 12 to 15 months. During this period they remained in good health. They then underwent acute experiments by the same methods to redetermine the size of the area of innervated gastric mucosa. Postmortem dissections were done to verify the anatomic accuracy of the type of vagotomy and also to examine the sites of vagotomy for any evidence of restoration of continuity of the divided nerves. The stomach was then removed and the percentage of residually innervated mucosa was calculated by the planemetric and pattern-weight method.[16]

RESULTS

The postmortem dissections verified the anatomic type of vagotomy performed in all six dogs. No restoration of continuity of the divided nerves was found in any dog.

The size of the area of residually innervated mucosa remained the same in all six dogs. In the three dogs with an intact branch of the esophageal plexus, the large areas of residual innervation of the posterior mucosal surface varied from 35 to 45 percent of the stomach. In the three dogs with an intact fundic branch, the small areas of residually innervated fundic mucosa varied from 10 to 16 percent of the stomach. No increase in the size of residually innervated mucosa was observed in any dog after 12 to 15 months (Fig. 1).

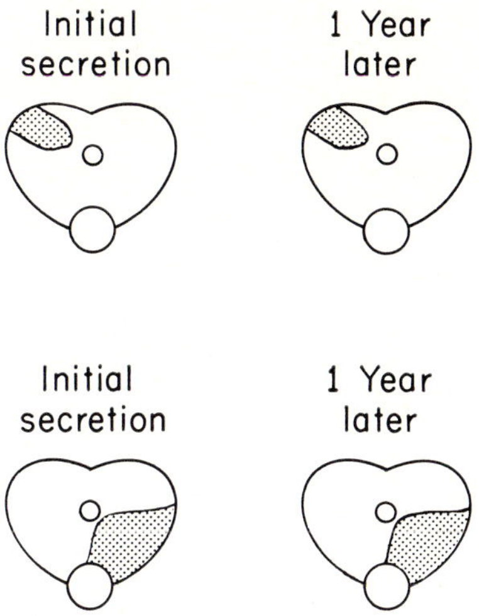

Fig. 1. Areas of secretion before (left) and 12 to 15 months after (right) incomplete vagotomy of an intact fundic branch (top) and an intact esophageal plexus branch (bottom). These diagrams represent the mucosal surface of the stomach opened along the greater curve and laid flat. The smaller upper circles represent the esophageal opening, and the larger lower circles the antrum. The shaded areas represent the residually innervated mucosa.

DISCUSSION

The results of no increase in the size of the residually innervated mucosa, and presumably no recovery of gastric secretion, are contrary to Clark's[4] findings with gastric motility. In one group of cats Clark[4] observed an immediate and significant decrease in intragastric pressure from gastric contraction consequent to electric vagal stimulation after an incomplete vagotomy of an intact branch of the esophageal plexus. In another group of cats without initial control studies, the contractile response at 4 to 6 weeks after the same type of incomplete vagotomy equaled the preoperative response in the first group. Both Clark[3] and Murray[15] explained this apparent recovery of gastric motility to one of us (C. A. G.) as follows: On the basis of the findings of Agostoni and associates,[1] they assumed that the residual vagal innervation of the stomach with an incomplete vagotomy due to one branch of the esophageal plexus was approximately 10 percent. And on the basis of Edds'[6, 7] reports of the patchy distribution of residual innervation in skeletal muscle after its partial denervation at the level of spinal nerve roots, Clark[3] and Murray[15] further assumed that this 10 percent residual vagal innervation was distributed throughout the gastric muscle in a patchy or shot-gun pattern, i.e., small islands of innervated muscle in a sea of denervated muscle. By the phenomenon of sprouting the small innervated islands were supposed to have enlarged until they coalesced with consequent reinnervation of all of the gastric muscle.

Explanation of the discrepancy between the apparent reinnervation of the gastric muscle in Clark's[4] study and the lack of reinnervation of the gastric mucosa in our study is impossible because the anatomic distribution of the vagal fibers to the gastric muscle has not been demonstrated as it has to the gastric mucosa. However, the vagi to the gastric muscle are most probably distributed in the same segmental pattern as to the gastric mucosa because a correlation exists between the amounts of the secretory and motile responses.[11] The less the amount of residual innervation, the lower are both the secretory and motile responses. In regard to the mucosa and secretion, two points seem clear. First, rather than a patchy shotgun pattern of residual innervation, the incomplete vagotomy studied by Clark[4] results in one large area of innervated mucosa in the posterior wall of the stomach that comprises 35 to 45 percent of the entire mucosal surface (Fig. 1). Second, Sebus and Charbon[19] showed that this amount of innervated mucosa after transection of any three of the four branches of the esophageal plexus has a high secretory potential, and this anatomic type of incomplete vagotomy is, therefore, inadequate in the beginning.

In subsequent discussions with Murray[15] at the beginning of this study, he predicted no significant increase in the size of a small localized area of residually innervated mucosa by sprouting. The less the amount of residual innervation, the less is the amount of sprouting. Microscopic sprouts are incapable of extending from the border of innervated tissue to reinnervate a significant area of denervated tissue. Murray[15] also stated on the basis of his and others' experience that sprouting is no longer effective after 1 year. Supportive evidence has been obtained in another study of 383 rats.[10] In rats with an incomplete vagotomy of an intact trunk, a very small amount of mucosa was gradually reinnervated during the first 9 months, but no further reinnervation was noted at 12 months. In rats with an intact fundic branch no reinnervation occurred. These findings in rats support not only Murray's[15] predictions but the present findings in dogs as well. The 12 to 15 month period of observation, therefore, seems valid.

Conventional reinnervation by restoration of continuity of the divided nerve ends was not seen in any of the six dogs studied, nor was it seen in the other study of 383 rats. Evidence by other investigators is conflicting. For example, Dragstedt and co-workers[5] observed negative insulin tests and no increase in gastric secretion for 3 years after merely crushing the vagi with a hemostat. On the other hand, Jefferson and associates[9] observed restoration of continuity of divided nerve ends and a return of the gastric motile response to electric vagal stimulation 1 to 2 years after vagotomy. Whether the gastric muscle becomes reinnervated and the gastric mucosa does not remains conjectural. Results of another study[11] showed that both the motile and secretory responses remained low after incomplete vagotomy of an intact fundic branch.

The evidence for vagal reinnervation in man by either sprouting or restoration of continuity of divided nerves is also conflicting. Many clinical observations of an increase in gastric secretion and conversion of negative insulin tests into positive tests have been reported. We cannot explain these findings, and can only state that we[8] and others[2, 18] have not observed them. Nor have we[6] and others[2, 18] seen a small and delayed insulin response indicative of an adequate incomplete vagotomy[12] convert into a large and early response indicative of an inadequate vagotomy with recurrent ulcer.

In conceding the evidence for vagal reinnervation by recovery of gastric motility, we note that no experimental study to date has demonstrated any recovery of gastric secretion. And in conceding the clinical evidence for vagal reinnervation by recovery of gastric secretion, we also note this evidence is by no means clear-cut and leaves room for doubt. From our own experimental and clinical findings we believe that vagal reinnervation of the stomach is insignificant and that either a complete or an adequate incomplete vagotomy remains permanently complete and adequate in both animals and man.

SUMMARY AND CONCLUSIONS

The size of the area of residually innervated gastric mucosa was determined by the method of electric vagal stimulation in the presence of circulating neutral red after an incomplete vagotomy of one intact branch of the esophageal plexus in three dogs and an intact branch to the gastric fundus in three other dogs. The areas of residually innervated mucosa did not increase in size but remained the same for 12 to 15 months. It was concluded that vagal reinnervation of the gastric mucosa is insignificant and that an initially adequate incomplete vagotomy remains permanently adequate.

REFERENCES

1. Agostoni, E., Chinnock, J. E., Daly, M. de Burgh, and Murray, J. G.: Functional and histological studies of the vagus and its branches to the heart, lungs and abdominal viscera in the cat, J. Physiol. **135:** 182, 1957.
2. Bell, P. R. F.: The insulin test after vagotomy, *in* Thomson, T. J., and Gillespie, I. E., editors: Postgraduate gastroenterology, London, 1966, Baillière, Tindall & Cassell, Ltd., p. 241.
3. Clark, C. G.: Personal communication, 1962.
4. Clark, C. G.: Recovery of gastric function after incomplete vagotomy, Brit. J. Surg. **51:** 539, 1964.
5. Dragstedt, L. R., Woodward, R. R., and Camp, E. H.: Question of the return of gastric secretion after complete vagotomy, Arch. Surg. **61:** 775, 1950.
6. Edds, M. V.: Experiments on partially deneurotized nerves, J. Exper. Zool. **112:** 29, 1949.
7. Edds, M. V.: Collateral nerve regeneration, Quart. Rev. Biol. **28:** 260, 1953.
8. Griffith, C. A.: Completeness of gastric vagotomy by the selective technic, Am. J. Digest. Dis. **12:** 333, 1967.
9. Jefferson, N. C., Geisel, A., Lott, P., Jr., and Necheles, H.: Vagus regeneration in the dog, SURGERY **61:** 808, 1967.
10. Jones, W. M., and Griffith, C. A.: A correlation of gastric motile and secretory responses after incomplete vagotomy. Submitted for publication.
11. Jones, W. M., and Griffith, C. A.: On the question of vagal reinnervation of the stomach. Submitted for publication.
12. Legros, G., and Griffith, C. A.: The anatomic basis for the variable adequacy of incomplete vagotomy, parts I and II, Ann. Surg. **168:** 1030, 1968.
13. Legros, G., and Griffith, C. A.: The abdominal vagal system in rats, J. S. Res. **9:** 183, 1969.
14. Murray, J. G.: The consequences of injury and disease of nervous tissue: Recent advances in knowledge, J. Roy. Coll. Surgeons, Edinburgh **4:** 199, 1959.
15. Murray, J. G.: Personal communications, 1962 and 1965.
16. Olch, P. D., and Harkins, H. N.: Quantitative assessment of extent of gastric resection, SURGERY **48:** 655, 1960.
17. Pritchard, G. R., Griffith, C. A., and Harkins, H. N.: The insulin response of vagally innervated gastric pouches following selective gastric vagotomy, J. S. Res. **8:** 68, 1968.
18. Ross, B., and Kay, A. W.: The insulin test after vagotomy, Gastroenterology **46:** 397, 1964.
19. Sebus, J., and Charbon, G. A.: Partial vagotomy and gastric secretion in dogs, Gastroenterology **44:** 311, 1963.

Circulating lymphocyte depletion: Effect on lymphoid tissue

JAY C. FISH, M.D.
GERALD BEATHARD, M.D.*
HARRY E. SARLES, M.D.
AUGUST R. REMMERS, Jr., M.D.
STEPHAN E. RITZMANN, M.D.**
GALVESTON, TEXAS
From the Departments of Surgery, Pathology, and Medicine, The University of Texas Medical Branch, and the Shriners Burns Institute

The establishment of chronic thoracic duct fistulas in calves and humans permits the removal of large numbers of circulating lymphocytes.[1, 6, 7, 11] Fluid and protein homeostasis are maintained by reinfusion of the cell-free lymph. Lymphocytes in lymph can be removed by continuous flow centrifugation[5] and destroyed by irradiation[2] or hypotonic lysis.[12]

The calf was chosen as an experimental animal because long-term lymph fistulas can be maintained under sterile conditions in this animal. In addition, depletion of circulating lymphocytes is accelerated in time because of the very high concentration of lymphocytes in lymph. In man the lymphocyte count in lymph is about the same as in the blood.[7, 11] In the calf the lymph contains an average of 10 times as many lymphocytes per cubic millimeter as does the blood. The mean blood lymphocyte count in calves was 4,152 per cubic millimeter, while the mean initial lymph lymphocyte count was 35,776 per cubic millimeter.

Lymph flow ranged from 4 to 20 L. per day in these animals. After 5 days of removing lymphocytes with reinfusion of the cell-free lymph, there was a 94 percent reduction in the lymph lymphocyte count and a 57 percent reduction in the blood lymphocyte count.

When long-term depletion of circulating lymphocytes, via a thoracic duct fistula, was used in man in preparation for cadaveric renal transplants, a very beneficial effect was noted on allograft survival.[7] No other form of immunosuppressive therapy was necessary for the first 3 to 10 weeks and only maintainance azathioprine and prednisone were employed after that. Extensive examination of the lymphoid tissues after lymphocyte depletion has not been possible in man. For this reason, the following studies were performed in the calf. These observations suggest that extensive depletion of the thymic-dependent areas of the peripheral lymphoid tissue occurs with removal of the circulating lymphocytes from lymph.

METHODS

Twenty-three calves were used in this study. The technique of sterile thoracic duct lymph collection, centrifugation, and reinfusion of cell-free lymph in calves has been described in separate reports.[3, 5] Supraclavicular lymph nodes were removed prior to thoracic duct cannulation in each animal. Complete autopsy material of lymphoid

Supported in part by Public Health Service Grants AM-11143--02 and HE 09955-02 (AI) from the National Institutes of Health and the Moody Foundation.

Received for publication April 18, 1969.

*United States Public Health Service Special Fellow, Grant No. 1-F3-6M-40, 802-01 (APA).

**Leukemia Society Scholar.

tissues was obtained in two normal animals. Lymph nodes were also obtained when the thoracic duct fistula was discontinued. Specimens of thymus, spleen, intestine, and additional lymph node material were removed at the killing or deaths of nine animals.

The tissues were fixed in 10 percent formalin and stained with hematoxylin and eosin.

RESULTS

Complete autopsy material was obtained in nine calves after varying periods of thoracic duct drainage and lymphocyte depletion. Three animals were autopsied immediately after terminating the lymph fistula. In the other six calves, killing or death occurred from 2 to 49 days after the lymph fistula ceased to drain. The animals were observed after stopping the lymph fistula in order to follow the survival of skin or renal allografts and to determine the time necessary to repopulate the lymphoid tissues with lymphocytes. Table I summarizes the duration of the lymph fistulas, number of lymphocytes removed, and length of time after discontinuing lymphocyte depletion before killing or death of the animal.

Lymph nodes. In those animals with satisfactory lymph flow for at least 5 days, the histologic appearance of the lymph nodes was comparable regardless of how many additional days the fistula functioned. The degree of change appeared to vary somewhat according to location of the node. Changes in cervical and aortic nodes were more severe than those in the mesenteric nodes. The general characteristics included a marked loss of lymphocytes from the medullary and paracortical regions (Fig. 1). The subcapsular area was uniformly spared. Germinal centers remained, but the surrounding mantle of small lymphocytes was often lost. The medullary cords were stripped of small lymphocytes, but plasma cells and histocytes remained.

Repopulation of lymph nodes with small lymphocytes apparently occurs quite slowly. In the animal killed 49 days after occlusion of the thoracic duct, the mesenteric nodes were partially repopulated, but little recovery was present in the aortic nodes (Fig. 2).

Spleen. No grossly discernible changes were present in the spleens. As with the lymph nodes, lymph drainage beyond 5 days did not influence the histologic appearance of the spleen up to the time of termination of lymphocyte depletion.

The number of lymphoid follicles appeared to be the same, but the follicles were decreased in size in the lymphocyte-depleted animals (Fig. 3). The general effect was a gross decrease in lymphocytes around the central arterioles, a reduction in the density of lymphocytes in the red pulp, and a miniaturization of the follicles.

Compared to the lymph node tissue, the splenic lymphoid follicles repopulated progressively with time after discontinuing lymph drainage. Follicle size and density of lymphocytes were increased in those animals in which killing was delayed.

Intestine. Large numbers of lymphoid follicles were present in the submucosa of the calf ileum. Follicles of lymphocytes were also found at random in the mucosa. The submucosal follicles were stripped of lymphocytes leaving the germinal center uncovered after lymphocyte depletion (Fig. 4). Repopulation with small lymphocytes occured more rapidly than in the other lymphoid tissues. In the calf autopsied 49 days after the cessation of lymphocyte de-

Table I

Calf No.	*Lymph flow (days)*	*Lymphocytes removed ($\times 10^9$)*	*Autopsy—No. of days after stopping TDF**
6	23	843	3
10	15	817	8
11	7	451	3
12	11	1,559	49
15	5	532	12
16	14	1,011	0
20	6	803	0
22	13	905	15
23	14	786	0

*TDF = Thoracic duct fistula.

A

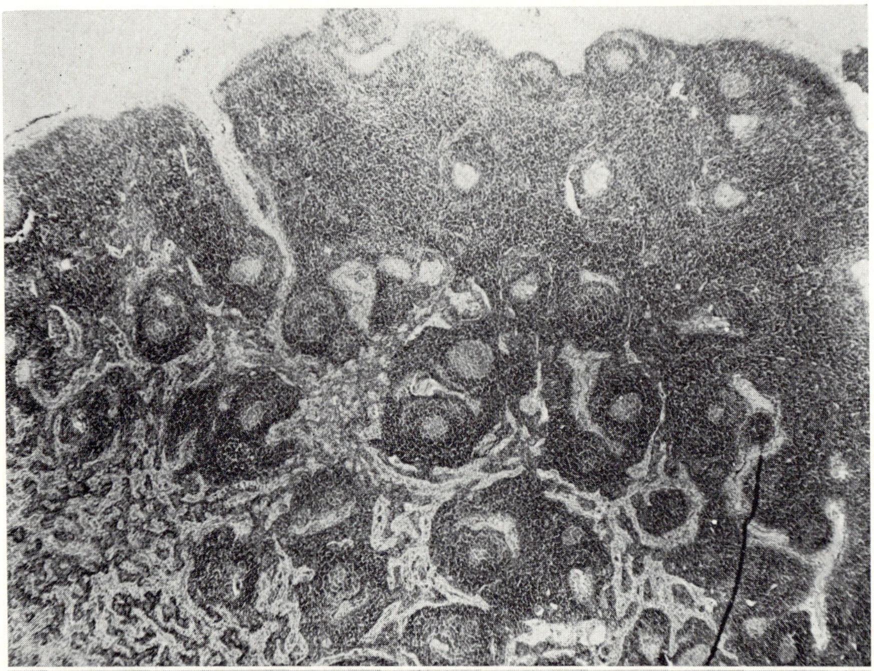

B

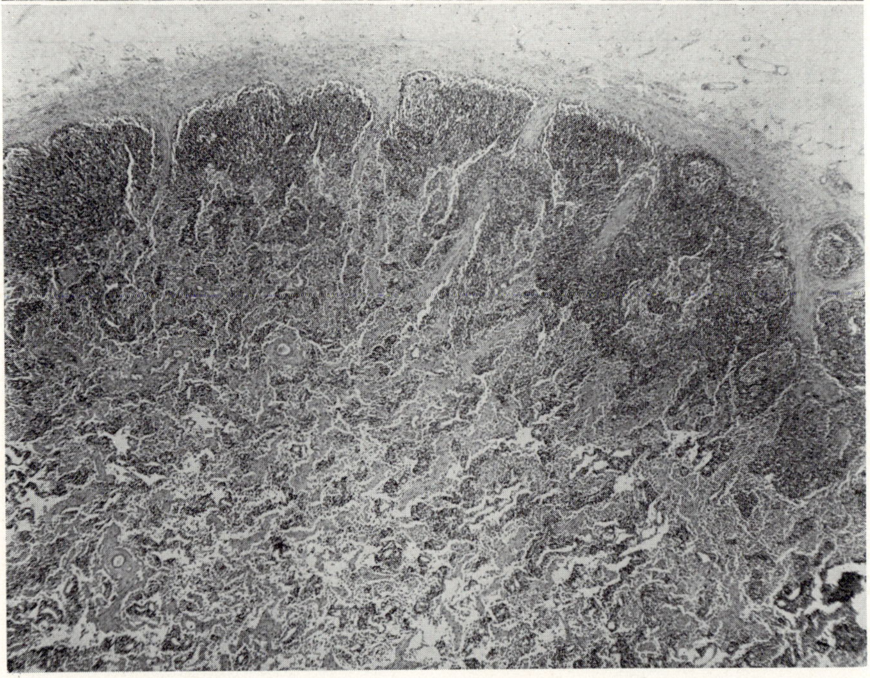

Fig. 1. Aortic lymph nodes. Comparison of normal *(A)* and lymphocyte depleted nodes *(B)* shows marked loss of lymphocytes from the paracortical and medullary areas. (Original magnification ×40.) Higher magnification (Original magnification ×125) of cortical follicles in the normal *(C)* and depleted *(D)* nodes illustrates the loss of lymphocytes from the mantle zone around the germinal center.

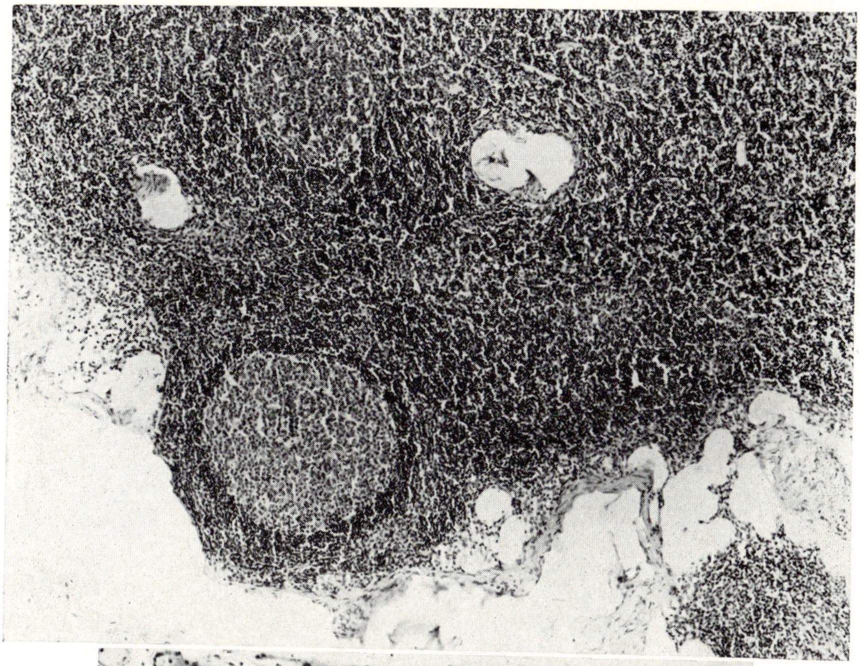

C

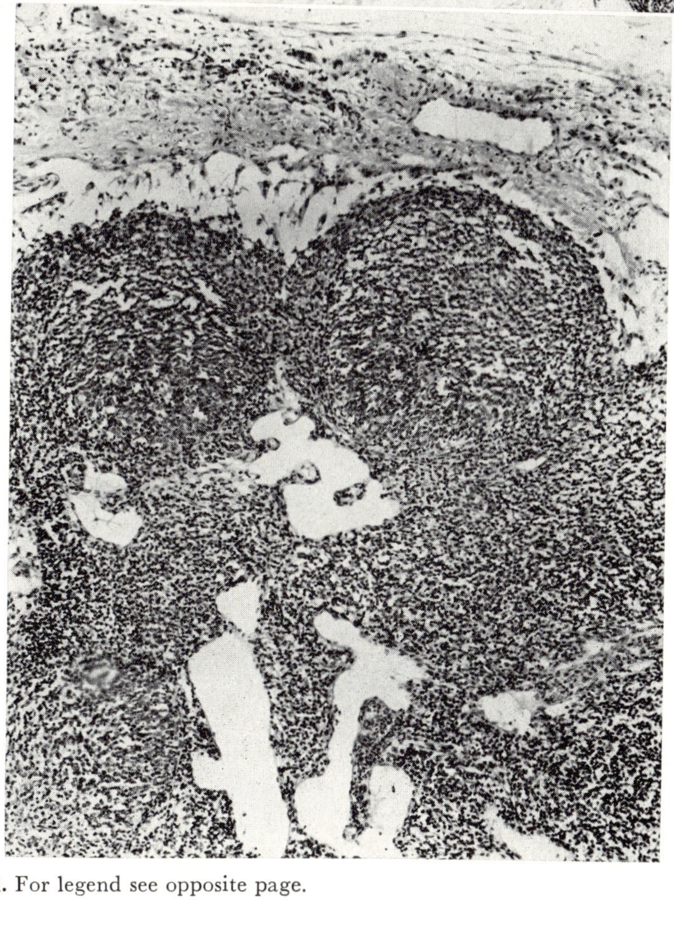

D

Fig. 1—cont'd. For legend see opposite page.

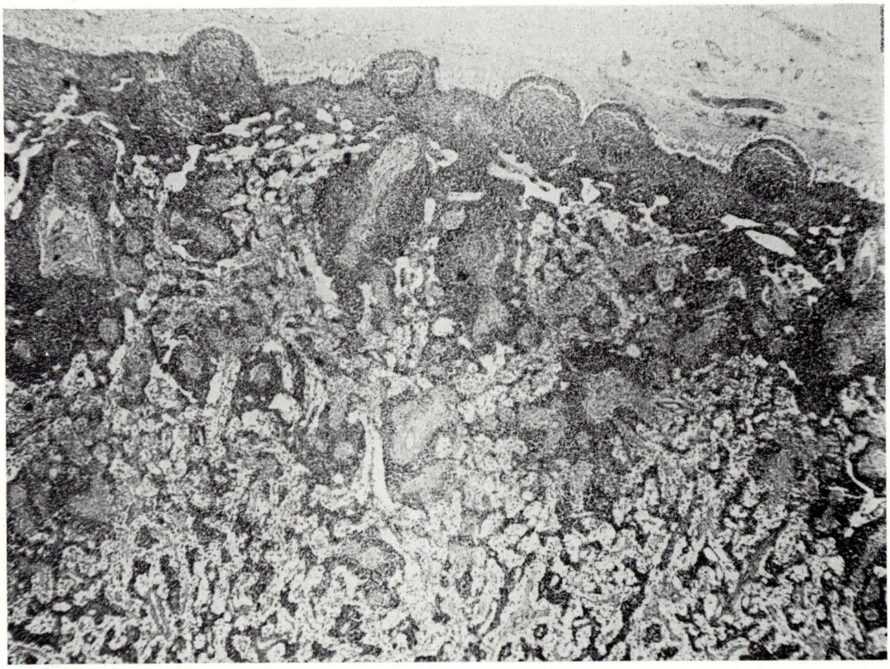

Fig. 2. Section of an aortic lymph node removed 49 days after cessation of lymph lymphocyte depletion. Note the absence of any significant repopulation by lymphocytes in the paracortical region. (Original magnification ×40.)

pletion, the submucosal lymphoid follicles had almost returned to pre-depletion appearance.

Before lymphocyte depletion the calf thymus was characterized by cortical areas of densely packed small thymocytes surrounding relatively large medullary areas of epithelial cells. A number of variables known to affect the thymus existed in the test animals, e.g. infection, fluctuations in plasma and extracellular fluid volumes, surgery, etc. These conditions may lead to cellular depletion or even atrophy of the thymus. While many remarkable changes were noted in the thymus of the lymphocyte-depleted calves, it is not possible to attribute all these alterations to lymphocyte depletion.

Grossly the thymus was quite small following depletion. There was a marked decrease in the numbers of thymocytes and in the density of the cortex. The medullary areas were reduced to only a small cluster of epithelial cells.

DISCUSSION

Because the calf's lymph flow is profuse and contains a high concentration of lymphocytes, it is possible to produce a rapid and massive depletion of circulating lymphocytes. This depletion is dramatically illustrated by monitoring the lymph lymphocyte concentrations, but it is less apparent in the blood lymphocytes. A significant depletion of total body lymphocytes is confirmed by examination of the lymphoid tissues. The sites of depletion are, in general, in the thymic-dependent areas of the lymphoid tissue.

In the lymph nodes, the subcapsular cortical areas are not depleted. Presumably, cells in these areas are sessile and do not circulate, or if they do, it is only after new cells are formed to replace them. Plasma cells and sinus histiocytes remain in the paracortical and medullary areas. This general picture is seen after neonatal thymectomy[8] and following treatment with antilymphocytic serum.[10, 13] McGregor and

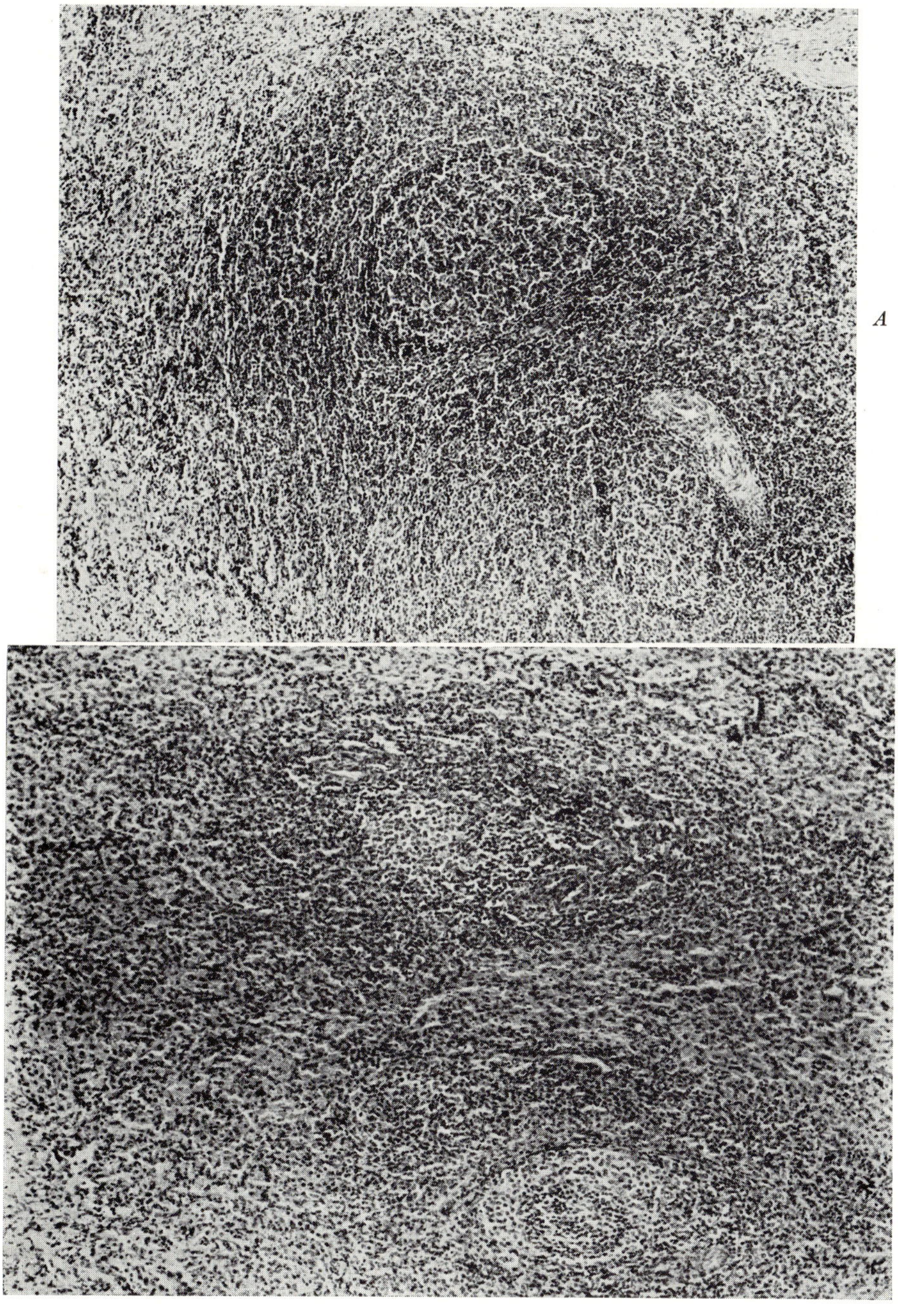

A

B

Fig. 3. Normal calf spleen *(A)*. Note the arteriole (lower right) and the well-developed follicle with distinct mantle of lymphocytes and the large numbers of surrounding lymphocytes. After lymphocyte depletion *(B)*, two follicles and arterioles are seen. There is marked diminution of lymphocytes in the mantle zone and follicle. (Original magnification ×125.)

A

B

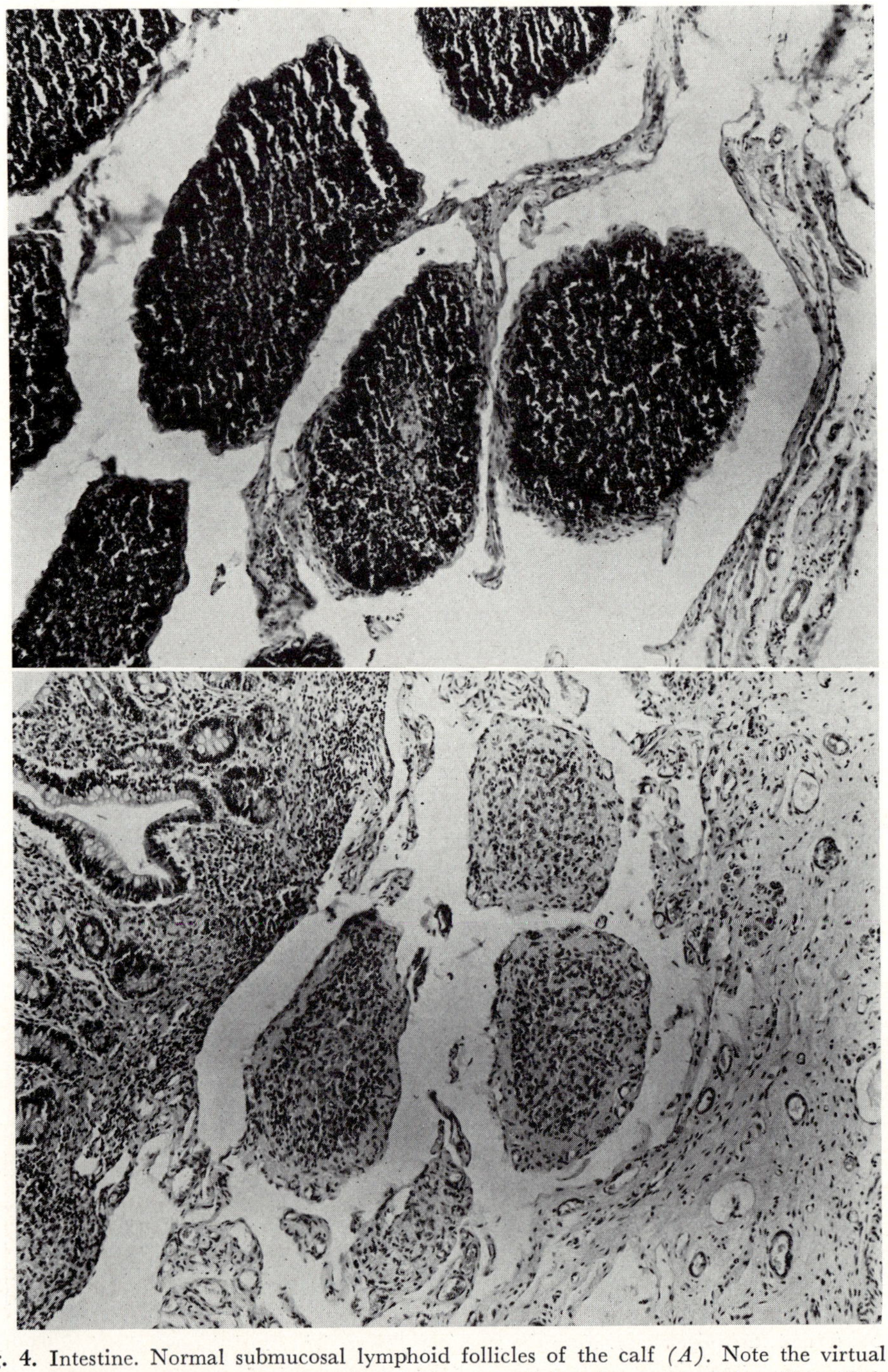

Fig. 4. Intestine. Normal submucosal lymphoid follicles of the calf *(A)*. Note the virtual absence of small lymphocytes in the follicles after lymph lymphocyte depletion *(B)*. (Original magnification ×125.)

Gowans[9] drained the thoracic duct of rats for 5 days. The lymph was discarded. Circulating lymphocyte depletion was produced, and the thymus, spleen, and lymph nodes were decreased in weight as compared with controls.

The delayed repopulation of lymph nodes in the calves may indicate that the life span of lymphocytes residing in these areas is quite long and that rapid formation of new cells does not occur.

There is quite possibly some variation in the degree of depletion according to the anatomic location of the nodes. Adequate data are not available to evaluate this question fully.

While there is little question that the spleen is affected by the lymphocyte depletion, the results are different from those in the lymph nodes. Follicles of lymphocytes were always present although the follicles were dwarfed in size after depletion. The longer the delay between cessation of lymph flow and tissue examination of the spleen, the larger the follicles. This may indicate that the splenic follicles are populated by cells other than those traversing the thoracic duct.

The intestinal follicles were severely stripped of lymphocytes but repopulated after lymphocyte depletion had ceased. It is interesting that this tissue reflected the highest degree of depletion, but the fastest repopulation.

Interpretation of changes in the thymus should be viewed with caution. The marked alterations of both cortical and medullary cells could be due to causes other than lymph lymphocyte depletion. Whatever the cause, the effect persisted throughout the longest follow-up period of 49 days.

These studies demonstrate that selective lymphocyte depletion is possible via a well-functioning thoracic duct fistula in the calf. They demonstrate further evidence for the circulation of lymphocytes from lymph to blood to lymphoid tissues. Furthermore, removal of thoracic duct lyomphocytes results in depletion of the thymic-dependent areas of the peripheral lymphoid tissues. The effect of total body lymphocyte depletion upon immunoglobulin levels is reported elsewhere for man,[7] and data on gamma globulin and other proteins will be reported subsequently for calves.[4] Assessment of the effect of lymphocyte depletion upon cellular and humoral immune systems will be the subject of later studies.

SUMMARY

Removal of lymphocytes from the lymph of calves with thoracic duct fistulas results in a rapid decrease in the circulating lymphocytes. Lymph nodes, spleen, and intestine are also severely depleted. The germinal center cells are not affected and the subcapsular region of lymph nodes as well as portions of the splenic follicle persist despite prolonged lymphocyte depletion. In general, thoracic duct lymphocyte removal results in depletion of the thymic-dependent areas of the peripheral lymphoid tissues. The most complete depletion occurred in intestinal follicles and was followed by the most rapid repopulation. The splenic follicles also recovered somewhat within 49 days after terminating lymphocyte depletion. Profound depletion of both cortical and medullary cells of the thymus was demonstrated. Because of the numerous variables that are known to affect the thymus which were present in these animals, no cause and effect relationship can be established.

REFERENCES

1. Chanana, A. D., Brecher, G., Cronkite, E. P., Joel, D., and Schnappauf, H.: The influence of extracorporeal irradiation of the blood and lymph on skin homograft rejection, Radiation Res. **27:** 330, 1966.
2. Cronkite, E. P.: Extracorporeal irradiation of the blood and lymph in the treatment of leukemia and for immunosuppression, Ann. Int. Med. **67:** 415, 1967.
3. Fish, J. C., Mattingly, A. T., Ross, M. V., Abston, S., Ritzmann, S. E., Sarles, H. E., and Remmers, A. R., Jr.: Circulating lymphocyte depletion in the calf. Effect on blood and lymph lymphocytes, Arch. Surg. In press.
4. Fish, J. C., Ritzmann, S. E., Sarles, H. E., Mattingly, A. T., and Remmers, A. R., Jr.:

Circulating lymphocyte depletion. Effect on serum proteins. Submitted for publication.

5. Fish, J. C., Ross, M. V., Sarles, H. E., and Remmers, A. R., Jr.: Separation of lymphocytes from lymph by continuous flow centrifugation, SURGERY **65:** 789, 1969.
6. Fish, J. C., Sarles, H. E., Mattingly, A. T., Ross, M. V., and Remmers, A. R., Jr.: Preparation of chronic thoracic duct lymph fistulas in man and animals, J. S. Res. **9:** 101, 1969.
7. Fish, J. C., Sarles, H. E., Remmers, A. R., Tyson, K. R. T., Canales, C. O., Beathard, G. A., Fukushima, M., Ritzmann, S. E., and Levin, W. C.: Circulating lymphocyte depletion in preparation for renal allotransplantation, Surg. Gynec. & Obst. **128:** 777, 1969.
8. Good, R. A., Dalmasso, A. P., Martinez, C., Archer, O. K., Pierce, J. C., and Papermaster, B. W.: The role of the thymus in development of immunological capacity of rabbits and mice, J. Exper. Med. **116:** 773, 1962.
9. McGregor, D. D., and Gowans, J. L.: Antibody response of rats depleted by lymphocytes by chronic drainage from the thoracic duct, J. Exper. Med. **117:** 303, 1963.
10. Parrott, D. M. V., deSousa, M. A. B., and East, J.: Thymus-dependent areas in the lymphoid organs of neonatally thymectomized mice, J. Exper. Med. **123:** 191, 1966.
11. Sarles, H. E., Smith, G. H., Fish, J. C., and Remmers, A. R., Jr.: Observations concerning human lymphocyte homeostasis during lymphatic diversion, Texas Rep. Biol. & Med. **25:** 573, 1967.
12. Sarles, H. E., Smith, G. H., Fish, J. C., and Remmers, A. R., Jr.: Further observations concerning the use of lymph for extracorporeal dialysis, Tr. Am. Soc. Artif. Int. Organs **12:** 33, 1966.
13. Turk, J. L., and Willoughby, D. A.: Central and peripheral effects of anti-lymphocyte sera, Lancet **1:** 249, 1967.

The immunologic response to intravascular skin allografts

WILLIAM J. DONAWICK, D.V.M.*
ARTHUR E. BAUE, M.D.**
KENNETT SQUARE AND PHILADELPHIA, PA.
From the Department of Clinical Studies, School of Veterinary Medicine, University of Pennsylvania, and the Harrison Department of Surgical Research and Graduate Hospital, School of Medicine, University of Pennsylvania

The host immunologic response and fate of viable cardiac valve allografts are uncertain. Allovital cardiac valves have been thought by various investigators to be only weakly antigenic,[12] to be rejected,[8, 9] not to be rejected,[2, 4, 6] to occupy an immunologically privileged site within the vascular system, and to persist as donor tissue within the host indefinitely[4] or to be replaced by host tissue.[11, 13]

In a previous study, Baue and associates[2] established that calf heart valve leaflets have an antigenicity comparable to skin as indicated by the fact that allogenic valve leaflets transplanted to subcutaneous sites in untreated calves were rejected within 14 days. In hosts presensitized to the donor with orthotopic skin grafts, the valve leaflets underwent an accelerated rejection, typical of second-set rejection. However, allovital aortic and pulmonic valves transplanted to the pulmonic valve area in presensitized and nonsensitized hosts did not undergo classical immunologic rejection. The authors suggested that the intravascular location of the allovital cardiac valves might account for the lack of classical rejection, the prolonged survival of the allovital valve leaflets, and the discrepancy in results reported by various investigators.

The purpose of the present study with intravascular skin autografts and allografts was to determine the influence of the intravascular site on the survival of allovital cardiac valves.

METHODS

Full-thickness pinch skin grafts, 1.5 cm. in diameter, were prepared from the dorsum of the ear of seven pairs of unrelated Holstein-Friesian calves, 3 to 4 months of age, weighing 65 to 100 kilograms. The method of preparing the grafts was that described by Anderson and co-workers.[1]

Recipient calves underwent cardiopulmonary bypass procedures as described previously.[7] With total bypass, the pulmonary artery was opened distally to the pulmonic valve with a 5 cm. longitudinal incision. The skin autografts and allografts were sutured in place circumferentially to the intact intima of the pulmonary artery as close to the pulmonic valve as feasible with a simple continuous Teflon-impregnated Dacron suture, or to the tunica media and edge of intima of the vessel after removal of the intima by blunt dissection.

Two skin autografts and two skin allografts were sutured inside the pulmonary artery of three calves. One skin autograft and one skin allograft were sutured to the intact intima of the pulmonary artery, and

Supported by United States Public Health Service Grant No. RO1-HE-09396 and a grant from the Delaware Heart Association.

Received for publication April 29, 1969.

*United States Public Health Service postdoctoral research trainee, Grant No. 5-T01-GM-00957.

**Recipient of Research Career Development Award, HE-28, 429. Present address: Department of Surgery, Jewish Hospital of St. Louis and the Washington University School of Medicine, St. Louis, Mo.

Table I. *Percent survival of intravascular and orthotopic skin autografts and allografts in calves*

Calf No.	Days from operation to necropsy	Skin grafts within pulmonary artery				Simultaneous orthotopic skin grafts	
		Intima intact		Intima removed			
		Autograft	Allograft	Autograft	Allograft	Autograft	Allograft
534	10	—	—	100	G.R.*	100	G.R.
177	10	—	I.N.†	—	G.R.	100	G.R.
793	10	I.N.	I.N.	100	75	—	—
693	12	—	—	100	25	—	—
533	14	—	—	100	25	—	—
966	20	—	—	100	G.R.	—	—
135	21	100	I.N.	100	G.R.	—	—

*G.R. = Graft rejected.
†I.N. = Ischemic necrosis of graft.

the remaining grafts were sutured to the pulmonary artery after a portion of the intima corresponding with the size of the grafts was removed.

To determine the mean survival time of a single orthotopic skin allograft, 10 calves each received a 1.5 cm. diameter full-thickness graft placed in a bed prepared over the thorax following the technique of Chanana and co-workers,[5] with the exception that the grafts were secured in place with four to six interrupted sutures. Initial inspection of these orthotopic skin grafts was begun 7 days after grafting, and they were evaluated daily until the epidermis was judged to be broken down, at which time they were removed for histologic study to confirm the gross observations.

Two orthotopic skin autografts and two allografts were placed on two calves (Calves No. 534 and 177) immediately after completion of the intravascular grafting procedure.

The calves were killed 10 to 21 days after operation. Histologic sections of all skin grafts were prepared and examined to determine the fate of the grafts. The skin grafts were scored from 0 to 100 based on the percentage of epidermal survival. A skin graft was judged to have been rejected if there was intense mononuclear cell infiltration of the dermis, dilatation and thrombosis of blood vessels, and epidermal necrosis. Ischemic necrosis of the skin graft was judged to have occurred when there was epidermal necrosis but no evidence of rejection or vascular union between the graft and the host.

RESULTS

The mean survival time of a single orthotopic skin allograft on calves was 9.7 ± 1.2 days.

At necropsy, the epidermis of the intracardiac skin grafts was covered with a 1 mm. friable layer of fibrin that was easily separated from the epidermis. Skin grafts placed on the intact tunica intima of the pulmonary artery had little or no fibrous union with the host. In contrast, skin transplanted to the tunica media of the pulmonary artery was firmly healed by 10 days.

The histologic results of intravascular and orthotopic skin grafts are summarized in Table I. With one exception, allogenic and autologous skin grafts that were sutured to the intact intima underwent ischemic necrosis (Fig. 1). The exception was an autograft which was viable at 21 days (Calf No. 135). On histologic section of this autograft, a vascular connection with the host was observed where the intimal layer had been disrupted by a suture.

All autologous skin grafts sutured to the pulmonary artery devoid of intima survived. An intravascular skin autograft 21 days after grafting is shown in Fig. 2.

When recipient calves were grafted with both an intravascular allograft placed on the pulmonary artery devoid of intima and an orthotopic allograft, both grafts underwent rejection within 10 days. At 10 days the in-

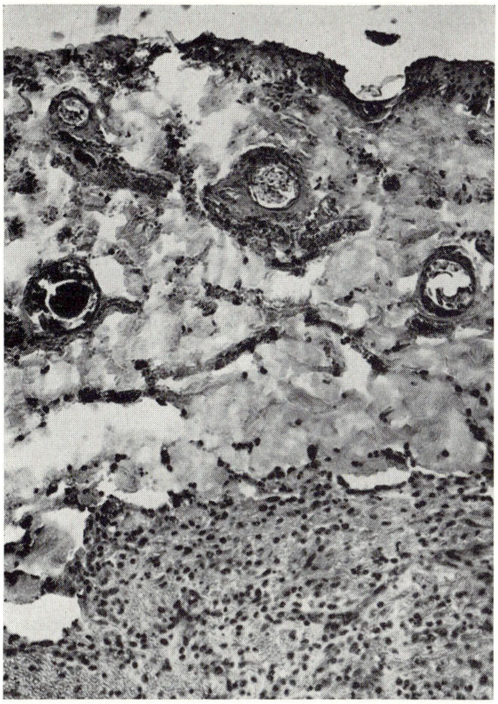

Fig. 1. Ischemic necrosis of a skin allograft 10 days after grafting to the intact tunica intima of the pulmonary artery. Note the absence of mononuclear cell infiltration and blood vessels with complete necrosis of the epidermis. (Hematoxylin and eosin. Original magnification ×400.)

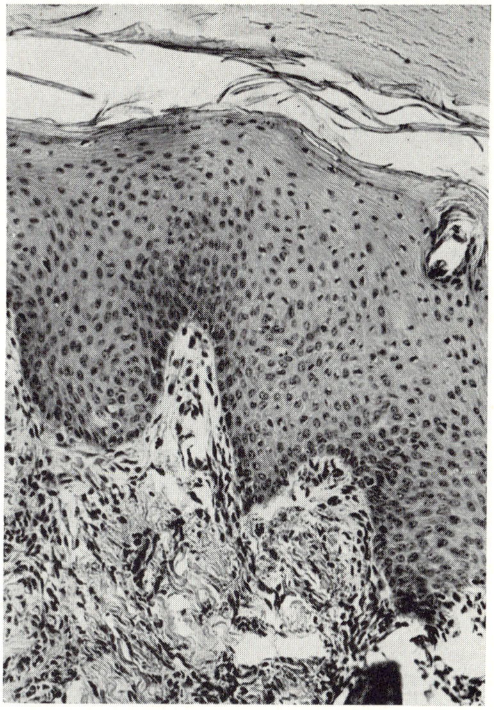

Fig. 2. Viable skin autograft 21 days after grafting to the tunica media of the pulmonary artery. (Hematoxylin and eosin. Original magnification ×400.)

travascular allograft transplanted to a calf that did not receive a simultaneous orthotopic allograft was viable and there was only slight mononuclear cell infiltration (Fig. 3). The skin allografts from calves killed 12 and 14 days after grafting had some viable epidermis, but many epidermal cells had vacuolated cytoplasm and pyknotic nuclei and there was intense infiltration of the graft with mononuclear cells—signs suggestive of impending rejection. By 20 and 21 days, rejection of intravascular allografts transplanted to the media was complete with complete loss of the epidermis (Fig. 4).

DISCUSSION

The fate of allovital heart valve transplants and the host response to them have been uncertain because of the difficulty in assessing the degree of destruction of the valve by the host, the inability to determine the relative numbers of donor and host cells populating the graft, and the difficulty in differentiating ischemic necrosis from immunologic rejection of the valve transplant. For these reasons, skin was chosen for the experiments instead of cardiac valve leaflets.

These experiments establish that the survival of intravascular skin autografts and allografts depends on the presence or absence of the tunica intima. The tunica intima composed of endothelium, elastic and collagenous fibers, fibroblasts, and small bundles of smooth muscle cells, when intact, is a barrier that prevents early vascular, fibrous, and, presumably, lymphatic union between the graft and the host. As a result, even with continuous bathing of the graft by blood flowing through the pulmonary artery, the skin grafts underwent ischemic necrosis. However, when the intima was disrupted or removed, vascular and lymphatic union between graft and host was established and the grafts survived until, in the case of allografts, immunologic rejection occurred.

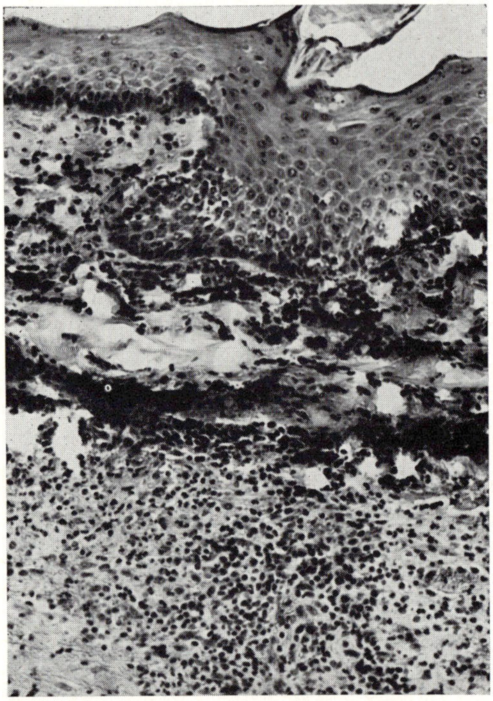

Fig. 3. Skin allograft 10 days after grafting to the tunica media of the pulmonary artery. Note the slight mononuclear cell infiltration, but viable epidermis. (Hematoxylin and eosin. Original magnification ×400.)

Barker and Billingham[3] recently demonstrated the importance of afferent lymphatic union between skin allografts and the host as a prerequisite to immunologic recognition and rejection. In guinea pigs, a skin allograft grafted on a skin pedicle having intact blood vessels but no lymphatic union with its host enjoyed a privileged survival. If guinea pigs with such isolated allografts were sensitized to the donor with a second orthotopic skin graft, or the isolated allograft was allowed to establish a lymphatic union with the host, the allografts were rejected in the usual manner.

Networks of thin-walled lymphatics are present in the vessel walls of the larger arteries and veins. They connect with the perivascular lymphatics and may be traced to the media of blood vessels.[10] Thus, an intravascular allograft transplanted to the media of the vessel would establish afferent lymphatic and vascular union with the host which, according to the work of Barker and Billingham,[3] should result in sensitization of the host and rejection. The slightly prolonged survival of intravascular skin allografts compared with orthotopic skin allografts was probably due to delayed sensitization of the host through the affer-

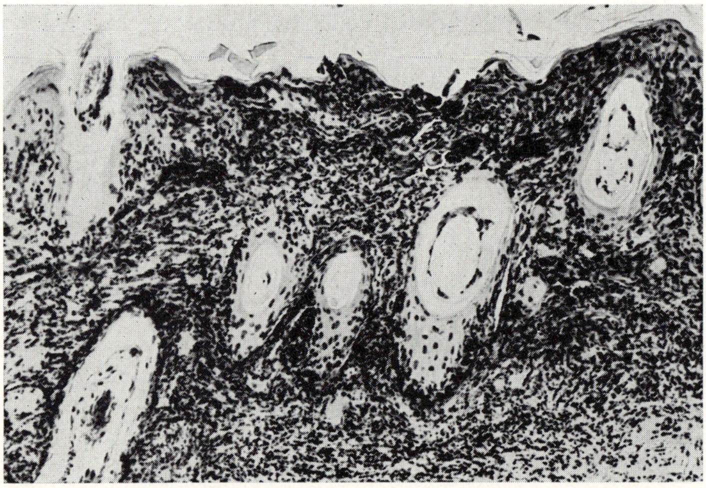

Fig. 4. Immunologic rejection of a skin allograft 21 days after grafting to the tunica media of the pulmonary artery. Note the intense mononuclear cell infiltration and complete loss of epidermis. (Hematoxylin and eosin. Original magnification ×100.)

ent lymphatics. This could be due to less lymphatic drainage of the tunica media of the pulmonary artery compared to skin. The fact that the intravascular grafts were promptly rejected when the host was sensitized with an orthotopic graft provides further evidence that delayed sensitization of the host was responsible for the prolonged survival of the intravascular allografts.

The discrepancy of results reported by investigators regarding the fate of allovital valve transplants can be explained on a "barrier" hypothesis. The tunica intima is not routinely removed before insertion of an allovital valve and, therefore, would act as a barrier to vascular and lymphatic connection with the host. As a result, the thick annulus or sleeve of the allograft valve undergoes early ischemic necrosis and, later, calcification. The leaflets probably survive initially because of their thin structure, their position within the bloodstream, small nutritional requirements, and failure, at least initially, to establish vascular and lymphatic connection with the host. Thus, the transplant heart valve leaflets would appear to be in an immunologically privileged site and would not be rejected. However, if the intima is disrupted during insertion of the allovital valve or the intima is removed intentionally during placement, one would expect immunologic rejection after establishment of vascular and lymphatic union with the host.

SUMMARY

Allografts and autografts of skin were grafted to the intact intima or to the tunica media of the pulmonary artery distal to the pulmonic valve to determine the host's immunologic response to intravascular grafts. With the intima removed, autografts were vascularized and survived. The allografts were vascularized but underwent immunologic rejection between 15 and 20 days after grafting. With the intima intact, both intravascular skin autografts and allografts underwent early ischemic necrosis.

These experiments establish that intravascular grafts are not in a privileged site and that such grafts are capable of sensitizing and eliciting a host response if the tunica intima is removed. They suggest a "barrier" hypothesis in which the intact tunica intima and transplanted valve annulus prevents immunologic rejection of allovital heart valve leaflets by the host.

REFERENCES

1. Anderson, D., Billingham, R. E., Lampkin, G. H., and Medawar, P. B.: The use of skin grafting to distinguish between monozygotic and dizygotic twins in cattle, Heredity **5:** 379, 1951.
2. Baue, A. E., Donawick, W. J., and Blakemore, W. S.: The immunologic response to heterotopic allovital aortic valve transplants in presensitized and nonsensitized recipients, J. Thorac. Cardiov. Surg. **56:** 775, 1968.
3. Barker, C. F., and Billingham, R. E.: The role of afferent lymphatics in the rejection of skin homografts, J. Exp. Med. **128:** 197, 1968.
4. Barnes, R. W., Mohri, H., and Merendino, K. A.: An experimental method for the study of the homologous aortic valve, Surg. Forum **18:** 122, 1967.
5. Chanana, A. D., Brecher, G., and Cronkite, E. P.: Histologic observations on skin autographs, isografts and allografts in cattle, Amer. J. Path. **49:** 1125, 1966.
6. Cleveland, R. J., Madge, G. E., and Lower, R. R.: Homovital graft replacement of the aortic valve, Surg. Forum **18:** 124, 1967.
7. Donawick, W. J., Nara, Y., and Baue, A. E.: Techniques for successful cardiopulmonary bypass in the calf, J. Surg. Res. **9:** 79, 1969.
8. Howard, H. S., Willman, V. L., and Hanlon, C. R.: Mitral valve replacement, Surg. Forum **11:** 256, 1960.
9. Kwong, K. H., Paton, B. C., and Hill, R. B., Jr.: Experimental use of immunosuppression in aortic valve homografts and heterografts, J. Thorac. Cardiov. Surg. **54:** 199, 1967.
10. Maximow, A. A., and Bloom, W.: A textbook of histology, ed. 7, Philadelphia, 1957, W. B. Saunders Company, p. 243.
11. McKenzie, M. B., Titus, J. L., Ellis, F. H., Jr., and Pappas, G.: Experimental semilunar valve homografts: Morphologic features, J. Thorac. Cardiov. Surg. **50:** 410, 1965.
12. Mohri, H., Nelson, R. J., Sands, M. P., and Merendino, K. A.: Homotransplantation of the aortic valve, Surg. Forum **17:** 173, 1966.
13. Van Vliet, P. D., Titus, J. L., Berghuis, J., and Ellis, F. H., Jr.: Morphologic features of homotransplanted canine mitral valves, J. Thorac. Cardiov. Surg. **49:** 504, 1965.

Experimental studies on the effect of dimethyl sulfoxide on pedicle flaps

H. E. KOEHNLEIN, M.D.
G. LEMPERLE, M.D.
FREIBURG, GERMANY
From the Division of Plastic Surgery, Department of Surgery, University of Freiburg

There are only a few medications, like low molecular weight dextran, which are able to improve the circulation in pedicle flaps. In 1966 Adamson, Horton, and Crawford[2] published a report on the effects of local dimethyl sulfoxide (DMSO) treatment of pedicle flaps. They observed a marked improvement of the circulation after daily local treatment with a 70 percent solution. This improvement disappeared if the animals were treated with an antihistamine at the same time. The authors, therefore, came to the conclusion that the action of DMSO was similar to histamine. We thought that this observation was important enough to justify further investigation.

If DMSO is applied locally to human skin, 15 to 30 percent of the applied amount is absorbed within 2 hours. Ten percent of the substance appears in the urine within 5 days. If DMSO is given intravenously, it accelerates the coagulation of fibrinogen and other plasma proteins and causes hemolysis. Large doses of DMSO can cause skin irritation and allergic reactions; they may be liver toxic, and very large doses may cause changes of the lense in the eye. DMSO has a lytic effect on collagen, demonstrable by an increased hydroxyproline excretion in the urine. Several changes in cell metabolism were described.

EXPERIMENTS

We operated on 130 Sprague-Dawley rats. The same operation was performed on 10 animals, five of which were treated with daily local application of 3 Gm. DMSO gel (89 percent), while the other five received no treatment. The resulting sloughs were measured daily.

In the first group of animals 1.5 by 2.5 inch full-thickness skin flaps were lifted off the underlying tissue, leaving them attached at the neck and sutured back into position. After 1 week 5 $cm.^2$ sloughed in the control group, but 16 $cm.^2$ in the DMSO group. If the grafts were completely severed and turned around their axis before suturing them back, the sloughs in the control group developed faster, but not as fast as in the DMSO–treated group (Figs. 1 and 2).

These differences were less impressive if DMSO was applied before the operation only. In the next group we formed tubed pedicle flaps, based on the neck. The free distal end of the tube was attached to the skin with a metal clip in order to avoid mechanical irritation. The result was not different from the previous experiments. The DMSO–treated flaps sloughed much faster than the others. In the last group bipedicle tubed flaps were formed from the skin on the back (Figs. 3 and 4). Even though the blood supply was much better, the sloughs developed considerably faster in the DMSO–treated group.

CONCLUSION

There were no macroscopic changes on the first postoperative day, but the flaps felt cooler than the surrounding tissue because of the insufficient circulation. The DMSO–treated animals started to show mottling of

Received for publication May 2, 1969.

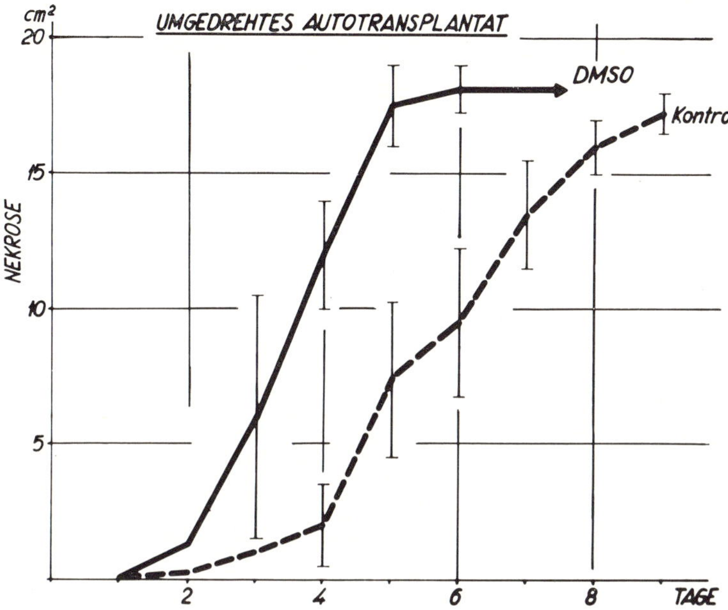

Fig. 1. Autograft, turned around its axis. Percentage of slough, in square centimeters, developing after the operation. The solid line illustrates the results in the DMSO-treated group and the deviations; the interrupted line illustrates the control group.

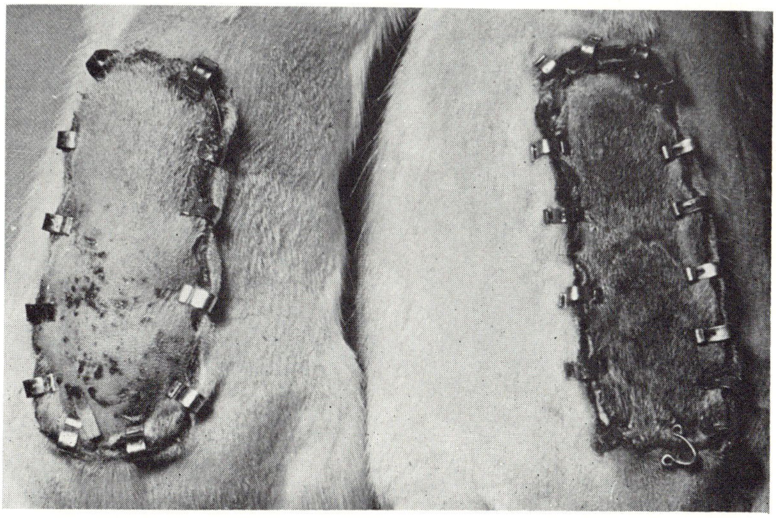

Fig. 2. Left side: untreated control animal, 6 days postoperatively; right side: graft of an animal that was treated locally and daily with 3 Gm. DMSO, 6 days postoperatively.

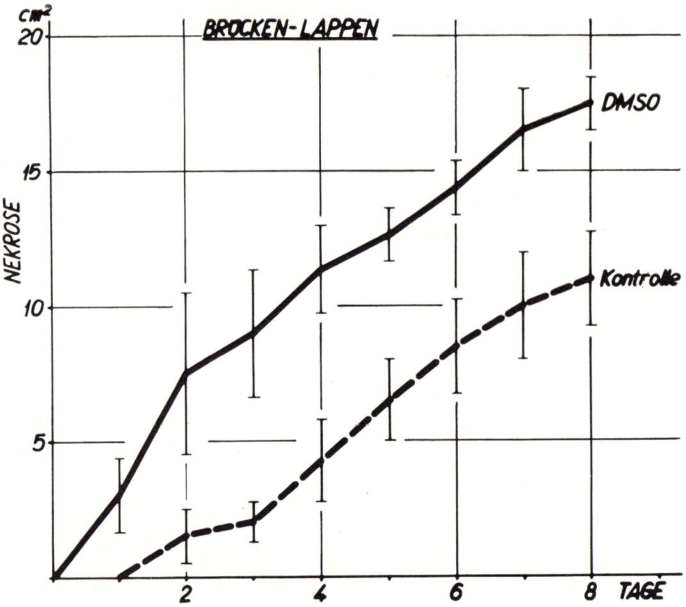

Fig. 3. Slough developing in bipedicle flaps, measured in square centimeters. Solid line: DMSO-treated group; interrupted line: control group.

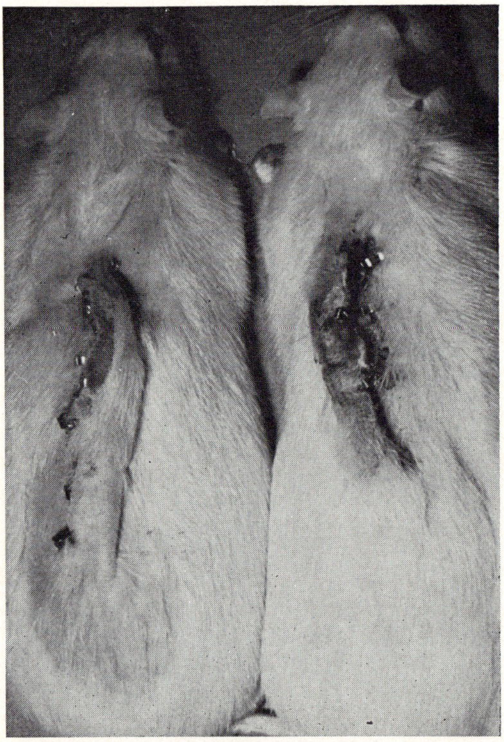

Fig. 4. Animals 8 days after bipedicle tubed flaps were formed from the back skin. The donor site was closed with clips. Left side: untreated control animal; right side: appearance of tube flap after daily treatment with 3 Gm. DMSO.

the grafts on the second postoperative day, the control animals not until the third day. The discolored spots grew larger and became confluent on the third and fourth days. On the fifth day about one third of the flaps started to slough in the control group, while it was already two thirds in the DMSO-treated group. There were only slight differences between the different types of grafts and flaps. The sloughs in the treated group were complete by the seventh postoperative day and began to show demarcation, while this was not the case in the control group until the tenth postoperative day. All the flaps were too long to have sufficient circulation through the pedicles. There was definite venous congestion. We therefore believe that the effective tissue concentration of DMSO after local treatment in flap tissue is much higher than after treatment of normal skin. Since a DMSO concentration of 30 percent can already cause fibrinogen coagulation and hemolysis, we believe that this is what happens in the pedicle flaps. The increased permeability of the cell membranes after DMSO treatment did possibly cause a faster distribution of autolytic enzymes which furthered the sloughing.

SUMMARY

Full-thickness grafts, pedicle flaps, bipedicle flaps, and tubed flaps were formed on the back skin of 130 Sprague-Dawley rats. Half of the animals were treated daily and locally with 3 Gm. of an 89 percent dimethylsulfoxide gel. The treated animals showed much more extensive sloughing than did the untreated control group, in contrast to the observations by Adamson, Horton, and Crawford.[2] These authors used 70 percent liquid DMSO. Our expectation, to improve the circulation in pedicle flaps by local treatment with DMSO, proved to be false.

REFERENCES

1. Adamson, J. E., Crawford, H. H., and Horton, C. E.: The action of dimethyl sulfoxide on the experimental pedicle flap, Surg. Forum **17:** 491, 1966.
2. Adamson, J. E., Horton, C. E., Crawford, H. H., and Ayers, W. T., Jr.: The effects of dimethyl sulfoxide on the experimental pedicle flap: A preliminary report, Plast. Reconstr. Surg. **37:** 105, 1966.
3. Ansel, H. C., and Leake, W. F.: Hemolysis of erythrocytes by antibacterial preservatives. III. Influence of dimethyl sulfoxide on the hemolytic activity of phenol, J. Pharm. Sci. **55:** 685, 1966.
4. Ashwood-Smith, M. J.: Low temperature preservation of mouse lymphocytes with dimethyl sulfoxide, Blood **23:** 494, 1964.
5. Ashwood-Smith, M. J.: Radioprotective effect of combinations of AET or cysteamine with dimethyl sulphoxide, Int. J. Radiat. Biol. **5:** 201, 1962.
6. Ashwood-Smith, M. J.: Viability of mouse bone marrow frozen to –79° C. in the presence of dimethyl sulfoxide, J. Physiol. **155:** 26P, 1961.
7. Barron, J., Veall, N., and Arnott, D. G.: The measurement of the local clearance of radioactive sodium in tubed skin pedicles, Brit. J. Plast. Surg. **4:** 16, 1951.
8. Bloch, J. H.: Preservative solutions for the freezing of whole organs in vitro, Fed. Proc. **22:** 170, 1963.
9. Bradham, G. B., and Sample, J. J.: The vascular and thermal effects of dimethyl sulfoxide, Ann. N. Y. Acad. Sci. **141:** 225, 1967.
10. Braithwaite, F.: Preliminary observations on the vascular channels in tubed pedicles, Brit. J. Plast. Surg. **3:** 40, 1950.
11. Bridges, B. A.: Protection of Pseudomonas sp. against gamma-radiation by dimethyl sulphoxide, Int. J. Radiat. Biol. **5:** 101, 1962.
12. Brown, J. H.: Klinische Erfahrungen mit DMSO bei akuten Erkrankungen des Muskel-Skelet-Systems, DMS–Symposium at Vienna, 1966, pp. 115-120.
13. Burri, C., and Matter, P.: Die Beeinflussung der Durchblutung im Rundstiellappen durch niedermolek. Dextran, Z. Ges. Exp. Med. **140:** 170, 1966.
14. Cavins, J. A.: Preservation of dog bone marrow at low temperatures in dimethylsulphoxide, Blood **20:** 635, 1962.
15. Cohen, E., and Rowe, A. W.: Detection of leukoagglutinins with dimethylsulfoxide (DMSO) protected leukocytes frozen with liquid nitrogen, Vox. Sang. **10:** 543, 1965.
16. Collins, W. E., and Jeffery, G. M.: The use of dimethylsulfoxide in the low temperature frozen preservation of experimental malarias, J. Parasit. **49:** 524, 1963.
17. Conway, H., Stark, R. B., and Joslin, D.: Cutaneous histamine reaction as a test of circulatory efficiency of tubed pedicles and flaps, Surg. Gynec. & Obst. **93:** 185, 1951.
18. Davis, H. L., Davis, N. L., and Clemons, A. L.: Procoagulant and nerve-blocking effects of DMSO, Ann. N. Y. Acad. Sci. **141:** 310, 1967.
19. Day, P. L.: Auswertung der Behandlungsergebnisse von annähernd 1000 mit DMSO behandelten Fällen in der orthopädischen Praxis, DMSO–Symposium at Vienna, 1966, pp. 107-109.
20. Distefano, V., and Borgstedt, H. H.: Reduction of dimethylsulfoxide to dimethylsulfide in the cat, Science **144:** 1137, 1964.
21. Fasske, E.: Zur Frage der Verwendbarkeit von DMSO als Lösungsmittel für Zytostatica, DMSO–Symposium at Vienna, 1966, pp. 43-51.
22. Formanek, K., and Kovać, W.: Die Wirkung von DMSO auf die Bildung des reparativen Granulationsgewebes bei Ratten, DMSO–Symposium at Vienna, 1966, pp. 24-26.
23. Franz, T. J., and Van Bruggen, J. T.: A possible mechanism of action of DMSO, Ann. N. Y. Acad. Sci. **141:** 302, 1967.
24. Gerhards, E., Gibian, H., and Raspé, G.: Stoffwechsel und Stoffwechselwirkungen von Dimethylsulfoxid, Arzneimittelforschung **15:** 1295, 1965.
25. Gottlob, R., and Zinner, G.: Die Bestimmung der endothelschädigenden Wirkung injizierbarer Lösungen. Der Einfluss des osmotischen Druckes und des pH, Wien. Klin. Wschr. **77:** 149, 1965.
26. Gries, G., Bublitz, G., Freytag, G., and Lindner, J.: Die Wirkung von DMSO auf das Bindegewebe, DMSO–Symposium at Vienna, 1966, pp. 26-32.
27. Horita, A., and Weber, L. J.: Skin penetrating properties of drugs dissolved in dimethyl

sulfoxide (DMSO) and other vehicles, Life Sci. **3:** 1389, 1964.
28. Hucker, H. B., Ahmad, P. M., Miller, E. A., et al.: Metabolism of dimethyl sulphoxide to dimethyl sulphone in the rat and man, Nature **209:** 619, 1966.
29. Hynes, W.: The blood-vessels in skin tubes and flaps, Brit. J. Plast. Surg. **3:** 165, 1950.
30. Hynes, W.: The use of fluorescein in estimating the blood flow in pedicled skin flaps and tubes Brit. J. Plast. Surg. **2:** 4, 1950.
31. Jacob, St. W., Bischel, M., and Herschler, R. J.: Dimethyl sulfoxide: Effects on the permeability of biologic membranes (preliminary report), Curr. Ther. Res. **6:** 193, 1964.
32. Jacob, St. W., and Rosenbaum, E. E.: The toxicology of dimethyl sulfoxide (DMSO), Headache **6:** 127, 1966.
33. John, H.: Therapeutische Erfahrungen mit Dimethylsulfoxyd in der orthopädischen Praxis, Arzneimittelforschung. **15:** 1298, 1965.
34. John, H.: Zweijährige Erfahrungen mit der DMSO–Therapie bei einem grossen orthopädischen Krankengut, DMSO–Symposium at Vienna, 1966, pp. 113-114.
35. Kamiya, S., Wakao, T., and Nishioka, K.: Studies on improvement of eye drops. III. Bacteriological consideration of DMSO, Rinsho Ganka (Jap. J. Clin. Ophthal.) **20:** 143, 1966.
36. Kharasch, N., and Thyagarajan, B. S.: The chemistry of dimethyl sulfoxide for the period 1961-1965, Quart. Rep. Sulfur Chem. **1:** 1, 1966.
37. Kleberger, E.: Zur Toxikologie von DMSO am Auge, DMSO–Symposium at Vienna, 1966, p. 56.
38. Klingenström, P., and Nylén, B.: Timing of transfer of tubed pedicles and cross-flaps, Plast. Reconstr. Surg. **37:** 1, 1966.
39. Kolb, K. H., Jänicke, G., et al.: Das Verhalten von 35 S markiertem Dimethylsulfoxid im menschlichen und tierischen Organismus, Arzneimittelforschung **15:** 1292, 1965.
40. Leake, Ch. D.: Einiges zur Vorgeschichte von DMSO, DMSO–Symposium at Vienna, 1966, pp. 2-5.
41. Lovelock, J. E., and Bishop, M. W. H.: Prevention of freezing damage to living cells by dimethyl sulfoxide, Nature **183:** 1934, 1959.
42. Lüth, H. F.: DMSO in der orthopädischen Praxis und bei Sportverletzungen, DMSO–Symposium at Vienna, 1966, pp. 105-107.
43. Misch, D. W.: The penetration of lysosomes by dimethyl sulfoxide, J. Cell Biol. **27:** 67A, 1965.
44. Murray, W.: The effect of delay on the circulatory efficiency of pedicled tissue, Plast. Reconstr. Surg. **33:** 16, 1964.
45. Myers, M. B., and Cherry, G.: Augmentation of tissue survival by delay: An experimental study in rabbits, Plast. Reconstr. Surg. **39:** 397, 1967.
46. Panuska, J. A., Malinin, T. I., and Mentz, R. J.: Der Einfluss von DMSO auf den Abfall der Körpertemperatur bei Ratten, Cryobiology **2:** 345, 1966.
47. Paul, M. M.: Vergleich von Dimethylsulfoxyd und konventioneller Behandlung bei Sportverletzungen, DMSO–Symposium at Vienna, 1966, pp. 101-105.
48. Peterson, C. G., and Robertson, R. D.: A pharmacodynamic study of dimethyl sulfoxide, Ann. N. Y. Acad. Sci. **141:** 273, 1967.
49. Pottz, G. E., Rampey, J. H., and Benjamin, F. A.: Method for rapid staining of acid-fast bacteria in smears and sections of tissue, Techn. Bull. Regist. Med. Techn. **34:** 552, 1964.
50. Prokop, L.: Erfahrungen mit DMSO bei sportbedingten Überlastungsschäden des Bindegewebes, DMSO–Symposium at Vienna, 1966, pp. 95-96.
51. Raettig, H.: Möglichkeiten des DMSO in der experimentellen Immunologie, DMSO–Symposium at Vienna, 1966, pp. 51-56.
52. Rammler, D. H.: The effect of DMSO on several enzyme systems, Ann. N. Y. Acad. Sci. **141:** 291, 1967.
53. Rosenbaum, E. E., and Jacob, St. W.: DMSO in acute musculoskeletal injuries and inflammations. I. Dimethyl sulfoxide in acute subdeltoid bursitis, Northwest Med. **63:** 167, 1964.
54. Saytzeff, A.: Über die Einwirkung von Salpetersäure auf Schwefelmethyl und Schwefeläthyl, Ann. Chem. Pharm. **144:** 148, 1867.
55. Scherbel, A. L., McCormack, L. J., and Poppo, M. J.: Alteration of collagen in generalized scleroderma (progressive systemic sclerosis) after treatment with dimethyl sulfoxide: Preliminary report, Cleveland Clin. Quart. **32:** 47, 1965.
56. Sciuchetti, L. A., and Born, A. E.: Effect of dimethylsulfoxide alone and combined with N-dimethylamino succinamic acid (B995) or (2-chloroethyl)trimethylammonium chloride (CCC) on the growth and alkaloid biosynthesis of Datura tatula, J. Pharm. Sci. **54:** 285, 1965.
57. Sciuchetti, L. A., and Connors Mingis, N.: The effect of dimethylsulfoxide (DMSO) and tributyl 2, 4-dichlorobenzylphosphonium chloride (Phosphon) on growth and alkaloid synthesis in Datura ferox, Lloydia **28:** 230, 1965.
58. Smith, E.: Diskussion, DMSO–Symposium at Vienna, 1966, pp. 74-75.
59. Störig, E.: Allgemeine Lehre von den Plas-

tiken und Transplantationen in der Wiederherstellungschirurgie, *in* Zetkin, M., and Kühtz, E. H., editors: Die Chirurgie des Traumas, Berlin, 1958, Veb Fischer, Band III/2, pp. 1055-1076.
60. Stoughton, R. B.: Percutaneous absorption, Toxicol. Appl. Pharmacol. **7:** 1, 1965. (Suppl.)
61. Suckert, R.: Klinische Erfahrungen mit DMSO bei Verletzungen und chronischen Schäden am Bewegungsapparat, DMSO–Symposium at Vienna, 1966, pp. 91-95.
62. Thomas, R., Brink Shoemaker, C., and Eriks, K.: The molecular and crystal structure of dimethyl sulfoxide, $(H_3C)_2SO$, Acta Crystallogr. **21:** 12, 1966.
63. Wodniansky, P.: DMSO–Behandlung bei Dupuytren und Sklerodermie, DMSO–Symposium at Vienna, 1966, pp. 158-160.
64. Wood, D. C., and Wirth, N. V.: Weitere Untersuchungen zur Wirkung von DMSO am Kaninchenauge, DMSO–Symposium at Vienna, 1966, pp. 58-67.

Auxiliary homotransplantation of the porcine liver into the retroperitoneal space

V. NOVAK
L. HILL
R. ROTHWELL-JACKSON
A. VELASQUEZ
R. WRIGHT
B. EISEMAN
DENVER, COLO.
From the Department of Surgery, University of Colorado Medical Center

Because of the regenerative capacity of the liver, hepatic failure during hepatitis or following acute toxicity is potentially reversible. Temporary extracorporeal hepatic assist perfusing the patient's blood through a heterologous liver is of limited clinical value.[7] Temporary liver transplantation might be of benefit in such patients.

Original experimental trials with auxiliary heterotopic liver transplantations were performed by Welch[38] and Goodrich and associates.[11] The problem, however, remains unsolved. Clinical trials have been unsuccessful.[13, 20, 32] To date, no such heterotopically transplanted liver has survived more than three weeks. With the current knowledge gained from Starzl and associates'[33, 34] successful clinical use of liver orthotopic transplants, the subject bears re-examination. This investigation explores techniques for the insertion of homologous livers for temporary auxiliary support.

Because in its clinical setting insertion and early removal of an auxiliary liver should represent a minimum operative insult, the following principles were adopted: (1) placement of the graft in the extraperitoneal space; (2) vascularization of the graft via hepatic artery only; (3) external biliary drainage; and (4) no immunosuppression.

METHODS

The donor pigs were prepared and hepatectomy was performed, as described previously,[21] in this laboratory. Small donor pigs (body weight, 9 to 16 kilograms) were paired with large recipients (body weight, 30 to 36 kilograms). Mean weight of the drained donor whole livers was 280 grams. Ischemic time between harvest and revascularization in the recipient was 44 to 48 minutes. One liter or more of Ringer's lactate supported the donor during operation.

In the recipient, the right retroperitoneal space was widely exposed through a transrectal abdominal incision. Occasionally the graft bed was enlarged by right nephrectomy.

Group I: Vascular combinations, whole liver (10 experiments). The eight various arterial and venous attachments used in these preliminary studies are illustrated in Fig. 1. In all but one instance, washout of the donor liver was done with buffered, heparinized Ringer's lactate solution. Right nephrectomy was performed in three experiments. A 2 cm. cuff of abdominal aorta adjacent to the celiac axis formed the vascular pedicle of the donor liver. In one of these experiments, the portal vein was as shown in Fig. 1, *H*.

Group II: Arterialized whole liver (6 ex-

Supported by grants from the United States Public Health Service and the Colorado Division of the American Cancer Society.

Submitted for publication June 2, 1969; resubmitted Aug. 18, 1969.

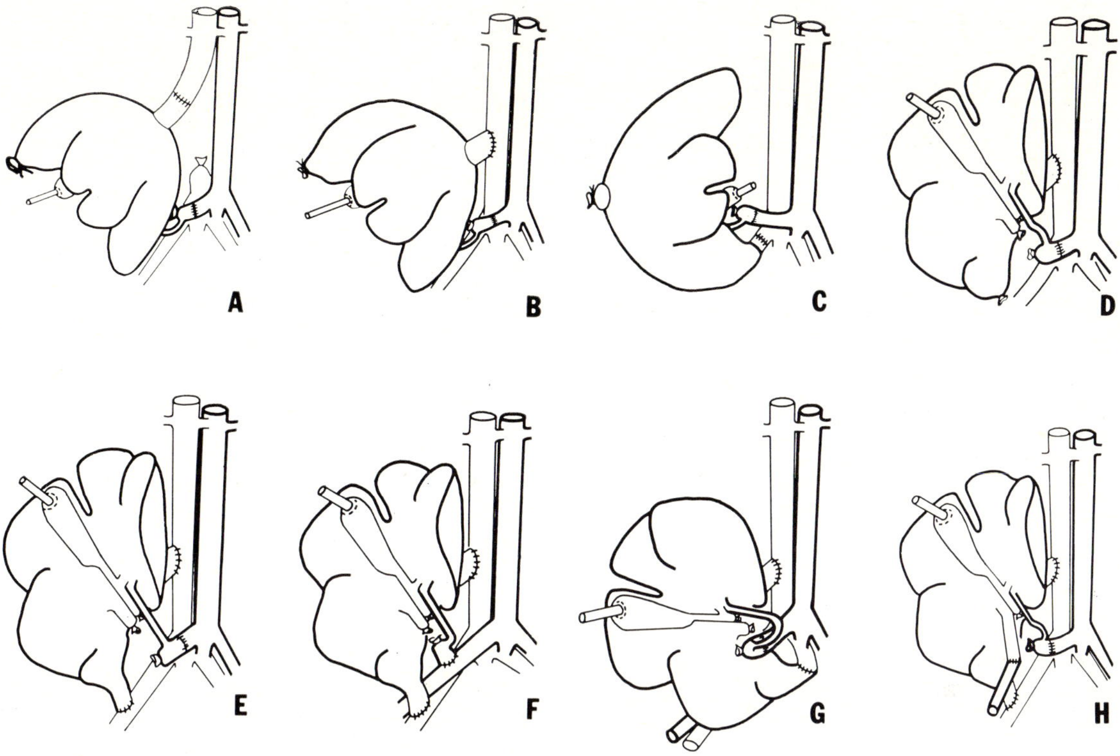

Fig. 1. Anastomotic techniques used for whole auxiliary liver transplantation.

periments). As illustrated in Fig. 1, *E,* the whole, unrinsed, donor liver was placed in the right retroperitoneal area. The graft was arterialized through the hepatic artery from the severed proximal right common iliac artery of the recipient. The portal vein was not vascularized. Donor effluence via the suprahepatic cava was end to side into the abdominal cava of the recipient. Auxiliary liver function was quantitated after ligating the recipient common duct at the time of grafting by collecting bile from the cannulated donor cholecystostomy in a Fenwall Laboratory Model TA-2 Blood Transfer Plastic Bag sutured to the recipient's skin. Bile volume and bilirubin concentration were measured daily. The serum bilirubin concentration, alkaline phosphatase, and serum glutamic oxalacetic transaminase (SGOT) were measured daily in the recipient. Arteriography and technetium scanning[25] of the donor liver were performed five to ten days following insertion of the graft.

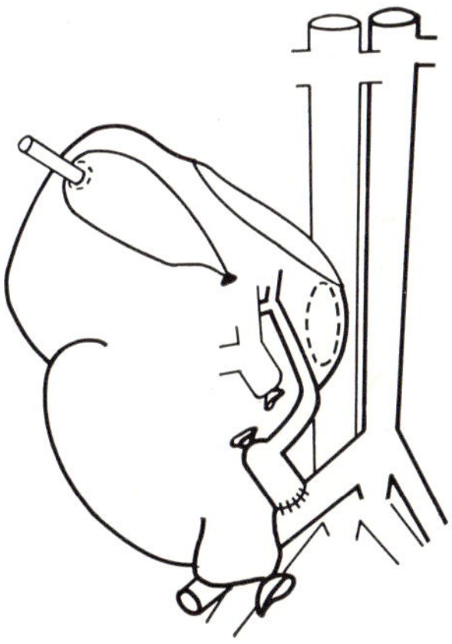

Fig. 2. Anastomotic technique with the use of right and right medial lobe of the liver. The common duct, portal vein, and intrahepatic cava are ligated. The graft is vascularized solely through the hepatic artery. Effluence is through the suprahepatic cava cut flush with the superior portion of the liver.

In 12 control animals, the effect of common duct ligation alone was evaluated by biochemical studies performed on the third and seventh postoperative days.

Group III: Arterialized right lateral and right medial lobes (8 experiments). Transplantation of the entire liver, even from small donors, resulted in impaired venous outflow from the left side of the graft. Therefore, the right half of the liver (right lateral and right medial lobes) was used as a graft. Branches of the portal vein, hepatic artery, and bile ducts were meticulously isolated, ligated, and severed as they entered the left medial and lateral lobes. Fig. 2 demonstrates the anastomoses in the recipients. The common duct, intrahepatic cava, and portal vein were ligated. Afferent supply was through the hepatic artery, and outflow was through the suprahepatic cava to the side of the host abdominal vena cava. The only difference between the techniques shown in Fig. 1, *D* and Fig. 2 is that in the latter the suprahepatic cava was cut flush with the top of the liver to avoid kinking. The common duct of the recipient was ligated at the time of transplantation. Postoperative studies followed as in Group II. Daily blood sampling was from an intravenous catheter containing a stylet, placed in the internal jugular vein. This usually functioned for a week. The pigs received 1.2 million units of Bicillin and 0.5 Gm. of streptomycin daily.

Group IV: Arterialized right lateral and right medial lobes, jaundiced recipients (7 experiments). In these animals, the recipient common duct was ligated five to fourteen days prior to insertion of the right half of a donor liver as an auxiliary graft. The recipients (mean body weight, 32 kilograms) lost an average of 2.3 kilograms between common duct ligation and insertion of the auxiliary liver.

RESULTS

Controls. The effect of common duct ligation alone is summarized in Table I. It illustrates the anticipated prompt elevation in serum bilirubin, alkaline phosphatase, and SGOT.

Group I: Vascular combinations, whole liver. Of the ten recipients in this preliminary study group, five died of technical complications within six hours of operation. Five pigs survived at least four days, but only two produced bile. Obstruction of the suprahepatic cava was the limiting factor in this operation. Pressures within this long segment of cava, which was variously stretched, compressed, or kinked, were markedly elevated above those recorded in

Table I. *Serum bilirubin, alkaline phosphatase, and SGOT after common bile duct ligation in 21 control pigs*

Time	*Bilirubin (mg. % ± S.D.)*	*Alk. phosphatase (Sigma U. ± S.D.)*	*SGOT (U. ± S.D.)*
Before operation	0.136 ± 0.048	3.12 ± 0.72	47.6 ± 13.96
Postop. day 3	7.185 ± 4.758	6.40 ± 2.30	71.1 ± 30.40
Postop. day 7	4.213 ± 1.959	4.29 ± 1.87	85.1 ± 28.81

Table II. *Function of heterotopic liver grafts*

	Group							
	I		*II*		*III*		*IV*	
	No.	*Percent*	*No.*	*Percent*	*No.*	*Percent*	*No.*	*Percent*
Death within 6 hr. after operation	5	50	2	33	0	0	1	14
Grafts never excreting bile	3	30	2	33	2	25	1	14
Functioning grafts	2	20	2	33	6	75	5	71

the recipients' vena cava (10 to 20 cm. H_2O). Such an auxiliary liver was severely cramped and often was folded on itself and hugely engorged following vascular attachment. Ascites, bleeding, or thrombosis resulted. An additional anastomosis between donor infrahepatic cava and recipient external iliac vein was only of minor additional benefit. Anastomosis of the portal vein to the distal end of the severed external iliac artery (type *H,* Fig. 1) considerably magnified engorgement of the liver. Anastomotic patterns *E* and *F* (Fig. 1) became the most convenient and successful. Type *E* was standardized for the subsequent experiments: The sole afferent blood supply was from the host external iliac artery attached to the hepatic artery of the graft via an abdominal aortic cuff. Effluence was via the suprahepatic cava connected end to side to the infrarenal recipient vena cava. The donor infrahepatic cava was also connected end to side to the host external iliac vein.

Group II: Arterialized whole liver. Two of these six pigs died within the first six hours after operation because of bleeding and insufficient fluid replacement during the operation (Table II). The remaining four survived 7, 15, and 29 days, and one was killed on the eleventh postoperative day. Only two pigs secreted bile, one of them until the sixth postoperative day in amounts of 125, 170, 295, 270, 110, and 5 ml., respectively, and the other only until the fourth day in smaller amounts.

As in Group I, where the entire liver was used as a graft, obstruction to the suprahepatic cava was the limiting factor. In all three animals that spontaneously succumbed, the donor cava was found thrombosed. In the two cases that never produced bile, the hepatic artery was thrombosed.

Group III: Arterialized right lateral and right medial lobes As shown in Tables II and III, all animals survived at least eight days after this technically acceptable procedure.

Bile was produced by six of the eight heterotopic grafts. One animal was still producing bile when killed on the fifteenth day.

As demonstrated in Table IV and Table V, bilirubin clearance by the auxiliary liver was most efficient on the second post-transplant day and bile volume greatest on the third day. The functioning graft cleared sufficient bilirubin to maintain a normal plasma bilirubin concentration for five days. Thereafter, hyperbilirubinemia ensued. The difference between the control animals with a ligated common duct but without the support of an auxiliary liver is graphically illustrated in Fig. 3.

Table III. *Bile secretion, survival periods, and causes of deaths in Groups III and IV*

	Cessation of bile production (days)	Death (days)	Cause of death
Group III			
NWH 18	7	14	Killed
NWH 19	5	23	Killed
NWH 20	6	19	Yellow hepatodystrophy
NWH 21	0	14	Killed
NWH 22	0	8	Killed
NWH 23	15	15	Killed
NWH 24	8	8	Hemorrhagic enterocolitis
NWH 26	3	17	Pneumonia
Group IV			
L 76	0	2 hr.	Bleeding due to venous outflow obstruction
L 80	2	2	Pneumonia
L 82	6	6	Aspiration and suffocation
L 83	2	2	Hemorrhagic enterocolitis, yellow hepatodystrophy
L 84	0	6	Secondary bleeding from vena cava anastomosis
L 86	4	9	Killed
L 87	7	9	Pneumonia

Table IV. *Function of right lobes used as auxiliary liver in hosts with common ducts ligated at transplant (Group III)*

	*Serum**			*Bile**		
Time	*Bilirubin (mg. %)*	*Alk. phosphatase (Sigma U.)*	*SGOT (U.)*	*Volume (ml.)*	*Bilirubin† (mg. %)*	*Bilirubin output (mg.)*
Beginning of operation	0.25	2.92	32.3			
End of operation	0.16	2.67	61.3			
Day 1	0.86	6.37	89.7	93.6	60.04	56.2
Day 2	1.48	7.67	87.0	116.7	77.40	90.3
Day 3	2.16	7.50	64.3	147.0	45.45	66.8
Day 4	1.33	7.05	85.0	118.3	50.82	60.1
Day 5	1.83	4.08	70.0	45.0	17.75	8.0
Day 6	6.15	5.27	62.7	19.4	6.75	1.3
Day 7	6.58	8.10	61.0	12.2	3.03	0.4
Total				552.2		283.1

*All values are mean.

†The values are weighted mean.

Alkaline phosphatase and SGOT concentrations rose slightly on the first postoperative day but remained practically unchanged thereafter during the first week.

Group IV: Arterialized right lateral and right medial lobes, jaundiced recipients. Three of these seven animals died within 48 hours of technical problems not pertinent to graft function, as shown in Table III. Another animal failed to secrete bile and bled from an anastomotic site on the sixth postoperative day. The other auxiliary liver grafts secreted bile for four, six, and seven days (Tables VI and VII). The plasma bilirubin concentrations decreased during surgery, presumably because of hemodilution resulting from supportive intravenous fluid administration. Graft function maintained bilirubin concentration within a normal range as long as efficient bile production persisted. By the fourth post-transplant day, decreased auxiliary liver function was reflected by a rising concentration of plasma bilirubin.

Arteriography and technetium visualization of the grafts. Arteriography did not correlate with function in the seven animals in which it was employed. Five displayed normal visualization, but in three of the five, no bile was being produced.

Technetium scanning was used in eight animals. In only two was there significant visualization of the donor organ on the fourth and fifth day following transplant. Both were producing bile at the time. In four experiments, lack of technetium visualization corresponded with lack of bile production. Minimal technetium visualization in two grafts on the eighth and ninth day corresponded to slight bile production in one animal.

Table V. *Bilirubin excretion—8 auxiliary half-livers (Group III)*

	Bile		*Serum*
Postop. day	*Volume (c.c.)*	*Bilirubin output (mg.)*	*Bilirubin (mg. %)*
1	93.6	56.2	0.86
3	147.0	66.8	2.16
5	45.0	8.0	1.83
7	12.2	0.4	6.58

Technetium scan thus proved to be of both qualitative and quantitative value in appraising gross graft function.

It is of interest that the porcine lung concentrates almost as much technetium as does the liver (Fig. 3). The human lung, in contrast, normally demonstrates no traces of this isotope.

DISCUSSION

Clinical use of an auxiliary liver is envisioned in a desperately ill patient who will not well tolerate a formidable opera-

Table VI. *Function of right lobes used as auxiliary liver in hosts with common ducts ligated before transplant (Group IV)*

	*Serum**			*Bile**		
Time	*Bilirubin (mg. %)*	*Alk. phosphatase (Sigma U.)*	*SGOT (U.)*	*Volume (ml.)*	*Bilirubin† (mg. %)*	*Bilirubin output (mg.)*
Beginning of operation	5.71	3.39	52.7			
End of operation	3.49	2.70	91.7			
Day 1	1.24	2.59	78.7	111.0	188.53	209.3
Day 2	1.83	2.53	61.7	102.6	69.84	71.6
Day 3	1.51	2.27	70.3	101.0	76.12	76.9
Day 4	2.54	2.33	125.3	48.3	82.23	39.7
Day 5	4.21	2.78	132.0	10.0	32.00	3.2
Day 6	6.29	2.85	56.0	4.7	18.84	0.9
Day 7	6.16	4.54	125.0	1.5	14.90	0.1
Total				379.1		401.7

*All values are mean.
†The values are weighted mean.

Table VII. *Bilirubin excretion—7 auxiliary half-livers (Group IV)*

	Bile		*Serum*
Postop. days	*Volume (c.c.)*	*Bilirubin output (mg.)*	*Bilirubin (mg. %)*
1	110	209	1.24
3	101	77	1.51
5	10	3.2	4.2
7	1.5	0.1	6.16

tive procedure. Both the technique of insertion and subsequent removal of the temporary graft should therefore be simplified.

In previous studies, auxiliary livers have been variously placed within the peritoneal cavity, usually in the right hypogastrium.[1, 3-5, 8-11, 13, 15-18, 22, 23, 30, 31, 36-38] Mehrez and associates[19] and Sicular and associates[28] used the left, rather than the right, hypogastric region. Hagihara and Absolon[12] and Dagradi and associates[4] in experiments and Absolon,[12] Hermann,[32] and Halgrimson and associates[13] in clinical transplantations used the left upper quadrant following splenectomy. Absolon[12] put the grafted liver in the left thorax, and Sigel and associates[29] placed the lobe of a liver in the neck. We placed the auxiliary liver in the retroperitoneal space primarily to minimize operative trauma.

Disagreement abounds as to the best way to vascularize an auxiliary liver homograft. Duplication of the arrangement in life is obviously beyond challenge. Argument exists whether arterial supply to the hepatic artery alone will suffice. Many investigators[8, 10, 13, 14, 37] suggest that a liver graft can survive with this single supply. We have chosen this simple arterialization in these experiments.

Marchioro and associates[18] believe that prolonged liver function requires nutrients from the portal venous drainage. Tretbar and associates[37] and Price and associates[27] agree with this concept, but Heyde[15] does not.

External biliary drainage of the graft was used both because it was simpler than internal drainage and because it would be appropriate for potential use in temporary human auxiliary transplantation. It also enables measurement of bile production.

Graft function was accurately reflected both by bilirubin clearance in the bile and technetium visualization of the auxiliary liver. Total bile excretion—not only bile volume—was the more accurate indication of graft function.[6, 35] The bilirubin concen-

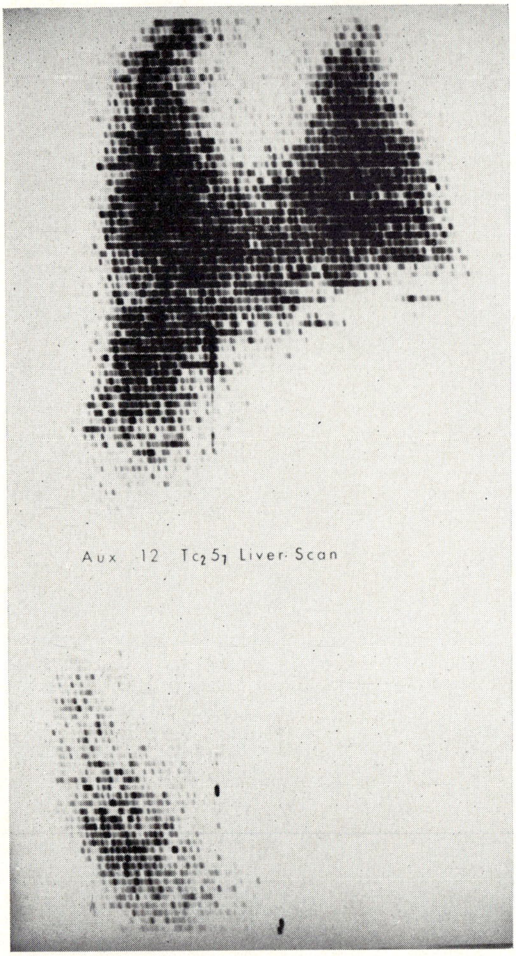

Fig. 3. Technetium-99m scan of the graft in the right retroperitoneal space. Note concentration of isotope in the porcine lung.

tration in the bile during the first few days following grafting was equivalent to that in normal pig gallbladder bile.[26]

These studies demonstrate effective auxiliary liver function for five to seven days without immunosuppression. This corresponds to equivalent findings in dogs.[11, 19, 28] Hagihara and Absolon[12] and Tretbar and associates[37] achieved somewhat longer function with the use of immunosuppression, but they were dealing with the more vigorous and immediate canine immune response. Peacock and Terblanche[24] and, subsequently, Calne and associates[2] have demonstrated that rejection of a porcine liver homograft was relatively less severe than in the dog.

Graft failures in the current study were not due to rejection. They occurred too soon after transplantation. Orthotopic transplants have worked efficiently in both experimental animals and clinical trials. Furthermore, microscopic study of these auxiliary livers also did not provide evidence of rejection. Characteristically, the pattern was one of lethal outflow obstruction and venous engorgement—not rejection.

Outflow venous obstruction caused by mechanical obstruction is, therefore, an immediate limiting factor in our studies as it has been in others.[1, 9, 10, 14, 19] This is not the intrinsic outflow block characteristic of a poorly preserved or insulted dog liver. In the pig, it is due to squeezing an oversized auxiliary liver into a limited space with resultant segmental or lobar obstruction of the liver. The right half of the liver fits more appropriately into the infrarenal retroperitoneal space. Use of a portion of a liver as an auxiliary graft has previously been employed experimentally and suggested clinically by others.[3, 9, 15, 17, 22, 29]

If rejection is not a limiting factor, two questions remain: (1) Can a better means be found for inserting an auxiliary liver and (2) will there be a place for temporary use of an auxiliary liver in patients with potentially severe hepatic failure? The techniques described are simple for both insertion and removal of the liver and allow effective function for from five to seven days.

SUMMARY

1. Thirty-one auxiliary livers were transplanted into the right retroperitoneal space of pigs in an effort to find a simple method for temporary support of patients in potentially reversible hepatic failure. Function of the heterotopic graft was monitored by bilirubin clearance and technetium concentration within the graft.

2. The right half of the liver vascularized solely via the hepatic artery was the most effective model. These grafts functioned five

to seven days without immunosuppression.

3. The limiting factor of graft function was hepatic venous hypertension, not rejection.

4. Possible clinical use of such a temporary auxiliary liver graft for potentially reversible liver failure is discussed. Although not suitable for permanent heterotopic homograft, this heterotopic technique meets the criteria for temporary use.

REFERENCES

1. Bengoechea-Gonzales, E., Yasuki, A., and Reemtsma, K.: Experimental auxiliary liver homotransplantation, Arch. Surg. **94:** 1, 1967.
2. Calne, R. Y., White, H. J. D., Yoffa, D. E., Binns, R. W., Maginn, R. R., Herbertson, R. M., Hillard, J. R., Molina, V. J., and Davis, D. R.: Prolonged survival of liver transplants in the pig, Brit. Med. J. **4:** 645, 1967.
3. Dagradi, A., Marzoli, G. P., Serio, G., Pinter, L., Piscitelli, M., Radin, S., Dagradi, V., Zannini, M., Dal Santo, F., and Puchetti, V.: Omotrapianti di lobo epatico, Chir. Pat. Sper. **13:** 295, 1965.
4. Dagradi, A., Marzoli, G. P., Serio, G., Fusaroli, P., Bano, A., Zannini, M., Radin, S., Pinter, L., Pandolfo, J., and Dagradi, V.: Omotrapianti ausiliari di fegato intero con arterializzazione dell'albero portale, Chir. Ital. **18:** 97, 1966.
5. Daloze, P. M., Huguet, C., Porter, K. A., and Starzl, T. E.: Auxiliary homotransplantation of the canine liver with the use of a "reverse" Welch technique, SURGERY **64:** 935, 1968.
6. Eiseman, B., Liem, D. S., and Raffucci, F.: Heterologous liver perfusion in treatment of hepatic failure, Ann. Surg. **162:** 329, 1965.
7. Eiseman, B., and Novak, V.: Die extrakorporale Leberperfusion bei Patienten mit schwerer Lebererkrankung. In press.
8. Faris, T. D., Dickhaus, A. J., Marchioro, T. L., and Starzl, T. E.: Radioisotope scanning in auxiliary liver transplantation, Surg. Gynec. Obstet. **123:** 1261, 1966.
9. Fonkalsrud, E. W., Ono, H., Shafey, O. A., Joseph, W. L., Tocornal, J., and Longmire, W. P.: Allogenic canine liver transplantation with cadaver donors, SURGERY **62:** 333, 1967.
10. Gliedman, M. L., Pangan, J., Minkowitz, S., Popowitz, L., and Karlson, K. E.: Heterotopic liver transplantation after liver damage, Trans. Amer. Soc. Artif. Intern. Organs **11:** 205, 1965.
11. Goodrich, E. O., Welch, H. F., Nelson, J. A., Beecher, T. S., and Welch, C. S.: Homotransplantation of the canine liver, SURGERY **39:** 244, 1956.
12. Hagihara, P., and Absolon, K. B.: Experimental studies on homologous heterotopic liver transplantation, Surg. Gynec. Obstet. **119:** 1297, 1964.
13. Halgrimson, C. G., Marchioro, T. L., Faris, T. D., Porter, K. A., Peters, G. N., and Starzl, T. E.: Auxiliary liver transplantation: Effect of host portocaval shunt, Arch. Surg. **93:** 107, 1966.
14. Heyde, M. N. v. d.: Auxiliary liver-graft without portal blood. Experimental autotransplantation of left liver lobes, Brit. J. Surg. **55:** 114, 1968.
15. Heyde, M. N. v. d., Cooper, J. R., Carter, J. H., and Welch, C. S.: Survival of hepatectomized dogs with partial liver transplants, SURGERY **59:** 1079, 1966.
16. Leger, L., Marcenac, N., Mathé, G., Patel, J.-C., Neveux, J. Y., Chapuis, Y., Lenriot, J.-P., Tubiana, M., Leroy, G., Lamaigre, G., and Frenoy, P.: État actuel de notre expérience de la transplantation hépatique chez l'animal, Mém. Acad. Chir. **91:** 289, 1965.
17. Mallet-Guy, P., Michoulier, J., Bernard, L., et al.: Documents expérimentaux sur le transplantation supplétive du foie en régime portal, Lyon Chir. **62:** 481, 1966.
18. Marchioro, T. L., Porter, K. A., Dickinson, T. C., Faris, T. D., and Starzl, T. E.: Physiologic requirements for auxiliary liver transplantation, Surg. Gynec. Obstet. **121:** 17, 1965.
19. Mehrez, I. O., Nabseth, D. C., Kekis, B. P., Apostolou, K., Gottlieb, L. C., and Deterling, R. A., Jr.: Homotransplantation of the canine liver: A new technique, Ann. Surg. **159:** 416, 1964.
20. Mersheimer, W. L., Cree, J. C., et al.: A liver transplant, Minn. Med. **50:** 1523, 1967.
21. Mieny, C. J., Moore, A. R., Homatas, J., and Eiseman, B.: Homotransplantation of the liver in pigs, S. Afr. J. Surg. **5:** 109, 1967.
22. Mito, M., Ackroyd, F. W., Covelli, V. H., Eyskens, E., Katayama, I., and McDermott, W. V., Jr.: Partial heterotopic liver homograft in dogs utilizing portal arterialization, Ann. Surg. **165:** 20, 1967.
23. Mouzas, G. L., Heeckeren, D. van, and Matano, I.: Auxiliary liver transplantation in dogs with arterialization of the portal vein, Int. Surg. **47:** 220, 1967.
24. Peacock, J. H., and Terblanche, J.: Orthotopic homotransplantation of the liver in the

pig, *in* Read, A. E., editor: The liver, London, 1967, Butterworth & Co., Ltd. pp. 333-365.

25. Petasnick, J. P., and Gottschalk, A.: Spleen scintiphotography with technetium-99m sulfur colloid and the gamma ray scintillation camera, J. Nucl. Med. **7:** 733, 1966.
26. Polonovski, M., and Bourillon, R.: Étude sur la composition des biles dans la série animale, Bull. Soc. Chim. Biol. **34:** 703, 1952.
27. Price, J. B., Voorhees, A. B., and Britton, R. C.: Partial hepatic autotransplantation with complete revascularization in the dog, Arch. Surg. **95:** 59, 1967.
28. Sicular, A. F., Paronetto, F., Kark, A. E., Dreiling, D. A., Burrows, L., and Popper, H.: Rejection of the homotransplanted dog liver in the absence of hepatic insufficiency, Proc. Soc. Exp. Biol. **112:** 760, 1963.
29. Sigel, B., Balvia, L., and Dunn, M. R.: Studies on liver lobes autotransplanted outside the abdominal cavity, Surg. Gynec. Obstet. **124:** 525, 1967.
30. Starzl, T. E., Marchioro, T. L., Huntley, R. T., Rifkind, D., Rowlands, D. T., Jr., Dickinson, T. C., and Waddell, W. R.: Experimental and clinical homotransplantation of the liver, Ann. N. Y. Acad. Sci. **120:** 739, 1964.
31. Starzl, T. E., Marchioro, T. L., Rowlands, D. T., Kirkpatrick, C. H., Wilson, W. E. C., Rifkind, D., and Waddell, W. R.: Immunosuppression after experimental and clinical homotransplantation of the liver, Ann. Surg. **160:** 411, 1964.
32. Starzl, T. E., Marchioro, T. L., and Porter, K. A.: Progress in homotransplantation of the liver, *in* Welch, C. E., editor: Advances in surgery, Chicago, 1966, Year Book Medical Publishers, Inc., vol. 2, pp. 295-370.
33. Starzl, T. E., Groth, C. G., Brettschneider, L., Penn, I., Fulginiti, V. A., Moon, J. B., Blanchard, H., Martin, A. J., and Porter, K. A.: Orthotopic homotransplantation of the human liver, Ann. Surg. **165:** 392, 1968.
34. Starzl, T. E., Porter, K. A., Brettschneider, L., Penn, I., Bell P., Putnam, C. W., and McGuire, R. L.: Clinical and pathologic observations after orthotopic transplantation of the human liver, Surg. Gynec. Obstet. **128:** 327, 1969.
35. Tait, I., and Eiseman, B.: Perfusion dynamics for extracorporeal hepatic assist, Arch. Surg. **93:** 131, 1966.
36. Thomford, N. K., Shorter, R. G., and Hallenbeck, G. A.: Homotransplantation of the canine liver. Survival and histology with and without Imuran, Arch. Surg. **90:** 527, 1965.
37. Tretbar, L. L., Beven, E. G., and Hermann, R. E.: The effects of portocaval shunt and portal flow occlusion on canine auxiliary liver homotransplants, SURGERY **61:** 733, 1967.
38. Welch, C. S.: A note on transplantation of the whole liver in dogs, Transplantation **2:** 54, 1955.

Adaptation of functioning and bypassed segments of ileum during compensatory hypertrophy of the gut

M. DAVID TILSON, M.D.
HASTINGS K. WRIGHT, M.D.
NEW HAVEN, CONN.
From the Department of Surgery, Yale University School of Medicine

Many investigators have described hypertrophy of the epithelium in small bowel remnants following massive gut resections. Flint[8] was among the first to note the appearance of villus hypertrophy in dogs, while Nygaard[14] and Bochov[3] have more recently documented the phenomenon in rats. Dowling and Booth[5] have suggested that the mechanism inducing growth in gut remnants is the local stimulus of ingested nutrients upon a reduced absorptive surface, whereas Lansky and associates[13] have suggested that growth is a consequence of work against partial obstruction. However, our finding that ileal hypertrophy occurs after colectomy[18] is not explained satisfactorily by either of these theories since (1) resection of gut downstream would not be expected to alter the intraluminal contents upstream and (2) there was no evidence of partial obstruction in the patients studied.

If either nutritional factors or partial obstruction provides the stimulus for hypertrophy, an unobstructed and bypassed ileal segment would not be expected to show epithelial growth after either jejunectomy or colon bypass. However, if the stimulus for hypertrophy were of a systemic nature, then growth in a bypassed segment would be anticipated after either of these procedures. Experiments were performed in rats to test both possibilities.

Reported in part in abstract form in Surgical Forum, 20:401, 1969.
Received for publication July 28, 1969.

METHODS

All experiments were performed upon female albino rats of identical age, maintained on a uniform pellet diet and weighing 200 to 220 Gm. Intraperitoneal Nembutal (2.5 mg. per 100 Gm. of body weight) was used for anesthesia. All bowel anastomoses were performed with a single layer of interrupted No. 6-0 silks. Rats were deprived of solid food for 12 hours prior to operation and 18 hours after operation.

Experiment I. Eight Lewis rats underwent jejunectomy with excision of approximately 40 cm. of proximal gut (Fig. 1). Continuity was restored by end-to-end jejunoileostomy. The ileum was divided and biopsied as "normal ileum" 10 cm. proximal to the ileocecal junction; the distal stoma was closed creating a defunctionalized remnant, and the proximal stoma was anastomosed end to side with the cecum creating a functioning ileocecostomy. On the thirteenth day, the eight experimental rats and eight normal control rats were given 100 μc of tritiated thymidine intraperitoneally. They were killed 21 hours later on the fourteenth day. Biopsies were taken of the defunctionalized remnant 1 cm. from the ileocecal junction and of the functioning remnant 10 cm. proximal to the ileocecostomy.

Experiment II. Twelve Sprague-Dawley rats underwent distal ileal bypass by division of the ileum 10 cm. proximal to the ileocecal junction with closure of the distal stoma (Fig. 1). The proximal stoma was anastomosed end to side with the cecum.

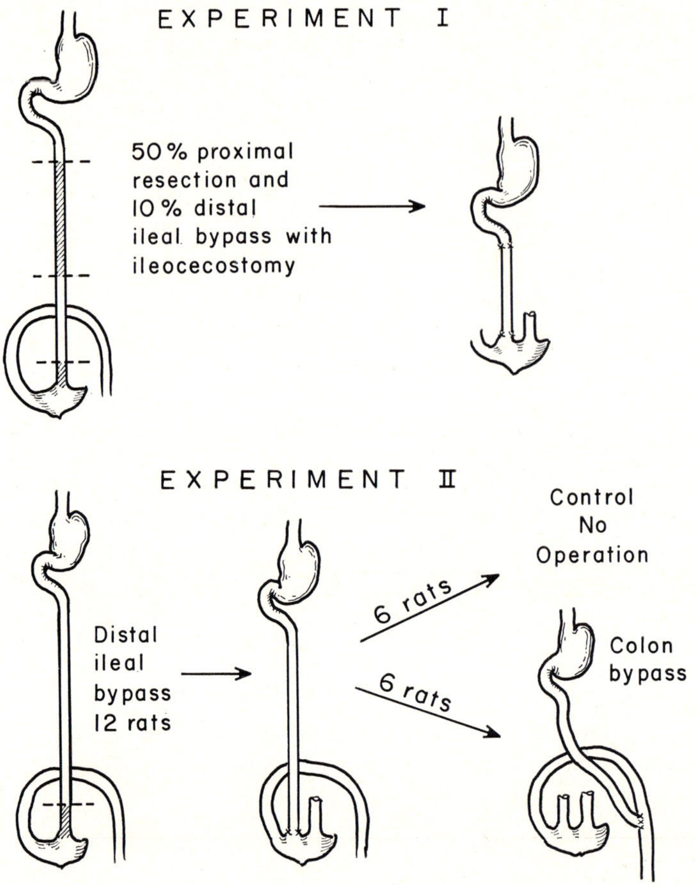

Fig. 1. Experiment I: Combined 50 percent proximal small bowel resection and distal 10 percent bypass. Experiment II: Ten percent distal ileal bypass followed by colon bypass.

All animals recovered well and gained weight. After two months, six rats underwent laparotomy with division of the ileocecostomy and anastomosis of the ileum end to side with the rectum. Five of the six animals survived this procedure. After one additional month, the eleven animals remaining in the study were killed. The "functioning ileum" specimen was taken 10 cm. proximal to the ileoproctostomy in the five rats with colon bypass. The "defunctionalized ileum" specimens were taken 1 cm. proximal to the ileocecal junction in both groups.

All animals were killed with ether. The specimens were fixed in 10 percent formalin, sectioned transversely to the lumen at 5 μ, and stained with hematoxylin and eosin. Radioautographs were prepared by coating with Kodak NTB3 emulsion, exposing for four weeks, and counterstaining with nuclear fast red. The slides were coded and examined "blind" to eliminate bias on the part of the microscopist. Villus length of the five tallest well-oriented villi in each section was measured at ×100 with an eyepiece micrometer; the unit (U.) measurement is 10 μ. The height of labeled cells in the radioautographs was similarly measured. Cell counts were made of the three tallest villi in each section from villus tip to base of crypt. Mean values for villus length, cell count, and migration rate were analyzed by Student's t test for significant differences.

RESULTS

All bypassed segments were unobstructed and devoid of gross intraluminal contents.

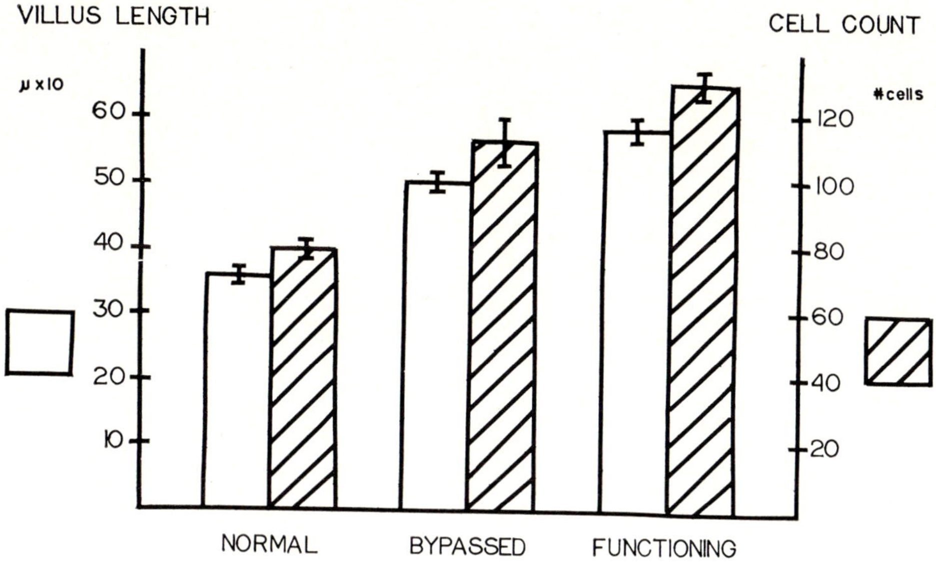

Fig. 2. Experiment I: Villus length and villus cell count in functioning and bypassed ileum after jejunectomy.

Table I. *Villus length, villus cell count, and migration rate per 21 hours in functioning and defunctionalized remnants of ileum after 50 percent resection*

Type of specimen	*No. of animals*	*Villus length (U. ± S.E.M.)*	*Cell count (No. of cells ± S.E.M.)*	*Migration rate/21 hours (U. ± S.E.M.)*
Normal ileum	8	36 ± 0.9	80 ± 2.3	29 ± 0.8
Defunctionalized ileum	8	50 ± 2.1*	113 ± 6.9*	42 ± 2.4*
Functioning ileum	8	58 ± 2.0*	128 ± 3.5*	42 ± 1.2*

S.E.M. = Standard error of the mean.

*Represents a statistically significant difference from normal ($p < 0.001$).

Experiment I. The mean length of villi in defunctionalized and functioning remnants after 50 percent proximal resection was increased over normal by 39 percent ($p < 0.001$) and 61 percent ($p < 0.001$), respectively. The mean cell counts were increased by 54 percent ($p < 0.001$) and 73 percent ($p < 0.001$), respectively. The migration rates at 21 hours were increased by 45 percent in both remnants ($p < 0.001$). The data are presented in Table I and Fig. 2. Photomicrographs at identical magnification illustrate the changes two weeks after jejunectomy in Fig. 3.

Experiment II. The villus length and cell count of both bypassed and functioning ileum were increased in the rats with colon bypass. The increases in cell count of 13 percent ($p < 0.05$) and 23 percent ($p < 0.01$) for the bypassed and functioning segments were statistically significant. The data are presented in Table II and Fig. 4.

DISCUSSION

The finding that unobstructed and defunctionalized ileum out of continuity with the intestinal stream shows villus growth after either jejunectomy or colon bypass is not explained satisfactorily by the theories that adaptive growth is produced by either partial obstruction or intestinal contents alone. Instead, the results suggest that a systemic stimulus may be present. Before this conclusion is reached, however, the evidence

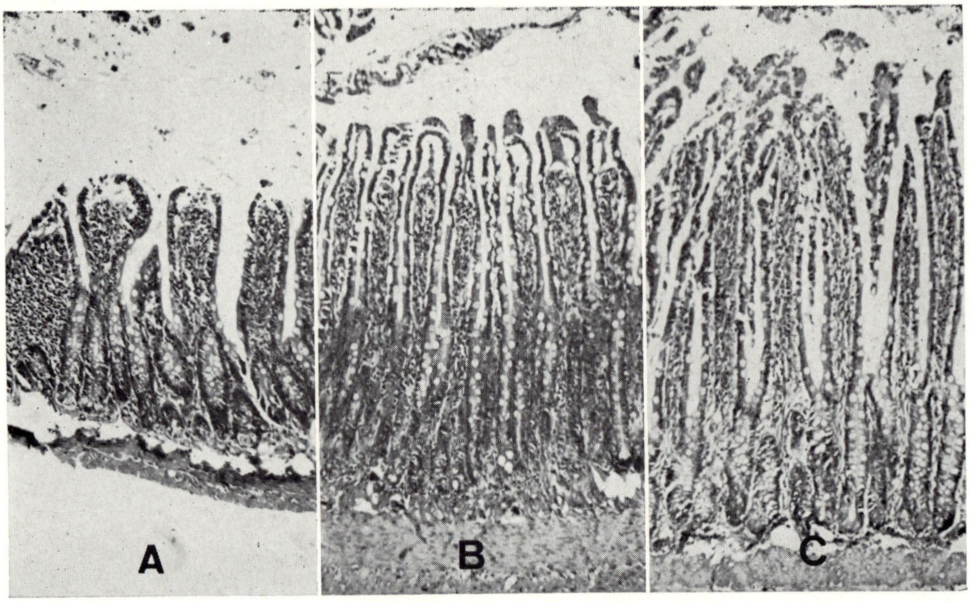

Fig. 3. *A,* normal ileum. (×25.) *B,* bypassed ileum after jejunectomy. (×25.) *C,* functioning ileum after jejunectomy. (×25.)

Table II. *Villus length and villus cell count in functioning and defunctionalized segments of ileum with and without colon bypass*

	Villus length (U. ± S.E.M.)			*Villus cell count (No. of cells ± S.E.M.)*		
Ileum segments	*No colon bypass*	*With colon bypass*	*p**	*No colon bypass*	*With colon bypass*	*p**
Defunctionalized ileum	38 ± 1.5	41 ± 1.3	ns	77 ± 1.8	88 ± 1.8	.05
Functioning ileum	45 ± 2.3	48 ± 1.4	ns	92 ± 4.3	119 ± 3.6	.01

S.E.M. = standard error of the mean; ns = not significant.

*Value of p by Student's t test.

supporting several methodological assumptions implicit in the experimental design should be reviewed.

First, the experimental results would be influenced if normal villi grew with the passage of time. However, Dowling and Booth[5] found no growth of villi during 24 weeks of observation of rats of similar age and weight.

Second, the local hypertrophy at the site of an anastomosis must not be taken to represent a systemic influence. Nygaard[14] found that this local effect was limited to within 5 to 6 cm. of an anastomosis in rats. Care was exercised that our biopsies were made 9 to 10 cm. from suture lines.

Third, the normal decrease in villus length along an aboral gradient should not influence the experimental design. Altmann and Enesco[2] showed that mean villus length decreases linearly from about 60 U. at the ligament of Treitz to 40 U. at the ileocecal junction in the rat. Thus villus length decreases about 2.5 U. per 10 cm. aborally. The presence of this gradient does not affect the interpretation of Experiment II, since comparison is made of biopsies taken from the same site in each gut. However, in Experiment I, the effect must be considered. The defunctionalized remnant was biopsied 10 cm. downstream from the site of the normal biopsy. Thus, the finding of an increase in villus length in bypass over normal

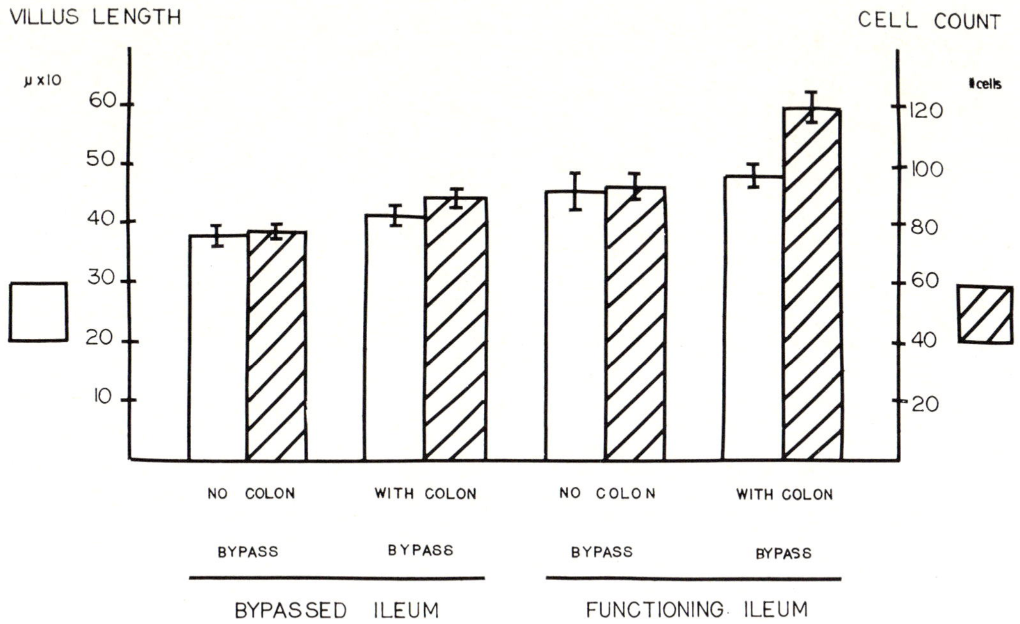

Fig. 4. Experiment II: Villus length and villus cell count in functioning and bypassed ileum with and without colon bypass.

is in the *opposite* direction to that predicted by the normal gradient.

Fourth, if the flow of intraluminal contents assists mechanically in the extrusion of cells at the villus tip, the observed increase in the length of bypassed villi might only represent an absence of abrasion of distal cells and not an actual increase in cell proliferation. The finding in this study that cell migration is enhanced in the bypassed ileum supports the thesis that cellular proliferation is indeed increased. Moreover, preliminary experiments in our laboratory showed no significant change in villus length one month after 10 percent distal bypass alone.[16]

Fifth, although it cannot be stated on the basis of measurement of villus length alone that an absolute increase in mucosal absorptive surface occurred, Hromadkova and Skala[11] found a statistically significant correlation between the height of villi and the ratio of the mucosal surface area corresponding to an adjacent area of serosal surface.

Our finding that hypertrophy is more pronounced in functioning than in bypassed remnants supports the hypothesis that intraluminal contents have a role in the production of growth, although these contents are not the sole stimulus. The evidence for the intraluminal nutrient theory stems from two sources. First, it has been shown that hyperphagia in rats with hypothalamic lesions,[4] lactation,[7] or diabetes[12] is associated with villus hypertrophy. Second, Dowling and Booth[5] observed that ileum transposed into the proximal position undergoes hypertrophy, which suggests that the absence of proximal bowel had affected the intraluminal environment to which the ileum was exposed. Increased dietary bulk alone does not produce villus hypertrophy, as shown by Friedman,[9] which suggests that the nutritional component of the diet and not its mere bulk plays the significant role.

The results of this study are compatible with four possible mechanisms acting in concert with intraluminal factors to produce growth.

A. The epithelium may secrete its own circulating growth inhibitor. Resection of a portion of gut would lower the concentration of inhibitor by decreasing the amount produced. As the concentration of inhibitor fell, the remaining gut would begin to grow until sufficient tissue mass was restored to raise the inhibitor concentration to a normal level. Then growth would cease. This concept, as related to the growth of any organ, was elaborated in terms of several variables by Weiss and Kavanau[17] in 1957. However, this theory does not explain the observation that compensatory changes occur in small bowel after colon bypass without the loss of any tissue mass.

B. The gut remnant may elaborate its own growth stimulatory product, perhaps in response to injury. Preliminary experiments in our laboratory with parabiotic animals have suggested that such a factor may be cross-circulated.

C. The whole gut may be stimulated by its autonomic innervation, which remains intact to functioning and defunctionalized remnants. Splanchnicectomy was shown by Padula and Camishion[15] to increase mesenteric blood flow, and if a period of parasympathetic predominance were to follow partial resection, a similar increase in blood flow might occur. It is possible that such an increase might wash out and thereby reduce the concentration of a local growth inhibitory factor present in the crypts.

D. The demand of the organism for increased absorption of salt, water, and other essential nutrients may be communicated to the gut by some known hormone (for example, aldosterone) with growth stimulatory properties as yet unrecognized. If a feedback mechanism existed to adjust the size of villi to the functional demand for absorptive surface, the evidence for a systemic stimulus and the known effect of dietary factors might be integrated. For example, the lactating rat may have larger villi, not because it eats more, but because of an increased functional demand for absorption. The intermittently starving rat has been found by Fabry and Kujolova[6] to have larger villi, even though it fails to gain weight normally.

The possibility that adaptive growth is related to the demand for function rather than to increased function itself is consistent with a large body of biological knowledge as outlined by Goss.[10] For example, Alho[1] was unable to produce hypertrophy of salivary glands by evoking increased function with pilocarpine, but adaptive growth begins rapidly after partial resection when the organism has a functional need for increased secretion of the remnant tissue. Finally, endocrine organs do not regenerate if their secretory products are replaced by exogenous hormones which eliminate the demand for increased function.

The findings of this study support the hypothesis that a systemic factor plays a role in the adaptive growth of the small bowel. Although no hormone is known at present to enhance epithelial growth, the existence of such a factor may be postulated.

SUMMARY

Functioning and bypassed segments of ileum were examined after either jejunectomy or colon bypass. Compensatory villus hypertrophy and radioautographic evidence of increased cellular proliferation were observed in defunctionalized segments as well as functioning segments. These findings suggest the presence of a systemic stimulus for epithelial growth.

REFERENCES

1. Alho, A.: Regeneration capacity of the submandibular gland in rat and mouse, Acta Path. Microbiol Scand. Suppl. **149:** 1, 1961.
2. Altmann, G. G., and Enesco, M.: Cell numbers as a measure of distribution and renewal of epithelial cells in the small intestine of growing adult rats, Amer. J. Anat. **121:** 319, 1967.
3. Bochov, N. P.: Morphological changes in the jejunum and ileum of rats after wide resection of the small intestine, Bull. Exp. Biol. Med. **47:** 339, 1959.
4. Brobeck, J. R., Tepperman, J., and Long, C. N. H.: Experimental hypothalamic hyperphagia in the albino rat, Yale J. Biol. Med. **15:** 831, 1943.
5. Dowling, R. M., and Booth, C. C.: Structural and functional changes following small intestinal resection in the rat, Clin. Sci. **32:** 139, 1967.

6. Fabry, P., and Kujolova, V.: Enhanced growth of the small intestine in rats as a result of adaptation to intermittent starvation, Acta Anat. **43:** 264, 1960.
7. Fell, B. F., Smith, K. A., and Campbell, R. M.: Hypertrophic and hyperplastic changes in the alimentary canal of the lactating rat, J. Path. Bact. **85:** 179, 1963.
8. Flint, J. M.: The effect of extensive resection of the small intestine, Bull. Hopkins Hosp. **23:** 127, 1912.
9. Friedman, M. H. F.: The response of different regions of the gastrointestinal tract to normal and abnormal stimuli (influence of feeding inert bulk material and of hypophysectomy), J. Nat. Cancer Inst. **13:** 1035, 1953.
10. Goss, R. J.: Adaptive Growth, London, 1964, Logos Press.
11. Hromadkova, V., and Skala, I.: Factors influencing the assessment of size of the mucosal surface and length of the small intestine in rats, Digestion **1:** 149, 1968.
12. Jervis, E. L., and Levin, R. J.: Anatomic adaptation of the alimentary tract of the rat to the hyperphagia of chronic alloxan diabetes, Nature **210:** 391, 1966.
13. Lansky, Z., Dodd, R. M., and Stahlgren, L. H.: Regeneration of the intestinal epithelium after resection of the small intestine in dogs, Amer. J. Surg. **116:** 8, 1968.
14. Nygaard, K.: Resection of the small intestine in rats. 3. Morphological changes in the intestinal tract, Acta Chir. Scand. **133:** 233, 1967.
15. Padula, T. H., and Camishion, R. C.: Mesenteric vascularity after vagotomy and splanchnicectomy, Surg. Gynec. Obstet. **127:** 41, 1968.
16. Tilson, M. D., and Wright, H. K.: Unpublished observations.
17. Weiss, P., and Kavanau, J. L.: A model of growth and growth control in mathematical terms, J. Gen. Physiol. **41:** 1, 1957.
18. Wright, H. K., Cleveland, J. C., Tilson, M. D., and Herskovic, T.: Morphology and absorptive capacity of the ileum after ileostomy in man, Amer. J. Surg. **117:** 142, 1969.

Vena cava catheter for asanguineous liver resection

FEDERICO CHÁVEZ-PEÓN, M.D.*
EDUARDO GONZALEZ, M.D.**
RONALD A. MALT, M.D.
BOSTON, MASS.
From the Surgical Services, Massachusetts General Hospital, and the Department of Surgery, Harvard Medical School

Lacerations of the hepatic veins at their junction with the vena cava are major contributors to the mortality from hepatic trauma and from elective hepatic resection.[1] Hemorrhage in that location is hard to control, and air embolism is difficult to prevent. To provide for return of blood through the inferior vena cava while excluding the hepatic veins temporarily from the circulation, Schrock and colleagues[3] have successfully employed a cannula inserted through the right atrium into the superior vena cava and thence into the inferior cava. In our experiments with liver transplantation and resection in dogs, we have employed a bypass constructed of material readily available and capable of being inserted through the inferior vena cava alone. Its ready adaptability to the human cadaver suggests that it may find clinical usefulness as well. An endocaval shunt for other purposes has been described by Buckberg and colleagues.[4]

TECHNIQUE

For dogs weighing about 20 Kg., a No. 28 Fr. Bardic or Silastic catheter is fitted with an inflatable cuff made to fit a pediatric endotracheal tube of similar size (Fig. 1). For use in human beings, a cuff of the standard adult size and a No. 36 to 40 Fr. catheter appear suitable.

After the retroduodenal inferior vena cava is exposed by Kocher's maneuver, inflow to the liver is stopped by cross-clamping the portal triad. A longitudinal incision 1 cm. long is made in the suprarenal vena cava, previously encircled with umbilical tapes placed with care to avoid damaging the lumbar veins. The catheter with the balloon partially inflated is guided through the venotomy and the tip positioned well above the liver with the aid of the left hand, which palpates the vena cava above the liver (Fig. 2). Once the balloon is above the diaphragm, it is inflated enough to prevent its slipping downstream. The lower umbilical tape is released to permit placing the lower end of the catheter within the cava and then tightened again to hold the catheter securely. A little blood is lost during placement of the catheter. Air embolism is prevented by having the catheter filled with saline and clamped, by inserting it during a phase of prolonged positive pressure respiration, and by maintaining the balloon fully inflated.

The region of the intrahepatic vena cava and the hepatic veins may then be inspected and operated upon in a dry field. The safe period of occlusion of the portal triad is estimated to be perhaps 20 to 25 minutes in the normothermic human being, but the limit can be extended either by intermittently restoring the circulation or by regional hypothermia.[2] At the end of the procedure, the

This study was supported by the Shriners Burns Institute.
Received for publication Sept. 15, 1969.
*Fellow of the Lilly Foundation.
**Advanced Research Fellow of the American Cancer Society.

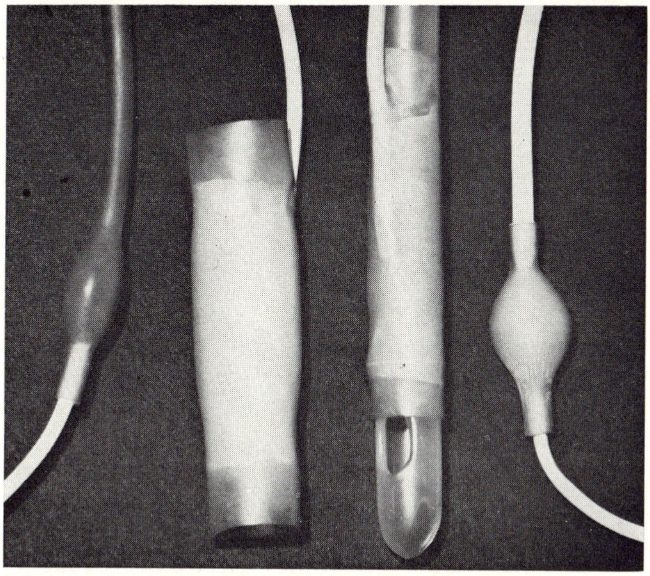

Fig. 1. Assembled catheter with balloon for use in the dog. Cuff for larger tube is alongside.

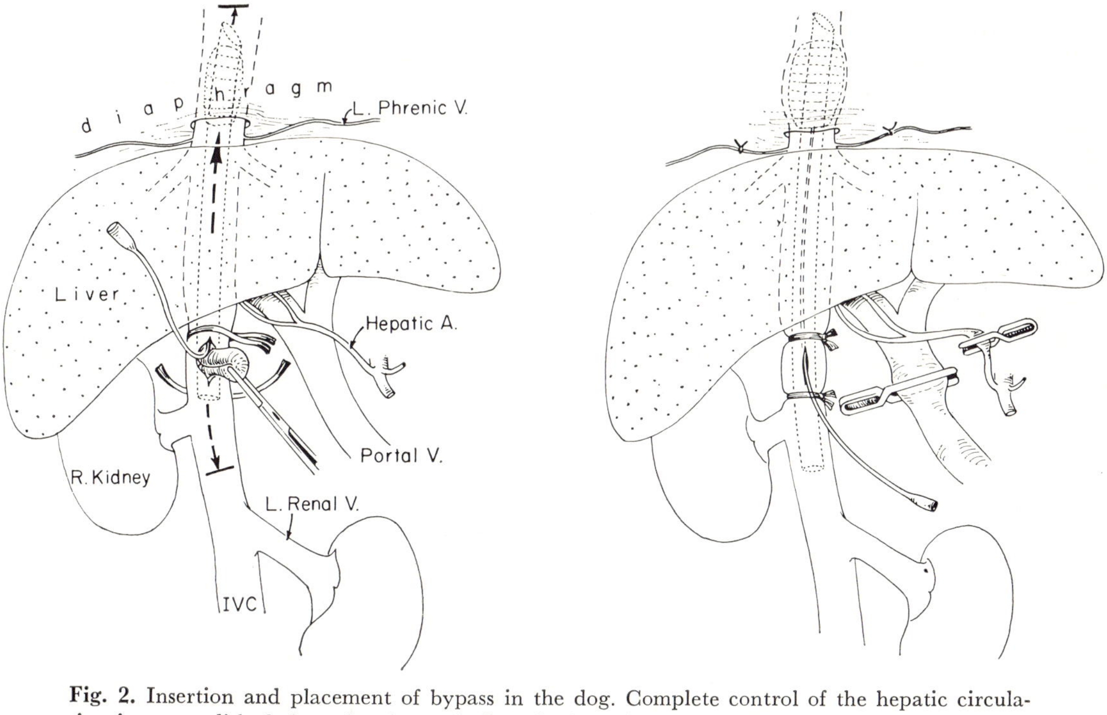

Fig. 2. Insertion and placement of bypass in the dog. Complete control of the hepatic circulation is accomplished thereafter by occluding the hepatic artery and portal vein *(right)*.

tube is removed with precautions to avoid air embolism. A Satinsky-type sidewall clamp provides isolation of venotomy for repair. Systemic heparinization has not been required in dogs and probably will not be in human beings, if a Silastic catheter is used and if the period of its use is brief.

Partial hepatectomies in the dog are accomplished in 20 minutes with almost no bleeding from the hepatic veins or liver substance. Liver function tests show no abnormality during this period nor after longer times of circulatory occlusion punctuated by intermittent periods during which blood flow is restored. Since placement of the catheter in the human cadaver is easy, we think that the technique may well be applied to improve the management of liver trauma and hepatic resection in surgical patients.

REFERENCES

1. Ackroyd, F. W., Pollard, J., and McDermott, W. V.: Massive hepatic resection in the treatment of severe liver trauma, Amer. J. Surg. **117:** 442, 1969.
2. Huggins, C. E., and Carter, E. L.: Partial hepatectomy employing differential hypothermia, Arch. Surg. **74:** 189, 1957.
3. Schrock, T., Blaisdell, F. W., and Mathewson, C.: Management of blunt trauma to the liver and hepatic veins, Arch. Surg. **96:** 698, 1968.
4. Buckberg, G., Ono, H., Tocornal, J. A., O'Connell, T., Wilkerson, J. A., and Longmire, W. P.: Results following hypothermic asanguineous liver perfusion in dogs, Ann. Surg. **167:** 51, 1968.

Emergency separation of thoracopagus (twins conjoined at thorax) in the newborn period: Importance of careful preoperative cardiac evaluation

JAMES S. SIMPSON, M.D.*
W. T. MUSTARD, M.D.
C. A. F. MOES, M.D.
T. IZUKAWA, M.D.
TORONTO, ONTARIO, CANADA
From the Departments of Surgery, Radiology, and Pediatrics, The Hospital for Sick Children, and the University of Toronto

Ideally, separation of conjoined twins should be undertaken at an age most favorable for survival and only after the exact extent of organ union has been determined. But life-endangering anomalies or the poor condition of one twin may necessitate early emergency surgery. Since 75 percent of thoracopagus (twins conjoined at thorax) have serious cardiac anomalies[2, 3] that may prevent separation or affect survival, the cardiovascular system should be investigated immediately.

Of the three sets of thoracopagus treated by us, the first[2] had separate hearts contained within a common pericardial sac, the second shared a common heart, and the third, the present case, had two hearts enclosed in a single pericardium and joined by a vascular channel between the right atria. One heart had additional abnormalities.

There are few reports of conjoined twins operated on in the newborn period. This paper describes such a case and discusses the indications for emergency separation and the problems associated with accurate preoperative cardiac assessment.

Received for publication Oct. 11, 1969.

*Reprint requests: The Hospital for Sick Children, 555 University Ave., Toronto 2, Ontario, Canada.

CASE REPORT

Male twins conjoined at the thorax (Fig. 1) were born on January 20, 1969, to a 24-year-old North American Indian mother, who was gravida 2, para 1. The infants were the product of a 33 week gestation and had a total birth weight of 2,630 grams. An abdominal roentgenogram of the mother (Fig. 2) had shown the presence of twins, and in retrospect, their conjoined state might have been suspected, as they were positioned with the ventral aspect of the thorax of each apposed and the heads presenting; their spines were relatively straight and roughly parallel. They were born by cesarean section, were slow to breathe, and required resuscitation.

When transferred to this hospital at two hours of age, the infants were cyanosed, hypotonic, and breathed irregularly. They were joined from the upper sternum to the umbilicus. One observer thought he heard two distinct heart beats and palpated separate femoral pulses. This was unconfirmed. The infants had separate respiratory rates and on auscultation both had good air entry into the lungs. The common umbilicus contained two umbilical veins and three arteries. Twin B, the smaller twin, was intubated shortly after admission because of respiratory distress. On admission Twin A had a blood pH of 6.9, a Pco_2 of 52, and a base excess of minus 25. Twin B had a pH of 6.97, a Pco_2 of 48, a Po_2 of 50, and a base excess of minus 20. Sodium bicarbonate was given intravenously to correct their marked acidosis, and just before operation the blood pH values were 7.47 and 7.41, respectively. Electrocardiograms obtained by connecting the left arm and left leg of Twin A with the right arm and

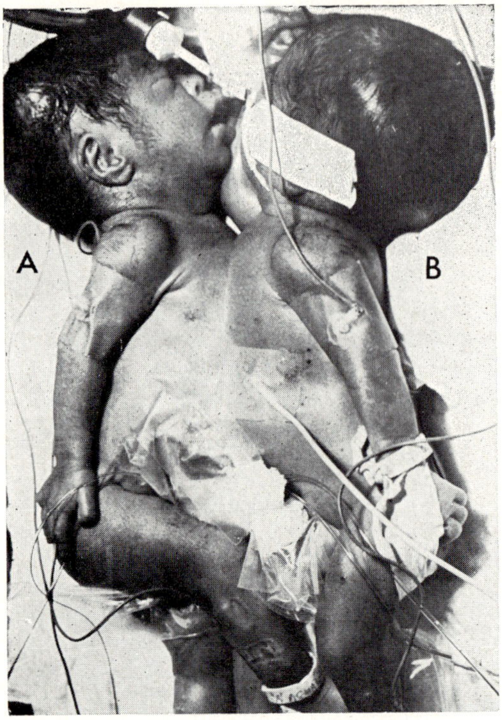

Fig. 1. Thoracopagus twins at two hours of age. Twin B was intubated and received assisted ventilation.

right leg of Twin B (Fig. 3) and from the limb leads of the twins separately (Fig. 4) showed a single QRS complex. This complex recorded in every lead was wide (0.09 seconds) and of bizarre configuration. The possibility of two completely separate conducting systems firing at different rates was thus excluded.

With the presence of independent hearts being doubtful, angiography was undertaken. An angiocatheter was inserted through the right femoral vein of Twin A and passed into the right atrium and right ventricle. Three milliliters of 75 percent Hypaque injected at the junction of the inferior vena cava and right atrium revealed a wide channel passing from the right atrium of Twin A to the right atrium of Twin B. Subsequently, there was opacification of a ventricle and pulmonary artery of Twin A, and following circulation of the contrast medium through the lungs, the heart and the aorta and its branches were visualized (Fig. 5).

The angiocatheter was then passed form the right atrium of Twin A through the connecting channel into the right atrium of twin B. Three milliliters of contrast medium injected into this atrium again demonstrated the communication between the atria (Fig. 6). From the atrium of Twin B, contrast medium passed into a ventricle anterior to the ventricles of Twin A and protrud-

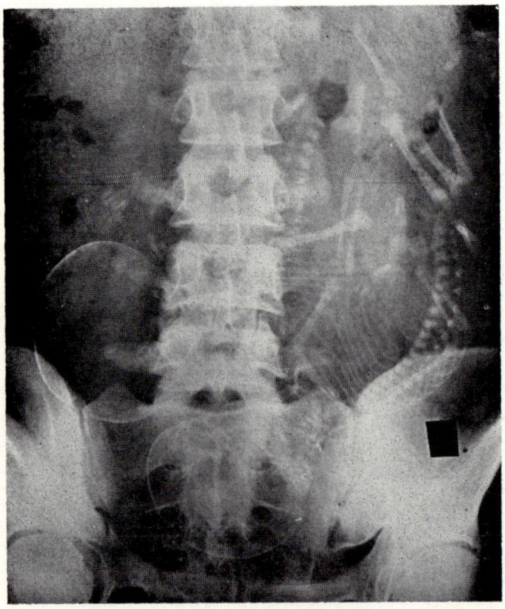

Fig. 2. Abdominal roentgenograms of mother taken prior to cesarean section showing face to face position of the twins.

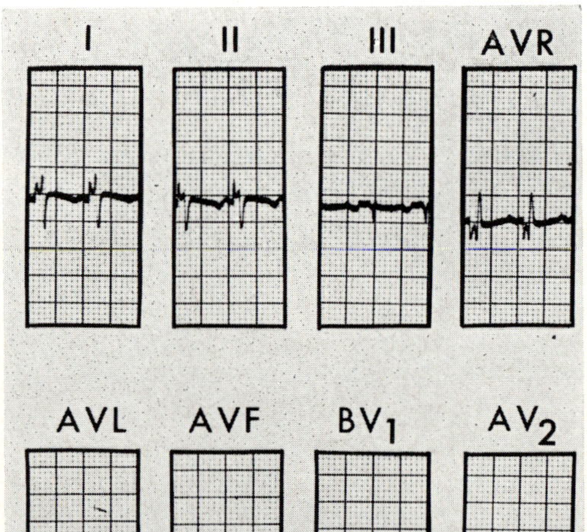

Fig. 3. Combined Twin A left arm and leg; Twin B right arm and leg. Electrocardiogram obtained by attaching limb leads to both twins. Note the wide, bizarre QRS complex.

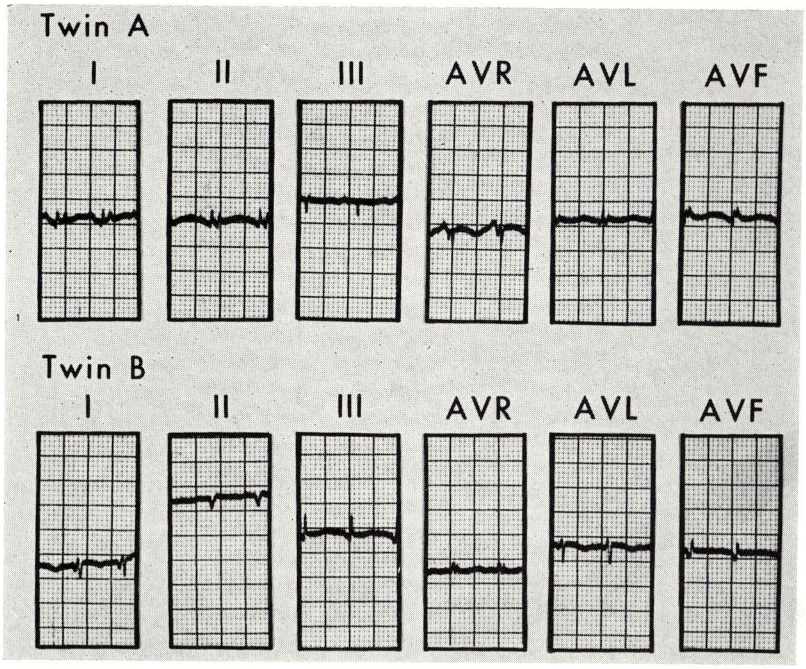

Fig. 4. Electrocardiogram obtained separately from limb leads of the twins. The distortion of the QRS complex is less apparent.

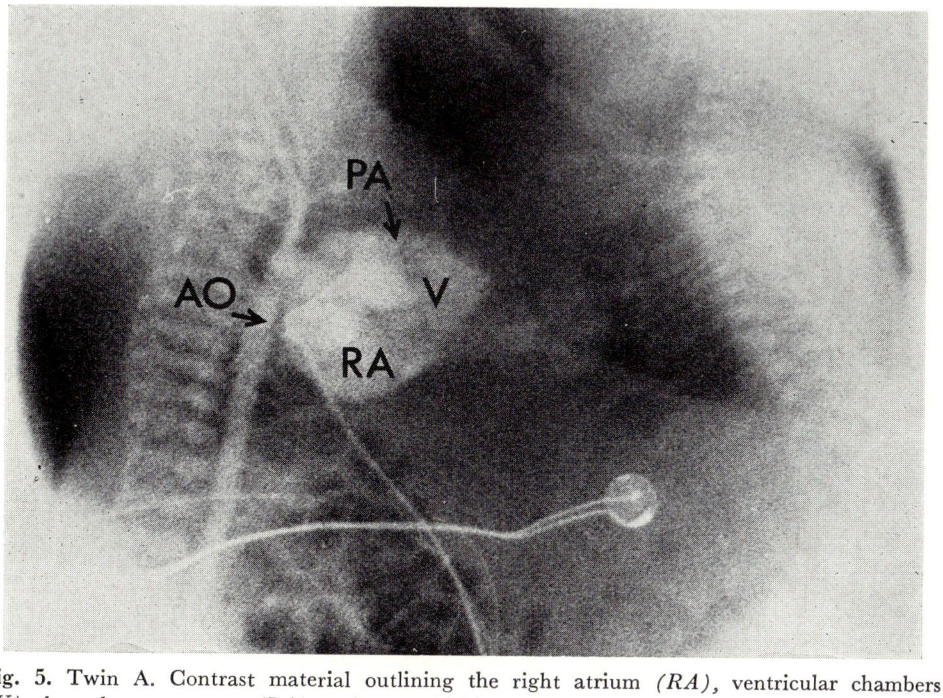

Fig. 5. Twin A. Contrast material outlining the right atrium *(RA)*, ventricular chambers *(V)*, the pulmonary artery *(PA)*, and aorta *(AO)*.

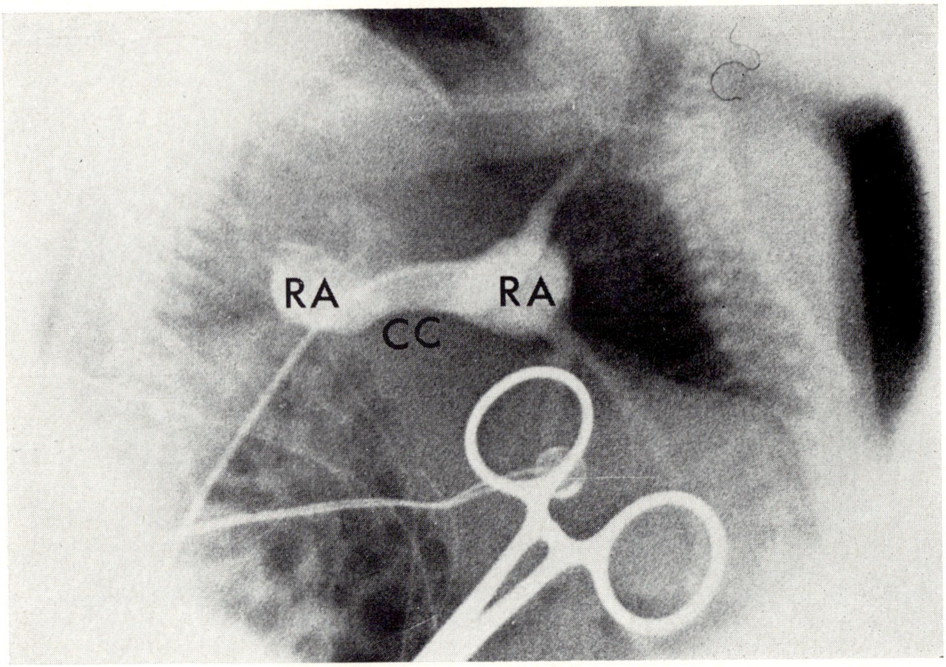

Fig. 6. Contrast material outlining the right atria *(RA)* of both infants and the venous connecting channel *(CC)*. Some contrast material has blown retrogradely into the superior vena cava and hepatic veins of Twin B on the right side.

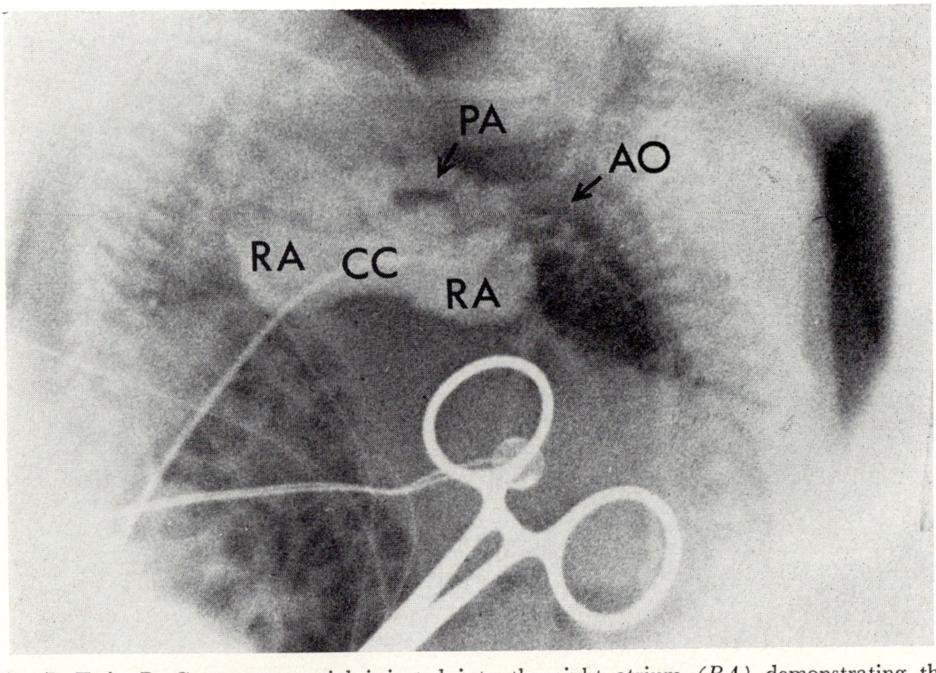

Fig. 7. Twin B. Contrast material injected into the right atrium *(RA)* demonstrating the venous connecting channel *(CC)*, the pulmonary artery *(PA)*, and aorta *(AO)*. The ventricles are obscured by the connecting channel.

ing into the thoracic cavity of Twin A. Subsequent opacification of the pulmonary artery and aorta of Twin B occurred (Fig. 7). Angiocardiography demonstrated no connection between the ventricles or great vessels of the twins; the sole communication was between the atria.

The condition of Twin B continued to deteriorate and emergency separation was undertaken when the babies were fourteen hours old.

The same operating room procedure, which employed two teams of surgeons, anesthetists, and nurses and the same draping, monitoring, and anesthetic techniques previously described were employed.[2, 5]

An incision in the midline of the junction revealed that the peritoneal cavities communicated freely. The livers were fused in the midline, but there were two falciform ligaments and two gallbladders. The gastrointestinal tracts were separate. The incision was extended to include the cartilaginous union of the sternum. The common liver was then divided by scalpel, with the use of digital compression to control hemorrhage, while vessels and bile ducts were ligated. The liver was friable, and hemostasis was more difficult to obtain than at the operation on the thoracopagus twins separated at three months of age.[5]

The common pericardial sac was then divided anteriorly and the hearts inspected. Although it was difficult to determine all the cardiac anomalies, the hearts appeared separate, except for a communicating channel joining the right atria. This vessel was ligated and divided. At this point Twin B's heart stopped and could not be restarted. The separation was completed and Twin A's chest and abdomen were closed using polypropylene mesh covered with silicone rubber sheeting.[5] Twin A died eight hours after operation.

NECROPSY FINDINGS

Twin A. Position of the heart and the relationship of the great arteries were normal. Veins from the head and neck drained through the left superior vena cava into the coronary sinus and right atrium (Fig. 8). The right superior vena cava was absent, but the inferior vena cava was normally inserted. The orifice of the channel connecting the atrium to that of the other twin was adjacent to the entrance of the coronary sinus into the right atrium. A small patent foramen ovale was present. The immediate cause of death was a massive subarachnoid hemorrhage.

Twin B. After fixation the heart appeared smaller than the heart of Twin A. The systemic and pulmonary veins drained nor-

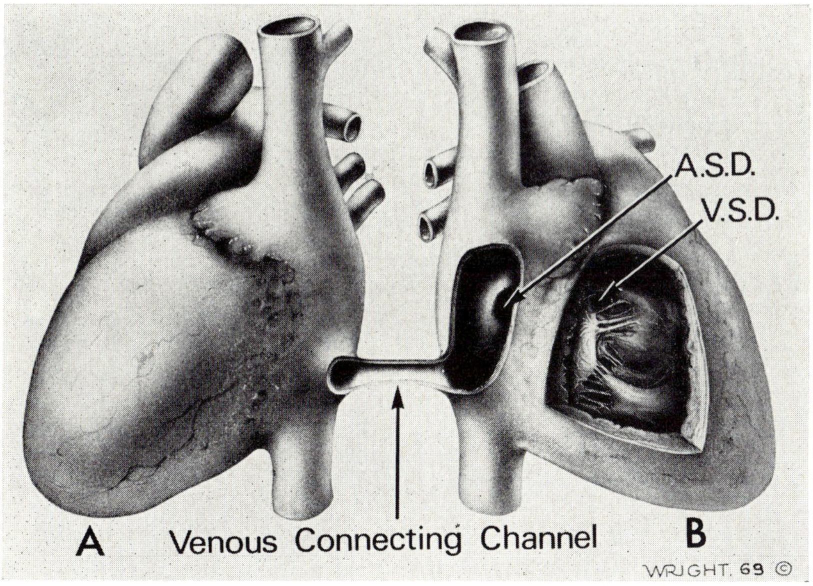

Fig. 8. Drawing showing venous channel connecting the right atria of both hearts. Twin A's heart also had a persistent left superior vena cava, right superior vena cava absent, and a small patent foramen ovale. Twin B's heart contained a small atrial septal defect (A.S.D.) and ventricular septal defect. (V.S.D.)

mally. The great arteries were equal in size and normally related. The channel joining the right atrium with that of Twin A originated near the inferior vena cava. A small atrial septal defect or patent foramen ovale 3 by 2 mm. was present. A membranous ventricular septal defect 4 by 3 mm. was located below the aortic valve. Cause of death was stated as massive right temporal lobe hemorrhage.

DISCUSSION

At the initial examination, palpation of femoral pulses suggested the possibility of separate hearts. The electrocardiographic examination, however, failed to corroborate this. Angiocardiography provided a more accurate assessment of the cardiac anatomy and suggested that separation would be feasible. The rapid deterioration of Twin B made it imperative.

Gans and associates[1] recently documented the indications for separation in the newborn period of nine sets of twins previously reported and one additional set in their care. A further set so treated was reported by Oberniedermayr and associates.[4] Ours is the twelfth.

Indications for separation in the newborn period resolve themselves into either the critical condition of one twin threatening the life of the other or the presence of life-endangering congenital anomalies that can be corrected.

Survival depends largely upon: the extent of union of organs, particularly the hearts; the general condition of the infants; co-existing lesions resulting from birth trauma, such as intracranial hemorrhage; and later in the postoperative period, infection.

CONCLUSIONS

Emergency separation of thoracopagus in the neonatal period may be necessary to preserve life. The cardiovascular systems at least should be investigated before operation, since approximately three quarters of these infants have serious cardiac anomalies that complicate or negate successful division. The value of angiocardiographic examination is well demonstrated in this case.

REFERENCES

1. Gans, S. L., Morgenstern, L., Gettelman, E., Zukow, A. H., and Cooperman, H.: Separation of conjointed twins in the newborn period, J. Pediat. Surg. **3:** 565, 1968.
2. Leachman, R. D., Latson, J. R., Kohler, C. M., and McNamara, D. G.: Cardiovascular evaluation of conjoined twins, *in* Bergsma, Daniel, editor: Conjoined twins, Birth Defects Original Article Series **3:** (No. 1) 52-62, 1967.
3. Nichols, B. L., Blattner, R. J., and Rudolph, A. J.: General clinical management of thoracopagus twins, *in* Bergsma, Daniel, editor: Conjoined twins, Birth Defects Original Article Series **3:** (No. 1) 38, 1967.
4. Oberniedermayr, A., Bühlmeyer, K., Fendel, H., and Georgü, A.: Report of operation on newborn thoracopagi, and of another inviable thoracopagus (in German), Z. Kinderchir. **6:** 162, 1968.
5. Simpson, J. S.: Separation of conjoined thoracopagus twins, with the report of an additional case, Canad. J. Surg. **12:** 89, 1969.
6. Simpson, J. S., Pelton, D. A., and Swyer, P. R.: The importance of monitoring during operations on conjoined twins, Canad. Med. Ass. J. **96:** 1463, 1967.

Torsion of the testis in the newborn infant

MELVYN J. MICHAELIAN, M.D.
G. H. MAHOUR, M.D., M.S. (SURGERY)*
PAUL W. JOHNSTON, M.D.
LOS ANGELES, CALIF.
From the Department of Surgery, Childrens Hospital of Los Angeles and the University of Southern California School of Medicine

Torsion of the testis in the newborn infant is rare but must be promptly diagnosed and treated to prevent testicular necrosis. Taylor,[18] in 1897, reported the first case of neonatal torsion. Reeves and associates[14] tabulated twenty-four additional cases by 1965. Since then, eight additional cases have been reported in the English literature.[3-6, 8, 10, 11, 16] The purpose of this paper is to emphasize the clinical manifestations and surgical management.

CASE REPORT

A 7 pound 3 ounce boy was delivered on March 20, 1969, after a normal full-term pregnancy. A hard, smooth, nontender mass was felt in the left scrotum at the time of delivery. The mass could not be transilluminated, and there was bluish discoloration of the overlying skin. The right testis seemed normal. After nine days of observation, the child was transferred to the Childrens Hospital of Los Angeles and was operated upon.

There was an extravaginal torsion of the spermatic cord, with three complete clockwise turns. The testis was purplish-black (Fig. 1), and the gubernaculum testis was absent. After the cord was untwisted, the testicular mass was decompressed by incising the tunica vaginalis. The testicle was biopsied and replaced in the scrotum. Through a small scrotal incision, a contralateral testicular fixation was performed. Microscopic examination of the affected testis showed hemorrhagic infarction.

Received for publication Sept. 12, 1969.

*Reprint requests: Department of Surgery, Childrens Hospital of Los Angeles, 4650 Sunset Boulevard, Los Angeles, Calif. 90027.

Convalescence was uneventful. When the patient was last seen, the left testicle was soft but definitely smaller than the right.

DISCUSSION

There are two types of testicular torsion: (1) intravaginal, more commonly found in older patients; (2) extravaginal, more common in infants. We have limited our discussion of symptoms and management to include only those cases in neonates less than twenty-four hours of age.

Several authors[4, 5, 8, 13, 14] have listed congenital abnormalities which predispose to intravaginal torsion, including: (1) a "roomy" scrotum, (2) high investment of tunica vaginalis on the cord with elongation of the intravaginal portion of the cord (known as the "bell and clapper defect"), and (3) absence or elongation of the gubernaculum testis. However, the exact mechanism of torsion of the spermatic cord in the newborn infant is not known. Campbell[2] credits Sir Astley Cooper with observing that the entire scrotal contents of a newborn infant can be lifted out of the scrotum without the tearing of tissue. The dense adhesions surrounding the damaged testis in several cases[1, 5] suggest that torsion can occur antenatally.

The infants usually do not have pain, vomiting, or fever. Swelling is the main presenting symptom. The testicle is usually firm and nontender, with discoloration of the overlying scrotum. Transillumination of

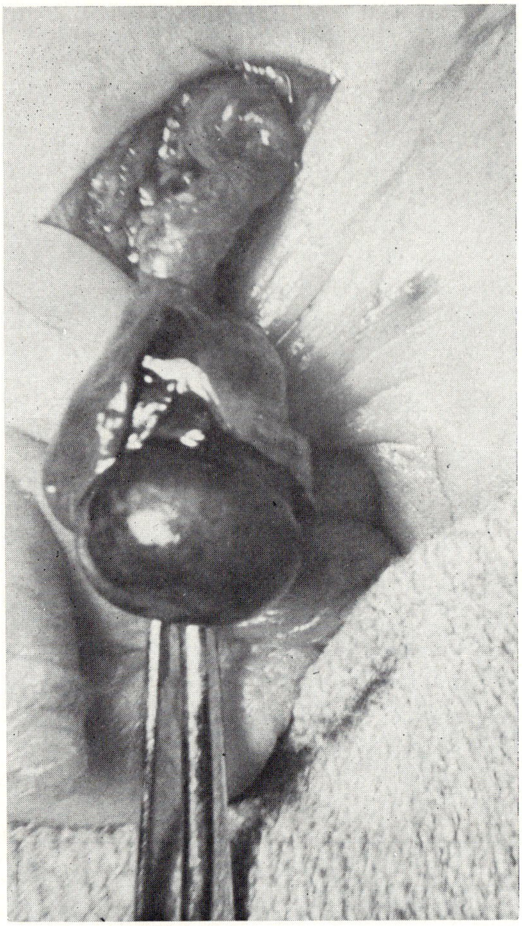

Fig. 1. Left testicle delivered through an inguinal incision and showing torsion of the cord and infarcted testis.

the testis is usually not of much value, but Hyams[8] recently reported a case of extravaginal torsion in a newborn infant presenting as a hydrocele.

The differential diagnosis includes hematoma secondary to trauma, hydrocele, strangulated hernia, torsion of epididymal appendices, tumor, epididymo-orchitis, and purulent infection in the tunica vaginalis.

There is controversy as to treatment. Glaser and Wallis[7] do not feel that operative management has brought any particular benefit, although most disagree and stress the necessity for immediate operative correction. Smith[15] found that seminiferous tubules are not viable after six hours of infarction, and Leydig's cells are not viable after twelve. Because of this observation and the differential diagnosis of a testicular mass which includes tumor, we feel that when the initial discovery of a testicular mass is made, operative intervention should be undertaken immediately in the hope of salvaging some testicular function. Several authors[6, 13, 14, 17, 19] advise orchidectomy if infarction has occurred. However, Longino and Martin[10] report that two out of seven apparently infarcted testes left in place have not developed significant atrophy. Reeves and associates[14] state that no complications have been observed when a grossly necrotic testis was left in place. Because of the chance of survival of some testicular function and the absence of complications, we would oppose orchidectomy. In view of the correctness of Sir Astley Cooper's observation and of the fact that cases of bilateral testicular torsion in the newborn infant have been reported,[4, 11] we advise contralateral fixation of the tunica albuginea to the dartos.

SUMMARY

A case of extravaginal torsion of the spermatic cord in a newborn infant is reported. Clinical signs, differential diagnosis, and treatment are discussed. An exploratory operation should be performed immediately, the infarcted testes should be left in place, and contralateral testicular fixation should be carried out.

REFERENCES

1. Bjorn, C. L., and Davis, J. R.: Torsion of the spermatic cord in the newborn, J. A. M. A. **145:** 1236, 1951.
2. Campbell, M. F.: Torsion of the spermatic cord in the newborn infant, J. Pediat. **33:** 323, 1948.
3. Donaldson, A. N., and Pearlman, C. K.: Torsion of the spermatic cord, Amer. Surg. **33:** 68, 1967.
4. Frederick, P. L., Dushker, N., and Eraklis, A. J.: Simultaneous bilateral torsion of the testes in a newborn infant, Arch. Surg. **94:** 299, 1967.
5. Gelband, H., and Wulfsohn, M. A.: Torsion of the spermatic cord in utero: Case report, J. Urol. **98:** 506, 1967.
6. Gilleinwater, J. Y., and Burros, H. M.: Tor-

sion of the spermatic cord in utero, J. A. M. A. **198:** 1123, 1966.
7. Glaser, S., and Wallis, H. R. E.: Torsion or spontaneous hemorrhagic infarction of testicle in newborn infant, Brit. Med. J. **2:** 88, 1952.
8. Hyams, B. B.: Torsion of the testis in the newborn, J. Urol. **101:** 192, 1969.
9. Lester, D. B., and Gummess, G. H.: Torsion of the spermatic cord in the newborn infant, J. Urol. **86:** 631, 1961.
10. Longino, L. A., and Martin, L. W.: Torsion of the spermatic cord in the newborn infant, New Eng. J. Med. **253:** 695, 1955.
11. Papadatos, C., and Moutsauris, C.: Bilateral testicular torsion in the newborn, J. Pediat. **71:** 249, 1967.
12. Pinto, P. S., and Kiefer, J. N.: Infarction of the testicle in the newborn infant, J. Pediat. **51:** 80, 1947.
13. Ravich, R.: Hemorrhagic infarction of the testicle in the newborn infant, J. Urol. **57:** 875, 1947.
14. Reeves, H. H., Sigler, R. M., Hahn, H. B., Jr., and Lynn, H. B.: Torsion of the spermatic cord in the newborn, Amer. J. Dis. Child. **110:** 676, 1965.
15. Smith, G. I.: Cellular changes from graded testicular ischemia, J. Urol. **73:** 355, 1955.
16. Sonneland, J. E.: Pain-free testicular torsion in the newborn, case description, Clin. Pediat. **8:** 289, 1969.
17. Tankin, L. H., and Robbins, M. A.: Hemorrhagic infarct of the testis in the newborn, J. Urol. **79:** 119, 1958.
18. Taylor, M. R.: A case of testis strangulated at birth, Brit. Med. J. **1:** 458, 1897.
19. Whittlesey, H.: Intrauterine torsion of the spermatic cord, Amer. J. Surg. **102:** 699, 1961.
20. Yunen, J. R.: Testicular torsion in the newborn: Report of a case, J. Urol. **97:** 318, 1967.

Complete transposition of the great vessels: Surgical results of emergency Blalock-Hanlon operation in infants

ROLANDO ZAMORA, M.D.
JAMES H. MOLLER, M.D.
RUSSELL V. LUCAS, Jr., M.D.
ALDO R. CASTANEDA, M.D.
MINNEAPOLIS, MINN.
From the Departments of Surgery and Pediatrics, University of Minnesota Medical Center

Corrective operative procedures for complete transposition of the great vessels (TGV) can be accomplished at present with a relatively low mortality rate and acceptable late functional results.[3, 4, 6] However, since more than 50 percent of infants with TGV die within the first month of life and 85 percent do not survive the first six months of life,[5] palliative treatment in early infancy continues to be of importance.

In TGV, the pulmonary and the systemic circulation are in parallel and palliation consists primarily of creating an atrial septal communication to enhance mixing between these two circuits. In 1950, Blalock and Hanlon[1] described a technique of atrial septectomy which has been used, with minor modifications, in the 28 patients reported in this study. In eight instances of coexisting ventricular septal defect (VSD), the pulmonary artery was also banded. Two infants with TGV and reduced pulmonary flow secondary to subpulmonary stenosis subsequently required a systemic to pulmonary artery anastomosis.

MATERIALS AND METHODS

Since June of 1964, 28 infants, 18 males and 10 females, with TGV had emergency Blalock-Hanlon operations performed at the University of Minnesota Medical Center (Table I). All operations were carried out under normothermic and normobaric conditions. Sixteen infants (57 percent) were operated upon within the first month and 75 percent of all infants within the first two months of life (Table II).

The diagnosis was substantiated preoperatively by right heart catheterization in 13 patients and by forward angiography in 15 patients. Eighteen infants had an intact ventricular septum and 16 required the Blalock-Hanlon operation within the first two months of life (Fig. 1). Rashkind balloon septotomy was attempted in nine of these infants during the course of right heart catheterization, but a continuously deteriorating clinical course made emergency surgical septectomy necessary within a few hours.

Fourteen infants had additional malformations, including VSD in eight, VSD and pulmonary stenosis in one, subpulmonary stenosis with intact ventricular septum in two, persistent ductus arteriosus (PDA) in two (less than 10 days of age), and VSD and PDA in one infant (Table III). Of the nine patients with VSD, pulmonary artery banding was performed on eight at the time of the Blalock-Hanlon operation. The other child had a large VSD and therefore banding was performed as an initial procedure. However, this patient required a Blalock-Hanlon operation eight months later.

Prior to operation the majority of infants were oxygenated and then intubated while awake. Anesthesia was induced and maintained with nitrous oxide and halothane.

Supported by Cardiovascular Clinical Research Program Project Budget No. 0685-5200.
Received for publication Nov. 14, 1969.

Table I. *Distribution of infants with transposition of the great vessels and Blalock-Hanlon operation according to age and operative mortality rate*

Age at operation (days)	*No. of patients*	*Operative deaths*	*Late deaths*
1 - 10	8	1	0
11 - 30	8	1	1
31 - 60	5	1	0
61 - 90	3	0	0
> 90	4	0	0
Totals	28	3 (10.7%)	1 (4%)

Table II. *Age distribution of infants at the time of Blalock-Hanlon operation. Most of the cases were operated in the first two months of life*

Age at operation (days)	*No. of patients*	*%*	
1 - 10	8	57 (1 - 10, 11 - 30)	75 (1 - 10 to 31 - 60)
11 - 30	8		
31 - 60	5		
61 - 90	3		
90	4		
	Total 28		

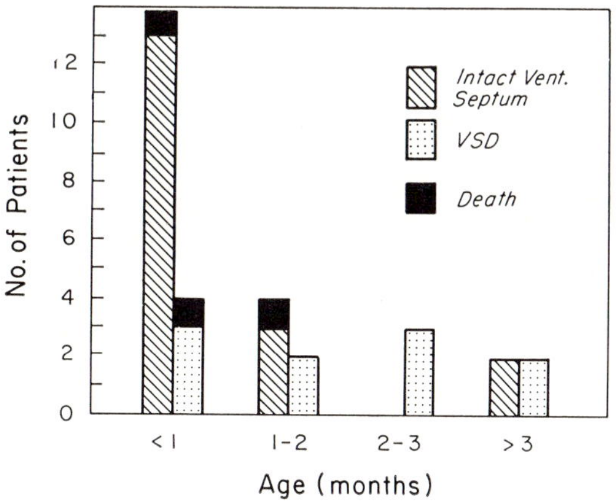

Fig. 1. Age distribution of infants with transposition of the great vessels at time of Blalock-Hanlon operation. Note high incidence of septectomy within the first two months of life in TGV with intact ventricular septum.

Table III. *Associated intracardiac malformations in 28 infants with transposition of the great vessels*

Anatomic classification	*No.*	
Intact ventricular septum	16	
Isolated		14
PDA		2
Associated VSD	9	
Isolated		8
PDA		1
Associated subpulmonary stenosis	3	
Intact septum		2
VSD		1
Total	28	

PDA = persistent ductus arteriosus; VSD = ventricular septal defect.

During operation temperature was checked by a rectal thermometer and normothermia was maintained with a thermoblanket. In the few instances in which transfusions were required during the procedure, the blood was passed through a warming coil.[9] All operations were carried out through the right fourth intercostal space or the bed of the resected fifth rib. Septectomy followed essentially the technique described by Blalock and Hanlon.[1] Resection of a generous portion of the atrial septum, including the limbus of the fossa ovalis, was sought. Following septectomy all infants, with the exception of two, tolerated extubation and were returned to the incubator and the infant intensive care unit.

RESULTS

In the group of 28 infants, there were three operative deaths (10.7 percent) (Table I). One 60-day-old child had two preoperative cardiorespiratory arrests and required external cardiac massage during transportation to the operating room. He died in irreversible metabolic acidosis shortly after atrial septectomy. At autopsy, the diagnosis of TGV was confirmed. In addition, a cleft in the anterior leaflet of the mitral valve was found. Part of this leaflet was attached via chordae tendineae to the ventricular septum, causing not only mitral insufficiency but also significant subpulmonary stenosis. The atrial defect, created under less than optimal conditions, measured only 7 mm. in diameter.

The other two deaths occurred in infants two and 20 days of age, respectively. They both died of respiratory failure and metabolic acidosis on the second postoperative day. In fact, these two infants were the only ones who required postoperative tracheal intubation and mechanical ventilatory assist. In the 20-day-old infant (intact ventricular septum), the autopsy showed patchy atelectasis of both lungs. The atrial defect measured 1 × 1 cm. The two-day-old infant showed bilateral pulmonary edema, marked intraparenchymal hemorrhage, and areas of acute pneumonia of the right lung. The atrial defect in this instance measured 1 × 2 cm. A pulmonary artery band (TGV and VSD), which had been placed at the same time, seemed well positioned.

There was one late death, 22 months following the original Blalock-Hanlon operation and pulmonary artery banding. The initial operation had been performed at age 20 days. The child died suddenly at home, while sleeping. The preoperative hemoglobin level of 17.5 Gm. percent had decreased to 15 Gm. percent two months following operation. One month prior to death, however, hemoglobin had reportedly risen to 21.5 Gm. percent. Since the child died at home, no postmortem examination was performed.

With the exception of one child, all other infants improved clinically immediately after operation. Cyanosis became less noticeable and indeed in most cases was difficult to discern at rest. Twenty-five infants were kept on digitalis postoperatively for 6 to 24 months. Hemoglobin dropped from an average preoperative level of 20 Gm. percent (range 15.5 to 26) to an average of 16.5 Gm. percent (range 13 to 19). This fall in hemoglobin lasted for about 15 months. Thereafter a slow, but steady rise in hemoglobin was uniformly noted.

Of particular interest is a group of 13 infants who were recatheterized at an average of two years following the original Blalock-Hanlon operation. Unfortunately, 10 of these patients had only forward angiograms prior to the shunt operation. In all 13 patients, however, mean aortic oximetry values were 73 percent (range 66 to 88 percent) following the Blalock-Hanlon operation, while the mean preoperative values were 42 percent (range 40 to 45 percent). Eleven patients who had recatheterization have undergone Mustard operations and are the subject of a separate report.[4] The twelfth patient had a Blalock-Taussig operation 3 years after the Blalock-Hanlon procedure because of demonstrated subpulmonary stenosis with VSD. This child had a 41 percent aortic oxygen saturation prior to the surgical septectomy. Three years after this procedure the saturation was 70 percent.

The other infant is the only one who failed to improve clinically immediately following the atrial septectomy which was done at age eight weeks of life. This infant had a hemoglobin level of 23.5 Gm. percent 12 months following operation, and repeated heart catheterization demonstrated a significant subpulmonary stenosis with an intact ventricular septum. The mean pulmonary artery pressure was 14 mm. Hg. This child died after a Blalock-Taussig operation.

DISCUSSION

Operative mortality rate in this group of 28 infants with TGV after a Blalock-Hanlon operation was 10.7 percent. One of the three operative deaths occurred in a moribund infant who had suffered two preoperative cardiorespiratory arrests. After reaching a state of irreversible metabolic acidosis, this infant was beyond surgical therapy. At postmortem examination, an associated partial form of endocardial cushion defect, subpulmonary stenosis, and an intact ventricular septum were identified. It is interesting to note that the only other child in this series with subpulmonary stenosis and intact ventricular septum died following a Blalock-Taussig operation. The second death must be ascribed to a technical problem requiring prolonged interruption of the circulation to the right lung leading to massive intrapulmonary hemorrhage. This complication occurred in the second operation of this series. The third infant had a very large VSD and therefore had additional banding of the pulmonary artery. The child died 2 days following operation in severe pulmonary edema. Perhaps under these circumstances, the Edwards and associates'[2] modification of the Blalock-Hanlon operation (with suturing of the septum behind the right pulmonary veins) would have provided a more favorable palliation by reducing pulmonary blood flow more effectively.

Careful follow-up of these children should be stressed. Although the hemoglobin levels fell to very acceptable values in all but one of the infants following atrial septectomy, in most instances, they tended to rise again within 15 months. For example, the one late death could probably have been prevented by following the hemoglobin levels more closely and bringing the child back at an earlier date for recatheterization and corrective surgical treatment. Also, in the only infant in whom increasing cyanosis was noted following a short initial improvement after septectomy, the eventual cardiac catheterization diagnosis of coexistent subpulmonary stenosis with intact ventricular septum should have been suspected earlier and systemic artery to pulmonary artery shunt performed before hemoglobin levels had reached 23.5 Gm. percent. In one infant, despite a large VSD, a Blalock-Hanlon procedure became necessary following initial pulmonary artery banding. In the presence of significant subpulmonary stenosis, with or without an intact ventricular septum, adequate mixing at the atrial level is important to allow hemodynamic adjustment following a systemic artery to pulmonary artery shunt (Waterston or Blalock-Taussig). We therefore make an atrial septal defect either by a Rashkind[8] balloon septotomy or a Blalock-Hanlon operation in all infants with TGV, irrespective of the associated lesions.

Hyperbaric oxygenation has been reported to improve operative survival substantially.[7] The results presented here, with the use of conventional operating room facilities, are comparable to those in which the Blalock-Hanlon procedure was performed within a hyperbaric chamber. The authors believe that a dedicated team (available day and night) of pediatric cardiologists, anesthesiologists, full-time cardiovascular surgeons, and an infant intensive care unit with specialized nursing care, add considerably more to the eventual survival of infants operated upon for TGV than any specific technical surgical innovation.

The reported improvement in results with Blalock-Hanlon operations in infants with complete transposition of the great vessels, particularly in infants within the first two months of life, is ascribed to early diagnosis and immediate (emergency) creation of an atrial septal communication before significant hemodynamic deterioration and irreversible metabolic acidosis occurs. The present approach includes right heart catheterization as soon as the cyanotic infant with a suspected diagnosis of TGV is admitted to the hospital. In the presence of TGV and intact ventricular septum, a Rashkind balloon septotomy is attempted. Although in this series nine of these infants had Blalock-Hanlon operations following an inadequate balloon septotomy, good palliation with this procedure has been achieved by us and by others.[8, 10] Balloon septotomy has the advantage of allowing initial palliation during diagnostic cardiac catheterization. Furthermore, by obviating thoracotomy and pericardiotomy, some of the technical difficulties encountered during dissection of the adhesed pericardium for use as an intra-atrial baffle (à la Mustard) are eliminated. On the other hand, in our experience, the Blalock-Hanlon technique has proved extremely reliable in the management of infants with this complex malformation. The low operative mortality rate (there have been no deaths in the last 15 consecutive patients) and the adequate palliation, lasting a minimum of 15 months and as long as 30 months, justifies the continued use of the Blalock-Hanlon technique, not only in cases of TGV with intact ventricular septum and failure of the Rashkind procedure, but electively in infants with

TGV and VSD who require a pulmonary artery banding. The addition of the Blalock-Hanlon operation to the banding procedure has not increased the operative risk. Also, the balloon septotomy has caused some complications. Two infants had thrombotic occlusion of the inferior vena cava which required placement of a third caval catheter (superior vena cava, inferior vena cava [transcardiac], and femoral vein) during the Mustard operation.

SUMMARY

In 28 infants with TGV, the operative mortality rate following a Blalock-Hanlon procedure was 10.7 percent (3 patients). There was one late death 22 months after operation. With the exception of one infant who had associated subpulmonary stenosis with intact ventricular septum, all patients showed immediate clinical improvement. The average preoperative hemoglobin level of 20 Gm. percent fell to 16.5 Gm. percent after operation. Aortic oxygen saturation rose from 42 to 73 percent. These values remained stable for at least 15 months after the Blalock-Hanlon operation when a gradual but steady deterioration began.

The present policy consists of creating an atrial communication as soon as the diagnosis of TGV is established, regardless of the associated defects. In case of intact ventricular septum, a Rashkind balloon septotomy is attempted. In this group of patients a Blalock-Hanlon operation is required only in case of the failure of or the inability to perform a Rashkind procedure. In infants with TGV and VSD, a Blalock-Hanlon procedure is added at the time of pulmonary artery banding.

A Blalock-Hanlon procedure is also carried out either simultaneously or prior to systemic artery to pulmonary artery shunts (Waterston or Blalock-Taussig) in case of TGV and subpulmonary stenosis.

The intimate collaboration of pediatric cardiologists, radiologists, anesthesiologists, and cardiac surgeons and the need for an infant intensive care unit are stressed.

REFERENCES

1. Blalock, A., and Hanlon, C. R.: The surgical treatment of complete transposition of the aorta and pulmonary artery, Surg. Gynec. Obstet. **90:** 1, 1950.
2. Edwards, W. S., Bargeron, L. M., and Lyons, C.: Reposition of right pulmonary vein in transposition of the great vessels, J. A. M. A. **188:** 522, 1964.
3. Haller, J. A., Jr., Crisler, C., Brawley, R., Cameron, J., and Rowe, R.: Operative correction and postoperative management of transposition of the great vessels in nine children, Ann. Thorac. Surg. **7:** 212, 1969.
4. Indeglia, R. A., Moller, J. H., Lucas, R. V., Jr., and Castaneda, A. R.: Treatment of transposition of the great vessels with an intra-atrial baffle (Mustard procedure). In preparation.
5. Keith, J. D., Rowe, R. D., and Vlad, P.: Heart disease in infancy and childhood, ed. 2, New York, 1967, The Macmillan Company.
6. Mustard, W. T., Keith, J. D., Trusler, G. A., Fowler, R., and Kidd, L.: The surgical management of transposition of the great vessels, J. Thorac. Cardiovasc. Surg. **48:** 953, 1964.
7. Plauth, W. H., Nadas, A. S., Bernhard, W. F., and Gross, R. E.: Transposition of the great arteries. Clinical and physiological observations of 74 patients treated by palliative surgery, Circulation **37:** 316, 1968.
8. Rashkind, W. J., and Miller, W. W.: Transposition of the great arteries: Results of palliation by balloon atrioseptotomy in thirty-one infants, Circulation **38:** 453, 1968.
9. Salmon, P. A., Buckley, J. J., and Assimacopoulos, C. A.: A simple disposable heat exchanger for blood transfusion purposes, SURGERY **52:** 784, 1962.
10. Tynan, M., Carr, I., Graham, G., and Carter, R. E.: Subvalvular pulmonary obstruction complicating the postoperative course of balloon atrial septotomy in transposition of the great arteries, Circulation **39** (Suppl.): 223, 1969.

The current status of immunosuppressive therapy

JOHN A. MANNICK, M.D.
BOSTON, MASS.
From the Department of Surgery, Boston University School of Medicine

The possibility of controlling the rejection of foreign tissue grafts was inherent in the classic report of Medawar[42] in 1944, which demonstrated that the rejection of transplanted foreign tissue was an immunological process. However, it was not until 15 years later that Schwartz and his co-workers[57, 58] described a clinically feasible means of inhibiting the transplantation-immune response reporting that 6-mercaptopurine (6-MP) would suppress both antibody formation and the rejection of skin allografts in rabbits. Billingham and associates[13] earlier reported that cortisone which inhibited the rejection of skin allografts had failed to launch the field of clinical organ transplantation when Persky and Jacob[55] and Dempster[20] reported that cortisone treatment did not prolong the survival of kidney allografts in dogs. However, following the report of Schwartz and his associates, [57, 58] it was quickly found that 6-MP and its analogues, particularly when administered in conjunction with adrenal corticosteroids, would permit the prolonged survival of renal allografts in animals and man.[14, 27, 51, 74, 76]

STANDARD CLINICAL IMMUNOSUPPRESSION

The immunosuppressive regimen used by most groups engaged in clinical kidney transplantation has remained remarkably standardized over the past five years. The basic drug is azathioprine, an analogue of 6-MP, which is administered daily, beginning shortly before or at the time of kidney transplantation in maximum tolerable doses, which are determined by the patient's ability to maintain an adequate circulating white blood count. The usual dose is 2 to 3 mg. per kilogram of body weight.

The second basic drug is a cortisol-like steroid, usually prednisone, which is ordinarily started in relatively high doses (from 60 to 200 mg. per day), beginning at the time of transplantation and then gradually tapered down to a maintenance dose, which varies widely depending upon the antigenic disparity between the donor and the recipient of the transplant and the practices of the individual transplantation group. At the first evidence of attempted rejection of the transplanted organ, the prednisone dosage is briefly raised again to high levels and is then tapered as the rejection crisis is successfully combated.

The third major tool employed by many groups in clinical kidney transplantation today is local irradiation of the organ graft. At first glance, this appears to be illogical therapy because little might be expected to be gained by the treatment of a systemic response by local measures. However, the work of Kauffman and Hume and their associates[36, 37] has clearly shown that local irradiation of an organ allograft is temporarily effective in delaying graft rejection by destroying those immunologically competent cells which are locally engaged in attack

Received for publication Dec. 12, 1969.

upon the transplanted organ and also by interfering with the sensitization of the host by the foreign organ graft, which is ordinarily mediated, at least in part, by lymphoid cells from the host which pass through the transplanted organ.[68] The statistics compiled by the kidney transplant registry[50] at first suggested that the administration of several small doses of local irradiation (about 150 rads per dose) early in the post-transplant period significantly improved the chances of survival of an organ graft from an unrelated cadaver donor. However, more recent reports from the registry question the validity of this earlier conclusion.[2, 3] The necessity for this form of treatment in transplants donated by close relatives of the recipient is even less clear.

There are a number of minor adjuncts to the standard immunosuppressive regimen which have been used clinically.[11, 46] The most widely employed adjuncts are the actinomycins,[31] which have been administered in modest doses at the time of rejection crises for a number of years but have gradually gone out of favor in many transplant centers.

Another drug, the alkylating agent cyclophosphamide, has been shown to be immunosuppressive in experimental animals and has received some clinical use in organ transplantation.[24] Its myelotoxicity has, however, prevented its widespread acceptance. It has recently found a major role in the preparation of patients for transplantation of bone marrow from sibling donors.[6]

RESULTS OF STANDARD IMMUNOSUPPRESSIVE THERAPY

While the standard immunosuppressive regimen outlined above has been utilized in heart, liver, and lung transplants in man, the efficacy of this therapy can best be judged by reviewing the results obtained in kidney transplantations, which have been performed much more frequently and with greater success than transplantations of any other organ. The figures from the kidney transplant registry indicate that current immunosuppressive therapy will permit the survival of slightly more than 80 percent of kidneys transplanted from sibling donors one year from the time of surgical treatment,[2, 3] and also show that there is very little additional kidney loss in the second year following transplantation. The results are slightly less good for kidneys transplanted from parental donors. However, results are far different with kidneys from unrelated cadaver donors. Here, one-year survival is approximately 45 percent and there is an additional loss of surviving kidneys between the first and the second year.[2, 3] These figures emphasize the fact that the results of immunosuppressive therapy are markedly dependent upon the antigenic similarity between the kidney donor and recipient.

The complications of conventional immunosuppressive therapy are now well known. The first of these, of course, is the increased susceptibility of the patient to infection by environmental pathogens.[31, 35, 66] This risk is particularly marked if the patient has received sufficient azathioprine to depress the bone marrow and to produce a granulocytopenia. Certainly, one of the major causes of death following kidney transplantation has been a combination of relentless transplant rejection in the face of excessive immunosuppressive therapy, which in turn has produced overwhelming infection.[31, 66] The second major complication of immunosuppressive therapy includes all of the toxic side effects of continued steroid administration,[31, 66] which has proved necessary in nearly every patient receiving a cadaver kidney transplant and in many patients who have received living donor transplants. Third, it is now apparent that there is an increased incidence of malignancy in patients receiving chronic immunosuppressive therapy.[40, 54] Malignancies of the lymphoid system are particularly likely to occur in such individuals at a greater rate than would be expected in the normal population of similar age and sex.

A good deal of progress has been made during the past three years in typing kidney donors and recipients for histocompatibility antigens by means of lymphoagglutination or lymphocytotoxicity techniques. The results of these and other studies have indicated that in man, as in many other mammalian species, there is a single genetic locus with multiple alleles and several subloci which determines the antigens which induce strong rejection reactions; these reactions are difficult to control with immunosuppressive drugs.[7, 17, 59] These strong antigens have been termed HL-A antigens, a number of which can now be reliably recognized on human lymphocytes by panels of antisera.[17, 44, 59]

The clinical course of a patient who has received a kidney transplant from an HL-A identical sibling donor is ordinarily remarkably benign. Rejection of the transplant can be averted with modest doses of conventional immunosuppressive drugs, and steroid therapy can often be discontinued without precipitating a rejection episode. However, because of the multiplicity of alleles at the HL-A locus and their random distribution in the population at large, the chances of finding an HL-A identical cadaver donor for any given recipent are poor and would remain poor even if a nationwide cadaver kidney distribution and typing system could be organized.[5] Consequently, the vast majority of cadaver kidney donors and recipients are HL-A incompatible.

This is clearly reflected in the reduced early survival of kidney transplants from cadaver donors as compared with those from related living donors[2, 3] and is, moreover, undoubtedly responsible for the progressive loss of cadaver kidney transplants over the second and third years following transplantation from a process termed "chronic rejection." Chronic rejection is manifested chiefly by vascular lesions in the transplanted kidney and has been remarkably resistant to most currently available forms of immunosuppressive therapy.[28, 31, 56] Because of this process, few kidney transplants from cadaver donors survive four years.[2, 3] Patient survival is, of course, better than this, and a number of indiviluals have had second, third, and fourth kidney transplantations.[31]

There are two logical means available for improving the average survival of organ transplants from unrelated cadaver donors. The first is improved matching of cadaver donors and recipients by histocompatibility typing techniques. This is being attempted in many cooperative cadaver kidney procurement programs throughout the world.[10, 48, 53] The second is the application of new and, hopefully, improved techniques of immunosuppressive therapy.

THE ROLE OF ANTILYMPHOCYTE SERUM

The addition to clinical immunosuppressive therapy which has aroused the most interest over the past two years is antilymphocyte serum (ALS) or antilymphocyte globulin (ALG). For human use, this material, as the name suggests, is an antiserum raised in a foreign species, usually the horse, against human lymphocytes. The crude serum is ordinarily absorbed with human erythrocytes in order to remove hemagglutinating activity and is then further purified by separating out the gamma globulin fraction containing the antibodies.

ALS or ALG has been shown in the experimental laboratory to be the most potent immunosuppressive material yet discovered, as indicated by its ability to prolong survival of skin allografts in rodents.[41, 73] These substances have also prolonged the survival of kidney transplants in a number of animal species.[1, 26, 32, 45, 47]

The mechanism of the immunosuppressive action of ALS and ALG is not known with certainty, although the current evidence suggests that these substances act by inhibiting or destroying thymus-dependent lymphocytes, which are the cells chiefly responsible for initiating transplant rejection.[33, 39, 41, 69] The antibodies in ALS, however, are by no means specific for lymphocytes, thymus derived or otherwise, and cross-react with most other tissues of the species used to immunize the ALS donor.[41]

Despite the myriad evidence of the efficacy of ALS in laboratory animals, the role of ALS or ALG therapy in the transplantation of human organs is not entirely clear.

One of the first reports of the clinical use of ALG by Starzl and his associates[64, 65] in 1967 indicated that the administration of ALG in the early post-transplant period had markedly simplified the control of rejection in a series of kidney transplants from related living donors. The impressions of this experienced and astute group cannot be discounted; however, a number of clinical transplant teams have subsequently reported equally good results with related, living donor kidney transplants achieved with conventional immunosuppressive drugs without the aid of ALG.[2, 3, 31] There is, unfortunately, no evidence that the use of ALG has altered the one-year survival rate of kidney transplants from cadaver donors, even though it is in this group of organ recipients that improvement in immunosuppressive therapy is urgently needed.

Starzl and his associates[63] have also reported that ALG therapy has eased the immunosuppressive management of patients receiving liver transplants. The experience of other groups with liver transplants has been very limited.

It was initially believed that ALG therapy was the key to successful cardiac transplantation. However, despite the use of this material, early acute rejection of heart transplants has, on the whole, apparently been more difficult to control than the rejection of kidney transplants from unrelated cadaver donors.[15, 67]

Interpretation of the results of the clinical use of ALG has been difficult for two reasons. First, in clinical transplantation, ALG has almost invariably been used in conjunction with conventional immunosuppressive therapy. Since conventional therapy is at least moderately successful by itself in most instances, the contribution of ALG is often difficult to ascertain. Second, it is now a well-established fact that it is difficult to predict the immunosuppressive potency of a given ALG preparation by most in vitro tests.[41] While it is generally agreed that all potent preparations of ALG contain relatively high titers of leukoagglutinating or leukocytotoxic antibodies, not all preparations with high antibody titers are potent. Since ethical and legal considerations prevent the testing of each ALG preparation designated for clinical use on a panel of human volunteers, the true immunosuppressive potency of a number of the ALG preparations currently used remains in doubt.

Bach and associates[8] have recently reported that inhibition of rosette formation may be one in vitro test, the results of which correlate with the immunosuppressive potency of ALG preparations in experimental animals. Attempts to match the results of the rosette inhibition test with the immunosuppressive potency of human ALG preparations have already been initiated. Moreover, Balner and his associates[9] have presented evidence that the immunosuppressive potency of human ALG preparations may be satisfactorily ascertained by studying the ability of these preparations to prolong the survival of skin allografts in monkeys. Both of these assay methods have indicated that several ALG preparations currently in clinical use have very different immunosuppressive potencies, and this fact may account for certain inconsistencies in reported clinical results.

Davis and associates[19] have recently noted that ALS raised in rabbits against mouse lymphocytes reaches maximum immunosuppressive potency after the first booster immunization and thereafter declines progressively in potency with each subsequent immunizing injection. These workers have also reported that, in ALS preparations harvested early in the course of immunization, the leukoagglutination titer does correlate with immunosuppressive effect. These studies suggest that potent ALG may be reliably prepared, in the rabbit at any rate, by an initial immunization followed by a single booster injection and that the antibody titer in such preparations is a reliable index of suppressive potency. Since many of the preparations of human ALG currently in use have been prepared in horses which have received multiple booster immunizations,[32, 52, 64] it would appear desirable to determine whether or not horse ALG also declines in potency following a certain optimum number of immunizing injections.

A number of adverse side effects of ALG administration have been documented both clinically and in the experimental laboratory. These include pain and inflammation at the site of subcutaneous or intramuscular injections[32, 62, 65] and a marked febrile response which accompanies intravenous administration of ALG as well. Thrombocytopenia has also been reported following prolonged use of ALG.[62] Most ALG preparations appear to induce an antibody response against the foreign serum proteins which they contain, and the problem of serum sickness may be encountered with repeated injections of this material.[62] Moreover, laboratory evidence indicates that there is a real danger of causing nephritis following the intravenous administration of ALG preparations.[32]

While the myelotoxicity of ALG appears to be minimal when compared with a number of immunosuppressive drugs, including azathioprine, ALG administration does appear to depress the natural immunological defenses, particularly those which work against viruses.[4, 29] It is also of interest that several lymphomas have been reported in patients who have received ALG therapy.[21, 40]

Based upon a rationale similar to that which has prompted the use of ALS, the depletion of circulating lymphocytes by thoracic duct drainage has been suggested as an adjunct to current immunosuppressive therapy. This procedure has been shown in experimental animals to delay the rejection of skin allografts[73] and similar findings have also been reported in one series of human subjects.[71] However, there is evidence that thoracic duct drainage is not nearly as effective in prolonging the survival of kidney allografts in experimental animals.[22] Nevertheless, at least two groups have utilized thoracic duct drainage in conjunction with other immunosuppressive drugs in managing patients with kidney allografts. Both groups have presented evidence suggesting that thoracic duct drainage has improved allograft survival in their patients.[23, 70] Whether the effectiveness of this means of lymphocyte depletion, as weighed against the technical problems associated with keeping a thoracic duct fistula open for a length of time sufficient to produce a real reduction in the circulating lymphocyte pool, will make this maneuver popular in many clinical transplant centers remains to be determined.

FUTURE PROSPECTS

While a wide variety of anticancer drugs have been shown to have immunosuppressive properties over the last ten years, most of these agents have myelotoxic side effects similar to those of azathioprine. However, two agents currently undergoing investigation in the experimental laboratory are demonstrably immunosuppressive without significant myelotoxicity and may, therefore, find a clinical role in future attempts to increase immunosuppressive effectiveness without increasing the danger of toxic side effects. The first of these is phytohemagglutinin (PHA), which is known to stimulate lymphocytes to proliferate in tissue culture. Apparently somewhat similar effects can be produced by this drug in vivo, and it has been shown to have definite immunosuppressive properties, presumably as a result of nonspecific stimulation of cells otherwise capable of mounting a specific immune response.[61]

Second, there has been considerable research interest recently in an immunosuppressive alpha globulin fraction of normal mammalian blood. Mowbray[49] in 1963 described the immunosuppressive properties of alpha globulin fractions isolated from the serum of several species. This work was more recently confirmed by Mannick and Schmid,[38] who isolated an active alpha globulin fraction from normal human plasma. This material has been termed "immunoregulatory alpha globulin" (IRA) by Cooperband and his associates.[16] IRA has been shown to inhibit the proliferative response of lymphocytes to specific antigens and to block delayed hypersensitivity responses, including the rejection of skin allografts in experimental animals. The clinical applicability of this material remains in doubt. However, its lack of any apparent systemic toxicity and the fact that it can be prepared from normal human serum suggest that IRA may have a place in clinical immunosuppressive therapy in the future.

Perhaps the most significant role that immunosuppressive agents may play in the future of clinical organ transplantation will be as tools to facilitate the induction of true immunologic tolerance to foreign tissue antigens in adult human beings. Although it has been demonstrated that adult tolerance may ultimately be achieved after repeated and massive doses of foreign tissue antigens in experimental animals, even across rather strong histocompatibility barriers,[25, 60] the use of a number of immunosuppressive agents has been demonstrated to facilitate markedly the induction of tolerance under these circumstances and to permit a reduced dose of antigen to be used.[30, 43] One of the major drawbacks to any attempt at induction of adult tolerance in human beings has been the fact that tolerance is ordinarily successfully induced in animals only by living lymphoid cells. The specter of graft versus host disease,[12, 72, 75] that is, an attack of the administered lymphoid cells against the new host, is enough to dampen enthusiasm for such maneuvers in clinical transplantation. However, since it has recently become possible to extract soluble antigenic preparations from lymphoid cells of several species including man,[18, 34] use of such soluble subcellular histocompatibility antigens, coupled with immunosuppressive therapy, may ultimately permit induction of a useful degree of immunological tolerance to organ allografts in man and thus may permit the transplantation of organs between suitably typed donor and recipient pairs without the necessity for continual immunosuppressive therapy.

REFERENCES

1. Abaza, M. H., Noland, B., Watt, J. G., and Woodruff, M. F. A.: Effect of antilymphocyte serum on the survival of renal homotransplants in dogs, Transplantation **4:** 618, 1966.
2. Advisory Committee of the Human Kidney Transplant Registry: Sixth report of the Human Kidney Transplant Registry, Transplantation **6:** 966, 1968.
3. Advisory Committee of the Human Kidney Transplant Registry: Seventh report of the Human Kidney Transplant Registry, Transplantation **8:** 728, 1969.
4. Allison, A. C., and Law, L. W.: Effect of antilymphocyte serum on virus oncogenesis, Proc. Soc. Exp. Biol. Med. **127:** 207, 1968.
5. Bach, F. H.: Transplantation: Problems of histocompatibility testing, Science **159:** 1196, 1968.
6. Bach, F. H., Albertini, R. J., Joo, P., Anderson, J. L., and Bortin, M. M.: Bone marrow transplantation in a patient with the Wiskott-Aldrich syndrome, Lancet **2:** 1364, 1968.
7. Bach, F. H., and Amos, D. B.: Hu-1: Major histocompatibility locus in man, Science **156:** 1506, 1967.
8. Bach, J. F., Dardenne, M., Dormont, J., and Antoine, B.: A new *in vitro* test evaluating antilymphocyte serum potency, Transplant. Proc. **1:** 403, 1969.
9. Balner, H., Eysvoogel, V. P., and Cleton, F. J.: Testing of anti-human lymphocyte sera in chimpanzees and lower primates, Lancet **1:** 16, 1968.
10. Batchelor, J. R., and Joysey, V. C.: Influence of the HL-A incompatibility on cadaveric renal transplantation, Lancet **1:** 790, 1969.
11. Berenbaum, M. C.: Immunosuppressive agents and allogeneic transplantation, J. Clin. Path. **20:** 471, 1967.
12. Billingham, R. E., and Brent, L.: Acquired tolerance of foreign cells in newborn animals, Proc. Roy. Soc. (Biol.) **146:** 78, 1957.
13. Billingham, R. E., Krohn, P. L., and Medawar, P. B.: Effect of cortisone on survival of skin homografts in rabbits, Brit. Med. J. **1:** 1157, 1951.
14. Calne, R. Y.: The rejection of renal homografts: Inhibition in dogs by 6-mercaptopurine, Lancet **1:** 417, 1960.
15. Cooley, D. A., Bloodwell, R. D., Hellman, G. L., Leachman, R. D., Nora, J. J., and Milam, J. D.: Cardiac transplantation. General considerations and results, Ann. Surg. **169:** 892, 1969.
16. Cooperband, S. R., Davis, R. C., Schmid, K., and Mannick, J. A.: Competitive blockade of lymphocyte stimulation by a serum immunoregulatory alpha globulin (IRA), Transplant. Proc. **1:** 516, 1969.
17. Dausset, J., Walford, R. L., Colombani, J., Legrand, L., Feingold, N., Barge, A., and

Rapaport, F. T.: The HLA-A system subloci and their importance in transplantation, Transplant. Proc. **1:** 331, 1969.
18. Davies, D. A. L.: Transplantation antigens *in* Rapaport, F. T., and Dausset, J., editors: Human transplantation, New York, 1968, Grune & Stratton, Inc., pp. 618-634.
19. Davis, R. C., Cooperband, S. R., and Mannick, J. A.: Preparation and in vitro assay of effective and ineffective antilymphocyte sera, SURGERY 66: 58, 1969.
20. Dempster, W. J.: The effects of cortisone on the homotransplanted kidney, Arch. Int. Pharmacodyn. **95:** 253, 1953.
21. Deodhar, S. E., Kuklinca, A. G., Vidt, D. G., Robertson, A. L., and Hazard, J. B.: Development of reticulum-cell sarcoma at the site of antilymphocyte globulin injection in a patient with renal transplant, New Eng. J. Med. **280:** 1104, 1969.
22. Ellis, F.: Renal homograft response following thymectomy and thoracic duct drainage in goats, Transplantation **5:** 21, 1967.
23. Fish, J. C., Sarles, H. E., Remmers, A. R., Tyson, K. R. T., Canales, C. O., Beathard, G. A., Fukushima, M., Ritzmann, S. E., and Levin, W. C.: Circulating lymphocyte depletion in preparation for renal allotransplantation, Surg. Gynec. Obstet. **128:** 777, 1969.
24. Fox, M.: Suppression of tissue immunity by cyclophosphamide, Transplantation **2:** 475, 1964.
25. Guttman, T. D., and Aust, J. B.: Acquired tolerance to homografts produced by homologous spleen cell injection in adult mice, Nature **192:** 564, 1961.
26. Guttman, T. D., Carpenter, C. B., Lindquist, R. R., and Merrill, J. P.: Renal transplantation in the inbred rat. III. A study of heterologous anti-thymocyte seras, J. Exp. Med. **126:** 1099, 1967.
27. Hamburger, J., Vaysse, J., Crosnier, J., Auvert, J., Lalanne, C. M., and Hooper, J.: Renal homotransplantation in man after radiation of the recipient: Experience with six patients since 1959, Amer. J. Med. **32:** 854, 1962.
28. Harlan, W. R., Holden, K. R., Williams, G. M., and Hume, D. M.: Proteinuria and nephrotic syndrome in rejection of kidney transplants, New Eng. J. Med. **277:** 769, 1967.
29. Hirsch, M. S.: Effects of antilymphoid sera on viral infections, Lancet **2:** 37, 1968.
30. Hoehn, R. J.: Induction of tolerance to mouse tail skin homografts by combining paired immunosuppressive agents and cellular antigens, Transplantation **3:** 131, 1965.
31. Hume, D. M.: Kidney transplantation, *in* Rapaport, F. T., and Dausset, J., editors: Human transplantation, New York, 1968, Grune & Stratton, Inc., pp. 110-150.
32. Iwasaki, Y., Porter, K. A., Amend, J. R., Marchioro, T. L., Zuhlke, V., and Starzl, T. E.: The preparation and testing of horse antidog and antihuman plasma or serum and its protein fractions, Surg. Gynec. Obstet. **124:** 1, 1967.
33. Jeejeebhoy, J. F., and Vela-Martinez, J. M.: Studies on the mode of action of heterologous antilymphocyte plasma, Transplantation **6:** 149, 1968.
34. Kahan, B. D.: Isolation of a soluble transplantation antigen, Proc. Nat. Acad. Sci. **53:** 153, 1965.
35. Kanich, R. E., and Craighead, J. E.: Cytomegalovirus infection and cytomegalic inclusion disease in renal homotransplant recipients, Amer. J. Med. **40:** 874, 1966.
36. Kauffman, H. M., Cleveland, R. J., Dwyer, J. J., Lee, H. M., and Hume, D. M.: Prolongation of renal homograft function by local graft radiation, Surg. Gynec. Obst. **120:** 49, 1965.
37. Kauffman, H. M., Cleveland, R. J., Robertshaw, G. E., Graham, W. H., and Hume, D. M.: Inhibition of the afferent arc of the immune response to renal homografts by local graft radiation, Surg. Gynec. Obstet. **123:** 1052, 1966.
38. Mannick, J. A., and Schmid, K.: Prolongation of allograft survival by an alpha globulin isolated from normal blood, Transplantation **5:** 1231, 1967.
39. Martin, W. J., and Miller, J. F. A. P.: Site of action of antilymphocyte globulin, Lanset **2:** 1285, 1967.
40. McKhann, C. F.: Primary malignancy in patients undergoing immunosuppression for renal transplantation, Transplantation **8:** 209, 1969.
41. Medawar, P. B.: Biological effects of heterologous antilymphocyte sera, *in* Rapaport, F. T., and Daussett, J., editors: Human transplantation, New York, 1968, Grune & Stratton, Inc., pp. 501-509.
42. Medawar, P. B.: The behaviour and fate of skin autografts and skin homografts in rabbits, J. Anat. **78:** 176, 1944.
43. Medawar, P. B.: Use of antigenic tissue extracts to weaken immunological reaction against skin homografts in mice, Transplantation **1:** 21, 1963.
44. Mickey, M. R., Singal, D. P., and Terasaki, P. I.: Serotyping for homotransplantation. XXV. Evidence for three HL-A subloci, Transplant. Proc. **1:** 347, 1969.
45. Mitchell, R. M., Sheil, A. G. R., Slafsy, S. F., and Murray, J. E.: The effect of het-

erologous immune serum on canine renal homografts, Transplantation **4:** 323, 1966.
46. Mitchell, M. S., Wade, M. E., DeConti, R. C., Bertino, J. R., and Calabresi, P.: Immunosuppressive effects of cytosine arabinoside and methotrexate in man, Ann. Intern. Med. **70:** 535, 1969.
47. Monaco, A. P., Abbott, W. M., Othersen, H. B., Simmons, R. L., Wood, M. D., Plaz, M. H., and Russell, P. S.: Antiserum to lymphocytes: Prolonged survival of canine renal allografts, Science **153:** 1264, 1966.
48. Morris, P. J., Kincaid-Smith, P., and Marshall, V. C.: Leukocyte antigens in cadaver transplantation, Transplant. Proc. **1:** 376, 1969.
49. Mowbray, J. F.: Ability of large doses of an $alpha_2$ plasma protein fraction to inhibit antibody production, Immunology **6:** 217, 1963.
50. Murray, J. E., Barnes, B. A., and Atkinson, J.: Fifth report of the Human Kidney Transplant Registry, Transplantation **5:** 752, 1967.
51. Murray, J. E., Merrill, J. P., Dammin, G. J., Dealy, J. B., Alexandre, G. W., and Harrison, J. H.: Kidney transplantation in modified recipients, Ann. Surg. **156:** 337, 1962.
52. Najarian, J. S., Merkel, F. K., Moore, G. E., Good, R. A., and Aust, J. C.: Clinical use of anti-lymphoblast serum, Transplant. Proc. **1:** 460, 1969.
53. Patel, R., Mickey, M. R., and Terasaki, P. I.: Serotyping for homotransplantation. XVI. Analysis of living transplants from unrelated donors, New Eng. J. Med. **279:** 501, 1968.
54. Penn, I., Hammond, W., Brettschneider, L., and Starzl, T. E.: Malignant lymphomas in transplantation patients, Transplant. Proc. **1:** 106, 1969.
55. Persky, L., and Jacob, S.: Effect of ACTH and cortisone on homogenous kidney transplants, Proc. Soc. Exp. Biol. Med. **77:** 66, 1951.
56. Porter, K. A., Dossetor, J. B., Marchioro, T. L., Peart, W. S., Rendall, J. M., Starzl, T. E., and Terasaki, P. I.: Human renal transplants, Lab. Invest. **16:** 153, 1967.
57. Schwartz, R., and Dameshek, W.: The effects of 6-mercaptopurine on homograft reactions, J. Clin. Invest. **39:** 952, 1960.
58. Schwartz, R., Eisner, A., and Dameshek, W.: The effects of 6-mercaptopurine on primary and secondary immune responses, J. Clin. Invest. **38:** 1394, 1959.
59. Scientific Forum on Transplantation Genetics: Proceedings of the Second International Congress of the Transplantation Society, Transplant. Proc. **1:** 331, 1969.
60. Shapiro, F., Martinez, G., Smith, J. M., and Good, R. A.: Tolerance of skin homografts induced in adult mice by multiple injections of homologous spleen cells, Proc. Soc. Exp. Biol. Med. **106:** 472, 1961.
61. Spreafico, F., and Lerner, E. M.: Suppression of the primary and secondary immune response of the mouse by phytohemagglutinin, J. Immun. **98:** 407, 1967.
62. Starzl, T. E., Brettschneider, L., Penn, I., Schmidt, R. W., Bell, R., Kashiwagi, N., Townsend, G. M., and Putman, C. W.: A trial with heterologous antilymphocyte globulin in man, Transplant. Proc. **1:** 448, 1969.
63. Starzl, T. E., Groth, C. G., Brettschneider, L., Penn, I., Fulginiti, V. A., Moon, J. B., Blanchard, H., Martin, A. J., and Porter, K. A.: Orthotopic transplantation of the human liver, Ann. Surg. **168:** 392, 1968.
64. Starzl, T. E., Groth, C. G., Terasaki, P. I., Putman, C. W., Brettschneider, L., and Marchioro, T. L.: Heterologous antilymphocyte globulin, histoincompatibility matching and human renal homotransplantation, Surg. Gynec. Obstet. **126:** 1023, 1968.
65. Starzl, T. E., Marchioro, T. L., Hutchison, D. E., Porter, K. A., Cerilli, G. J., and Brettschneider, L.: The clinical use of antilymphocyte globulin in renal homotransplantation, Transplantation **5:** 1100, 1967.
66. Starzl, T. E., Marchioro, T. L., Porter, K. A., Moore, C. A., Rifkind, D., and Waddell, W. R.: Renal homotransplantation. Late function and complications, Ann. Intern. Med. **61:** 470, 1964.
67. Stinson, E. B., Dong, E., Schroeder, J. S., Harrison, D. C., and Shumway, N. E.: Initial clinical experience with heart transplantation, Amer. J. Cardiol. **22:** 791, 1968.
68. Strober, S., and Gowans, J. L.: The role of lymphocytes in the sensitization of rats to renal homografts, J. Exper. Med. **122:** 347, 1965.
69. Taub, R. N., and Lance, E. M.: The effect of heterologous antilymphocyte serum on the distribution of 51-Cr-labeled lymph node cells in mice, Immunology **15:** 633, 1968.
70. Tilney, N. L., and Murray, J. E.: The thoracic duct fistula as an adjunct to immunosuppression in human renal transplantation, Transplantation **5:** 1024, 1967.
71. Tunner, W. S., Carbone, P. P., Blaylock, W. K., and Irvin, G. L.: Effect of thoracic duct man, Surg. Gynec. Obstet. **121:** 334, 1965.
72. Woodruff, M. F. A.: Can tolerance to homologous skin be induced in the human infant at birth? Transplant. Bull. **4:** 26, 1957.
73. Woodruff, M. F. A., and Anderson, N. A.: Effect of lymphocyte depletion by thoracic duct fistula and administration of antilympho-

cyte serum on survival of skin homografts in rats, Nature **200:** 702, 1963.

74. Woodruff, M. F. A., Robson, J. S., Nolan, B., Lambie, A. T., Wilson, T. I., and Clark, J. G.: Homotransplantation of kidney in patients treated by preoperative local irradiation and postoperative administration of an antimetabolite (Imuran): Report of six cases, Lancet **2:** 675, 1963.

75. Woodruff, M. F. A., and Sparrow, M.: Further observations on the induction of tolerance of skin homografts in rats, Transplant. Bull. **4:** 157, 1957.

76. Zukoski, C. F., Lee, H. M., and Hume, D. M.: The effect of 6-mercaptopurine on renal homograft survival in the dog, Surg. Gynec. Obstet. **112:** 707, 1961.

Surgical techniques

Conducted by WILLIAM S. BLAKEMORE, M.D.

Control of the hepatic parenchyma by direct compression: A new instrument

DONALD B. DOTY, M.D.
HEINZ W. KUGLER
ROGER V. MOSELEY, M.D.
WASHINGTON, D. C.
From the Division of Surgery and the Division of Instrumentation, Walter Reed Army Institute of Research, Walter Reed Army Medical Center

Control of hemorrhage from the cut surface of the liver remains an unsolved technical problem in surgery. None of the accepted methods for hemostasis during resection of the liver is uniformly successful, and large volumes of blood may be lost as the parenchyma is divided or when a liver wound is inspected and debrided prior to suture repair. Many of these methods require temporary interruption of blood supply to the entire liver, with the possible consequences of ischemia. In addition, air embolism is a constant hazard during division of hepatic veins.

Application of a hemostatic instrument directly to the liver parenchyma eliminates these problems and offers a logical approach to control of the divided hepatic surface. A new instrument has been designed, tested in animals and humans, and found to be effective for this purpose. This report describes the instrument and its clinical application.

DESCRIPTION OF INSTRUMENT

The instrument consists of a stainless steel frame with blades of a size and shape that conform to the coronal section of the adult liver (Fig. 1). For convenience, a hand grip is attached to the frame. The two blades, which actually compress the hepatic parenchyma, are made of stainless spring steel or plastic (Lexan). A material of sufficient tensile strength to retain a uniform bend and to return to its original shape is necessary for proper blade function. The blades are covered with a removable foam rubber sheath to allow atraumatic application and to provide sufficient friction to prevent slipping on the liver surface.

The instrument is placed across the interlobar plane of the liver after the right lobe of liver has been mobilized completely. One of the blades will then be on the superior surface and the other on the inferior surface of the liver (Fig. 2). In this position, the instrument isolates the right lobe of the liver from its blood supply. Conformity to the shape of the liver and coarse tension adjustment are accomplished by drawing the superior blade into firm contact with the liver while depressing the spring loaded thumb catch and then releasing the catch into an appropriate hole in the superior blade. A steel guide insures alignment of the blade.

The compression of the hepatic parenchyma is achieved by turning the screw of the slide mechanism in the handle of the instrument. This moves the inferior blade forward and, since it is fixed at the opposite end, forces it to buckle, achieving greatest elevation in the middle of the blade (Fig. 1).

Received for publication July 24, 1969.

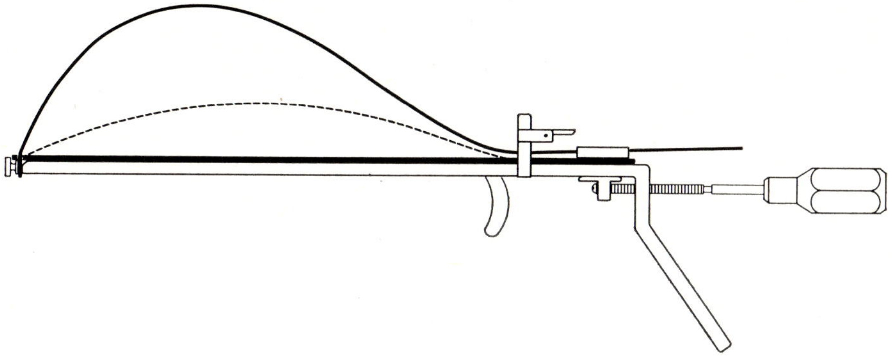

Fig. 1. The instrument for control of the hepatic parenchyma is shown in diagrammatic form. Its shape is similar to the coronal section of the liver. Conformity to the liver is achieved by adjustment of the superior blade by use of the thumb catch. Compression of the hepatic parenchyma is accomplished by turning the screw of the slide mechanism which moves the inferior blade forward, causing it to buckle as illustrated by the broken line.

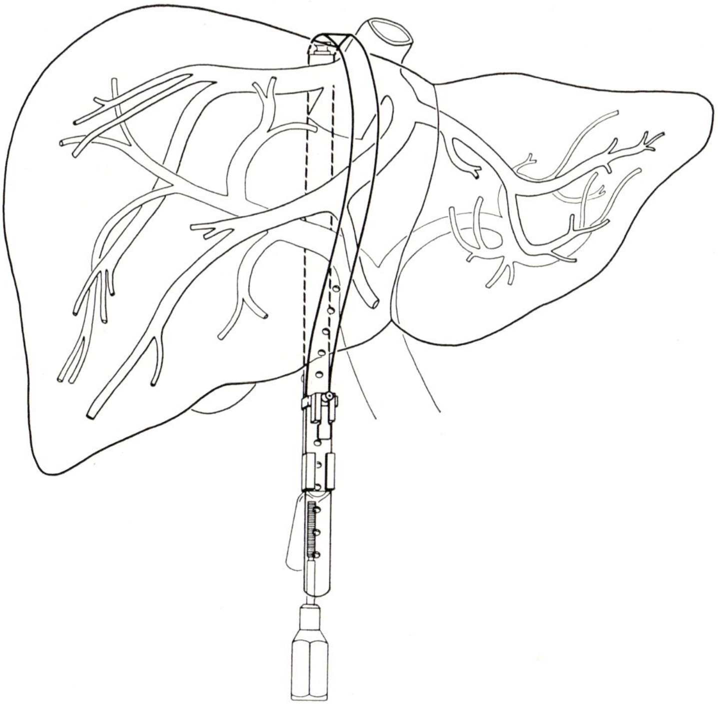

Fig. 2. The instrument is placed across the interlobar plane of the liver, thereby isolating the right lobe of the liver from its blood supply.

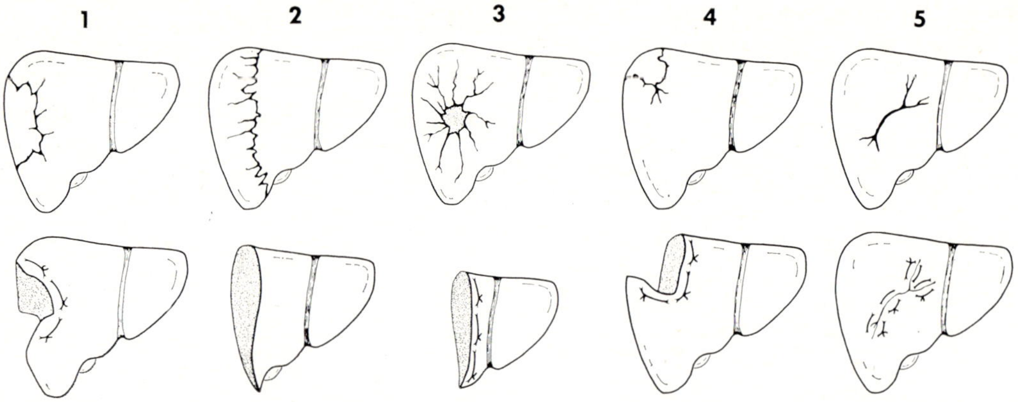

Fig. 3. The hepatic injury and operative repair in five battle casualties is illustrated.

CLINICAL USE

The instrument was initially tested on animals and found to be effective in achieving hemostasis. Autopsy room trials insured that atraumatic application of the instrument to the liver was possible.

The instrument was used in five patients who had severe trauma to the liver resulting from combat injury in Viet Nam. The procedures performed were two major resections of the right lobe of the liver, two large wedge resections, and one debridement and suture repair (Fig. 3).

CASE REPORTS

Case 1. The patient had a wedge-shaped fracture located laterally in the right lobe of the liver resulting from a mortar fragment. There was devitalized tissue in the margin of the defect but no active bleeding. The hemostatic instrument was placed medial to the wound, and debridement by wedge resection was performed. The nylon blades which were used at that time were not sufficiently resilient to apply sufficient hepatic compression to achieve hemostasis, and therefore hepatic inflow occlusion was necessary. The instrument, however, helped in positioning, handling, and exposure of the liver. Parenchymal hemostasis was achieved with suture ligature and n-butyl cyanoacrylate tissue adhesive. Recovery was uncomplicated.

Case 2. The patient had a mortar fragment wound with a linear fracture deep into the hepatic parenchyma, extending from the anterior to posterior margin slightly lateral to the gallbladder fossa. The liver was devitalized lateral to the injury. Excellent hemostasis was achieved during resection of the devitalized parenchyma with the instrument equipped with plastic (Lexan) blades. The divided surface was sprayed with n-butyl cyanoacrylate following suture ligation of large vessels and bile ducts. A T tube placed in the common bile duct did not prevent a bile fistula which eventually closed spontaneously.

Case 3. A high-velocity bullet wound completely disrupted the parenchyma of the right lobe of the liver. There was also a severe contusion of the lower lobe of the right lung. Hemostasis was achieved during total right hepatic lobectomy by use of the instrument. More medial placement of the instrument was achieved by preliminary ligation of the right hepatic vein. Individual blood vessels and bile ducts were ligated as they were encountered during the resection supplemented by sutures deep through the parenchyma. Bleeding from the contused lung and pulmonary edema with severe respiratory insufficiency resulted in death on the sixth postoperative day.

Case 4. The patient had a defect in the extraperitoneal surface of the liver caused by a fragment wound. Wedge resection of the injured area was accomplished with excellent hemostasis with use of the instrument. Mattress sutures were used in the margin of the resection. A subphrenic abscess complicated the postoperative course.

Case 5. Mortar fragments caused a deep linear fracture of the dome of the right lobe of the liver. Excellent hemostasis was achieved through use of the instrument during debridement of the depth of the wound and approximation of the wound edges with mattress sutures. The postoperative course was uncomplicated.

COMMENT

The plastic blades selected for trial in the initial patient were too malleable to compress the liver adequately and were discarded in favor of more rigid plastic. Following this

Table I. *Operation, incision, and total blood replacement during surgery in five patients using the new hepatic surgery instrument*

Case	Operation	Incision	Total blood replacement
1	Wedge resection	Abdominal	Not evaluated
2	Subtotal right lobectomy	Abdominal	2,000
3	Total right lobectomy	Thoraco-abdominal	4,000
4	Wedge resection	Abdominal	1,000
5	Suture repair	Abdominal	1,500

modification, the instrument was successful in controlling both arterial and venous hemorrhage in every case. Blades made of stainless spring steel, which may be more ideal in terms of tensile strength, durability, and ease of sterilization, are being evaluated. The proper function of the instrument is almost entirely dependent on the resilient properties of the material used in the lower blade. The deficiency of the instrument is a tendency for somewhat unequal distribution of compression if the lower blade does not maintain a uniform bend with its highest point centrally located.

In addition to effective control of blood loss as shown in Table I, the threat of air embolism was eliminated. Improved ability to manipulate the liver and better exposure were unexpected benefits. The instrument served as a mechanical grip on the liver, making movement and positioning of this large organ easier. With gentle traction on the instrument, the liver was easily exposed by abdominal incision in four of the five patients.

DISCUSSION

Control of hemorrhage during hepatic surgery is a formidable problem to the surgeon during both emergency and elective operations. Baker and associates[2] emphasized the need for immediate availability of large amounts of blood and showed that the average volume required in treatment of patients with nonpenetrating liver injuries was 2,700 ml. One thousand to 10,000 ml. of blood were required during major hepatic resection for trauma in a series of patients studied by Foster and associates.[3] A mean volume of 4,750 ml. for blood transfusions during operative procedures for trauma was compared with a mean volume of 2,500 ml. required during elective operations. These are typical figures for operative blood loss during major hepatic resections in which currently accepted techniques for hemostasis are used.

Each of the available methods for control of blood loss during hepatic surgery has its inherent limitations. As pointed out by Adson,[1] different techniques are appropriate in different situations, and acquaintance with all suitable methods will minimize their individual limitations.

Hepatic inflow occlusion by digital or mechanical compression of the porta hepatis has no effect on bleeding from hepatic efferent vessels. It is generally successful in controlling blood loss from parenchyma injured at a sublobar level but is ineffective if major hepatic veins are involved. Also, the hepatic cells in the uninjured portion of the liver are subjected to a period of arterial ischemia. It is generally accepted that without adjuvant hypothermia, the liver cannot be deprived of arterial blood flow for more than fifteen minutes if irreversible hepatic cell damage is to be avoided.

Preliminary ligation of appropriate primary hepatic arterial, portal venous, and hepatic venous branches to the injured segments of the liver is time consuming and may be only partially effective in controlling blood loss. Major anastomotic channels from the middle hepatic vein remain uncontrolled and may cause serious hemorrhage during division of the hepatic parenchyma.

The total inflow-outflow hepatic occlusion has been described by Heaney and associates.[4] Occlusion of aorta, porta hepatis, and vena cava above and below the liver offers a method of emergency control of blood loss from the hepatic vein or retrohepatic vena cava. Modifications of this technique using internal vena cava shunts have been employed by Schrock and associates[6] and by Timmis and associates[7] in an attempt to decrease the danger of cardiac arrest caused by vena cava occlusion. This is an effective and possibly the only way to prevent air embolus when the vena cava or hepatic veins are injured. The danger of hepatic cellular ischemia, as well as ischemia to the intestine, kidney, and lower half of the body, however, make this method unsatisfactory for elective use during resection of the liver.

Direct compression of the hepatic parenchyma by the assistant is probably an important aspect of hemostasis in nearly every hepatic resection. Uniform manual compression, however, is exceedingly difficult to apply and to maintain, and none of the several instruments devised for this purpose have been sufficiently effective to become widely employed.[5] The instrument described in this report has successfully achieved hemostasis during hepatic resection by direct compression of the hepatic parenchyma. This approach has the advantages of reducing blood loss, avoiding ischemia to uninvolved liver, preventing air embolization, improving exposure, and facilitating manipulation of this bulky organ. A dry operating field can be maintained during division of liver tissue, adding precision to the procedure. Improved exposure by direct retraction of the liver usually allows major resection to be accomplished through an abdominal incision, thus eliminating the pulmonary complications associated with the thoracoabdominal approach. If mobilization of the liver is complete prior to application, the instrument can be placed on the interlobar plane, even in the critical area of the hepatic vein–vena cava junction. Prior division of the right hepatic vein allows the instrument to be placed medial to the entire anatomic right lobe of the liver.

SUMMARY

A new instrument for direct compression of the hepatic parenchyma has been described. It was found to be effective in controlling arterial and venous hemorrhage from the divided liver surface. It also eliminated threat of air embolism and provided mechanical advantage for improved exposure during resection of the liver.

Illustrations by Mrs. Leesy McDonnell, Armed Forces Institute of Pathology, are greatly appreciated.

REFERENCES

1. Adson, M. A.: Major hepatic resections: Elective operations, Mayo Clin. Proc. **42:** 791, 1967.
2. Baker, R. J., Taxman, P., and Freeark, R. J.: An assessment of the management of nonpenetrating liver injuries, Arch. Surg. **93:** 84, 1966.
3. Foster, J. H., Lawler, M. R., Welborn, M. B., Holcomb, G. W., and Sawyers, J. L.: Recent experience with major hepatic resection, Ann. Surg. **167:** 651, 1968.
4. Heaney, J. P., Stanton, W. K., Halbert, D. S., Seidel, J., and Vice, T.: An improved technique for vascular isolation of the liver: Experimental study and case reports, Ann. Surg. **163:** 237, 1966.
5. Madding, G. F., and Kennedy, P. A.: Trauma to the liver. Major problems in clinical surgery, vol. III, Philadelphia, 1965, W. B. Saunders Co.
6. Schrock, T., Blaisdell, F. W., and Mathewson, C.: Management of blunt trauma to the liver and hepatic veins, Arch. Surg. **96:** 698, 1968.
7. Timmis, H. H., Rosanova, A. R., and Larkin, W. B.: Bloodless hepatic resection with an internal caval shunt, Surgery **65:** 109, 1969.

Editorial

Conducted by EDWIN H. ELLISON, M.D.

Experiments in delivery of surgical care

B. EISEMAN, M.D.
M. POMERANTZ, M.D.
F. MERKEL, M.D.
D. COWEN, M.D.
DENVER, COLO.
From the Denver General Hospital and the University of Colorado Medical School

Surgeons characteristically are more interested in a single patient than they are in means of delivering surgical care "en masse." Ready to devote untold hours to a patient needing surgical care, we, as a specialty, have not been notable pioneers in social medicine! Times are changing and, as socially sensitive physicians and citizens, surgeons are being challenged to devise new, more efficient, and more economic means of delivering surgical care to all economic levels of society.

Recognizing the need for better delivery of medical care to the underprivileged, the Denver Department of Health and Hospitals in 1966 pioneered a system for furnishing first-class comprehensive health care at a reasonable cost to the economically underprivileged.

In brief, the system at its grass-roots level has established nine Neighborhood Health Stations, located throughout the low-income areas of the city. These facilities have a staff of about 20 and are manned by two to five physicians who are generalists and pediatricians.

Patients requiring surgical consultation are referred from these health stations to one of two Neighborhood Health Centers. One is located in the heart of the Negro community; the other is in a Spanish-American area. Each building is a low-cost, cinder-block structure of approximately 20,000 square feet. Although not spacious, they are air-conditioned, carpeted, and each contains well-equipped areas for emergency care, for outpatient work-up, and for minor surgery. Equipment backup is adequate for laboratory work-up, bacteriologic and diagnostic radiographic studies, and all but the most sophisticated laboratory procedures.

Employees from the surrounding neighborhood are used extensively as paramedical personnel in the health stations and centers; this is economical and permits easy identification of the patient with the physician and his assistant, as well. The physician staff numbers 65, along with 17 dentists. The number of nonphysician personnel is greater than one is accustomed to in an ordinary outpatient hospital setting—it includes 45 registered nurses, 64 public health nurses, 62 visiting nurses, 25 licensed practical nurses, and 258 paramedical personnel of all degrees of training.

All surgical consultations are performed in the Neighborhood Health Centers, four afternoons per week by members of the full-time medical school surgical faculty based at the Denver General Hospital.

Patients requiring hospitalization are referred directly from the Neighborhood Health Center through a surgery secretary at the Denver General Hospital who simultaneously can record anticipated hospital admission,

Received for publication Dec. 5, 1969.

preoperative laboratory studies, and schedule the patient for the operating room. Many days of hospitalization are thus saved.

The program is financed by a grant of 5 million dollars per year from the Office of Economic Opportunity, as well as additional support from numerous other local, state, and federal sources, amounting to 1.9 million dollars per year. Annual operating costs are 7 million dollars. The over-all cost per patient visit is difficult to compare to other systems, but apparently is competitive with a classic hospital outpatient department.

As surgeons we were, at first, much less enthusiastic than our internist and pediatric colleagues to embrace this new facility. Gradually, however, we have recognized this as a logical, simple, and efficient extension of our hospital outpatient department facilities. The prime difference is that we, as surgeons, travel a few minutes across town to the Neighborhood Health Centers, rather than have the patients come to our own hospital. Generalists, internists, and pediatricians screen patients for referral to our surgery and surgical specialty clinics, with traditional appointment scheduling. Housed all in one building, the atmosphere is similar to a private clinic with consultations immediately available and easy communication between the specialist and his referring physician.

As with any outpatient department, the index of physician frustration is obviously higher than in caring for a population captive within hospital beds where our orders are law. The key fact is, however, that this is an economically efficient means for providing better surgical service to an underprivileged segment of our community. It also has been of enormous benefit as a source of patient referral for the university teaching program. These twin benefits should serve as a stimulus to the interest of the academic surgical community, both as it benefits surgical teaching and as it puts surgeons where we belong as socially sensitive citizens—where the action is.

Delivery of health care is not the prime role of a medical school; it is education and research. Discovering new and more efficient ways to deliver surgical care is, however, a valid objective for academic departments of surgery. When such systems improve surgical teaching, there is added reason for continued experimentation.

Volume 67 Number 5 SURGERY

MAY, 1970

Clinical surgery

Perforated duodenal ulcer: Long-term follow-up

GEORGE J. NEMANICH, M.D.
DEMETRE M. NICOLOFF, M.D., PH.D.
MINNEAPOLIS, MINN.
From the Departments of Surgery, University of Minnesota Health Sciences Center and Veterans Administration Hospital

Over the past 15 to 20 years, considerable controversy has arisen concerning the optimal treatment of perforated duodenal ulcer. Until recently, most attention has been focused on hospital deaths; little attention has been paid to the relatively high incidence of morbidity in the form of recurrent symptoms, complications of therapy, and subsequent operations necessary to control additional complications of the ulcer diathesis.

There are essentially three methods of treatment for acute perforation: Simple closure, introduced by Mickulicz[13] in 1880, has been widely used. Conservative or nonoperative management was first used by Redwood[17] in 1870. Wangensteen,[25] Taylor,[21] and others later proposed continuous nasogastric suction and use of antibiotics for the treatment of perforated duodenal ulcers.[8] A third method, definitive gastric surgery, employing either subtotal gastrectomy or vagotomy and pyloroplasty, has been used to manage the perforation while at the same time treating the peptic ulcer diathesis responsible for the perforation. In general, American surgeons have been reluctant to utilize primary gastrectomy for treatment of acute duodenal perforation. However, in the past 10 to 15 years, numerous reports of fairly large series of carefully selected patients treated by primary gastrectomy or vagotomy and pyloroplasty with mortality rates as low as that for elective gastric surgery have appeared in the literature.[2, 7, 10, 23]

Most of the clinical studies on perforated peptic ulcer include both gastric and duodenal perforations in their statistics. Because gastric and duodenal ulcers are two distinct entities in regard to their pathogenesis and clinical features, gastric ulcer perforation has been eliminated from our study in an attempt to arrive at a better concept of the various factors influencing the mortality and morbidity rates of perforated duodenal ulcer.

CLINICAL DATA

An effort has been made to evaluate, on a retrospective basis, methods of treatment used on patients with a perforated duodenal

Submitted for publication Jan. 24, 1969; resubmitted Dec. 5, 1969.

ulcer at the Minneapolis Veterans Administration Hospital during the ten-year period of 1953 through 1962.

This series concerns a total of 104 patients. Three additional patients who had no treatment were found to have a perforated duodenal ulcer at autopsy. Two of the three patients had far-advanced metastatic cancer; the remaining patient died of a massive cerebral embolus from a mural thrombus.

Eleven patients were treated nonsurgically with nasogastric suction, intravenous fluids, and antibiotics. Seven patients in this group died during the period of treatment. Of the remaining four patients, two have been followed for seven and eight years, and have required no surgical treatment for their peptic ulcer disease. Nearly all of the seven patients who were treated conservatively and died were felt to be too debilitated for surgical therapy.

The remaining 90 patients in this series were divided into several subgroups depending on the initial treatment for their perforated ulcer (Table I).

Eighty-five patients were treated surgically initially. Seventy-nine of these patients were treated with simple closure. Five patients had primary subtotal gastrectomy and one patient underwent vagotomy and pyloroplasty.

Five patients initially had conservative management for periods of from five days to five weeks followed by surgical treatment. One patient was treated by simple closure and four patients had subtotal gastrectomies. Two of these patients died in the postoperative period of peritonitis from the perforation. Three patients had subtotal gastrectomies and are doing well with no recurrent symptoms, five, nine, and ten years after perforation.

Twenty-one of the 104 patients died—an over-all hospital mortality rate of 20 per cent. Of the 79 patients who underwent

Table I. *Perforated duodenal ulcers treated at the Minneapolis Veterans Administration Hospital Jan. 1, 1953, through Dec. 31, 1962*

	No. of patients
Found at autopsy	3
Treated conservatively	11
Surgically treated patients:	
Simple closure	79
Subtotal gastrectomy	5
Closure with vagotomy and pyloroplasty	1
Total	85
Initial conservative management and subsequent surgery:	
Simple closure	1
Subtotal gastrectomy	4
Total	5
Grand total	104

Table II. *Postoperative complications in 79 patients treated with simple closure for perforated duodenal ulcer*

Complication	*No.**
Right upper quadrant abscess	3
Subphrenic abscess	3
Closure leak with abscess formation	2
Bilateral subphrenic abscess	1
Pelvic abscess	1
Duodenocutaneous fistula	1
Evisceration	1
Bronchopneumonia	1
Total	13

*Complication rate, 16.3 per cent.

Table III. *Postoperative complications in nine patients who died in the postoperative period, showing the interval between perforation and treatment*

Patient	*Time interval*	*Local problem**
F. N.	18 hr.	None
L. R.	24 hr.	Subphrenic abscess
E. W.	9 hr.	Bronchopneumonia
W. L.	17 days	Bilateral subphrenic abscesses
G. B.	16 hr.	Closure leak and abscess
R. T.	60 hr.	Right upper quadrant abscess
E. F.	8 hr.	Closure leak and peritonitis
T. C.	2-3 hr.	None
L. B.	10 hr.	Duodenocutaneous fistula

*Seven of the nine patients who died in the postoperative period had contributory local problems.

simple closure of the perforation, nine died—a hospital mortality rate of 11.4 percent, very similar to that of other reported series.[1, 3, 8, 18, 19]

COMPLICATIONS

There were no postoperative complications or deaths in the six patients treated initially with definitive surgery—subtotal gastrectomy in five and vagotomy and pyloroplasty in one. A total of 13 postoperative complications occurred in the simple closure group of 79 patients with a 16.3 percent complication rate in patients undergoing simple closure (Table II). More than half (7 of 13) of the postoperative complications occurred in the nine patients who died postoperatively. Two of the nine postoperative deaths were directly due to a condition unrelated to the patient's perforated peptic ulcer (Table III): one died of congestive heart failure and the other of cerebrovascular accident. Of the remaining seven patients, six died of peritonitis secondary to their perforation. The remaining patient died of aspiration pneumonia in the immediate postoperative period.

FACTORS INFLUENCING MORTALITY AND MORBIDITY

Several factors are thought to influence the number of deaths due to perforated duodenal ulcer, such as age, duration of interval between perforation and treatment, location of perforation, and presence of severe concurrent disease. In this series, the age range varied from 25 to 85 years, and the average age was 53 years. The over-all and postoperative mortality rates for perforated duodenal ulcer increased with age (Fig. 1). In patients more than 60 years of age, the number of deaths due to perforated duodenal ulcer was discouragingly high (31.7 percent).

In our group of duodenal perforations, the mortality rate increased progressively with the length of the interval between perforation and treatment up to an 18 to 24 hour interval (Fig. 2). Four of the nine patients who died in the postoperative period had an interval between perforation and treatment of less than 12 hours, but two of these deaths were due to medical causes not related to the perforation. If these two patients are eliminated, the mortality rate for perforated

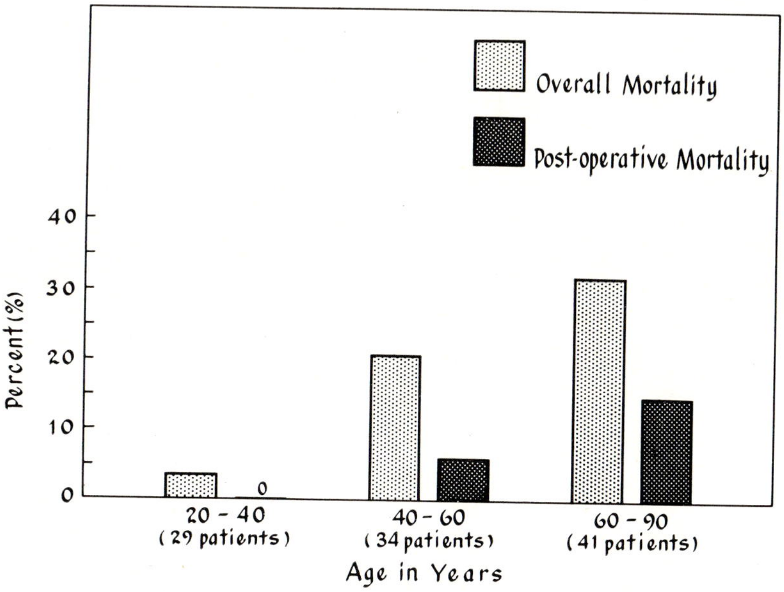

Fig. 1. The over-all and postoperative mortality rates of patients with perforated duodenal ulcer increase with age.

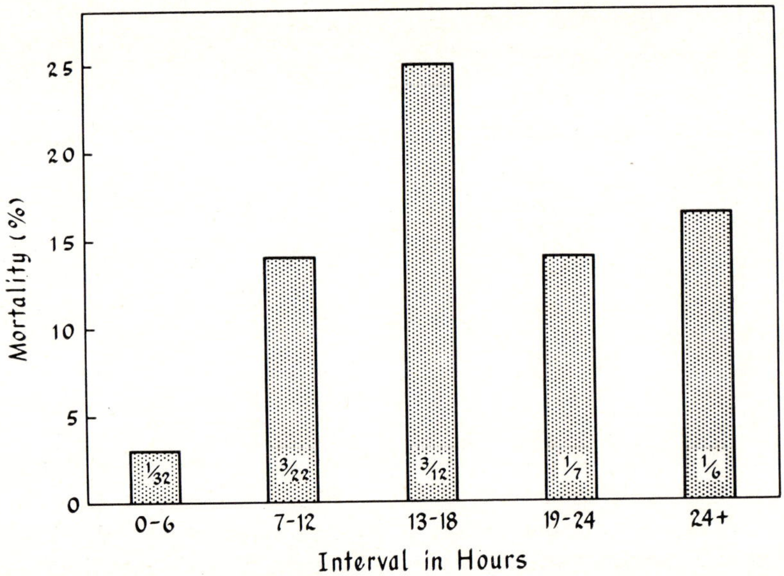

Fig. 2. There is a dramatic increase in mortality rates when the interval of perforation exceeds six hours. There was no increase with an interval of perforation greater than 18 hours.

Table IV. *Types of severe concurrent medical diseases*

	No. of patients
Pulmonary emphysema	8
Tumor with metastasis	7
Severe arteriosclerotic heart disease	6
Congestive heart failure	6
Diabetes mellitus	4
Severe hypertension	3
Laennec's cirrhosis	2
Collagen diseases treated with steroids	
Polymositis	1
Rheumatoid arthritis	1
Tuberculosis	2
Pancreatitis	2
Polycythemia vera	1
Cerebral emboli	1
Buerger's disease	1
Enterocutaneous fistula secondary to gunshot wound	1

Table V. *Relationship of deaths to site of perforations*

	No. of perforations	*No. dead*	*Percent dead*
Anterior duodenum	87	14	16
Posterior duodenum	9	6	67
Pylorus	3	0	0

duodenal ulcers treated within 12 hours after perforation is 3.7 percent versus a mortality rate of 20 percent for those with an interval of more than 12 hours between perforation and treatment.

Another factor of considerable importance regarding the mortality rate is the presence or absence of serious concurrent disease (Table IV). The most common concurrent diseases found in this study were pulmonary emphysema, tumor with metastases, severe arteriosclerotic heart disease, congestive heart failure, and diabetes. Of the entire group of 104 patients, 35 percent had severe concurrent disease. One half of these patients died following the perforation. The large series of perforated ulcers reported by Rogers[18] had a postoperative mortality rate similar to that observed in our study. However, only 14 percent of Rogers' patients had concurrent disease and he noted a 35 percent mortality rate in patients with perforated ulcer who had concurrent disease. The relatively high rate of concurrent disease in our series suggests that our patients

Table VI. *Perforated peptic ulcer: Late results of simple closure*

Author	Follow-up (yr.)	No. of cases	Symptomatic (%)	Subsequent operation (%)
Tovee[22]	5–20	78	69.0	35.0
Troell[23]	4–13	69	70.0	50.0
Stabins[20]	2–26	169	65.1	36.5
Noordijk[14]	3–19	826	61.0	35.4
Glenn and Harrison[5]	1–19	115	69.5	40.9
Illingworth, Scott, and Jamison[9]	5	773	70.0	—
Turner[24]	20	143	75.5	38.5
Carneveli and ReMine[2]	1–17	91	65.9	46.1
Minneapolis Veterans Administration Hospital	1.5–14.5	60	61.6	43.0

may have been more debilitated than the average patient population in other reports.

The location of the perforation as well as its size are important factors. In this series, the site of perforation was known in 99 of 104 cases (Table V). The anterior duodenum was the most common location of the perforation (88 percent). The mortality rate for posterior duodenal perforation was much higher than that for anterior duodenal perforation.

The incidence of bleeding with perforation in various series ranges from 12 to 20 percent. In this series, 16 patients with perforations out of 104, or 15.4 percent, had associated gastrointestinal bleeding and, of this group, 56 percent died of ulcer perforation. These figures compare well with the report by Rogers,[18] who noted gastrointestinal bleeding in 14 percent of the perforations. The mortality rate in that group in whom associated bleeding attended perforation was 60 percent.

In the present series, in 67 of the 98 patients, or 68 percent, free air was demonstrated under the diaphragm on scout and upright abdominal films. This incidence of free air with perforation is similar to other series of perforated ulcers.[18] We observed no significant difference in incidence of free air in patients in whom perforation occurred 6, 12, 18, and 24 or more hours prior to abdominal x-rays. In a few cases, a Gastrografin gastrointestinal study demonstrated a perforation when no free air was noted.

Most recent reports on the late results of simple closure show a very high rate of recurrent ulcer symptoms and a high incidence of subsequent operations (Table VI). Of the 79 patients with perforated duodenal ulcer treated by simple closure, 70 left the hospital and 88 percent of these were followed for periods of 1.5 to 14.5 years. Thirty-seven of the 60 patients followed had significant peptic ulcer symptoms following simple closure—an incidence of 61.6 percent. Twenty-six of the 60 patients, or 43 percent, had subsequent operations either for intractable pain, as in 21 of them, and/or because of complications of their ulcer diathesis such as obstruction, bleeding, or reperforation. In 11 of the 26 patients who underwent subsequent operations, intractable pain was the essential or primary indication for operation.

It is interesting to note that only two of the 26 patients who required subsequent operations had a prior ulcer history of less than six months' duration. Of the 60 patients with simple closure who were followed, 57 percent of those with a chronic ulcer history needed subsequent surgical treatment whereas only 11 percent of those with a preperforation ulcer history of less than six months needed it. This correlates well with Cassell's[3] large retrospective study of acute and chronic duodenal ulcers.

An interesting aspect in the follow-up of these 60 patients with simple closure was an increased incidence of subsequent operations as length of follow-up increased (Fig. 3).

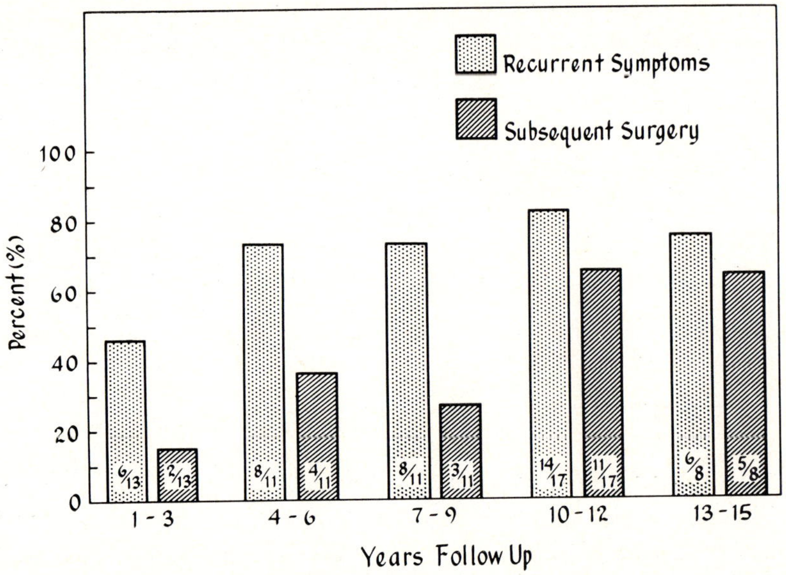

Fig. 3. Follow-up, 1.5 to 14.5 years, of 60 patients with simple closure. Subsequent surgery increased to a level of 66 percent at ten or more years. Symptoms recurred in 46 percent in the first three years and in 75 percent after four years.

The incidence of subsequent operations increased progressively to a level of 65 percent at ten or more years after perforation. The incidence of recurrent symptoms following simple closure of a perforation was 46 percent in the first three years after perforation and then rose to a level of approximately 75 percent for the remainder of the 15 year follow-up period.

Four patients treated initially with simple closure of a perforation during the ten-year period of study had subsequent reperforation. This represents an incidence of 6 percent for reperforation in our series of simple closure of duodenal perforations.

DEFINITIVE SURGERY

In our series of 104 patients with duodenal perforations, only six were treated initially with definitive surgery. Five of the six patients had a subtotal gastrectomy and the sixth had a vagotomy and pyloroplasty. The interval between perforation and treatment was 12 hours or less in all six. Only one patient, who had a subtotal gastrectomy, did not have a chronic ulcer history. None of these patients had concurrent disease. The average age was 59 years, which was slightly higher than the average age of the simple closure group—52.4 years. Follow-up data, ranging from five to ten years, was available for all six patients. There were no postoperative complications and no postoperative deaths. Only one patient, who had subtotal gastrectomy, has mild ulcer symptoms which are relieved by antacids.

Though this is admittedly a very small and select group, the results compare quite well with those in previous reports. Carneveli and ReMine[2] in 1962 gathered from the literature 888 cases of perforated peptic ulcer treated by primary subtotal gastrectomy and noted a combined mortality rate of only 2.4 percent, which is comparable with mortality rates of elective gastrectomy. Pierandozzi and associates[15] reported on 75 patients in whom vagotomy and pyloroplasty were performed as the initial treatment for the perforation; the postoperative mortality rate was 1.3 percent.

RETROSPECTIVE ANALYSIS

When we eliminate from the simple closure group those patients who have an interval

Table VII. *Fifty-five patients treated with simple closure, with interval between perforation and treatment of 24 hours or less (no concurrent disease)*

	No.
Complications:	
Intra-abdominal abscess	3
Closure leak	1
Duodenocutaneous fistula	1
Bronchopneumonia	1
	6
Complication rate	9.1%
Postoperative mortality rate	3 (5.4%)

Table VIII. *Fifty-five patients treated with simple closure, with interval between perforation and treatment of 24 hours or less (no concurrent disease)*

	No.	Percent
Recurrent symptoms	31	56.4
Indications for subsequent surgery:		
Reperforation	4	
Rebleeding	4	
Obstruction	4	
Pain	18	
Subsequent surgery:		
Subtotal gastrectomy	12	
Segmental resection	6	
Closure and segmental	1	
Gastroenterostomy and vagotomy	1	
	20	36.3

between perforation and treatment of more than 24 hours and those who have severe concurrent disease, we are left with 55 patients whose average age is 48 years. This group of patients would satisfy the criteria required by most surgeons who advocate definitive surgical therapy in the manner of vagotomy and pyloroplasty. Results in this group of 55 patients treated with simple closure revealed that complications occurred in 9.1 percent and the mortality rate for this group was 5.4 percent (Table VII). In addition, follow-up revealed that recurrent symptoms developed in 56.4 percent and subsequent operations were necessary in 36.3 percent (Table VIII).

CONCLUSION

Although a prospective randomized study is necessary, it would appear from our retrospective analysis that a patient with a chronic ulcer history who has an interval of less than 12 hours between perforation and treatment, has no concurrent disease, and is less than 60 years of age should tolerate a definitive procedure such as vagotomy and pyloroplasty for treatment of the perforation and the peptic ulcer diathesis with minimal risk of morbidity and death. There were many patients in our study who fell into this category who were treated by simple closure and, as a consequence, were exposed to a high risk of complications and required subsequent operations to control their peptic ulcer diathesis. Conversely, it would be equally wrong to treat all patients with perforated duodenal ulcers with gastric resection or vagotomy and pyloroplasty because a number of these patients would have had no further ulcer symptoms after simple closure. Hopefully, with careful selection of patients and an increased use of definitive surgery, especially vagotomy and pyloroplasty, the immediate and long-term mortality and morbidity rates of perforated duodenal ulcer can be further decreased.

SUMMARY

A retrospective study was made of 104 patients who had a perforated duodenal ulcer treated at the Minneapolis Veterans Administration Hospital. Eighty-five patients were treated surgically initially. Seventy-nine patients had simple closure of the duodenal perforation. A recurrence rate of peptic ulcer symptoms was noted in 61.6 percent and subsequent operations were required in 43 percent of the 60 patients followed. The rate of recurrent symptoms and subsequent operations was directly proportional to the length of follow-up. A high postoperative mortality rate occurred in the group treated with simple closure and reasons for this were reviewed. Six patients had definitive surgery initially for their duodenal perforation and the results in this group were excellent.

Simple closure in a group of patients selected retrospectively to include only those less than 60 years of age, whose perforation was of less than 12 hours' duration and who did not have severe concurrent disease, still resulted in a high rate of recurrent symptoms, complications, subsequent operations, and postoperative deaths. It would appear from the findings in this study that there is sufficient reason to utilize a definitive procedure such as a vagotomy and pyloroplasty in selected cases of perforated duodenal ulcer. Final proof, however, will depend on a randomized prospective study.

REFERENCES

1. Burdette, W., and Rasmussen, B.: Perforated peptic ulcer, SURGERY **63:** 576, 1968.
2. Carneveli, J. F., and ReMine, W. H.: Radical versus conservative surgical management of acute perforated peptic ulcer, Postgrad. Med. **32:** 119, 1962.
3. Cassell, P.: The prognosis of the perforated acute duodenal ulcer, Gut **10:** 572, 1969.
4. De Bakey, M. E.: Acute perforated gastroduodenal ulceration: Statistical analysis and review of the literature, SURGERY **8:** 852, 1940.
5. Glenn, F., and Harrison, C. S.: Acute free perforation of pepetic ulcer: Complications of ulcer diathesis: 139 consecutive cases, Arch. Surg. **65:** 795, 1952.
6. Graham, R. R.: The treatment of perforated duodenal ulcers, Surg. Gynec. Obstet. **64:** 235, 1937.
7. Hodfield, J. I. H., and Watkins, D. F. L.: Vagotomy in the treatment of perforated duodenal ulcer, Brit. Med. J. **5400:** 12, 1964.
8. Hastins, N., and Mochida, R.: Simple closure of perforated peptic ulcer, Am. J. Surg. **102:** 136, 1961.
9. Illingworth, C. F. W., Scott, L. D. W., and Jamison, R. A.: Progress after perforated peptic ulcer, Brit. Med. J. **1:** 787, 1946.
10. Jordon, G. L., De Bakey, M. E., and Cooley, D. A.: The role of resective therapy in the management of acute gastroduodenal perforation, Am. J. Surg. **105:** 396, 1963.
11. Kincannon, W. M., McLenathen, C. W., and Weinberg, J. W.: Vagotomy and pyloroplasty for acute perforated duodenal ulcer, Amer. Surg. **29:** 692, 1963.
12. Kozall, D. D., and Meyer, K. A.: Effect of surgery on morbidity and mortality in acute gastroduodenal perforations, Am. J. Surg. **103:** 577, 1962.
13. Mikulicz, J.: Sur operativen Behandlung des stenosirenden Magengeschwurs, Verh. Deutsch. Ges. Chir. **16:** 337, 1887.
14. Noordijk, J. A.: Perforated peptic ulcer: The results of treatment in the Netherlands (1934–1950). An analysis of 2,551 cases, Arch. Chir. Neerl. **5:** 262, 1953.
15. Pierandozzi, J. S., Hinshaw, D. B., and Stanford, C. E.: Vagotomy and pyloroplasty for acute perforated duodenal ulcer: A report of 75 cases, Am. J. Surg. **100:** 245, 1960.
16. Postlethwait, R. W., and others: Results of surgery for peptic ulcer: A cooperative study of 12 V.A. hospitals, Philadelphia, 1963, W. B. Saunders Company.
17. Redwood, T. H.: Two cases of perforation of the stomach. One recovery, Lancet **1:** 647, 1870.
18. Rogers, F. A.: Factors affecting the mortality from acute gastroduodenal perforation, Surg. Gynec. Obstet. **111:** 771, 1960.
19. Shippey, S. H., and Amerson, J. R.: Acute gastroduodenal perforation—Report of 192 patients and review of recent literature, Am. Surg. **32:** 870, 1966.
20. Stabins, S. J.: The aftermath of perforated duodenal ulcer, SURGERY **34:** 614, 1953.
21. Taylor, H.: Perforated peptic ulcer treated without operation, Lancet **2:** 447, 1946.
22. Tovee, E. B.: Late results of surgery in perforated duodenal ulcer, Arch. Surg. **63:** 408, 1951.
23. Troell, L.: To what extent should gastric resection be resorted to in perforating ulcer? Acta Chir. Scand. **107:** 19, 1954.
24. Tumer, F. P.: Acute perforations of stomach, duodenum, and jejunum: Analysis of 224 cases with late follow-up data on 147 cases of acute perforated peptic ulcer, Surg. Gynec. Obstet. **92:** 281, 1951.
25. Wangensteen, O. H.: Nonoperative treatment of localized perforations of the duodenum, Minn. Med. **18:** 477, 1935.

Studies of the "gastroesophageal sphincter mechanism": The role of the phrenoesophageal membrane

CEDRIC G. BREMNER, M.CH., F.R.C.S.
JERRY F. SCHLEGEL, B.S.
F. HENRY ELLIS, JR., M.D., PH.D.
ROCHESTER, MINN.
From the Mayo Clinic and Mayo Foundation: Section of Physiology (Mr. Schlegel) and Section of Surgery (Dr. Ellis). Mayo Graduate School of Medicine (University of Minnesota), Rochester, Fellow in Surgical Research (Mr. Bremner)

Although the mechanism responsible for gastroesophageal competence remains controversial, most evidence suggests an important role for the inferior esophageal sphincter. Recent studies[1-5] suggest that the phrenoesophageal membrane may be an important component of this sphincter. The evidence depends largely on experimental studies which have relied on the development of esophagitis as the main criterion for measuring impaired sphincteric function. The purpose of our study is to assess the influence of the phrenoesophageal membrane (1) on the length and amplitude of sphincteric pressure, by means of esophageal manometry, and (2) on sphincteric competence, by cinefluoroscopy and not on the development of reflux esophagitis.

MATERIAL AND METHODS

Nineteen adult mongrel male dogs weighing 9 to 11 kilograms were used. Preoperative esophageal manometric studies were made on each animal and were repeated two and four weeks after operation; each dog was also examined cinefluoroscopically between three and six weeks after operation. At the end of the study the animals were killed and autopsies were performed. Sodium pentobarbital anesthesia (15 mg. per kilogram of body weight), endotracheal intubation, and controlled respiration were used for all operations, which were performed via a left thoracotomy through the seventh or eighth interspace. There were three experimental preparations (Fig. 1).

Group I. Circumferential division of the phrenoesophageal membrane. Several experimental models were prepared while developing a satisfactory permanent separation of the phrenoesophageal membrane from the esophagus. Circumferential division alone resulted in spontaneous reattachment. When a collar of Teflon fabric was used to prevent reattachment in other animals, excessive fibrous tissue response resulted in prompt reattachment of the membrane to the esophagus. Finally, a series of five animals was prepared in which the esophagogastric junction was loosely encircled with Silastic sheeting (Dow-Corning No. 0108, 0.005 mm. thick) after circumferential division of the phrenoesophageal membrane (Fig. 1, *I*). This technique insured permanent separation of the esophagus from the phrenoesophageal membrane. A gastropexy via a radial diaphragmatic incision prevented the postoperative development of a hiatal hernia.

Group II: Division of the phrenoesophageal membrane and subsequent reattachment. The phrenoesophageal membrane

This investigation was supported in part by Research Grants AM-5457 and AM-2015 from the National Institutes of Health, United States Public Health Service.
Submitted for publication May 11, 1969; resubmitted Nov. 5, 1969.

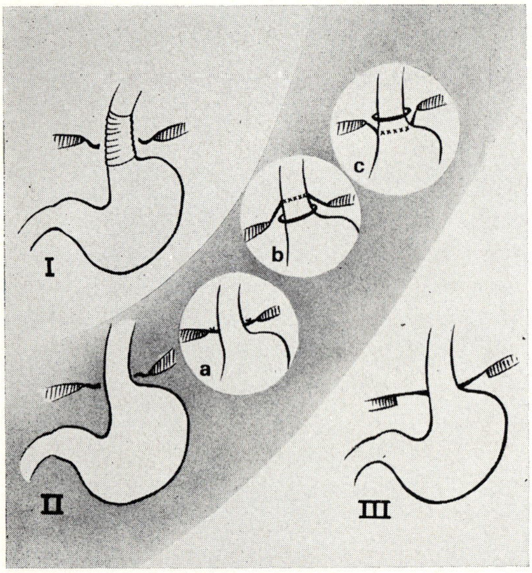

Fig. 1. Experimental procedures. *I,* Division of phrenoesophageal membrane. *II,* Division and reattachment of phrenoesophageal membrane *(a)* at original site, *(b)* proximally, and *(c)* distally. *III,* Excision of hiatal muscle. Dark circle around esophagus in *II, b* and *c,* indicates original site of membrane attachment to esophagus.

was divided circumferentially in nine dogs and immediately reattached with silk sutures at different levels (Fig. 1, *II*): (*a*) in three dogs the membrane was sutured to the original site of attachment, *(b)* in three dogs it was sutured to the esophageal wall 3 cm. proximal to the original site of attachment, and *(c)* in three dogs it was sutured 1 cm. distal to the original site of attachment.

Group III: Excision of hiatal muscle. Five dogs underwent complete excision of a strip of diaphragmatic crural muscle 1.5 cm. wide which encircled the distal esophagus (Fig. 1, *III*).

Manometric tests. Pre- and postoperative resting and swallowing studies were performed without anesthesia and with the animals lying on their backs, using methods similar to those described by Schlegel and Code.[12] Three polyethylene tubes were tied together; a spherical water-filled balloon, 5 mm. in diameter, was tied to the end of one tube and served as the most distal pressure probe, while lateral openings were made at 5 and 10 cm. proximal to the balloon in the second and third tubes, respectively. All tubes were filled with water and were connected to water-filled strain gauges. A pneumograph belt was tied about the dog's thorax, and a pneumograph was fixed around the neck at the level of the thyroid cartilage to detect swallowing. Recordings were made photokymographically via galvanometers.

The pressure-detecting units were withdrawn from the stomach at 0.5 cm. distances, and pressures were recorded at each level during three respiratory cycles. Deglutitory responses were obtained at 1 cm. distances. Swallowing was induced by injecting 1 to 2 ml. of water via a separate tube placed in the pharynx. The recordings were assessed according to the method described by Fyke and associates.[6] Both end-inspiratory and end-expiratory pressures were measured and used for calculation of mean values. For ease of graphic representation, a mean of the open-tip end-inspiratory and end-expiratory values was used.

RESULTS

Group I: Division of phrenoesophageal membrane. The postoperative course was normal in the five dogs which had simple division of the phrenoesophageal membrane and Silastic wrapping of the esophagus. The resting pressures, as determined by the balloon tip detector, were significantly increased after division of the membranes (Table I), but by open-tip detection, neither the pressures nor the length of the sphincter were significantly altered (Fig. 2). Peristalsis and sphincteric relaxation were normal although repetitive responses to swallowing did occur in two dogs. There was no radiographic evidence of reflux.

Group II. Division and reattachment of phrenoesophageal membrane.

Resuture at the same site. In all three animals in which the membrane was resutured at its original site on the esophagus, the postoperative course was normal. Deglutitory responses were not altered. Sphinc-

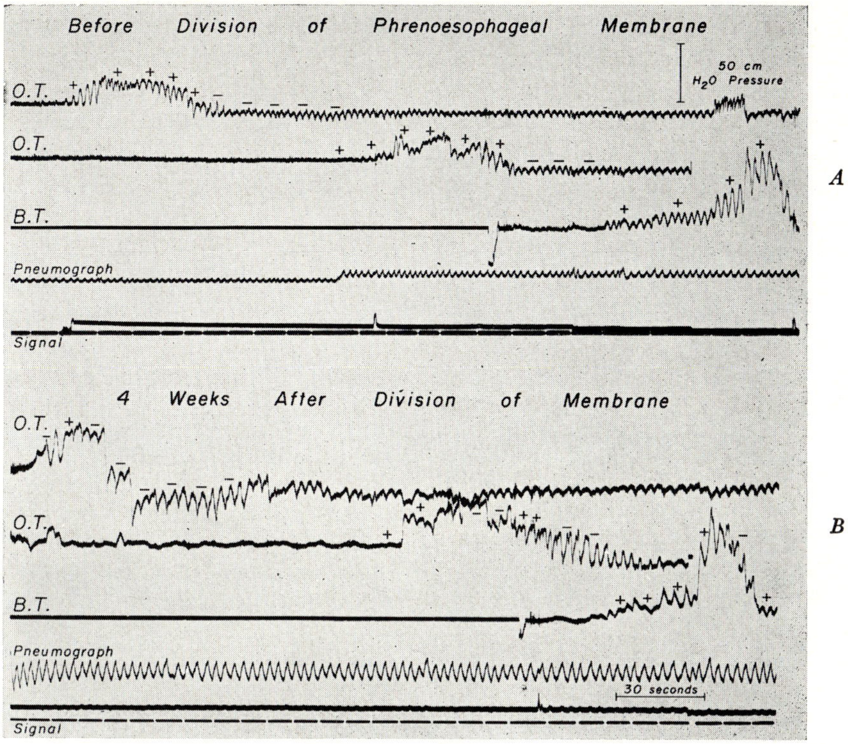

Fig. 2. Resting gastroesophageal pressures in dog before *(A)* and after *(B)* division of phrenoesophageal membrane (Group I). There is no significant change in sphincteric pressure. *OT* = Open-tip catheter; *BT* = balloon-covered catheter.

Table I. *Mean maximal gastroesophageal pressures*

		Before operation				*4 Weeks after operation*			
		Balloon		*Open-tip*		*Balloon*		*Open-tip*	
Operation	*No. of dogs*	*EE**	*EI**	*EE*	*EI*	*EE*	*EI*	*EE*	*EI*
Group I. Detachment and Silastic interposition	5	29.2† ± 7.7‡	34.1 ±12.0	20.0 ±5.0	13.6 ±2.4	61.0 ± 8.4	67.0 ± 9.2	14.9 ±3.3	19.2 ±3.5
Group II. Detachment and reattachment:									
(a) Same site	3	21.5 ±11.1	30.1 ± 8.1	12.7 ±3.8	12.7 ±4.1	21.7 ± 8.8	26.6 ± 8.8	16.7 ±5.6	11.8 ±2.0
(b) 3 cm. higher	3	39.2 ± 8.7	55.1 ±13.9	14.9 ±4.4	13.4 ±4.9	104.5 ±24.4	52.9 ±20.0	15.2 ±3.7	8.7 ±2.7
(c) 1 cm. lower	3	73.9 ±16.0	39.3 ±22.7	16.8 ±2.8	21.7 ±8.2	96.0 ±19.2	62.8 ±16.7	22.2 ±6.5	19.9 ±2.9
Group III. Excision of hiatal muscle	5	40.7 ± 6.0	56.6 ± 9.7	15.5 ±2.6	11.57 ±2.6	52.2 ± 5.7	45.3 ±13.0	15.6 ±2.9	9.3 ±1.7

*EE, end-expiratory; EI, end-inspiratory.

†Pressures in cm. H_2O.

‡Standard error.

teric pressures were unchanged (Table I) as was the length of the zone of elevated pressure. Cineradiographic studies were normal.

Reattachment of membrane 3 cm. proximally. When the divided membrane was sutured to the esophagus 3 cm. proximally, the postoperative course of the three animals so treated was normal. Resting-pressure studies showed a change in the elevated-pressure zone in relation to the respiratory reversal level (diaphragm); the zone was at a more distal level than before operation, due to the proximal attachment of the membrane. The end-expiratory balloon pressures were greater, but the open-tip values were not significantly altered (Table I). The length of the zone was decreased 0.5 cm. by this operation. Deglutition studies were normal. Gastroesophageal reflux was detected radiographically in two animals. There was no gross or histologic evidence of esophagitis.

Reattachment of phrenoesophageal membrane 1 cm. distally. Regurgitation of food was a constant feature in one dog following suture of the divided membrane at a more distal point on the esophagus. There was evidence of vagus nerve damage in this dog as demonstrated by simultaneous esophageal contractions and failure of the inferior esophageal sphincter to relax normally after swallowing. The length and height of the resting pressure profile were not altered in any of the dogs after four weeks, although the zone of elevated pressure was located more proximally after operation in relation to the point of respiratory reversal, as would be expected after the downward displacement of the membrane. Cinefluoroscopy studies revealed tertiary contractions and delayed sphincteric relaxation in a second animal.

Group III. Excision of the hiatal muscle. One animal which underwent excision of a ring of crural muscle from around the distal esophagus regurgitated food after meals, but

A

B

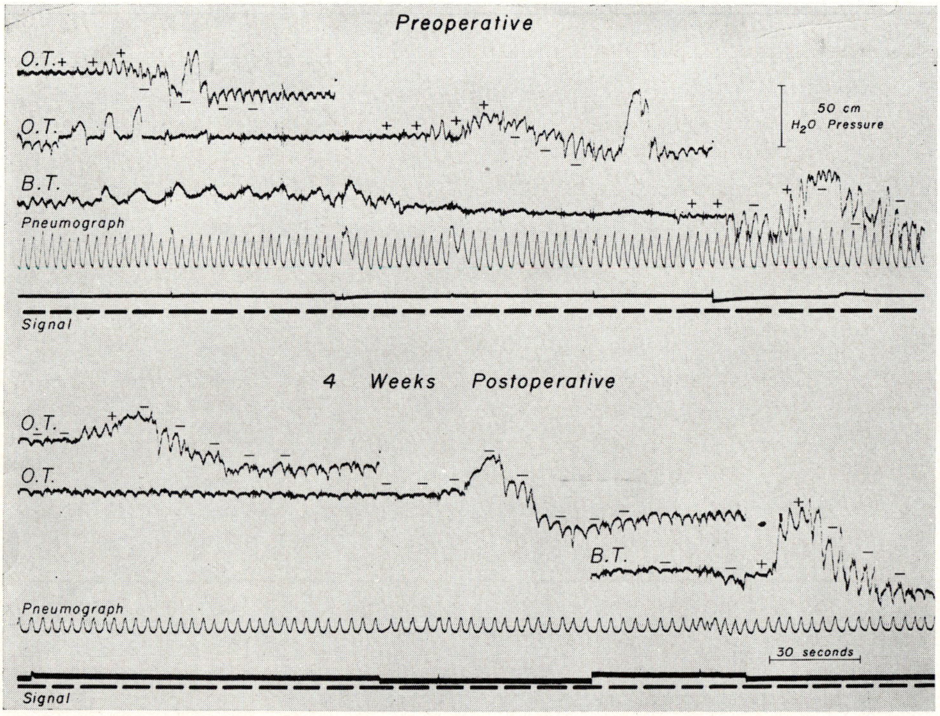

Fig. 3. Resting gastroesophageal pressures in a dog before *(A)* and after *(B)* excision of a ring of hiatal muscle encircling the lower esophagus. Peak sphincteric pressures are not altered.

improved after two weeks. The pressure profile after four weeks showed shortening of the zone of elevated pressures on both balloon and open-tip studies by 0.5 to 1.0 cm. The peak pressure values were unaltered, though located at a slightly higher than normal level in relation to the point of respiratory reversal (Table I and Fig. 3). Although the exact site of respiratory reversal was difficult to locate, there was no manometric or cinefluorographic evidence of a hiatal hernia. Deglutitory studies were normal.

COMMENT

The results suggest that the amplitude of the zone of elevated pressure at the gastroesophageal junction in the dog is not dependent on the phrenoesophageal membrane and the site of its esophageal attachments. As in previous studies,[10, 13] the results suggest that the intrinsic musculature at the lower end of the canine esophagus is mainly responsible for maintaining sphincteric pressure. These findings are contrary to those of Michelson and Siegel,[11] who found lowered sphincteric pressures after experimental division of the phrenoesophageal membrane. Our results are also in conflict with those of Dillard and Anderson[5] and Anderson and associates,[1] who believe that sphincteric failure is the result of malposition of the phrenoesophageal membrane to a point lower on the esophagus than normal. They assessed sphincteric function from pathologic findings, and such interpretations are notoriously inaccurate. Even so, reflux esophagitis developed only occasionally after alterations of phrenoesophageal membrane attachment in their dogs, even when gastric secretion was stimulated with histamine.

Sphincteric pressure and sphincteric competence may not always be directly related. In this study, competence was evaluated by cinefluoroscopy, and reflux was observed in only two dogs that had resuture of the phrenoesophageal membrane to a more proximal point on the esophagus.

While the phrenoesophageal membrane and its esophageal attachments seemed to play no direct role in producing sphincteric pressure in the dog, the length of the zone of elevated pressure varied with changes in the anatomic relationships of sphincter to diaphragm. Thus, the zone was shorter when the diaphragm was reattached at a higher level on the esophagus and when a ring of hiatal musculature was excised, suggesting that the length of the elevated pressure zone may be related to normal diaphragmatic relations.

Mann and co-workers[9] described similar findings after reapproximation of the membrane to the esophagus 6 cm. proximally in dogs. The procedure also resulted in decreased sphincteric pressures. However, as they mention, there was some evidence of vagal nerve damage as shown by premature contractions and a reduced incidence of relaxation at the sphincter. Excision of the diaphragmatic crura has produced conflicting results. Esophagitis has been reported by some[1, 2, 7] while manometric assessment of lower esophageal pressures in monkeys showed no change after excision of the left crus of the diaphragm.[8] As already mentioned, the only result of this procedure in our experiments was slight shortening of the sphincter.

The clinical implications of these experiments are not entirely clear for it is difficult to relate findings in the dog directly to the human state because of known species differences. They do, however, cast doubt on the role of the phrenoesophageal membrane in the gastroesophageal sphincteric mechanism. The role of the phrenoesophageal membrane (of potential importance in hiatal hernia repairs) may well be more that of a supportive anatomic structure than a physiologic one.

SUMMARY

The role of the phrenoesophageal membrane in maintenance of inferior esophageal sphincteric pressure and competence was studied manometrically and cinefluorographically after a series of experimental procedures on dogs; these procedures included division of the membrane, its division and reattachment at different levels, and excision of a ring of diaphragmatic crural musclc.

Sphincteric pressures were not altered significantly by the experimental procedures. The sphincter was shortened when surgically separated from the diaphragm and when a ring of hiatal muscle was excised. Gastroesophageal reflux was detected radiographically in only 2 of the 19 animals.

The phrenoesophageal membrane does not play a significant role in the function of the inferior esophageal sphincter in the dog, although it does provide structural support for maintenance of its normal anatomic position.

REFERENCES

1. Anderson, H. N., May, K. J., Jr., Steinmetz, G. P., Ofstun, M., Harrison, H. G., Leyse, R. M., and Dillard, D. H.: The lower esophageal intrinsic sphincter and the mechanism of reflux: Experimental observations supporting a new concept, Ann. Surg. **166:** 102, 1967.
2. Bombeck, C. T., Aoki, T., and Nyhus, L. M.: Anatomic etiology and operative treatment of peptic esophagitis: An experimental study, Ann. Surg. **165:** 752, 1967.
3. Bombeck, C. T., Dillard, D. H., and Nyhus, L. M.: Muscular anatomy of the gastroesophageal junction and role of phrenoesophageal ligament: Autopsy study of sphincter mechanism, Ann. Surg. **164:** 643, 1966.
4. Dillard, D. H.: Esophageal sphincter and reflux, Surg. Clin. N. Amer. **44:** 1201, 1964.
5. Dillard, D. H., and Anderson, H. N.: A new concept of the mechanism of sphincteric failure in sliding esophageal hiatal hernia, Surg. Gynec. Obstet. **122:** 1030, 1966.
6. Fyke, F. E., Jr., Code, C. F., and Schlegel, J. F.: The gastroesophageal sphincter in healthy human beings, Gastroenterologia (Basel) **86:** 135, 1956.
7. Giuseffi, V. J., Grindlay, J. H., and Schmidt, H. W.: Canine esophagitis following experimentally produced esophageal hiatal hernia, Proc. Staff Meet. Mayo Clin. **29:** 399, 1954.
8. Karas, L. M., Stern, H., Bloom, D., Binder, H. J., Poindexter, R., Thayer, W., and Spiro, H. M.: The gastroesophageal junction in the monkey and its relation to reflux, J. Surg. Res. **6:** 469, 1966.
9. Mann, C. V., Ellis, F. H., Jr., Schlegel, J. F., and Code, C. F.: Abdominal displacement of the canine gastroesophageal sphincter, Surg. Gynec. Obstet. **118:** 1009, 1964.
10. Meiss, J. H., Grindlay, J. H., and Ellis, F. H., Jr.: The gastroesophageal sphincter mechanism. II. Further experimental studies in the dog, J. Thorac. Cardiovasc. Surg. **36:** 156, 1958.
11. Michelson, E., and Siegel, C. I.: The role of the phrenico-esophageal ligament in the lower esophageal sphincter, Surg. Gynec. Obstet. **118:** 1291, 1964.
12. Schlegel, J. F., and Code, C. F.: Pressure characteristics of the esophagus and its sphincters in dogs, Amer. J. Physiol. **193:** 9, 1958.
13. Vandertoll, D. J., Ellis, F. H., Jr., Schlegel, J. F., and Code, C. F.: An experimental study of the role of gastric and esophageal muscle in gastroesophageal competence, Surg. Gynec. Obstet. **122:** 579, 1966.

The value of pneumoperitoneum in the diagnosis of hernia in the inguinal region

ORED ARNER, M.D.
INGMAR FERNSTRÖM, M.D.
STOCKHOLM, SWEDEN
From the Department of Surgery and the Radiological Institution, Karolinska Sjukhuset

Injection of gas into the peritoneal cavity, pneumoperitoneum, is a well-known radiologic technique. It is used as a method of examination in cases of tumors and inflammatory processes within the abdominal cavity. If a radiograph of the true pelvis is taken after inducing pneumoperitoneum, the technique is called "pneumopelvography" (gynecography) and is employed quite often for investigating gynecologic cases.

In 1967 we performed pneumopelvography on a patient, aged 57 years, with a history of pain for 9 years in the right side of the lower abdomen and right groin. She had consulted several physicians who all failed to make the correct diagnosis. Nor did repeated physical examinations and radiography of various organs, including the colon and urinary tract, give any information of diagnostic value.

As adhesions in the true pelvis were suspected, pneumoperitoneum was induced. This disclosed a gas-filled peritoneal bulge in the inguinal region which resembled a sac and was believed to represent a hernia (Fig. 1). The physical examination carried out by one of us (O. A.) after the induction of pneumoperitoneum supported the tentative diagnosis. The findings at operation confirmed the presence of an inguinal hernia which was repaired. At the time of writing the patient has been followed for 2 years and has been free from symptoms since the operation.

The observations made in this case prompted the idea that pneumoperitoneum might be of diagnostic value in supplementing the physical examination in cases in which the site of the pain suggests a hernia but the lesion is not perceptible on palpation.

CASE MATERIAL

During the year from 1967 to 1968 pneumoperitoneum was induced in 21 patients in the X-ray Department of this hospital. Eighteen of these were men and three were women. Their ages ranged from 19 to 67 years, the average age being 42 years.

In three cases an inguinal hernia was demonstrated on palpation, the bulging hernial sac being distinctly perceptible.

In 10 cases the clinical symptoms such as the site of the pain, a dilated superficial inguinal ring, and an "impulse" on coughing indicated an inguinal hernia but its presence could not be conclusively proved.

In two cases the pain was suspected to be due to femoral hernia, but the lesion was not demonstrated on palpation.

In six cases with a history of pain in the groin, hernia was not suspected, the induction of pneumoperitoneum being one step in the investigation of the cause of the pain. The causative factors in these cases were later found to be prostatitis, an abscess in the inguinal region, and various neuropathies.

METHOD

With the patient supine and under local anesthesia and x-ray television control, the

Received for publication June 18, 1969.

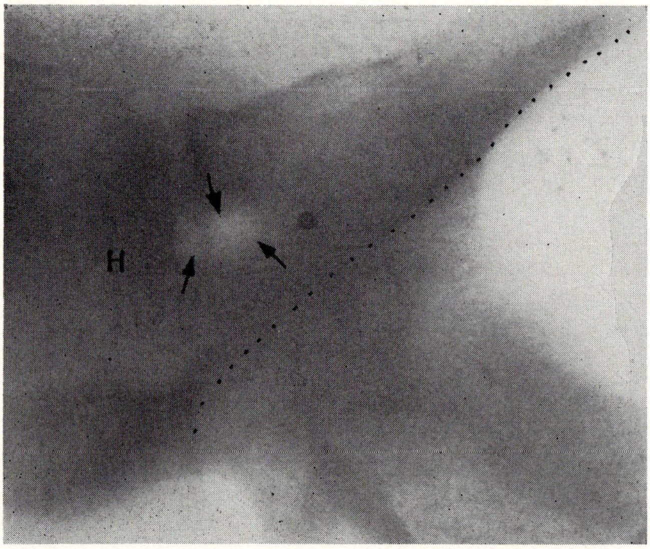

Fig. 1. Femoral hernia in a 57-year-old woman with a history of obscure pain in the right groin for 3 years. Pneumoperitoneum showed a hernial sac, 1 cm. by 2 cm. in size. Arrows point toward the gas-filled hernial sac; the dotted line indicates the lower lateral margin of the peritoneum. *H* = hip joint. The patient was free from symptoms following repair of the hernia.

anterior abdominal wall is punctured on the left side, a few centimeters below the umbilicus, with a needle fitted with a stylet. The length of the needle is 12 cm., its outer diameter being 1.3 mm. When the needle is assumed to have transversed the abdominal wall, a few millimeters of a water-soluble opaque medium is instilled. This makes it possible to check the position of the needle and to adjust it if necessary. Thereafter 1,200 ml. of oxygen is injected. The foot of the table is raised 30 to 35 degrees, and the exposures are made. As a rule, four coned-down views are taken, with a horizontal beam directed toward the affected side. The first two views are taken in anteroposterior projection, one with the patient lying on the unaffected side and the other with the patient tilted 30 to 40 degrees backward. The other two views are taken with the tube angled 20 degrees toward the feet and with the patient tilted 30 to 40 degrees and 70 degrees backward, respectively. In male patients the gonads are shielded. The patient is requested to strain during the exposures because the abdominal pressure is thereby increased and this results in better visualization of a hernia if one is present. Most of the gas is usually absorbed within 24 hours. With the exception of a feeling of fullness in the upper abdomen, which is experienced during the first day after the examination, the procedure does not involve any noteworthy discomfort for the patient.

RESULTS

The radiographs were considered to be positive if a gas-filled peritoneal sac in the inguinal region was seen.

Clinically proved cases of inguinal hernia. Of the three cases in which a hernia was perceptible on palpation, the radiographs were positive in two and negative in the third. All these patients had an operation. In the case in which the radiographs were negative, operation disclosed that the hernial sac contained omentum which was adherent to the bottom of the sac.

Clinically suspected cases of inguinal hernia. Of the 10 cases in which the history suggested an inguinal hernia but palpation failed to demonstrate it, the radiographs were positive in seven cases and negative in three. In five of the seven positive cases a

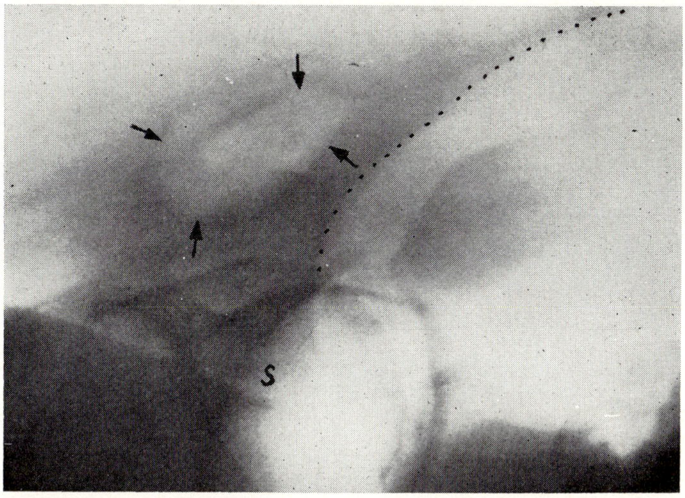

Fig. 2. Inguinal hernia in a 32-year-old woman with a history of obscure pain for 6 years in the left groin. Pneumoperitoneum showed a hernial sac, 2 cm. by 3 cm. in size. Arrows point toward the gas-filled sac; the dotted line indicates the lower lateral margin of the peritoneum. *S* = symphysis. The patient was free from symptoms following the repair of the hernia.

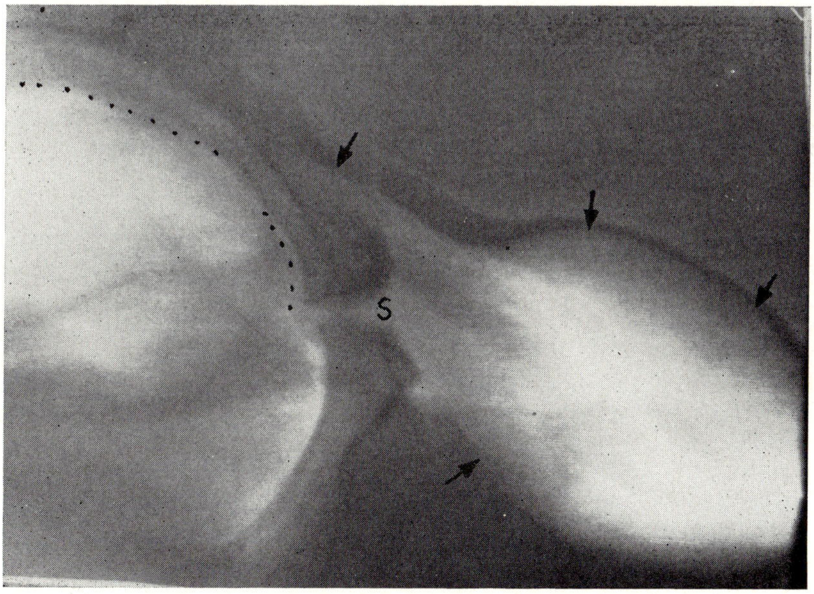

Fig. 3. Congenital, oblique hernia in a 21-year-old man with a history of pain in the right groin. A swelling of the spermatic cord was perceptible on palpation but no hernia. Pneumoperitoneum disclosed a hernial sac, 6 cm. by 12 cm. in size. Arrows point toward the gas-filled hernial sac. The dotted line indicates the lower lateral margin of the peritoneum. *S* = symphysis. The patient was free from symptoms following the repair of the hernia.

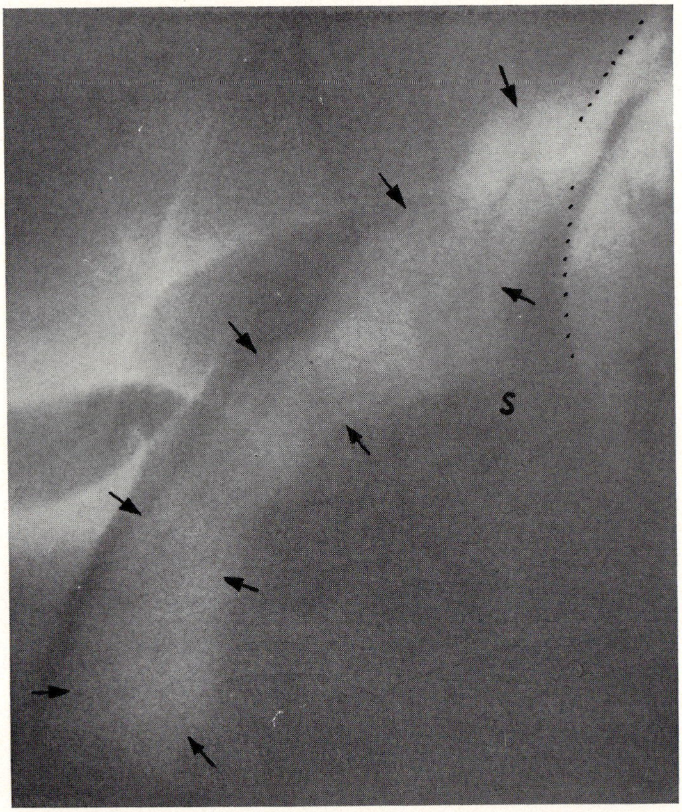

Fig. 4. Acquired hernia in a 55-year-old man with a history of pain in the left groin. No hernia was perceptible on palpation but there was an impulse on coughing. Pneumoperitoneum showed a hernial sac. The dotted line indicates the lateral lower margin of the peritoneum. *S* = symphysis. Following the repair of the hernia the patient was free from symptoms.

small hernial sac, 1 to 3 cm. by 2 to 3 cm. in size, was shown. The radiographic findings were confirmed at operation in all these 5 cases. One of these patients was a woman, aged 32 years, with a history of pain for 6 years in the left groin. She had consulted several physicians and surgeons who all failed to establish the cause of the pain. After the repair of the hernia the patient was free from symptoms (Fig. 2).

In the other two positive cases there was radiographic evidence of a large hernial sac which was seen to descend into the scrotum. Although x-ray examination had conclusively proved the presence of an inguinal hernia the lesion could not be demonstrated on subsequent palpation. In one of these cases a congenital hernia with a narrow neck (Fig. 3) and in the other an acquired hernia with a wide neck (Fig. 4) was found at operation.

In two of the cases which the radiographs were negative, inguinal hernias 1 cm. by 2 cm. and 1 cm. by 3 cm., respectively, were found at operation. The third patient had no operation. It is planned to re-examine this last patient by pneumoperitoneum after about 1 year.

Clinically suspected cases of femoral hernia. In the two cases in this group in which the history suggested a femoral hernia but palpation failed to demonstrate its presence, x-ray examination disclosed a hernial sac which was 1 cm. by 2 cm. in size. In the case described in more detail earlier in this paper, pneumoperitoneum disclosed a gas-filled peritoneal sac, the site of which indicated the presence of a femoral hernia (Fig.

Table I. *Comparison of the findings at operation with radiographs obtained following induction of pneumoperitoneum*

Diagnosis	No. of cases	Radiographs: Positive	Radiographs: Negative	Findings at operation (No. of cases of hernia)
Inguinal hernia	3	2	1*	3
Suspected inguinal hernia	10	7	3†	9
Suspected femoral hernia	2	2	—	2
Absence of hernia	6	—	6	—

*Hernial sac occluded by omentum.
†One patient had no operation.

1). Both patients were operated on and a femoral hernia, the size of the tip of the small digit, was found in both cases.

Absence of inguinal hernia. In six cases in this series a hernia was not suspected, the induction of pneumoperitoneum being one step in the investigation of the cause of the pain in the groin. The radiographs were negative in all these cases. None of these patients had an operation. Nor did the physical examination carried out about 6 months after the induction of pneumoperitoneum disclose an inguinal hernia.

The findings at operation in the cases in this series are compared with the radiographic appearances as observed after the induction of pneumoperitoneum in Table I.

DISCUSSION

Conditions associated with pain in the groin are common and the cause of the pain may be difficult to establish. The pain may be due to factors such as inflammatory processes involving abdominal and pelvic organs or the external genitals, diseases of the hip joint, neuropathies, and inguinal or femoral hernia. In an earlier paper[1] the difficulties associated with the differential diagnosis between inguinal hernia and prostatitis were discussed. Several cases of prostatitis were encountered in the Department of Surgery of this hospital in which the symptoms were wrongly interpreted to be due to an inguinal hernia with unnecessary exploration of the inguinal canal being performed as a result. On the other hand, pain in cases in which the patient is treated for conditions other than hernia may actually be due to a hernia, despite the fact that the lesion is not diagnosed on palpation. In cases in which a hernia is suspected, the patient should be followed up by palpation on several occasions as the findings in some form of hernia may be deceiving and may easily be misinterpreted or the lesion may easily be overlooked even by the experienced examiner. This applies particularly to incipient hernia which, at an early stage, is extremely difficult to recognize on physical examination.

Pneumoperitoneum appears to be of diagnostic value in patients with a history of obscure pain in the groin. Radiographic evidence of a gas-filled peritoneal bulge resembling a sac is positive proof of the presence of a hernia. In 12 of the cases in this series the history suggested an inguinal or femoral hernia but palpation failed to confirm the presence of the lesion. With the exception of one patient, all these patients did have an operation, the presence of a hernia being confirmed at operation. The radiographs were positive in 9 of these 11 patients.

It is interesting to note that little attention has so far been given to the diagnostic possibilities of pneumoperitoneum in cases of abdominal hernia. Farr[2] described two cases of hernia in which the patient was examined by pneumoperitoneum. In one the patient was a woman with a well-established incisional hernia, pneumoperitoneum being induced to clarify the cause of the latter. The other patient was a man with a history of pain in the upper part of the abdomen. On palpation a swelling in the scrotum was felt which was believed to be due to an accumulation of gas in a hernial sac. The swelling was tympanitic on percussion and could be reduced in size by compression. Farr[2] expressed the view that pneumoperitoneum might be helpful in demonstrating a "potential hernia," i.e., a nonobliterated part of the processus vaginalis. On the other hand, he discussed the possibility that the patient might later claim that the introduction of gas into the peritoneal cavity was involved in the production of the hernia. In his opinion, this factor was one of the contraindications to pneumoperitoneum.

White, Parks, and Haller[3] described a radiologic method, herniography, that permits the diagnosis of inguinal hernia to be made in infants and children. With the patient supine they injected 10 to 15 ml. of 60 percent Renografin-60 intraperitoneally. Thereafter, the patient was held erect until an upright anteroposterior radiograph of the lower abdomen and upper thigh had been taken. This technique resulted in filling of the hernial sac, i.e., a herniogram was obtained. They used this method in 50 children who were less than 5 years old and reported that a hernia was found at operation when it was indicated by the herniogram. Experience in their series of cases showed that the physical examination does not result in a correct diagnosis in many cases of children.

Naturally, the diagnosis of hernia in the inguinal region should rest principally on the findings on palpation but in questionable cases pneumoperitoneum, possibly induced on several occasions, is preferable to the exploration of the inguinal canal. It is interesting to note that in two of the cases here presented in which the radiographs were positive and the patients did have an operation, the resident, although quite experienced, was unable to detect the lesion at operation. A senior surgeon was summoned and he succeeded in demonstrating and repairing the hernia.

Pneumoperitoneum will probably be of value in the diagnosis of the cause of incisional hernia, of obturator hernia and of Spigelian hernia which may be very difficult to recognize.

No complications were observed in the cases in this series. We have so far induced pneumoperitoneum on about 300 occasions in patients suffering from conditions other than hernia without any complications occurring. This leads us to assume that the procedure does not involve any danger to the patient, provided it is carried out under x-ray television control and the position of the needle is carefully checked before gas is injected into the peritoneal cavity.

As we have no experience with herniography which White and co-workers[3] have performed in infants and children, using an opaque medium, it is difficult to say whether gas or an opaque medium should be used in the radiologic diagnosis of hernia. Moreover, we have so far only examined adults by pneumoperitoneum. Both methods afford information of diagnostic value. As it is well known that opaque media may cause a local reaction of the peritoneum as well as an allergic reaction, we feel that gas should be the medium of choice.

It is hoped that with increasing skill and experience the radiodiagnostic possibilities following the induction of pneumoperitoneum will be further developed in cases of hernia in the inguinal region.

SUMMARY

Pneumoperitoneum was induced in 21 patients and was followed by radiography of the inguinal region.

In three of these cases an inguinal hernia was perceptible on palpation; in two of them a gas-filled peritoneal bulge resembling a hernial sac was shown in the radiographs. In the third case there was no radiographic evidence of a hernial sac. At operation the latter was found to contain omentum which was adherent to the bottom of the sac.

In 12 cases the history and the findings on palpation indicated the presence of inguinal or femoral hernia; in 9 of these cases there was radiographic evidence of a hernia, the radiographic findings being confirmed at operation.

In 6 of the 21 patients in this series with a history of pain in the inguinal region, a hernia was not suspected, the induction of pneumoperitoneum being one step in the investigation of the cause of the pain. The radiographs of all these patients were negative.

Pneumoperitoneum appears to aid in the diagnosis of inguinal hernia in cases in which the presence of the lesion is suspected from the history but the physical examination fails to demonstrate its presence.

REFERENCES

1. Arner, O.: Misdiagnosis of incipient inguinal hernia in prostato-vesiculitis, Nord. Med. **59:** 912, 1958.
2. Farr, R. E.: Pneumoperitoneum as an aid in the diagnosis of hernia, J. A. M. A. **82:** 1774, 1924.
3. White, J. J., Parks, L. D., and Haller, J. A.: The inguinal herniogram: A radiologic aid for accurate diagnosis of inguinal hernia in an infant, SURGERY **63:** 991, 1968.

Role of mammography with palpable breast lesions

EZRI S. SOKOL, M.D.
BARRY WALKER, M.D.
JOSE J. TERZ, M.D.
WALTER LAWRENCE, Jr., M.D.
RICHMOND, VA.
From the Divisions of Surgical Oncology and Diagnostic Radiology, Medical College of Virginia, Health Sciences Division of the Virginia Commonwealth University

Mammography has been particularly impressive as a diagnostic tool when breast cancer has been identified in the absence of a palpable mass, but the patient who presents with a palpable breast mass is usually subjected to surgical excision of this mass for pathologic diagnosis despite radiologic findings. A concerted effort has been made by the Division of Surgical Oncology at this institution over the past 2 years to determine the role of mammography in this type of patient by subjecting all of our patients to mammography prior to surgical biopsy. This report is a summary of the findings of both the radiologic examinations and the biopsies in this group of patients. An attempt was made to assess the accuracy of both the radiologic and clinical examinations and to evaluate the variables that might influence the mammographic diagnoses obtained. The study was also designed to evaluate the importance of clinical information to the radiologist in his interpretation, the variability in mammographic diagnosis by different radiologists, and the importance of the patient's age in terms of our ability to identify, and correctly diagnose, a palpable breast mass.

METHODS

The radiologic technique employed for the mammograms to be described was essentially the same as that described by Egan,[2] namely, a high milliamperage-seconds and low kilovoltage procedure using a special fine-grain industrial type M film emulsion. The radiologist carrying out this procedure had an opportunity to examine the patient in order to obtain optimal film coverage. All mammograms were taken under the supervision of, and interpreted by, one of three radiologists in the Division of Diagnostic Radiology who were experienced in this technique.

The mammograms from 128 breast lesions that were eventually subjected to biopsy and pathologic study form the basis of this report. The clinical diagnosis recorded at the time of admission for surgical biopsy was classified as (1) benign breast mass, (2) a possible cancer, or (3) definite carcinoma. The mammographic interpretations were classified in three similar categories or the additional category of "no lesion identified." The pathologic diagnoses were based on the review of the histologic material by one of the staff members of our Division of Surgical Pathology.

DESIGN OF STUDY

Three classes of mammographic data were recorded and tabulated for the purpose of the comparisons to be described:

1. The first tabulations were those original readings by one of three radiologists performing these studies.

Received for publication June 19, 1969.

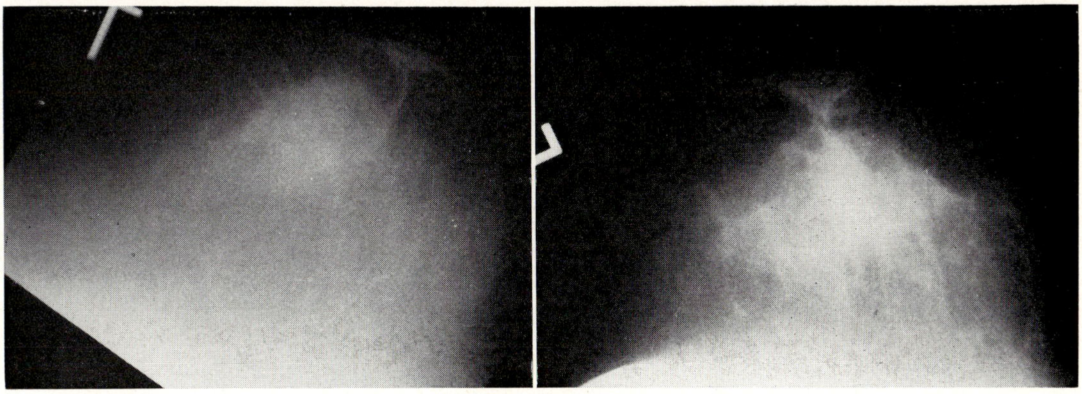

Fig. 1. Mammogram of a clinically suspected breast cancer showing minute calcifications and irregular borders.

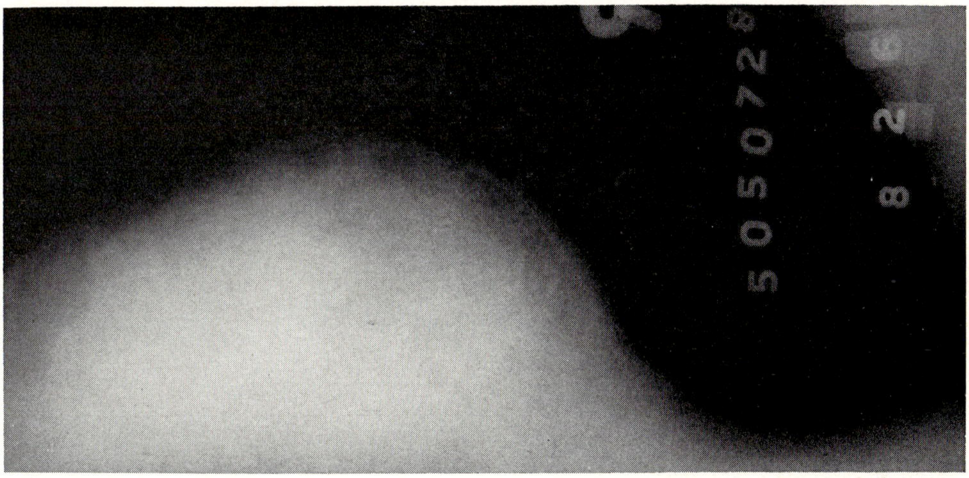

Fig. 2. Mammogram of inflammatory breast cancer showing marked thickening of the skin and homogeneous density of breast.

2. All films were read "cold" at a later date by a single radiologist (B. W.) without benefit of any clinical information.

3. All films were reread by this same radiologist after receiving pertinent preoperative clinical data regarding age and physical findings.

The criteria utilized by the single radiologist in analyzing the films in categories 2 and 3 were obviously uniform. The diagnostic features of mammograms that led to an interpretation of malignancy were (Figs. 1 and 2): (1) irregular versus regular borders of the visible breast lesion; (2) the size of the lesion radiographically versus the size on clinical examination (Lesions clinically larger than the radiographic lesion were considered to favor cancer.); (3) the presence of minute calcification; (4) thickening of the overlying skin.

RESULTS

Of the 128 lesions comprising this study, 34 proved to be carcinomas, and 94 were benign breast lesions that were proved by surgical biopsy and pathologic examination. Of the 34 cancers, 27 were correctly diagnosed by mammography prior to surgical biopsy (79 percent). When these same mammograms were reviewed by one radiologist without benefit of clinical information (category 2), accuracy of interpretation was similar (26 were correct). Review of the same x-rays with description of preoperative clinical findings changed the diagnosis (correctly) in only one instance.

The preoperative diagnosis on clinical examination was correct in 29 of the 34 cancers (85 percent), an accuracy similar to that achieved with radiologic examination; however, the clinician made the correct diagnosis of cancer in five patients in whom the mammographic diagnosis was that of a benign process, while the opposite situation was true in three instances. Thus, in only two of the 34 cancers was the lesion thought to be benign both on clinical examination and radiologic study.

In a study of the 94 benign breast lesions the initial diagnosis by mammography was correct (i.e., benign lesions or "no identifiable lesion") in 80 instances (85 percent). When uniform diagnostic criteria were employed by means of review by a single radiologist, the accuracy of the examination was increased to 88 of the 94 cases (94 percent). When these same films had been reviewed by this radiologist without the benefit of clinical information, only 83 lesions were correctly interpreted. In an attempt to correlate both the clinical and radiologic diagnoses in this group of benign lesions, it was found that there was correct diagnostic agreement in 81 of 94 cases. The mammograms were correct in seven cases when the preoperative clinical diagnosis was in error, whereas the opposite situation was true in only two instances.

Viewed as a whole, the incidence of correct diagnoses, whether benign or malignant,

Table I. *Over-all accuracy of mammographic interpretation (128 cases)*

Source of data	*No. correct*	*No. read malignant*	*% Correct*	*No. read benign*	*% Correct*
Original reading	107 (83.6%)	41	65.9	87	92.0
Single "interpreter"					
Without clinical data	109 (85.2%)	37	70.3	91	91.2
With clinical data	115 (90.0%)	33	81.8	95	92.6

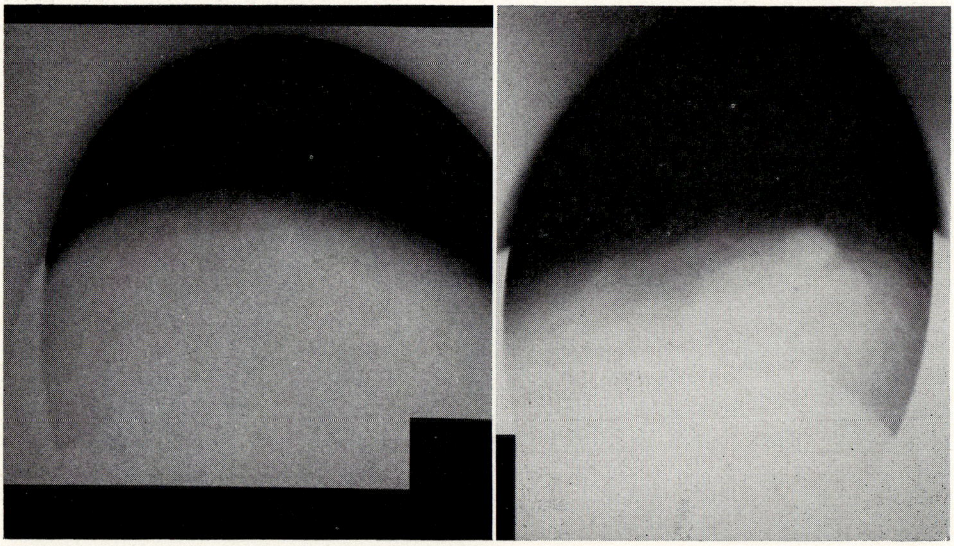

Fig. 3. Mammograms of breast abscess showing the radiologic features of inflammatory cancer.

was calculated for the three types of mammographic data (Table I). Calculated in this fashion it is apparent that the over-all accuracy was slightly greater when a single radiologist (B. W.) reviewed all the films with all clinical data available to him. This small diagnostic advantage was due entirely to a smaller number of benign lesions being incorrectly diagnosed as cancer.

One finding of interest in review of the entire group of mammograms was that the palpable lesion was identified radiographically in only 15 of 36 lesions in patients who were under 30 years of age. In patients over 30, the palpable lesion was identified radiographically in 84 of the 92 cases.

DISCUSSION

In Egan's[3] study of 2,522 mammograms interpreted without the benefit of clinical findings, 501 of 518 proved carcinomas (96.7 percent) were diagnosed correctly. In 383 proved benign lesions the correct diagnosis was made in 351 (91.6 percent). Unfortunately, several other studies have not been able to reproduce this diagnostic accuracy. In a study by Clark and co-workers[1] on the reproducibility of the Egan technique, prebiopsy mammography of 1,580 breast lesions produced 475 radiographic diagnoses of malignant neoplasm. This was verified pathologically in 376 patients for an accuracy of 79 percent, with a false positive rate of

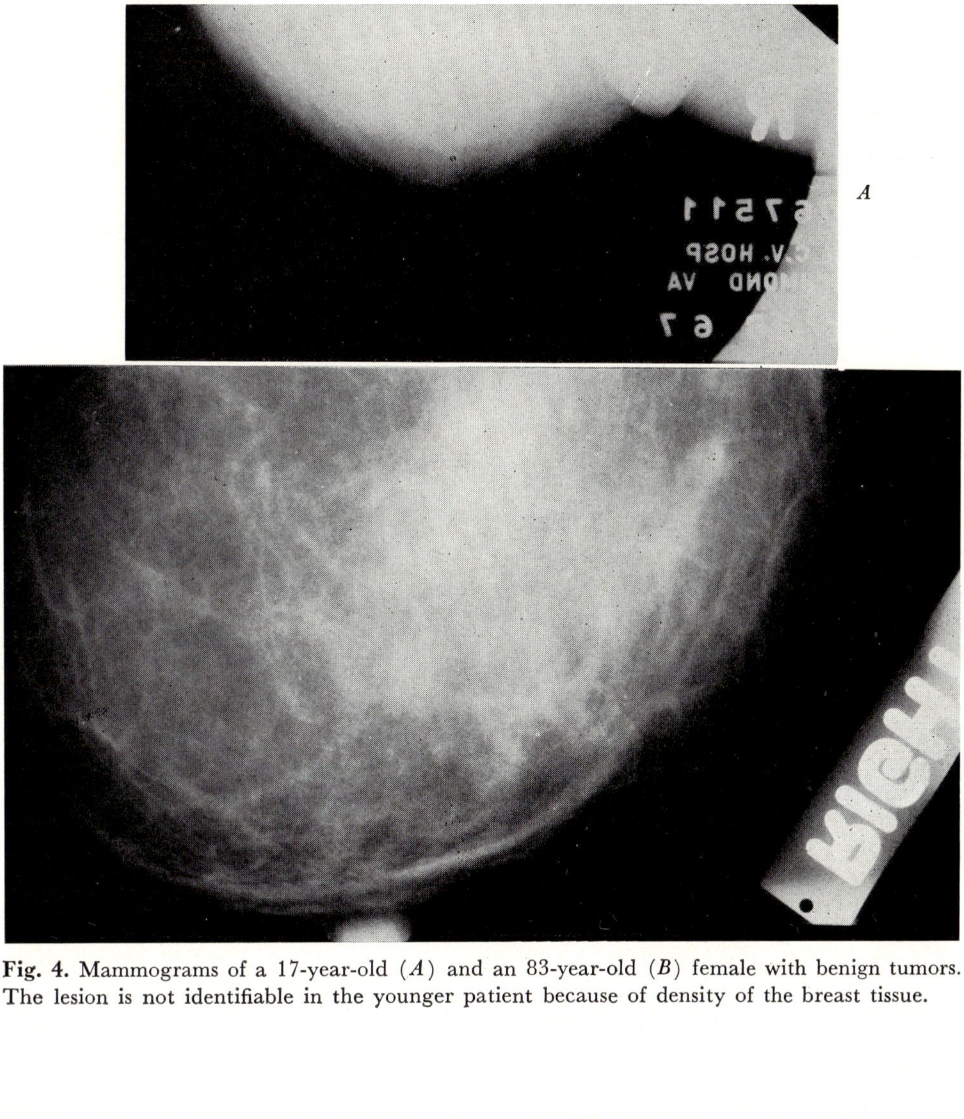

A

B

Fig. 4. Mammograms of a 17-year-old (*A*) and an 83-year-old (*B*) female with benign tumors. The lesion is not identifiable in the younger patient because of density of the breast tissue.

10 percent. Our accuracy of diagnosis in the carcinoma group was similar, but, in contrast, there was only a 6.4 percent incidence of false positives in our benign group when one radiologist reviewed all films with clinical data available.

In our assessment of mammography for palpable lesions, we found our ability to make a diagnosis of cancer was greater than we suspected. However, the correct clinical diagnosis of cancer was made in five of the 34 patients in whom the mammographic interpretation was that of a benign lesion. Mammography, therefore, adds little to our diagnostic accuracy of a palpable breast cancer.

In the benign group diagnostic accuracy of mammography was somewhat higher. Occasionally a radiologic diagnosis of cancer proved to be a "false positive" (Fig. 3), but this leads to no major problems if histologic diagnosis is routinely established before definitive treatment of a breast cancer is instituted. Nevertheless, the fact that a few cancers were incorrectly interpreted as benign lesions still places the surgeon in the position of being unable to avoid surgical biopsy of a palpable breast mass.

The clinical situation in which a diagnostic tool that would avoid operation would be most helpful is in the younger age group. The incidence of breast cancer in this group is considerably lower than in patients who are over 30 years of age, and there are many lesions, particularly fibroadenomas, that appear to be definitely benign on clinical examination. Unfortunately, this age group is also the group in which the characteristics of normal breast tissue lead to interference with radiologic identification of palpable breast lesions (Fig. 4). We were unable to identify the palpable lesion on film in 21 of the 36 palpable breast masses in patients less than 30 years of age. The only cancer in this group of young patients was identified and correctly diagnosed by mammography, but the value of this study in this age group was definitely curtailed by this frequent difficulty. On the basis of these findings, we plan to discontinue preoperative mammography in patients with palpable lesions in this age group.

One finding in this study that was surprising to us was the relatively small advantage afforded the radiologist by having clinical data available to him. Many surgeons have secretly attributed the high diagnostic accu-

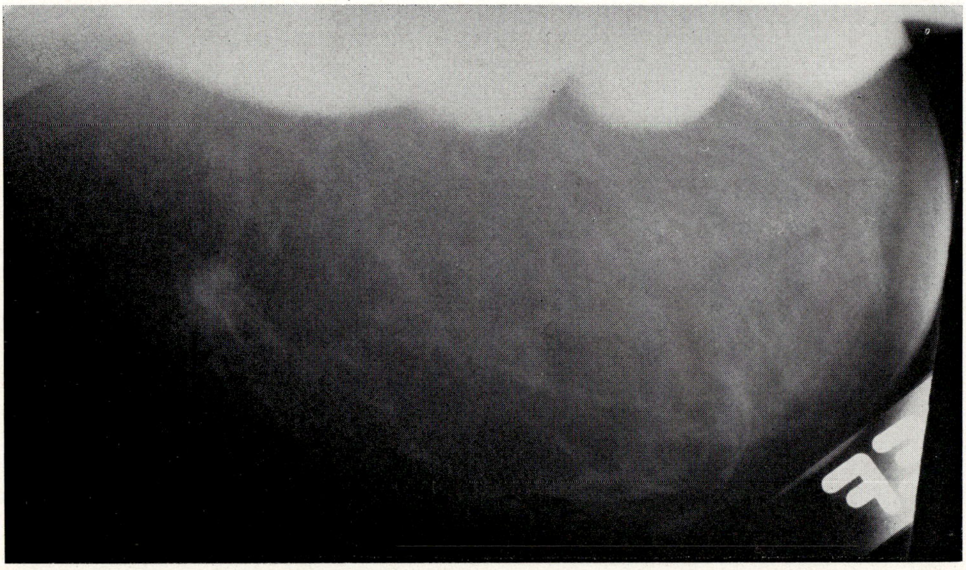

Fig. 5. Mammogram in a clinically negative breast showing occult carcinoma (patient of Dr. H. F. Conquest).

racy of mammography that has been reported to the fact that the radiologist examines the patient's breast as a means of outlining ideal radiologic procedure. This concept is in error, since only a small increase in accuracy occurred when the radiologist was given pertinent clinical findings. The variability in diagnostic accuracy when several trained radiologists are involved as opposed to a single radiologist is also small.

There seems to be no question that mammography occasionally detects a cancer when no lesion is actually palpable in the breast (Fig. 5). There are studies underway to determine whether or not this is a frequent enough finding to justify mammography as a periodic screening technique.[4, 5] For the present, general opinion favors radiologic assistance for periodic examinations in the high-risk populations, particularly women with prior radical mastectomy for cancer, or women with strong familial histories of breast carcinoma. The detection of an occult cancer of the breast does occasionally occur, however, in patients being investigated radiographically for another clinically benign tumor in the same or opposite breast.

After demonstrating a small but significant incidence of false negative diagnoses with mammography, as well as a higher degree of correlation between the clinical examination and pathologic findings than with mammography, what should be the role of mammography in a patient who has a palpable breast mass? It must first be assumed from this analysis that mammography cannot eliminate the need for biopsy when a palpable mass is present. However, mammography does add to the diagnostic accuracy of clinical examination of breast cancer, and in this regard it might produce some advantage in terms of preoperative preparation of the patient. More important, however, is the fact that an unsuspected lesion may be found in the opposite breast or the same breast of a patient who presents with either a cancer or a benign breast lesion. Of further importance is to have a base-line study of the normal breast so that at a future date the detection of a lesion may be facilitated. For these reasons, we plan to continue mammography prior to biopsy of the breast mass in question if the patient is over 30 years of age. In the younger patient, the possibility of adding useful information by this technique is reduced enough to consider omission of this diagnostic aid prior to routine surgical biopsy of the palpable mass.

REFERENCES

1. Clark, R. L., Copeland, M. M., Egan, R. L., Gallager, H. S., Geller, H., Linday, J. P., Robbins, L. C., and White, E. C.: Reproducibility of the technic of mammography (Egan) for cancer of the breast, Amer. J. Surg. **109:** 127, 1965.
2. Egan, R. L.: Mammography, Amer. J. Surg. **106:** 421, 1963.
3. Egan, R. L.: Mammography, an aid to early diagnosis of breast carcinoma, J. A. M. A. **182:** 839, 1962.
4. Gershen-Cohen, J., Hermel, M. B., and Berger, S. M.: Detection of breast cancer by periodic x-ray examination—five year survey, J. A. M. A. **176:** 114, 1961.
5. Strax, P., Venet, L., and Shapiro, S.: Mammography and clinical examination in mass screening for cancer of the breast, Cancer **20:** 2184, 1967.

Hemodynamic alterations in acute cardiac tamponade after penetrating injuries of the heart

W. C. SHOEMAKER, M.D.
J. S. CAREY, M.D.
S. T. YAO, M.D.
P. A. MOHR, M.D.
J. J. AMATO, M.D.
K. J. PRINTEN, M.D.
R. D. CORLEY, M.D.
D. O. MONSON, M.D.
S. YOUSSEF, M.D.
N. J. SHOEMAKER, R.N.
NEW YORK, N. Y., AND CHICAGO, ILL.
From the Department of Surgery, Mount Sinai Hospital, New York, and the Department of Surgical Research, Hektoen Institute, Cook County Hospital, Chicago

Cardiac tamponade incident to penetrating wounds of the chest is a rare but catastrophic occurrence. We encountered an average of 16 cases of clinical tamponade in 800 admissions for stab and gunshot wounds of the chest per year. Of 80 patients in whom the diagnosis of cardiac injury was established at operation, one or more of the usual signs of cardiac tamponade were present in 87 percent, but the classic Beck's triad was seen in only 35 percent.[9] The experience of others has been similar.[1, 6, 8]

Cardiac tamponade after stab or gunshot wounds may develop in a subtle and unsuspected manner. Cardiac wounds are easily suspected from precordial and anterior chest wall injuries, but we have observed penetration of the cardiac chambers with tamponade from wounds of the right midaxillary region, the left posterior chest wall, and the epigastrium. Transfusions and plasma expanders return vital signs toward normal values and mask the presence of cardiac injury. Pericardial injury may permit partial or complete decompression of intrapericardial blood when it is under pressure; this may occur before or after there is hemodynamic evidence of tamponade.

Clotted blood is frequently found in the pericardial cavity. Large clots which weighed up to 300 Gm. were observed in 65 percent of our series.[9] These clots, in part, may explain the relatively high (15 percent) incidence of negative pericardiocenteses. Moreover, clots may produce localized compression on the myocardium and thereby limit myocardial blood flow and function.

Many factors may lead to a delay in diagnosis in the patient with stable arterial pressure. Ideally, it would be advantageous to have more precise criteria for evaluation of the primary hemodynamic derangements and their physiologic compensations. Moreover, it would be helpful to predict when sudden decompensation is likely to occur.

Lange and associates[5] studied seven patients with acute cardiac tamponade; cardiac output was measured in four of these patients and found to average 1.8 L. per minute per square meter. These authors observed that a reduced cardiac index did not allow

Submitted for publication May 26, 1969; resubmitted July 28 and Sept. 8, 1969.

good diagnostic discrimination because a cardiac index of less than 2.5 was also present in some of their patients with constrictive pericarditis, in patients with pericardial fluid not under significantly increased pressure, and in a miscellaneous group of patients with clinical findings suggestive of compressive cardiac disease. However, the low cardiac index increased to normal values after pericardiocentesis in three of four cases.

In a study of experimental hemopericardium in unanesthetized dogs, it was found that arterial and venous pressures did not change markedly until 6 ml. of blood per kilogram of body weight was injected into the pericardial cavity.[4] Apparently considerable volumes of blood could accumulate within the pericardial cavity before significant hemodynamic alterations occurred. Increased systemic vascular (peripheral) resistance, heart rate, and venous pressures occurred early in response to reduced stroke volumes and cardiac outputs. In spite of severe tamponade, volume expansion alone returned cardiac output and arterial pressure to normal values and further increased venous pressures.[4]

The present study was undertaken to investigate some of these mechanisms in man. Sequential measurements of hemodynamic events were made in a series of patients with hemopericardium from penetrating cardiac wounds. The clinical and hemodynamic data suggest possible diagnostic criteria which may be useful when blood pressure is normal and pericardiocentesis is negative. The hemodynamic effects of volume expansion and isoproterenol infusion during tamponade were also investigated. From these studies a hemodynamic classification of cardiac tamponade has evolved which reflects the pathophysiologic stages of the disease.

METHODS

Nine patients from a larger series of 80 penetrating cardiac injuries[9] were monitored; observations began shortly after admission and were continued at intervals until surgical exploration. A central venous catheter was inserted into the right atrium and a plastic catheter was placed in the femoral artery by the percutaneous route. Arterial and venous pressures were measured with Statham P23Db transducers and recorded continuously on an Offner Dynograph recorder. The cardiac output was measured in eight patients by the dye dilution technique with the use of indocyanine green as the indicator. The concentration of the dye in arterial blood was measured by a Gilford photodensitometer. The method for estimation of cardiac output, various derived calculations, and their reproducibility have been described previously.[3]

Correlation of pericardial volume changes produced with progressive increments of pericardial blood with physiologic sequential hemodynamic measurements during graded cardiac tamponade in the unanesthetized dog[4] has provided a basis for categorization of patients with tamponade. Three grades of tamponade are suggested, as follows:

Grade I tamponade (less than 200 ml. of blood in the pericardial cavity) is characterized by normal or elevated cardiac output, normal systemic arterial pressure, tachycardia, and increased central venous pressure.

Grade II tamponade (more than 200 ml. of blood in the pericardial cavity) is characterized by decreased cardiac output, normal or slightly decreased systemic arterial pressure, tachycardia, and increased venous pressure.

Grade III tamponade (more than 200 ml. of blood in the pericardial cavity) is characterized by severe hypotension, distended neck veins, muffled heart sounds, severely depressed cardiac output, markedly elevated venous pressure, and decreasing heart rate.

Because of the labile nature of the cardiovascular defect, it was possible for patients to pass from one grade to another, depending on relief or recurrence of tamponade. The hemodynamic data are presented at the stage most closely related in time to the operation.

During the period of preoperative study

the hemodynamic responses to administration of dextran-40 and isoproterenol as well as pericardiocentesis were investigated. Dextran-40, 500 ml. of 10 percent solution, was infused over a one-hour period. Isoproterenol was infused continuously at a rate of 5 to 10 micrograms per minute.

RESULTS

Clinical data. The clinical information on nine patients included in this study is given in Table I. Most of the patients were relatively young and were known to have been in good health prior to the injury. Seven of the nine injuries were stab wounds of the left parasternal area, one was a stab wound of the back in the left interscapular area, and another was a gunshot wound of the left parasternal area. Seven of the nine patients either were hypotensive on admission or had given a history of hypotension when examined at another hospital prior to admission. Two patients were not hypotensive at any time during the course of their disease. Beck's triad (Grade III tamponade) was clearly present on admission in only one patient. Chest x-ray, when taken, was unrevealing in most patients. Pericardiocentesis was positive in four of six patients and equivocal or negative in the other two. Pericardiocentesis was not performed in two patients and rapid thoracotomy was performed in lieu of pericardiocentesis in another. Transfusion therapy was given to most patients with beneficial results, as judged by clinical criteria. Major blood loss (greater than 20 percent of blood volume) was encountered only in the patient with the gun-

Table I. *Clinical data*

Patient	Age	Sex	Injury	Initial findings: Blood pressure	Initial findings: Pulse	Initial findings: Neck veins
Grade I tamponade						
1. S. B.	27	F	Stab wound, left second intercostal parasternal	60/40	120	Flat
2. E. G.	21	M	Stab wound, left fourth intercostal parasternal	40/20	130	Distended
3. W. B.	22	M	Stab wound, back, left interscapular area	140/98	100	
4. H. H.	49	M	Stab wound, left intercostal parasternal	125/70	105	
Grade II tamponade						
5. J. F.	41	M	Stab wound, left fourth intercostal parasternal	80/50	120	Distended
6. L. B.	45	M	Stab wound, left fourth intercostal parasternal	Unobtainable	110	Normal
7. J. N.	21	M	Stab wound, left fourth intercostal parasternal	90/60	96	
8. S. S.	22	M	Gunshot wound, left fifth intercostal parasternal	100/60	110	Slightly distended
Grade III tamponade						
9. C. S.	37	M	Stab wound, left sixth intercostal, parasternal	60/40	120	

*Anterior mediastinum.

shot injury. Findings at operation revealed injury of the right ventricle in seven of the nine patients, of the left atrium in one, and of the left ventricle in one. Large clots were found in the pericardial cavity in six of the nine patients. Frequently these clots were removed as a single mass of gelatinous blood covered by a thin, fibrinous membrane.

Several aspects of individual cases are of significance.

In Patient 1 the diagnosis was delayed because of the high position of the stab wound on the chest, the alertness of the patient, and the absence of Beck's triad. Initial hypotension accompanied by increased systemic vascular (peripheral) resistance may have led to the patchy necrosis of the small bowel which was found at operation.

The classic Beck's triad (Grade III tamponade) was present on admission in Patient 2. Initial pericardiocentesis was productive of 40 ml. of nonclotting blood and led to rapid clinical improvement. Subsequent hemodynamic studies revealed Grade I tamponade; at operation 400 ml. of blood was found in the left pleural cavity but only 125 ml. in the pericardial cavity; this suggests that the major portion of the intrapericardial blood had decompressed through the pericardial laceration.

The presence of pneumopericardium led to the diagnosis of cardiac injury in Patient 3, who was not hypotensive at any time. At operation minimal hemopericardium was noted; the presence of air in the pericardium was thought to have occurred from the stab wound through the pericardium and lung tissue which was adherent to it.

		Pericar-diocen-tesis		Surgical findings		
Heart tones	*Chest x-ray*	*(ml.)*	*Fluid and transfusion therapy*	*Cardiac injury*	*Hemopericardium*	*Hemothorax (ml.)*
Normal	Negative	Neg.	1,500 ml. blood, 500 ml. dextran-70	Stab wound, right ventricle, necrosis of small bowel	100 ml. clot	200*
Distant		40		Stab wound, right ventricle	100 ml. liquid, 25 ml. clot	200
Normal	Pneumopericardium	Neg.		Stab wound, left atrium	60 ml. liquid, air	
Normal	Left hemothorax	9		Stab wound, right ventricle	150 ml. liquid	700
Normal	Clear	20	750 ml. plasma, 750 ml. saline	Stab wound, right ventricle	300 ml. clot, 100 ml. liquid	
Normal	Clear		2,000 ml. saline, 500 ml. dextran-40	Stab wound, right ventricle	200 ml. clot, 150 ml. liquid	
Normal	Enlarged heart	7	Saline	Stab wound, right ventricle	250 ml. clots, liquid blood	
Normal	Bullet in pericardium		750 ml. plasma, 500 ml. blood	Gunshot wound, left ventricle	200 ml. clot, 250 ml. liquid	650
Normal				Stab wound, right ventricle	250 ml. liquid blood, clots	

Patient 4 also was not hypotensive at any time in his hospital course. A chest x-ray revealed the presence of left hemothorax; 700 ml. of blood was evacuated from the chest by closed thoracostomy. After pericardiocentesis, which was productive of 9 ml. of nonclotting blood, the pericardial area was explored; 150 ml. of liquid blood was evacuated from the pericardium.

In Patient 5 an equivocal hemodynamic response was seen on two occasions after pericardiocentesis which were productive of 20 ml. of partially clotting blood. Administration of 1,500 ml. of plasma and saline produced moderate improvement. The sequence of hemodynamic changes observed is illustrated in Fig. 1. Arterial pressure and vascular resistance deteriorated rapidly; it was felt that mechanical limitation of blood flow was the primary hemodynamic abnormality and an exploratory operation was performed. When the pericardium was opened, a clot estimated at 300 Gm. and 100 ml. of liquid blood were removed; the blood pressure returned to normal over a period of several minutes. The femoral artery pressure response to the opening of the pericardium is illustrated in Fig. 2. The recovery of arterial pressure in Patient 5 was much more gradual than that of Patient 9 (Fig. 2), probably because of the slower onset, the more prolonged time course of

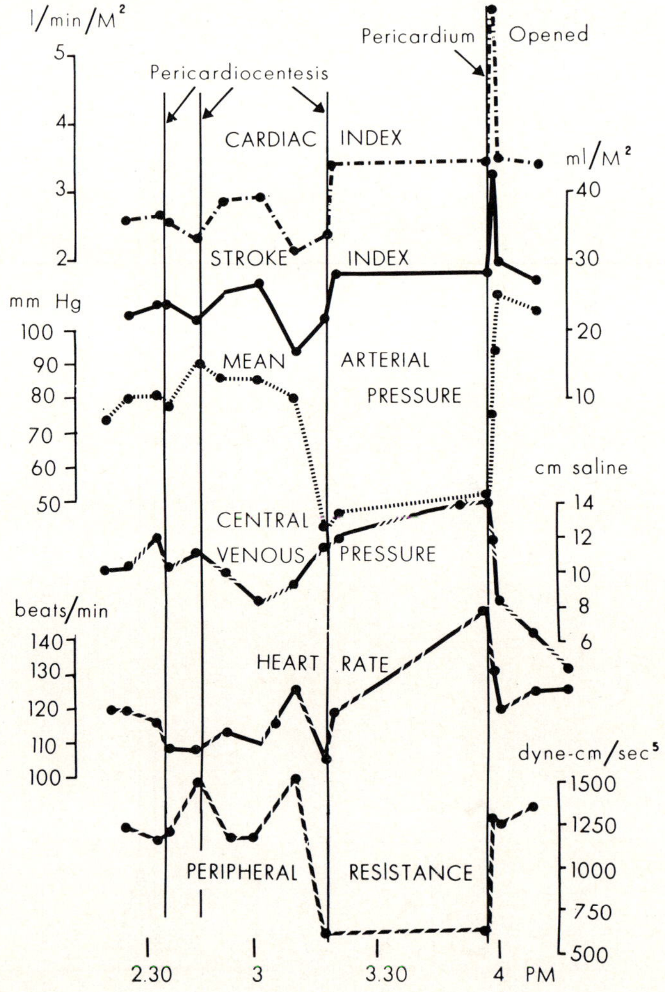

Fig. 1. Hemodynamic values of Patient 5.

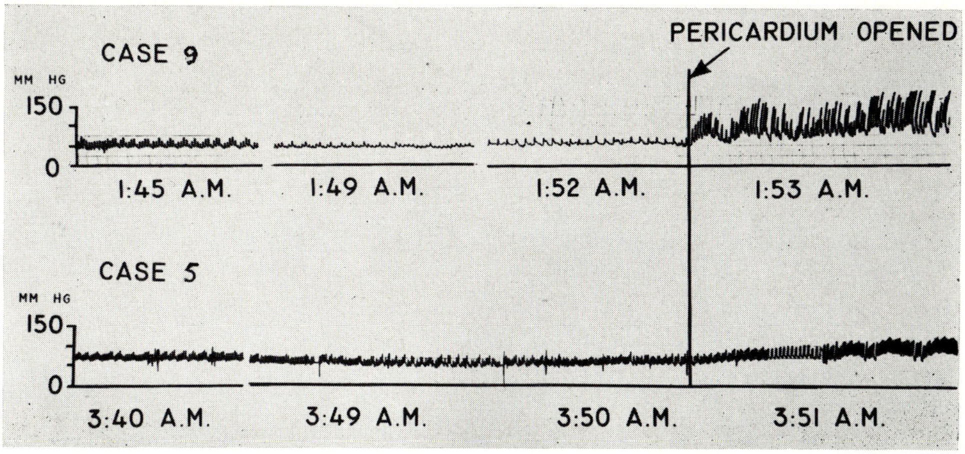

Fig. 2. Arterial pressures in Patients 9 and 5 obtained at the time the pericardium was opened. The upper section illustrates pressures in a case in which severe hypotension developed rapidly and pressures rapidly returned to normal after the pericardiotomy. The lower section illustrates a case in which the syndrome developed more slowly and restoration of pressure was more gradual.

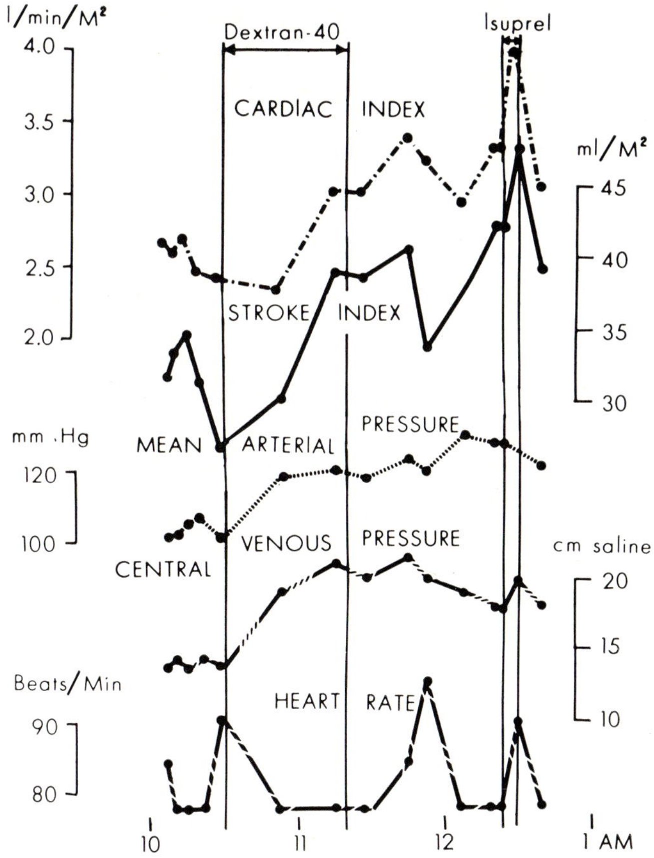

Fig. 3. Hemodynamic values of Patient 6.

the disorder, and the delay in diagnosis.

In patient 6 the blood pressure was unobtainable on admission but rose to 100 mm. Hg after rapid administration of 2,000 ml. of saline. Then hemodynamic monitoring was instituted (Fig. 3). After administration of 500 ml. of dextran-40, the cardiax index and the stroke index rose to normal levels and the venous pressures increased to about 20 cm. of saline. Administration of isoproterenol resulted in a further rise of the cardiac index and the stroke index. At operation a 200 ml. clot and 150 ml. of liquid blood were removed from the pericardium. In spite of this degree of tamponade, normal cardiac output values were produced by plasma volume expanders alone.

In Patient 7 pericardiocentesis yielded only 7 ml. of nonclotting blood. The hemodynamic values remained low. At operation the hemopericardium consisted entirely of a large clot. This patient's case illustrates the futility of nonoperative therapy in the face of a massive pericardial clot.

In Patient 8 a gunshot wound of the left fifth intercostal space 1 cm. lateral to the midclavicular line gave rise to a left hemothorax; 650 ml. of blood was removed by a chest tube. Transfusion of 750 ml. of plasma and 500 ml. of blood restored the blood pressure to 100/60 and the cardiac output to normal. Sixteen hours after admission cardiac index and the stroke index were markedly decreased; this was accompanied by increased vascular resistance and central venous pressure. A moderate increase in the cardiac output was observed after infusion of 500 ml. of 10 percent dextran-40, and an even greater increase in the cardiac output occurred during isoproterenol infusion. At operation 200 ml. of clotted and 250 ml. of liquid blood was removed from the pericardial cavity. A through-and-through gunshot wound of the left ventricle was repaired. This report illustrates the hemodynamic changes that occur with nonoperative therapy and reaccumulation of hemopericardium.

Patient 9 was transferred to the operating room immediately after admission for hemodynamic monitoring. However, rapid deterioration to Grade III tamponade necessitated early thoracotomy before hemodynamic studies could be obtained. Recording of femoral artery pressure during rapid deterioration, thoracotomy, and decompression by opening the pericardium are illustrated in Fig. 2. Pulsus paradoxus is clearly evident in the initial section of the tracing. The blood pressure returned toward normal more rapidly after opening of the pericardium than did that of Patient 5.

Hemodynamic data. In four patients with Grade I tamponade, the cardiac index was normal or high; it ranged from 3.3 to 5.9 (average 4.4) L. per minute per square meter. The stroke index was normal or slightly decreased; it ranged from 30 to 52 (average 41) ml. per square meter. The central venous pressure increased to an average of 22 cm. of saline. Changes of mean transit times were not remarkable; the heart rate varied between 102 and 124 beats per minute. The mean systematic arterial pressure was essentially normal in two patients and slightly decreased in two. Peripheral resistance was somewhat decreased in all patients; the average was 1380 dynes · sec./cm.^{5}/M.^{2}.

In four patients with Grade II tamponade the estimated volume of hemopericardium varied between 250 and 450 ml. The hemodynamic findings were similar to those noted in experimental studies.[4] The cardiac index and the stroke index were markedly decreased (mean values, 1.75 ± 0.2 L. per minute per square meter and 17.5 ± 1.8 ml. per square meter, respectively). Peripheral resistance increased to 3,834 dynes · sec./cm.^{5}/M.^{2}, and mean transit time increased to 25.7 seconds; these elevations were statistically significant. The central venous pressures averaged 17 cm. of saline. The heart rate varied between 90 and 114 beats per minute. The mean arterial pressure was normal in one patient and slightly decreased in the other three.

The hemodynamic responses to an infusion of 500 ml. of dextran-40 were observed in four patients. In two patients with Grade I tamponade there were further increases in the cardiac index and the central venous pressures after infusion. The mean arterial pressure, heart rate, and peripheral resistance did not change significantly. Two patients with Grade II tamponade were given dextran-40 infusion; the cardiac index, stroke index, central venous pressure, and arterial pressure increased; peripheral resistance decreased. The response of mean transit times to dextran administration was variable.

Hemodynamic responses during infusion of isoproterenol were studied in four patients. In one patient with Grade I tamponade the cardiac index doubled and the stroke index increased significantly during infusion. In this patient the mean arterial pressure increased while peripheral resistance and mean transit time decreased. The central venous pressure and the heart rate increased. In two patients with Grade II tamponade the cardiac index and the stroke index increased significantly during isoproterenol infusion; the central venous pressure and the mean arterial pressure showed little change; peripheral resistance and mean transit time decreased; the heart rate increased.

DISCUSSION

Data from the present clinical series of cardiac tamponade closely resemble those from prior experimental findings during graded production of hemopericardium in unanesthetized dogs.[4] Three grades of tamponade are recognizable, depending on the volume of intrapericardial blood and the rapidity with which it accumulates. With hemopericardia of 200 ml. or less (Grade I tamponade) hemodynamic abnormalities consisted primarily of tachycardia, slightly decreased stroke volumes, and elevated venous pressures. Hemopericardium of up to 450 ml. in patients with Grade II tamponade was associated with increased central venous pressure, heart rate, and vascular resistance, as well as reduced stroke index and cardiac index; the central venous pressures were less elevated in patients with Grade II tamponade than in patients with Grade I tamponade. This suggests that the absolute level of venous pressure reflects both the adequacy of the transfusion therapy and the severity of the cardiac tamponade. Elevation of systemic vascular resistance may be thought of as a compensatory response which tends to maintain arterial pressures in the face of severely reduced stroke index and cardiac index. Experimentally, it was noted that systemic arterial pressure was maintained until rather late in the course of events by marked vasomotor activity, even in the face of severe degrees of tamponade.[4] The data of the present clinical studies support these observations. In Patient 1 apparently vasomotor activity was severe enough to produce intestinal necrosis. Increased heart rate and central venous pressure compensate for reduced stroke volume and increased ventricular filling pressure.

In these studies Beck's triad was present only in Grade III tamponade. With Grade I or Grade II tamponade, systemic arterial pressure may be normal or only slightly reduced and venous pressure may be elevated depending on the adequacy and rate of transfusion therapy. Chest x-rays and physical findings were not generally helpful. Thus, the diagnosis of tamponade may be based on serial observations of arterial and venous pressures. However, more definitive cardiovascular patterns may be elucidated by hemodynamic monitoring.

The monitoring of intra-arterial and right atrial pressure alone may be of considerable assistance. A graphic representation of femoral arterial and right atrial pressures in Patient 5 is illustrated in Fig. 4. Pulsus paradoxus is clearly evident on the femoral artery tracing, when the changes were too subtle to be felt by palpation of the peripheral arteries. At peak inspiration arterial pressures fall and right atrial pressures simultaneously rise; spikes in the A waves of the atrial pressures are evident. Immediately after inspiration the femoral arterial pressures reached maximum values and atrial pressures decreased. These findings are con-

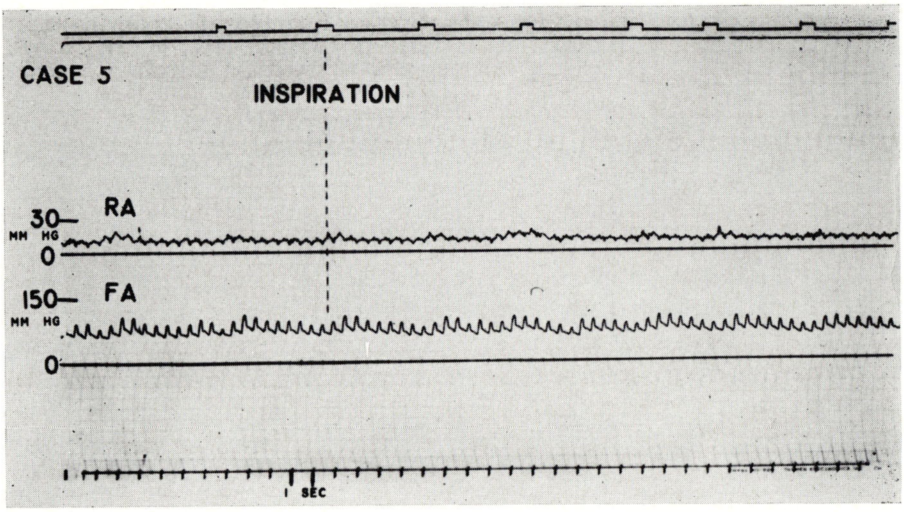

Fig. 4. Right arterial *(RA)* and femoral arterial *(FA)* pressure tracings in Patient 5, showing exaggerated respiratory variation with low, arterial pressure at peak inspiration, and with maximal arterial pressure immediately after inspiration.

sistent with those of Shabetai and colleagues,[7] who noted that, during inspiration, right ventricular pressure and volume rise as venous return to the right heart increases. This results in increased intrapericardial pressure and decreased left atrial filling. Thus systemic arterial pressures are lowest at peak inspiration. Immediately after inspiration venous return to the left side of the heart increases and systemic arterial pressure rises. Pulsus paradoxus, which is suggestive of cardiac tamponade, represents an exaggeration of the normal respiratory variation in systemic arterial pressure.

The response to volume expansion was clearly beneficial in the patients studied. The cardiac index increased approximately 1 L. per minute per square meter in three of four patients; the central venous pressures increased in all. In Patient 6 the blood pressure was initially unobtainable but rose to normal following infusion of 2 L. of normal saline; the cardiac index rose to normal values after the administration of 500 ml. of dextran-40.

Administration of sympathomimetic agents during cardiac tamponade is reported to produce variable effects. Binion and coworkers[2] believed that infusion of vasopressor agents could improve ventricular function during cardiac tamponade by improving the coronary blood flow. We studied the effects of the inotropic agent, isoproterenol, on the hemodynamic patterns of tamponade. The results show that, with Grade I tamponade, where there was essentially no mechanical limitation to blood flow, the isoproterenol response was similar to that observed in normal patients.[3] In Grade II tamponade, where there was significant but not severe limitation of cardiac output, the two patients showed somewhat lesser increases in cardiac index and stroke index during isoproterenol infusion. It would appear that the influence of isoproterenol depends upon the severity of tamponade. It is unlikely that isoproterenol would have a beneficial effect in Grade III tamponade, where severe mechanical limitation to blood flow may militate against the expected inotropic response. The effects of this agent also are dose related; with the use of an infusion rate of 0.103 micrograms per kilogram per minute, there were significant cardiac output responses, arterial pressures increased or were maintained at normal levels, and there were only modest degrees of peripheral vasodilatation in the patients studied.

Pericardiocentesis has been shown to improve hemodynamics both experimentally and clinically.[3, 5, 9] However, in the present series two patients had only modest increases in cardiac output and the third patient had a marked hemodynamic improvement from pericardiocentesis (Patient 2). This patient presented with a Grade III tamponade; following the removal of 40 ml. of liquid blood from the pericardium arterial pressures returned toward normal. It is likely that many a patient with Grade II tamponade has a clotted hemopericardium, which limits the diagnostic and therapeutic effectiveness of pericardiocentesis.

Clinical and hemodynamic observations suggest that compensatory mechanisms do not follow a fixed time course. Patient 2 presented with Grade III tamponade which became Grade I tamponade after removal of a small amount of blood by pericardiocentesis. By contrast, initial monitoring in Patient 8 suggested that Grade I tamponade was present, but over a period of 17 hours there was gradual deterioration to the Grade II stage in which the mean arterial pressure remained normal but the cardiac index and the stroke index decreased markedly.

The effects of volume expansion, decompression into the chest, and myocardial functional changes resulting from prolonged tamponade all serve to illustrate the dynamic nature of acute hemopericardium from penetrating injuries of the heart. In this unstable environment, accurate diagnosis with suitable monitoring techniques, followed by definitive surgery when indicated, would appear to be the most prudent course of action.

SUMMARY

Hemodynamic studies were performed in nine patients with acute cardiac tamponade after penetrating wounds of the heart. The studies were correlated with operative findings. Three grades of tamponade were identified. Grade I tamponade had less than 200 ml. of blood in the pericardial cavity and was characterized by normal or elevated cardiac index, normal or decreased stroke index, normal mean arterial pressure, increased heart rate, and elevated central venous pressure. Grade II tamponade had more than 200 ml. of blood in the pericardial cavity and was characterized by decreased cardiac index and stroke index, normal or slightly decreased mean arterial pressure, and increased central venous pressure. Grade III tamponade had more than 200 ml. of blood in the pericardial cavity and was characterized by severe hypotension, markedly elevated central venous pressure, and the appearance of imminent circulatory arrest. In four patients with Grade I tamponade, the cardiac index averaged 4.4 L. per minute per square meter and the stroke index averaged 41 ml. per square meter. In four patients with Grade II tamponade, the cardiac index and the stroke index averaged 1.75 L. per minute per square meter and 17.5 ml. per square meter, respectively. Pulsus paradoxus was demonstrated on arterial pressure tracings in Grade II and Grade III tamponade, but Beck's triad was present only in Grade III cases. Plasma volume expansion converted Grade III to Grade I tamponade. Infusion of dextran-40 increased the cardiac index significantly in two patients with Grade I and in two patients with Grade II tamponade. Isoproterenol administration was beneficial in Grade II tamponade, particularly when prolonged, but may be deleterious when mechanical limitation to blood flow is severe. Pericardiocentesis was of limited value because of the high incidence of clotted hemopericardium. Diagnosis was facilitated by graphic observation of arterial and venous pressure tracings and hemodynamic monitoring of sequential changes and responses to therapy. In view of the unstable nature of the disease, definitive surgical repair is recommended.

REFERENCES

1. Beall, A. C., Jr., Ochsner, J. L., Morris, G. C., Jr., Cooley, D. A., and De Bakey, M. E.: Penetrating wounds of the heart, J. Trauma 1: 195, 1961.
2. Binion, J. T., Morgan, W. J., Welch, G. H., and Sarnoff, S. J.: Effects of sympathomimetic

drugs in acute experimental cardiac tamponade, Circ. Res. **4:** 705, 1956.
3. Carey, J. S., Brown, R. S., Mohr, P. A., Monson, D. O., Yao, S. T., and Shoemaker, W. C.: Cardiovascular function in shock; responses to volume loading and isoproterenol infusion, Circulation **35:** 327, 1967.
4. Carey, J. S., Yao, S. T., Kho, L. K., Tasche, C., and Shoemaker, W. C.: Cardiovascular responses to acute hemopericardium, compression by balloon tamponade, and acute coronary artery occlusion, J. Thorac. Cardiovasc. Surg. **54:** 65, 1967.
5. Lange, R. L., Botticelli, J. T., Tsagaris, T. J., Walker, J. A., Garni, M., and Bustanante, R. A.: Diagnostic sign in compressive cardiac disorders, Circulation **33:** 763, 1966.
6. Naclerio, E. A.: Penetrating wounds of the heart: Experience with 249 patients, Dis. Chest **46:** 1, 1964.
7. Shabetai, R., Fowler, N. O., Fenton, J. C., and Masangkey, M.: Pulsus paradoxus, J. Clin. Invest. **44:** 1882, 1965.
8. Wilson, R. F., and Bassett, J. S.: Penetrating wounds of the pericardium and its contents, J. A. M. A. **195:** 513, 1966.
9. Yao, S. T., Vanecko, R. M., Printen, K. J., and Shoemaker, W. C.: Penetrating wounds of the heart: A review of 80 cases, Ann. Surg. **168:** 67, 1968.

Hypoxemia during the first twelve hours after battle injury

ROGER V. MOSELEY, M.D.
DONALD B. DOTY, M.D.
WASHINGTON, D. C.
From the Division of Surgery, Walter Reed Army Institute of Research, Walter Reed Army Medical Center

Respiratory insufficiency is often seen after severe trauma even when the lung is not directly injured. Progressive pulmonary failure is an all too familiar experience after the apparently successful treatment of a severe injury, and is the principal cause of in-hospital death in battle casualties in Vietnam.[13] The importance of this problem has been emphasized in a recent symposium of the National Academy of Sciences[5] and a recent book.[8] Our experience with the problem of respiratory insufficiency in battle casualties with chest injury[10] and aspiration pneumonitis[9] has been reported previously.

Arterial hypoxemia occurring soon after injury is evidence of pulmonary insufficiency and may be a premonitory sign of lethal respiratory failure. This report describes observations made on patients who developed arterial hypoxemia within the first 12 hours after combat injury. It is an attempt to identify the causes, characterize the pathophysiologic mechanisms, and evaluate the therapeutic implications of this hypoxemia.

METHODS

During the period of study several thousand patients were admitted to the Third Surgical and Twenty-fourth Evacuation Hospitals in the Republic of Vietnam after combat injury. The more seriously wounded were studied as a guide to treatment, and to obtain further understanding of respiratory insufficiency in battle casualties. These studies were usually performed as soon as the patient arrived in the receiving ward, though in some instances, because of the exigencies of patient care, they were not done until the period after resuscitation. All patients who were found to have a partial pressure of oxygen in arterial blood of less than 80 mm. Hg during the first 12 hours after wounding are included in this report.

Received for publication June 30, 1969.

Blood was drawn from the femoral or brachial artery, and from a catheter placed at the level of the right atrium, for determination of pH and partial pressure of oxygen and carbon dioxide. Expired air samples were collected through a two-way valve into a specially constructed bag and analyzed for oxygen and carbon dioxide tension, and minute volume was measured with a Wright respirometer. These data allowed calculation of the dead space to tidal volume ratio (VD/VT) from the Bohr equation. One hundred percent oxygen was then administered for 15 minutes and arterial and central venous blood again obtained for analysis of gas tension. Physiologic intrapulmonary shunting was calculated as a percentage of cardiac output by a modification of the Fick principle.[10] Studies were repeated throughout the patient's hospital course at appropriate intervals depending on the clinical status. Blood volume was measured by isotope dilution technique with I^{125}-albumin and Cr^{51}-tagged O-negative red blood cells.[12]

RESULTS

There were 58 patients who had a partial pressure of oxygen in arterial blood of less

Table I. *Principal causes of hypoxemia during first 12 hours after wounding in 58 patients*

Type of injury	*No. of patients*
Chest injury	
Penetrating	26
Nonpenetrating	3
Aspiration	
Gastric, definite	4
Gastric, probable	3
Blood	7
Fat embolism	
Probable	3
Possible	3
Overtransfusion	
Without spinal cord injury	1
With spinal cord injury	3
Brain injury	5

than 80 mm. Hg during the first 12 hours after wounding, and they are grouped according to the principal cause of hypoxemia in Table I. It is emphasized that this is a select group of severely injured patients, often with manifest respiratory insufficiency, and these figures must be interpreted accordingly.

Chest injury. The most common cause of early arterial hypoxemia was direct injury to the lung, and a detailed study of these patients has been previously reported.[10] Twenty-six patients had hypoxemia caused by penetrating chest injuries, while three had tangential high velocity missile wounds of the chest wall which produced severe damage to underlying pulmonary parenchyma. The important functional deficit in these patients was physiologic intrapulmonary shunting of blood, which often exceeded 30 percent of the cardiac output and which was related to the extent of pulmonary contusion. Tachypnea, hyperpnea, and increased dead space ventilation were also seen. When the injury was severe enough to warrant it, the most effective treatment was tracheostomy and assisted ventilation, which decreased shunting to such an extent that 40 percent inspired oxygen often produced a higher arterial oxygen tension than the spontaneous breathing of pure oxygen. As the patient recovered there was a progressive decrease in shunt and VD/VT ratio, and an increase in arterial oxygen tension which accompanied radiologic improvement of the lungs.

Comment. There are two principal types of chest injury: hemopneumothorax and pulmonary contusion. From a physiologic point of view these injuries are quite distinct, although in clinical practice they often occur together. The former, exemplified by the small penetrating fragment wound, could be rapidly fatal because of impairment of respiratory mechanics, yet is easily managed with a tube thoracostomy, resulting in minimal physiologic insult. The latter is associated with hemorrhagic atelectasis, and the insult may appear less significant at first. Later, with progressive consolidation, severe hypoxemia may result from intrapulmonary shunting of blood. Tracheostomy and assisted ventilation, by clearing the airway and decreasing the number of nonventilated alveoli, proved most effective in decreasing shunting and improving arterial oxygen tension. Despite rapid initial improvement, however, significant hypoxemia and shunt may persist in some patients for several weeks.

Fat embolism. There were six patients who had arterial hypoxemia attributable to pulmonary fat embolism. Table II shows the findings in these patients, three of whom were considered on clinical grounds to have definite fat embolism (Nos. 1 to 3) and three in whom the diagnosis was considered probable (Nos. 4 to 6). Severe hypoxemia, hypocarbia, increased VD/VT ratio, and cerebral symptoms were seen in all patients thought to have definite fat embolism, and two had petechiae. Fever rising to 103° on the second day was noted in four patients. Of particular interest is the progressive increase of intrapulmonary shunt shown in each patient with definite fat embolism in Fig. 1. This rising shunt paralleled increasing hypoxemia and deteriorating clinical status in these patients, two of whom died. The shunt then slowly decreased in the single survivor, as he recovered. All six patients

Table II. *Respiratory function studies following presumed fat embolism*

Patient	*Injury*	*Arterial pO_2 (mm. Hg)*	*Resp. rate (breath/min.)*	*Min. vol. (L./min.)*	*Shunt (%)*	*VD/VT*	*Temp. (max. °F.)*	*Petechia*	*Cerebral symptoms*
1	Fracture femur and tibia, bilateral	50	44	25.7	21	0.55	103	−	+
2	Fracture right femur and tibia	42	44	58.4	15	0.50	103	+	+
3	Traumatic amputation legs, bilateral	50	30	11.3	17	0.48	103	+	+
4	Traumatic amputation left arm and leg	51	12	—	31	—	103	−	+
5	Fracture femur and ulna	70	15	—	—	—	100	−	−
6	Fracture pelvis with extensive soft tissue destruction	66	26	—	30	—	101	−	−

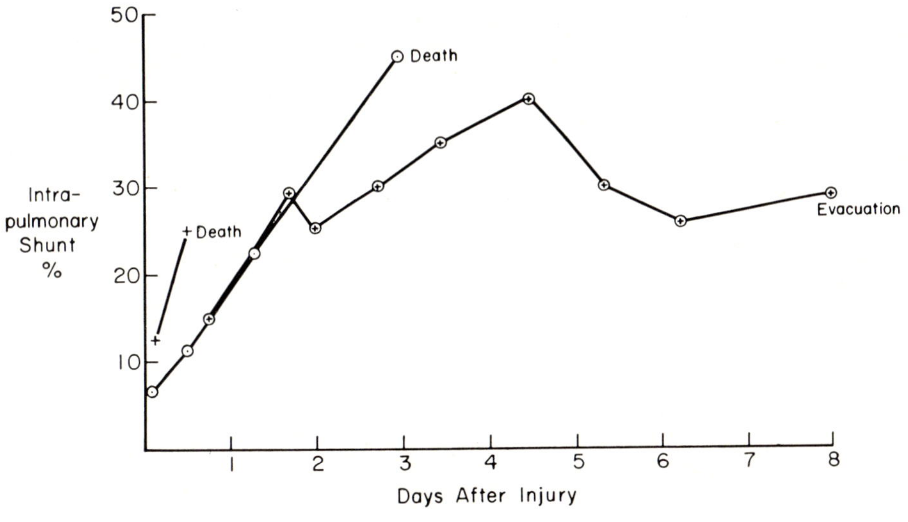

Fig. 1. Intrapulmonary shunting after fat embolism.

had a normal chest x-ray at first, even though hypoxemia was already present. Eventually, a characteristic pulmonary infiltrate occurred in all patients except No. 2, who died before a follow-up chest x-ray was obtained.

Comment. The syndrome of fat embolism is easily recognized in a patient with fever, petechiae, respiratory insufficiency, cerebral symptoms, and a major long bone fracture. Such cases are rare, however, compared with the large number in which the diagnosis is considered, but rejected because of lack of evidence. There were undoubtedly instances of fat embolism overlooked in this study of early posttraumatic hypoxemia since the most marked effects of embolic fat often occur 24 to 48 hours after injury. Collins and associates,[3] in an earlier report from the Surgical Research Team in Vietnam, and Peltier[11] have drawn attention to the existence of arterial hypoxemia, often occult, in patients with major fractures or blast amputations. Most of the patients studied by Collins and associates[3] survived and, as in this study, arterial hypoxemia was often the first clue to the presence of fat embolism. The increasing intrapulmonary shunt and progressive radiologic evidence of pulmonary consolidation are consistent with the concept of fat embolism as a form of "hematogenous lipid pneumonia," in which embolic fat or its breakdown products cause a direct chemical insult to the alveolar-capillary membrane.[11] Eventually, chemically induced edema produces complete alveolar obstruction.

Aspiration. There were 14 patients with hypoxemia attributable to aspiration of foreign substances into the airway: seven that were due to aspiration of gastric contents and seven that were due to blood. Initial observations on the seven patients with aspiration of gastric contents (Table III) showed severe arterial hypoxemia, tachypnea, hyperpnea, increased VD/VT ratio, and significant intrapulmonary shunting of blood. Fever developed in all patients except those treated with corticosteroids. All seven were critically ill and had severe respiratory distress which necessitated tracheostomy and assisted respiration. All showed an initial response to treatment, and except for two who died (one of pneumonia and one of associated wounds) physiologic abnormalities disappeared and chest x-ray cleared over the course of a week.

Seven patients with severe maxillofacial wounds were thought to have aspirated blood. The average pO_2 in this group of patients was 66 mm. Hg, and the average physiologic intrapulmonary shunt was 25

Table III. *Respiratory function studies following aspiration of gastric contents*

Patient	*Arterial pO_2 (mm. Hg)*	*Resp. rate (breath/min.)*	*Min. vol. (L./min.)*	*Shunt (%)*	*VD/VT*	*Typical x-ray changes*
1	42	28	17.7	46	0.49	+
2	43	25	21.1	24	—	+
3	31	36	17.7	51	0.65	+
4	26	46	23.0	55	0.90	+
5	45	36	—	25	—	+
6	53	18	8.1	12	0.42	+
7	39	26	16.0	38	0.45	+

Table IV. *Respiratory function and blood volume studies following overtransfusion*

Patient	*Diagnosis*	*Arterial pO_2 (mm. Hg)*	*Resp. rate (breath/min.)*	*Min. vol. (L./min.)*	*Shunt (%)*	*CVP* (cm. saline)*
1	Brain wound	34	48	20	67	13
2	C_8 spinal cord with chest wound	44	39	13.5	58	17
3	C_4 spinal cord injury	58	32	22	—	16
4	C_7 spinal cord injury and chest wound	59	30	—	45	—

*CVP = central venous pressure.
†TBV = total blood volume.

percent of cardiac output. The physiologic insult appeared minimal, however, as none of these patients had symptomatic respiratory insufficiency, and all recovered rapidly except one who had a severe brain injury.

Comment. It was extremely difficult to be sure when aspiration had actually occurred under the circumstances of combat injury. There were only four patients in whom this could be documented with certainty. One patient gave a reliable history of aspiration, and in one patient food particles were found in the airway at the time of tracheostomy. The other two patients had severe respiratory distress, and one developed cardiac arrest. The cause of their symptoms was unknown and unsuspected until microscopic examination of bronchial fluid demonstrated food particles. The other three patients with presumed aspiration of gastric contents presented only circumstantial evidence of aspiration; vomitus found on clothing and x-ray changes was considered to be quite characteristic. In those patients with maxillofacial wounds the evidence for aspiration of blood was also circumstantial except in one instance where bronchoscopy was needed to remove clots from the bronchi. All had severe bleeding and coughed up blood, and except for one patient with a small chest wound no other explanation for the observed hypoxemia was apparent.

Overtransfusion and quadriplegia. Overtransfusion as the sole cause of hypoxemia was unusual, occurring in only one patient (Table IV, Patient No. 1). Three instances of overtransfusions were associated with quadriplegia, with chest injuries in two, and these factors alone would be expected to produce hypoxemia. However, two of these patients developed bubbling pulmonary edema and another developed bilateral crepitant râles. Evidence of massive bleeding was absent, but all received large volumes of blood and fluid during attempts to restore blood pressure to normal. Measured blood volume averaged 900 c.c. greater than predicted. The volume changes and severe hypoxemia and increased physiologic intrapulmonary shunt associated with the development of pulmonary edema in these patients are seen in Table IV. Although all four patients responded well initially to phlebotomy of 500 to 1,000 ml. and controlled positive-pressure ventilation, the quadriplegic patients subsequently died from complications of their primary wounds and also had progressive pulmonary failure despite respiratory assistance.

Comment. The first patient was a small man who appears to have been the victim of overenthusiastic blood replacement following a relatively small wound. This was a unique situation, for undertransfusion is the rule in these patients when restoration of normal blood pressure and urine output are used as guidelines for volume replacement.[12] Following the total sympathectomy of quadriplegia, however, restoration of nor-

Blood pressure after resuscitation (mm. Hg)	*Pulse (beat/min.)*	*Pulmonary edema, overt*	*Blood infused (ml.)*	*Other fluid infused (ml.)*	*TBV† predicted (ml.)*	*TBV measured (ml.)*
106/78	98	+	4,000	3,500	4,250	5,700
90/75	148	+	4,000	6,000	4,711	5,465
75/—	92	+	1,500	1,500	4,300	5,000
100/70	100	–	3,000	3,500	5,300	6,600

Table V. *Respiratory function studies following severe head injury*

Patient	*Arterial* pO_2 *(mm. Hg)*	*Resp. rate (breath/min.)*	*Min. vol. (L./min.)*	*Shunt (%)*	*VD/VT*
1	40	30	10.0	27	0.52
2	65	35	20.4	26	0.63
3	36	15	9.4	30	—
4	55	25	20.8	50	0.34
5	60	5	6.4	40	0.62

mal blood pressure is clearly an unrealistic objective. In each of these patients the correct clinical diagnosis was at first uncertain, and persistent hypotension was inevitably attributed to hypovolemia. It is noteworthy that the quadriplegic patients continued to have blood volumes ranging from 400 to 1,400 ml. greater than predicted normal for several days after injury, even though the pulmonary edema had cleared. Whether this was a physiologic response to sympathectomy or persistence of the iatrogenic disturbance is uncertain.

Brain injuries. Five patients with hypoxemia had severe brain injuries and died within a few hours of admission to the hospital (Table V). Arterial pO_2 ranged from 36 to 63 mm. Hg and physiologic intrapulmonary shunt from 26 to 50 percent of cardiac output.

Comment. The cause of hypoxemia is hard to ascertain in these patients. In only one instance (Patient No. 5) could it be attributed to hypoventilation resulting from brain injury; all the other patients were hyperventilating and had hypocapnia. Similar observations of hypoxemia and hypocapnia after head injury have been made by Froman.[6] One patient developed pulmonary edema with frothy pink mucus bubbling from the endotracheal tube suggesting that hemodynamic aberrations induced by the brain injury may be a factor.[2] An alternative explanation for the hypoxemia in these unconscious patients is unrecognized aspiration of blood or gastric contents. Although all five patients eventually died of their brain injuries, the very severe hypoxemia was noteworthy because it was clinically unsuspected and in itself a threat to life.

DISCUSSION

It was hoped that by screening patients with blood gas studies on admission it would be possible to identify those with potentially lethal respiratory insufficiency and distinguish characteristic pathophysiologic mechanisms. But, despite the variety of underlying causes, the functional deficits in each group of patients seemed similar, differing in degree rather than kind, and often making it difficult to ascribe a specific cause to the observed symptoms. Respiratory function studies provided an indication of the severity of injury but little indication of its etiology. Apparently, the lung with its simple, fragile architecture, and phylogenetically primitive function of transfer of gases from air to liquid phase, has only limited ways in which it can respond to injury. In virtually all patients described here, the fundamental defect was the filling of alveoli with foreign material with resultant impairment of gas exchange. Persistent perfusion of nonventilated alveoli permitted unoxygenated venous blood to enter the left side of the heart, and produced arterial hypoxemia.

This uniformity of response, regardless of underlying cause, may be the reason for the persistence of the term "traumatic wet lung." Though regarded with universal disdain because of its vagueness, the expression is useful because it describes quite accurately features seen in all patients with posttraumatic respiratory insufficiency, when the lungs become filled with fluid and cease to function effectively. For example, after direct injury to the lung, airway obstruction results from hemorrhage into the alveoli and bronchioles, and is compounded by aspiration of blood into uninjured portions of the lung. Aspiration of gastric contents causes not only mechanical blockage, but an acid-induced inflammatory response with edema and exudation of plasma into the alveoli. Similarly, in fat embolism the demonstrable alveolar obstruction appears to be the result of chemical irritation of the alveolar-capillary membrane by embolic fat. Overtransfusion also fills the alveoli with plasma, once the hydrostatic pressure in the pulmonary capillaries exceeds plasma oncotic pressure. Even after fatal head injury, nonventilation of perfused alveoli is the functional pulmonary defect.

Other changes in pulmonary function, common to all groups of patients, such as increased respiratory rate, minute volume, and dead space ventilation, may be largely a response to arterial hypoxemia or a nonspecific response to severe injury. Contributing factors of varying importance in each group include the rapid shallow antalgic respiration of the patient with chest injury, and the hyperpnea of cerebral dysfunction following head injury or fat embolism.

The common objective of treatment is improvement of arterial oxygenation, and in the light of the above discussion it is apparent why the most effective methods are those which relieve airway obstruction. Even when 100 percent oxygen is breathed spontaneously, the venous admixture resulting from perfusion of nonventilated alveoli is sometimes of such magnitude as to preclude obtaining normal arterial oxygenation. On the other hand, an endotracheal tube or tracheostomy followed by mechanical removal of blood or fluid and assisted ventilation are often dramatically effective. These methods reduce shunting and improve arterial oxygenation by clearing the airway and by forceful insufflation of oxygen into previously nonventilated alveoli. The usefulness of a volume-cycled respirator in the treatment of early pulmonary edema whether it is due to overtransfusion, aspiration or fat embolism, may be the result of alteration of the hydrostatic pressure relationships in the lung decreasing the transudation of fluid into the alveoli.[1] When the alveolar ventilation can be improved by such direct mechanical methods, as is the case in direct lung injury or aspiration, rapid recovery is the rule. Early hypoxemia, caused by fat embolism or a head wound, is usually a manifestation of a severe underlying injury and the mortality rate is high, despite initial improvement in pulmonary function with treatment.

Of interest in this study is the absence of patients with "shock lung." The most likely explanation is that rapid aeromedical evacuation eliminated prolonged episodes of hypotension and, thus, no patients were in shock long enough to develop changes in the lungs. The acute fall in venous oxygen tension which results from decreased cardiac output after hemorrhage may also, theoretically, result in arterial hypoxemia even when pulmonary function is normal.[7] We did not have to invoke this mechanism, although it could have contributed to the hypoxemia of some of the patients described here. Also noteworthy for its absence is pulmonary interstitial edema caused by fluid overload which is often incriminated as a cause of respiratory insufficiency. We have reported[4] that, although severely wounded patients usually receive large sodium and water loads, significant expansion of the extracellular fluid space does not take place until 24 to 48 hours after injury. We observed two patients in whom iatrogenic hypervolemia and pulmonary edema produced severe hypoxemia, but both instances occurred several days after wounding. In limiting this study to instances of hypoxemia occurring within 12 hours after injury, such slowly evolving causes of hypoxemia are excluded.

SUMMARY

Patients with arterial hypoxemia in the first 12 hours after combat injury have been studied. Hypoxemia could be attributed to a variety of familiar causes including direct pulmonary injury, aspiration, fat embolism, overtransfusion, and brain injury, but the underlying functional deficit was the same, i.e., failure of ventilation of perfused alveoli with resultant admixture of venous to arterial blood. Common associated physiologic responses included increase of respiratory rate, minute volume, and dead space/tidal volume ratio.

Chest injury was the most common cause of early arterial hypoxemia, while patients with "shock lung" and electrolyte fluid overload were notable by their absence. Despite the widespread use of large volumes of blood, overtransfusion was rare except in patients with quadriplegia in whom arterial blood pressure was an unreliable guide to blood volume replacement. Aspiration of gastric contents may be easily overlooked and more common than is usually appreciated in critically wounded individuals. Microscopic study of fluid from the trachea or bronchus may establish this critical diagnosis on a firm basis. Fat embolism was also common and, in some instances, the first clue was arterial hypoxemia. Severe head injury may be associated with unsuspected hypoxemia, and once again the only clue is provided by measurement of the gas tension of arterial blood. The most effective treatment for severe hypoxemia, regardless of the primary deficit, was timely use of tracheostomy, attention to removal of fluid and secretions in the airway, and positive-pressure breathing. This reduced the number of nonventilated alveoli and, as a result of the decrease in intrapulmonary shunting, produced improved blood oxygen tensions.

REFERENCES

1. Ashbaugh, D. G., Petty, T. L., Bigelow, D. B., and Harris, T. M.: Continuous positive pressure-breathing (CPBB) in adult respiratory distress syndrome, J. Thorac. Cardiov. Surg. **57:** 31, 1969.
2. Berman, I. R., Ducker, D. B., and Simmons, R. L.: The effects of increased intracranial pressure on the oxygenation of blood, J. Neurosurg. **30:** 532, 1969.
3. Collins, J. A., Gordon, W. C., Jr., Hudson, T. L., Irvin, R. W., Jr., Kelly, T., and Hardaway, R. M., III: Inapparent hypoxemia in casualties with wounded limbs: Pulmonary fat embolism, Ann. Surg. **167:** 511, 1968.
4. Doty, D. B., Hufnagel, H. V., and Moseley, R. V.: The distribution of body fluids following hemorrhage and resuscitation in battle casualties, Surg. Gynec. Obstet. Accepted for publication.
5. Eiseman, B., and Ashbaugh, D. B., editors: Pulmonary effects of nonthoracic trauma, Division of Medical Sciences, National Academy of Sciences, National Research Council, J. Trauma **8:** 621, 1968.
6. Froman, C.: Alterations of respiratory function in patients with severe head injuries, Brit. J. Anaesth. **40:** 354, 1968.
7. Kelman, G. R., Nunn, J. F., Prys-Roberts, C., and Greenbaum, R.: The influence of cardiac output on arterial oxygenation: A theoretical study, Brit. J. Anaesth. **39:** 450, 1967.
8. Moore, F. D., Lyons, J. H., Jr., Pierce, E. C., Jr., Morgan, A. P., Jr., Drinker, P. A. MacArthur, J. D., and Dammin, G. J.: Post traumatic pulmonary insufficiency, Philadelphia, 1969, W. B. Saunders Company.
9. Moseley, R. V., and Doty, D. B.: Physiologic changes due to aspiration pneumonitis, Ann. Surg. Accepted for publication.
10. Moseley, R. V., Doty, D. B., and Pruitt, B. A., Jr.: Physiologic changes following chest injury in combat casualties, Surg. Gynec. and Obstet. Accepted for publication.
11. Peltier, L. F.: Fat embolism: A pulmonary disease, SURGERY **62:** 756, 1967.
12. Simmons, R. L., Heisterkamp, C. A., III, Doty, D. B., and Moseley, R. V.: Post resuscitative blood volumes in battle casualties, Surg. Gynec. Obstet. **128:** 1193, 1969.
13. USARV Surgery Consultants Report 1967-1968.

A simple and accurate manometer for monitoring central venous pressure

GERALD MOSS, PH.D., M.D.
TROY AND ALBANY, N. Y.
From the Biomedical Engineering Curriculum, Rensselaer Polytechnic Institute, and the Department of Surgery, Albany Medical College

Central venous pressure monitoring is now an accepted clinical technique. We developed an instrument that simplifies measurement, while improving accuracy and decreasing the risk of complications.

We previously described a closed-system apparatus for direct intra-arterial pressure monitoring.[1] Fluid pressures are transmitted to an air-filled chamber, averaged, and this latter pressure sensed by a standard sphygmomanometer-type aneroid gauge. It was obvious that venous pressure could be measured with the same device by substituting a more sensitive (by a factor of ten) gauge to detect these lower pressures. Initially, commercially available, sensitive units monitored the venous pressures well. Invariably, they were subjected to excessive pressure, and all were irreparably damaged within days (if not hours). A new aneroid manometer was developed for this application with 1 cm. accuracy over the entire scale of –5 to +50 cm. H_2O. The 1 cm. gradations are easily read. The unit will not malfunction despite high vacuum or ten times "full-scale" overpressure* (Fig. 1).

The right atrium reference level is marked with ink or tape on the patient's lateral chest wall. With the patient horizontal and the unit hand held at the reference level, mean venous pressure is read directly from the dial (Fig. 2). This eliminates inaccuracies related to (1) variations in the "0" refer-

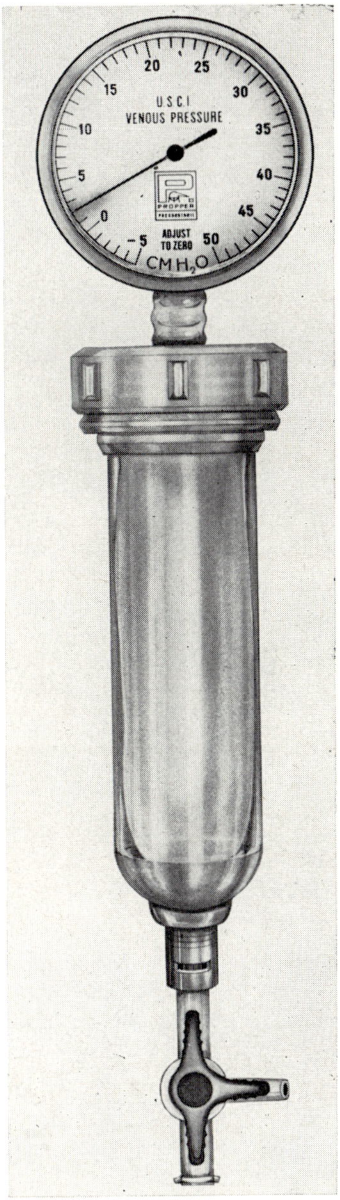

Fig. 1.

Received for publication June 25, 1969.

*Available from United States Catheter & Instrument Corporation, Glens Falls, N. Y.

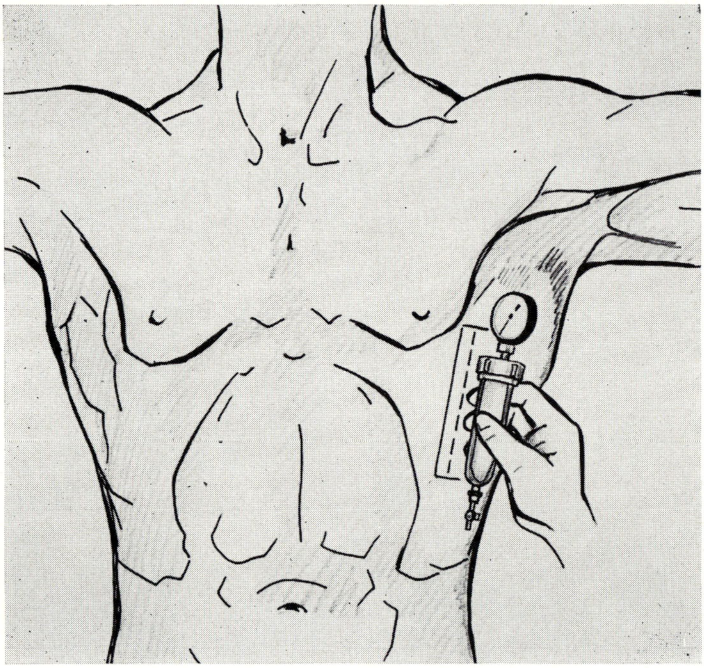

Fig. 2.

ence level; (2) pressure fluctuations with respiration, etc.; (3) misreading the fluid level against a vertical scale.

This closed unit provides additional advantages over conventional techniques that utilize a vertical column of saline, open to the atmosphere. Blood or fluid cannot overflow with subsequent bacterial entry. Similarly, air embolism is obviated. The device is compact, and need not be mounted in any fixed position. A self-contained spring clip fastens it to the bed sheet between readings.

The full hydrostatic head of pressure developed by inflow from an I.V. bottle can be 100 cm. H_2O. Because there is no overflow or gauge damage, a four-way disposable stopcock can be set to interconnect all three ports (I.V. bottle, venous catheter, and pressure monitor). This permits continuous intravenous infusion, minimizing risk of stasis, clotting within the catheter, and expression of an embolus, or the inconvenience of catheter replacement. The fluid inflow line is momentarily occluded. Saline leaves the monitor until its pressure matches that of the vein, the reading is taken, and the infusion resumed.

The device has had extensive use in our experimental laboratories and in community hospitals. It has proved to be a stable "workhorse," well accepted by the medical and nursing personnel.

REFERENCE

1. Moss, G.: A simple, inexpensive unit for direct arterial pressure monitoring, SURGERY **61:** 711, 1967.

Extra-abdominal management of late aortofemoral graft thrombosis

LAWRENCE H. COHN, M.D.
WESLEY S. MOORE, M.D.
ALBERT D. HALL, M.D.*
SAN FRANCISCO, CALIF.
From the Surgical Services, Veterans Administration Hospital and the University of California School of Medicine

Aortofemoral bypass has proved to be an effective method of re-establishing blood flow in cases of aortoiliac occlusive disease. Although the long-term patency of these grafts is greater than 90 percent,[5] late thromboses do occur. In the past the standard approach to this problem has been transabdominal graft replacement.[2] This report presents our experience in eight patients with an extra-abdominal technique for the management of this complication.

CLINICAL MATERIAL

Eight male patients, in whom thrombosis of one limb of an aortofemoral bypass graft occurred, are the subjects of this study (Table I). Their ages ranged from 40 to 70 and averaged 56 years. All were originally operated upon for severe intermittent claudication with angiographic demonstration of extensive aortoiliofemoral arteriosclerosis. Graft occlusions presented 10 days to 6 years after the original graft insertion. Five patients (Cases 1 to 5) presented with a recurrence of claudication and were seen 7 days, 8 days, 6 weeks, 3½ months, and 6 months following graft thrombosis. Three patients (Cases 6 to 8) presented within 48 hours of thrombosis because of threatened limb loss, probably because of extension of thrombus into the distal femoral vessels.

Received for publication June 9, 1969.
*Reprint requests: Veterans Administration Hospital, 4150 Clement St., San Francisco, Calif. 94121.

OPERATIVE TECHNIQUE

All occlusions are documented by translumbar aortography. The distal portion of the thrombosed graft limb and femoral bifurcation is exposed through the previous inguinal incision (Fig. 1, *A*). Systemic heparin is administered. A transverse incision in the distal graft is made, and thrombectomy of the graft limb and femoral vessels is performed with a Fogarty arterial embolectomy catheter (Fig. 1, *B* and *C*). During the initial passage of the catheter, compression of the opposite femoral artery with the palm of the hand minimizes the chance of contralateral embolization. Several passes with the catheter are made until good inflow occurs and no further fragments of thrombi can be obtained. An arteriogram of the graft limb is obtained. If there is residual thrombus this can be loosened by passing a flexible wire loop endarterectomy stripper toward the aorta and then making an additional passage of the embolectomy catheter. The endarterectomy stripper was described in a previous report.[4] This technique can be employed only if one is confident of the strength of the proximal anastomosis. It is not advisable to use undue traction on the graft, particularly if the anastomosis was originally performed with silk suture. The femoral anastomosis is carefully evaluated with intraoperative angiography, and angioplastic procedures are performed when indicated. In the current series this consisted

Table I. *Summary of clinical and operative data*

Case No.	*Age*	*Time after aortofemoral graft*	*Time after thrombosis*	*Outflow procedure*	*Results*
1	56	3 years	3½ months	Interposition of Dacron graft, distal graft limb to profunda femoris artery	Graft opened, relief of claudication
2	40	10 days	8 days	None	Graft opened, relief of claudication
3	52	4 months	6 weeks	Interposition of vein graft between the distal graft limb and the superficial femoral artery	Graft opened, relief of claudication
4	48	3 years	7 days	Profundaplasty	Graft opened, relief of claudication
5	70	6 years	6 months	Excision of false aneurysm	Graft opened
6	66	3 years	48 hours	None	Graft opened, limb salvaged
7	55	8 months	48 hours	Anastomosis to profunda femoris artery reconstructed	Graft opened, limb salvaged
8	66	5 years	48 hours	Anastomosis to profunda femoris artery reconstructed	Graft opened, limb salvaged

of either an end-to-side interposition graft or a reconstruction of the anastomosis to the profunda femoris artery (Table I). Graft patency, the quality of the distal anastomosis, and runoff vessels are then documented by intraoperative angiography.

RESULTS

All thrombosed graft limbs were successfully reopened by the described technique, including the prostheses that had been occluded for 3½ and 6 months. Runoff was re-established in all cases as documented by intraoperative and postoperative arteriography.

In the five patients with claudication the symptoms were ameliorated, and all five have returned to normal activity. Successful thrombectomy avoided the need for amputation in the three patients with threatened limb loss. There were no postoperative deaths or complications.

CASE REPORTS

The following two case histories illustrate the management of delayed graft thrombosis and the relative simplicity and effectiveness of this operative approach.

Case 1. A 56-year-old man had an aortofemoral bypass graft performed at another hospital for severe intermittent claudication 7 years previously. Three years before admission he had an intra-abdominal replacement of a thrombosed right graft limb with an end-to-side anastomosis to the common femoral artery which included the orifice of the profunda femoris. Although in retrospect an intraoperative arteriogram demonstrated persistent stenosis at the distal anastomosis, this was not appreciated at the original operation (Fig. 2, *A*). He was asymptomatic until 3½ months before the current admission, when he developed symptoms of ½ block claudication in his right leg.

Physical examination on admission showed absence of pulses in the right extremity, and aortography documented complete occlusion of the right graft limb.

Reoperation was performed through a right inguinal incision. The graft and profunda femoris artery were dissected free. Old organized thrombus was completely removed with a No. 6 Fogarty embolectomy catheter through a distal transverse incision in the graft. Because the superficial femoral artery had an arteriosclerotic occlusion, an interposition Dacron graft was used to connect the side of the distal graft to the end of the profunda

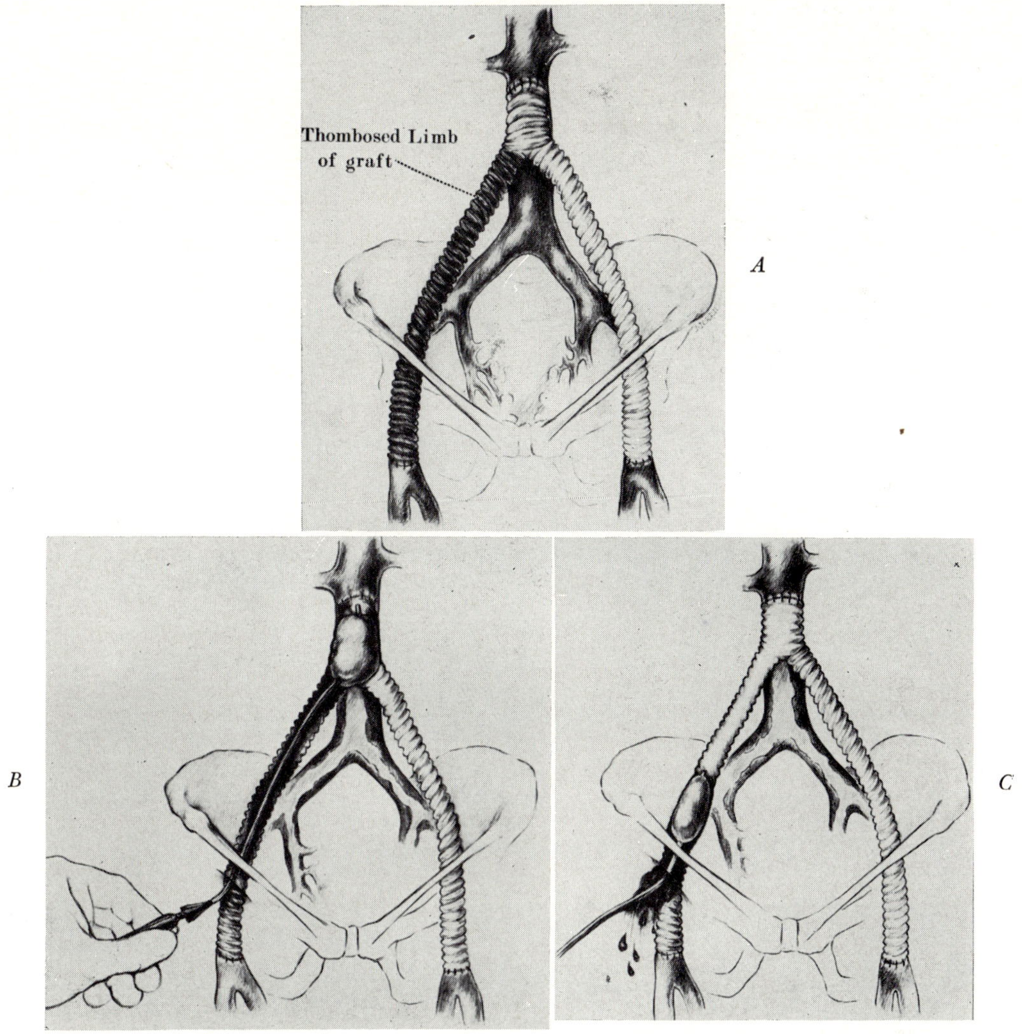

Fig. 1. The technique of extra-abdominal thrombectomy of an aortofemoral bypass graft. *A,* A thrombosed right limb of an aortofemoral bifurcation graft. *B,* Insertion of a Fogarty catheter through thrombus into the patent portion of the bifurcation graft. *C,* Inflated Fogarty balloon; withdrawal of balloon and thrombus through graft incision.

femoris artery. Operative angiography demonstrated excellent runoff (Fig. 2, *B*).

The patient had complete remission of symptoms, developed a collateral pedal pulse on the operated side, and has returned to full-time employment.

Case 2. A 40-year-old man had an aortofemoral bypass graft performed for ½ block claudication. Intraoperative angiography showed a filling defect in the midportion of the left limb, which was not recognized at the time of operation (Fig. 3, *A*). Eight days after the procedure, studies were repeated because of persistent claudication on his left side. Arteriography showed an occluded left graft limb.

Ten days after initial graft insertion, his left groin was re-explored and a thrombectomy of the graft limb was performed. Operative and postoperative angiography demonstrated an open-graft limb without residual thrombus (Fig. 3, *C*). His symptoms were completely relieved.

DISCUSSION

Late thrombosis of a prosthetic graft limb may present either as a recurrence of claudi-

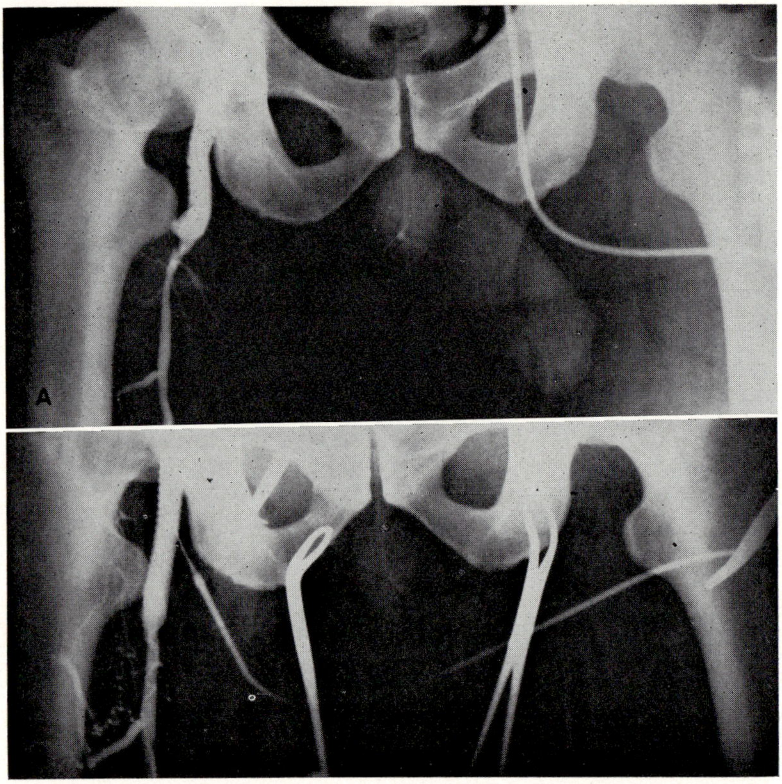

Fig. 2. *A,* Intraoperative arteriogram of aortofemoral graft illustrating stenotic profunda femoris artery. *B,* Intraoperative arteriogram after thrombectomy and interposition graft from distal limb to profunda femoris artery.

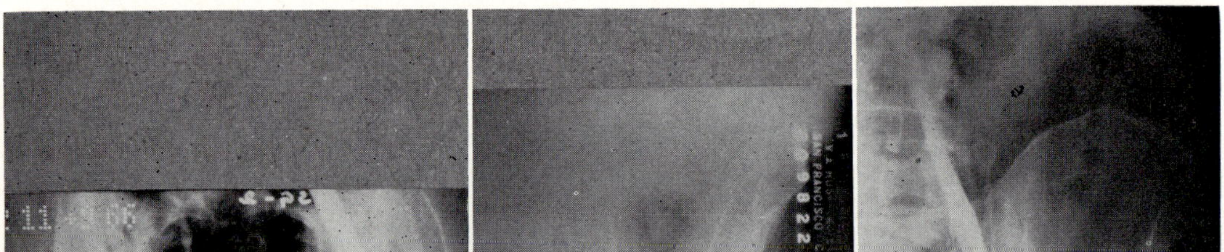

A *B* *C*

Fig. 3. *A,* Intraoperative aortogram of aortofemoral graft. Arrow points to residual unrecognized thrombus in graft limb. *B,* Postoperative aortogram demonstrating thrombosed graft limb. Dye column outlines the external iliac artery. *C,* Intraoperative aortogram after thrombectomy demonstrating open-graft limb.

cation or as threatened limb loss if the thrombus extends into the femoral artery. Characteristically, symptoms and signs of ischemia are so severe on the affected side that surgical revascularization should be carried out without undue delay. Anticoagulation and nonoperative treatment is not a satisfactory form of therapy. With the development of the Fogarty embolectomy catheter,[1] an effective tool is available for the removal of graft thrombus, thus obviating the need for laparotomy and graft replacement. This series of patients demonstrates that the extra-abdominal approach to the revascularization of an occluded graft limb is capable of re-establishing flow, even when the occlusion is as old as 6 months. This technique was successfully used with both Dacron and Teflon grafts, suggesting that the type of graft material is not important to the success of the procedure.

Lyons and Weismann[3] have reported successful blind thrombectomy of late graft thrombosis in 13 of 18 patients, although the thrombectomy technique utilized in their series was not described. They were unable, however, to open grafts occluded 1 to 4 months. In three patients in our series the grafts were successfully opened 6 weeks, 3½ months, and 6 months after thrombosis. That chronically occluded arteries can be reopened has been well shown by the experience with retrograde thrombectomy of the occluded common carotid artery.[4]

One theoretical objection to this technique is the possibility of sending thrombotic fragments down the open contralateral graft limb. This is prevented by external manual compression of the opposite side during passage of the embolectomy catheter. Once the catheter is in the common channel of the bifurcation graft, inflation of the balloon successfully occludes the contralateral limb as the catheter is withdrawn, thus preventing contralateral embolization (Fig. 1, *B*). In addition, as flow is re-established arterial pressure will preferentially propel any fragments of thrombus through the opened distal graft limb.

The causes of graft thrombosis in almost every case were related to technical errors at the original operation, some of which were seen in retrospective analysis of operative angiography. Outflow obstruction was relieved in four of six patients by revising the distal graft anastomosis. Lyons and Weismann[3] concluded that deterioration of distal runoff was responsible for graft thrombosis in 12 of 18 patients. Simple graft thrombectomy without correcting the existing outflow lesions would probably have restored flow for only a short time before the graft rethrombosed. Evaluation of the femoral outflow at the operating table by careful palpation and operative angiography are useful techniques in avoiding both early and late graft thrombosis.

SUMMARY

Eight patients with late thrombosis of aortofemoral graft limbs underwent graft thrombectomy through an extra-abdominal approach with a Fogarty embolectomy catheter. All grafts were successfully opened, including a prosthesis occluded for 6 months. In five patients concomitant reconstruction of stenotic femoral outflow vessels was performed in order to prevent rethrombosis. This technique avoids transabdominal graft replacement and also provides the opportunity to correct existing lesions in femoral outflow vessels.

REFERENCES

1. Fogarty, T. J., and Cranley, J. J.: Catheter technic for arterial embolectomy, Ann. Surg. **161:** 325, 1965.
2. Keshishian, J. M.: Sudden arterial thrombosis occurring in a bypass graft, Surg. Gynec. Obstet. **114:** 763, 1962.
3. Lyons, J. H., Jr., and Weismann, R. E.: Surgical management of late closure of aortofemoral reconstruction grafts, New Eng. J. Med. **278:** 1035, 1968.
4. Moore, W. S., Blaisdell, F. W., and Hall, A. D.: Retrograde thrombectomy for chronic occlusion of the common carotid artery, Arch. Surg. **95:** 664, 1967.
5. Moore, W. S., Cafferata, H. T., Hall, A. D., and Blaisdell, F. W.: In defense of grafts across the inguinal ligament: An evaluation of early and late results of aorto-femoral bypass grafts, Ann. Surg. **168:** 207, 1968.

Metabolic changes in surgical delirium tremens

E. TRUMAN MAYS, M.D.
HERBERT T. RANSDELL, M.D.
BOB M. DeWEESE, M.D.
LOUISVILLE, KY.
From the Department of Surgery and The Price Institute of Surgical Research, University of Louisville, School of Medicine

Delirium following major surgery or trauma is a dreaded complication. Multiple factors contribute to the high mortality rate universally reported. The term delirium tremens has generally been used in discussion of this entity because the symptoms and signs are similar to those seen in alcoholic withdrawal syndromes. It has yet to be demonstrated whether they are the same from a biochemical and physiologic standpoint or whether they are two different entities with common symptomatology. We are using the term posttraumatic delirium to include a broad range of patients on the surgical ward who develop delirium. This terminology refers to patients who have major elective surgical procedures and patients admitted following various forms of trauma who may or may not require surgical treatment in the management of their injury. The symptoms and signs are the same as those seen in the nonsurgical patients with delirium tremens (i.e., severe anxiety, tremulousness, visual and auditory hallucinations, and hyperpyrexia).

The mortality rate of patients with multiple injuries and severe trauma has been greatly reduced by a better understanding of shock and the application of principles gleaned from the research laboratory. Extensive surgical procedures are becoming more and more a part of routine surgical practice. In both these groups it is awesome to stand by helplessly and watch many of these well-managed patients develop delirium and die.

It seemed wise to investigate the biochemical alterations occurring in these patients in order that a more rational approach to the management of this complication can be adopted. Therefore, we began a prospective study of this problem at the University of Louisville Hospitals on the basis of the following observations.

PATHOPHYSIOLOGIC BASIS FOR STUDY

The brains of the patients who are dying with this disease are relatively unremarkable. Except for congestion and varying degrees of edema, there are no anatomic lesions to explain the basis of the cerebral dysfunction.[3, 34] In individuals surviving this complication the delirious state is spontaneously reversible within a short period of time. Full recovery without residual neurologic or psychiatric sequelae is the rule.

The failure to find organic lesions in the brains of patients dying from this disease and the spontaneous and rapid reversibility of the delirium in survivors suggest a dynamic biochemical derangement as the cause of the cerebral dysfunction. It seemed logical to direct our thinking to biochemical processes that are rapidly changeable and that are consistent with the following facts concerning patients with this syndrome.

There is an increased incidence of liver

Supported by Public Health Service Department of Health, Education, and Welfare, Grant GM 13400-01.
Submitted for publication June 4, 1969; resubmitted July 3, 1969.
Reprint requests: 511 South Floyd Street, Louisville, Ky. 40202.

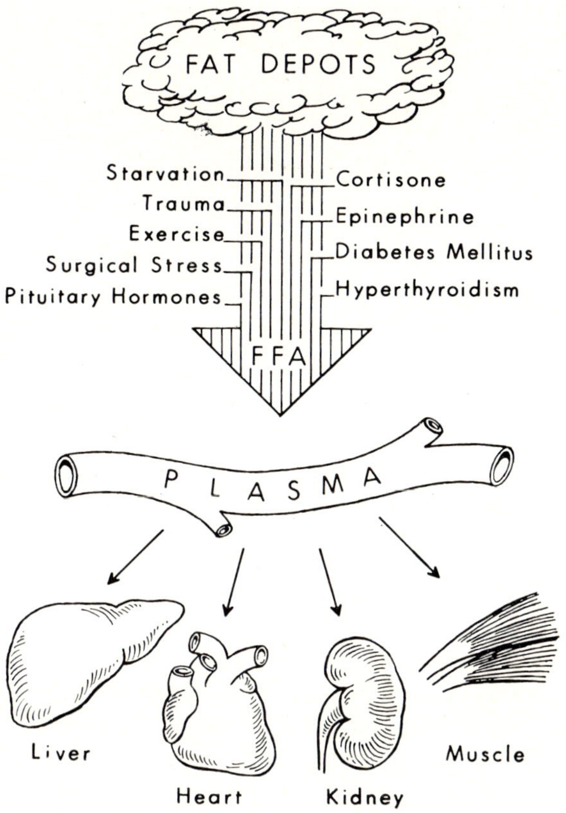

Fig. 1. Fatty acids are mobilized from fat depots to plasma in response to various stimuli.

disease among alcoholics who develop delirium tremens as compared with those who do not.[24] Hepatic abnormalities are common in patients dying with delirium tremens. Tavel and associates[34] found the liver uniformly abnormal in 39 fatal cases. The liver plays a major role in lipid metabolism. The most dynamic fraction of lipid metabolism is the plasma free fatty acid (FFA). One of the important regulatory mechanisms of the liver is the removal of FFA from the plasma and incorporation into hepatic triglycerides.[17, 23, 27, 33]

Chronic alcohol ingestion produces significant alterations in plasma lipids. Beard and Barboriak[2] report a marked decrease of plasma free fatty acids (FFA) and a significant and sustained increase in plasma concentrations of triglycerides, lipid phosphorus, and total cholesterol.

Urinary norepinephrine and epinephrine are significantly elevated in patients with delirium tremens.[14] One of the most potent FFA mobilizers is epinephrine.[18, 31, 32] Catecholamines induce increased lipolysis in adipose tissue with a concomitant increase of plasma FFA.

Plasma FFA also increase after trauma[25, 26, 36, 56] and are mobilized from fat depots by many adipokinetic substances and neurohumoral stimuli (Fig. 1). Plasma FFA are lowered by glucose, insulin, nicotinic acid,[4] and ethanol.[2]

The plasma FFA fulfill the criteria of dynamic biochemical factors that change rapidly with stress and are largely dependent upon hepatic function for their removal from the blood. On the basis of these observations we decided to evaluate plasma FFA levels in patients who develop delirium after operative or traumatic stress, to correlate these with hepatic function, and to compare these FFA levels with those in patients who undergo similar stress but do not develop delirium.

MATERIALS AND METHODS

The clinical material utilized for this study consisted of patients on the surgical and psychiatric wards of the University of Louisville Hospitals. Ninety-one patients were admitted to this prospective study and divided into the following groups.

Group 1, normal controls (24 patients). These were patients with minor problems, medical students, and laboratory technicians who had normal liver function.

Group 2, normal operative controls (24 patients). This group consisted of patients who were admitted for major elective operations and whose liver function was normal. The purpose of this control group was to determine the effect of major surgical stress on plasma FFA levels (e.g., gastric resections, abdominal aortic aneurysmectomy, thoracotomy, etc.).

Group 3, suspect group (38 patients). These patients were admitted to this study group on the basis of past medical histories and physical findings. They had either sustained major trauma or were admitted for elective operation. The presence of one or more of the following criteria was necessary for admission to this group: (1) signs of intoxication on admission, (2) cirrhosis, (3) past episodes of delirium tremens, and (4) continuous heavy ethanol intake prior to admission. None of these patients had delirium at the time of admission and so were considered as potential delirium patients.

Group 4, delirium tremens group (5 patients). This control group consisted of patients admitted directly to the psychiatric ward and who were in overt delirium tremens at the time of admission. Before admission to this group, patients had to have all of the following: (1) heavy alcoholic ingestion and withdrawal, (2) tremulousness, auditory or visual hallucinations, (3) hypermetabolism, (4) rapid and complete recovery without residual mental disorders (i.e., Korsakoff's syndrome, schizophrenia, chronic brain syndrome, etc.).

Liver function was evaluated in the clinical laboratory by standard methods and included the following: serum bilirubin and alakaline phosphatase, total serum protein, albumin and globulin, serum glutamic oxalacetic transaminase, serum glutamic pyruvic transaminase, thymol turbidity, cephalin flocculation, cholesterol, prothrombin time, and Bromsulphalein excretion. Fasting blood glucose, serum ammonia, serum calcium, and electrolytes were determined in appropriate instances to exclude these factors as a cause of cerebral dysfunction. Serum magnesium levels were determined in a small number of cases in which the dietary history was suspicious . After blood samples for FFA were drawn, dehydration was corrected with glucose infusions and serum electrolyte abnormalities corrected as indicated. Patients with elevated blood glucose or family histories of hyperlipemia and hypercholesterolemia were excluded before final analysis of data.

Plasma FFA were determined in the biochemistry section of the Price Surgical Research Laboratories at the University of Louisville. Venous blood was drawn in the fasting state at approximately the same time of day except in those instances in which serial specimens were taken at frequent intervals in the postoperative period. Because a number of these patients had increased blood lactate levels secondary to decreased tissue perfusion, a modification of the Dole and Meinertz[10] technique described by Trout and co-workers[35] to wash out interfering lactate ions and improve specificity was utilized in determining plasma FFA.

RESULTS

The patients in Group 1 ranged in age from 15 to 75 years with an average age of 37. Their plasma FFA ranged from 115 to 661 μEq per liter with a mean of 358 μEq per liter. This corresponds well with fasting venous blood FFA reported in normal individuals.[27, 28]

Group 2 patients ranged in age from 30 to 79 years with an average age of 56. Liver function studies in this group were normal. The purpose of this group was to determine the response of the plasma FFA to surgical stress. The mean elevation between 2 and 6 hours postoperatively is statistically significant ($t = 2.6$, d.f. $= 38$) when compared with the mean plasma FFA of the group preoperatively and is explained by mobilization of lipid in the form of FFA from the fat depots of the body in response to stress. When liver function is normal, the FFA are rapidly incorporated into hepatic triglycerides and the plasma levels return to normal. The heart skeletal muscle and kidney also utilize the excess FFA mobilized during periods of stress.

There were 38 patients admitted to Group 3, the suspect group, on the basis of criteria outlined above. The age range in this group was 24 to 74 years. Twenty patients developed some form of confusion or delirium, and 18 patients recovered without evidence of delirium. We divided this group into subgroups on the basis of delirium.

The first is the suspect group with delirium. Of these 20 patients, nine were eliminated because of associated factors that could be responsible for the delirium (e.g., head injuries, hypoglycemia, cerebral ischemia, etc.). Eleven patients with posttraumatic delirium remained for final statistical analysis.

Table I. *Postoperative serum albumin (mean concentrations) in suspect groups, with and without delirium, and in normal operated control group*

Group	No. of patients	Mean serum albumin (Gm./100 ml.)	S.D.
Operated control patients	14	3.9	0.563
Suspect patients with delirium	10	2.5	0.574
Suspect patients without delirium	11	4.1	0.625

Table II. *Similarity between histologic lesions in lungs of patients dying with elevated FFA and the cytotoxic effect of FFA on lung tissue of animals*

Pathologic changes in lungs of humans dying with elevated plasma FFA and delirium tremens	Pathologic changes in lungs of animals infused with FFA[1, 21]
Focal atelectasis	Alveolar atelectasis
Intra-alveolar hemorrhage	Intra-alveolar hemorrhage
Hyaline membranes	Hyaline membranes
Edema and congestion	Edema

Most of the patients developed delirium some time between the first and fourth days postoperatively. One patient did not develop delirium until the eleventh postoperative day. The mean serum albumin levels are shown in Table I. Serum electrolytes were maintained in normal range with balanced salt solutions. Serum calcium was within normal range. Serum magnesium levels were determined in selected cases and were normal.

There were five deaths in this group. Permission for necropsy was obtained in only two of the five deaths. The pathologist listed massive hyaline membrane disease as the cause of death in both patients. Unfortunately, examination of the brain was not done in either of these two fatal cases. Hepatic abnormalities were present in both: One had acute hepatitis, focal liver cell necrosis, fatty liver, and hepatomegaly, while the other had infarction, acute passive congestion, and fatty infiltration. The most remarkable findings were in the lungs. They are listed in Table II and compared with pathologic changes in the lungs of experimental animals infused with fatty acids.[1, 21] Tavel and colleagues[34] have observed similar pulmonary changes in patients dying in delirium tremens.

When the mean plasma FFA of delirious patients who died are compared with the mean plasma FFA of the survivors (Fig. 2), it can be seen that during the first 24 to 48 hours the plasma FFA of the two groups closely parallel each other, but after this period of time there is a remarkable difference between the survival group and those who died.

The second subdivision is the suspect group without delirium. Of the 18 patients admitted to this study group, seven were excluded either because of diabetes mellitus or insufficient data for statistical analysis. The mean plasma FFA levels in this group are compared with mean FFA in those patients who developed delirium after surgery and in turn both are compared with the normal operated controls after major surgery (Fig. 3). The suspect group with delirium differed from the suspect group without delirium at the 0.01 level of significance ($F = 18$) in regard to mean plasma FFA levels over the first 5 posttraumatic days. The mean plasma FFA levels of patients who developed delirium were significantly elevated ($t = 3.1$, d.f. $= 23$ and $t = 2.9$, d.f. $= 25$, respectively) above the operated control group 24 and 48 hours after major surgery. Mean serum albumin in these patients is compared with the delirious group in Table I. The mean serum albumin of the suspect group with delirium was significantly lower than the normal operated control group ($t = 5$, d.f. $= 22$), and the suspect patients who did not develop delirium tremens ($t = 5$, d.f. $= 17$). The normal operated control group did not differ significantly from the nondelirious sus-

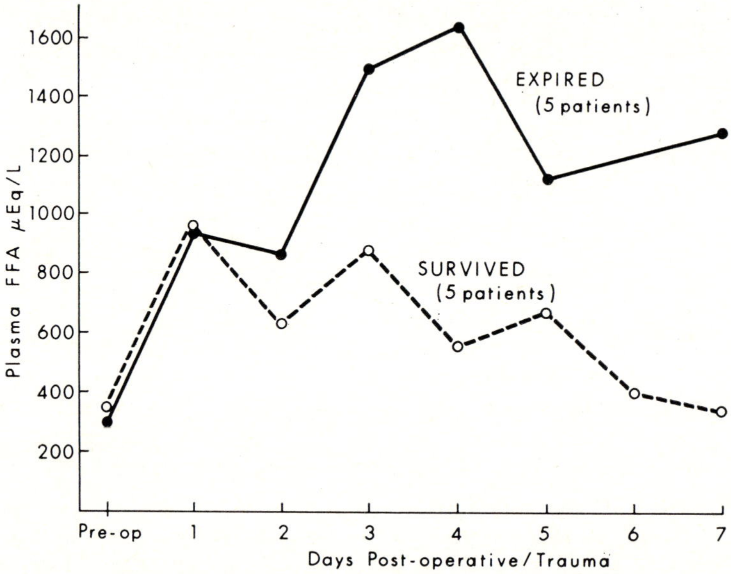

Fig. 2. Mean plasma FFA after operation in three study groups. The normal range is shown by vertical striped lines.

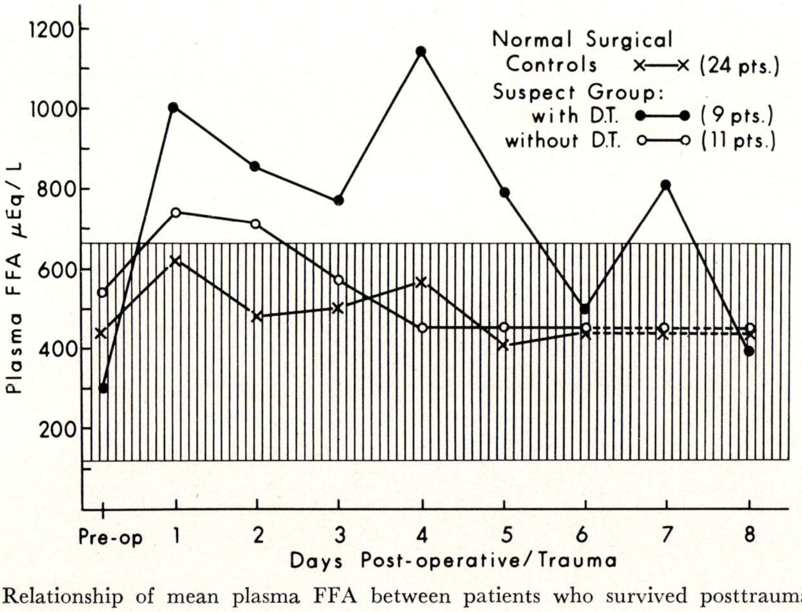

Fig. 3. Relationship of mean plasma FFA between patients who survived posttraumatic delirium and those who died in delirium.

pect patients (t = 1, d.f. = 21) in regard to mean serum albumin.

The patients in the suspect group who developed delirium had a prolongation of the physiologic elevation of FFA that normally follows operative or traumatic stress. That this prolonged elevation of plasma FFA is partially due to failing liver function is seen by the significantly lower serum albumin levels in the delirious group when compared to the nondelirious group and the normal operative control group.

The patients in Group 4 were in overt delirium tremens at the time of admission to the hospital. They had, for various reasons, experienced withdrawal from alcohol and were admitted directly to the psychiatric ward. The five patients in this group ranged in age from 31 to 52 years with an average age of 41. The mean plasma fatty acids upon admission to the psychiatric ward was 1,233 μEq per liter (S.D. = $\pm$390). The third day of hospitalization the mean plasma FFA in this group subsided to 587 μEq per liter (S.D. = $\pm$329) and on the fourth hospital day had decreased even further to a mean of 213 μEq per liter.

The delirium had usually cleared in these patients by the third hospital day, and this corresponded to a return of plasma FFA to normal range. The liver function studies in these patients were not as seriously deranged as those in the surgical group who developed delirium postoperatively. This is probably explained by the fact that hepatic function is decreased significantly by surgery and anesthesia.[13]

The delirium was rapidly reversible in all patients and there was no underlying mental or neurologic disease. One patient had a questionable diagnosis of schizophrenia, but his symptoms and signs of delirium tremens were so classic and so rapidly and completely reversible that he was included in this study.

DISCUSSION

Delirium tremens was first described in 1813, yet for so ancient a disease very little is known of the causative factors and hence of specific methods of treatment. Bowman and Jellinek[3] in 1941 reviewed extensively the theories common at that date relating to the pathogenic mechanisms and the biochemical studies on which they were based. In a classic paper in 1955, Isbell and colleagues[20] clearly demonstrated in humans that at least one of the precipitating factors was the withdrawal of alcohol after chronic intake. Still, the physiologic pathways through which this results in a delirious state are not known.

This study had demonstrated two definite metabolic alterations in patients who develop delirium tremens after operation or trauma. The mean serum albumin is low, and there is a prolonged elevation of plasma FFA. An important function of plasma protein is transporting substances from one part of the body to another in much the same manner that hemoglobin transports oxygen. The affinity of the plasma proteins for a variety of small molecules strongly suggests that this function is extremely useful to the survival of the organism. In particular, the unique affinity of albumin for fatty acids reinforces this view. Albumin prevents some chemotherapeutic agents from exerting their cytotoxic effects on bacteria in the host or in the test tube. The notion of a similar action of albumin with fatty acids in protecting the body's own cells is reasonable.

In plasma systems, fatty acids are not free anions but circulate as an albumin-FFA complex. Some authors prefer the term nonesterified fatty acids (NEFA) or unesterified fatty acids (UFA).[12] Each albumin molecule bears a discrete number of sites to which fatty acids are bound.[15, 16] This unique property of serum albumin serves a useful physiologic function in safely transporting a cytotoxic substance in the blood to various tissues in the body. This mechanism protects cellular function against the toxic effects of FFA.

Plasma free fatty acids are a ready source of energy for cell metabolism. They are utilized through B-oxidation by the myocardium, kidneys, and skeletal muscle.[12, 26] In albumin or plasma free systems they are cytotoxic. FFA uncouple oxidative phosphorylation and lyse erythrocytes. At certain levels of concentration, FFA are thrombogenic.[8, 30]

In addition to these cytotoxic effects there is growing evidence in medical literature of their disruptive effects on living tissue, particularly the lungs. Jefferson and Necheler[21] and Ashbaugh and Uzawa[1] demonstrated intra-alveolar hemorrhage, edema, alveolar atelectasis, and hyaline membranes in the lungs of animals infused with FFA. Similar findings in the lungs of two of our patients who died with elevated plasma FFA were noted, and others have reported similar pulmonary histopathology in patients dying from delirium tremens.[34] Peltier[29] has emphasized the role of FFA in producing the pulmonary lesion of patients and experimental animals dying from fat embolism.

Helinski and Cooper[19] demonstrated a relationship between FFA and albumin on mitochondrial function. They showed that albumin enhances the ability of aged rat mitochondria to carry out oxidative phosphorylation and demonstrated that this function is diminished when the binding sites of albumin are saturated by fatty acids. Davis and Dubos[9] observed that fatty acids were necessary in promoting growth of certain bacteria but, in the absence of albumin, fatty acids inhibited growth. The albumin binds the FFA and prevents its cytotoxic effect, then releases the FFA as needed for nutrition. This combination of cytotoxic and nutritive properties of FFA and the modification of this balance by serum albumin is a rather unique biochemical principle essential for cell function.

The failure of this study to correlate clearing of delirium with lowering of plasma FFA does not exclude this anion as a causative factor. The degree of elevation may not be so important as the time of exposure of the central nervous system and the level of serum albumin. In other instances of cerebral dysfunction, the degree of elevation of plasma constituents cannot always, hour by hour, be correlated with the degree of cerebral dysfunction (e.g., serum ammonia levels in patients with hepatic coma[11]).

The finding of prolonged elevations of FFA in surgical delirium may simply reflect increased catecholamines circulating in these patients as a result of stress. The infusion of norepinephrine produces elevated FFA and increased liver glycerides in animals.[4-6, 32] Increased adrenocortical activity in alcoholics with delirium tremens has also been demonstrated.[22] Both cortisol and trauma increase plasma FFA. The patient with normal liver function assimilates this influx of FFA quite easily, and plasma levels return to normal within 24 hours. However, in patients with liver disease, surgery and trauma further reduce hepatic function and the influx of FFA from adipose tissue causes prolonged elevations. Whether the low serum albumin and the elevated plasma FFA in alcoholics are factors in producing delirium in the postoperative patient is not definitely established by this inchoative study. In any case, the albumin–FFA complex must be thought of as an entity with considerable biological significance.

A number of therapeutic implications are suggested by this study. The first is the administration of serum albumin to correct deficiencies and provide adequate binding sites for the increased plasma FFA, thereby avoiding the cytotoxic properties of these anions. Serum albumin with open binding sites is then available to exert its salubrious effect on mitochondrial function. A second therapeutic consideration is the use of sympathetic blocking agents to prevent the increased mobilization of FFA from adipose tissue and, third, generous quantities of agents that are known to lower plasma FFA levels (that is, glucose, insulin, ethanol, and nicotinic acid) should be administered intravenously.

SUMMARY

Serum albumin is decreased and plasma FFA increased over a prolonged period of time in patients developing delirium after surgical stress as compared with a similar group of patients who do not develop delirium. Hepatic abnormalities are common in both groups. Plasma FFA were also elevated in nonsurgical patients admitted to the psychiatric ward for delirium tremens. FFA have a dual nutritive and cytotoxic role in cellular function and serve as a transport form of lipid. Serum albumin serves a useful physiologic function in safely transporting cytotoxic FFA in the blood to various tissues of the body.

In addition to the usual sedation therapy, sympathetic blocking agents to prevent FFA mobilization and serum albumin to provide binding sites for FFA are suggested in the management of this complication. Generous quantities of substances that lower plasma

FFA (i.e., glucose, insulin, and ethanol) should be administered intravenously.

The technical help of Mrs. Dorothy Anderson is gratefully acknowledged.

REFERENCES

1. Ashbaugh, D. G., and Uzawa, T.: Respiratory and hemodynamic changes after injection of free fatty acids, J. Surg. Res. **8:** 417, 1968.
2. Beard, J. D., and Barboriak, J. J.: Plasma lipids of dogs during and after chronic ethanol administration, Proc. Soc. Exp. Biol. Med. **118:** 1151, 1965.
3. Bowman, K. M., and Jellinek, E. M.: Alcoholic mental disorders, Quart. J. Stud. Alcohol **2:** 312, 1941.
4. Carlson, L. A.: Inhibition of the mobilization of free fatty acids from adipose tissue, Ann. N. Y. Acad. Sci. **131:** 119, 1965.
5. Carlson, L. A., and Liljedahl, S. O.: Lipid metabolism and trauma. I. Plasma and liver lipids during 24 hours after trauma with special reference to the effect of guanethidine, Acta. Med. Scand. **173:** 25, 1963.
6. Carlson, L. A., and Liljedahl, S. O.: Lipid metabolism and trauma. II. Studies on the effect of nicotinic acid on norepinephrine induced fatty liver, Acta. Med. Scand. **173:** 787, 1963.
7. Carpenter, D., Engberg, I., and Lundberg, A.: Blood glucose and plasma unesterified fatty acid changes induced by the stress of an emergency situation, Experientia **18:** 451, 1962.
8. Connor, W. E., Hoak, J. C. M., and Warner, E. D.: Massive thrombosis produced by fatty acid infusion, J. Clin. Invest. **42:** 860, 1963.
9. Davis, B. D., and Dubos, R. J.: The binding of fatty acids by serum albumin, a protective growth factor in bacteriological media, J. Exp. Med. **86:** 215, 1947.
10. Dole, V. P., and Meinertz, H.: Microdetermination of fatty acids, J. Biol. Chem. **235:** 2598, 1960.
11. Egense, J.: Ammonia and hepatic coma, Acta. Med. Scand. **173:** 7, 1963.
12. Fredrickson, D. S., and Gordon, R. S.: Transport of fatty acids, Physiol. Rev. **38:** 585, 1958.
13. French, A. B., Barss, T. P., Fairlie, C. S., Bengle, A. L., Jones, C. M., Linton, R. R., and Beecher, H. K.: Metabolic effects of anesthesia in man, Ann. Surg. **135:** 145, 1952.
14. Giacobini, E., Izikowitz, S., and Wegmann, A.: Urinary norepinephrine and epinephrine excretion in delirium tremens, Arch. Gen. Psychiat. **3:** 289, 1960.
15. Goodman, D. S.: The interaction of human serum albumin with long chain fatty acid anions, J. Amer. Chem. Soc. **80:** 3892, 1958.
16. Goodman, D. S.: Preparation of human serum albumin free of long chain fatty acids, Science **125:** 1296, 1957.
17. Havel, R. J.: Conversion of plasma free fatty acids into triglycerides of plasma lipoprotein fractions in man, Metabolism **10:** 1031, 1961.
18. Havel, R. J.: Some influences of the sympathetic nervous system and insulin in mobilization of fat from adipose tissue: Studies of the turnover rates of free fatty acids and glycerol, Ann. N. Y. Acad. Sci. **131:** 91, 1965.
19. Helinski, D. R., and Cooper, D.: Studies on the action of bovine serum albumin on aged rat liver mitochondria, J. Biol. Chem. **235:** 3573, 1960.
20. Isbell, H., Fraser, H. F., Wikler, A., Belleville, R. E., and Eisenman, A. J.: An experimental study of the etiology of "rum fits" and delirium tremens, Quart. J. Stud. Alcohol **16:** 1, 1955.
21. Jefferson, N. C., and Necheler, H.: Oleic acid toxicity and fat embolism, Proc. Soc. Exp. Biol. Med. **68:** 248, 1948.
22. Kissin, B., Schenker, V., and Schenker, A. C.: Adrenal cortical function and liver disease in alcoholics, Amer. J. Med. Sci. **238:** 344, 1959.
23. Laurell, S.: Recycling of intravenously injected palmitic acid 1-C^{14} as esterified fatty acid in the plasma of rats and turnover rates of plasma triglycerides, Acta. Physiol. Scand. **47:** 218, 1959.
24. Leevy, C. M., Patrylo, I., and Doody, W.: Hepatic abnormalities in alcoholics with delirium tremens, Quart. J. Stud. Alcohol **14:** 568, 1953.
25. Mallov, S., and Witt, P.: Effect of prolonged stress on plasma unesterified fatty acids, Fed. Proc. **19:** 229, 1960.
26. Mayes, P. A.: Blood glucose and plasma unesterified fatty acid changes induced by the stress of an emergency situation, Experientia **18:** 451, 1962.
27. Mayes, P. A., and Fetts, J. M.: Regulation of fat metabolism in the liver, Nature **215:** 716, 1967.
28. Mueller, P.: Free fatty acid concentration (FFA) in chronic schizophrenia before and after insulin stimulation, J. Psychiat. Res. **1:** 106, 1962.
29. Peltier, L. F.: Fat embolism. III. The toxic properties of neutral fat and free fatty acids, SURGERY **40:** 665, 1956.
30. Poole, J. C. F.: Effect of certain fatty acids on the coagulation of plasma in vitro, Brit. J. Exp. Path. **36:** 248, 1955.
31. Rudman, D.: The mobilization of fatty acids

from adipose tissue by pituitary peptides and catecholamines, Ann. N. Y. Acad. Sci. **131:** 102, 1965.

32. Salvador, R. A., Colville, K. I., and Burns, J. J.: Adrenergic mechanisms and lipid mobilization, Ann. N. Y. Acad. Sci. **131:** 113, 1965.
33. Stein, Y., and Shapire, B.: Assimilation and dissimilation of fatty acids by the rat liver, Amer. J. Physiol. **196:** 1238, 1959.
34. Tavel, M. E., Davidson, W., and Batterton, T. D.: A critical analysis of mortality associated with delirium tremens, Amer. J. Med. Sci. **242:** 18, 1961.
35. Trout, D. L., Estes, H. E., Jr., and Friedberg, S. J.: Titration of free faty acids of plasma: A study of current methods and a new modification, J. Lipid Res. **1:** 199, 1959.
36. Wadstrom, L. B.: The effect of trauma on plasma lipids, Acta. Chir. Scand. **115:** 409, 1958.

Antibody localization in horse, rabbit, and goat antilymphocyte sera

NOBORU KASHIWAGI, M.D.
DAVID SHERER, M.D.
COURTNEY M. TOWNSEND, M.D.
ROBERTA JACOBS, M.A.
KEIJI ONO, M.D.
BRIJ KAPUR, M.D.
THOMAS E. STARZL, M.D., PH.D.
DENVER, COLO.
From the Department of Surgery, University of Colorado School of Medicine, and the Veterans Administration Hospital

During the last 3 years, there has been an increasing clinical use of heterologous antilymphocyte sera (ALS) or various globulin fractions (ALG) of these antisera.[4, 15, 17-19, 21, 22] The most commonly used serum donor has been the horse. Numerous efforts have been made to refine the globulin removed from the raw serum for eventual injection so that the ratio of desired equine antibodies to irrelevant protein would be increased. These attempts at purification were based upon evidence from many sources that the immunosuppressive activity of ALS is heavily concentrated in IgG or 7S gamma globulin.[6, 8, 9, 23]

In our own institution, a highly purified horse IgG (ALGG) was given a clinical trial in early 1968 with extremely disappointing results. The ALGG, which was administered in combination with azathioprine and prednisone, appeared to have a reduced ability to mitigate the rejection of renal homografts.[11, 19] A similar loss of efficacy of refined horse ALGG was noted by Clunie and associates[3] in canine experiments.

Supported by United States Public Health Service Grants AM-06344, AM-07772, FR-00051, AI-04152, FR-00069, AM-12148, and AI-AM-08898.

Received for publication June 16, 1969.

As a consequence of these findings, the present study was undertaken to re-evaluate the location of various antibodies as well as the immunosuppressive effect in horse ALS. In addition, the same information about antibody localization was sought for ALS raised in rabbits and goats.

METHODS

Immunization. The immune serum obtained from the three different animals was initially treated in the same way. It was sterilized by millipore filtration, inactivated by heating at 56° C. for 30 minutes, and then stored at 4° C. until testing. However, there were some differences in the details of the prior immunization.

Horse. One horse received subcutaneous injections of 2.5 to 5 $\times$ 10^{10} canine splenic lymphocytes approximately once a week for 9 weeks before bleeding. Two other animals were immunized with human spleen lymphocytes for 6 and 9 weeks, respectively, following the same schedule.

Rabbit. Six New Zealand white rabbits were injected intraperitoneally once a week for 4 weeks with an average of 5 $\times$ 10^9 human spleen lymphocytes per injection. One week after the last immunizing dose, they were bled by heart puncture. The sera from the six rabbits were pooled for analysis.

Goat. Before being bled, one goat was immunized for 12 weeks by the same technique as that described for the horse except that the individual cell doses were 1×10^{10}.

Analysis of proteins. The proteins were separated by DEAE-cellulose column chromatography. Five to 6 ml. of raw ALS were brought to pH 8.0 by dialyzing against 0.01M sodium phosphate; the sera were then applied to a 2 by 20 cm. column containing 20 Gm. of activated DEAE-cellulose* that had been prebuffed to pH 8.0 with 0.01M sodium phosphate and packed under 10 pounds of pressure. The samples were followed through the column by gradient elution with a solution of sodium phosphate that began at pH 8.0 (0.01M) and finished after 900 ml. with pH 4.5 (0.3M). The flow rate through the column was about 1 ml. per minute; 5 ml. were collected in each test tube. The optical densities of the eluates were measured spectrophotometrically at 280 mμ. The collecting tubes containing protein "peaks" were pooled and designated fractions I to VII (horse and rabbit) and I to VI (goat); for subsequent analyses these fractions were lyophilized and reconstituted at 50 times their original concentration.

The total protein concentrations of the raw sera and the various fractions were determined by the biuret method of Henry and co-workers.[7] The presence and quantity of IgG in any of the fractions was detected by the agar immunodiffusion technique† of Fahey and McKelvey.[5] In addition, protein constituents were identified with cellulose acetate membrane electrophoresis‡ and by microimmunoelectrophoresis§ with commercial antisera.||

*Whatman DE32, H. Reede Angel Inc., London, England.

†The antirabbit IgG and antigoat IgG were obtained from Hyland Laboratories, Los Angeles, Calif. The antihorse IgG was raised in rabbits with pure horse IgG.

‡Beckman Instruments, Inc., Fullerton, Calif.

§LKB-Producter AB, Stockholm, Sweden.

||Hyland Laboratories, Los Angeles, Calif.

Lymphocytotoxicity, leukoagglutination, hemagglutination, and thromboagglutination activities of the sera and the protein fractions were determined as described previously,[10] except for one modification in the thromboagglutinin titration. The incubation period for the thromboagglutination was for 6 hours without agitation, instead of for 20 minutes with agitation.

Ammonium sulfate fractionation.

Rabbit and goat ALS. Twenty milliliters of each of the two raw antisera were precipitated with 33, 36, and 40 percent saturated ammonium sulfate (SAS). After reconstituting the sediment to 20 ml. with normal saline, a second precipitation was carried out with the same concentration of SAS as before. The final sediment was then reconstituted to 10 ml. and dialyzed against normal saline before being submitted to analysis by the techniques described in the preceding section.

Horse ALS. The differential ammonium sulfate fractionation of Allen and associates[1] was used to obtain two kinds of horse protein that were rich, respectively, in gamma globulin and T-equine (also known as gamma$_1$ or beta$_2$) globulin. Sixty milliliters of horse ALS were added to the same volume of normal saline and precipitated with 33 percent SAS. The sediment was reconstituted to 60 ml. with normal saline and again precipitated with 33 percent SAS. The final precipitate was reconstituted with normal saline to one third the original serum volume and dialyzed against normal saline. The product was designated as Fraction G.

The supernatant from the first 33 percent SAS precipitation step was precipitated with 50 percent SAS. The precipitate obtained was reconstituted to 60 ml. with normal saline, and a second 33 percent SAS precipitation was performed. This sediment was discarded, and the supernatant was again precipitated with 50 percent SAS. The last precipitate was reconstituted to one third the volume of the original serum and dialyzed against normal saline. The end product was designated as Fraction T.

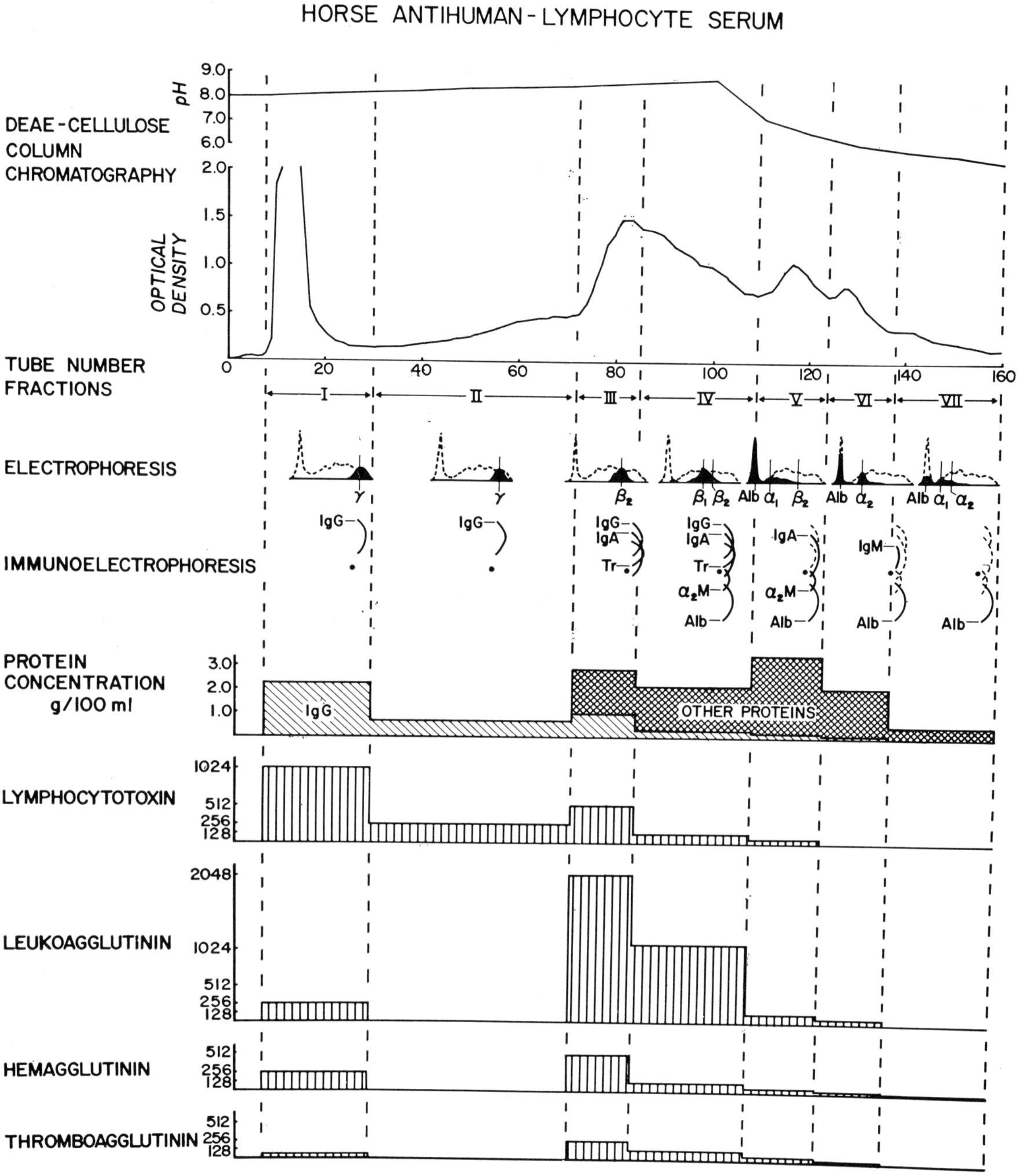

Fig. 1. Analysis of the location of antibodies in the serum of a horse that had been immunized for 6 weeks with weekly subcutaneous injections of human splenic cells. Adjuvant was not used in this or any of the other heterologous serum donors. The multiple analytic techniques shown were used to determine the varieties, concentrations, and activities of the proteins in the different fractions. *Alb* = albumin; α_1 = alpha$_1$ globulin; α_2 = alpha$_2$ globulin; α_2M = alpha$_2$ macroglobulin; β_1 = beta$_1$ globulin; β_2 = beta$_2$ globulin or T-equine; γ = gamma globulin; *IgA* = immunoglobulin A; *IgG* = immunoglobulin G; *IgM* = immunoglobulin M; *Tr* = Transferrin.

In vivo testing. Serum was obtained from the horse that had been immunized for 9 weeks against canine splenic lymphocytes; preliminary absorption was carried out with dog erythrocytes, thrombocytes, and plasma. The above described Fractions G and T were then prepared and either diluted or concentrated so that the gamma globulin and T-equine concentrations, respectively, were equal to those in the original absorbed serum. They were then tested for their ability, when given subcutaneously, to induce

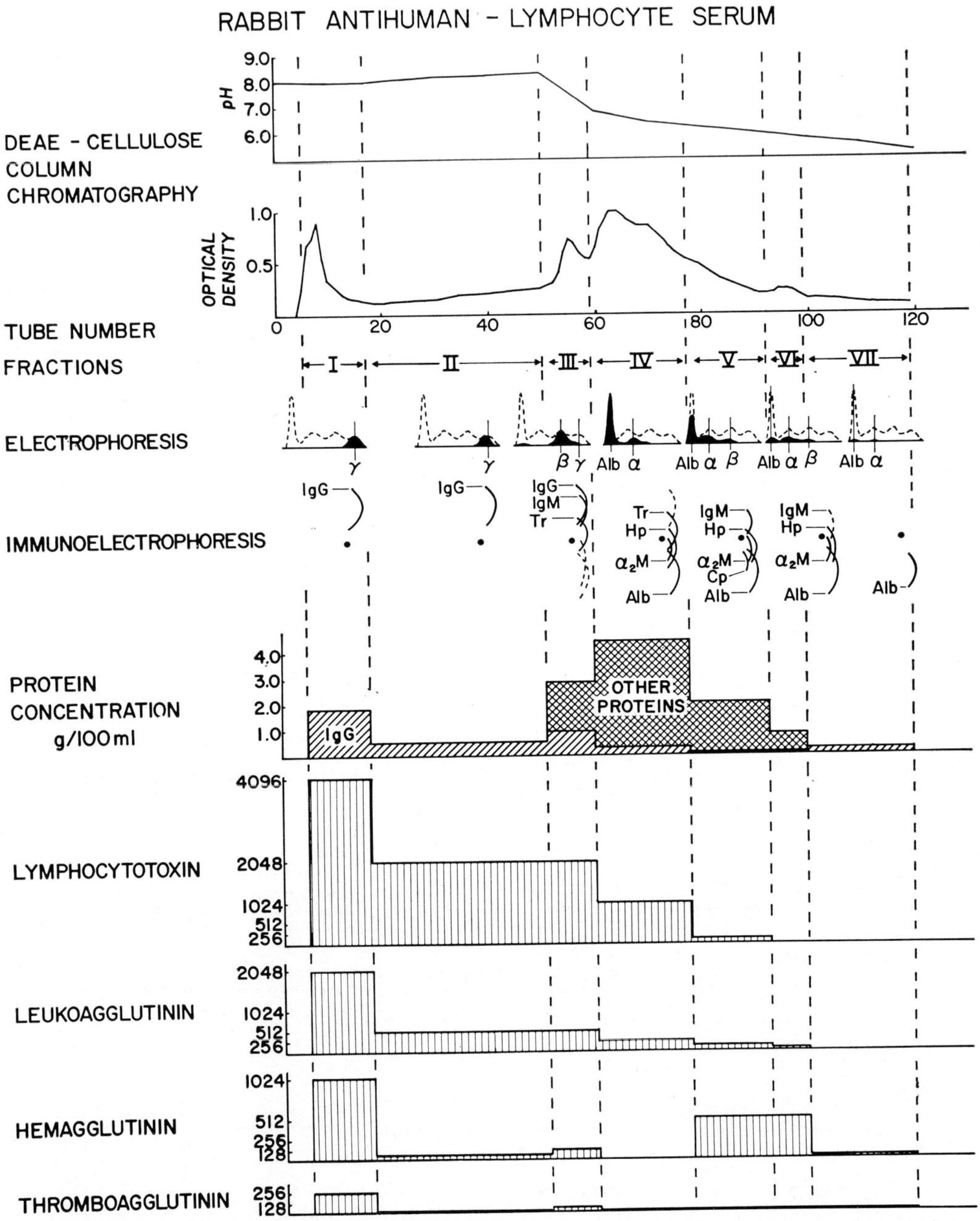

Fig. 2. The localization of antibodies in the pooled sera of six rabbits that had been immunized weekly for 4 weeks with human spleen cells subcutaneously. The protein constituents for which abbreviations were not given in Fig. 1 are *Cp* = ceruloplasmin and *Hp* = haptoglobin.

lymphopenia and to mitigate rejection of renal homografts. The results were compared with those obtained with the use of the absorbed ALS from which the fractions were obtained. Another group of control animals was untreated. All recipient dogs in the three test series were injected daily with 0.5 ml. per kilogram of the appropriate material, beginning 1 day before transplantation and continuing until the day of death.

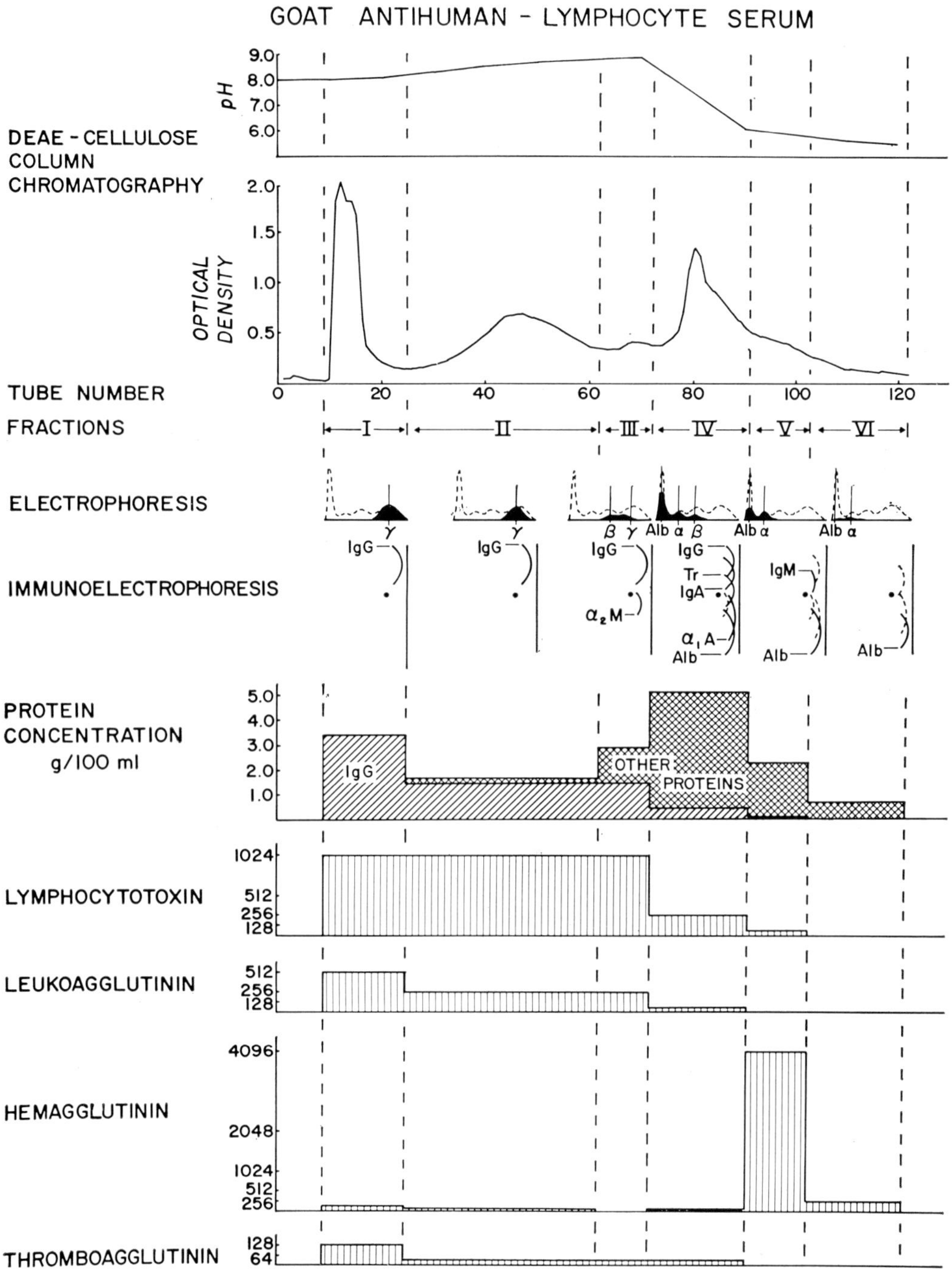

Fig. 3. The antibodies in goat ALS raised with human splenic cells over a period of 12 weeks. The only abbreviation not used in Figs. 1 and 2 is $\alpha_1 A$ = alpha$_1$ A globulin.

Table I. *The protein concentrations and titers of crude globulin obtained by double precipitation with different proportions of saturated ammonium sulfate (SAS)**

	Volume (ml.)	Protein concentration (Gm.%)		Antibodies	
		Total	Gamma	Leukoagglutinin	Lymphocytotoxin
Rabbit ALS	20.0	7.3	3.2	1:1,024	1:4,096
33% SAS	10.5	2.2	1.9	1:1,024	1:2,048
36% SAS	11.8	2.5	2.0	1:1,024	1:4,096
40% SAS	11.7	2.6	1.9	1:1,024	1:4,096
Goat ALS	20.0	7.7	3.6	1:512	1:2,048
33% SAS	11.5	4.9	4.4	1:512	1:1,024
36% SAS	12.5	5.4	4.7	1:512	1:1,024
40% SAS	13.2	5.4	4.5	1:512	1:2,048

*The gamma contribution to the total protein was calculated from electrophoresis scans.

The peripheral lymphocytes were frequently counted.

RESULTS

Chromatography and antibody localization.

Horse ALS. The results were essentially the same in the two horses that were given human splenic tissue as well as in the horse immunized with canine spleen. There were seven protein peaks. The lymphocytotoxic activity was very heavily, if not exclusively, concentrated in the IgG (Fig. 1). This was particularly evident in the pooled Fractions I and II in which only IgG was represented. The lymphocytotoxins in the Fractions III and IV were probably also contained in the IgG which contributed to these heterogenous collections.

In contrast, more than 80 percent of the leukoagglutinins were in the Fractions III and IV which consisted predominantly of IgA (also known as "fast" gamma G, or IgG(T). The hemagglutinins and thromboagglutinins were mostly in the same location, although these antibodies were also detectable in the IgG (Fig. 1).

Rabbit ALS. This antiserum was also separable into seven fractions. However, almost all the measured antibodies were in the IgG (Fig. 2). The only significant spread was of the hemagglutinins which were found in the IgM as well (Fig. 2).

Goat ALS. This goat ALS was separable into six fractions (Fig. 3). The distribution was very similar to that in the rabbit except that the hemagglutinins were almost exclusively in the IgM. The other antibodies were in the IgG.

Ammonium sulfate fractions.

Rabbit and goat ALS. The properties of the crude globulin obtained in both species by double precipitation with 33, 36, or 40 percent SAS are shown in Table I and Fig. 4. With 40 percent SAS, the antiwhite cell titers were fully retained. At 33 percent SAS, there was some loss of lymphocytotoxicity, but the precipitated protein was much less heterogeneous.

Horse ALS. The properties of the Fractions G and T removed by differential ammonium sulfate precipitation were essentially the same with the use of the serum of the two horses immunized with human splenic lymphocytes and with the use of the serum of the third animal which was given canine spleen. Fraction G had a very high proportion of IgG compared with the T-equine content. The Fraction T also contained IgG (Fig. 5), but the predominant immunoglobulin was IgA. Before testing Fraction G for its immunosuppressive effect (see below), it was diluted to give the same gamma globulin content as in the ALS. A similar adjustment was made for the T-equine content of Fraction T. The protein concentrations and the antibody activities of the adjusted fractions are shown in Table II.

In vivo testing. Both the absorbed horse

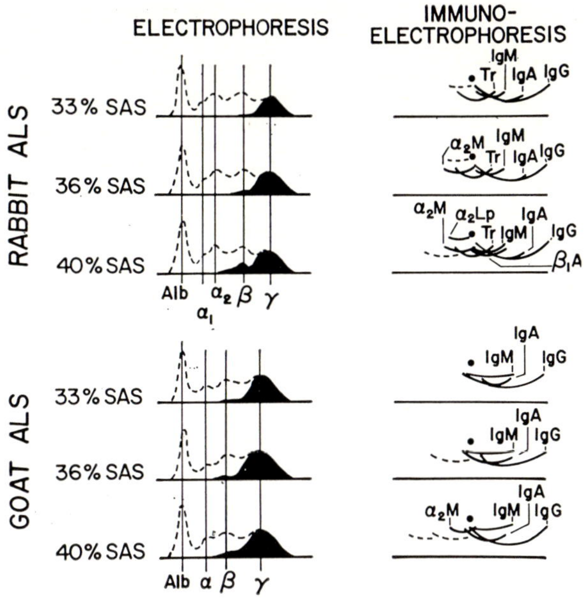

Fig. 4. The electrophoretic and immunoelectrophoretic features of the crude globulin precipitated from rabbit and goat ALS with different percentages of saturated ammonium sulfate (SAS). The only abbreviations not used in Figs. 1 to 3 are $\alpha_2 Lp$ = alpha₂ lipoprotein and $\beta_1 A$ = beta₁ A globulin.

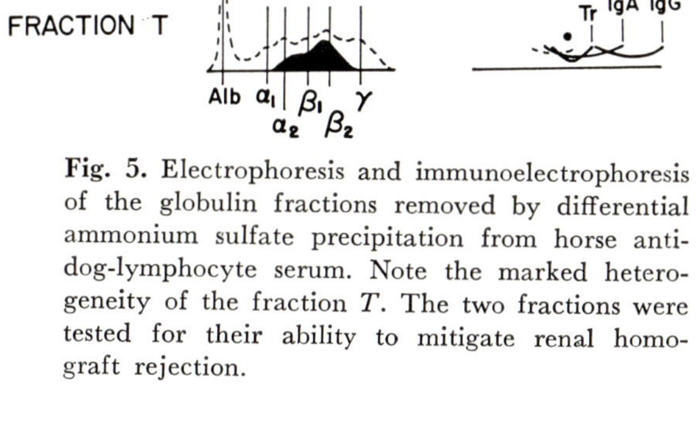

Fig. 5. Electrophoresis and immunoelectrophoresis of the globulin fractions removed by differential ammonium sulfate precipitation from horse anti-dog-lymphocyte serum. Note the marked heterogeneity of the fraction *T*. The two fractions were tested for their ability to mitigate renal homograft rejection.

antidog-lymphocyte serum and the Fraction T removed from it caused prompt lymphopenia with declines of the peripheral lymphocyte counts in dogs to 1,500 mm.^{3} or less. There was a delayed lymphopenia with the administration of Fraction G but to a lesser degree and only after 10 days of continuous treatment.

The results of canine renal homotransplantation between nonrelated mongrel donors and recipients are shown in Table II. Of the 43 transplantations performed, six were eliminated from the analysis because of technical accidents which spoiled the experiments.

The dogs treated with ALS and the Fractions G and T had a significantly longer survival than the animals given no therapy. There seemed to be no difference when ALS and Fraction T ($p > 0.1$) were used, whereas the animals injected with Fraction G lived for somewhat shorter periods ($p < 0.01$).

DISCUSSION

The two animals that have been most commonly used as sources for ALS have been the rabbit and the horse. In the immunized rabbit, there has been little doubt that the antiwhite cell antibodies and the immunosuppressive effect reside in the gamma-G globulin.[9, 12-14, 20] The findings in the pres-

Table II. *Results of canine renal transplantation with whole horse ALS or globulin fractions being*

	Protein concentration (Gm. %)				Antibodies	
	Gamma	T-equine	Beta$_1$, alpha, and albumin	Total	Leukoagglutinin	Lymphocytotoxin
Absorbed ALS	1.7	1.6	3.8	7.1	1:2,048	1:512
Fraction G	1.9	0.7	0.4	3.0	1:512	1:512
Fraction T	0.7	1.6	2.6	4.9	1:2,048	1:256
No treatment						

*By concentration or dilution, it was attempted to give the Fraction G injections the same gamma globulin content as that in the the Fraction T with extraneous protein.

cnt study were in agreement with these earlier investigations in that both the leukoagglutinins and lymphocytotoxins of the rabbit serum were in the IgG. Moreover, essentially all the undesirable thromboagglutinins and the preponderance of the hemagglutinins were in the same location; some hemagglutinin activity also appeared to be in the IgM. The analysis of goat ALS provided almost identical results except that the hemagglutinins were exclusively found in the IgM.

In the horse, a greater spread of the various antibodies has been reported by several authors during the first few months after beginning immunization.[2, 8, 9, 16, 19] Most of these publications contained data indicating that leukoagglutinins or cytotoxins or both were present not only in the IgG ("slow" gamma G) but also in the T-equine globulin of which the principal constituent is IgA or "fast" gamma G; the skin graft experiments of James and Medawar[9] suggested that a Sephadex-separated 7S globulin that may have contained IgA was immunosuppressive. At a later time, after 3 to 11 months of immunization, Pichlmayer and associates[16] showed a shift of the antiwhite cell antibodies to the IgM fraction.

The three horses in the present study which had received splenic cells for 6 to 9 weeks were considered to be early serum donors. Essentially no leukoagglutinins or lymphocytotoxins were in the IgM. However, abundant antibodies were present in the T-equine globulin and, in fact, most of the leukoagglutinins were in this location whereas the lymphocytotoxins were primarily in the IgG. The patterns of localization and the separability of these two kinds of activity were similar to the findings described by Carraz and co-workers.[2]

If, as appears to be the case, there are two distinct kinds of antiwhite cell antibodies in horse ALS, both apparently have immunosuppressive qualities as judged by the canine kidney transplantation experiments that were done using the ALG prepared by differential ammonium sulfate precipitation. The IgA-rich Fraction T which contained high leukoagglutinin but relatively low lymphocytotoxin titers was at least as effective as the IgG-rich Fraction G which had a greater lymphocytotoxicity relative to its leukoagglutinating properties.

The results of these studies have not weakened the generally held proposition that most of the active portion of equine ALS in the first months after the beginning of immunization is 7S gamma globulin. However, they do provide a possible explanation for the loss of potency seen with highly refined horse IgG since this fraction ("slow" gamma G) represents only part of the total activity. The other portion consists of the "fast" gamma G (IgA), so called because of its slightly greater electrophoretic mobility. The IgA, which is buried in the T-equine globulin, is discarded in the process of refinement of IgG. Separation of the IgA from the other components of the heterogenous T-equine globulin and retention of it with the more easily removable IgG is a practical problem which has not yet been satisfactorily solved for mass production.

Such difficulties can be avoided in a num-

*used**

Hemag-glutinin	Thrombo-agglutinin	No. dogs	Survival Mean	Survival Range	Survival S.E.(I)	P value To control	P value To ALS
1:128	1:32	6	20.6	10-50	7.5	<0.01	—
1:128	1:16	10	16.3	9-34	3.3	<0.01	<0.01
1:128	1:32	10	19.4	11-35	3.3	<0.01	>0.1
		11	9.9	5-21	3.5	—	—

ALS doses. A similar adjustment was made for the T-equine content of the Fraction T. Note the high degree of contamination of

ber of other species. For example, the desired immunoglobulins in both the rabbit and goat are in the IgG and in a condensed and relatively isolated segment of the serum, thereby greatly simplifying the methodology for their nearly complete removal in an unadulterated form. The main disadvantage is that large amounts of ALS cannot be so easily raised because of the limiting factor of low blood volume in small serum donors.

SUMMARY

The localization of antibodies was studied in rabbit, goat, and horse ALS raised by weekly immunization with canine or human spleen cells for 4 to 12 weeks. A combination of analytic techniques was used including column chromatography, electrophoresis, immunoelectrophoresis, determination of protein concentration, and measurement of antibody titers.

In the rabbit and goat ALS, virtually all of the leukoagglutinins and lymphocytotoxins were in the easily separable IgG; accidentally induced thromboagglutinins were in the same location. In the rabbit hemagglutinins were found in both the IgG and IgM, whereas in the goat these were almost exclusively in the IgM.

The antiwhite cell antibodies were most widely distributed in the horse. The cytotoxins were primarily in the IgG, but the leukoagglutinins were most heavily concentrated in the T-equine globulin which consists mostly of IgA. By differential ammonium sulfate precipitation of a horse antidoglymphocyte serum, fractions were prepared that were rich in IgG and IgA. Both were able to delay the rejection of canine renal homografts, the IgA-rich preparation to a somewhat greater degree. The findings in this study have been discussed in relation to the refining techniques that have been used for the production of globulin from heterologous ALS.

REFERENCES

1. Allen, P. Z., Sirisinha, S., and Vaughan, J. H.: Immunochemical studies on equine antibodies to human γ_2-globulin, J. Immun. **95:** 918, 1965.
2. Carraz, M., Traeger, J., Fries, D., Perrin, J., Saubier, E., Brochier, J., Veysseyre, C., Prevot, J., Bryon, P., Jouvenceaux, A., Archimbaud, J. P., Bonnet, P., Manuel, Y., Bernhardt, J. P., and Traeger Fouillet, Y.: Préparation, proprietet et activite d'immunoglobulines de cheval antilymphocytes humains, Revue de l'Institut Pasteur de Lyon **1:** 17, 1967.
3. Clunie, G. J. A., Nolan, B., James, K., Watt, J. G., and Woodruff, M. F. A.: Prolongation of canine renal allograft survival with antilymphocytic serum, Transplantation **6:** 459, 1968.
4. Cooley, D. A., Bloodwell, R. D., Hallman, G. L., and Nora, J. J.: Transplantation of the human heart, J. A. M. A. **205:** 479, 1968.
5. Fahey, J. L., and McKelvey, E. M.: Quantitative determination of serum immunoglobulins in antibody-agar plates, J. Immun. **94:** 84, 1965.
6. Fateh-Moghadam, A., Pichlmayr, R., von Schweder, H. W. J., and Knedel, M.: Isolierung immunologisch wirksamer γ-Globuline eines Pferdantihundelymphocytenserums, Klin. Wschr. **45:** 578, 1967.
7. Henry, R. J., Sobel, C., and Berkman, S.: Interferences with biuret methods for serum proteins. Use of Benedict's qualitative glucose

reagent as a biuret reagent, Anal. Chem. **29:** 1491, 1957.

8. Iwasaki, Y., Porter, K. A., Amend, J. R., Marchioro, T. L., Zuhlke, V., and Starzl, T. E.: The preparation and testing of horse antidog and antihuman antilymphoid plasma or serum and its protein fractions, Surg. Gynec. Obstet. **124:** 1, 1967.
9. James, K., and Medawar, P. B.: Characterization of antilymphocytic serum, Nature **214:** 1052, 1967.
10. Kashiwagi, N., Groth, C. G., Amend, J. R., Gecelter, L., Blanchard, H., and Starzl, T. E.: Improvements in the preparation of heterologous antilymphocyte globulin with special reference to absorption and dicthylaminoethyl cellulose batch production, SURGERY 65: 477, 1969.
11. Kashiwagi, N., Groth, C. G., Gecelter, L., Amend, J. R., Blanchard, H., and Starzl, T. E.: A DEAE-cellulose batch technique for antilymphocyte globulin preparation, Surg. Forum **19:** 196, 1968.
12. Mandel, M. A., and Asofsky, R.: The effects of heterologous antithymocyte sera in mice. II. Quantitative evaluation of IgM, IgG, and their subunits in suppressing homograft reactions, J. Immun. **100:** 1259, 1968.
13. Monaco, A. P., Wood, M. L., Gray, J. G., and Russell, P. S.: Studies on heterologous antilymphocyte serum in mice. II. Effect on the immune response, J. Immun. **96:** 229, 1966.
14. Monaco, A. P., Wood, M. L., van der Werf, B. A., and Russell, P. S.: Effects of antilymphocytic serum in mice, dogs, and man, *in* Wolstenholme, G. E. W., and O'Connor, M., editors: Antilymphocytic serum, London, 1967, J. & A. Churchill, Ltd., pp. 111-134.
15. Najarian, J. S., Mcrkcl, F. K., Moore, G. E., Good, R. A., and Aust, J. C.: Clinical use of antilymphoblast serum, Transplantation Proc. **1:** 460, 1969.
16. Pichlmayr, R., Brendel, W., Mikaeloff, P. H., Wiebecke, B., Rassat, J. P., Pichlmayr, I., Bomel, J., Fateh-Moghadam, A., Thierfelder, S., Messmer, K., Descotes, J., and Knedel, M.: Survival of renal and liver homografts in dogs treated with heterologous antilymphocyte serum, *in* Dausset, J., Hamburger, J., and Mathe, G., editors: Advance in transplantation, Baltimore, 1968, The Williams & Wilkins Company, pp. 147-154.
17. Pichlmayr, R., Brendel, W., Tsirimbas, A., Bock, E., Thierfelder, S., Fateh-Moghadam, A., Hornung, B., and Pfisterer, H.: Use of heterologous antilymphocyte sera in man, J. Cardiov. Surg. VIII Congress of the International Cardiovascular Society: 57, 1968.
18. Shorter, R. G., Hallenbeck, G. A., Nava, C., O'Kane, H. O., DeWeerd, J. H., and Johnson, W. J.: Antilymphoid sera in renal allotransplantation, Arch. Surg. (Chicago) **97:** 323, 1968.
19. Starzl, T. E., Brettschneider, L., Penn, I., Schmidt, R. W., Bell, P., Kashiwagi, N., Townsend, C. M., and Putnam, C. W.: A trial with heterologous antilymphocyte globulin in man, Transplantation Proc. **1:** 448, 1969.
20. Thierfelder, S., Moller, D., Fulitz, M., Dormer, P., and Kimura, I.: Antikorperpopulationen im heterologen Antilymphozytenserum des Kaninchens, Klin. Wschr. **46:** 277, 1968.
21. Traeger, J., Carraz, M., Fries, D., Perrin, J., Saubier, E., Bernhardt, J. P., Revillard, J. P., Bonnet, P., Archimbaud, J. P., and Brochier, J.: Studies of anti-lymphocyte globulins made from thoracic duct lymphocytes, Transplantation Proc. **1:** 455, 1969.
22. Woodruff, M. F. A.: Antilymphocyte serum as an immunosuppressive agent, *in* Seiffert, K. E., and Geisendorffer, editors: Transplantation von Organen und Geweben, Stuttgart, 1967, Thieme Verlag, pp. 93-97.
23. Woodruff, M. F. A., James, K., Anderson, N. F., and Reid, B. L.: *In vivo* and *in vitro* properties of antilymphocytic serum, *in* Wolstenholme, G. E. W., and O'Connor, M., editors: Antilymphocytic serum, London, 1967, J. & A. Churchill, Ltd., pp. 57-68.

Hemodynamics and blood gas exchange in allografted canine lungs. I. Immediate effects

KAZUO MOMMA, M.D.
LEONARD M. LINDE, M.D.
ERIC W. FONKALSRUD, M.D.
GARY H. STEVENS, M.D.
DECIO M. RANGEL, M.D.
YOZO YAKEISHI, M.D.
LOS ANGELES, CALIF.
From the Departments of Pediatrics and Surgery, UCLA School of Medicine

Transplantation of the lung is a possible means of therapy for advanced widespread lung disease.[15, 17, 27] In animals, techniques of lung transplantation have been established[4, 17, 19] and long-term survivors over one year have been reported,[5, 17, 22] but data on the functioning of the transplanted lung are still incomplete.

Interruption of the Hering-Breuer reflex[17, 18] is the severe and usually fatal complication of bilateral lung transplantation. Following unilateral lung transplantation, pulmonary edema,[6, 10, 16] venous thrombosis,[12] hemorrhage,[8] and infection[6, 11] are common causes of early death. Total circulatory occlusion time of the transplanted lung has been related to these complications and deaths.[2, 3]

The present studies were undertaken to evaluate pulmonary hemodynamics and blood gas exchange in the dog immediately after left lung transplantation.

MATERIALS AND METHODS

Twenty-two unrelated adult mongrel dogs were used in eleven pairs. The animals were anesthetized with pentobarbital and methoxyfluorane, and respiration was maintained through an endotracheal tube with a Bird respirator. Fifty percent oxygen in room air was used for ventilation. Eight cadaver dogs and three live dogs served as donors (Table I). Cadaver donor dogs were killed by injection of magnesium sulfate prior to removal of the lung. The left lung of the recipient was removed, leaving cuffs of the pulmonary artery, bronchus, and atrium to receive the graft. Simultaneously, the left lung of the donor was removed after systemic heparinization. The anastomosis between the donor and recipient pulmonary veins was performed by means of the atrial cuff technique.[17] The pulmonary artery was then sutured to the cuff of the homologous structure in the recipient by the use of a continuous stitch. For the bronchial anastomosis, continuous everting mattress sutures were placed posteriorly and interrupted mattress stitches anteriorly.

Systemic arterial pressure (SAP), pulmonary arterial pressure (PAP), and left atrial pressure (LAP) were measured through polyvinyl catheters (internal diameter of 1 mm.) connected to pressure transducers.* The zero heights were adjusted to the middle of the chest of the dog. Pulmonary artery pressure and SAP were recorded continuously on a Beckman Type R polygraph recorder. Mean pressure was calculated by the following formula:

$$\text{mean pressure} = \frac{\text{systolic pressure} + 2\ \text{diastolic pressure}}{3}.$$

Blood samples were drawn from the pulmo-

Supported by funds from the United States Public Health Service and the Los Angeles County Heart Association.
Received for publication July 16, 1969.

*Model P23AA, Statham Instrument Co., Los Angeles, Calif.

Table I. *Clinical data in recipient dogs*

Dog No.	*Donor*	*Ischemia time (min.)*	*Survival (days)*	*Autopsy findings in the transplanted lung*
64	Cadaver	92	51	Emphysematous lung; thick scar tissue around PA; scar tissue closed PV*
65	Cadaver	124	0	Pulmonary edema
67	Cadaver	117	1	All vessels patent; cause of death unknown
68	Cadaver	151	26	Atrial thrombosis occluding upper PV; scar-thickening of veins
69	Cadaver	71	14	PA, patent; superior PV obliterated by proximity with suture line; middle vein stenosed; cause of death—rejection
70	Living	62	5	All vessels patent; bronchus disrupted
71	Cadaver	46	5	Atrial thrombosis with incomplete obstruction of PV; cause of death—infection
72	Cadaver	95	43	All PV patent but narrowed by fibrous tissue
73	Cadaver	115	18	PV all occluded by thrombosis
74	Living	120	8	All vessels patent; probably died of bronchial air leak
75	Living	76	> 160	Alive 160 days after transplantation

*PA = pulmonary artery; PV = pulmonary vein.

nary artery and systemic artery catheters simultaneously for measurement of P_{O_2}, P_{CO_2} and pH.* Oxygen saturation of the blood was calculated from P_{O_2} and pH, with reference to the P_{O_2}, pH, and saturation diagram.[23] Pressures and blood samples were measured immediately after thoracotomy in the recipient dog with bilateral normal lungs. Prior to removal of the recipient's left lung, his right pulmonary artery was clamped for one minute and measurements were repeated with all blood flowing through the dog's own left lung. A third measurement was done ten minutes after removal of the recipient left lung, while all blood flowed through the dog's own right lung. The fourth measurement was done ten minutes after completion of the transplantation, while blood flowed through both right and transplanted left lung. Then, the right pulmonary artery was clamped for one minute and, with all blood flowing through the transplanted left lung, pressures and blood gas measurements were repeated. Lungs were hyperinflated frequently to avoid atelectasis, especially after opening anastomoses

*Model 113, pH/Gas Analyzer, Instrumentation Laboratory, Inc., Boston, Mass.

to the transplanted left lung. Total circulatory occlusion time (ischemia time) of the transplanted left lung ranged from 46 to 151 minutes. Postoperatively, azathioprine, 3 mg. per kilogram of body weight, and prednisone, 1 mg. per kilogram, were given initially and these were gradually tapered to 0.25 and 0.50 mg. per kilogram, respectively. Procaine penicillin and kanamycin or chloromycetin were given intramuscularly for one week.

RESULTS

Ischemia time, survival, and pathologic findings. Donor types, ischemia time, survival, and autopsy findings in these 11 dogs are listed in Table I. Ischemia time ranged from 46 to 151 minutes. Survival of ten dogs ranged from zero to 43 days and one dog still survives at the time of writing. Autopsy findings were variable. Pulmonary edema was severe in a dog which died a few hours after operation. Occlusion of pulmonary veins resulting from thrombosis or scar tissue was apparent in six dogs. No case showed stenosis of pulmonary artery or pulmonary veins at the suture lines.

Hemodynamic findings. Pulmonary artery

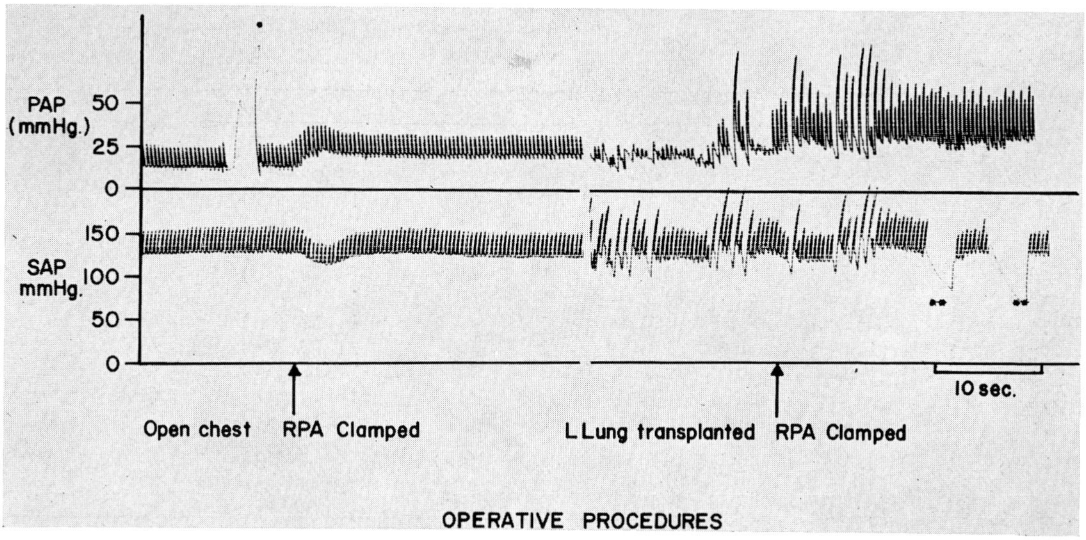

Fig. 1. Pulmonary and systemic arterial pressures (*PAP* and *SAP*) during lung transplantation. Right pulmonary artery was clamped temporarily before and after transplantation of the left lung. •, PAP catheter was flushed; ••, blood sampled from SAP catheter.

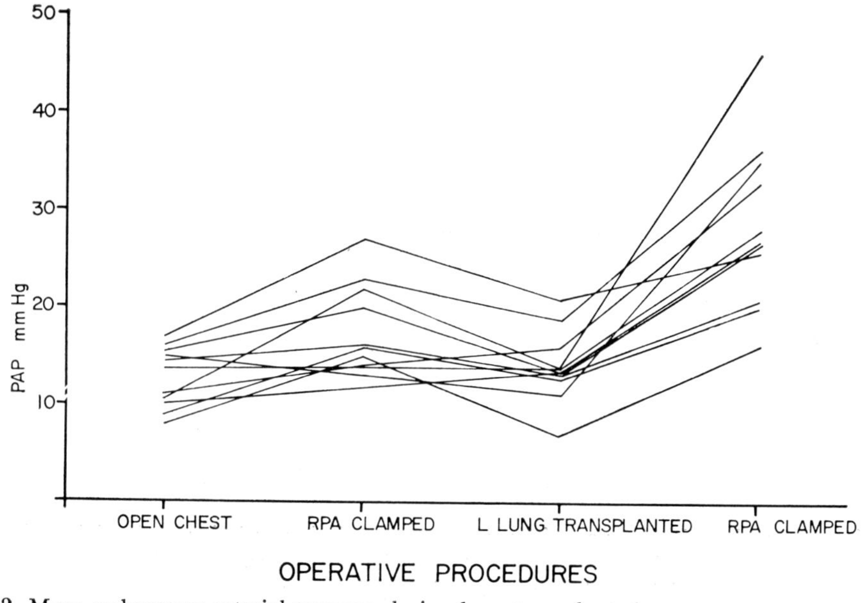

Fig. 2. Mean pulmonary arterial pressure during lung transplantation.

pressures are shown in Figs. 1 and 2 and in Table II. Initially, with bilateral pulmonary blood flow, mean PAP averaged 13 mm. Hg and increased to 19 mm. Hg when the right pulmonary artery was clamped and all blood flowed through the left lung. Pressure returned to the control level after release of the clamp and stayed at the same level after clamping the left pulmonary artery. After the anastomosis, the left pulmonary artery was opened, and PAP was 14 mm. Hg but increased to 29 mm. Hg when the right pulmonary artery was clamped and all blood flow went through the transplanted left lung

Table II. *Main pulmonary arterial pressures in lung homotransplantation experiments*

Dog No.	Before transplantation			After transplantation	
	*Intact PA**	*Clamped right PA*	*Clamped left PA*	*Open PA*	*Clamped right PA*
64	15/7 (10)†		18/8 (11)	24/8 (13)	
65	22/12 (15)		27/11 (16)	16/9 (11)	65/20 (35)
67	15/8 (10)	35/15 (22)	32/9 (17)	22/10 (14)	70/34 (46)
68	17/13 (14)		12/5 (7)	17/12 (14)	45/20 (28)
69	18/13 (15)	27/16 (20)	14/9 (11)	20/10 (13)	38/21 (27)
70	13/5 (8)	25/10 (15)	16/4 (8)	12/5 (7)	26/11 (16)
71	14/7 (9)	21/13 (16)	16/8 (11)	18/11 (13)	25/17 (20)
72	17/8 (11)	20/10 (14)	13/4 (7)	21/13 (16)	43/27 (33)
73	25/13 (17)	40/20 (27)	35/14 (21)	31/16 (21)	44/17 (26)
74	25/9 (14)	27/10 (16)	24/12 (16)	18/11 (13)	33/15 (21)
75	25/12 (16)	32/18 (23)	26/15 (19)	25/16 (19)	54/27 (36)
Average	19/10 (13)	28/14 (19)	21/9 (13)	20/11 (14)	44/21 (29)
S.D.	5/3 (3)	7/4 (5)	8/4 (5)	5/3 (4)	15/7 (9)

*PA = pulmonary artery.
†Numbers in parentheses = mean pressure.

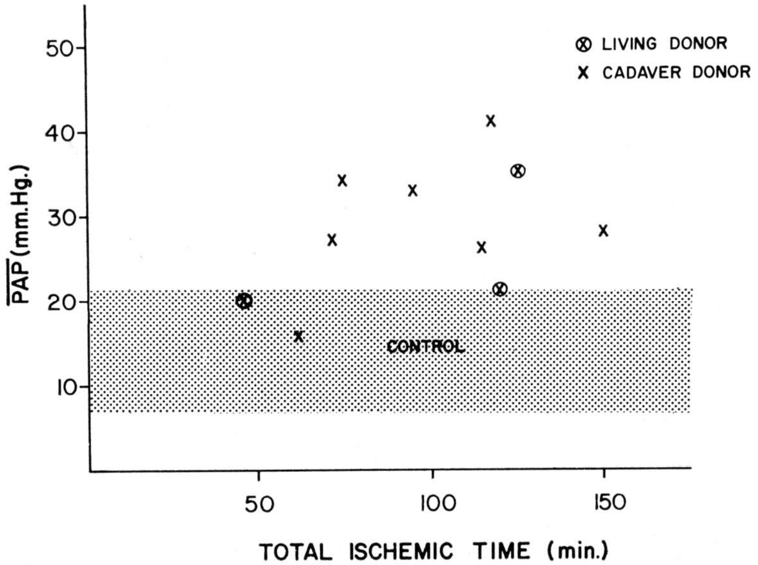

Fig. 3. Mean main pulmonary arterial pressure *(PAP)* during occlusion of the right pulmonary artery after transplantation plotted against total ischemia time. Control pulmonary arterial pressures were obtained by occlusion of the right pulmonary artery before transplantation of the left lung.

(Table II and Fig. 2). Mean PAP in each dog was plotted against ischemia time, or the time the left lung was without perfusion (Fig. 3). The two cases with ischemia time less than 70 minutes showed expected increases in PAP with right pulmonary artery clamping, but the others showed a greater increase in PAP. A regression line between mean PAP with clamping and ischemia times had a positive slope ($Y = 0.1X + 19$), although the correlation coefficient was small ($\gamma = 0.38$).

Systemic arterial pressure was recorded in all studies. The average of these 11 was

Table III. *The Po_2 in arterial and venous blood in lung homotransplantation experiments*

	Pao_2					Pvo_2				
	Before transplant			After transplant		Before transplant			After transplant	
Dog No.	Intact PA	Clamped RPA	Clamped LPA	Open PA	Clamped RPA	Intact PA	Clamped RPA	Clamped LPA	Open PA	Clamped RPA
64	138		94	192	210					
65	180		185	275	350					
67	175	92	210	179	250					
68	260		64	79	70					
69	249	80			130	22	17			24
70	152	53	66	64	220	31	26		33	20
71	181	219	79	75	59	25	28	23	30	26
72	59	31	200	255	265	32	27	41	56	53
73	108	128	230	175	139	37	36	53	42	36
74	56	96	121	145	156	30	40	35	36	38
75	260	235	240	330	295	34	24		36	49
Average	165	117	149	177	195	30	28	38	39	37
S.D.	73	74	71	90	93	5	8	12	9	11

Table IV. *The Pco_2 in arterial and venous blood in lung homotransplantation experiments*

	$Paco_2$					$Pvco_2$				
	Before transplant			After transplant		Before transplant			After transplant	
Dog No.	Intact PA	Clamped RPA	Clamped LPA	Open PA	Clamped RPA	Intact PA	Clamped RPA	Clamped LPA	Open PA	Clamped RPA
64	39		55	47	37	41		58	52	48
65	40		42	32	40	44		47	48	47
67	24	26	21	29	30	27	30	25	34	35
68	21		42	38	41	37		53	50	50
69	19	16			24					29
70	29	33	58	62	40	40	55		66	59
71	24	28	31	40	44	28	28	31	51	52
72	50	54	36	44	43	51	55	36	60	49
73	26	23	19	28	36	29	32	54	34	36
74	36	29	32	24	25	39	33	32	28	27
75	32	40	49	57	55	39	45		60	55
Average	30	31	39	40	38	38	40	42	48	44
S.D.	10	12	13	13	9	8	12	13	13	15

128/98 with standard deviation of ± 18/16 initially. During the operation, four dogs showed mild hypotension with systolic pressure below 100 mm. Hg, but others had stable pressure. Systemic arterial pressure dropped slightly for a few seconds following clamping of the right pulmonary artery but recovered to the original level (Fig. 1). Average SAP in these 11 studies was 103/78 when the right pulmonary artery was clamped and all blood flowed through the recipient's normal left lung, 115/87 when the left pulmonary artery was clamped and all blood flowed through the recipient's right lung, 103/76 when the anastomosis to the transplanted left lung was opened, and 102/74 when the right pulmonary artery was clamped and all blood flowed through the transplanted left lung.

Left atrial pressure was measured in four

dogs. It ranged from 1 to 5 mm. Hg and stayed at the same level during all procedures.

Blood gas and pH measurements. Arterial Po_2 was highly variable from one measurement to another in the same dog, reflecting variable conditions of each lung (Table III). Pao_2 was usually over 130 and in many instances over 200 mm. Hg, when the right pulmonary artery was clamped and all blood flowed through the transplanted left lung. Arterial oxygen saturation was over 98 percent in these cases. In two dogs, Pao_2 was 59 and 70 mm. Hg, and corresponding oxygen saturation was 87 and 88 percent, respectively. The Po_2 in mixed venous blood ranged from 17 to 56 mm. Hg and showed only a small change during these procedures in each dog (Table III).

The Pco_2 in arterial blood and venous blood is listed in Table IV. No particular trend was noticed during the course of transplantation. $Pvco_2$ did not increase with the one-minute occlusion of the right pulmonary artery after transplantation, and adequate venoarterial Pco_2 difference was maintained. Arterial pH, measured in all 11 dogs, fell below 7.20 in two dogs (Dog Nos. 64 and 68) but was fairly constant and between 7.28 and 7.51 in the other nine.

DISCUSSION

Comparison of PAP following right pulmonary artery clamping before and after left lung transplantation gives a rough estimate of the pulmonary vascular resistance (PVR) of the transplanted lung. Although we did not measure cardiac output, minimal changes in SAP and arteriovenous oxygen saturation difference during the operation suggest little change in cardiac output. Left atrial pressure was stable during the operation. Therefore, a greater increase in PAP reflects higher PVR. From an average PAP of 19 mm. Hg with all blood flowing through the dog's own left lung and 29 mm. Hg with all blood flowing through the transplanted left lung, a relative increase of 50 percent in PVR of this transplanted lung can be calculated, constant LAP and cardiac output being assumed. Since PVR decreases as PAP rises,[6, 24] PVR of the transplanted lung would be much higher when exposed to normal PAP. Referring to Rudolph and Auld's data[24] on the relationship of PVR to PAP at fixed levels of pulmonary venous pressure, increase in PAP from 19 to 29 is expected to decrease the PVR about 30 percent passively. Therefore, the net increase in PVR in the transplanted lung is probably much more than 50 percent. Blood flow through the transplanted left lung may be about 20 to 25 percent of the total, instead of 45 percent as in the normal left lung.

This study does not establish the exact cause of the increase in PVR. Stenosis of the pulmonary artery or pulmonary veins at the site of anastomosis was not found in any case at autopsy. Obstruction of pulmonary veins by thrombosis or scar tissue surrounding them was frequently observed at autopsy, but these are probably terminal events and do not play a significant role in the early observations comprising this study. Correlation between higher PAP and longer ischemia time has been reported by several authors.[2, 3] Daly and associates[9] noticed that pulmonary vascular response to hypoxia decreased after lung ischemia longer than 25 minutes. Production of lung surfactant was decreased in the transplanted lung if ischemia time was longer than 70 minutes.[31] The frequency of pulmonary edema and death increased following lung ischemia of more than 30 minutes.[2, 3, 6, 10, 16] Although these data do not elucidate the exact cause of increased PVR, all suggest that increase in vascular resistance is related to changes associated with prolonged ischemia of lung. Persistence of ischemic pulmonary vasoconstriction would be unlikely after ten minutes of 60 percent oxygen ventilation.[26] Perhaps atelectasis[1, 10, 27] and mild pulmonary edema[30] may exist. Rigor mortis of vascular smooth muscle is probably not a significant etiologic factor.[20]

One early complication of lung transplantation in the experimental animal is pulmonary edema, and this proved fatal in one of our dogs. Several factors associated with Starling's[28] hypothesis of edema are probably operative. In the transplanted lung, lymphatic drainage is impaired, as all lymph vessels around the bronchus are disrupted. Vascular permeability may be increased because of ischemic damage.[14] Pulmonary venous obstruction, if present, causes pulmonary edema and hemorrhage.[12] Pulmonary arterial pressure following transplantation usually stays normal in unilateral pulmonary transplantation in a healthy animal,[21, 25, 29] but is increased more or less before transplantation in many clinical candidates for lung transplantation. In cases with preoperative severe pulmonary hypertension, postoperative PAP would be determined mainly by the PVR of the transplanted lung. With pulmonary hypertension with PAP at systemic levels, most blood would flow through the transplanted lung, and pulmonary edema would readily develop.[21] Our data suggest that shorter ischemia time may result in maintenance of the normal vascular resistance of the transplanted lung and may help prevent lung edema.

Measurement of arterial Po_2 is a sensitive method of detecting intrapulmonary arteriovenous shunt. Under our experimental conditions, alveolar Po_2 was about 380 mm. Hg. The difference between alveolar Po_2 and arterial Po_2 is due to intrapulmonary shunts and varied over a wide range in this study. Anesthesia and thoracotomy cause small airway obstruction and atelectasis[3, 27] and probably explain variable arterial Po_2. Pao_2 during the second clamping of the right pulmonary artery with all blood flowing through the transplanted lung was usually higher than Pao_2 with the first clamping of the right pulmonary artery and all blood flowing through the recipient's own left lung. Therefore, the transplanted lung had less intrapulmonary shunting than the recipient's original left lung. This may be due to more frequent, careful inflation of the lung after transplantation and suggests that intrapulmonary shunting can be decreased following lung transplantation by careful inflation of the lung and by administration of oxygen in adequate concentration.

Arterial Pco_2 is an indicator of ventilation. According to our data, carbon dioxide exchange by the transplanted lung was excellent. This is predictable because carbon dioxide is highly diffusible through the alveolar-capillary membrane.

Late studies of hemodynamics and gas exchange in the transplanted lung of long-term survivors are in progress.

SUMMARY

Pulmonary function was studied in 11 dogs subjected to homologous left lung transplantation. Vascular resistances of the recipient's own left lung and transplanted lung were compared by measurement of pulmonary arterial pressure and transient clamping of the right pulmonary artery before and after transplantation. Arterial and venous blood were sampled at each stage for measurement of Po_2, Pco_2, and pH.

Vascular resistance of the transplanted lung was generally increased compared to the recipient's own lungs. A positive correlation was noticed between ischemia time and pulmonary arterial pressure with clamping of the right pulmonary artery after left lung transplantation, and pulmonary arterial pressure was within control levels when ischemia time was less than 70 minutes. Systemic arterial pressure and left atrial pressure were stable during all procedures.

Arterial and venous Po_2, Pco_2, and pH were not significantly altered by homologous lung transplantation in the immediate postoperative period.

REFERENCES

1. Barer, G. R.: Reactivity of the vessels of collapsed and ventilated lungs to drugs and hypoxia, Circ. Res. **18:** 366, 1966.
2. Blades, B.: Ischemia of the lungs, Arch. Surg. **69:** 529, 1954.
3. Blades, B., Pierpont, H. C., Samadi, A., and Hill, R. P.: The effect of experimental lung ischemia on pulmonary function, Surg. Forum **4:** 255, 1963.
4. Blumenstock, D. A., and Kahn, D. R.: Replantation and transplantation of the canine lung, J. Surg. Res. **1:** 40, 1961.
5. Blumenstock, D. A., Collins, J. A., Thomas, E. D., and Ferrebee, J. W.: Functioning

homografts of the lung in dogs, Ann. N. Y. Acad. Sci. **99:** 882, 1962.
6. Blumenstock, D. A., Collins, J. A., Thomas, E. D., and Ferrebee, J. W.: Homotransplants of the lung in the dog, SURGERY **21:** 541, 1962.
7. Borst, H. G., McGregor, M., Whittenberger, J. L., and Berglund, E.: Influence of pulmonary arterial and left atrial pressures on pulmonary vascular resistance, Circ. Res. **4:** 393, 1956.
8. Christiansen, K. H., Buck, A. S., Fanfera, F., Gross, R., Pinch, L. W., Stainback, W. C., and Trummer, C. M. J.: Homologous transplantation of canine lungs, Arch. Surg. **90:** 38, 1965.
9. Daly, I. de B., Michel, C. C., Ramsay, D. J., and Waaler, B. A.: Conditions governing the pulmonary vascular response to ventilation hypoxia and hypoxemia in the dog, J. Physiol. **196:** 351, 1968.
10. Davis, H. A., Gordon, W. B., Hayes, E. W., and Wasley, M. T.: Effects upon the lung of varying periods of temporary occlusion of the pulmonary artery, Arch. Surg. **64:** 464, 1952.
11. Faber, L. P., Kenwell, J. M., and Beattie, E. J.: Homologous lung transplantation, Arch. Surg. **83:** 491, 1961.
12. Fonkalsrud, E. W., Stevens, G. H., and Rangel, D. M.: Physiologic evaluation of allogeneic canine lung transplants from living donors. J. Thorac. Cardiovasc. Surg. **57:** 607, 1969.
13. Gago, O. B.: Proceedings of the International Committee on Lung Transplantation, Dis. Chest **55:** 66, 1969.
14. Hankinson, H. W., and Edwards, F. R.: The effect of pulmonary ischemia on lung function, Thorax **14:** 122, 1959.
15. Hardy, J. D.: Proceedings of the International Committee on Lung Transplantation, Dis. Chest **55:** 66, 1969.
16. Hardy, J. D., Eraslan, S., and Dalton, M. L., Jr.: Autoplantation and homotransplantation of the lung. Further studies, J. Thorac. Cardiovasc. Surg. **46:** 606, 1963.
17. Hardy, J. D., and Alican, F.: Lung transplantation, Advances Surg. **2:** 235, 1966.
18. Hardy, J. D., Eraslan, S., Dalton, M. L., Jr., Alican, F., and Turner, M. D.: Reimplantation and homotransplantation of the lung, Ann. Surg. **157:** 707, 1963.
19. Juvenelle, A. A., Citret, C., Wiles, C. E., Jr., and Stewart, J. D.: Pneumonectomy with replantation of the lung in the dog for physiologic study, J. Thorac. Cardiovasc. Surg. **21:** 111, 1951.
20. Lundholm, L., and Lundholm, E. M.: Length at inactivated contractile elements, length-tension diagram, active state and tone of vascular smooth muscle, Acta Physiol. Scand. **68:** 347, 1966.
21. Nigro, S. L., Riemann, A. F., Mock, L. F., Fry, W. A., Benfield, J. R., and Adams, W. E.: Dogs surviving with a reimplanted lung. Bronchospirometric and pulmonary artery pressure study, J. A. M. A. **183:** 854, 1963.
22. Nigro, S. L., Evans, R. H., Benfield, J. R., Gago, O., Fry, W. A., and Adams, W. E.: Physiologic alterations of cardiopulmonary function in dogs living one and one-half years on only a reimplanted right lung, J. Thorac. Cardiovasc. Surg. **46:** 598, 1963.
23. Rossing, R. G., and Cain, S. M.: A nomogram relating pO_2, pH, temperature, and hemoglobin saturation in the dog, J. Appl. Physiol. **21:** 195, 1966.
24. Rudolph, A. M., and Auld, P. A. M.: Physical factors affecting normal and serotonin-constricted pulmonary vessels, Amer. J. Physiol. **198:** 864, 1960.
25. Rudolph, A. M., Neuhauser, E. B. D., Golinko, R. J., and Auld, P. A. M.: Effects of pneumonectomy on pulmonary circulation in adult and young animals, Circ. Res. **9:** 856, 1961.
26. Rudolph, A. M., and Yuan, S.: Response of the pulmonary vasculature to hypoxia and H^+ ion concentration changes, J. Clin. Invest. **45:** 399, 1966.
27. Sinoi, K., Hayata, Y., Aoki, H., Kozaki, M., Yoshioka, K., Shinoda, A., Iwahashi, H., Ito, M., and Endo, M.: Pulmonary lobe homotransplantation in human subjects, Amer. J. Surg. **111:** 617, 1966.
28. Starling, E. H.: The fluid of the body, Chicago, 1909, W. T. Keener & Company, p. 186.
29. Unpublished data.
30. West, J. B., Dollery, C. T., and Heard, B. E.: Increased pulmonary vascular resistance in the dependent zone of the isolated dog lung caused by perivascular edema, Circ. Res. **17:** 91, 1965.
31. Yakeishi, Y., Nozaki, M., Rangel, D. M., Stevens, G. H., Adams, F. H., and Fonkalsrud, E. W.: Effect of allotransplantation of the canine lung on pulmonary surfactant, Surg. Gynec. Obstet. **128:** 1264, 1969.

The value of dextrans in the treatment of experimental pancreatitis

PHILIP W. WRIGHT
BERNARD GOODHEAD*
TORRANCE AND LOS ANGELES, CALIF.
From the Department of Surgery, Harbor General Hospital, Torrance, and the School of Medicine, University of California, Los Angeles.

Many studies have emphasized the importance of vascular factors in the pathogenesis of acute hemorrhagic pancreatitis.[2, 5] Vascular injury and impaired pancreatic blood flow are considered to be important secondary factors which determine the absorption of enzymes and enzyme products into the circulation and the susceptibility of the pancreas to enzymatic injury.[2] It has been demonstrated that increased and prolonged enzymatic activity is an integral factor in the vascular damage in pancreatitis, which ranges from an alternation of capillary permeability in edematous pancreatitis to a severe necrotizing vasculitis in hemorrhagic pancreatitis.[2, 5]

The vascular abnormalities in edematous pancreatitis are undoubtedly reversible, but under certain circumstances which are not well understood, tissue perfusion may become grossly impaired and hemorrhagic necrosis develops. It seems reasonable to suggest that if stasis and thrombosis within the pancreatic microcirculation were prevented and a satisfactory blood flow maintained, enzymes would continue to be absorbed into the systemic circulation, and the pancreatic injury should then be minimized.

A substance capable of increasing or maintaining tissue perfusion should theoretically be of therapeutic value in pancreatitis. Low molecular weight dextran (Rheomacrodex, Pharmacia Ltd.) with an average molecular weight of 40,000 has aroused considerable interest recently in the treatment of a variety of disorders characterized by stasis and defective circulation.[8]

The results of infusion of this substance are complex but consist essentially of three principal effects, namely, improvement in blood flow by a specific erythrocyte disaggregating effect,[8] increase in plasma volume,[1] and an antithrombotic effect.[7] Initial experiments demonstrated that administration of this substance prevented hemorrhagic pancreatitis from developing, and, therefore, in an attempt to elucidate the relative importance of these three factors, further groups of animals were treated with clinical dextran and with plasma.

METHODS AND MATERIALS

Fifty-eight healthy mongrel dogs weighing from 13 to 19 Kg. were used and each was fasted for 18 hours prior to the experimental procedure. The operations were carried out aseptically under pentobarbital (25 mg. per kilogram of body weight) anesthesia. The duodenum and pancreas were mobilized through an upper midline abdominal incision, and the greater and lesser pancreatic ducts were identified at their site of entry into the duodenum. The lesser duct was ligated. The greater duct was cannulated through a small duodenotomy, and 0.75 ml. per kilogram of a mixture of equal volumes of autologous whole blood and crystallized trypsin (Tryptar, Armour Pharmaceutical,

Submitted for publication July 21, 1969; resubmitted Aug. 26, 1969.

*Reprint address: Department of Surgery, the University of Texas, Medical School at San Antonio, 7703 Floyd Curl Dr., San Antonio, Texas 78229.

Ltd.) 25,000 units per milliliter normal saline, which had been allowed to incubate for 24 hours at 37° C. under sterile conditions, were injected into the duct at a pressure of 140 mm. Hg.[10] Following injection, the greater duct was ligated as the catheter was removed. The duodenotomy and abdominal incisions were closed and the animal was permitted to recover. No antibiotics were administered. Each animal was given a daily maintenance intravenous infusion of 60 ml. per kilogram of dextrose-saline and allocated to one of the following five groups:

Control (normal saline-treated) group (20 dogs). These animals received 10 ml. per kilogram normal saline immediately after operation and every 8 hours subsequently for 3 days, or until death.

Plasma group (11 dogs). These animals received 10 ml. per kilogram of canine plasma immediately after operation and every 8 hours subsequently for 3 days, or until death.

Clinical dextran group (10 dogs). These animals received 1 Gm. per kilogram of clinical dextran (Don Baxter, Inc.), (6 percent in normal saline) immediately after operation and every 8 hours subsequently for 3 days, or until death.

Low molecular weight dextran group (12 dogs). These animals received 1 Gm. per kilogram low molecular weight dextran (10 percent in normal saline) immediately after operation and every 8 hours subsequently for 3 days, or until death.

Delayed treatment with low molecular weight dextran group (5 dogs). These animals received 10 ml. per kilogram normal saline immediately after pancreatitis had been induced. Twelve hours later, treatment with 1 Gm. per kilogram of low molecular weight dextran every 8 hours was started and continued until they either died or were killed at 72 hours.

An autopsy was done on each animal as soon as possible after death or, if survival occurred, 72 hours after pancreatitis had been induced. The gross appearance of the pancreas, the presence of fat necrosis, and the character and amount of peritoneal fluid were noted. Specimens of the head, body, and tail were taken for histological study.

RESULTS

Control (normal saline treated) group. These animals became gravely ill within 8 to 12 hours of induction of pancreatitis. Frequent vomiting and progressive prostration leading to death within 30 hours occurred in over 75 percent. All animals died within 72 hours, with a mean duration of survival of only 26 hours.

At autopsy, a variable amount of dark purple serosanguinous fluid (150 to 300 ml.) was present in the peritoneal cavity. The peripancreatic tissues showed marked edema and often fat necrosis. Hemorrhagic pancreatitis, often severe in degree and affecting mainly the head and body, was present in each animal (Table I). Edema of the gland was usually a prominent feature.

Upon histological examination, a common finding was extensive areas of hemorrhagic

Table I. *Histological character of the pancreatitis and mortality*

		Histological character of pancreatitis					
		Edematous			*Hemorrhagic*		
Group	*No. of dogs*	*Mild*	*Moderate*	*Severe*	*Mild*	*Severe*	*Mortality*
Control	20	0	0	0	2	18	20 (100%)
Plasma	11	0	1	2	3	5	4 (36%)
Clinical dextran	10	2	2	1	3	2	2 (20%)
L.M.W. dextran	12	8	2	2	0	0	0 (0%)
Delayed treatment with L.M.W. dextran	5	1	1	1	2	0	0 (0%)

L.M.W. = low molecular weight.

necrosis, often extending throughout the gland. Edema of the interlobular spaces was present and associated with leukocytic infiltration. Hemorrhage was often a marked feature. The arteries and veins showed a severe vasculitis with perivascular edema, infiltration with leukocytes, and necrosis of the wall (Fig. 1). The arteries showed loss of elastic tissue in the adventitia and less frequently in the media. The changes in the veins were more pronounced. Intraluminal thrombi were visible clearly in many cases. Capillary congestion and hyaline necrosis were common findings.

Plasma group. The postoperative course of these animals varied considerably. Four animals were very ill with profuse vomiting and prostration and died 48, 56, 60, and 64 hours, respectively, after pancreatitis had been induced. Another 4 animals had quite severe systemic signs but nevertheless survived for 72 hours. The remaining animals had mild or moderate systemic signs and were eating and drinking at the time that they were killed.

At autopsy, hemorrhagic pancreatitis was present in 8 dogs (Table I). There was marked edema and fat necrosis of the peripancreatic tissues with free peritoneal serosanguinous fluid. Hemorrhage and necrosis, often severe in degree, were present in the pancreas. Three dogs had edematous pancreatitis; the edema was variable in degree but severe in two.

Upon histological examination, the five dogs with severe hemorrhagic pancreatitis had changes identical with those found in the control animals treated with normal saline. In the three animals with mild hemorrhagic pancreatitis, the histological appearance was characterized by prominent vascular congestion and marked interstitial edema with numerous acute inflammatory cells (Fig. 2). Small scattered foci of parenchymal necrosis and interlobular hemorrhage were present. In the dog with severe edematous pancreatitis, there was evidence of circulatory stasis in the smaller intrapancreatic blood vessels.

Clinical dextran group. These animals

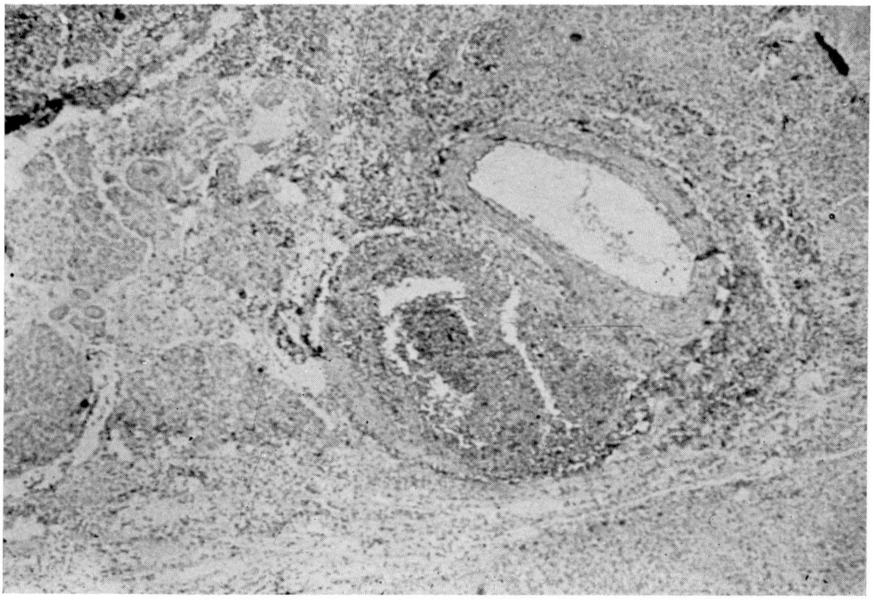

Fig. 1. Control (normal saline treated) group. Extensive parenchymal necrosis with moderate interstitial edema and massive leukocytic infiltration. Severe arteritis and phlebitis with perivascular edema, infiltration with leukocytes, and necrosis of the wall. Intraluminal thrombus in the vein. (Hematoxylin and eosin. ×100.)

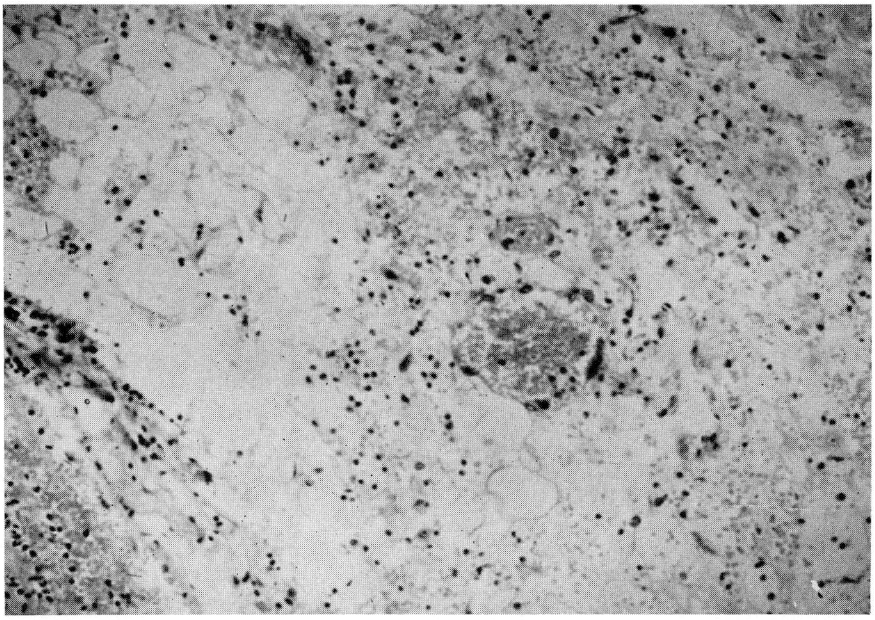

Fig. 2. Plasma group. Severe interstitial edema with numerous inflammatory cells and prominent vascular congestion and stasis. Parenchymal necrosis present in some areas. (Hematoxylin and eosin. ×200.)

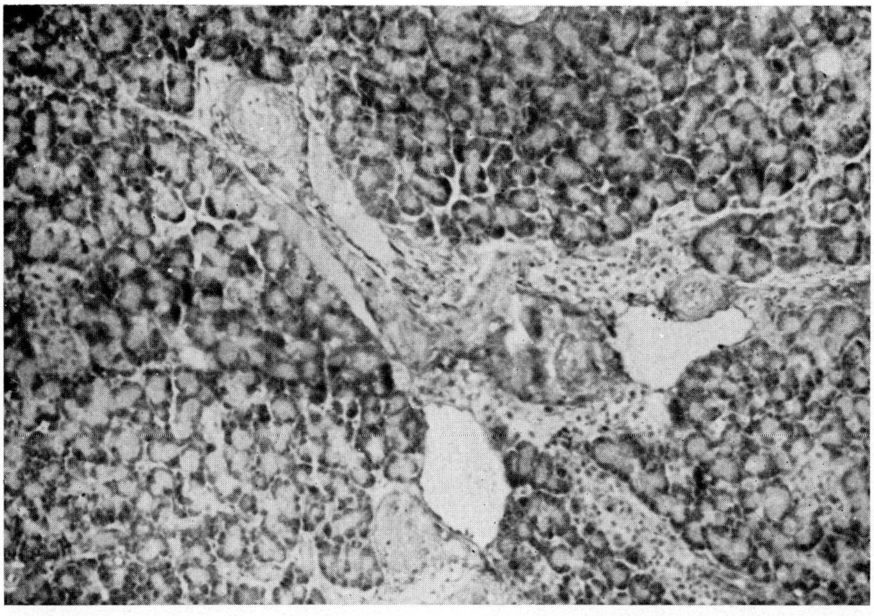

Fig. 3. Clinical dextran group. Mild interlobular edema associated with moderate leukocytic infiltration and vascular congestion. No parenchymal necrosis present. (Hematoxylin and eosin. ×100.)

had a very variable postoperative course. Two animals became very ill with profuse vomiting and marked prostration and died 60 to 70 hours after pancreatitis had been induced. Fairly severe systemic signs were present also in the three animals who eventually rallied and survived for 72 hours. The remaining dogs had only mild symptoms and all were eating and drinking at the time that they were killed.

At autopsy, hemorrhagic pancreatitis was present in five animals and these had the usual macroscopic appearances. Fat necrosis was occasionally present. In the remaining animals with edematous pancreatitis (Table I) small quantities of serous peritoneal fluid were present in association with fat necrosis and variable edema of the gland.

The pancreas of the animals with edematous pancreatitis showed, upon histological examination, a variable amount of interlobular edema associated with moderate leukocytic infiltration. Vascular congestion was present in two glands (Fig. 3). Five animals had hemorrhagic pancreatitis and this was severe in two. In these animals, intravascular thrombosis was found in association with vasculitis and severe interstitial edema. In some areas, the walls of the veins had disappeared completely and the arteries showed loss of elastic tissue in the adventitia and also occasionally, loss in the media. There was extensive parenchymal necrosis in 2, whereas in the other 3 only small foci were present.

Low molecular weight dextran group. In contrast with the control group treated with normal saline, these animals showed only mild or moderate systemic disturbances during the first 24 hours. After this period, they improved rapidly and all were eating and drinking on the second day. No deaths occurred in this group.

At autopsy, in some animals, a small quantity of serous fluid was present in the peritoneal cavity and the majority of the animals showed only mild pancreatic edema (Table I). In a few, the pancreas appeared macroscopically almost normal. Hemorrhage and fat necrosis were noted to be absent.

Upon histological examination, the pancreas showed minimal interlobular edema

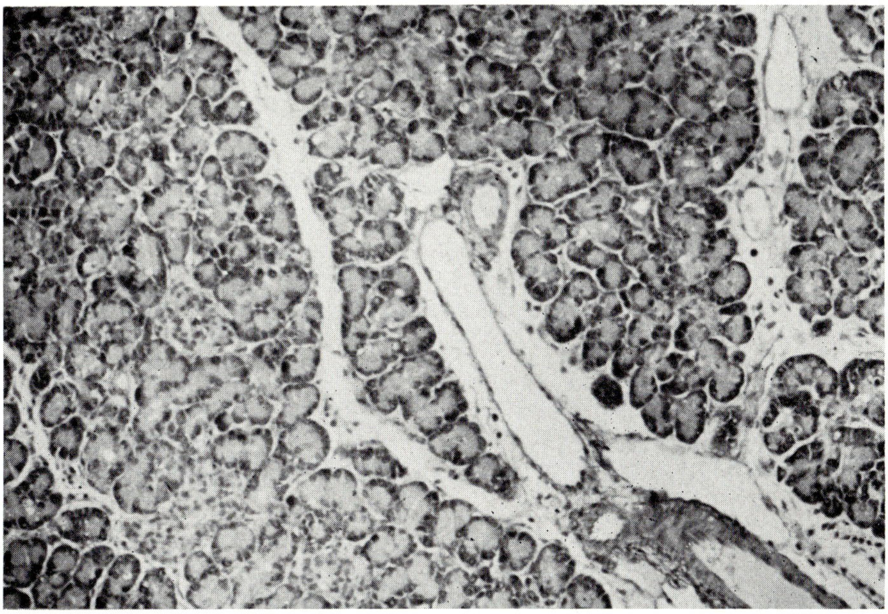

Fig. 4. Low molecular weight dextran group. Mild interstitial edema and leukocytic infiltration. No evidence of parenchymal necrosis or vasculitis. (Hematoxylin and eosin. ×100.)

with only occasional leukocytes in the interstitium (Fig. 4). The parenchymal cells were normal, and careful study of the blood vessels failed to show any evidence of vasculitis, elastolysis, congestion, or thrombi.

Delayed treatment with low molecular weight dextran group. The general condition of each animal was poor at the time treatment was started and frequent vomiting and marked prostration were prominent features. Within 12 hours of the commencement of treatment, considerable improvement occurred and all animals were in good condition and eating and drinking at the time that they were killed. There were no deaths in this group.

A variable amount of serous fluid was present in the peritoneal cavity at autopsy. The pancreas in 3 animals showed severe edema and in 2 of these there were small focal areas of necrosis in the head. In the remaining animals, the edema was mild or moderate in extent. Fat necrosis was a common finding.

In general, histological study confirmed the above finding. Parenchymal necrosis was present in 2 dogs, and this was associated with evidence of vasculitis and some loss of staining of the elastic fibers. In the other dogs, a little more interstitial edema and leukocytic infiltration was present than in the low molecular weight dextran group. The vascular congestion was minimal and necrosis, vasculitis, and hemorrhage were not seen.

DISCUSSION

The etiology of acute pancreatitis is complex and it is apparent that many different factors may play a role.[13] Despite these complexities, however, there is considerable evidence to suggest that, once the process of inflammation has been initiated, the response of the pancreas to injury is relatively stereotyped.

Edematous pancreatitis results in an illness of varying severity, but with a low mortality rate and complete resolution in most cases. In approximately 20 percent, however, edematous pancreatitis progresses to hemorrhagic necrosis of the gland. This complication is associated with high mortality and morbidity rates.[13]

The progression of pancreatic edema to necrosis is thought to be determined principally by vascular changes.[2, 5] An attack of pancreatic edema is associated with an increase in capillary permeability, which results in extravasation of a few erythrocytes into the interstitium of the gland. Trypsin is known to produce these changes.[3] Additional edema formation may result in venous compression and interference with local blood flow. Under these circumstances, and especially if the blood flow is insufficient to remove digestive products, trypsin may react with the extravasated blood to form a vasotoxic substance. Further vascular damage now ensues, and an arteritis, phlebitis, and additional capillary damage occur. Aggregation of intravascular erythrocytes results in the formation of hemagglutination thrombi. Additional erythrocytes are now exposed to the action of enzymatic activity and more vasotoxic substance is formed. A vicious circle is created. Further vascular damage and stasis occur and, if these processes are not reversed rapidly, thrombosis and tissue necrosis are initiated.[2]

A logical conclusion from this hypothesis is that maintenance of an adequate blood flow through the pancreatic microcirculation would be of great importance in the prevention of pancreatic necrosis. If this occurred, the interstitial concentration of enzymes and their digestive products would be kept to a minimum, since absorption into the systemic circulation would continue. Optimal conditions for the formation and action of the vasotoxic substance would be absent under these circumstances.

The studies reported in this paper were done to evaluate this hypothesis, since it seems reasonable to conclude that treatment with therapeutic agents given with the objective of maintaining blood flow through the pancreatic microcirculation should prevent the development of hemorrhagic pancreatitis.

The initial studies were carried out with

low molecular weight dextran. The effects of intravenous infusion of this substance are complex[8] but consist essentially of three principal actions: improvement in peripheral blood flow,[12] increase in plasma volume,[1] and an antithrombotic action.[7] The increase in peripheral blood flow is due mainly to a decrease in blood viscosity. This has been demonstrated both in vitro and in vivo, and it has been shown that the dextran molecule becomes adherent to the surfaces of the erythrocytes which become more electronegative and actively repel each other.[7] This effect directly inhibits the formation of hemagglutination thrombi and, indirectly, the formation of arterial or venous thrombi. Infusion of low molecular weight dextran increases the plasma volume and each gram retains approximately 20 to 25 ml. of water.[1] This results in an increase in the venous return and cardiac output with consequent improvement in peripheral blood flow.[12]

In the present studies, it has been demonstrated conclusively that early and intensive treatment with low molecular weight dextran will prevent the development of hemorrhagic pancreatitis. The development of stasis and hemagglutination thrombi followed by thrombosis appear to be dominant factors which determine the development of this complication and presumably low molecular weight dextran acted by reversing these changes and thus maintained an adequate local blood flow through the pancreatic microcirculation.

Recently, Anderson and Lewis[4] have reported their experience in treating experimental pancreatitis with low molecular weight dextran. They were unable to prevent hemorrhagic pancreatitis from developing and considered that this substance had a detrimental effect. In their study however, each animal was only given a single injection of low molecular weight dextran, which is inadequate therapy, since it has been demonstrated that the level of low molecular weight dextran in the blood falls rapidly after an intravenous injection,[6] and repeated doses must be given to maintain a therapeutic level. With an adequate sustained therapeutic level in the blood, aggregation of erythrocytes is minimal, stasis is prevented, and local blood flow improved.

It will be recalled that the development of hemorrhagic pancreatitis is a continuous, self-perpetuating process which, in the experimental model used in this study, takes 12 to 36 hours to complete. It is extremely unlikely, therefore, that the processes could be reversed by a single injection of a substance which is only at a therapeutic level in the bloodstream for a few hours.

A group of dogs was treated with a comparable dose of clinical dextran in an attempt to determine whether the beneficial effect of low molecular weight dextran was specific or nonspecific. Clinical dextran is a polysaccharide with an average molecular weight of 75,000 and has both plasma expending[14] and antithrombotic actions.[11] This substance was much less effective than low molecular weight dextran in preventing hemorrhagic pancreatitis. Fifty percent of the animals developed this complication and 20 percent died. This does represent a significant reduction in mortality, however, and it is considerably better than the 74 percent mortality reported by Hara and associates,[9] who gave only a single injection of dextran to each animal.

Animals treated with plasma manifested the effect of pure plasma replacement without the complicating effects of changes in blood viscosity or specific antithrombotic effects. The results in this group were worse than in the clinical dextran group. Hemorrhagic pancreatitis developed in 73 percent, although mortality was reduced to 36 percent. It is concluded that the improved results in the clinical dextran group can be attributed to the additional antithrombotic effect of this substance.

It is apparent that there is a spectrum of changes which range from the most severe in the control animals, followed by the plasma group, then the clinical dextran group, and finally the low molecular weight dextran group, in which the least severe changes were found. The therapeutic efficacy of the latter substance is attributed to its ability to promote blood flow through the pancreatic microcirculation in edematous pancreatitis and thereby prevent the development of stasis of erythrocytes and the formation of hemagglutination thrombi.

The development of acute hemorrhagic pancreatitis is the end result of a continuous, and not abrupt, process, and there is evidence that, once initiated, the process is self-perpetuating. Therefore, the beneficial results obtained by immediate treatment with low molecular weight dextran may not have any practical significance, because it is acknowledged that acute pancreatitis in man is not seen until after the onset of the disease; as a consequence, treatment is always delayed to some extent. It was necessary, therefore, to determine if delayed treatment had any beneficial effect.

A reduction in the mortality rate from 100 percent to zero resulted when treatment with low molecular weight dextran was initiated 12 hours after the induction of pancreatitis. Although the clinical results of delayed therapy were remarkably good, it was apparent at autopsy that the delay had had its disadvantages. The pathological features of resolving mild hemorrhagic or severe edematous pancreatitis were present. These studies suggest, however, that effective treatment of humans with acute pancreatitis may still be possible, despite the fact that treatment cannot be initiated at the onset of the disease.

SUMMARY

The comparative value of low molecular weight dextran, clinical dextran, plasma, and normal saline in the treatment of experimental hemorrhagic pancreatitis in the dog has been studied.

Acute hemorrhagic pancreatitis induced by injecting trypsin digested blood into the pancreatic duct was fatal. Treatment with low molecular weight dextran prevented hemorrhagic pancreatitis from developing. Treatment with either clinical dextran or plasma resulted in a reduction in morbidity and mortality rates, but hemorrhagic or severe edematous pancreatitis was found at autopsy in all cases.

A twelve-hour delay in initiating treatment with low molecular weight dextran was still associated with a reduction in morbidity and mortality rates.

It is concluded that the development of hemorrhagic pancreatitis is dependent on changes which result in a reduced blood flow in the pancreatic microcirculation. Stasis of erythrocytes and thrombosis with subsequent parenchymal necrosis result. Prevention of these changes inhibits the development of hemorrhagic pancreatitis.

REFERENCES

1. Ahnefeld, F. W., Halmagyi, M., and Überla, K.: Untersuchungen zur Bewertung kolloidaler Volumenersatzmittel, Anaesthetist **14:** 137, 1965.
2. Anderson, M. C.: Venous stasis in the transition of edematous pancreatitis to necrosis, J. A. M. A. **183:** 534, 1963.
3. Anderson, M. C., and Bergan, J. J.: Effect of proteolytic enzymes on pancreatic blood vessels, Surg. Forum **13:** 304, 1962.
4. Anderson, M. C., and Lewis, M. B.: Low molecular weight dextran therapy in experimental pancreatitis, J. A. M. A. **192:** 398, 1965.
5. Anderson, M. C., Schoenfeld, F. B., Iams, W. B., and Suwa, M.: Circulatory changes in acute pancreatitis, Surg. Clin. N. Amer. **47:** 127, 1967.
6. Arturson, G., Granath, K., Thorén, L., and Wallenius, G.: The renal excretion of low molecular weight dextran, Acta Chir. Scand. **127:** 543, 1964.
7. Chopra, P. S., Sprinivasan, S., Lucas, T., and Sawyer, P. N.: Effect of low molecular weight dextran, heparin, and protamine on the surface charge of blood vessels, Surg. Forum **18:** 195, 1967.
8. Gelin, L.-E., and Ingelman, B.: Rheomacrodex—a new dextran solution for rheological treatment of impaired capillary flow, Acta Chir. Scand. **122:** 294, 1961.
9. Hara, M., Thompson, B. W., and Hudson, L. H.: The comparative effects of dextran and blood in lethal sterile hemorrhagic pancreatitis, Surg. Forum **6:** 377, 1955.
10. Nemir, P., Jr., and Drabkin, D. L.: The pathogenesis of acute necrotizing hemorrhagic pancreatitis: An experimental study, Surgery **40:** 171, 1956.
11. Sawyer, R. B., and Moncrief, J. A.: Dextran

specificity in thrombus inhibition, Arch. Surg. **90:** 562, 1965.
12. Schenk, W. G. J., Delin, N. A., Domanic, E., Hahnlaser, P., Hoyt, R. K., and Ny, B.: Blood viscosity as a determinant of regional blood flow, Arch. Surg. **89:** 783, 1964.
13. White, T. T.: Pancreatitis, London, 1966, Edward Arnold Ltd.
14. Witham, A. C., Fleming, J. W., and Bloom, W. L.: Effect of intravenous administration of dextran on cardiac output and other circulatory dynamics, J. Clin. Invest. **30:** 897, 1951.

Dissociation of the hyperglycemic and vascular effects of glucagon

STEN TIBBLIN, M.D.*
NILS G. KOCK, M.D.*
WORTHINGTON G. SCHENK, Jr., M.D.
BUFFALO, N. Y.
From the Department of Surgery, State University of New York at Buffalo, and the Surgical Research Laboratory, E. J. Meyer Memorial Hospital.

In 1959, Shoemaker and associates[10] reported an increase in hepatic blood flow in dogs following administration of glucagon. The increase in hepatic blood flow concurred with the elevation of glucose concentration in the hepatic vein, and the authors suggested that the increase in hepatic circulation could represent a response to increased metabolic activity of the liver incident to rapid glycogenolysis. In experiments in unanesthetized dogs, Shoemaker and Van Itallie[9] confirmed their previous findings concerning the effect of glucagon on hepatic blood flow. Depletion of glycogen stores induced by fasting was associated with a decreased or absent response in hepatic blood flow and hepatic glucose output to glucagon.

In recent publications, Kock and associates[4] and Tibblin and associates[12] found that the main cause of the increased hepatic blood flow after administration of glucagon was produced by a vasodilatory action of glucagon on the splanchnic vascular bed. There was no significant change of the vascular resistance on the portal venous side, suggesting that the flow increase was not a result of metabolic changes in the liver. It was also noted that the blood flow response to glucagon in some experiments could be evoked without any change in blood sugar concentration. The aim of the present investigation was to study the relationship between the responses in superior mesenteric artery flow and blood sugar concentration following glucagon.

MATERIALS AND METHODS

Twenty-one adult mongrel dogs of both sexes, weighing 15 to 26 Kg. (mean 20.5 Kg.) were used. Sodium pentobarbital (30 mg. per kilogram of bodyweight) was used for anesthesia. The animals breathed room air spontaneously. Plastic catheters were inserted into the superior caval vein via the external jugular vein, into the ascending aorta via the carotid artery, and into the inferior vena cava via the femoral vein. The catheter in the ascending aorta was used for recording of the arterial blood pressure with a Statham pressure transducer connected to a direct writing recorder. One of the caval catheters was used for injections and infusions and the other for sampling of blood for blood sugar determination.

The superior mesenteric artery was exposed retroperitoneally through a left subcostal incision. An electromagnetic flow probe was placed around the vessel approximately 5 mm. distally from the aorta. In order to obtain zero flow recordings by temporary occlusions, a nylon snare was located around the vessel. In some of the dogs, an additional flow probe was placed on the carotid artery. The blood flows were recorded

Supported in part by Grants-in-Aid from the Institute of General Medical Sciences (GM-15768) and the National Heart Institute (HE-03181) of the United States Public Health Service.

Received for publication June 28, 1969.

*Buswell Fellow in Surgical Research, State University of New York at Buffalo.

on a square-wave electromagnetic flowmeter (Carolina Medical Electronics, Inc., Winston-Salem, N. C.) and monitored on a Sanborn direct writing recorder (Schenk and Dedichen[8]). After the operation, the experiments were not started until stable blood flows had been recorded for at least 15 minutes. In some of the animals 200 to 300 c.c. of saline were infused prior to the experiments.

Every experiment included the recording of the superior mesenteric artery flow and the blood sugar concentration during the 35 min-

Table I

Group	*No. of dogs*	*Treatment prior to the injection of glucagon*	*Blood sugar level at the time of injection*
A	6	None	Normal
B	6	Glucose infusion (10% dextrose in saline) 200 ml. during 10 min.	Elevated
C	7	Glucagon infusion (0.1 μg/Kg./min. in saline) during 30 min.	Elevated
D	6	Insulin injection (40 I.U.) 20 min. prior to glucagon injection	Depressed
E	6	Glucagon administration in fractionated doses (approx. 3 mg.) during 2-4 hr.	Depressed

Table II. *The effect of a single injection of glucagon (10 μgs/Kg.) on the superior mesenteric artery flow*

Dog No.	*Control*	*Superior mesenteric artery flow (ml./Kg./min.) — Minutes after the injection*						*Peak after inj.*
		1	*5*	*10*	*15*	*25*	*35*	
3	23	39	53	39	29	25	21	58
4	16	39	39	35	30	23	16	42
49	13	25	27	27	26	20	13	28
55	13	27	28	20	18	16	13	30
64	13	34	41	34	27	23	14	46
66	20	70	84	76	72	51	33	84
Mean	16.3	39.0	45.3	38.5	33.7	26.3	18.3	48.0
S.E.	1.75	6.65	8.66	7.99	7.86	5.10	3.18	8.49

Table III. *The effect of a single injection of glucagon (10 μgs/Kg.) on the blood sugar concentration*

Dog No.	*Control*	*Minutes after the injection*					
		1	*5*	*10*	*15*	*25*	*35*
3	107	117	150	199	207	243	207
4	95	97	145	142	207	192	212
49	80	83	120	136	142	160	155
55	78	90	160	215	220	185	180
64	95	95	153	195	200	213	220
66	105	110	187	235	283	268	228
Mean	93	99	153	187	210	210	200
S.E.	5.0	5.2	8.9	16.3	18.4	16.2	11.3

utes following a single injection of glucagon (Eli Lilly and Co., Indianapolis, Ind.) in a dose of 10 μg/Kg. of body weight. The injection was always given into the superior caval vein. Blood sugar concentration was determined according to Folin-Wu before the injection of glucagon and subsequent to it at 1, 5, 10, 15, 25, and 35 minutes. In 25 of the experiments, various kinds of treatments were given prior to the single injection of glucagon in order to induce changes in the blood sugar concentration. The different groups of experiments are presented schematically in Table I.

One or two experiments were carried out in each individual dog. In one exceptional animal, three experiments were performed. For statistical analysis of the data, calculation of the means and the standard error of the means (S.E.) was performed. Statistical comparisons were carried out according to the Student's t test for paired observations.

RESULTS

A. The effect of a single injection of glucagon on superior mesenteric artery flow and blood sugar concentration. No previous treatment. The absolute data for all the individual dogs in this group are presented in Tables II and III. The mean results for the whole group are graphically depicted in Fig. 1. Immediately following the injection of glucagon, a rise in superior mesenteric artery flow was noted. A maximal flow response, 190 percent increase from control level, was reached approximately three minutes after the injection. Following the peak flow, a decline in the curve can be noted and control flow was reached about 35 minutes after the injection. The blood sugar concentration increased gradually during the first 15 minutes after the injection. A stable level was then maintained during the remaining period of observation.

B. The effect of a single injection of glucagon on superior mesenteric artery flow and blood sugar concentration after previous infusion of 10 percent dextrose. Fig. 2 illustrates one of these experiments. During the 10 minute period of glucose administration, an increase in superior mesenteric artery flow was recorded. The flow increase was moderate compared with the response to glucagon, and when the infusion was discontinued, the flow gradually returned toward basal level. During glucose infusion, the blood sugar concentration increased rapidly reaching a peak value when the infusion was completed. Glucagon (10 μgs/Kg.) injected 8 minutes after discontinuing the glucose infusion, when the blood sugar concentration was declining, produced a flow increase of about 130 percent but no rise in the blood sugar concentration. In Table IV, data from each individual experiment are presented. The mean control flow recorded in the superior mesenteric artery was 13.8 ml. per kilogram per minute. The mean flow value before glucagon injection was 23.2

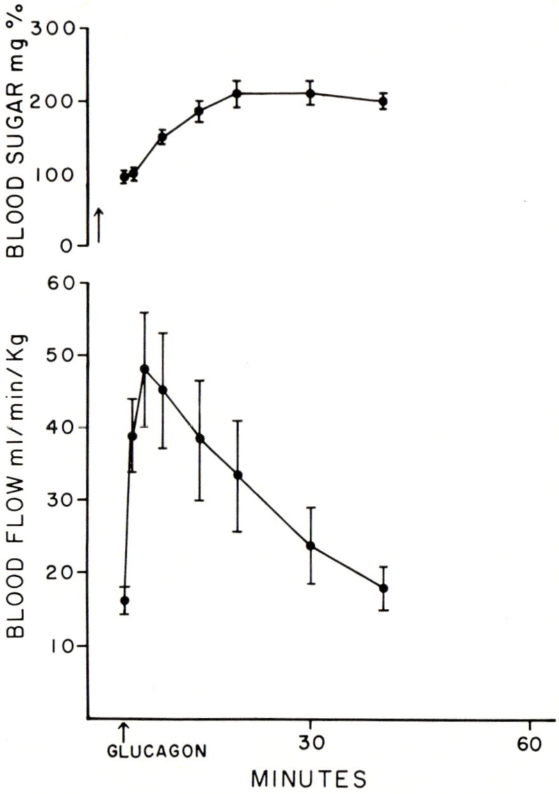

Fig. 1. The effect of a single injection of glucagon (10 μgs/Kg.) on the superior mesenteric artery flow and the blood sugar concentration. Each curve represents the mean result ± S.E. of 6 experiments.

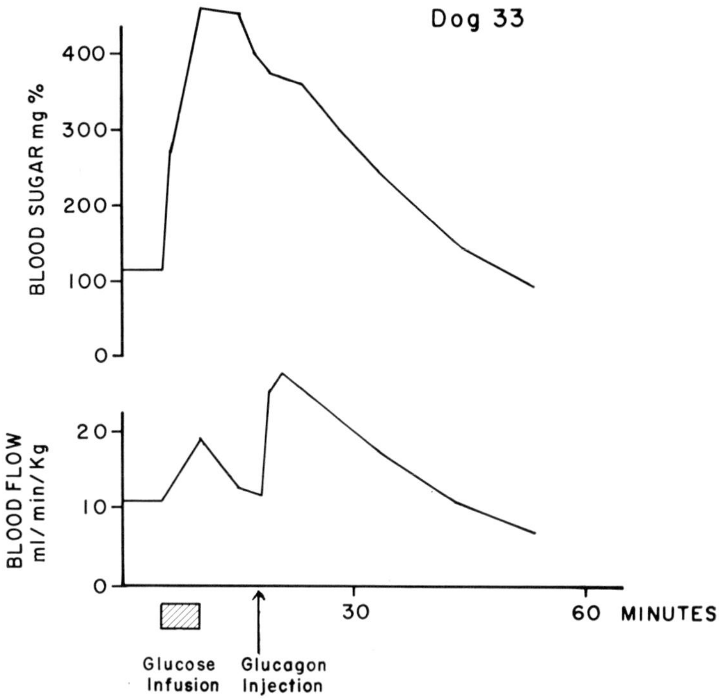

Fig. 2. The effect of a single injection of glucagon (10 μgs/Kg.) on the superior mesenteric artery flow and blood sugar concentration when the blood sugar level had been elevated by a previous glucose infusion (200 ml. 10 percent dextrose in saline).

Table IV. *The effect of a single glucagon injection on the superior mesenteric artery flow and the blood sugar concentration after glucose infusion*

	Superior mesenteric artery flow (ml./Kg./min.)			*Blood sugar (mg. %)*	
Dog No.	*Control*	*Before injection*	*Peak after injection*	*Before injection*	*At peak flow*
33	10	12	28	400	376
38	17	38	78	340	340
49	13	28	42	223	223
52	11	11	24	485	485
54	17	35	57	233	235
71	15	15	49	328	304
Mean	13.8	23.2	46.3	334	327
S.E.	1.22	4.91	8.12	40.7	39.7

ml./Kg./min. (this higher flow value was a consequence of the previous glucose infusion). The mean maximal flow following glucagon was 46.3 ml./Kg./min., a 100 percent increase from the flow before injection. The mean blood sugar concentration following glucose infusion was 334 mg. percent and after glucagon injection, when maximal flow response was obtained, was 327 mg. percent. In one animal, the effect of glucose infusion and subsequent glucagon injection was recorded simultaneously from the superior mesenteric artery and the common carotid artery (Fig. 3). Glucose infusion produced an 83 percent increase in superior mesenteric artery flow and a 52 percent increase in carotid artery flow. After discontinuing the infusion, the flows successively

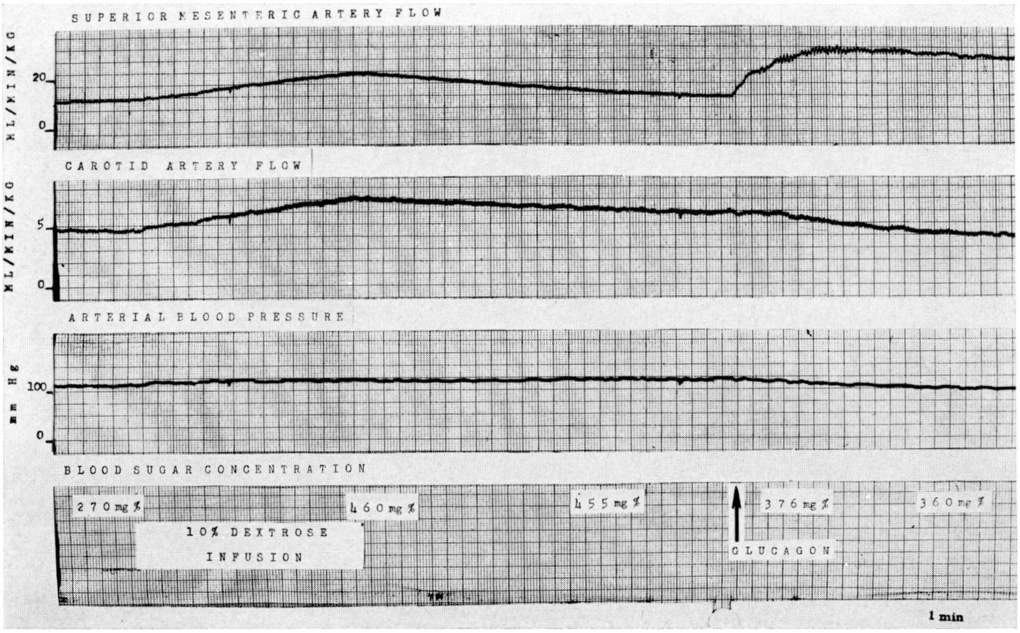

Fig. 3. The effect of a glucose infusion (200 ml. 10 percent dextrose in saline) and of a subsequent single injection of glucagon (10 μgs/Kg.) on the blood flow in the superior mesenteric artery and carotid artery and on the arterial blood pressure. Blood sugar concentration at different times is given in the lowest section. One minute = three squares.

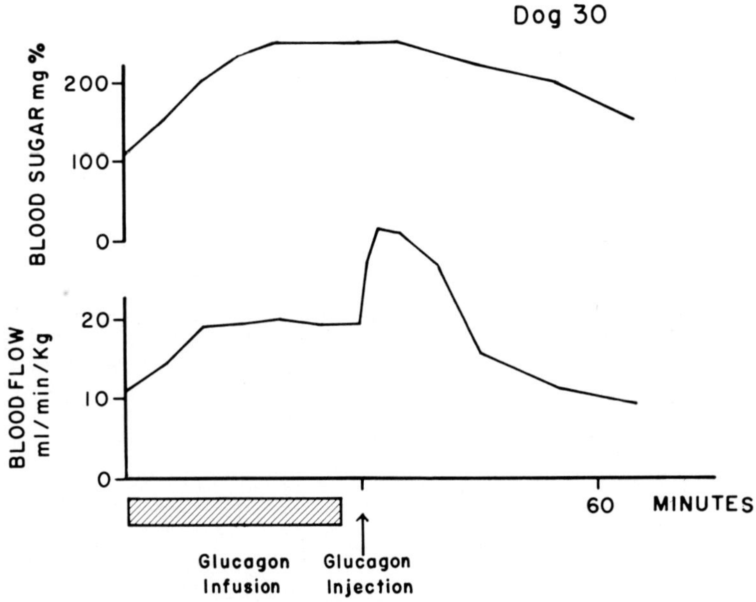

Fig. 4. The effect of a single injection of glucagon (10 μgs/Kg.) on the superior mesenteric artery flow and blood sugar concentration when the blood sugar level has been elevated by a previous glucagon infusion (0.1 μg/Kg./min.).

returned toward control values. Injection of glucagon (10 μgs/Kg.) evoked an increase in the superior mesenteric artery flow but a decrease in the carotid artery flow. Arterial blood pressure rose 15 mm. Hg during the infusion of glucose but declined subsequent to the glucagon injection. The blood sugar concentration was 270 mg. percent (because of a previous glucose injection) and increased following the glucose infusion to a peak value of 460 mg. percent. A subsequent glucagon injection did not increase the glucose concentration.

C. The effect of a single injection of glucagon on superior mesenteric artery flow and blood sugar concentration after previous glucagon infusion. A representative example of these experiments is depicted in Fig. 4. The infusion of glucagon in a dose of 0.1 μg per kilogram of body weight per minute induced a gradual increment of the superior mesenteric artery flow. Concomitantly, blood sugar concentration rose from 100 to 250 mg. percent. When a steady level in blood flow and blood sugar concentration was achieved, a single injection of glucagon (10 μgs/Kg.) was given. Within three minutes, a further elevation of the blood flow was recorded. This flow increase amounted to 160 percent calculated from the control flow and to 60 percent calculated from the flow during glucagon infusion. Following the single injection of glucagon, the blood sugar did not change significantly. In Table V, data from each individual dog are presented. Glucagon infusion (0.1 μg/Kg./min.) produced an increase in superior mesenteric artery flow from a mean control of 15.7 to 26.1 ml./Kg. /min. After the single injection of 10 μgs/ Kg. of glucagon, the mean maximal flow was 37.3 ml./Kg./min. ($P < 0.001$). The mean sugar concentration before the glucagon injection was 213 mg. percent and after the injection, when maximal flow response was recorded, was 216 mg. percent. The difference is not statistically significant ($P > 0.05$).

D. The effect of a single glucagon injection on superior mesenteric artery flow and blood sugar concentration after previous insulin administration. An illustrative example of these experiments is depicted in Fig. 5. Superior mesenteric artery flow did not change following the injection of 40 I.U. of insulin. The blood sugar concentration gradually decreased from 80 to 40 mg. percent after insulin. A single injection of glucagon (10 μgs/Kg.) produced a 180 percent increase in superior mesenteric artery flow. The maximal flow response was recorded within five minutes after the injection of glucagon. Blood sugar concentration increased from 40 mg. percent before the injection to 80 mg. percent 10 minutes after the injection. When the peak blood flow was recorded, the maximal increase in blood sugar had not been achieved.

In Table VI, individual data from the six

Table V. *The effect of a single glucagon injection on the superior mesenteric artery flow and blood sugar concentration after glucagon infusion*

	Superior mesenteric artery flow (ml./Kg./min.)			*Blood sugar (mg. %)*	
Dog No.	*Control*	*Before injection*	*Peak after injection*	*Before injection*	*At peak flow*
28	16	22	33	223	218
30	11	18	29	245	255
37	15	31	46	168	168
48	20	25	36	223	235
53	18	30	39	222	200
54	17	41	53	225	235
55	13	16	25	185	201
Mean	15.7	26.1	37.3	213	216
S.E.	1.15	3.26	3.67	10.1	11.0

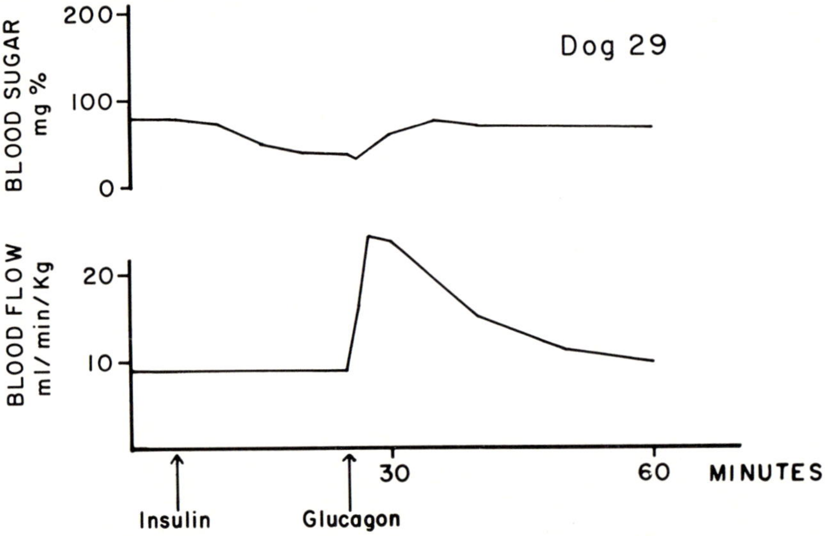

Fig. 5. The effect of a single injection of glucagon (10 μgs/Kg.) on the superior mesenteric artery flow and the blood sugar concentration when the blood sugar level had been depressed by an injection of insulin (40 I.U.).

Table VI. *The effect of a single glucagon injection on the superior mesenteric artery flow and the blood sugar concentration after insulin administration*

Dog No.	*Superior mesenteric artery flow (ml./Kg./min.)* Control	Before injection	Peak after injection	*Blood sugar (mg. %)* Before injection	At peak flow
29	9	9	25	38	45
38	17	21	60	105	95
52	11	8	17	52	52
54	17	14	31	13	60
57	18	18	30	53	53
71	10	11	26	75	69
Mean	13.7	13.5	31.5	56	62
S.E.	1.67	2.11	6.05	12.9	7.3

experiments are presented. The mean flow in the superior mesenteric artery before and approximately 20 minutes after insulin administration was 13.7 and 13.5 ml./Kg./min. respectively. The difference is not statistically significant ($P > 0.05$). After glucagon injection, the mean maximal flow was 31.5 ml./Kg./min. ($P < 0.01$), a flow increase of approximately 135 percent. The mean blood sugar concentration before and after glucagon injection was 56 and 62 mg. percent ($P > 0.05$). The latter value was at the peak flow.

E. The effect of a single injection of glucagon on superior mesenteric artery flow and on blood sugar concentration after repeated glucagon administration. One of these experiments is presented in Fig. 6. The animal had received 3 mg. glucagon in fractionated doses during the preceding three hours, resulting in a blood sugar concentration of 40 mg. percent. In this hypoglycemic situation when 10 μgs/Kg. of glucagon were injected, the blood glucose level gradually increased during 25 minutes to 55 mg. percent. Superior mesenteric artery flow increased 230

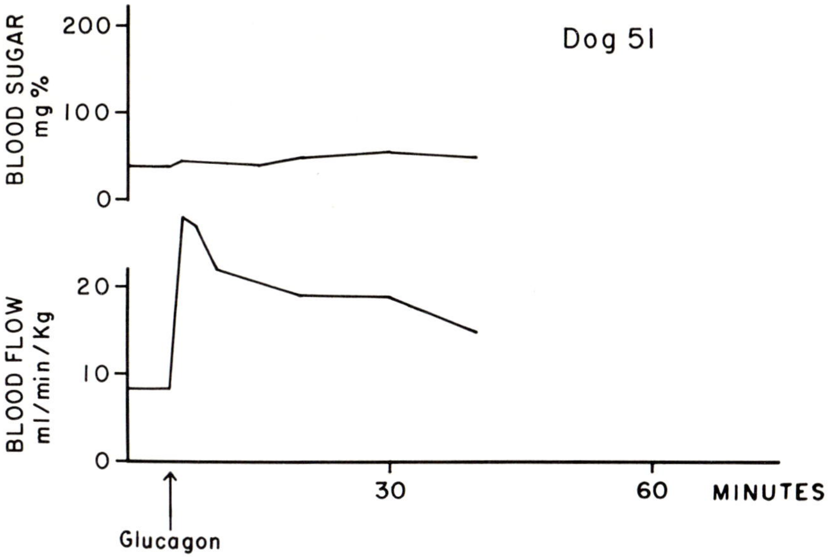

Fig. 6. The effect of a single injection of glucagon (10 µgs/Kg.) on the superior mesenteric artery flow and blood sugar concentration when the blood sugar level had been depressed by repeated glucagon administration (a total of 3 mg. was given in fractionated doses during 4 hours).

Table VII. *The effect of a single glucagon injection on the superior mesenteric artery flow and the blood sugar concentration after repeated glucagon administration*

	Superior mesenteric artery flow (ml./Kg./min.)			*Blood sugar (mg. %)*	
Dog No.	*Control*	*Before injection*	*Peak after injection*	*Before injection*	*At peak flow*
8	13	15	32	38	25
28	18	9	22	75	78
30	11	6	15	87	92
37	15	17	40	76	73
51	19	9	27	38	43
55	13	7	32	33	33
Mean	14.8	10.5	28.0	58	57
S.E.	1.28	1.82	3.57	9.8	11.1

percent within three minutes after glucagon injection.

In Table VII, the results from the six individual experiments are summarized. From a mean control flow of 14.8 ml./Kg./min., the blood flow decreased to 10.5 ml. per kilogram per minute after the repeated, fractionated administration of glucagon. This difference is not statistically significant ($P > 0.05$). The injection of glucagon elicited a mean increase in blood flow to 28.0 ml./Kg./min., which corresponds to 167 percent ($P < 0.001$). The mean blood sugar concentration was 58 mg. percent before the single injection of glucagon and 57 mg. percent when the peak flow value was recorded ($P > 0.05$).

DISCUSSION

The aim of the present study was to investigate whether an interrelationship exists between the changes in blood sugar concentration and splanchnic blood flow following glucagon injection.

In the first series of experiments, a single dose of glucagon was injected intravenously and the responses in superior mesenteric artery flow and blood sugar concentration were compared with regard to the time of maximum increase in blood sugar and flow. Peak flow was recorded within five minutes in all experiments whereas the blood sugar concentration reached its highest value approximately 20 minutes after the injection.

Shoemaker and associates[10] in 1959 reported that the time of the maximum hepatic vein glucose increase coincided with maximum increase in estimated hepatic blood flow. Peak values were achieved approximately 15 minutes after glucagon injection. As the Bromsulphalein method used by these authors does not permit a continuous recording of blood flow, it might well be possible that a peak flow had occurred earlier. The dissociation between the maximal responses in superior mesenteric artery flow and blood sugar concentration in our experiments suggests that the blood sugar concentration per se cannot be responsible for the enhanced blood flow in the splanchnic bed following the administration of glucagon.

In the second group of experiments, an elevation of the blood sugar concentration was produced by infusion of 10 percent glucose prior to the glucagon injection. The infusion of hyperosmolar glucose solution resulted in a marked elevation of the blood sugar concentration and also in a temporary increase in superior mesenteric artery flow, which is in accordance with findings reported by Tibblin and associates.[11] A single injection of glucagon did not further increase the elevated blood sugar concentration but was able to produce the usual flow response.

In the third series of experiments a hyperglycemic situation was created by continuous infusion of glucagon in small amounts. The glucagon infusion induced a moderate increase in superior mesenteric artery flow. At the end of infusion, a single injection of 10 μgs/Kg. of glucagon still evoked a marked flow increase without any rise in the blood sugar concentration.

In another series of experiments, a hypoglycemic situation was produced prior to the glucagon injection in one group of animals by insulin administration and in another group by repeated administration of glucagon. Insulin injection did not significantly affect the superior mesenteric artery flow but produced a hypoglycemia with a mean blood sugar concentration of 56 mg. percent. Glucagon injection evoked the usual flow response but only a slight increase in blood sugar concentration. In the animals which received approximately 3 mg. of glucagon in fractionated doses, the mean blood sugar concentration was 58 mg. percent after 2 to 4 hours. A single injection of glucagon (10 μgs per kilogram) produced a 180 percent mean increase in the superior mesenteric artery flow without any change in the blood sugar concentration.

These experiments have thus shown that changes in blood sugar concentration are not essential for the flow responses following glucagon to occur. This is in disagreement with Henneman and Shoemaker,[2] who suggested in 1961 that the effect of glucagon on blood flow appeared to be related to changes in blood glucose levels.

Glucagon has not previously been used deliberately to induce experimental hypoglycemia. Bondy and Cardillo[1] reported in 1956 hypoglycemic reactions in patients during a two-hour infusion of glucagon. In only one of them, however, were blood sugar values under 80 mg. percent observed. The reactions could be abolished by administration of glucose. Kibler and associates,[3] on the other hand, reported in 1964 that an elevated concentration of blood glucose could be maintained for 3½ hours by intravenous infusion of glucagon. The insulin stimulating capacity of glucagon was demonstrated in 1965 by Samols and associates.[7] In healthy individuals, these authors could show a rapid and significant rise in plasma insulin within the first four minutes following glucagon. Blood glucose rose more slowly and reached its maximal level 10 minutes after injection. The hypoglycemia following repeated, fractionated administration of glucagon observed in the present study might well be a consequence of prolonged insulin stimulation. The similarities between the plasma insulin concentration curve and the flow response to glucagon in the superior mesenteric artery could suggest a connection between the flow response and the liberation of insulin. Insulin injection did not, however, significantly affect the superior mesenteric artery flow. It has thus been found that neither blood sugar changes nor insulin liberation can be responsible for the blood flow response to glucagon.

Part of the splanchnic blood flow increase can probably be attributed to the enhancement of cardiac output following glucagon administration.[6] In a previous study,[5] it was demonstrated that ascending aortic flow increased 36 percent after glucagon in the same dose as in the present investigation. In order to achieve a blood flow increase of 190 percent, there must be a selective influence of glucagon on the mesenteric vascular bed. Whether this influence implies a direct action on the vascular smooth muscle cells, an interference with the neurogenic control of the vascular bed, or a release of some metabolic vasoactive substance remains to be investigated.

SUMMARY

Alterations in the superior mesenteric artery flow and the blood glucose concentration following intravenous injection of glucagon (10 μgs/Kg. of body weight) were studied in 21 anesthetized dogs. The electromagnetic technique was used for the blood flow measurements.

Glucagon induced a peak flow response to 190 percent, which appeared within five minutes after the injection. The increase in blood sugar concentration reached a maximum fifteen minutes after the injection of glucagon. A glucagon induced peak flow response of the same magnitude also appeared when the blood sugar concentration had been elevated by glucose or glucagon infusion or had been depressed by insulin injection or repeated administration of glucagon. It is concluded that the increase in superior mesenteric artery flow induced by glucagon is not an effect of the alterations in blood sugar concentration following glucagon.

REFERENCES

1. Bondy, P. K., and Cardillo, L. R.: The effect of glucagon on carbohydrate metabolism in normal human beings, J. Clin. Invest. **35:** 494, 1956.
2. Henneman, D. H., and Shoemaker, W. C.: Effect of glucagon and epinephrine on regional metabolism of glucose, pyruvate, lactate, and citrate in normal conscious dogs, Endocrinology **68:** 889, 1961.
3. Kibler, R. F., Taylor, W. J., and Myers, J. D.: The effect of glucagon on net splanchnic balances of glucose amino acid nitrogen urea, ketones, and oxygen in man, J. Clin. Invest. **43:** 904, 1964.
4. Kock, N. G., Roding, B., Hahnloser, P., Tibblin, S., and Schenk, W. G., Jr.: The effect of glucagon on hepatic blood flow, Arch. Surg. In press.
5. Kock, N. G., Tibblin, S., and Schenk, W. G., Jr.: Hemodynamic responses to glucagon. Ann. Surg. In press.
6. Parmley, W. W., Glick, G., and Sonnenblick, E. H.: Cardiovascular effects of glucagon in man, New Eng. J. Med. **279:** 12, 1968.
7. Samols, E., Marri, G., and Marks, V.: Promotion of insulin secretion by glucagon, Lancet **2:** 415, 1965.
8. Schenk, W. G., Jr., and Dedichen, H.: Electronic measurement of blood flow, Amer. J. Surg. **8:** 111, 1967.
9. Shoemaker, W. C., and Van Itallie, T. B.: The hepatic responses to glucagon in the unanesthetized dog, Endocrinology **66:** 260, 1960.
10. Shoemaker, W. C., Van Itallie, T. B., and Walker, W. F.: Measurement of hepatic glucose output and hepatic blood flow in response to glucagon, Amer. J. Physiol. **196:** 315, 1959.
11. Tibblin, S., Hahnloser, P., and Schenk, W. G., Jr.: Effect of hyperosmolar infusion on the superior mesenteric artery flow. To be published.
12. Tibblin, S., Kock, N. G., and Schenk, W. G., Jr.: Splanchnic hemodynamic responses to glucagon, Arch. Surg. In press.

Synthetic thromboresistant surfaces from sulfonated polyelectrolyte complexes

LITA NELSEN
ROBERT A. CROSS
MARY ANN VOGEL
VINCENT L. GOTT
A. MONIEM FADALI
LEXINGTON, MASS., AND BALTIMORE, MD.
From the Amicon Corporation and the Department of Surgery, the Johns Hopkins University School of Medicine

During the past few years, a great deal of attention has been devoted to the problem of producing a synthetic material which would not initiate thrombosis when placed in contact with the bloodstream. Considerable experimental success has been achieved with the use of synthetic polymers with heparin bonded to their surfaces, either ionically or covalently.[5, 7, 8, 12] However, the inherent problems of the leaching of heparin from the surfaces and of surface abrasion have given encouragement to the continued search for a homogeneous, totally synthetic (i.e., nonheparinized) thromboresistant material. This paper will report on the evaluation of such a material formed from charged, highly hydrated polymeric materials known as polyelectrolyte complexes under the Artificial Heart Program of the National Heart Institute.

It has been thought that the unique anticoagulant properties of heparin are caused by the sulfate and aminosulfate groups on the heparin molecule, a hypothesis supported by reports of anticoagulant activity of many other naturally occurring sulfated compounds in solution.[1-3, 6] It was also hypothesized that a synthetic surface with bound anionic groups, such as sulfate or sulfonate ions, might simulate the action of the heparinized surfaces and prevent thrombus formation. Some early investigations on the clotting of blood in contact with sulfonated polystyrene reported in the literature lent support to this theory.[9]

It was hypothesized that polyelectrolyte complexes might offer a unique way of forming a variety of surfaces with controllable charge density to achieve anionic thromboresistant surfaces, while the previously demonstrated lack of toxicity and resistance to chemical breakdown in vivo of these materials[10, 11] made them worthwhile candidates for investigation for use as permanent prosthetic materials. In the work to be reported here, a range of these materials, varying in both charge density and sign of the net charge, were subjected to both short-term and long-term in vivo testing of thromboresistance in the inferior vena cava of dogs. The results, to be reported below, showed anticoagulant activity of the sulfonated surfaces within certain ranges of sulfonation.

MATERIALS AND METHODS

Composition and properties of polyelectrolyte complexes. Polyelectrolyte complexes (or "polysalts") are synthetic, ionic materials formed from the coprecipitation of oppositely charged, linear polyelectrolytes.[11]

The studies performed at Johns Hopkins were supported by United States Public Health Service Grant No. H-5999 and Contract No. PH43-68-84 from the Artificial Heart Contract Office. Much of the Amicon work was supported by National Heart Institute Contract No. PH43-66-1129, Frank W. Hastings, M.D., Contracting Officer.

Received for publication July 7, 1969.

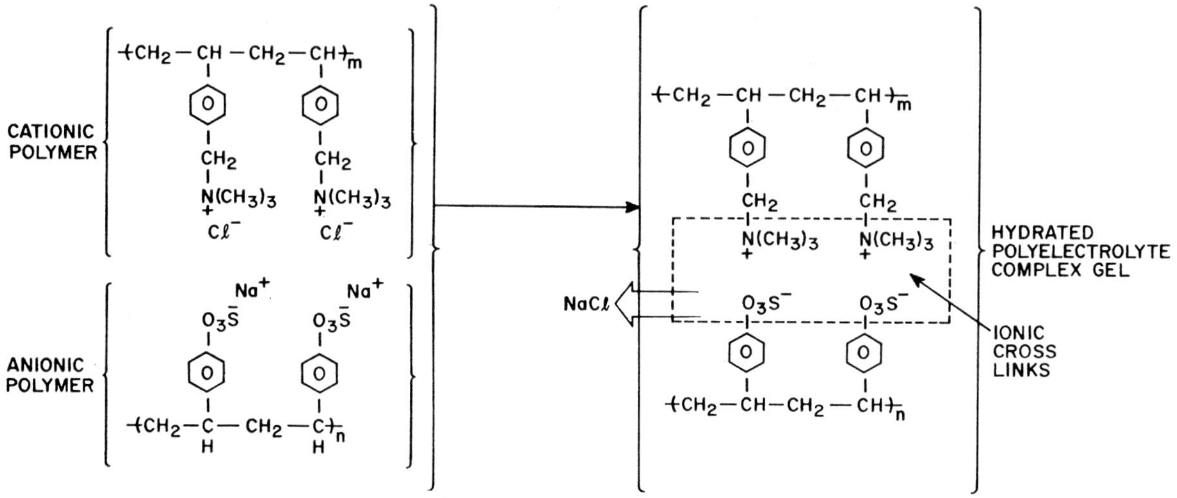

Fig. 1. Formation of polyelectrolyte complexes.

The resulting product, which is insoluble in water and in most organic solvents, contains both bound anionic and bound cationic groups in its structure, with the net charge density determined by the ratio of polyanion to polycation used in the formation of the complex. These materials can be formed into controllably hydrated structures (with water contents ranging from 1 part water per 2 parts of resin up to 9 parts water per 1 part resin). Certain forms of these materials have been used as ultrafiltration and dialysis membranes for several years, and others are currently under investigation as permeable contact lenses, corneal replacements, controlled-release encapsulants, and in other "biomaterials" applications.

The particular polyelectrolyte complex used in the experiments described here was made from the coreaction of two aromatic polyelectrolytes—poly (sodium styrene sulfonate) and poly (vinyl benzyltrimethylammonium) chloride (a schematic of the formation of the complex is shown in Fig. 1). This combination has been shown to be quite chemically stable in biological environments.

In vivo evaluation of ioplex materials. Polyelectrolyte materials that were felt to be theoretically thromboresistant were formed into small prosthetic tubes (9 mm. length, 7 mm. inside diameter with ½ mm. wall thickness). These tubes had streamlined leading and trailing edges and were suitable for implantation in the inferior vena cava of dogs weighing 17 to 20 pounds. This is a very severe screening test for potential thromboresistant materials and has been described in detail in previous publications.[4] It has ordinarily been found that caval implant rings of plain polymers and silicone rubber will be markedly thrombosed within a two-hour implantation period. Materials that demonstrate minimal or no thrombus after two hours in the vena cava are ordinarily considered to be moderately thromboresistant. Materials passing the two-hour implantation test are then implanted as prosthetic rings for two weeks. Materials free of thrombus at the end of this period are considered to have significant thromboresistance.

Ordinarily, the two-hour implants were not sterilized; however, the rings implanted for two weeks were sterilized in 10 percent hydrochloric acid and then equilibrated to body pH prior to implantation.

RESULTS

Charts IA and IB depict the pertinent in vivo results with the polyelectrolyte materials. It is apparent that the Type I rings,

Chart IA

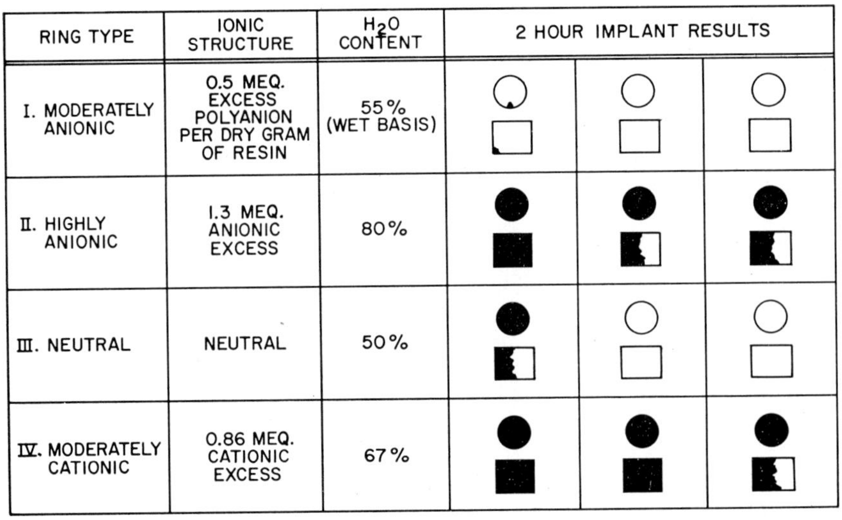

Chart IB

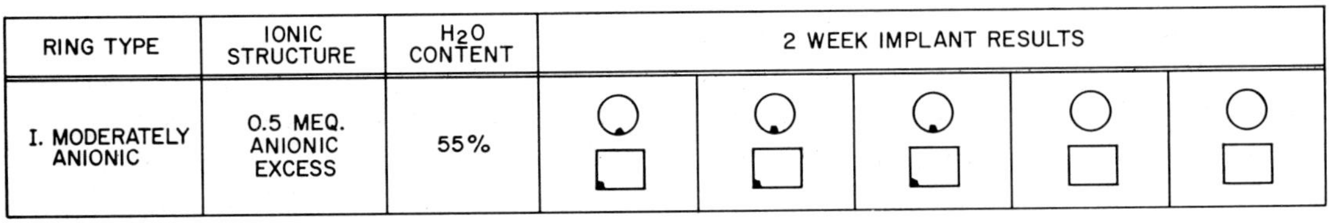

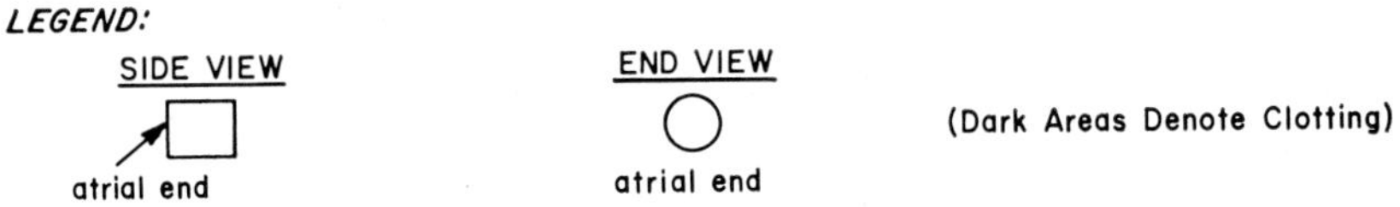

which were moderately anionic, demonstrated significant thromboresistance with five rings (Chart IB) almost completely free of thrombus at two weeks. Type II rings which were considered to be highly anionic, but having a much greater water content and thus lower negative-charge density on the surface, did not prove to be thromboresistant. As might be expected, rings which were moderately cationic (Type IV) demonstrated no thromboresistance. Type III rings which were considered to be approximately neutral in ionic structure had suggestive thromboresistance, but the results did not warrant two-week implantation of this type of ring.

Such a venous implantation as used in the screening of these materials is a very severe test of thromboresistance as evidenced by the data obtained previously in rings constructed of silicone rubber, Teflon, and polypropylene. In vivo results with these aforementioned materials are presented in Chart II. It is the experience of this laboratory that any plain polymer or plain silicone material, when molded into the small implant ring, will always be the site of severe thrombus within two hours after implantation in the vena cava.

The majority of the acute short-term studies performed with these polyelectrolyte materials were with nonsterilized rings; however, rings for all chronic long-term studies were sterilized. A number of different sterilization techniques were evaluated for the polyelectrolyte materials, and the method

Chart II

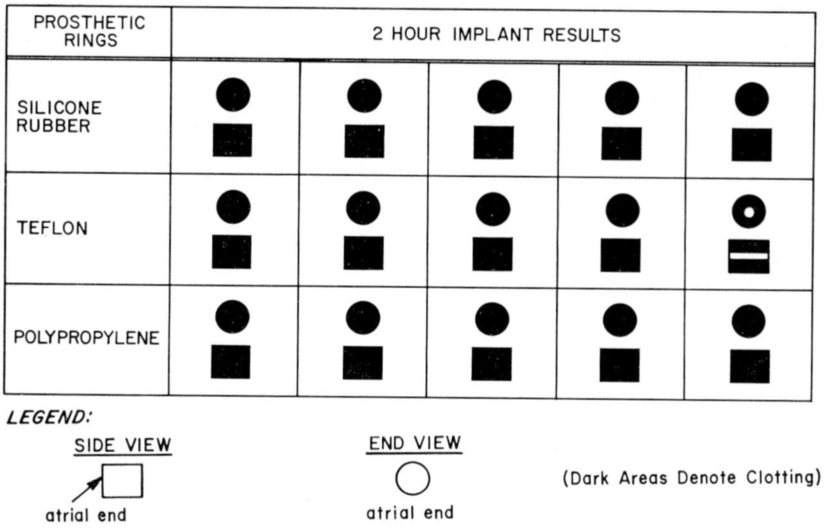

finally selected was sterilization with hydrochloric acid with neutralization to pH of 7.4. The Type I rings presented in Chart IB were sterilized in this manner.

The data presented on the polyelectrolyte rings have been selected from more than 100 implant studies of these materials. The majority of these studies were carried out in the attempt to find the most suitable method for sterilization of the materials.

DISCUSSION

The most important finding of this series of tests was the consistent nonthrombogenic behavior in both short-term and long-term tests of the polyelectrolyte complex containing a moderate excess of bound sulfonate groups, containing 0.5 mEq. excess polyanion per dry gram of resin and a water content of 55 percent. This nonthrombogenic activity is comparable to that displayed by the more successful heparinized materials and is far superior to the behavior of low-energy polymers, such as silicone rubber and Teflon (which were usually completely thrombosed within 2 hours as shown in Chart II). Considering the hypercoagulability of dogs' blood, the nonthrombogenic behavior displayed by this material in these series of tests is thought to be extremely significant, warranting investigation for long-term applications.

In marked contrast to the behavior of the moderately anionic materials is that of the polycation-excess complexes (Type IV). The latter showed rapid clotting; rings of this type usually become totally occluded within two hours. Since these rings are of approximately the same water content and of essentially the same chemical structure as the nonthrombogenic materials, except for the ratio of polyanion to polycation in the structure, the influence of surface charge is strongly shown. Neutral polyelectrolyte complexes, having an equal number of anionic and cationic groups bound to the matrix (Type IV), displayed behavior intermediate between that of the anionic and cationic complexes, which show only moderate thrombosis in two hours, with some neutral rings essentially clear of thrombus.

The highly anionic rings (1.3 mEq. excess polyanion per dry gram) are available only with high water contents (with a weight ratio of resin to water of about 1 to 9). This high water content, which results in a relatively low charge density (sulfonate groups per square centimeter) on the surface, may explain the rather poor behavior of these highly negative complexes in vivo (Type II).

It should be noted here in passing that modified Lee-White whole blood clotting times with the use of recalcified Blood Bank blood in contact with these complexes showed no prolongation of clotting times over those of blood in contact with conventional low surface energy polymers and that there was no significant difference between anionic and cationic complexes. These findings would appear to invalidate in vitro clotting tests as a measure of nonthrombogenic activity in vivo. These relatively short clotting times, however, are an indication that no substance is released from the polyelectrolyte complex that interferes with the intrinsic clotting mechanism.

CONCLUSIONS

Short-term and long-term chronic in vivo experiments in dogs have shown certain types of polyelectrolyte complexes to possess highly significant nonthrombogenic activity which is superior to that displayed by conventional low surface energy polymers and comparable to that displayed by heparinized surfaces. Consistently nonthrombogenic complexes contained a moderate excess of polyanion over polycation in the structure (0.5 mEq. excess polyanion per dry gram of resin) and a water content of approximately 55 percent (wet basis). Rings of this formulation ordinarily remained free of thrombus for two weeks in the inferior vena cava of dogs.

Formulations with a net bound positive charge (excess polycation) usually clotted within two hours, while neutral complexes displayed intermediate behavior. Highly anionic formulations usually clotted within two hours, possibly because their high water content (90 percent) reduced the over-all bound sulfonate density below a critical level.

The consistently nonthrombogenic moderately anionic complexes warrant further investigation as materials for long-term use in blood-contacting sites in vivo. Mechanical and fabrication properties of these complexes are not presently satisfactory and require further development. Further investigation of polyelectrolyte complexes differing in physical and chemical composition from those already tested is also warranted.

REFERENCES

1. Arge, E.: Dextran sulfate, comparison with heparin, Acta Med. Scand. **155:** 496, 1956.
2. Bhattacharya, B. K., and Singh, C.: A comparative biological and chemical study on the heparin-like action of polyanionic compounds, Arch. Int. Pharmacodyn. **155:** 326, 1965.
3. Doane, W., and Whistler, R. L.: Comparison of the anticoagulant activity of the polysaccharide sulfates, Arch. Biochem. **101:** 436, 1963.
4. Gott, V. L., Koepke, D. E., Daggett, R. L., Zarnstorff, W., and Young, W. P.: The coating of intravascular prostheses with colloidal graphite, SURGERY **50:** 382, 1961.
5. Gott, V. L., Whiffen, J. D., and Dutton, R. C.: Heparin bonding on colloidal graphite surfaces, Science **142:** 1297, 1963.
6. Hashimoto, K.: A dextrorotatory polysaccharide of very high anticoagulant activity newly isolated from the whale's lung and intestine, Tohoku J. Exp. Med. **81:** 93, 1963.
7. Leininger, R. I., Epstein, M. M., Falb, R. D., and Grode, G. A.: Preparation of nonthrombogenic plastic surfaces, Trans. Amer. Soc. Artif. Intern. Organs **12:** 151, 1966.
8. Lipps, B. L., Jr.: Antithrombogenic dialysis membranes for the artificial kidney, Sc.D. Thesis, Massachusetts Institute of Technology, February, 1966.
9. Lovelock, J. E., and Porterfield, J. S.: Blood coagulation: Its prolongation in vessels with negatively charged surfaces, Nature **167:** 39, 1951.
10. Markley, L. L., Bixler, H. J., and Cross, R. A.: Utilization of polyelectrolyte complexes in biology and medicine, J. Biomed. Mat. Res. **2:** 145, 1968.
11. Michaels, A. S.: Polyelectrolyte complexes, Industr. Engin. Chem. **57:** 32, 1965.
12. Whiffen, J. D., Dutton, R. C., Young, W. P., and Gott, V. L.: Heparin application to graphite-coated intravascular prosthesis, SURGERY **56:** 404, 1964.

The effect of epicardiectomy on the function and diastolic compliance of the normal canine left ventricle

HAMNER HANNAH, III, M.D.
LEE P. ENRIGHT, M.D.
ROBERT L. REIS, M.D.
BETHESDA, MD.
From the Clinic of Surgery, National Heart Institute

Previous studies in this laboratory have demonstrated that epicardiectomy significantly improves the performance of the acutely ischemic left ventricle.[4] The mechanism or mechanisms responsible for this improvement in function are, however, not understood. Vineberg[5] has theorized that epicardiectomy allows the heart to dilate and expand the sinusoidal bed, which permits blood to enter the myocardium directly from the lumen of the left ventricle during diastole. In our studies, however, improved ventricular performance was observed when there was no opportunity for blood to enter the myocardium from the left ventricular lumen, which suggests that this mechanism is not responsible for the functional improvement which occurred. An understanding of the effects of epicardiectomy on the contractile state of the normal heart might be helpful in defining the mechanism by which this procedure improves the performance of the acutely ischemic ventricle. The present study was therefore designed to determine the effects of epicardiectomy on the function and diastolic compliance of the normal canine left ventricle.

METHODS

Adult mongrel dogs, weighing 17 to 25 Kg., were anesthetized with intravenous pentobarbital (35 mg. per kilogram of body weight). A cuffed endotracheal tube was inserted, and ventilation was maintained by a positive pressure respirator supplying air. A bilateral transsternal thoracotomy was performed, and heparin (3 mg. per kilogram) was administered intravenously. The cannulations and extracorporeal circuit employed to obtain left ventricular function curves were identical to those described previously.[4] Blood temperature was monitored by a thermistor in the inferior vena cava and maintained at 36° to 37° C. by a heat exchanger in the extracorporeal circuit. The sinoatrial node was crushed, and the heart rate was maintained constant by electrical stimulation of the right atrium at a rate of 170 beats per minute. Aortic pressure was maintained constant during each study by infusing or withdrawing arterial blood through cannulas inserted into both femoral and carotid vessels. The left ventricular function curves were determined by relating left ventricular stroke work to left ventricular–end diastolic pressure. The first derivative of the left ventricular pressure (dp/dt max.) was computed from the full left ventricular pressure pulse by an electronic differentiating circuit. The ventricular epicardium, including the epicardium over the major coronary arteries, was removed. In some areas, the epicardium was peeled off in sheets, but in most areas it was removed with an epicardial abrader. Ventricular function curves were inscribed before and 30 minutes after epicardiectomy in 15 dogs.

In four animals, isovolumic left ventricular contractions were obtained by inserting a balloon attached to a metal cannula into

Received for publication July 9, 1969.

the left ventricle through a stab incision at its apex during cardiopulmonary bypass. The apparatus and technique of insertion have been previously described.[4] Ventricular volume was established by inflating the balloon with a measured volume of saline solution. The mitral valve orifice was occluded with a fenestrated plug which drained coronary blood returning directly to the left ventricular cavity. At constant aortic pressure and fixed heart rate, this preparation provided data from which force-velocity curves, length-tension curves, and diastolic pressure-volume curves were constructed. Each of these curves was determined before and 30 minutes after epicardiectomy in each animal. Left ventricular–end diastolic pressure, the full left ventricular pressure pulse, and the first derivative of left ventricular pressure (dp/dt) were simultaneously recorded as the volume of the intraventricular balloon was increased to 25 ml. in 5 ml. increments. Diastolic pressure-volume curves were inscribed by relating the intraventricular balloon volumes to left ventricular–end diastolic pressure. Length-tension curves were constructed by plotting the peak systolic force developed versus the increase in ventricular volume. Force was calculated from the equation:

$$F = \frac{P \times r_1^2}{r_o^2 - r_1^2} \times 1.36.$$

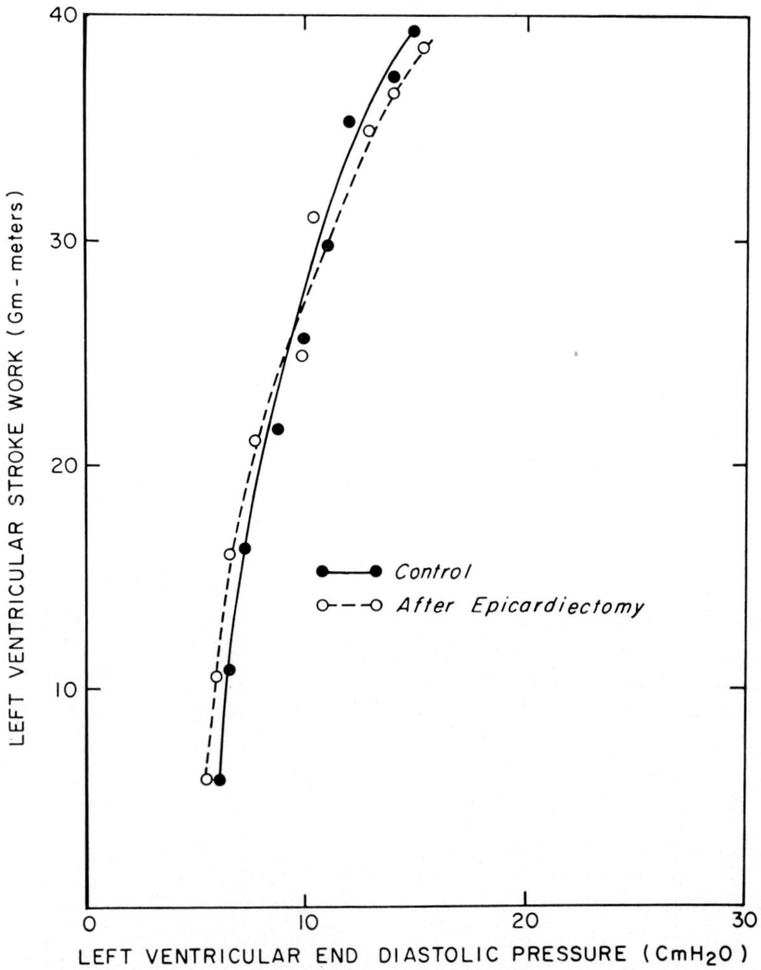

Fig. 1. Representative left ventricular function curves inscribed in an animal before and after epicardiectomy. No alteration of ventricular function is apparent.

Where F is force ($\frac{\text{gram-weight}}{\text{cm.}^2}$), P is peak systolic left ventricular pressure (mm. Hg), r_i is internal (endocardial) ventricular radius (cm.), and r_o is external (epicardial) ventricular radius (cm.). For these calculations, the ventricle was assumed to be a sphere, and the equation

$$\text{Volume} = 4/3\ \pi\ r_i^3$$

was solved for the radius. The external ventricular radius was determined from the sum of the volume of the left ventricular muscle mass and the intraventricular volume. The specific gravity of left ventricular muscle was assumed to be 1, and the left ventricular muscle volume was therefore determined by its weight.

Force-velocity curves were inscribed by determining the instantaneous relations between force and contractile element velocity at 10 msec. intervals during the course of single isovolumic beats. Force was determined as described above. Velocity was calculated from the equation

$$\text{Vc.e.} = \frac{\text{dp/dt}}{28\text{P}} \times 2\ \pi\ \text{r}$$

where $Vc.e.$ is velocity of the contractile element (cm. per second), P is ventricular pressure (mm. Hg), and r is the midventricular radius (mm.). The computations were facilitated by a digital computer.

RESULTS

In 14 of the 15 dogs there was no significant change in the ventricular function curve inscribed after epicardiectomy when compared to the control curve recorded in the same animal prior to the epicardiectomy (Fig. 1). In the remaining animal, the anterior descending coronary artery was injured during epicardiectomy, and moderate depression of ventricular function resulted. In this animal, maximum dp/dt was 1963 mm. Hg per second before epicardiectomy and decreased to 1,230 mm. Hg per second after epicardiectomy. In the remaining 14 dogs, maximum dp/dt was similar before and after epicardiectomy. Force-velocity relations, length-tension relations, and diastolic pressure-volume relations were also not changed by epicardiectomy (Figs. 2, 3, and 4).

DISCUSSION

The studies of Agrawal and associates[1] suggest that epicardiectomy adversely affects left ventricular function in normal dogs. In their studies, myocardial contractile force was measured before and following epicardiectomy; heart rate, systemic blood pressure, and ventricular volume were not controlled, however, and these variables may significantly influence contractile force. Vineberg[5] and Agrawal and his associates[1] have also suggested that ventricular volume is augmented following epicardiectomy, due to the release of constricting influences which the epicardium exerts on the myocardium. These observations, however, have also been

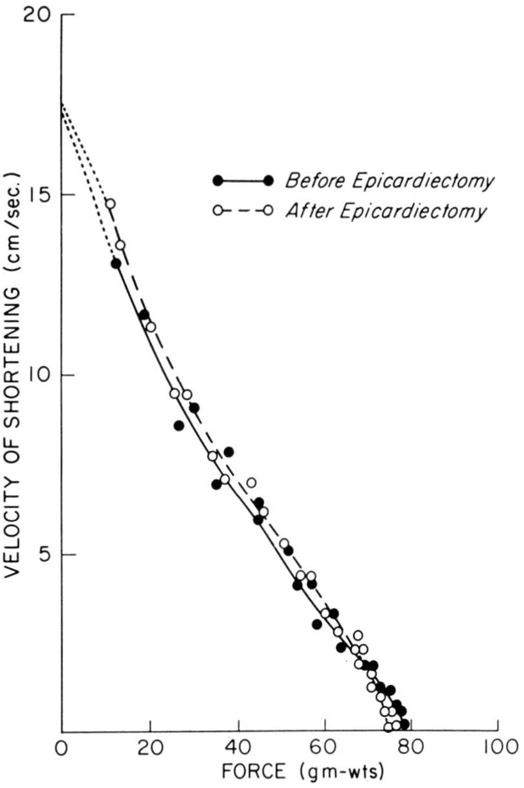

Fig. 2. Representative force-velocity curves inscribed in an animal before and after epicardiectomy. There is no change in myocardial contractility in that the instantaneous relations between force and velocity are unchanged.

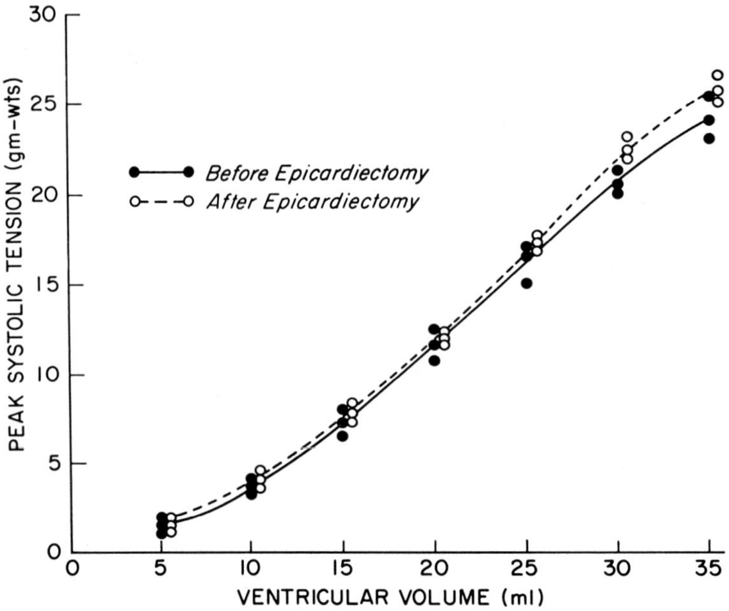

Fig. 3. Length-tension curves demonstrating no alteration in myocardial function after epicardiectomy. At similar myocardial fiber length (ventricular volumes), peak isometric wall tension is the same before and after epicardiectomy.

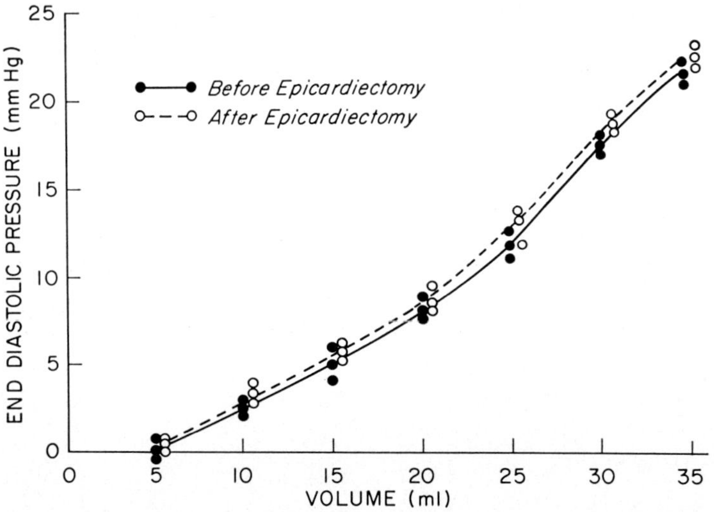

Fig. 4. Left ventricular–diastolic pressure volume curves inscribed in an animal before and after epicardiectomy. There is no change in left ventricular diastolic compliance.

made under circumstances in which heart rate was not controlled. It has been shown that heart rate decreases following epicardiectomy,[1] and an increase in ventricular volume could result from the slower heart rate alone. In the present experiments, when heart rate and systemic arterial pressure were kept constant, epicardiectomy did not produce any immediate alteration in the function or diastolic compliance of the normal canine ventricle.

The present study also provides information regarding possible mechanisms by which epicardiectomy improves the performance of the acutely ischemic ventricle. Epicardiectomy undoubtedly produces cardiac denervation, and although the contractile state of heart muscle is not altered by denervation,[2] its responsiveness to circulating catecholamines may be enhanced. If it is by this mechanism that epicardiectomy improves the performance of the acutely ischemic ventricle, epicardiectomy should also enhance the contractile state of the normal heart. The failure of epicardiectomy to do so in the present study excludes this possibility as the mechanism by which epicardiectomy improves the performance of the acutely ischemic ventricle.

Neural ablation may produce blood vessel dilation and thereby increase collateral blood flow to the ischemic myocardium. Indeed, King and associates[3] have shown by radioactive rubidium (Rb^{86}) uptake that an increase in myocardial blood flow following epicardiectomy occurs in the normal dog heart. Ischemia, however, is a most potent stimulus to coronary vasodilation, and any additional inhibition of constriction of coronary blood vessels that might be provided by sympathectomy would seem to be superfluous. It is possible, however, that the mechanism by which epicardiectomy improves cardiac performance during acute regional myocardial ischemia is related to augmentation of the contractile state of the ischemic muscle as a result of increased collateral blood flow to the ischemic area. Further studies are needed to define the mechanism by which epicardiectomy improves cardiac performance during acute regional myocardial ischemia.

SUMMARY

The effects of epicardiectomy on the function and diastolic compliance of the normal canine left ventricle were determined by ventricular function curves, length-tension curves, force-velocity curves, and pressure-volume curves inscribed at fixed heart rate and constant aortic pressure before and 30 minutes following epicardiectomy. Epicardiectomy produced no immediate alteration in the function or diastolic compliance of the normal canine left ventricle. The relevance of these findings to the still unknown mechanism by which epicardiectomy improves ventricular function during acute regional myocardial ischemia were discussed.

REFERENCES

1. Agrawal, G., Silk, P., Glotfelty, E., and Levowitz, B. S.: Effect of epicardiectomy on myocardial function, SURGERY **61:** 399, 1967.
2. Daggett, W. M., Willman, V. L., Cooper, T., and Hanlon, C. R.: Work capacity and efficiency of the autotransplanted heart, Circulation **35**(Suppl. 1)**:** 96, 1967.
3. King, R. D., Steiner, S. H., and Heimburger, I. L.: Effect of epicardiectomy on myocardial blood flow, J. Thorac. Cardiov. Surg. **51:** 660, 1966.
4. Reis, R. L., Enright, L. P., Hannah, H., and Morrow, A. G.: The effects of epicardiectomy on the performance of the acutely ischemic left ventricle, J. Thorac. Cardiov. Surg. **56:** 647, 1968.
5. Vineberg, A.: Experimental background of myocardial revascularization by internal mammary artery implantation and supplementary techniques, with its clinical application in 125 patients: A review and critical appraisal, Ann. Surg. **159:** 185, 1964.

Local irrigation with an antibiotic solution in the prevention of infection in vascular prostheses

JOHN W. D. DiGIGLIA, M.D.
GEORGE L. LEONARD, M.D.
JOHN L. OCHSNER, M.D.
NEW ORLEANS, LA.
From the Departments of Surgery and Pathology, Ochsner Clinic and Ochsner Foundation Hospital

Infection of a vascular prosthesis is one of the most dreaded complications of vascular surgery, and frequently it leads to a catastrophe. Fry and Lindenauer[5] described a series of 12 infected vascular prostheses with a 75 percent mortality rate. In Smith and Szilagyi's[13] series, 54 percent of the patients with infected wounds after vascular surgical procedures bled, with a resultant mortality rate of 37.5 percent.

Many methods[5, 11, 12] for the management of infected arterial prostheses have been suggested, but all have limitations. Prevention of infection should be of prime importance in vascular surgery where a prosthesis is used as a conduit. The role of prophylactic systemic antibiotic therapy in vascular surgery remains controversial. Some authors[1, 2, 8-10] have condemned routine use of systemic antibiotics prophylactically, but do recommend their use in high risk or contaminated cases. Other authors[3-7] advocate the use of prophylactic systemic antibiotics in all vascular surgical procedures. Topical antibiotics should be a useful adjunct in the prevention of infection where vascular prostheses are present. The purpose of this paper is to evaluate the effectiveness of topical kanamycin-bacitracin solution in the prevention of vascular graft infection.

PHASE I

Methods and materials. Twenty adult mongrel dogs, weighing between 15 and 25 kilograms, were anesthetized intravenously with 1 mg. of pentobarbital sodium per kilogram of body weight. The operative site was prepared with pHisoHex and tincture of Zephiran chloride and draped with sterile linen. A 6 cm. incision was made in each groin and the common femoral arteries isolated. Three centimeter arteriotomies were made in each artery, and a 3 cm. by 1 cm. knitted Dacron patch graft was sutured into place with a continuous 5-0 Tevdek (Fig. 1). Each wound was then inoculated with 1 c.c. of a standardized bacterial broth solution containing hemolytic *Staphylococcus aureus* coagulase positive, in a concentration of 8 million organisms per cubic centimeter. The wounds were held open for 30 minutes and then closed in an identical manner, with the

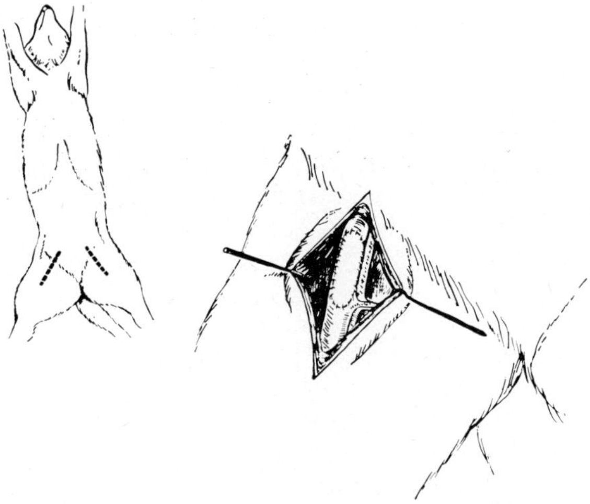

Fig. 1. Illustration of arteriotomy site and knitted Dacron patch graft sutured in place.

Supported in part by Grant FR 05518 from the National Institutes of Health and the William Loring Ferguson Cardiovascular Fund.
Received for publication July 14, 1969.

use of 3-0 chromic catgut on the deep layers and 4-0 Dermalon to approximate the skin. Prior to closure some wounds were irrigated with 100 c.c. of normal saline, or 100 c.c. of a bactericidal solution which contained 0.2 percent kanamycin and 5,000 units of bacitracin (Table I). The solutions were prepared daily, labeled A or B, and selected at random for irrigation. The type of irrigating solution used on each wound was not known to the surgeon until after the completion of the procedure, effecting a blind study. Table II illustrates the random sampling of irrigating solution for each individual wound.

No pre- or postoperative systemic antibiotics were used in any of the animals.

Seven days after operation each animal was again anesthetized, the femoral areas prepared with pHisoHex and tincture of Zephiran chloride and draped with sterile linen. The wounds were inspected for evidence of gross infection, reopened, and cultures of the Dacron patch grafts taken. Evaluations of the condition of the graft and the flow through this area of the femoral artery were made.

Table I. *Types of irrigation and number of wounds in which each was used*

Type of irrigation	*No. of wounds*
No irrigation (control)	6
100 c.c. normal saline	10
100 c.c. kanamycin-bacitracin	24

Table II. *Illustration of the random selection of irrigation solution for each wound*

Type of irrigation used on each wound	*No. of dogs*
One wound—no irrigation One wound—normal saline irrigation	1
One wound—no irrigation One wound—kanamycin-bacitracin irrigation	5
One wound—normal saline irrigation One wound—kanamycin-bacitracin irrigation	5
Both wounds—normal saline irrigation	2
Both wounds—kanamycin-bacitracin irrigation	7

Results. In all six control wounds which had no irrigation there was disruption of the suture line of the graft with hemorrhage, false aneurysm formation, and gross infection (Fig. 2). All of these wounds had abscess formation at the surgical site. All of the grafts in the control group were infected with *Staphylococcus aureus* of the type used in the wound inoculation.

In all 10 wounds washed with 100 c.c. of normal saline, there was evidence of gross infection. All of the saline-washed wounds had leakage of the graft suture lines with hemorrhage and false aneurysm formation. All of the grafts in these wounds were also infected with *Staphylococcus aureus* of the type used in the wound inoculation.

In all 24 wounds washed with 100 c.c. of kanamycin-bacitracin solution, there was primary wound healing. All arterial grafts were patent with good pulsation (Fig. 3). There was no evidence of grossly visible infection or leakage from the suture lines of the graft. There was no hematoma or false aneurysm formation. All of the grafts, however, when cultured, revealed *Staphylococcus aureus* of the type used in inoculation of the wounds.

Results of evaluation of the wounds 1

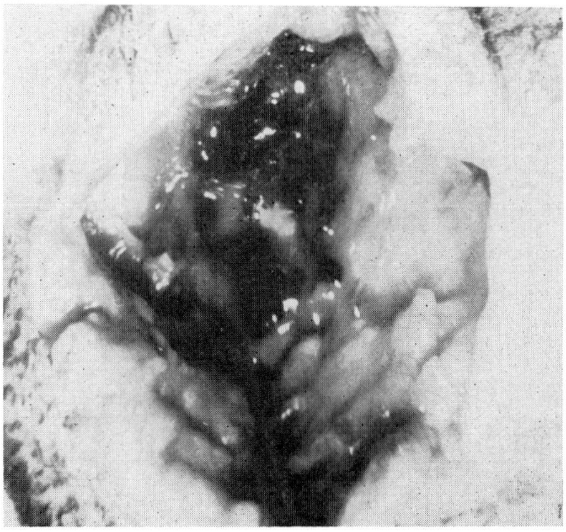

Fig. 2. Photograph of control wound taken 7 days after operation, showing hemorrhage from the suture line and gross infection.

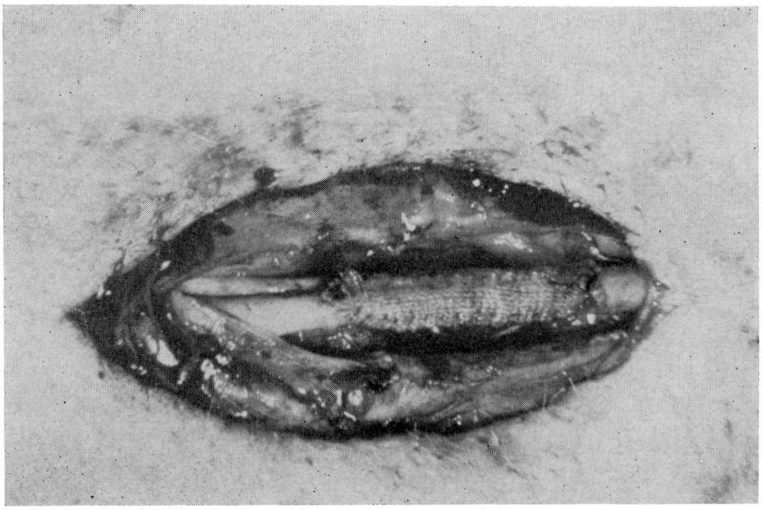

Fig. 3. Photograph of kanamycin-bacitracin–washed wound taken 7 days after operation, showing an intact suture line and no evidence of gross infection.

Table III. *Evaluation of the wounds in the Phase I experiments 1 week after operation*

	Control—no irrigation (6 wounds)		*Normal saline irrigation (10 wounds)*		*Kanamycin-bacitracin irrigation (24 wounds)*	
	No. of wounds	*%*	*No. of wounds*	*%*	*No. of wounds*	*%*
Gross infection	6	100	10	100	0	0
Leakage of arterial graft suture line	6	100	10	100	0	0
Hematoma formation	6	100	10	100	0	0
Staph. aureus cultured from graft	6	100	10	100	24	100
Primary wound healing	0	0	0	0	24	100
Patency of artery at site of graft	0	0	0	0	24	100

week after operation are shown in Table III.

PHASE II

Prompted by the fact that, although visibly clean, all 24 wounds washed with kanamycin-bacitracin solution housed *Staphylococcus aureus* on culture, a second phase of the experiment was undertaken.

Methods and materials. Five adult mongrel dogs, weighing between 15 and 25 kilograms, were anesthetized intravenously with 1 mg. of pentobarbital sodium per kilogram of body weight, the operative sites prepared with pHisoHex and tincture of Zephiran chloride, and draped with sterile linen. A 6 cm. incision was made in each groin and the common femoral arteries isolated. Three centimeter arteriotomies were made in each artery, and a 3 cm. by 1 cm. knitted Dacron patch graft was sutured into place with continuous 5-0 Tevdek. Each wound was then inoculated with 1 c.c. of a standardized bacterial broth solution containing hemolytic *Staphylococcus aureus,* coagulase positive, in a concentration of 8 million organims per cubic centimeter and held open for 30 minutes, as in Phase I. All 10 wounds were then irrigated with 100 c.c. of a bactericidal solution which contained 0.2% kanamycin and 5,000 units of bacitracin. The wounds were then closed identically, with 3-0 chromic catgut on the deep layers and 4-0 Dermalon to approximate the skin.

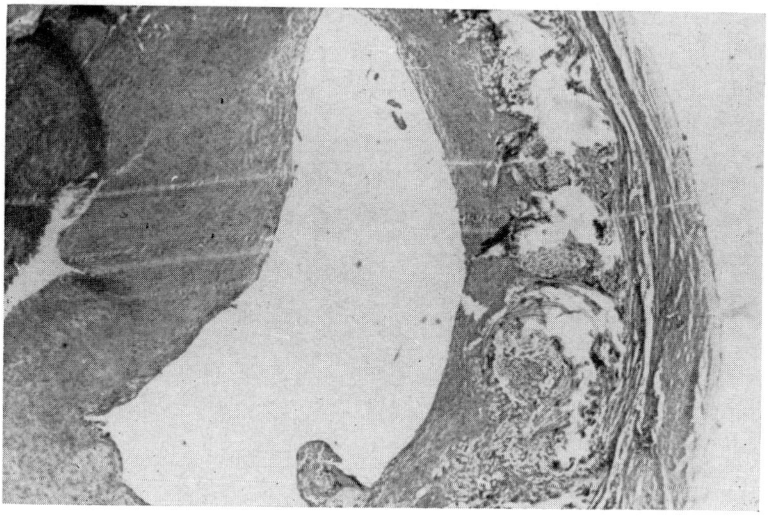

Fig. 4. Photomicrograph of femoral arterial segment, showing incorporation of the graft into the arterial wall by fibrous proliferation.

Six weeks postoperatively the dogs were reanesthetized, the femoral areas prepared with pHisoHex and tincture of Zephiran chloride and draped with sterile linen. The wounds were opened and cultures of the Dacron grafts taken. Segments of the femoral arteries, including the grafts, were taken for microscopic examination. As in Phase I, no pre- or postoperative antibiotics were used in the animals.

Results. All 10 wounds were well healed and showed no evidence of infection. There was no leakage from the arterial graft suture line, hematoma, or false aneurysm formation. In every case the arterial segment containing the Dacron patch graft was patent. All of the grafts were cultured and grew no organisms. Microscopic sections of the arterial segments containing the patch grafts showed incorporation of the graft into the arterial wall by fibrous proliferation (Fig. 4). The luminal diameter was not decreased by the fibrous proliferation in any of the arterial segments.

DISCUSSION

This study clearly demonstrates the value of antibiotic wound irrigation for the prevention of infection in vascular grafts. All of the untreated wounds in those irrigated with saline solution became grossly infected and broke down, whereas all of the treated wounds healed primarily. Although usually described as "prophylactic" antibiotic irrigation, it is obvious that the antibiotic solution is in reality used for the purpose of *treating* infection introduced at the time of operation. Since operative contamination is inevitable in a small but definite number of cases, and since there is no way to distinguish the contaminated wounds from the sterile ones at the time of operation, it is apparent that all wounds should be treated at the termination of the procedure.

Wound irrigation is a simple inexpensive procedure and carries no appreciable risk. It is a small price to pay to prevent a complication with as high a mortality rate as infection of a vascular prosthesis has.

It is of interest that the treated wounds in the present study yielded positive cultures at the end of the 7 day period, even though the vessels looked normal grossly. Identical wounds treated with the antibiotic solution were sterile at the end of a 6 week period. This may be a direct result of the extremely large dose (8 million per cubic centimeter) of bacteria in the original inoculum, perhaps too many bacteria for the antibiotic solution to kill in such a short-time interval. That these bacteria were effectively reduced in number and/or inhibited in their growth potential is well demonstrated by the sterile cultures obtained at the 6 week period. The fact that 10 of the 24 treated wounds were present in dogs with an infected contralateral wound (saline-washed or control wounds) may have contributed to the infection of the treated wound by cross contamination, either directly or by the bloodstream route. However, in seven animals both wounds were irrigated with the antibiotic solution and all 14 of these wounds grew *Staphylococcus aureus* when cultured at the end of 7 days. Nevertheless, the inoculum employed was far greater than the number of bacteria likely to be present in a contaminated wound at clinical surgery. The antibiotic solution used was of approximately the same volume and concentration as that employed routinely during clinical surgery, and is more than adequate to prevent clinical infection in all vascular grafts.

REFERENCES

1. Altemeier, W. A., Culbertson, W. R., Sherman, R., Cole, W., Elstun, W., and Fultz, C. T.: Critical re-evaluation of antibiotic therapy in surgery, J. A. M. A. **157:** 305, 1955.
2. Altemeier, W. A., Culbertson, W. R., and Vetto, M.: Prophylactic antibiotic therapy, Arch. Surg. **71:** 2, 1955.
3. Barker, W. F.: Peripheral arterial disease, Philadelphia, 1966, W. B. Saunders Company.
4. Burke, J. F.: Preoperative antibiotics, S. Clin. North America **43:** 665, 1963.
5. Fry, W. J., and Lindenauer, S. M.: Infection complicating the use of plastic arterial implants, Arch. Surg. **94:** 600, 1967.
6. Linton, R. R.: The prophylactic use of the antibiotics in clean surgery, Surg. Gynec. & Obst. **112:** 218, 1961.
7. Linton, R. R., and Darling, R. C.: Autogenous saphenous vein bypass grafts in femoropopliteal obliterative arterial disease, SURGERY **51:** 62, 1962.
8. Pulaski, E. J.: Discriminate antibiotic prophylaxis in elective surgery, Surg. Gynec. & Obst. **108:** 385, 1959.
9. Pulaski, E. J., Filler, R. M., and Dibbins, A. W.: Local and systemic antibiotic therapy of wounds and burns, Canad. M. A. J. **93:** 864, 1965.
10. Pulaski, E. J., and Shaeffer, J. R.: The background of antibiotic therapy in surgical infections, Surg. Gynec. & Obst. **93:** 1, 1951.
11. Schramel, R. J., and Creech, O., Jr.: Effects of infection and exposure on synthetic arterial prostheses, Arch. Surg. **78:** 271, 1959.
12. Seidenberg, B., Gitlitz, G. F., and Hurwitt, E. S.: Management of the infected arterial prosthesis, Surg. Gynec. & Obst. **120:** 585, 1965.
13. Smith, R. F., and Szilagyi, D. E.: Healing complications with plastic arterial implants, Arch. Surg. **82:** 34, 1961.

Pediatric surgery

Conducted by MARK M. RAVITCH, M.D.

Appendicitis in the newborn infant

JOHN M. PARSONS, M.D.
BRIAN G. MISCALL, M.D.
CHARLES K. McSHERRY, M.D.
NEW YORK, N. Y.
From the Department of Surgery, The New York Hospital–Cornell Medical Center

Acute appendicitis occurring in the first month of life is rare; by 1967 only 31 cases had been reported in the literature. The entity was first described by Diess,[3] who reported in 1908 a case of a 14-day-old patient who died following appendectomy for nonperforated gangrenous appendicitis. Single case reports appeared in the literature over the ensuing years, and by 1936 eight cases had been reported. Meigher and Lucas,[11] in 1952, described the first survivor, a 10-day-old female infant who at operation was found to have an acutely inflamed appendix without perforation. In 1960, Schaupp and associates[15] documented 5 cases of neonatal appendicitis from autopsy material, bringing the total to 24. Between 1963 and 1966, each of the reports prepared by Hardman and Bowers,[8] Fonkelsrud and associates,[6] Neve and Quenville,[12] and Parkhurst and Wagoner[13] added one case. Martin and Perrin[10] reported 3 cases, all associated with Hirschsprung's disease, to bring the total in 1967 to 31. We have recently had experience with a one-week-old infant with acute appendicitis and generalized peritonitis who survived appendectomy.

CASE REPORT

A 2,700 gram male infant was admitted to The New York Hospital–Cornell Medical Center on March 15, 1969, at age 7 days. Four days after normal delivery he developed jaundice, diarrhea, and bilious vomiting associated with poor feeding. On the fifth day, he was admitted to another hospital where he was hydrated and begun on antibiotics. A day later he was transferred to this institution. Temperature was 37.0° C., pulse 140 beats per minute, and respirations 40 per minute. Examination revealed a lethargic, jaundiced infant. There was erythema of the skin overlying the right lower quadrant of the abdomen as well as in the midline from the umbilicus to the xyphoid. The abdomen was distended, bowel sounds were hypoactive, and there was guarding in the right lower quadrant. No mass was palpable. Admission laboratory data revealed a hematocrit of 53 percent, a white blood cell count of 10,800 per cubic millimeter with a normal differential. Urinalysis was normal. Total bilirubin was 9.9 mg. percent with an indirect fraction of 8.8 mg. percent. Abdominal flat plate revealed abundant gas in the small and large intestine, but was otherwise normal. The diagnosis was sepsis with reflex ileus, and the patient was placed on parenteral penicillin and kanamycin. After 24 hours, erythema had increased in the right lower quadrant and right flank, and a 3 by 3 cm. mass was palpated in the right lower quadrant. Intravenous pyelogram was normal. The white blood cell count rose to 14,000 per cubic millimeter. At operation, there was generalized peritonitis with purulent fluid throughout the abdominal cavity. Cultures yielded *Klebsiella aerobacter*. In the right lower quadrant, one loop of small intestine was adherent to an acutely inflamed appendix that was gangrenous in its distal half. No perforation was demonstrated grossly or microscopically. Appendectomy with drainage was performed. The patient did well, and was discharged 2 weeks later. At follow-up examination six months later the patient was vigorous, healthy, and gaining weight.

Received for publication Oct. 27, 1969.

DISCUSSION

Acute appendicitis, common in childhood and adult life, is extremely rare in the neonatal period. Numerous large series of appendicitis in childhood have been reported by Abel and Allen[1] (1,165 cases), Deane[2] (777 cases), Hudson and Chamberlain[9] (848 cases), Penberthy and associates[14] (1,653 cases), Snyder and Chaffin[16] (1,051 cases), and Gross[7] (2,070 cases), none of which includes a patient in the neonatal period. Fields and Cole[4] reviewed 6,915 cases of acute appendicitis of all ages and was able to find only one patient in the newborn period. At The New York Hospital–Cornell Medical Center, 1,595 children under 15 years of age have undergone appendectomy during the years from 1940 through 1968. There had been no previous patients with appendicitis under one month of age.

Firor and Myers[5] attribute the rarity of appendicitis in the first 12 months of life to a wide-based, funnel-shaped appendix not prone to obstruction. A milk and soft food diet, the recumbent position of the infant, and the infrequent occurrence of intestinal and respiratory infections in infancy are additional factors cited by Walker[17] to account for the rare occurrence of appendiceal inflammation in the neonatal period. It is pointed out that if appendicitis does occur in the neonatal period, it is tolerated poorly by the infant because of the following factors: (1) The thin-walled appendix is prone to perforation; (2) the cecum is not distensible to decompress the appendix at its base; (3) the omentum is rarely of sufficient size to wall off a perforation; (4) there is a small abdominal cavity so that infection is easily, quickly, and widely disseminated; and (5) in the neonatal period, there is a generalized lack of physiologic reserve.

Of the 31 cases of acute appendicitis in children under one month of age, only 5 had not progressed to gangrene, an incidence of 16 percent. Assuming all perforated appendices were gangrenous, the incidence of gangrene in neonatal appendicitis is 84 percent. Frank perforation, invariably described as a gross pathologic finding, occurred in 19 of 31 cases, an incidence of 61 percent. Until Martin and Perrin[10] reported a patient with neonatal appendicitis with perforation who had survived, ruptured neonatal appendicitis was invariably associated with death.

The preoperative diagnosis of acute appendicitis in the neonate is difficult. The three most common symptoms are anorexia, vomiting, and abdominal distention. The duration of symptoms in previously reported cases has ranged from 7½ hours to 9 days. Anorexia and vomiting were present in 24 of the 31 cases, with abdominal distention present in 20 of 31 cases. Other symptoms that occur with irregular frequency are irritability, lethargy, constipation, diarrhea, and fever.

The most consistent and reliable finding on physical examination is abdominal distention which occurred in 67 percent of cases. As with other infections in the neonatal period fever is often absent. Findings occasionally present are abdominal tenderness or guarding, palpable mass, hyper- or hypoactive bowel sounds, and respiratory distress. Neve and Quenville[12] report finding cellulitis of the abdominal wall extending into the right flank in his patient and mentions this finding described in 3 other cases in the literature. This sign was also present in the patient described herein. The over-all incidence of abdominal wall cellulitis in the 31 patients was 16 percent.

Although there was a progressive rise in the leukocyte count in our patient, leukocytosis is rarely present in neonatal appendicitis or other neonatal infections. Abdominal x-rays usually show only dilated loops, confirming the clinical finding of ileus.

Other causes of the acute abdomen in the neonate must be considered in the differential diagnosis. Among these are intestinal atresias with proximal perforation, meconium ileus with perforation, intestinal infarction, trauma from enemas and thermometers, gastric perforation, primary peritonitis and Hirschsprung's disease. History, physical findings, and ancillary diagnostic aids will either establish the diagnosis in many of the above entities or at least indicate the need for laparotomy. Martin and Perrin[10] reported 3 cases of neonatal appendicitis with perforation, all associated with Hirschsprung's disease, and the coexistence of these two entities should be borne in mind. Colon perforation in congenital megacolon is well known, occurring most frequently in the cecum, although it may occur closer to the site of obstruction. Following appendectomy and survival these patients should be observed for signs or symptoms of Hirschsprung's disease. If congenital megacolon is suspected at the time of laparotomy, Martin and Perrin[10] suggest that the ileum be exteriorized. Rectal biopsy can be performed when the patient's condition permits.

Twenty-five of the 31 patients with neonatal appendicitis died, a mortality rate of 81 percent. All but 1 of 19 patients with perforation succumbed, a mortality rate of 95 percent. In the absence of perforation, the mortality rate is less. There were 7 fatalities in the series of 12 reported cases, for a mortality rate of 58 percent. It would appear, then, that it is perforation that accounts for the lethality of this disease and that delay in diagnosis or exploration must be avoided if the neonate is to survive this threat to life.

SUMMARY

Acute appendicitis in the first month of life is rare. There have been 31 patients under one month of age previously reported in the literature. The management of a seven-day-old infant surviving appendectomy for acute appendicitis and generalized peritonitis is reported. The most common presenting findings are anorexia, vomiting, and abdominal distention. Cellulitis of the abdominal wall is an infrequent finding but may aid in the preoperative diagnosis. Delay in diagnosis is largely responsible for the high mortality rate of 81 percent.

REFERENCES

1. Abel, W. J., III, and Allen, P. D.: Acute appendicitis in children: A review of 1,165 cases, Ann. Surg. **132:** 1093, 1950.
2. Deane, J. M.: Acute appendicitis in children, Ann. Surg. **136:** 243, 1952.
3. Diess, F.: Die appendizitis im Basler Kinderspitel, Basle Dissertations, 1908, case No. 36, p. 63. As cited in Schaupp and associates.[15]
4. Fields, I. A., and Cole, N. M.: Acute appendicitis in infants 36 months of age or younger, Amer. J. Surg. **113:** 269, 1967.
5. Firor, H. V., and Myers, H. A. P.: Perforating appendicitis in premature infants, SURGERY **56:** 581, 1964.
6. Fonkelsrud, E. W., Ellis, D. G., and Clatworthy, H. W.: Neonatal peritonitis, J. Pediat. Surg. **1:** 227, 1966.
7. Gross, R. E.: The surgery of infancy and childhood, Philadelphia, 1953, W. B. Saunders Company, p. 255.
8. Hardman, R. P., and Bowers, D.: Appendicitis in the newborn, Amer. J. Dis. Child. **105:** 99, 1963.
9. Hudson, H. W., Jr., and Chamberlain, J. W.: Acute appendicitis in childhood: Statistical study of 848 cases from Children's Hospital, Boston, J. Pediat. **15:** 408, 1939.
10. Martin, L. W., and Perrin, E. V.: Neonatal perforation of the appendix in association with Hirschsprung's disease, Ann. Surg. **166:** 799, 1967.
11. Meigher, S. C., and Lucas, A. W.: Appendicitis in the newborn: Case report, Ann. Surg. **136:** 1044, 1953.
12. Neve, R., and Quenville, N. F.: Appendicitis with perforation in a 12-day-old infant, Canad. Med. Ass. J. **94:** 447, 1966.
13. Parkhurst, G. F., and Wagoner, S. C.: Neonatal acute appendicitis, New York J. Med. **69:** 129, 1969.
14. Penberthy, G. C., Benson, C. D., and Weller, C. N.: Appendicitis in infants and children: A 15 year study, Ann. Surg. **115:** 945, 1942.
15. Schaupp, W., Clausen, E. G., and Ferrier, P. K.: Appendicitis during the first month of life, SURGERY **48:** 805, 1960.
16. Snyder, W. H., Jr., and Chaffin, L.: Appendicitis in the first two years of life: Report of 21 cases and review of 477 cases from the literature, Arch. Surg. **64:** 549, 1952.
17. Walker, R. H.: Appendicitis in the newborn infant, J. Pediat. **51:** 429, 1957.

Traumatic pseudodiverticulum of the esophagus in the newborn infant

RAYMOND G. ARMSTRONG, Lieutenant Colonel, USAF (MC)
EVAN F. LINDBERG, Lieutenant Colonel, USAF (MC)
WILLIAM STANFORD, Lieutenant Colonel, USAF (MC)
ROBERT M. TAKAMOTO, Major, USAF (MC)
RICHARD D. WOLFE, Lieutenant Colonel, USAF (MC)
JAMES W. DIETZ, Major, USAF (MC)
LACKLAND AIR FORCE BASE, TEXAS
From the Thoracic Surgery Service of the Department of Surgery and the Departments of Radiology and Pediatrics, Wilford Hall USAF Medical Center

Vigorous resuscitative maneuvers in newborn infants with respiratory distress may inadvertently cause perforation of the cricopharyngeal wall and development of a mediastinal pseudodiverticulum of the esophagus. Such cases are rarely reported[2] but are probably more common than are generally realized. These infants tend to regurgitate all feedings and present a picture of esophageal fistula.

Nasogastric intubation is generally difficult because of the cricopharyngeal spasm which tends to cause an erroneous diagnosis of congenital anomaly. Contrast x-ray studies in these infants disclose abnormal mediastinal channels suggestive of esophageal duplication or diverticulum. Thoracotomy is undertaken because of these objective signs, and the clinical problem of dysphagia discloses the true nature of the defect.

We recently managed an infant in whom the correct diagnosis was not made preoperatively. This infant was suspected of having a duplication of the esophagus which communicated with the true esophageal lumen.

Received for publication Oct. 13, 1969.

CASE REPORT

A 3-day-old female infant, product of an uncomplicated term vaginal delivery, was referred to Wilford Hall Medical Center with a diagnosis of tracheoesophageal fistula, on the basis of regurgitation of all feedings, coarse rhonchi, and suspected aspiration penumonia. At birth, the infant was noted to be cyanotic and in respiratory distress, and she was given an Apgar rating of 4. Immediate aspiration of the nares and oropharynx was carried out, and endotracheal intubation was attempted and abandoned because of inability to visualize the vocal cords. With aspiration and positive pressure ventilation via a face mask, the general condition promptly improved and within 4 minutes the Apgar rating was upgraded to 8. Subsequently, feeding and respiratory difficulties were noted.

Upon admission to the Pediatric Service, a nasogastric tube was passed with difficulty. At this point, the working diagnosis was H type tracheoesophageal fistula. Plain chest films showed no pneumonia and contrast x-ray studies (Fig. 1), carried out by injection through the nasogastric tube, suggested a duplication of the esophagus with communication between the true and false esophageal lumens at an indeterminate point in the upper esophagus. The contrast material seen in the bronchial tree was thought to be the result of aspiration, for no evidence of a tracheoesophageal communication was seen at fluoroscopy. The significance of an ill-defined, retrocardiac,

A

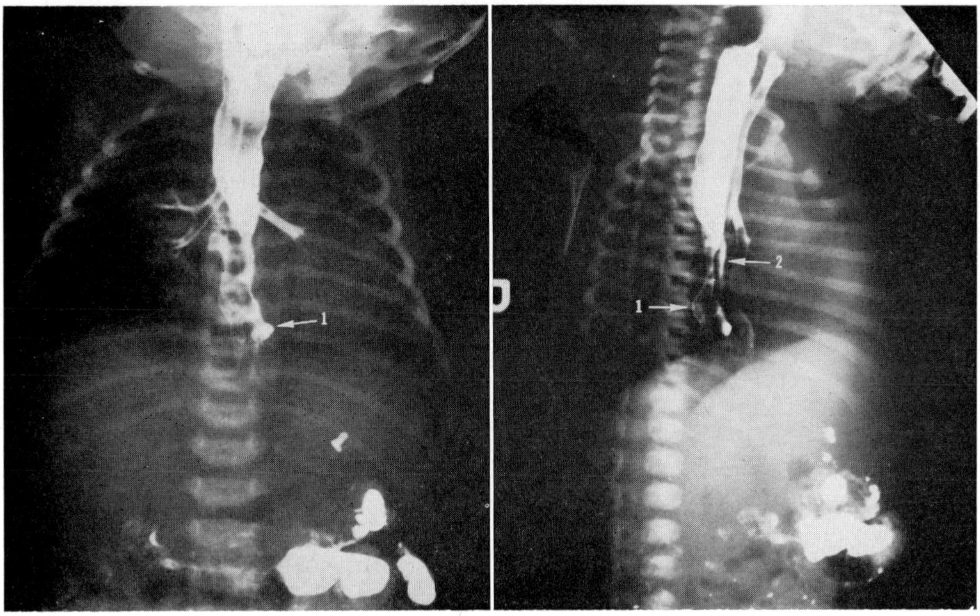

B

Fig. 1. Anteroposterior *(A)* and right anterior oblique *(B)* preoperative barium contrast studies showing pseudodiverticular pouch *(1, A* and *B)* adjacent to the esophageal lumen *(2, B)*.

vertical sliver of radiolucency at the mid- and left paraspinal area (Fig. 2) was unappreciated preoperatively.

On the fifth day of life, exploratory right thoracotomy was undertaken. Preliminary esophagoscopy disclosed at the level of the distal cricopharyngeal muscle only flecks of barium, presumed to represent retained contrast material in the true esophageal lumen. The hypopharyngeal tissue was friable; however, no evidence of perforation could be appreciated during this study, and because of difficulty in adequately visualizing the lumen, the procedure was abandoned.

The patient then underwent a right thoracotomy through the fifth intercostal space. There was a minimal degree of pneumomediastinum. After division of the azygous vein, mediastinal pleura was opened from the thoracic inlet to just above the diaphragm. A whitish, friable, thin-walled structure was found extending from the neck to its bilobed terminus just above the diaphragm. The intact esophagus lay anterior to this abnormal structure. The latter was resected and found to have a small lumen containing bile-stained fluid at its distal end. The proximal lumen of the structure was probed with a small catheter which easily passed into the hypopharynx and exited from the mouth, establishing the presence of a cervical esophageal perforation. The rubber catheter was left in place to aid in cervical exploration of the esophagus. The mediastinal

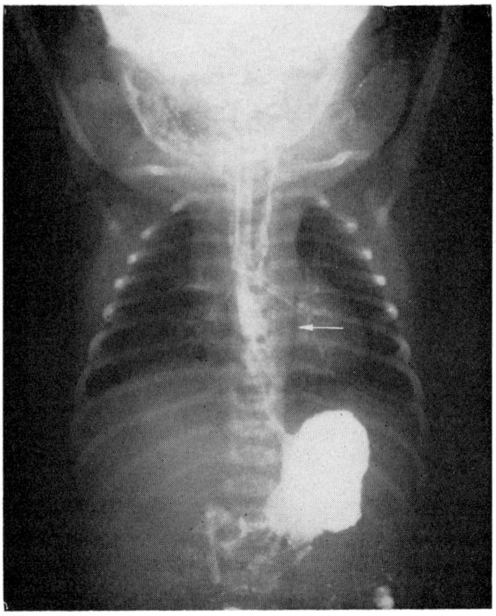

Fig. 2. Preoperative barium contrast film showing iatrogenic bronchogram and mediastinal emphysema (arrow).

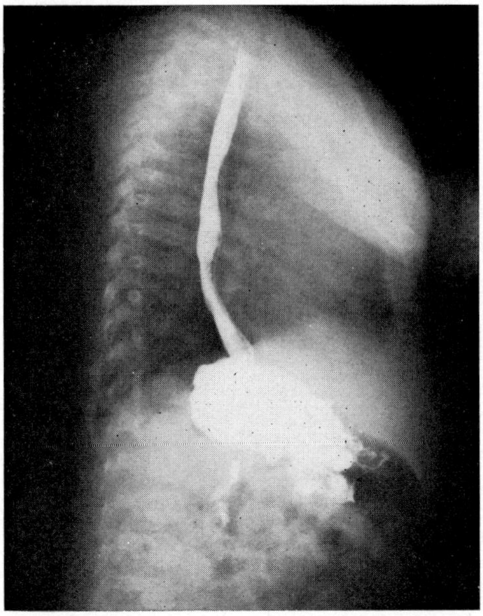

Fig. 3. Normal barium swallow 4 months after surgery when the infant was clinically well.

pleura was left open, the chest was drained, and the thoracic incision closed.

In the cervical esophagus explored through the right side of the neck, there was an 8 mm., axial, posterior, midline perforation. The rubber catheter was removed through the mouth, the nasogastric tube retained, and the paraesophageal area drained through the neck incision. No attempt was made at primary esophageal closure. Mediastinal and cervical cultures showed no growth.

The patient remained afebrile. However, for the first 5 postoperative days, she had continual coarse rhonchi without pneumonia. She was continued on broad-spectrum antibiotics which had been started two days preoperatively. Oral instillation of methylene blue on the second postoperative day disclosed no cervical esophageal leak and the diet was advanced to full-strength formula. At discharge, all wounds were healed. Follow-up barium swallows at two weeks and four months (Fig. 3) were normal. The histologic sections of the resected fistulous tract were consistent with a barium granuloma.

DISCUSSION

Cricopharyngeal perforation in the newborn infant may result from traumatic aspiration of the upper airway and has also resulted from perforation by the obstetrician's finger during extraction of a breech presentation.[2]

In a recent report, Eklöf and associates[1] indicate that a lack of awareness of this entity may lead to an erroneous diagnosis of cervical esophageal diverticulum or duplication of the esophagus. They recommend a conservative, nonoperative approach for the infant in whom the extravasation is shown to be localized to the cervical paraesophageal level. Girdany and associates[2] report that in one of their two cases, the proper diagnosis was made preoperatively and the perforation was managed with transcervical drainage alone. In the present case, since the pseudodiverticulum extended to just above the level of the diaphragm, cervical drainage might not have sufficed. The small size of the perforation and the absence of leakage made gastrostomy unnecessary.

SUMMARY

An instance is presented of traumatic perforation of the posterior cricopharyngeal wall leading to mediastinal extravasation in a newborn infant. Excision of the mediastinal drainage tract and drainage of the cervical esophagus led to cure.

REFERENCES

1. Eklöf, O., Löhr, G., and Okmian, L.: Submucosal perforation of the esophagus in the neonate, Acta Radiol. (Diag.) **8:** 187, 1969.
2. Girdany, B. R., Sieber, W. K., and Osman, M. Z.: Traumatic pseudodiverticulum of the pharynx in newborn infants, New Eng. J. Med. **280:** 237, 1969.

Idiopathic edema of scrotum in young boys

J. L. NICHOLAS, F.R.C.S.
A. MORGAN, F.R.C.S.
R. B. ZACHARY, F.R.C.S.
SHEFFIELD, ENGLAND
From The Children's Hospital, Western Bank

There have been several reports of a clinical condition in young boys which has been labeled "idiopathic edema of scrotum."[2, 3, 5] It occurs frequently enough to be important in the differential diagnosis of scrotal swellings, although its existence is not widely appreciated. This report of 15 cases is presented in order to draw attention to the condition once again and to discuss its pathological nature and diagnosis.

CLINICAL FEATURES

There is usually a 1 to 2 day history of discomfort in the groin or scrotum, and on examination the boy is found to have redness and swelling affecting the scrotum, groin, and perineum, mainly of one side. There is no evidence of conditions which more commonly cause acute swelling of the scrotum, such as incarceration of a hernia, torsion of the testis, or epididymitis. In most cases, the cord, testis, and epididymis can be felt to be normal through the edematous skin. Occasionally, the surgeon is unable to satisfy himself that the testis is not twisted and therefore proceeds to operative examination. Whatever the treatment, resolution is rapid and recurrence is rare.

These cases form a distinct clinical entity, the cause of which is uncertain. It is therefore difficult to give it a satisfactory name.

CASE HISTORIES

Fifteen cases have been seen at Sheffield Children's Hospital during the last 8 years. The ages of these boys ranged from 2 to 7 years, except for one boy who was 4 months old. The mode of presentation was similar in many of them. Usually the boy had suffered discomfort in the groin or scrotum for a few hours, and the parents had been alarmed to find his scrotum swollen and red. In no case was the pain severe and most of these boys showed little distress. One boy, two years old, had vomited once, but otherwise, the rest had suffered no gastrointestinal upset. None had dysuria. The only boy in whom trauma might have been a factor had been horseback riding on the day of onset, but he was only 2 years old and it seemed unlikely that this could have been responsible.

The redness of the skin was unilateral with a variable degree of extension across the midline in some cases. The red area was usually clearly demarcated and affected the skin of the scrotum, groin, and perineum on the same side. In 5 cases, it was not recorded whether or not the perineum was affected.

In most cases, the cord, testis, and epididymis were thought to be normal on palpation. Two boys, aged 4 months and 5 years, respectively, had retractile testes palpable in the superficial inguinal region. Five of them were diagnosed as having torsion of the testis and underwent operation (see below). In 2 cases, enlarged tender nodes were palpable in the groin of the affected side.

Six were thought to have either a break in the perianal skin or a frank anal fissure, although only one of them gave a definite history of painful defecation.

The temperature was often raised though rarely above 38° C.

Investigations. Peripheral blood white cell count, not determined in all, was never found to be above 7,000 per cubic millimeter. Urinalysis was normal in the 5 cases in which it was done. Antistreptolysin titer was measured only once and was 200 units (normal). Bacteriological swabs were taken from the perineal skin in 4 instances; one grew beta hemolytic streptococci, the rest

Received for publication Oct. 16, 1969.

grew skin commensals. Swabs taken from the incision in 2 of the cases which underwent operation grew beta hemolytic streptococci.

Treatment. Of the 10 boys treated conservatively, 8 were given penicillin and 2 sulphadimidine. All recovered within 48 hours.

Five boys underwent exploration of testis, 4 via an inguinal incision and 1 via the scrotum. In each case, the cord, testis, and epididymis were normal, but the striking feature was edema of the skin and subcutaneous tissues. In 2 of these boys, swabs of the incision grew beta hemolytic streptococci and the wound in one subsequently broke down as the result of infection and had to be resutured. Of the other 3 patients, 2 were given pencillin and the incisions of all 3 healed by first intention.

Follow-up. There were no undesirable sequelae; the testis in every case apparently remained normal with no instance of atrophy.

We know of only one case of recurrence. This boy was seen with an attack at the age of 3 years and again with a similar attack at 6 years.

DISCUSSION

Qvist[5] reviewed 158 cases of swelling of the scrotum in boys. Of these, 61 were due to incarcerated hernia, 42 to torsion of appendix testis, 9 to torsion of testis, and 14 to either epididymitis or orchitis. In 32 cases he described a state of "edema," which was unilateral and extended "down into the perineum and up into the groin." The testis and epididymis could be felt to be normal. Onset was acute and resolution occurred in a few hours. Qvist thought the condition was generally caused by infection together with regional lymphangitis, but in some cases, it could be allergic when it was bilateral and associated with other allergic manifestations in other parts of the body.

Hanstead and John[3] reviewed 7 cases of scrotal edema. They were boys between the ages of 3 and 9 years. The findings were similar to those above with redness and swelling of the scrotum, usually unilateral but in 2 cases bilateral and involving the groin and perineum. They described the affected area as being sharply demarcated posteriorly by the "origin of the perineal membrane." These authors favored an allergic cause, although they were unable to find a source of allergy. This conclusion was apparently strengthened when one of their patients made a rapid recovery following administration of an antihistamine drug. However, it is a feature of these cases that recovery is rapid whatever the treatment.

Essenghigh and Stewart[2] reviewed 7 cases of idiopathic scrotal swelling. Their findings were in many respects similar to ours except that they did not describe the redness and swelling as extending into the perineum in any of their cases. These authors favored an infective cause but were unable to suggest a portal of entry.

The nature of the condition. The clinical features described in this and previous papers are so similar that it seems reasonable to assume that they are all examples of the same pathological process, although the nature of this process is uncertain.

The redness and swelling present all the appearances of an inflammatory condition, the cause of which has in the past been a matter for discussion. Trauma would seem to be an unlikely cause in view of the absence of a history of injury in any of our cases. An allergic cause also seems unlikely since there is no obvious allergen and the unilateral distribution is difficult to explain on this basis. As Qvist[5] pointed out in those cases where allergy is obviously the cause, the signs are bilateral and associated with other allergic manifestations in other parts of the body. We have not included such cases in our series, regarding them as being a totally different entity.

The most likely cause therefore of idiopathic edema of scrotum is infection, and to support this theory, there is the evidence from 2 cases in our series in which the swabs taken at operation grew beta hemolytic streptococci. We therefore propose to use the term cellulitis rather than idiopathic edema in the discussion hereafter.

It is interesting to speculate on the relationship between our cases of cellulitis and another condition thought to be caused by beta hemolytic streptococci, namely idiopathic gangrene of the scrotum.[1] There are certain points of similarity; for example, both have sudden and obscure onset in apparently healthy individuals and both are often self-limiting. There are points of contrast. Cellulitis occurs in boys between 2 and 7 years of age; idiopathic gangrene is commonest between 20 and 50 years of age. The first is a low-grade superficial cellulitis; the second is a fulminating, subcutaneous infection causing endarteritis and gangrene, as well as having a significant mortality rate. The exact nature of both conditions is obscure.

Portal of entry of infection. There is little to indicate the portal of infection in these cases of cellulitis of the scrotum. However, this is not an uncommon observation in cases of cellulitis in other parts of the body, the break in the skin being often indiscernible. There is some evidence from our cases that the portal of entry may be through a break in the perianal skin. In one case, there was a frank anal fissure and in several others the skin of that region was cracked or soggy. As beta hemolytic streptococci are known to colonize the perineum in healthy subjects,[4] it is easy to imagine how they might enter and cause a spreading cellulitis. The direction of spread depends on the direction of lymph flow, which in this area is toward the groin nodes. A sequence of events can therefore be envisaged which explains the clinical features of these cases of cellulitis. The marked edema of the scrotum which is such a notable feature may be due merely to the lax nature of the skin in that part. It was not noted in any of our cases that the cellulitis was limited posteriorly by the origin of the perineal membrane, as was observed by Hanstead and John.[3] In fact, in many of our cases the cellulitis definitely "reached" the anus. It may, of course, have been "arising" there rather than reaching it.

Diagnosis and management. Cellulitis of the scrotum in boys is not a condition that requires operative treatment, and it seems to follow a benign course. To this extent it is relatively unimportant. Its significance, however, lies in the possibility of its confusion with conditions that do require operation, such as torsion of testis. Such confusion may result either in a boy with cellulitis having an unnecessary operation, or, more regrettably perhaps, in a boy with torsion of testis not having an operation because a diagnosis of cellulitis has been made. The former error is the more likely because the existence of idiopathic cellulitis is not widely recognized. We think it deserves wider recognition, since among other considerations its incidence is about the same as torsion of testis.

The diagnosis of cellulitis of the scrotum should only be made after the exclusion of incarcerated hernia, torsion of testis, and epididymo-orchitis. If this can be done with certainty in a boy with red swollen scrotum, a nonoperative course can be confidently followed. The surgeon need not fear that the redness and swelling indicate torsion of the testis, if the testis feels strictly normal. It must be stressed, however, that any acute scrotal swelling can also cause a remarkable degree of inflammation of the skin and the presence of redness and swelling of the skin itself does not justify a diagnosis of "cellulitis." The diagnosis must depend on the feel of the testis on palpation. If there is any doubt, the safest course is to resolve it in the operating theater. Making an incision through an area of cellulitis does not seem to be a particular hazard, although one of our patients who underwent operation had to have secondary wound suture as a consequence of gross infection.

These boys with cellulitis of scrotum are likely to be admitted to hospital to be sure of the diagnosis, and although many are likely to get better spontaneously, the finding of beta hemolytic streptococci in some cases suggests that a routine course of oral penicillin V is a reasonable precautionary measure.

SUMMARY

Fifteen cases of idiopathic edema of scrotum are described. It is suggested that the condition is in fact a cellulitis and that a possible portal of entry of the infection is a fissure in the perianal skin.

ADDENDUM

Since this paper was submitted for publication, a further case has come to our notice which supports the theory of etiology put forward in this paper.

A child of seven years had pain on defecation one morning and by afternoon had redness and swelling in the perineal region on one side, so that the General Practitioner diagnosed ischiorectal abscess. By evening there was a scrotal swelling. There was obvious cellulitis around the anus and at least one break in the epithelium at the mucocutaneous junction.

We wish to thank Mr. H. B. Eckstein for permission to quote the above case.

REFERENCES

1. Dunaif, C. B.: Fournier's gangrene. Report of a case and review of the literature, Plast. Reconstr. Surg. **33:** 84, 1964.
2. Essenhigh, D. M., and Stewart, J. S. S.: Idiopathic scrotal oedema, Brit. J. Surg. **53:** 419, 1966.
3. Hanstead, B., and John, H. T.: Idiopathic scrotal oedema of children, Brit. J. Urol. **36:** 110, 1964.
4. McKee, W. M., Di Caprio, J. M., Roberts, C. E., and Sherris, J. C.: Anal carriage as a probable source of streptococcal epidemic, Lancet **2:** 1007, 1966.
5. Qvist O.: Swelling of the scrotum in infants and children, and nonspecific epididymitis. Study of 158 cases, Acta Chir. Scand. **110:** 417, 1956.

Total prosthetic transplantation of the inferior vena cava, with venous drainage restoration of the one remaining kidney on the graft, successfully performed on a child with Wilms' tumor

LORENZO SARTI, M.D.
MILAN, ITALY
From the Thoracic and Cardiovascular Surgery Division, Children's Hospital

A total prosthetic transplantation of the inferior vena cava, with regrafting of the remaining renal vein on the Y-shaped caval graft, was performed on a girl suffering from a Wilms' tumor which required right nephrectomy and total resection of the inferior vena cava. The middle lobe of the right lung was simultaneously excised because of a metastatsis. Eighteen months later, the girl is apparently cured and leads a normal life.

While only one case of complete replacement of the inferior vena cava by a preserved aortic homograft has been reported,[1] there is no record of total caval transplantation with the use of a prosthesis.

The prognosis for preserved aortic homografts in part replacements of the subrenal inferior vena cava has not been very encouraging because of the well-known difficulties experienced in reconstruction of large veins.

The main obstacle in this kind of surgery is postoperative thrombosis resulting from both the low pressure of the blood flow through the graft and the lack of a vein substitute than can duplicate the properties of the natural walls of the vein. Complications are more serious and graft canalization troubles are more severe and frequent in the caval than in the aortic area.

Submitted for publication Aug. 11, 1969; resubmitted Sept. 11, 1969.

CASE REPORT

Clinical findings. A 5-year-old girl was hospitalized in February, 1968, for an abdominal swelling, mostly located on the right side of the abdomen, which lifted the corresponding costal arch. The swelling, hard and painless, extended beyond and approximately 2 inches to the left of the midline. No hematuria, fever, or signs of a urinary infection had been noticed within the 20 days since the discovery of the mass.

Urography. The urogram (Fig. 1) failed to demonstrate the right kidney. The left kidney eliminated satisfactorily and was virtually normal.

Phlebography. Inferior caval phlebography (Fig. 2) performed through the left saphenous showed a marked leftward displacement of the the cava. The inferior vena cava appeared to be flattened and rotated longitudinally around its axis by the mass and was incompletely filled by the contrast medium (70 per cent Urokon).

A well-developed collateral retroperitoneal venous circulation was noted at the level of the left iliohypogastric trunk, with many lumbar channels persistently visualized.

Chest x-rays showed a nodular metastasis, approximately ⅜ inch in diameter, in the parenchyma of the right lung.

Operative findings. At operation, on Feb. 28,

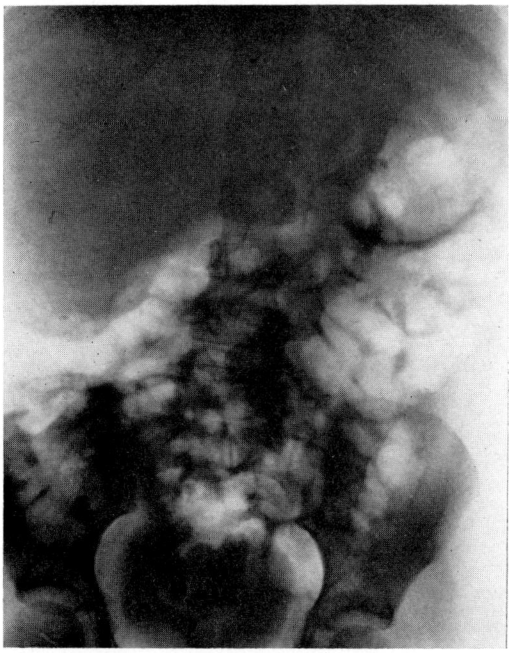

Fig. 1. Preoperative urogram.

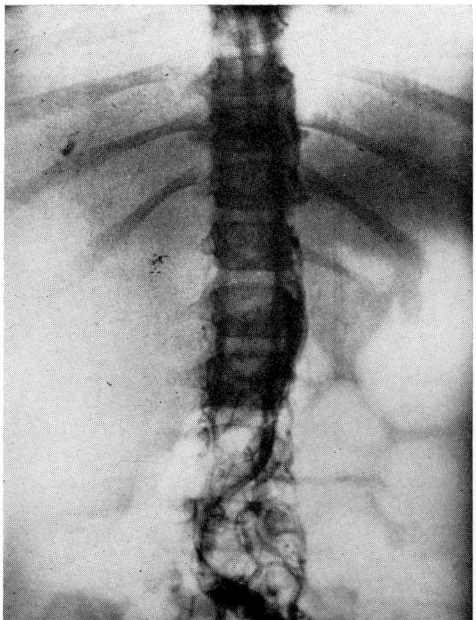

Fig. 2. Preoperative inferior cavagram.

1968, a Wilms' tumor was seen in the right kidney, compressing the inferior vena cava and metastatic to the middle lobe of the lung.

The operative field was exposed by a right thoracophrenolaparotomy through the eighth intercostal space. A huge malignant mass was seen, originating from the right kidney, extending beyond the midline, and infiltrating the inferior vena cava and the posterior, paravertebral portion of the right lobe of the liver.

The tumor could be excised from the anterior wall of the aorta and from both renal arteries without any particular trouble, along a subadventitious cleavage plane. The mass could not be separated from the whole inferior vena cava and the renal veins. To excise the retroperitoneal tumor mass and attempt a cure, it was necessary to remove (1) the right kidney, (2) 6 inches of the inferior vena cava, from the confluence of the common iliac veins up to the inferior hepatic veins, including the venous renal outlets and the last ⅜ inch of the renal vein, (3) the dorsal portion of the right lobe of the liver with the corresponding suprarenal gland, and (4) a marginal portion of the middle lobe of the lung, including the nodular metastasis of the malignancy.

The inferior vena cava was excised totally, in one piece with the tumor, and was replaced by a Y-shaped corrugated tubular Teflon prosthesis (Figs. 3*A* and 3*B*). The most proximal portion of the prosthetic tube was terminally anastomosed with the hepatic portion of the inferior vena cava, which had been prepared in advance by sectioning the inferior hepatic veins. One of the two smaller branches of the Y-shaped tube was anastomosed terminally with the most distal portion of the inferior cava, immediately after the confluence of the common iliac veins, while the other branch was anastomosed terminally with the stump of the left renal vein. A venous reimplantation of the remaining kidney on the inferior caval graft was thus performed.

During the performance of the renal venous anastomosis, the left renal artery was occluded with a bulldog clamp. The three anastomoses were performed with the use of an everting suture (No. 5-0 Teflon) interrupted at three equidistant points around each circumference. The temporary clamping of the inferior vena cava, which lasted 45 minutes in all, was well tolerated by the patient. The arterial blood pressure quickly reverted to normal after the venous flow was restored.

The right hemithorax was closed under continuous gravity suction. Layer reconstruction was used for the thoracolaparotomy. As the operation was completed, the child's hemodynamic condition was satisfactory.

Pathological anatomy. The portion removed as a single piece weighed 1,230 grams and its over-all dimensions were 22 by 14 by 9 cm. (approximately 9 by 6 by 4 inches). The wall of the inferior vena cava had been coarsely infiltrated by the malignancy from which the lung metastasis had apparently originated, proceeding through blood vessels. Histological examination confirmed the diagnosis of a Wilms' tumor.

Postoperative course. Approximately 20 hours postoperatively, there was a severe drop in the arterial blood pressure (60 mm. Hg systolic) but no sign of acute anemia. Systolic pressure values reverted to normal (around 100 mm. Hg) after approximately 6 hours of hypotension (metabolic acidosis). Excretion of urine, which had been normal during the first postoperative hours, before the hypotensive crisis began, changed rapidly to extreme oliguria and then anuria (which lasted approximately 4 hours) during the second postoperative day.

During this period, diffuse edema appeared on the face, arms, and thorax. Nitrogen blood values soared to very high levels (3.7 per cent) without sleepiness or impairment of consciousness. There was a shift of the electrolytic picture toward hyperchloremia and hyperpotassemia, with heavy creatinine retention. Cylinders were never found in the urinary sediment, the only findings being microscopic hematuria.

Hemodialysis was performed thrice as a remedy for the acute renal insufficiency that had set in.

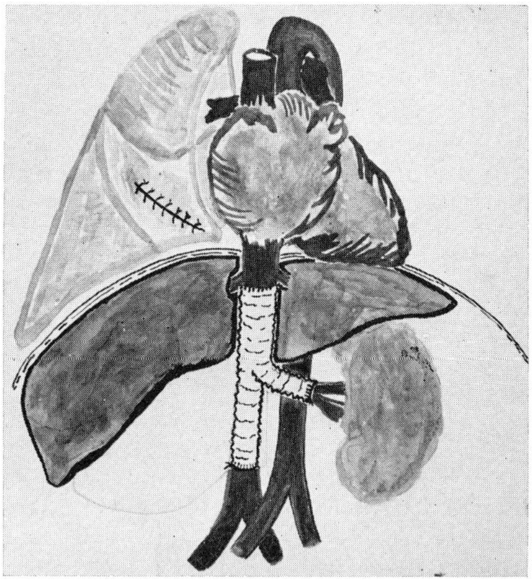

Fig. 3*A*. Schematic drawing of the prosthetic inferior vena cava transplantation with left venous renal drainage restoration after renal, caval, and pulmonary resections.

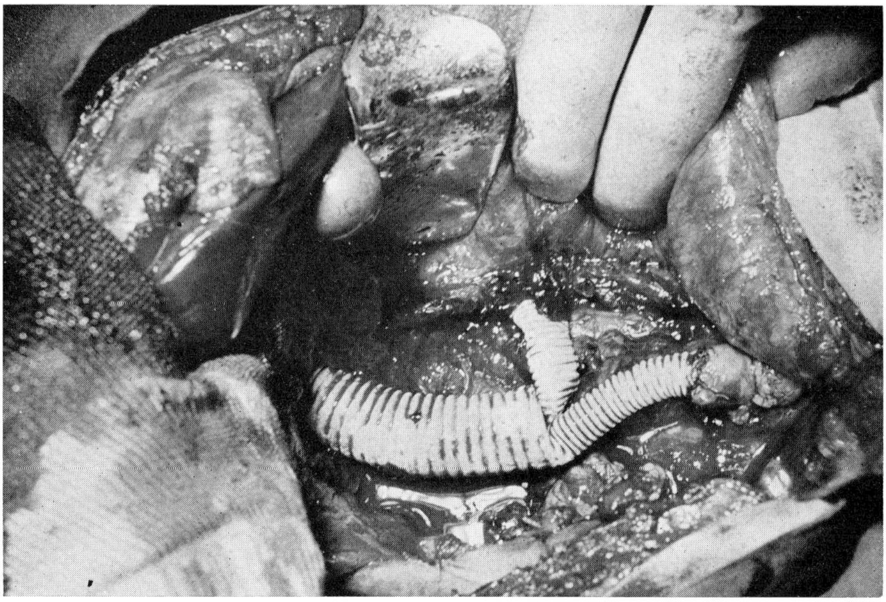

Fig. 3*B*. Operative photograph of the inferior vena cava Y-shaped graft at completion of operation. The upper caval anastomosis is behind the line; one limb of the Y serves for an end-to-end anastomosis to the left renal vein; the other for an end-to-end anastomosis to the distal cava.

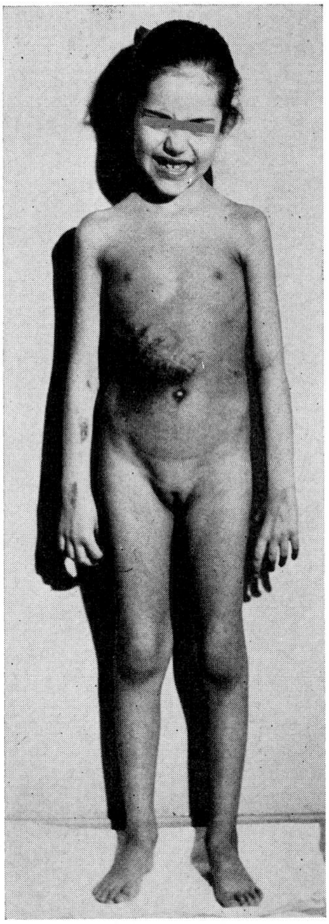

Fig. 4. The girl one month after operation.

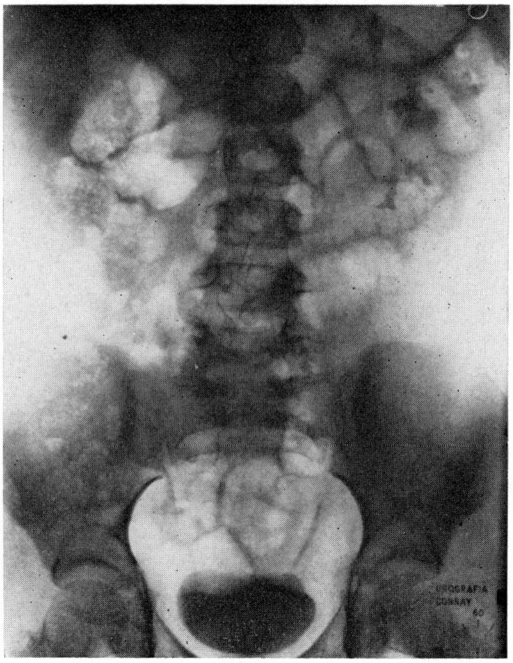

Fig. 5. Postoperative urogram. The left kidney functions normally.

Anticoagulant treatment with heparin was administered as evidence was gained that the clinical picture was a result of venous stagnation in the reimplanted kidney.

Resumption of urine excretion was slow, and normal values were not restored until the sixth postoperative day.

At no time did the legs exhibit any signs of venous overfilling or patching due to blood stagnation to indicate a thrombosis of the systemic branch of the caval graft.

As diuresis was restored, urinalysis findings, arterial blood pressure values, and biochemical blood data gave evidence that the remaining kidney was again operating normally.

The operative area received roentgen therapy (a total of 3,000 r). In the meantime the patient received actinomycin D (Cosmegen) at the rate of 0.1 mg. per kilogram of body weight during five consecutive days at a time, once a month for a four-month period and, after one year, once every six months.

The patient was discharged 50 days after operation. There were no signs of leg edema even after protracted standing or walking (Fig. 4).

Eighteen months after the operation, the patient's condition was still quite satisfactory. The kidney was functioning normally and urography showed normal elimination from the remaining left kidney reimplanetd on the caval graft.

A checkup by caval phlebography was withheld to avoid the risk of thrombophlebitis. Satisfactory elimination from the remaining kidney was regarded as reliable evidence of the functional permeability of the inferior caval graft (Fig. 5).

The child is very well two years after operation.

COMMENT

It is still too early to tell whether and to what extent complete excision of the inferior vena cava will cure a retroperitoneal tumor.

Thrombosis in the renal area is the development that can most seriously impair the successful outcome of a complete prosthetic replacement of the inferior cava. The restoration of the venous renal drainage is the most critical part of the operation and the main potential source of postoperative complications (kidney hemorrhagic infarction). Only a partial thrombosis of the renal branch on the graft, followed by recanalization, however, had resulted in the clinical picture presented by this patient.

Anticoagulant treatment is also advisable as a protection against lung embolism. This should not be regarded as a mere potential threat associated with the replacement of the inferior vena cava. There seems to be no need to continue the anticoagulant treatment over a long period of time: graft endothelialization may be assumed to have fully consolidated within two months of the operation.

The type of graft used is a highly important factor in inferior vena cava transplantations. So far, no solution to the problem has emerged that may be regarded as optimal. The vascular prostheses have been developed for artery replacements and are not particularly appropriate when large veins must be replaced. Yet, in certain cases, such as the one reported here, they must be regarded as the only solution currently available, and should therefore be taken advantage of.

The better results obtained in superior vena cava transplantations compared with those on the inferior vena cava can be explained on a hemodynamic basis. Superior caval grafts indeed are often exposed to a thrombosis unless the azygos vein's flow is interrupted by ligature of the channel. It is well known that the collateral circulation of the superior vena cava can be provided only by the azygos vein. The collateral circulation is far richer in the inferior vena cava and has a very substantial influence upon the failures that so often ensue when inferior caval replacements are attempted. Probably, the shorter the portion of inferior vena cava removed, and the larger the amount of collateral circulation undisturbed, the higher is the risk of failure.

After complete excision of the inferior vena cava just so much collateral circulation is re-established as is required for survival, reimplanting the vein of the remaining kidney onto the inferior caval graft. The massive blood flow thus available, although low in pressure, and the reduction of collateral circulation down to the bare minimum needed for survival, are likely to contribute materially to keeping the inferior caval transplantation permanently pervious.

SUMMARY

A case has been reported of total prosthetic graft of the inferior vena cava in a 5-year-old girl with Wilms' tumor which required removal of the right kidney, complete excision of the inferior vana cava, and marginal resection of the middle lobe of the lung. The remaining renal vein was reimplanted on one branch of the Y-shaped graft of the cava by a terminoterminal anastomosis. The patient has recovered and has been found normal from the hemodynamic standpoint 18 months after the operation.

REFERENCE

1. McPeak, C. J.: Resection of inferior vena cava and graft replacement (aortic homograft) for retroperitoneal sarcoma, SURGERY 50: 778. 1961.

Vascular obstruction of the superior renal infundibulum in children

PETER J. DECKERS, M.D.
ELWIN E. FRALEY, M.D.
DAVID F. PAULSON, M.D.
JOHN C. HARBERT, M.D.
BETHESDA, MD.
From the Surgery Branch, National Cancer Institute and the Department of Nuclear Medicine, National Institutes of Health

Roentgenographic evidence of arterial and venous impressions on the renal collecting system is a well-described finding.[1, 8, 9] A previously unrecognized syndrome of nephralgia caused by vascular obstruction of the superior infundibulum was recently described in adults.[3, 4, 9] Detailed studies showed that renal vessels can impinge upon the intrarenal collecting structures sufficiently to impede the flow of urine from the superior calyx into the renal pelvis. According to present concepts, pain in these patients is caused by periodic overdistention of the obstructed calyx. The purpose of this report is to present two additional cases of vascular obstruction of the superior infundibulum in children.

CASE REPORTS

Case 1. A ten-year-old Caucasian boy had had left flank pain for one year. He had been well until he developed recurrent episodes of sharp left upper abdominal pain radiating to his left flank. The pain was of sudden onset, was incapacitating, and usually lasted five to ten minutes. The patient could obtain partial relief by assuming the supine position. These episodes occurred two to three times each month and interrupted his educational and athletic activities.

With the exception of the flank pain, he was a healthy young boy. The results of all laboratory studies, including a urine culture, were negative.

Using excretory urography, we were able to demonstrate a persistent filling defect across the left superior infundibulum with dilatation and clubbing of the superior calyx. Impaired drainage from the superior calyx with the patient erect was also evident (Fig. 1*A*). However, delayed drainage films on the retrograde pyelogram, recorded while the patient was supine, failed to show delayed drainage from the superior calyx. Findings from scintillation camera renography, from which scintiphotos are simultaneously integrated, were also normal when the patient was in the supine position (Fig. 2*A*). A left renal arteriogram demonstrated several small arterial branches in the area of the left superior infundibulum, but these did not seem to be causing obstruction. These negative studies were perplexing because the symptomatology and the intravenous pyelogram (IVP) findings were characteristic of infundibular obstruction.

During the next six weeks, the patient had nine characteristic episodes of left upper abdominal pain which lasted five to ten minutes; most episodes were incapacitating in nature. The patient was admitted again; when the scintillation camera renogram was repeated with the patient standing erect, it showed prolonged transit time with flattening and elevation of the excretory phase of the tracings on the left. The late scintiphotos showed evidence of superior calyceal retention. These findings are consistent with functional impairment in the transit of urine from the superior calyx to the infundibulum (Fig. 2*B*). Thus the fact that the nature of the obstruction was dependent upon his position had been established. Review of the excretory urograms taken when he was in the erect position failed to reveal any evidence of left renal ptosis. By means of venography, a plexus of veins was seen surrounding and compressing the infundibulum.

At operation, the infundibulum was trapped between several veins and the artery to the middle vascular segment. Repair was accomplished by dividing the veins, rotating the kidney, and fixing it in a position so that the artery to the middle

Submitted for publication Jan. 21, 1969; resubmitted March 21, 1969.

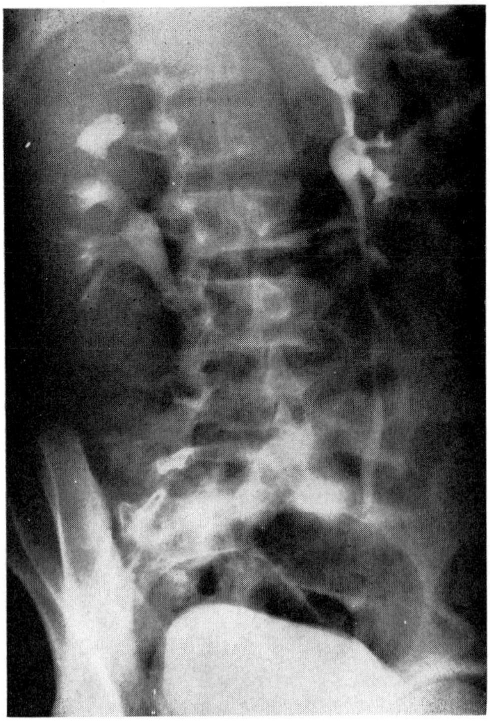

Fig. 1*A*. Case 1. Preoperative oblique excretory urogram showing filling defect over the left superior infundibulum with proximal superior caliectasis.

vascular segment remained away from the infundibulum (Fig. 3).

The postoperative IVP showed a definite decrease in the previously prominent superior caliectasis (Fig. 1*B*). Four months postoperatively, the patient has remained asymptomatic.

Case 2. A 15-year-old Caucasian boy had had right flank and right upper abdominal quadrant pain for four years. He had been well until he experienced recurrent episodes of colicky right flank pain which lasted ten to fifteen minutes and which were often severe enough to awaken him at night and to cause him to "double up" for relief. These attacks occurred two to three times each month. In 1963 an IVP showed right superior infundibular caliectasis. A retrograde pyelogram demonstrated poor drainage from the right superior calyx. The patient was told he had a slight urinary tract infection related to a congenital abnormality. An episode of severe right flank pain which incapacitated him for fourteen hours prompted his admission.

He was a normal, robust adolescent with moderate right costovertebral angle tenderness. Results of all laboratory studies, including urine culture, were normal.

The IVP showed a persistent, sharply circumscribed, transversely oriented filling defect in the right superior infundibulum with clubbing and dilatation of the associated calyx. The results of cystoscopy and a cinecystourethrogram taken while the patient was voiding were normal. Selective renal arteriography and venography identified in the anteroposterior projection the artery or veins responsible for the obstruction. In order to determine precisely whether the true obstructing

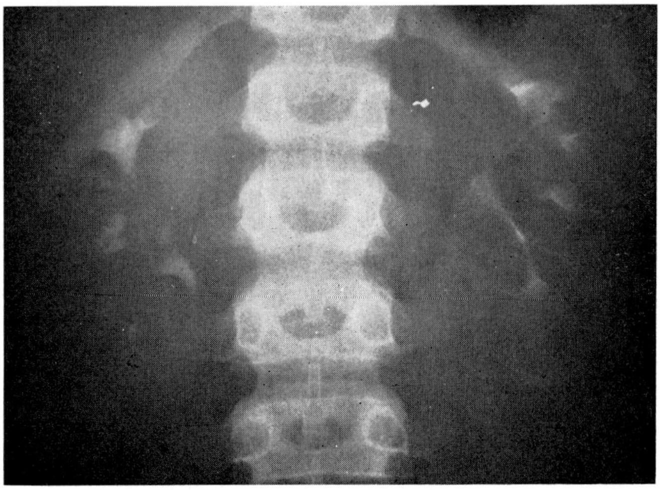

Fig. 1*B*. Case 1. Postoperative films showing decreased caliectasis and improved drainage on the left.

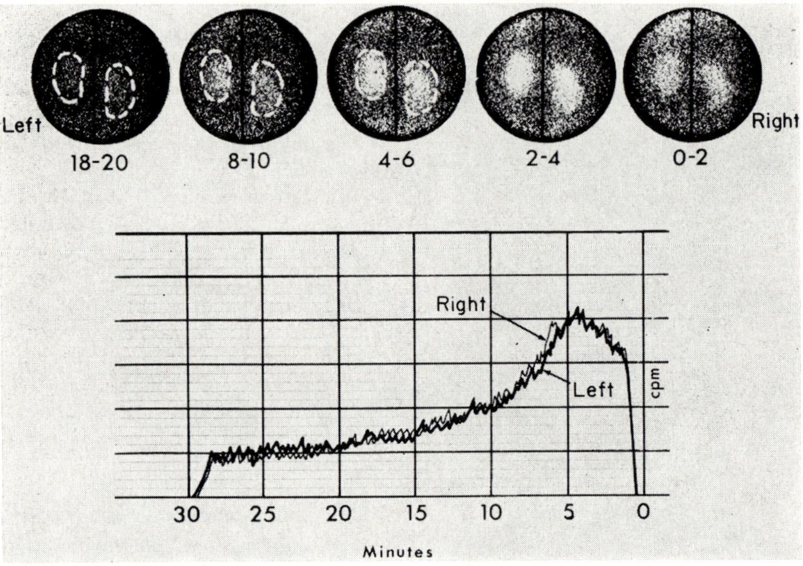

Fig. 2*A*. Case 1. Normal scintillation camera renogram and scintiphotos while patient is in the supine position. There is equal appearance and disappearance of the radioactivity in both kidneys in the scintiphotos above, and the renogram tracings are superimposed, indicating similar function.

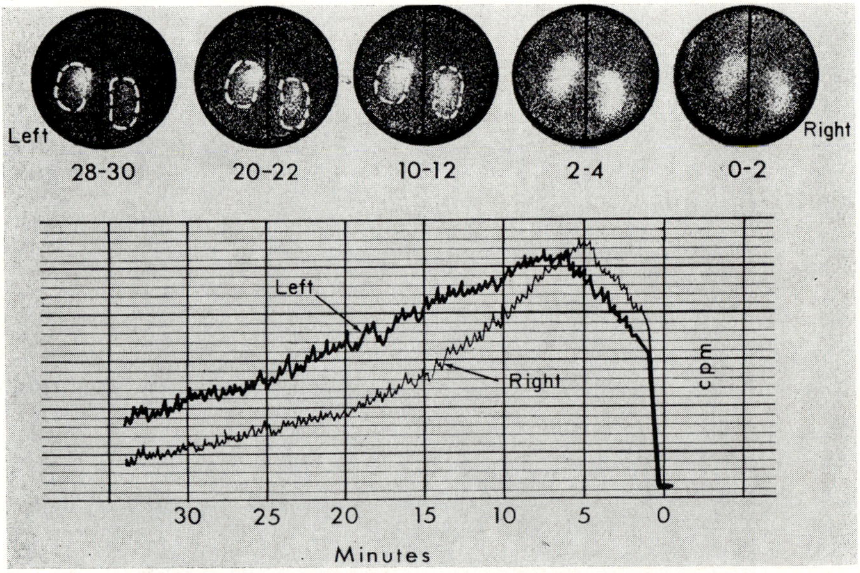

Fig. 2*B*. Case 1. Characteristic prolonged transit time with flattening and elevation of the excretory phase in the left renogram tracing below. Scintiphotos above from 10 to 30 minutes show retention of activity in the superior pole of the left kidney.

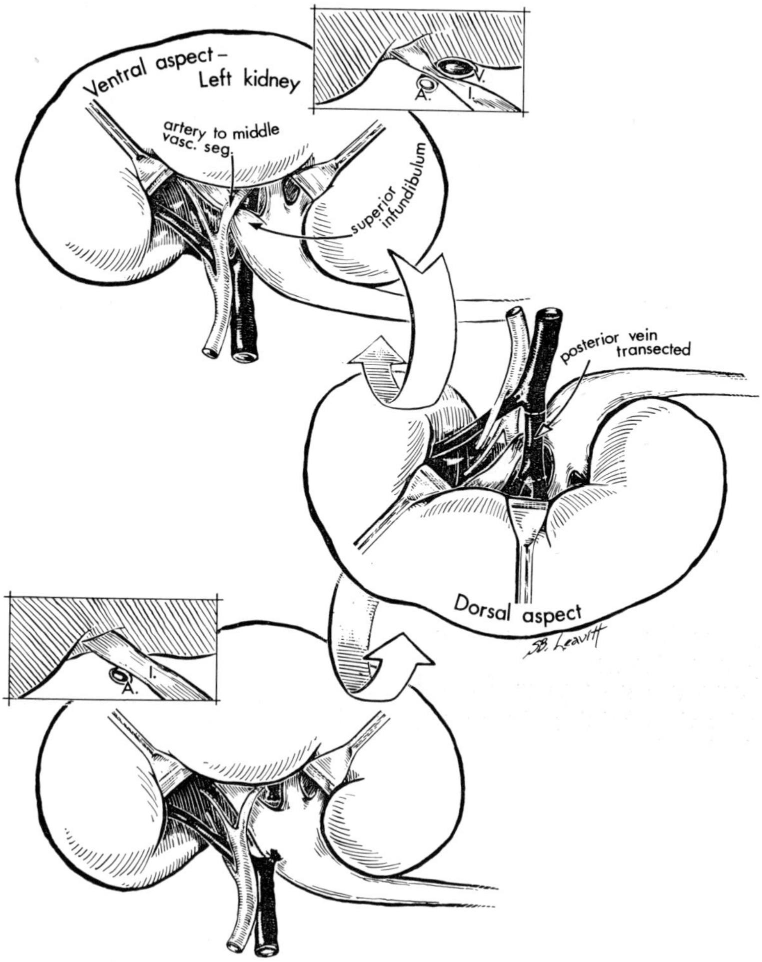

Fig. 3. Case 1. Infundibulum caught in vascular vise composed of several veins and artery to middle vascular segment. Correction by vein division and kidney rotation to position the artery away from the infundibulum.

vessel was located ventral or dorsal to the infundibulum, flexible guide wires were introduced through the selective catheter previously placed in the vessel via a transfemoral percutaneous approach.[2] Under fluoroscopic control, the wire was directed toward the infundibulum and into the vessel of interest. Simultaneous excretory urography was performed and a series of spot films taken while the patient was rotated under fluoroscopic control to the affected side. The technique enabled us to obtain a more true lateral view of the renal hilus and, in this case, established that the infundibulum was caught in a vascular vise consisting of the artery ventrally and several veins dorsally (Fig. 4).

An exploratory operation confirmed the radiographic findings. Repair was accomplished by division of the veins posteriorly as well as by transverse infundibuloplasty performed to increase the internal diameter of the infundibulum (Fig. 5).

Nine months postoperatively the patient was free of pain and his IVP showed considerable decrease in the previously prominent caliectasis.

DISCUSSION

Acute obstruction of the free flow of urine anywhere in the proximal urinary drainage system results in an overdistension of the affected part. The consequence of such obstruction may be pain, often severe or colicky, usually localized to the flank but occasionally felt vaguely in the upper abdominal quadrant. If the obstruction is per-

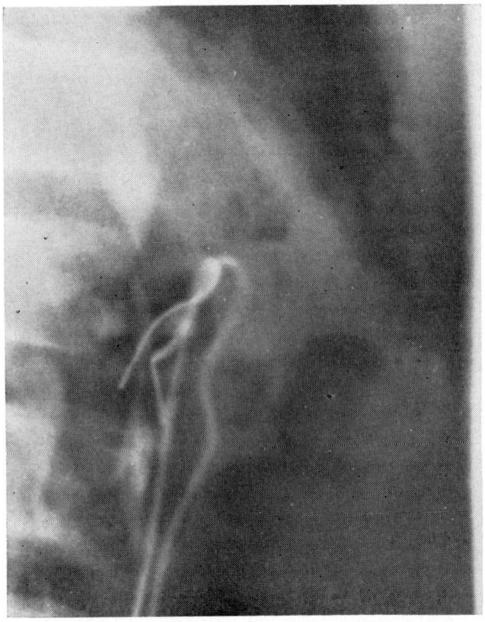

Fig. 4. Case 2. Guide wires in the obstructing vein and artery during simultaneous excretory urography to establish that the infundibulum was caught in a vascular vise consisting of the artery ventrally and vein dorsally.

sistent or its periodic occurrence frequent, then stagnation of urine can lead to urinary tract infection and possibly even stone formation.[3]

The occurrence of vascular obstruction of the superior infundibulum was first suggested by Wabrosch,[11] but precise definition of the clinical, diagnostic, and therapeutic aspects of this entity was only recently presented.[3, 5, 6, 9] Since the appearance of these original reports, an increasing awareness of the syndrome led to its description in a child.[10] The recognition of this abnormality in children reinforces our belief that when the disease occurs in adults it has been present since birth. Those factors which mediate the onset of acute symptoms in both adults and children are presently unknown.

Both of our patients had characteristic symptoms and IVP findings. In Case 1, the retrograde pyelogram failed to show selective entrapment of dye in the superior calyx and the results of the angiographic studies were somewhat equivocal. Furthermore, in the supine position, the findings from the renogram and the late scintiphotos were normal. The fact that the upright scintiphotos and radioactive renogram were consistent with obstruction of the superior infundibulum was accepted, along with the history, IVP, and venogram, as sufficient evidence to justify exploration. Case 2 presented little problem in diagnosis because there was delayed drainage from the obstructed calyx shown on the retrograde pyelogram and the angiographic studies demonstrated a vascular obstruction of the superior infundibulum.

The diagnostic evaluation of patients with this syndrome has undergone considerable evolution. A history of periodic colicky flank or upper abdominal pain has been the symptom that has most frequently brought these patients to a physician. The intravenous and retrograde pyelographic findings are characteristic, and the IVP must be performed in both the supine and erect positions, if position-dependent obstruction is not to be overlooked.

Presently, we are investigating the use of scintillation camera renography to determine the functional significance of vascular impressions on the superior infundibulum in both adults and children. Case 1 demonstrates the sensitivity of this technique, the precise details of which are soon to be described.[7] The renogram tracings and scintiphotos, the results of which were normal when the patient was in the supine position, showed the characteristic prolonged excretory phase and delayed excretion from the superior collecting system with the patient standing erect (Fig. 4). Scintillation camera renography has demonstrated significant functional obstruction in six patients to date. This technique may allow us to dispense with the intravenous cinepyelogram, as well as the anesthetic and technical hazards of retrograde pyelography. Another obvious advantage, especially in children, is the minimal radiation dose when compared with that necessary for other radiographic techniques.[7]

Although position-dependent nephralgia

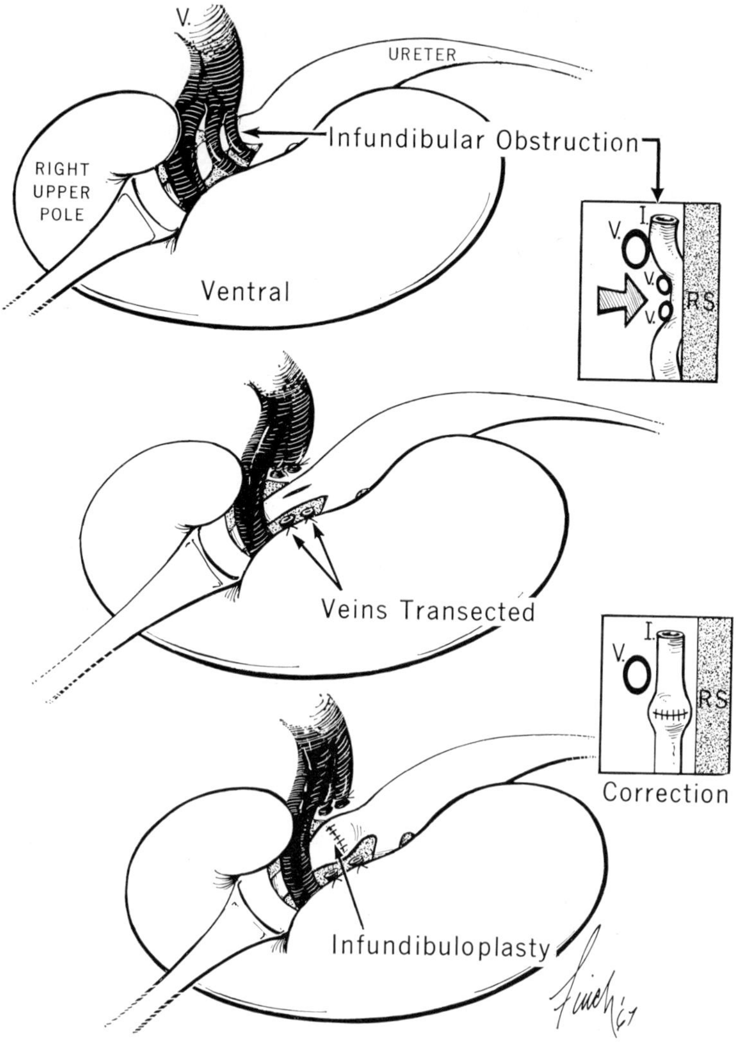

Fig. 5. Case 2. Infundibular compression between veins *(V)* and renal substance *(RS)* in the right kidney. Correction by division of veins and transverse infundibuloplasty.

due to obstruction of the superior infundibulum must be related to definite anatomic changes, the exact mechanism is unknown. Often the onset of symptoms has been related to generalized weight loss. This may lead to an increased renal mobility resulting from a decrease in perirenal and retroperitoneal fat.[3] As the ptotic kidney descends along the psoas muscle when the patient assumes the upright position, it undergoes a dorsolateral to ventromedial rotation about its long axis.[3] This movement may place increased tension on the renal vasculature with compression of the contiguous infundibulum. However, this mechanism could not explain the findings in Case 1. Therefore, we have postulated that, in this patient, infundibular obstruction occurring while the patient is in the erect position may have been caused by the superior pole of the kidney tipping ventrally, thereby increasing the compression of the infundibulum by the taut, overlying vasculature. Numerous attempts to prove this conjecture were unrewarding.

Mobilization of the renal pedicle and its

branches within the renal sinus must be done with care to avoid ischemic death of renal tissue. This dissection is greatly facilitated if the precise anatomical orientation of the obstructing vessel is known preoperatively. A new technique utilizing simultaneous excretory urography with wires placed in the offending vessels has been useful in obtaining this type of information.[2] Prior to development of this technique, the results of selective venography and arteriography often showed only the proximity of the offending vessel to the infundibulum. This procedure can demonstrate the contiguity of the vessels to the infundibulum and helps to establish precise three-dimensional relationships.

Division of the offending renal venous branches performed in both cases has not in any way compromised the venous drainage of the kidney. Division is never accomplished without prior cross-clamping of the vessel to determine if there is any significant morphologic change in the kidney parenchyma. This has not been observed, perhaps as the result of an extensive collateral intrarenal venous circulation. Postoperative studies have shown no evidence of infarction of renal tissue, and there has been no significant gross or microscopic hematuria.

SUMMARY

Two children with nephralgia caused by vascular obstruction of the superior infundibulum are presented. The clinical syndrome and principal roentgenographic findings are reviewed. Two new techniques, scintillation camera renography and selective renal angiography with guide wires, have allowed some modification and improvement of the original diagnostic evaluation. Both children have remained totally free of pain for nine and four months, respectively, after the obstruction was relieved by surgical operation.

REFERENCES

1. Baum, S., and Gillenwater, J. Y.: Renal artery impressions on the renal pelvis, J. Urol. **95:** 139, 1966.
2. Doppman, J. L., and Fraley, E. E.: Angiographic techniques in the syndrome of vascular obstruction of the superior infundibulum, Radiology **91:** 1039, 1968.
3. Fraley, E. E.: Vascular obstruction of superior infundibulum causing nephralgia, New Eng. J. Med. **275:** 1403, 1966.
4. Fraley, E. E.: Surgical correction of intrarenal disease. I. Obstruction of the superior infundibulum, J. Urol. **98:** 54, 1967.
5. Fraley, E. E.: Dismembered infundibulopyeloplasty: Improved technique for correcting vascular obstruction of the superior infundibulum, J. Urol. **101:** 144, 1969.
6. Graves, F. T.: Anatomy of intrarenal arteries and their application to segmental resection of the kidney, Brit. J. Surg. **42:** 132, 1954.
7. Harbert, J. C., and Fraley, E. E.: Scintillation camera renography in superior infundibular obstruction, J. A. M. A. **207:** 2433, 1969.
8. Kreel, L., and Pyle, R.: Arterial impressions on renal pelvis, Brit. J. Radiol. **35:** 609, 1962.
9. Nebesar, R. A., Pollard, J. J., and Fraley, E. E.: Renal vascular impressions, Amer. J. Roentgen. **101:** 719, 1967.
10. Starer, F.: Partial hydronephrosis due to pressure from normal renal arteries, Brit. Med. J. **1:** 98, 1968.
11. Wabrosch, C.: Observations on the symptoms and treatment of calyx obstruction caused by renal vessels, Orv. Hetil. **104:** 1204, 1963.

External iliac artery occlusion in a newborn infant

FELIX SALERNO, M.D.*
O. DALE COLLINS, M.D.
DANIEL C. REDMOND, M.D.
FORT HOOD, TEXAS
From the Departments of Surgery and Pediatrics, U. S. Darnall Army Hospital

Abdominal aortography and peripheral arteriography are performed infrequently during the neonatal period because of the unusual occurrence of peripheral vascular disease in this age group. Angiography during the neonatal period is usually performed as a diagnostic procedure for congenital heart disease and aortic arch anomalies. The various routes of performing aortography in newborn infants and children are: brachial artery; common carotid artery; radial artery; puncture of the interatrial septum; percutaneous puncture of the left atrium; percutaneous puncture of the left ventricle; and transumbilical retrograde aortography.

The present report deals with the problem of an external iliac artery occlusion in a newborn infant; the approach to diagnosis and management.

CASE REPORT

A 4 pound 10 ounce male infant was born after a gestation marred by exposure to rubella with subsequent administration of gamma globulin in the eleventh week of pregnancy. The mother was gravida 3 with a history of two stillbirths, each at eight months of gestation; autopsies of these children were uninformative. The estimated date of confinement was February 20, 1968, but the mother went into spontaneous labor on February 8. The delivery was uneventful, and the one minute Apgar was 9 in the delivery room with no abnormalities being noted; but a detailed physical examination was not done.

Received for publication Oct. 6, 1969.
*Present address: Veterans Administration Center, Temple, Texas 76501.

The infant had been in the nursery for eight hours when the nursing staff noted persistent dependent cyanosis of the left leg extending onto the left half of the scrotum and to the level of the umbilicus; a sharp midline demarcation was visible.

Examination of the baby revealed the left lower leg to be cool, without a palpable femoral pulse, blanched on elevation (Fig. 1), and with no apparent motor impairment. The remainder of the physical examination was unremarkable. The laboratory studies were reported as follows: complete blood count, normal; urinalysis, normal; platelets, normal; serum calcium, 9.8 mg. percent; phosphorous, 3.1 mg. percent; and the urine amino acid screening showed no abnormalities. The prothrombin time was 13 seconds with a control of 13 seconds and the partial thromboplastin time was 36 seconds (normal less than 45 seconds). The electrocardiogram and chest x-ray were normal.

The infant was kept in an incubator at a constant temperature and 30 percent oxygen over the next three days while the leg was being observed. There was a gradual improvement in the color of the leg. On the fifth day of life, transumbilical retrograde abdominal aortography was performed to determine the site and possible etiology of the vascular occlusion.

A complete obstruction of the left external iliac artery up to the level of the inguinal ligament with good collateral flow was demonstrated (Fig. 2). Over the following week, expectant management was continued with the gradual return of normal color to the extremity. At age eight days, the leg appeared normal except for the lack of pulses. The infant was followed on an outpatient basis and at six months a femoral pulse became palpable; there was good color and no apparent muscular atrophy or shortening of the extremity. When last seen at eighteen months, the infant was walking normally and the femoral pulse remained palpable.

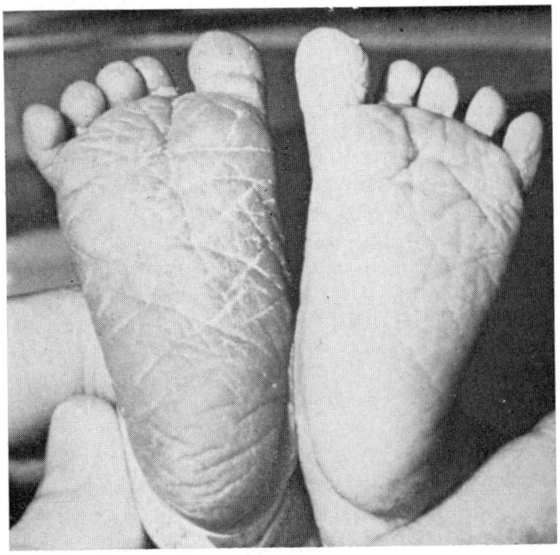

Fig. 1. On elevation, the left lower extremity became markedly ischemic.

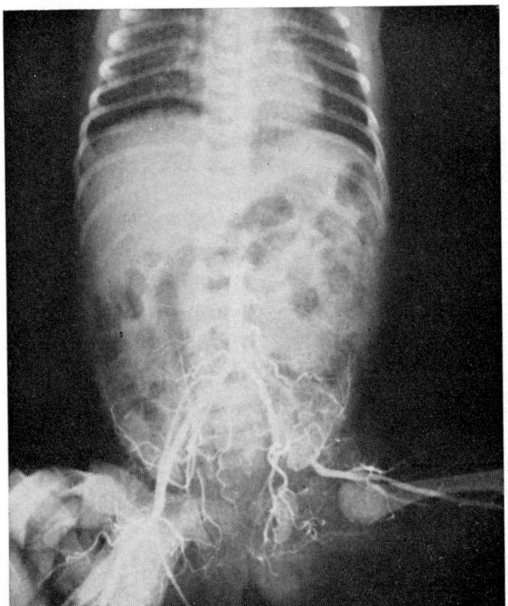

Fig. 2. The transumbilical retrograde abdominal aortogram illustrates the occluded left external iliac artery and the extent of collateral vessels.

DISCUSSION

Although peripheral vascular occlusive disease is an uncommon occurrence in the newborn period, when it does occur, the diagnostic procedures available to determine the etiology and occluded site are limited because of the size of the infant's vessels. A variety of vascular occlusive disease has been reported in the neonatal period and infancy, namely, cerebral artery occlusion,[5] coronary artery sclerosis,[14] aortic occlusion,[8] mesenteric artery occlusion,[13] renal artery stenosis,[16] and peripheral arterial embolism and thrombosis.[1-3, 6, 9, 10, 12, 15, 18-20]

The problem of gangrene in infants, as well as peripheral embolism and thrombosis, has been amply reviewed from 1934 to 1945 by Dohan,[3] and from 1945 to 1965 by Heller and Alvari,[9] Gross,[6] and Braly.[2] A total of over 65 cases of arterial occlusive disease has been reported in these reviews, but in none were arterial studies done to evaluate the occluded vessels.

The various possible etiological factors in vascular occlusion in the newborn infant are: sepsis; trauma; vasospasm; congenital heart disease; embolism from thrombus within the ductus arteriosus; thrombus extension from the umbilical artery into the peripheral circulation; hypercoagulability states. Of all the various possibilities, that postulated by Gross,[6] namely, embolism or propagation of thrombus from the ductus arteriosus or umbilical artery into the peripheral circulation, explains best the picture seen in the majority of newborn infants with a vascular occlusion. It explains readily the clinical situation encountered; a healthy newborn infant who suddenly develops a pulseless, cyanotic extremity which becomes pale with a progressive motor weakness and gangrene or gradually improves as collateral circulation is established. These theories are further substantiated by Gross' autopsy studies and the cases reported by Heggtveit and Hill[8] and Braly.[2] In Heggtveit and Hill's case study, an autopsy on a two-week-old infant revealed the ductus arteriosus partially occluded by a thrombus that extended into the descending thoracic aorta and completely occluded its lumen. Braly's case demonstrated the propagation of thrombus from the umbilical artery into the iliac system. These theories do not explain the occurrence of vascular occlusion in the upper extremities during the neonatal period, for as stated by Askue and Wong,[1] embolism would have to occur in a retrograde manner from the ductus arteriosus into the subclavian artery. Pathological studies on amputated extremities in several of the reported cases have failed to show evidence of arterial occlusion.[1, 3] Hardy and Alican[7] reviewed the problem of ischemic gangrene without major vascular occlusion and commented on the etiological factors in 1961. The possibility of congenital absence of vessels or hypoplastic vessels as the cause of arterial insufficiency in the extremities in infancy seems unlikely since its occurrence has been reported mainly in adults.[4, 11, 21]

TREATMENT

Peripheral occlusive disease in the newborn infant can be studied by transumbilical aortography, as described by Sapin and associates[17] in 1963. It should be performed to determine: (1) the site of occlusion, (2) the possible etiology of the occlusion (intraluminal thrombosis versus external compression), and (3) whenever operative intervention is anticipated. The time at which the study is performed is determined by the progression of the process and whether emergency surgery is being considered.

The majority of cases of arterial insufficiency in infants have exhibited various degrees of gangrene with either loss of tissue, function, or the extremity. Treatment has consisted of local supportive therapy, lumbar sympathetic block, anticoagulation, vasodilators, antibotics, and amputation when indicated. The value of these modalities is debatable and has not been proved to increase limb survival in the newborn period. Limb survival will depend upon the adequacy of collateral flow which will be evident within 12 to 24 hours after the acute occlusion. In addition, the use of such measures may masquerade the clinical picture or delay a necessary surgical procedure. Initial therapy therefore should consist of keeping the extremity warm and constant observation to determine the stability of the process and whether tissue loss or a motor deficit is occurring. The latter indicates a necessity for surgery.

Conservative therapy had been advocated by all until 1960, when Henry and associates[10] reported two cases of common iliac artery embolectomy in newborn infants. The initial patient died from postoperative complications. This was followed by Braly's[2] report in 1965 of a successful case of right common and external iliac artery thrombectomy. In many of the cases conservative treatment has been indicated because of the self-limitation of the process and lack of motor deficit. If a functional limitation of the limb occurs, surgery would definitely be indicated in order to salvage the extremity. Although the age of the infant and size of the vessels are limiting factors, salvage of such extremities can only be accomplished surgically. The two successful cases reported demonstrate that such procedures can technically be performed in this age group.

SUMMARY

A case of peripheral vascular occlusive disease in the newborn infant successfully studied by retrograde aortography along with a review of the literature on this problem is presented. The present case was managed conservatively with a good result. At the present time, it would appear that surgical intervention is indicated if the ischemic extremity progresses toward a motor deficit and salvage becomes necessary. Although the etiology remains debatable, it would appear that which is suggested by Gross[6] (embolism or propagation of thrombus from the ductus arteriosus or umbilical artery into the peripheral circulation) explains adequately the clinical picture seen. In the newborn period, the diagnosis of peripheral vascular occlusion should be suspected when a healthy newborn infant suddenly develops a pulseless cyanotic extremity which progresses to a pale ischemic state.

REFERENCES

1. Askue, W. E., and Wong, R.: Gangrene of the extremities in the newborn infant, J. Pediat. **40:** 588, 1952.

2. Braly, B. D.: Neonatal arterial thrombosis and embolism, SURGERY **58:** 769, 1965.
3. Dohan, C. F.: Gangrene of an extremity in a newborn infant, J. Pediat. **57:** 756, 1934.
4. Dumanian, A. V., Frahm, C. J., Benchik, F. A., and Wooden, T. F.: Intermittent claudication secondary to congenital absence of iliac arteries, Arch. Surg. **91:** 604, 1965.
5. Frantzen, E., Jacobsen, H. H., and Therkelsen, J.: Cerebral artery occlusions in children due to trauma to the head and neck, Neurology **11:** 695, 1961.
6. Gross, R. E.: Arterial embolism and thrombosis in infancy, Amer. J. Dis. Child. **70:** 61, 1945.
7. Hardy, J. D., and Alican, F.: Ischemic gangrene without major organic vascular occlusion: An enlarging concept, SURGERY **50:** 107, 1961.
8. Heggtveit, H. A., and Hill, D. P.: Thromboaortitis in the newborn, Arch. Path. **76:** 578, 1963.
9. Heller, G., and Alvari, G.: Gangrene of the extremities in the newborn, Amer. J. Dis. Child. **62:** 133, 1941.
10. Henry, W., Johnson, B. B., and Petersen, A. L.: Left common iliac arterial embolectomy in the newborn, Western J. Surg. **68:** 352, 1960.
11. Howard, J. M., Goudelock, W. J., and Couves, C. M.: Congenital atresia of the external iliac artery, Arch. Surg. **75:** 296, 1957.
12. Israels, S., and Stein, D.: Vascular occlusion in infancy, Lancet **70:** 190, 1950.
13. Kennard, K. G., Twyman, R. A., and Anderson, R. B.: Mesenteric arterial occlusion in the newborn, Missouri Med. **63:** 29, 1966.
14. Lev, M., Craenen, J., and Lambert, E. C.: Infantile coronary sclerosis with atrioventricular block, J. Pediat. **70:** 87, 1967.
15. Perlmutter, H. D., and Wagner, D. H.: Arterial thrombosis in the newborn infant, J. Pediat. **37:** 259, 1950.
16. Puyau, F. A.: Renal arteriography in infancy, Pediatrics **36:** 789, 1965.
17. Sapin, S. O., Linde, L. M., and Emmanouilides, G. C.: Umbilical vessel angiography in the newborn infant, Pediatrics **31:** 946, 1963.
18. Stadler, H. E.: Neonatal symmetrical pedal gangrene with complete recession, J. Pediat. **43:** 447, 1953.
19. Steiner, M. D.: Gangrene of an extremity in a newborn child, Amer. J. Obstet. Gynec. **49:** 686, 1945.
20. Stokes, G. E., and Shumacker, H. B.: Spontaneous gangrene in infancy, Angiology **3:** 226, 1952.
21. Stoll, W. M.: Surgical correction of congenital absence of abdominal aorta and iliac arteries, Wisconsin Med. J. **63:** 241, 1964.

Prevention of prosthetic cardiac valve detachment

NOEL H. FISHMAN, M.D.
JOHN C. HUTCHINSON, M.D.
BENSON B. ROE, M.D.
SAN FRANCISCO, CALIF.
From the Departments of Surgery and Medicine, University of California School of Medicine

Partial disruption of the suture line is a serious and potentially fatal complication of prosthetic valve replacement. Periprosthetic incompetence severe enough to produce death or require reoperation varies from 2.5 to 15 percent in several reported series.[2, 5, 6, 9, 10, 13, 14, 17] The characteristic pathologic finding is failure of the tissue to retain the sutures along a major portion of the valve annulus. Review of these reports suggests that detachment results from deficiency in the tissue's tensile strength which might be overcome by improvements in suture technique. We reviewed our own experience with prosthetic valve replacement to determine the relationship between surgical technique and severe periprosthetic incompetence.

MATERIAL AND METHODS

Clinical material. Between January, 1964 and December, 1968, 433 ball-valve prostheses were inserted into 367 patients. Prior to December, 1965, Starr-Edwards prostheses were used; since January, 1966, Cutter-Smeloff prostheses have been used exclusively.

Follow-up studies. After discharge, every patient was re-examined periodically either in the cardiac clinic or by one of the authors. Autopsies were performed on every patient who died in the hospital. Follow-up information was available on 100 percent of patients during the first postoperative year, but decreased to 80 percent by the end of the third year.

Diagnosis of detachment. Significant periprosthetic incompetence was suspected in all patients who failed to improve after operation. When the diagnosis of periprosthetic aortic incompetence was made on clinical grounds (murmur and signs of reversal of aortic blood flow during diastole), the magnitude of the leak was calibrated by angiocardiography.[1, 16] After mitral or tricuspid valve replacement, however, residual functional disability was the sole indication for restudy, including cardiac catheterization and angiocardiography.

MITRAL VALVE REPLACEMENT TECHNIQUE

The diseased valve is removed with its attached chordae tendineae and papillary muscles, leaving a 3 mm. rim of leaflet tissue (Fig. 1). Calcified deposits are removed except when they extend into the annulus or ventriculaı wall itself. The size of the prosthesis is based upon the estimated end-systolic volume of the ventricle rather than the area of the annulus. Four equally spaced mattress sutures are placed from below upward so that the cloth ring is placed beneath the valve remnant. The remaining 20 to 30 sutures (No. 2-0 Dacron) are placed radially as simple interrupted sutures at equal distances from each other and at equal depths through the host tissue (Fig. 2). Deep bites of the cloth sewing ring are

Received for publication Nov. 6, 1969.

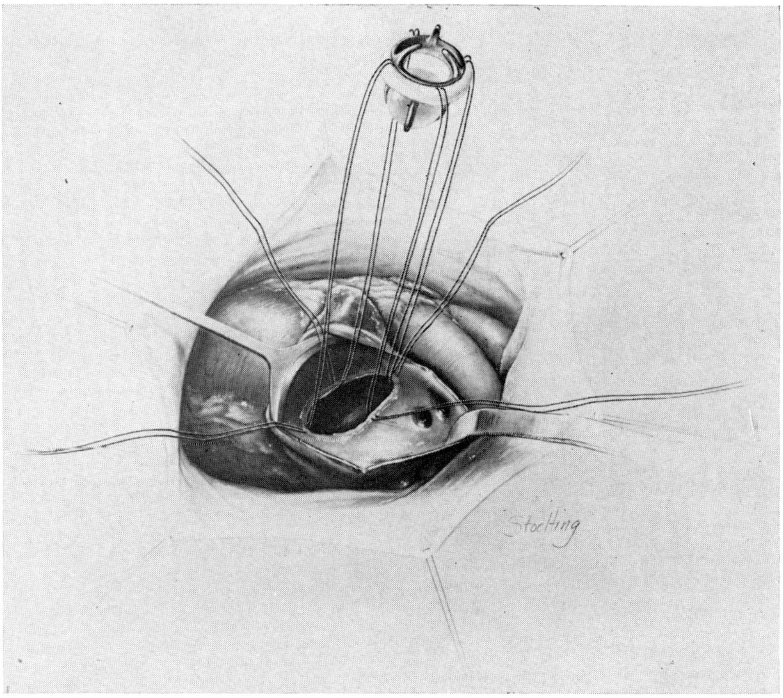

Fig. 1. Technique of mitral valve replacement. A Cutter-Smeloff prosthesis is being inserted into the mitral valve area through a left-sided approach. The diseased valve, chordae tendineae, and papillary muscles have been excised, leaving a 3 mm. rim of leaflet tissue. Four equidistant mattress sutures have been inserted into the sewing ring and through the tissue of the annulus.

incorporated into each suture. The sutures are tied and the knots are heat-sealed to prevent unraveling (Fig. 3).

AORTIC VALVE REPLACEMENT TECHNIQUE

A rim of leaflet tissue is left behind if possible. A prosthesis is chosen which is small enough to be pushed through the annulus into the left ventricle. Approximately 25 single interrupted sutures (No. 2-0 Dacron) are placed as nearly as possible into the same plane, avoiding the steep portion of the commissures (Fig. 4). The sutures at the deepest portion of each cusp are tied first, in order to seat the valve at the lowest level.

RESULTS

Of the 292 surviving patients, three developed significant paravalvular leaks, all within a few months of operation.

CASE REPORTS

Case 1. A 52-year-old woman had a Starr-Edwards mitral prosthesis inserted on Oct. 11, 1962, with a single *continuous* Mersilene suture. Three months later she was reoperated upon for repair of paravalvular insufficiency. The valve had become detached along an entire quadrant in the region adjacent to the aortic valve. The tissue was quite friable at the time and she died several months later from a second recurrent valve detachment.

Case 2. A 51-year-old man was reoperated upon for paravalvular mitral regurgitation. At operation it was discovered that an entire quadrant of sutures had pulled through the valve tissue in the region of the posterior commissure. Review of the records from his first operation disclosed that a suture in that same region had to be replaced after the valve was already tied into place.

Case 3. A 78-year-old woman had a mitral valve replacment with a Cutter-Smeloff prosthesis on Feb. 20, 1968. Her Class IV disability proved to be on the basis of ruptured chordae tendineae. She was reoperated upon twice during the next 24 hours for recurrent bleeding and tamponade resulting from a posteriorly located

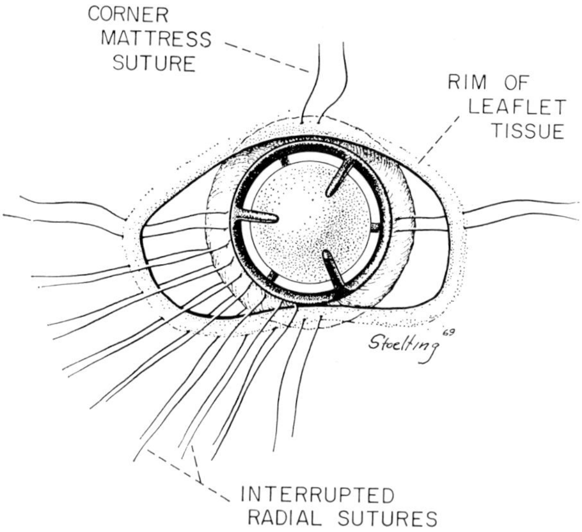

Fig. 2. Technique of mitral valve replacement. The prosthesis has been pulled beneath the annulus by traction on the four mattress sutures. Note that the remaining interrupted sutures are placed at equal distance from each other and at equal depths through the host tissue and that the largest possible amount of the cloth ring is incorporated into each suture.

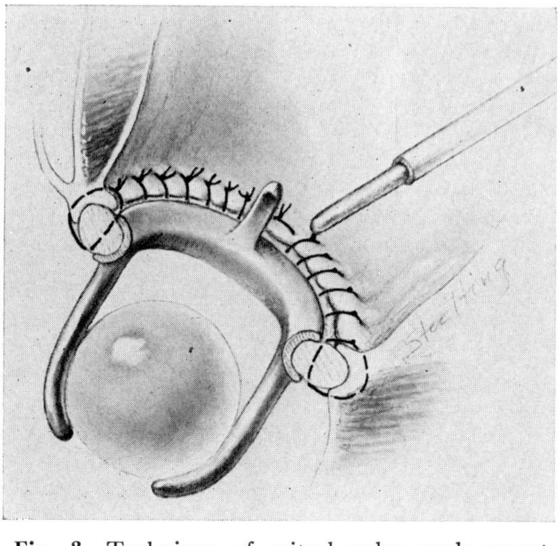

Fig. 3. Technique of mitral valve replacement. Except for the four "corner" mattress sutures, the sutures have all been placed in a radial direction. The knots of the polyester sutures are being heat fused. Note the small amount of visible cloth sewing ring and suture material.

left ventricular laceration. A postoperative left ventricular angiogram demonstrated significant paravalvular regurgitation, in association with an aneurysm of the atrioventricular groove. The patient has continued to have mild chronic congestive heart failure but has refused to have another operation.

AUTOPSY FINDINGS

One patient who died from an arrhythmia was found to have a small (5 mm.) paravalvular cleft defect at the base of the left coronary cusp, where two Tevdek sutures had become untied. Postoperative cardiac catheterization and angiography had been performed one year earlier to determine the course of the Grade III/VI aortic diastolic murmur, and hemodynamically insignificant aortic regurgitation (1+ on a scale of 4) was found.[3, 16] In two patients with aortic and four patients with mitral replacements who died of other causes it was possible at autopsy to pass only a 1 mm. probe through a single paravalvular defect, usually at a point where a suture had passed directly through a calcific deposit.

Five patients with aortic prostheses and six with mitral prostheses now have very soft murmurs which could be attributed to small paravalvular leaks. All are free from symptoms and have no clinical indications for restudy.

DISCUSSION

Diagnosis. Aortic periprosthetic incompetence is usually detected by its characteristic murmur and physical signs.[9, 10, 17] The presence of hemolytic anemia is another useful index.[18] The size of the paravalvular hole may be estimated by supravalvular aortography,[3, 11] left ventricular cineangiography,[16] and isotope dilution techniques.[8]

Mitral periprosthetic incompetence is more difficult to detect. Systolic murmurs are frequently absent.[5, 10, 14] Other criteria of paravalvular mitral leak, such as loss of systolic click[10] and "rocking" of the prosthesis on cinefluorography,[7] have been proposed. However, the diagnosis of mitral regurgitation cannot be established or ruled out except by left ventricular angiography;

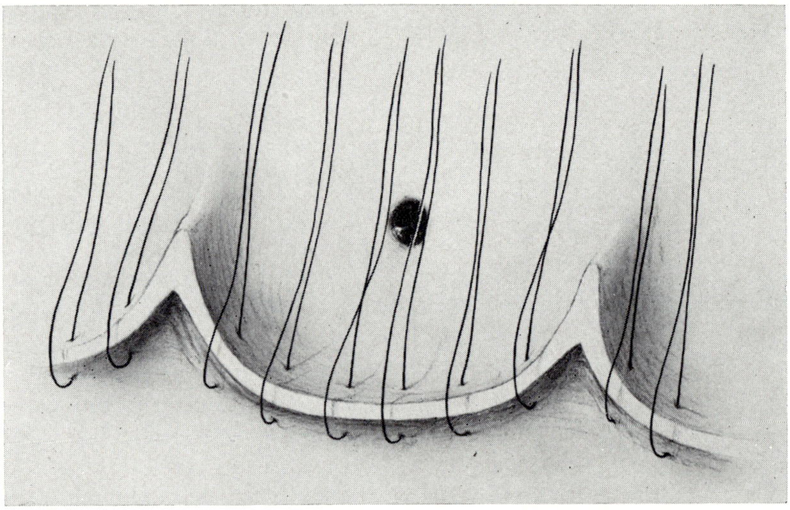

Fig. 4. Technique of aortic valve replacement. The cusps have been excised, leaving a 5 mm. rim of host tissue. The sutures have been placed as nearly as possible in the same plane, avoiding the steep portions of the commissures.

therefore, all patients who fail to improve satisfactorily after mitral valve replacement should be restudied.[13, 14]

Incidence. The true incidence of partial prosthetic detachment is unknown because few institutions perform as complete a postoperative follow-up as that described in the report of Rockoff and associates,[14] in which postoperative cardiac catheterization was performed upon every patient.

In order to compare our results with those from the institutions referred to earlier, we disregarded all subclinical lesions. The comparison was based upon only those cases of detachment severe enough to produce a poor result (i.e., failure of symptomatic improvement, intractable congestive failure, hemolytic anemia, or death).

Timing. The diagnosis of partial detachment is usually made within a few weeks of operation and nearly always during the first postoperative year.[5, 6, 9] Cases which occur later are probably related to subacute bacterial endocarditis.[9]

Etiology. The opportunity for suture disruption following implantation of a prosthetic valve is greater than in almost any other surgical circumstance because the ideal conditions for healing are necessarily violated. The suture line is subject to repeated and unevenly distributed impact stress, and fibrous union may only supplant the role of sutures to a limited degree.[17] Although suture breakage is now uncommon, Danielson and colleagues[4] documented a case in which two Tevdek sutures were fractured by calcific deposits in the annulus; significant valve detachment occurred when the then unsupported adjacent sutures pulled out of the annular tissue.

Failure of the host tissue to retain the sutures is the characteristic finding in most cases of paravalvular leakage. Rockoff and colleagues[14] have made the point that the so-called fibrous skeleton of the heart is devoid of firm collagen in the area adjacent to the aortic valve. Neville and colleagues[12] noted individual variations in the apparent tissue strength in mitral valve annuli. Kastor and colleagues[9] showed that the incidence of circumferential dehiscence was higher in patients who had mitral insufficiency from ruptured chordae tendineae, whereas individual radial tears were found more often in patients operated upon for calcific mitral stenosis. Although deficiencies of tissue tensile strength are obviously present in many patients, Wheat and colleagues,[17] Rockoff

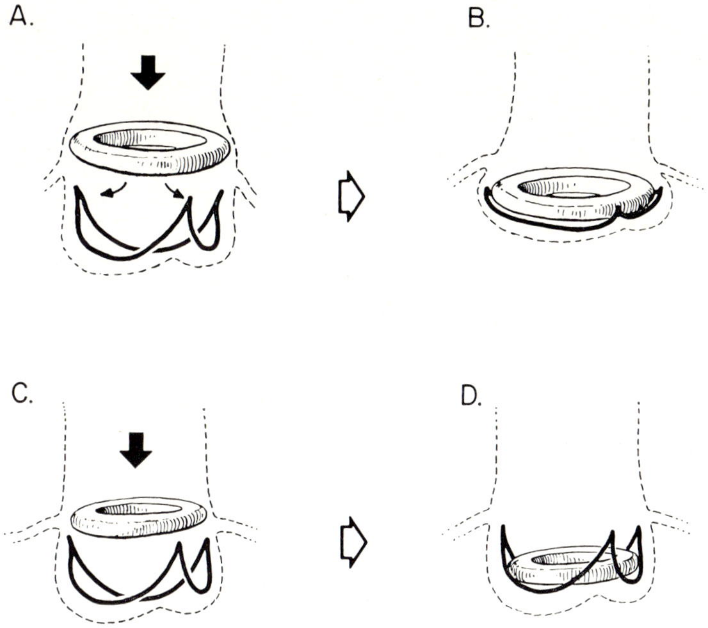

Fig. 5. Technique of aortic valve replacement. *A* and *B*, attempts to insert the largest possible valve into the aortic valve annulus produce distortion and increased tension on sutures. *C* and *D*. Use of a smaller prosthesis permits ready accommodation without distortion.

and colleagues,[14] and Neville and colleagues[12] have all reported improvement in detachment rates by altering their suture technique (using deep mattress or figure-of-8 sutures reinforced with Teflon bolsters) suggesting that technical factors are important.

In our opinion, the two factors that are most likely to promote tissue disruption are: (1) suture tension unequally distributed to the adjacent tissue and (2) impaired blood supply to the annulus because of the type of sutures used and their tension and spacing.

Unequal tension. The disparity in tensions in the aortic area results from attempts to insert an essentially planar sewing ring into a three-dimensional aortic valve annulus (Fig. 5).

To distribute tensions more evenly, the sutures should be placed as nearly as possible into the same plane (Fig. 4). For this reason, no sutures are placed into the commissure itself. The use of a slightly smaller prosthesis than is usually recommended avoids the distortion of the annulus depicted in Fig. 5, and permits greater tactile sensitivity while tying. The possibility of sutures being pulled forcefully through the tissue is thus reduced.

In the mitral valve area the disparity of tension results from attempts to insert a small round sewing ring into the much larger ellipsoidal valve bed. In addition, the rim of the prosthesis must be attached on one side to an area of contracting left ventricular muscle, and on the opposite side to the weakest portion of the fibrous skeleton.

The case report by Danielson and associates[4] provides an excellent description of the pathogenesis of major valve detachment. Breakage of one suture resulted in transmitting a greater burden to adjacent sutures, which in turn disrupted sequentially. A suture which has been placed more deeply than the others may carry a disproportionate share of the impact stress and may tear through the tissue to become as ineffective as if it had broken.

In an effort to distribute the stress equally to the tissue we place interrupted sutures at approximately 3 mm. intervals and at

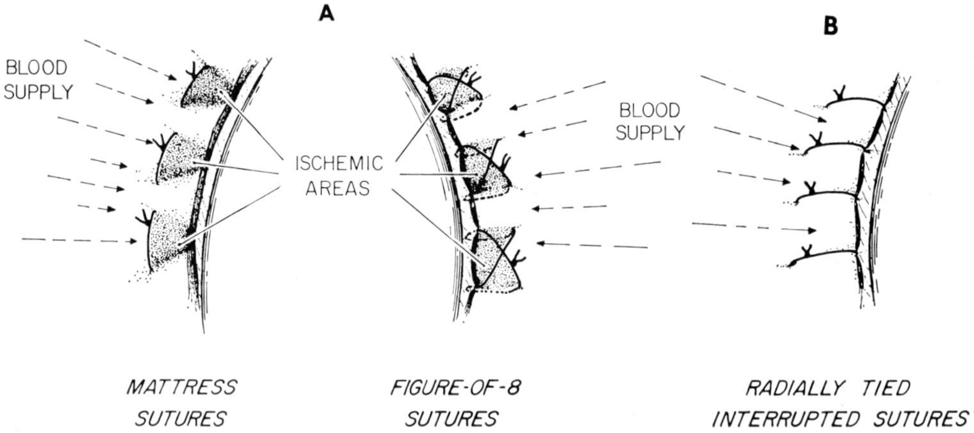

Fig. 6. Suture technique in prosthetic valve replacement. *A,* Mattress and figure-of-8 sutures produce tissue ischemia. *B,* Blood supply to the valve remnant may be preserved by placing interrupted sutures in a radial direction.

precisely equal depths into the tissue. As much as possible of the cloth sewing ring is incorporated into the suture to cushion the transmitted impact of valve closure to the tissue. When the mitral prosthesis is positioned on the ventricular side of the annulus, a portion of the systolic impact of valve closure is diffused around the entire annulus, whereas in supra-annular implantations the stress is borne only by the sutures.

Tissue ischemia. Mattress sutures or figure-of-8 sutures tend to obstruct the blood supply into the healing interface between tissue and cloth (Fig. 6). For this reason we have used simple interrupted sutures radially oriented so as not to interfere with centripetal blood flow.

We believe that technical errors were responsible for two of the three cases of suture line discontinuity in our series. The continuous suture (Case 1) is no longer used because of its ischemic effect. In this regard it is interesting to note the recent report of six major postoperative mitral valve detachments related to utilization of a continuous suture.[10] Furthermore, the technical difficulties of working around a seated prosthesis interfere with precise placement of sutures, especially as the procedure nears completion. The same problem exists when replacement of a broken interrupted suture is attempted after the prosthesis has already been secured in place (Case 2). (It may be preferable to remove several sutures in order to facilitate accurate placement.)

The untying of sutures, which occurred in one of our patients after aortic valve replacement, demonstrates the tendency for plastic sutures to regain their original (untied) shape. This episode preceded our present routine of fusing the knots of polyester sutures.[15]

SUMMARY AND CONCLUSIONS

Only three cases of hemodynamically significant prosthetic valve detachment occurred in 367 consecutive valve replacement operations at the University of California Medical Center, in which 433 ball valve prostheses were implanted: an incidence of less than 1 percent. In two of the three cases, partial prosthetic detachment is attributable to departure from the above described techniques.

On the basis of this experience we believe that prosthetic valve detachment is an avoidable complication. Equal distribution of tension and preservation of blood supply to the valve remnant can best be accomplished by use of frequent, evenly placed, radially oriented, interrupted sutures. Unequal tensions can be minimized by using a smaller aortic prosthesis, by "planar" placement of aortic sutures, subannular implantation of mitral prostheses, and incorporation of large portions of the cloth ring into each suture.

REFERENCES

1. Arvidsson, H., and Karnell, J.: Quantitative assessment of mitral and aortic insufficiency by angiocardiography, Acta Radiol. (Diagn.) Stockholm **2:** 105, 1964.
2. Attar, S., Saunders, E., Singleton, R., McLaughlin, J., Scherlis, L., and Cowley, R. A.: Prosthetic heart valve surgery in acquired valvular heart disease, Amer. Surg. **33:** 294, 1967.
3. Colapinto, R. F., Thorfinnson, P. C., and Holmes, R. B.: Aortic insufficiency. A cineradiologic assessment, J. Canad. Ass. Radiol. **13:** 112, 1962.
4. Danielson, G. K., Cooper, E., and Ifuku, M.: Severance of mitral prosthesis fixation sutures by annulus calcification, J. Thorac. Cardiovasc. Surg. **53:** 858, 1967.
5. Duvoisin, G. E., Wallace, R. B., Ellis, R. H., Jr., Anderson, M. W., and McGoon, D. C.: Late results of cardiac valve replacement, Circulation Suppl. 37 and 38, April, 1968.
6. Favaloro, R. G., Effler, D. B., Groves, L. K., Suarez, E., and Shirley, E. K.: Surgical repair of leaking prosthetic heart valves, Ann. Thorac. Surg. **3:** 503, 1967.
7. Gabriele, O. F.: Postoperative radiography of aortic valve prostheses, J. Thorac. Cardiovasc. Surg. **58:** 248, 1969.
8. Hildner, F. J., Pierson, W. R., Barold, S. S., Linhart, J. W., and Samet, P.: Isotope quantitation of aortic insufficiency compared to cineangiography in man, Ann. Thorac. Surg. **8:** 84, 1969.
9. Kastor, J. A., Akbarian, M., Buckley, M. J., Dinsmore, R. E., Sanders, C. A., Scannell, J. G., and Austen, W. G.: Paravalvular leaks and hemolytic anemia following insertion of Starr-Edwards aortic and mitral valves, J. Thorac. Cardiovasc. Surg. **56:** 279, 1968.
10. Leachman, R. D., and Cokkinos, D. V. P.: Absence of opening click in dehiscence of mitral-valve prosthesis, New Eng. J. Med. **281:** 461, 1969.
11. Lehman, J. S., Boyle, J. J., and Debbas, J. N.: Quantitation of aortic valvular insufficiency by catheter thoracic aortography, Radiology **79:** 361, 1962.
12. Neville, W. E., Leininger, B., and Pifarré, R.: Disruption of the mitral prosthesis following replacement for the "floppy valve syndrome," *in* Brewer, L., editor: Prosthetic heart valves, Springfield, Ill., 1969, Charles C Thomas, Publisher, chap. 48, p. 674.
13. Peterson, C. R., Herr, R., Crisera, R. V., Starr, A., Bristow, J. D., and Griswold, H. E.: The failure of hemodynamic improvement after valve replacement surgery. Etiology, diagnosis and treatment, Ann. Intern. Med. **66:** 1, 1967.
14. Rockoff, S. D., Ross, J., Jr., Oldham, N. N., Jr., Mason, D. T., Morrow, A. G., and Braunwald, E.: Ventriculo-atrial regurgitation following prosthetic replacement of the mitral valve, Amer. J. Cardiol. **17:** 817, 1966.
15. Roe, B. B., and Kelly, P. B., Jr.: Heat fusion of synthetic suture knots during prosthetic valve implantation, Ann. Thorac. Surg. **1:** 775, 1965.
16. Sadler, H., Dodge, H. T., Hay, R. E., and Rackley, C. E.: Quantitation of valvular insufficiency in man by angiocardiography, Amer. Heart J. **65:** 501, 1963.
17. Wheat, M. W., Jr., Linhart, J. W., Bartley, T. D., Taylor, W. J., Crevasse, L. E., and Green, J. R., Jr.: Aortic ball-valve (Starr-Edwards) prostheses. A follow-up evaluation, Ann. Thorac. Surg. **2:** 166, 1966.
18. Yacoub, M. H., and Keeling, D. H.: Chronic haemolysis following insertion of ball-valve prostheses, Brit. Heart J. **30:** 676, 1968.

Diagnostic peritoneal irrigation—a simple and reliable technique

JOSEPH M. CIVETTA, MAJOR, USAF (MC)
M. J. WILLIAMS, COLONEL, USAF (MC)
ROBERT E. RICHIE, LIEUTENANT COLONEL, USAF (MC)
KEESLER AIR FORCE BASE, MISS.
From the Department of Surgery, USAF Medical Center Keesler

A simple and reliable method for diagnosing hemoperitoneum has long been desired for the patient who is comatose, has multiple injuries, or is otherwise difficult to evaluate. To simplify the over-all plan of management of such patients, a technique was developed combining the simple, but inaccurate, diagnostic peritoneal needle aspiration[1, 2] with the reliable but more complicated peritoneal dialysis catheter lavage.[3-5] The resulting technique has proved to be highly accurate and easy to perform.

TECHNIQUE

Commercially available plastic cannulas with internal metal needle guides are readily obtainable in most emergency rooms. After the skin is prepared with alcohol and local anesthetic has been administered, two Nos. 14 or 16 needles are introduced into the peritoneal cavity through the abdominal wall (Fig. 1). Saline may be injected as the peritoneum is traversed in an attempt to avoid injury to the bowel (Fig. 2). The needle guides are aspirated and then withdrawn. No specific sites for needle placement need be chosen except to avoid the epigastric vessels and old incisions in order not to damage adherent viscera. If no blood has been obtained, physiologic saline or Ringer's solution is infused through intravenous tubing attached to one cannula hub until there is spontaneous outflow from the second cannula (Fig. 3). The patient may be rolled from side to side to facilitate mixing. The infusion is limited to 1,000 c.c., but outflow usually starts after much smaller amounts have been infused. The character of the

The views expressed herein are those of the authors and do not necessarily reflect the views of the United States Air Force or the Department of Defense.

Submitted for publication June 20, 1969; resubmitted Jan. 7, 1970.

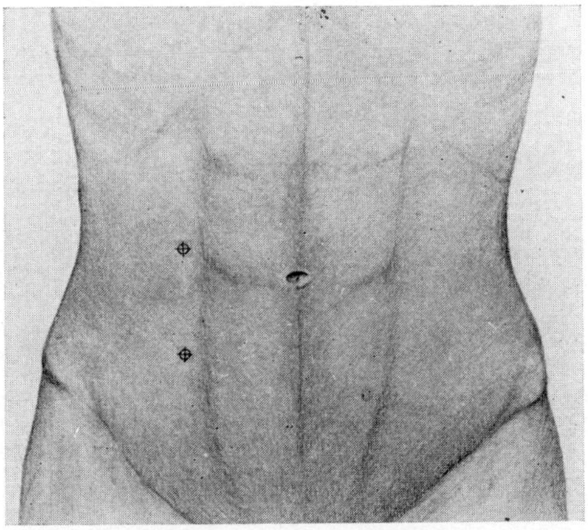

Fig. 1. Points lateral to rectus sheath to avoid inferior epigastric artery may be chosen. Old incisions should be avoided. Simple alcohol preparation and local anesthetic infiltration of immediate area performed.

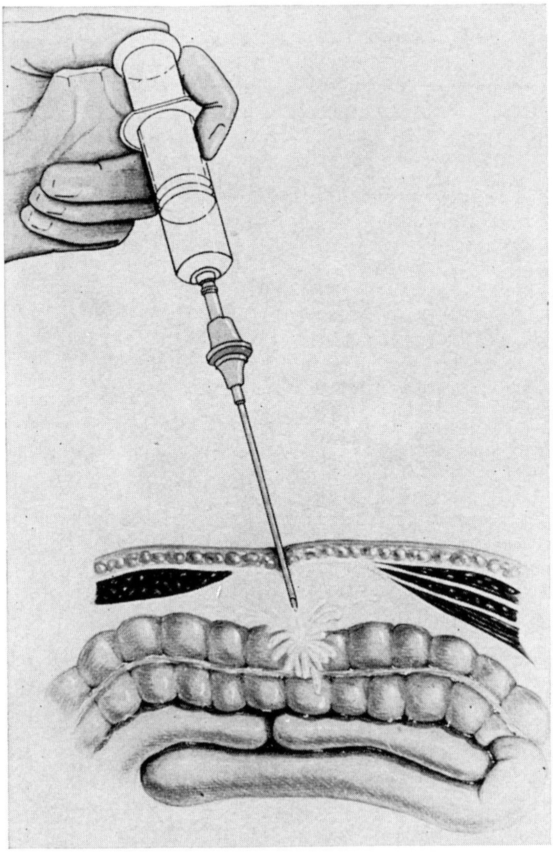

Fig. 2. Cannula with needle guide in place is introduced through the abdominal wall. Saline is injected as peritoneum is traversed in an attempt to avoid bowel injury.

effluent can be interpreted as a reliable indication of the presence or absence of free intraperitoneal blood. Bile, bowel contents, or other abnormal fluids can also be recovered, which expands the diagnostic capabilities of the test. This same technique may be used to recover peritoneal fluid as a diagnostic aid in other clinical settings, such as pancreatitis, mesenteric infarction, and peritonitis.

In an initial series of 50 patients in whom peritoneal aspiration was negative, diagnostic peritoneal irrigation was performed. Suspicion of internal injury on the part of the examining physician initiated utilization of peritoneal irrigation. In most patients, other diagnostic and therapeutic maneuvers could be simultaneously performed, expediting over-all patient management. If blood was found, a laparotomy was performed. Since a clear effluent was interpreted as reliable evidence that there was no intraperitoneal bleeding, the patient was treated for his other injuries and carefully observed.

RESULT

Of 50 patients, 13 had a positive irrigation (blood-tinged effluent) (Table I). Each patient was shown at laparotomy to have a

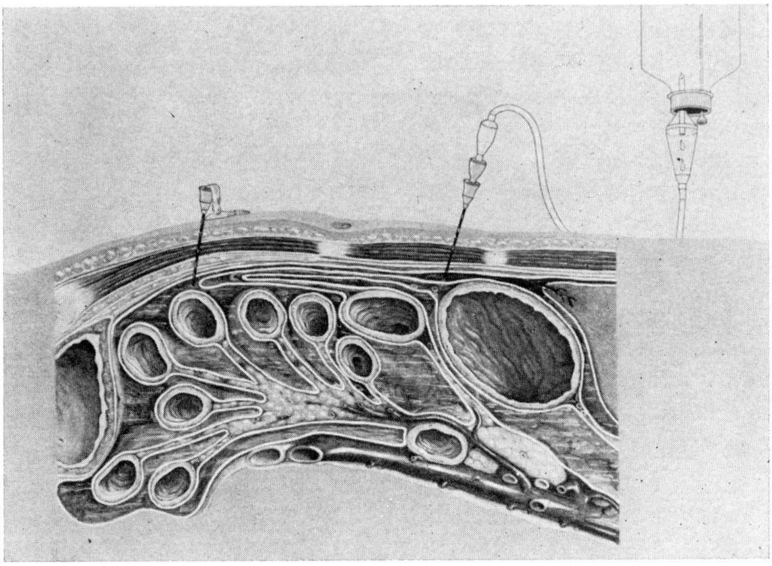

Fig. 3. Needle guides are removed. Fluid infusion is started through one cannula and continued until there is spontaneous outflow from the second.

Table I. *Positive peritoneal irrigations (13 patients)*

Diagnoses	*Indications*	*Operative findings*	*Comments*
Motorcycle accident; fractured wrist	Abdominal and chest abrasions, abdominal tenderness	Ruptured liver and spleen	Large amount of intraperitoneal blood, yet negative aspiration
Automobile accident	Abdominal symptoms and signs	Stellate laceration of liver	Negative aspiration
Motorcycle accident	Shock	Liver and hepatic vein laceration	
Automobile accident	Abdominal tenderness	Liver laceration	Less than 200 c.c. free blood in abdomen
Automobile accident	Abdominal tenderness; fractured right tenth and eleventh ribs	Liver laceration	
Infectious mononucleosis	Falling hematocrit; abdominal tenderness	Ruptured spleen	
Motorcycle accident	Abdominal contusion and tenderness	Ruptured spleen	
Automobile accident	Abdominal signs and symptoms	Lacerated spleen	Less than 200 c.c. free blood in abdomen
Bicycle accident	Abdominal signs	Lacerated spleen	Initial aspiration negative; irrigation later positive
Construction accident crushing patient	Abdominal contusion	Ruptured spleen	
Automobile accident	Abdominal pain and rigidity	Ruptured spleen	
Automobile accident	Abdominal symptoms and signs	Bleeding mesenteric vessel	
Laceration of scalp; cardiac arrest secondary to local anesthetic; flail chest postresuscitation	Shock; falling hematocrit	Lacerated inferior surface of massive fatty liver	

significant intra-abdominal lesion to account for the hemoperitoneum. In 37 patients, the irrigation was judged to be negative (clear effluent) (Table II). No patient who had an initially negative irrigation has required a later exploratory operation for possible intraperitoneal bleeding.

DISCUSSION

Abdominal paracentesis as a diagnostic aid has been in use since Salomon described the technique in 1906.[1] The validity and limitations of the technique have been well established.[2] The incidence of false negative taps has been reported to be as high as 18 percent in clinical series. In animal experiments, only 78 percent of the taps were positive in the presence of the equivalent of 500 c.c. intraperitoneal blood in an adult and no positive taps could be obtained if less than 200 c.c. were present. Perforations were made in the bowel and other viscera in 39 percent, but results of these perforations have been of no consequence either in the experimental animal or in clinical patients. Because of these clinical and laboratory findings, the unreliability of a negative aspiration has been repeatedly stressed. Aspiration, however, should be carried out since a positive aspiration precludes the need for irrigation. In seven patients with recent liver injuries in which aspiration had been carried out initially, irrigation was necessary and served to establish the presence of intraperitoneal blood in four of the patients.

The accuracy of the diagnostic peritoneal lavage has, on the other hand, been well established clinically. Animal experiments have

Table II. *Negative peritoneal irrigations—11 selected cases*

Diagnoses	*Indications*	*Course*
Infectious mononucleosis	Developed peritoneal signs; possible ruptured spleen	Explored in spite of negative irrigation; no blood found
Automobile accident	Semicomatose; abdomen difficult to evaluate	Obtundation cleared; no evidence of abdominal injury
Automobile accident; acute alcoholic intoxication	Abdominal tenderness	Abdominal signs cleared in 24 hours without evidence of visceral injury
Automobile accident; head injury	Unconscious patient	Slow neurologic recovery; no abdominal problems
Automobile accident; fractured femur and wrists, bilaterally	Abdominal tenderness; multiple injuries	Abdominal findings cleared
Automobile-train accident	Comatose; abdominal rigidity	Negative irrigation initially; perforation of stress ulcer at 3 wks.; no old injury or blood found
Motorcycle accident; dislocated hip, concussion, multiple abrasions	Multiple system injuries; combative, uncooperative patient; difficult to evaluate abdomen	Other injuries treated; no abdominal problems
Assault victim; multiple contusions	Severe abdominal tenderness	Recovered rapidly
Motorcycle accident	Ruptured thoracic aorta; abdominal signs	Did well after repair of thoracic aorta
Motorcycle accident; fat emboli, fractured femur	Persistent ileus and abdominal tenderness	Abdominal signs gradually cleared
Severely battered by hurricane water	Hypothermia, shock, abdominal tenderness	Abdominal signs cleared; shock and hypothermia related to severe bruises and long exposure

demonstrated that as little as 5 c.c. of blood could cause a significant increase in the number of red blood cells in the effluent and that as little as 75 c.c. of blood was ample to stain the fluid pink.[3] The usual technique is considerably more complicated and requires various sterile surgical instruments, a small surgical incision, peritoneal dialysis equipment, and a series of five steps to place the catheter.[5] Significant complications have also been reported.[4]

The technique herein described seems to combine the simplicity, safety, and rapidity of the needle aspiration with the proved reliability of the peritoneal dialysis technique. In particular, because the accuracy of a negative irrigation has been established, one can more readily and reliably formulate an initial plan of management of the severely injured or comatose patient.

ADDENDUM

This technique has been subsequently utilized as a diagnostic aid in mass casualty situations by one of us (M. J. W.) in a Vietnamese civilian hospital. The diagnostic method used there previously consisted of performing a laparotomy because of the lack of x-ray, laboratory, and virtually all support facilities. The rapidity and reliability of the technique described here facilitated proper and prompt triage of the daily load of 25 to 30 civilian war casualties handled by the two or three available surgeons.

REFERENCES

1. Chapman, N. D., Nyhus, L. M., and Harkins, H. N.: Abdominal paracentesis as a diagnostic aid, J. A. M. A. **170:** 1625, 1959.
2. Giacobine, J. W., and Siler, V. E.: Evaluation of diagnostic abdominal paracentesis with experimental and clinical studies, Surg. Gynec. Obstet. **110:** 676, 1960.
3. Gumbert, J. L., Frodermen, S. E., and Mercho, J. F.: Diagnostic peritoneal lavage in blunt trauma, Ann. Surg. **165:** 70, 1967.
4. Root, H. D., Hawser, C. W., McKinley, C. R., LaFarve, J. W., and Mendrela, R. P.: Diagnostic peritoneal lavage, SURGERY **57:** 633, 1965.
5. Veith, F. J., Webber, W. B., and Deysine, M.: Diagnostic peritoneal lavage in acute abdominal disease, Ann. Surg. **166:** 290, 1967.

Editorial

Conducted by EDWIN H. ELLISON, M.D.

A fork in the road: The geographic full-time system

RICHARD H. EGDAHL, M.D.
BOSTON, MASS.
From the Department of Surgery, University Hospital, Boston University Medical Center

It is common knowledge that research grant funds have helped support medical education during the past two decades. This was done with the at least tacit support of all involved individuals and was justified on the basis of the importance of training doctors and the unavailability of moneys to support education directly. It now appears that the next challenge to medical academia, with respect to fiscal accounting, centers around the current availability of patient care dollars. There are several reasons why diversion of care funds from their prime purpose—personalized patient care—to medical education is more hazardous than was the same action when it involved research funds. The purpose of this editorial is to explore this issue and provide one viewpoint as to how the surgical staff, organized on the "geographic" full-time basis, is better prepared to meet the community demand for personalized services than is a "full" full-time staff.

This editorial is *not* concerned with questions of the desirability of high quality research in a department of surgery, constant curriculum appraisal, concentration of attention on undergraduate and graduate medical education, funds specifically earmarked for medical education, or the necessity for a core of clinician-teachers geographically limited for the bulk of their activities to the teaching medical center. Most surgical educators are agreed on the importance of the latter issues. The debate centers around the simple question as to whether it is better to have fees or their equivalent in salary for patient care go to the surgeon who is responsible for the surgical care of the patient or to a central authority (department head, dean, etc.) who makes the decision as to final allocation of practice moneys. There is, of course, nothing to preclude payment by a central authority to the surgeon who delivers the care, either by salary or for individual services.

The basic point raised by the difference in the two methods, however, is that in one case the fee or salary money goes directly or indirectly through central collection to the provider and in the other it may find its way into a variety of pockets with a variety of goals and purposes. There is the very real chance in the full full-time system that patient care income could end up at least partially supporting the salary of a basic research worker who never sees patients, the travel fund for the department, or some other generally desirable purpose. Unlike the accounting situation in the past twenty years with research grants, we have two new and very active groups who are watching what we in the teaching medical centers work out with respect to patient care moneys—the federal auditors and the "community." Each will demand an accounting directed towards one key purpose—seeing that the money awarded to either individuals or groups in major medical centers ends up in identifiable services and improvements in patient care. Statements concerning "extra" care funds from departmental collections,

Received for publication Dec. 23, 1969.

funds to be "reinvested" from Medicare fees, and large accumulations of "general department funds" from Blue Shield cases (often with perfunctory "attending surgeon" participation) are red flags for auditors and the public alike.

Most clinicians are agreed that patients benefit from being treated by a "group" of doctors who interact with, consult, and educate each other. A mystique is growing up around the term "group," as if participation in a fraternity with that label automatically ensures both better patient care and savings in financial resources. One form of group consists of a number of doctors voluntarily banded together to take care of a mutual patient practice, with economic rewards commensurate with contributions in time and effort to patient care. The principle of this type of group seems unassailable. Another type of "group," however, exists when the department or other administrative unit collects income from patient practice and spends those moneys as it sees fit (and often allows a difference in "privateness" to exist between patients who pay directly and those who pay through third party payers, especially when the patient is an "unreferred" case).

We all are proud of our surgical housestaffs, both interns and residents, and achieve much satisfaction from our close and frequent contacts with them. Despite our high regard for their abilities, however, they are still in a period of training and are not qualified for board certification before *completing* the final year of residency. We must strive for excellence in their training so that their stipends truly recognize their future benefit to society, rather than their unsupervised patient care. Society permits us to continue to train house officers in a rapidly approaching all-private patient population but also demands both personalized supervision of the house officer and a responsible and personalized relationship between the private staff surgeon and his patient. To consider house officers as "deliverers of care" has dangerous moral, legal, and pedagogic aspects. The concept of a "team" of doctors taking care of a patient is all right only so long as it is understood that one doctor is responsible and the others are being trained or are helpers.

All of the above points lead to the conclusion that we must deliver the kind of personalized care that society is paying for, or it will penalize us if we fail to do so. Furthermore, it is likely that in any environment where there are alternate facilities, the public will choose the one with more personalized services. The geographic full-time system provides an incentive and a challenge to the academic surgeon-practicioner to continue to develop his facility in patient care, keeps him in the real world of surgical practice, and avoids the town-gown problem. Geographic and full full-time systems are similar in one respect, and that is a salary for administrative and teaching functions. In addition, the full full-time individual is assured an extra increment in income which depends on patient care activities by *someone*. In the geographic system, this patient care income is directly proportional to the amount of care delivered, and although there may be time or income limitations, care moneys go to the individuals who deliver personalized care. There is nothing to preclude donations by the deliverers of care from their personal income to the department for the salary of research workers or any other purpose upon which they and the department agree. Such donations will probably fall within the charitable deductions of the Internal Revenue Service and will compete with other charities of the private surgeon. In this case, the moneys are generated by personalized care and are freely given by the earner.

It is up to the departmental chairman to make available for his staff opportunities in private practice, either by rotating unreferred cases with third party coverage, emergency room duty, or some other device. An occasional individual will not desire to compete for referred practice and will not want to participate in clinical or emergency room activities. Other sources of support must be found for this man if he is particularly valuable to the department, and often clinical teaching assignments at a Veterans Administration or similar hospital will provide an outlet for clinical experiences.

Does the full full-time system provide the same incentive for that extra trip back to the hospital at night, the same extra attention to a distraught relative, and the same knowledge of the problems with forms, red tape, and fee schedules that concern the practicing surgeon? It is the thesis of this editorial that if we in academic surgery are, on the one hand, to fulfill the commitment to a society that has appropriated large sums of money for personalized care, and on the the other, to train the majority of our surgical housestaff for the world of surgical practice, the geographic full-time system provides the better environment. The advent of national health insurance, community involvement, expanded group practice, and a new health care system (preceded, of course, by a definition of what these terms mean in practice) does not change the issue but does make its solution more pressing. Because we have to train young surgeons for a health care system in which the public expects and demands personalized care for their investment of funds, they should receive their training in an environment where exposure to personalized services is maximized and where economic rewards are scrupulously directed toward the responsible providers of the care.

The stark reality of the situation is that the need to support teaching and administration in their own right and for their own sake must be recognized and met. The choice lies before us. Let us not be forced again down the road of subterfuge and misrepresentation.

The retrievable error

JOHN R. DERRICK, M.D.
GALVESTON, TEXAS
From The University of Texas Medical Branch

In any residency program, the faculty member has an important and sometimes overlooked responsibility. The staff surgeon must necessarily recognize and continually re-evaluate the capabilities of each resident. This re-evaluation would include the personality prototype, the strong and weak points, the comprehensive knowledge, the operative experience and ability, and the capability of cautious judgment on the part of the resident. Only after such recognition and evaluation is it possible in a planned program to place the residents in "supervised" situations in which to witness and literally to experience what could be called the operative retrieval of error. The retrievable error situation is an integral part of the judgment involved in the surgical procedure. First, the patient and, second, the resident and his ability to function in crisis must be considered.

In most teaching hospitals, the staff can be given a diagnosis susceptible to correction or, at least, qualified to the point of confusion. Can a surgeon honestly revise his judgment, make a rapid decision without his own supervision of the patient, and counsel the resident—by telephone? It is a question that should occur to every responsible practitioner in a faculty position.

The cavities of the human body can contain an unimaginable number of surprises. As a result, a predetermined technique may have to be discarded instantly and another substituted. Often, regrettable as it is, the real decisions can be made only during the actual surgical operation. Usually if a resident has difficulties, the staff surgeon can "bail him out" easily, but in other instances —in vascular surgery, for example—he would have to be close at hand, indeed, for his help to be received in time. This is true of much of thoracic surgery. In a number of cardiac situations, the retrievable error (or the chance of retrieving it) must be handled immediately.

Any surgeon can think of examples in which diagnoses must be changed and procedure decided in the operative situation when time is precious and perilously limited. Severe respiratory distress, internal hemorrhage, inexplicable bleeding from the gastrointestinal tract, an acute coronary attack—in all of these instances, time is a significant element, and in some cases, that time is limited to minutes. If the resident has insufficient experience, the casual ward rounds and encouragement by telephone cannot replace experienced on-the-spot judgment.

A Dominican friar and battle surgeon some seven hundred years ago is said to have advised observation of skilled surgeons during operation with diligence, "because all the things which are necessary to the art cannot be included in books, cannot easily be foreseen, and many of these frequently happen to the operator." It is the unforeseen problem that should concern the responsible staff surgeon. Whether he can properly supervise in absence is suspect.

To a degree, this can be a matter of communication. If the residents and interns are known individually, the surgeon has more chance of being helpful. If his supervisory function is to be discharged correctly, communication with the attending physician

Received for publication Jan. 17, 1970.

must be clear in both directions. In other words, the surgeon must know how that physician thinks and talks, whether he understates, whether he is an alarmist, and whether he says one thing and means another.

Obviously the first and major concern is the patient. Referred patients are an individual responsibility so that a faculty member must assume it. Although, in a brochure, current training programs appear thorough, meaningful, and solid, the trappings must not obscure the primary purpose, which is the welfare of the patients. Everything that can be done must be done, and it is the staff surgeon's duty to see that preparation is made for comprehensive care. This includes establishing clear communication with each resident, and, of paramount importance, putting that resident in a position in which he can gain experience in the crisis situation. The error can all too easily be irretrievable.

Volume 67 *Number* 6

SURGERY

JUNE, 1970

Clinical surgery

Arterialization of the liver with portacaval shunt in the treatment of portal hypertension due to intrahepatic block

JEAN-NOËL MAILLARD, M.D.
JEAN-PIERRE BENHAMOU, M.D.
BERNARD RUEFF, M.D.
CLICHY, FRANCE
From the Faculté de Médecine, Bichat-Beaujon, Université de Paris and the Hôpital Beaujon

A program of arterialization of the liver in association with end-to-side portacaval shunt in cases of portal hypertension resulting from intrahepatic block was initiated for two reasons. First, in a previous study,[7] the authors showed that there is a significant correlation between operative survival after portacaval shunt in cirrhosis and portal venous blood flow before anastomosis; when portal venous blood flow was over 800 ml. per minute, the operative risk was significantly higher than when the portal venous blood flow was below this value. It was concluded that the acute postoperative failure was probably of oligemic or ischemic origin. Second, arterialization of the distal stump of the portal vein after portacaval shunt has frequently been realized in the dog with normal liver,[1-4, 6, 8, 10] and longer postoperative survival with lowered incidence of hepatic encephalopathy has been found to result. Although these experimental results were not, of course, evidence of the usefulness of arterialization of the portal vein in the treatment of cirrhosis in man, they were encouraging. In order to maintain hepatic blood flow at preoperative level, it was decided to arterialize the distal stump of the portal trunk in all patients in whom portacaval shunt was indicated and arterialization was feasible.

Ten patients were operated on by two different techniques, and the purpose of the present paper is to compare these techniques.

Submitted for publication March 3, 1969; resubmitted Oct. 8, 1969.

Reprint requests: Dr. J.-N. Maillard, Hôpital Beaujon, 100 Bd. du Général Leclerc, 92, Clichy, France.

MATERIAL AND METHODS

Patients. Portal hypertension was present in all ten patients. In five, it was due to alcoholic cirrhosis, in two, to cirrhosis of unknown etiology, in one, to cirrhosis with carcinomatous nodules in the hepatic hilus, in one, to primary biliary cirrhosis, and in one, to stenosis of the intrahepatic branches of the portal vein with normal liver. In all ten patients, the performance of a portacaval shunt was indicated because of bleeding esophageal varices.

Table I. *Patients and techniques*

Patient No.	*Sex*	*Age (yr.)*	*Etiology of the hepatic block*
Aortoportal prosthesis			
1	M	58	Alcoholic cirrhosis
2	M	64	Cirrhosis of unknown etiology
3	M	49	Alcoholic cirrhosis
4	F	51	Alcoholic cirrhosis
5	M	45	Cirrhosis of unknown etiology
Splenic artery–portal vein anastomosis			
6	F	47	Primary biliary cirrhosis
7	F	45	Alcoholic cirrhosis
8	M	41	Alcoholic cirrhosis
9	M	57	Cirrhosis of unknown etiology; carcinomatous nodules in the gastro-duodenal ligament
10	M	52	Stenosis of the intra-hepatic branches of the portal vein

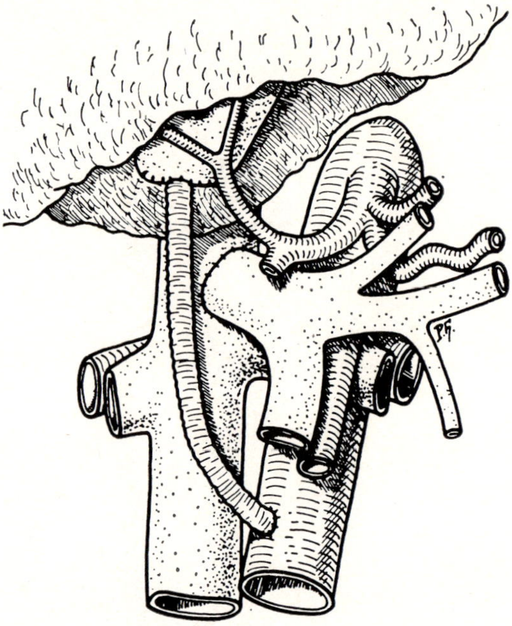

Fig. 1. Dacron prosthesis between inferior part of aorta and hepatic stump of portal vein.

Surgical techniques.

First technique: aortoportal prosthesis. The first technique, applied in Patients 1 to 5 (Table I), was the interposition of a knitted Dacron prosthesis, 5 or 6 mm. in diameter, between the aorta under the left renal vein and the distal stump of the portal trunk. The anastomosis was side to end between the aorta and the prosthesis and end to end between the prosthesis and the portal trunk (Fig. 1). The prosthesis was isolated from the portacaval anastomosis by suturing the right anterenal cellular tissue to the right border of the duodenum. Care was taken not to injure the preaortic lymph nodes and channels during dissection of the aorta and to prevent direct contact between prosthesis and duodenum.

Second technique: splenic artery–portal vein anastomosis. The second technique, applied in Patients 6 to 10 (Table I), was an end-to-end anastomosis between the splenic artery and the distal stump of the portal vein (Fig. 2). The artery was uncovered along the superior border of the body of the pancreas and stripped to its division in the splenic hilus. It was then severed, and the proximal end turned over to the right, behind the duodenohepatic ligament, obliquely recut, and anastomosed to the portal vein. Spasm of the artery frequently observed during stripping was alleviated by dilatation with a Fogarty's catheter before anastomosis. In two patients, thrombosis of the anastomosis occurred during operation and thrombectomy was performed. In one of the two patients (Patient 6), thrombectomy was unsuccessful and arterial obstruction was permanent. This second technique generally proved more difficult than the first, especially when the patient was obese and the artery was in a retropancreatic position. It was therefore not performed when conditions were unfavorable.

Before anastomosis, blood pressures were measured in the portal vein and in the inferior vena cava with an electromanometer (Telco, Gentilly, France); portal venous blood flow was measured with a square-wave electromagnetic flowmeter (Carolina Medical Electronics, Winston-Salem, N. C.). After anastomosis, blood pressures were measured in the inferior vena cava and in the splanchnic and hepatic stumps of the portal vein; blood flow was measured in the

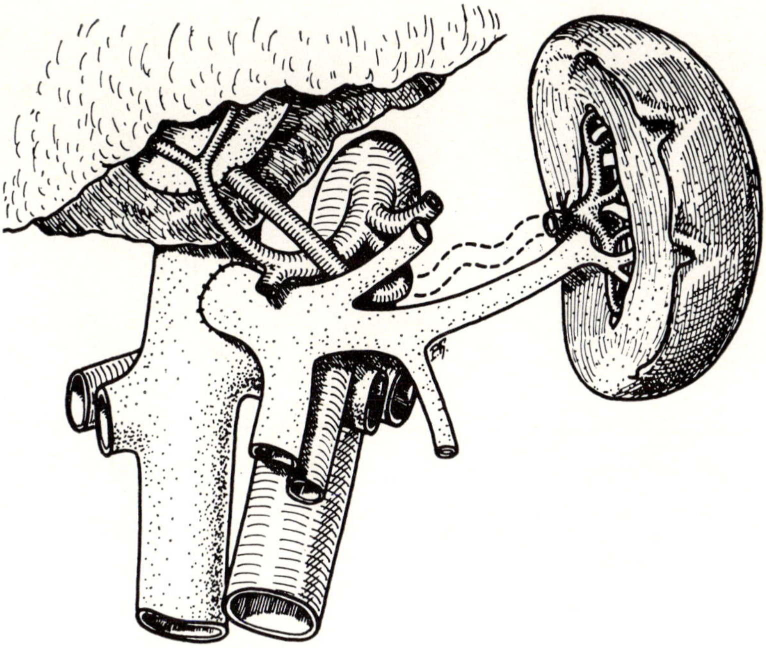

Fig. 2. End-to-end anastomosis between splenic artery and hepatic stump of portal vein.

Table II. *Aortoportal prosthesis: Blood flow (ml./min.)*

Patient No.	*Diameter of the prosthesis (mm.)*	*Portal vein before anastomosis*	*Prosthesis*	*Portal vein after anastomosis*
1	6	900	1,800	1,400
2	5	800	700	1,000
3	5	580	300	1,650
4	6	600	850	1,200
5	5	300	600	1,000

Table III. *Aortoportal prosthesis: Blood pressure (mm. Hg)*

Patient No.	*Diameter of the prosthesis (mm.)*	*Portal vein before anastomosis*	*Portal vein, hepatic stump*	*Portal vein, splanchnic stump*
1	6	20	28	13
2	5	17	20	5
3	5	19	8	10
4	6	22*	20*	3
5	5	18	18	10

*On reoperation after 11 days.

splanchnic stump of the portal trunk and either in the prosthesis (first technique) or in the splenic artery (second technique).

RESULTS

Hemodynamic results.

Aortoportal prosthesis. The hemodynamic results obtained in the five patients treated by the first technique are given in Tables II and III. Patients 1 and 2 had a preshunt portal venous blood flow superior or equal to 800 ml. per minute. Peripheral portal pressure fell to a value which can be considered normal. In Patients 1 and 4, the diameter of the prosthesis was 6 mm. and blood flow through the prosthesis was higher

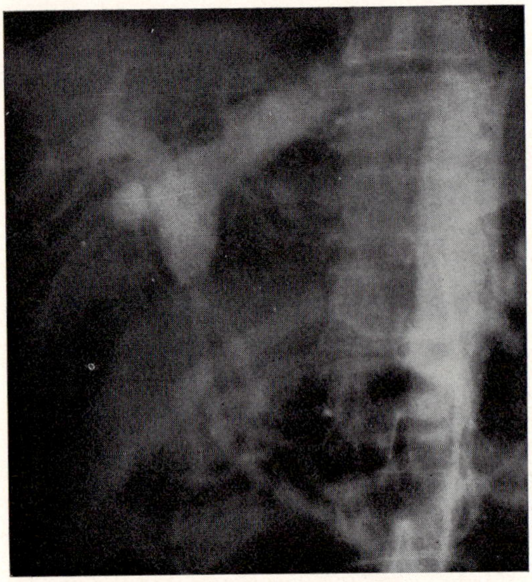

Fig. 3. (Patient 3). Aortography eight days after operation. Simultaneous opacification of the prosthesis, intrahepatic branches of portal vein, and hepatic artery.

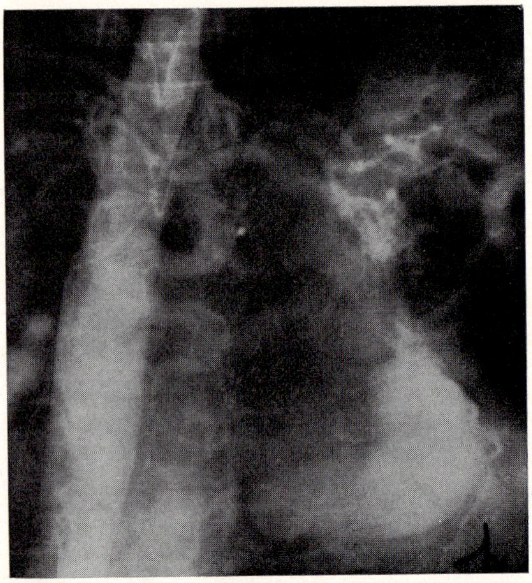

Fig. 4. (Patient 3). Aortography after 22 months. The prosthesis is patent. Portal vein caliber has increased.

Table IV. *Splenic artery–portal vein anastomosis: Blood flow (ml./min.)*

Patient No.	*Portal vein before anastomosis*	*Splenic artery after anastomosis*	*Portal vein after anastomosis*
6	—	200	1,000
9	400	400	1,000
10	200	200	350

Table V. *Splenic artery–portal vein anastomosis: Blood pressure (mm. Hg)*

Cases	*Portal vein before anastomosis*	*Portal vein, hepatic stump*	*Portal vein, splanchnic stump*
7	28	20	6
8	26	24	6
9	32	26	8
10	45	14	10

than the preshunt portal venous blood flow; in the other patients the diameter of the prosthesis was 5 mm. and blood flow through the prosthesis was less than the preshunt portal venous blood flow. Blood pressure in the hepatic stump of the portal vein did not rise markedly except in Patient 1. Evidence for the patency of the prosthesis was obtained in all cases: in Patients 1, 3, and 5 by aortography (Fig. 3), in Patient 2 during reoperation, and in Patient 4 by necropsy. In Patients 1 and 3, a second aortography was performed 18 and 22 months after operation, respectively: The prosthesis was still patent and the intrahepatic branches of the portal vein were markedly dilated (Fig. 4).

Splenic artery—portal vein anastomosis. In the patients treated by the second technique, blood flow (Table IV) through the anastomosis between the splenic artery and the portal vein was equal to and the intrahepatic portal blood pressure lower than the preshunt levels (Table V). Arteriography of the celiac axis was performed in four patients (Fig. 5). In one of them (Patient 8), the anastomosis was found to be thrombosed. Splenic vascularization was partially preserved in every case, the distal end of the splenic artery being supplied either through the left gastric artery and the short vessels of the greater curvature (Fig. 6) or directly through the right gastric arteries. In Patient

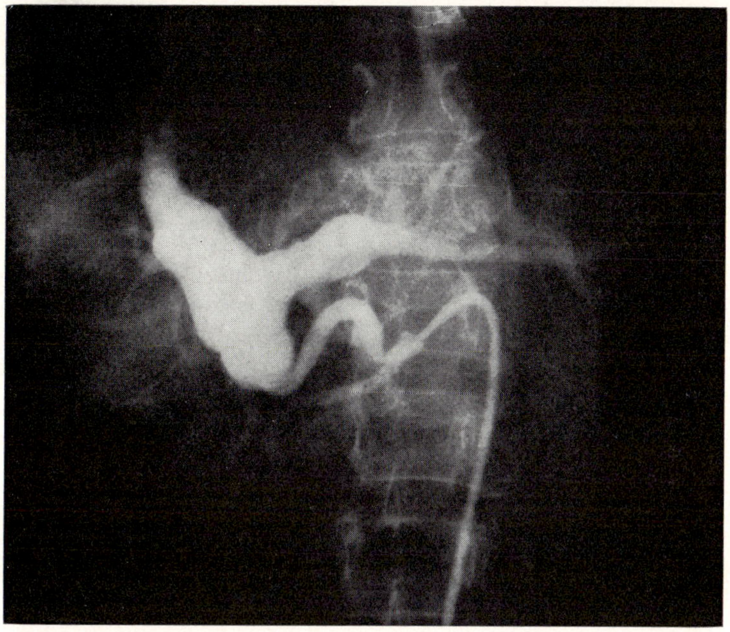

Fig. 5. (Patient 7). Selective celiac axis arteriography two months after operation. The hepatic and splenic arteries and the portal vein are simultaneously opacified.

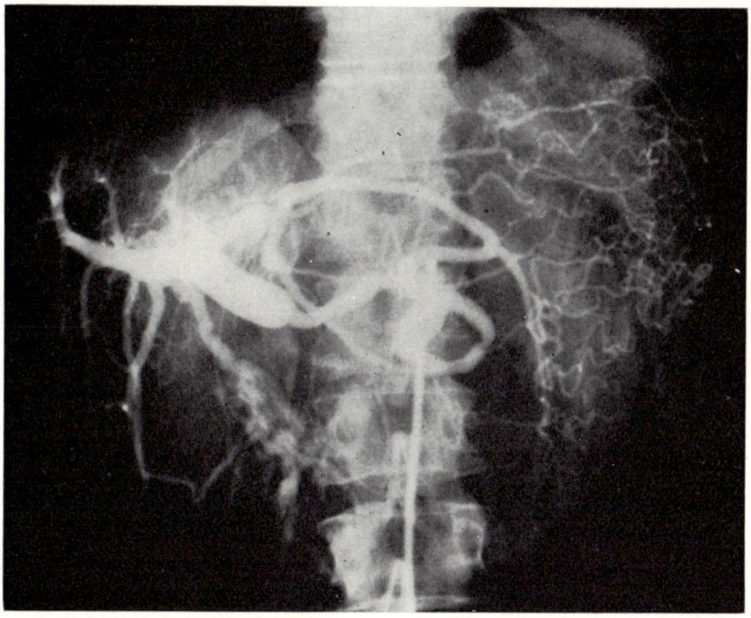

Fig. 6. (Patient 6). Selective celiac axis arteriography one month after operation. The splenic artery and the portal vein are injected. Only one left hepatic artery arising from the left gastric artery is opacified. The spleen is revascularized via the short vessels of the stomach.

10, opacification of the esophageal varices via gastric veins arising in the cavernoma could be demonstrated. In all cases in which a valid hepatography was obtained, it was similar in size and opacity to that obtained preoperatively by splenoportography.

Operative and late deaths. In the prosthesis group, Patient 4 died three weeks after the operation from progressive hepatic insufficiency and high protein content ascites (3.8 Gm. percent) which could not be controlled. In the days immediately preceding death, alimentary bleeding and hepatic coma developed; at necropsy, multiple ulcerations were found in the gastric mucosa. Patient 1 became anemic one year after operation. Three tests with ^{51}Cr-tagged red cells demonstrated fecal blood loss of approximately 50 ml. per day. Angiographic evidence of the patency of the portacaval anastomosis and of the prosthesis was obtained. There was no abnormality in the upper gastrointestinal series. This patient died from hematemesis. At necropsy, an erosion resulting from the prosthesis was discovered in the second portion of the duodenum.

There were no postoperative deaths in the splenic artery–portal trunk anastomosis group.

Other postoperative complications. Ascites with a high protein content (4.3 Gm. percent) developed after operation in Patient 3 and disappeared in five months. In Patient 2, a cholestatic-type jaundice appeared (bilirubin: 26 mg. per 100 ml.; alkaline phosphatase: 82 Bodansky units); this patient was operated on again on the eleventh day. Cholangiography performed through the gallbladder revealed a normal extrahepatic biliary system and faint opacification on the intrahepatic biliary ducts. Blood pressure in the prosthesis was 20 mm. Hg at the first operation and 40 mm. Hg at the second. Partial ligation of the prosthesis performed in order to lower the blood pressure to 25 mm. Hg was followed by thrombosis; thrombectomy was not attempted. Although the jaundice diminished rapidly, the serum bilirubin level did not return to normal until six weeks after the second operation.

In Patients 5 and 10, hematemesis occurred the day after the operation. Radiologic investigation revealed no abnormality. No explanation can be proposed for these hemorrhages.

In the prosthesis group, Patients 2 and 3 suffered episodes of transient hepatic coma attributable to faulty diet, excessive intake of sedative, or severe hypokalemia; between these episodes, clinical and electroencephalographic abnormalities disappeared completely. In the splenic artery–portal trunk anastomosis group, no evidence of hepatic encephalopathy was detected.

In Patient 8, thrombosis of the arteriovenous anastomosis was demonstrated by arteriography of the celiac axis. There were no clinical signs.

Pathologic results.

Action on hypersplenism. In all patients in whom hypersplenism was present (Table VI), it was unchanged after treatment by portacaval shunt and aortoportal prosthesis. In patients treated by portacaval shunt and splenic artery–portal vein anastomosis, on the other hand, hypersplenism disappeared without the thrombocytemia usually observed after splenectomy.

Action on liver parenchyma. Three pathologic controls of liver after arterialization were obtained, two by operative biopsy, 20 and 11 days, respectively, after the first

Table VI. *Effects of arterialization on the platelet count (platelets per cubic millimeter)*

Patient No.	*Preoperative value*	*Postoperative value*
Aortoportal prosthesis		
1	80,000	130,000
2	52,000	55,000
3	85,000	74,000
4	—	—
5	230,000	220,000
Splenic artery–portal vein anastomosis		
6	140,000	210,000
7	215,000	230,000
8	85,000	120,000
9	58,000	300,000
10	70,000	195,000

operation (Patients 2 and 4), and one at necropsy two years after operation (Patient 1). In the early controls, the portal spaces were enlarged and sclerous; in Patient 2, in whom reoperation on the twentieth day was necessary because of cholestatic-type jaundice, numerous thrombi were observed in the canaliculi, mainly in centrolobular areas. In the only late control available, the intrahepatic portal veins were the site of collagen fibrosis, dissociating the muscle fibers; the right branches of the portal vein were obstructed by recent thrombi which had probably immediately preceded death, since they were not apparent on arteriograms performed four days before. In the three cases, neither intra- nor extrahepatic iron deposition was visible; this is at variance with the observations of Zuidema and his colleagues[11] in dogs with arterialization of the portal vein.

DISCUSSION

Disadvantages of prosthesis. 1. Arterial prosthesis has on occasion been found to be associated with excessive arterial flow, which cannot be safely reduced by stenosing the prosthesis. In patients with high arterial flow intrahepatic cholestasis may occur. This complication can be paralleled with the observations of Schwartz and associates[10] in dogs with arterialization of the portal vein through prosthesis. When the prosthesis blood flow was high, phosphatasemia increased; it decreased when the prosthesis was thrombosed. The authors ascribed this intrahepatic cholestasis to compression of the canaliculi by distended sinusoids.

2. It could be assumed that ascites observed in two patients was secondary to sinusoidal hypertension caused by arterialization of the liver.[9] Indeed, in Patient 3, blood flow through the prosthesis was below the preshunt portal blood flow (Table II), and in Patients 3 and 4, intrahepatic portal pressure after arterialization was below the preshunt portal pressure (Table III). The high protein content of the ascites suggests a lymphatic origin; stripping of the portal vein in the hepatoduodenal ligament and stripping of the aorta may lead to severance of numerous lymphatic channels.

3. The duodenal erosion observed in one patient of this group is similar to the digestive complications described after aortic prosthesis.[5]

4. There is no action on hypersplenism.

These disadvantages appear to be major and to justify abandonment of prosthesis.

Disadvantages of anastomosis between splenic artery and portal vein. (1) Anastomosis is not always technically feasible, especially in obese patients; (2) spasm resulting from arterial stripping may lead to arterial thrombosis. These technical drawbacks can, however, be avoided, and arterialization of the portal trunk through the splenic artery is the technique of choice whenever practicable.

The benefits to be derived from arterialization of the cirrhotic liver cannot be evaluated in so small a series. Only the effect of splenic artery ligation on hypersplenism can be regarded as well established.

SUMMARY

The authors proposed to treat portal hypertension caused by intrahepatic block by end-to-side shunt associated with arterialization of the distal stump of the portal trunk to maintain hepatic blood flow. In the first group of five patients, a prosthesis was inserted between the aorta and the portal vein, whereas in the second group of five patients, anastomosis was effected between the splenic artery and the portal vein. Comparison of the two techniques favors the second. However, it is not always feasible. The value of arterialization of the cirrhotic liver remains questionable.

REFERENCES

1. Cohn, R., and Herrod, C.: Some effects upon the liver of complete arterialization of its blood supply, SURGERY 32: 214, 1952.
2. Fisher, B., Russ, C., Fedor, E., Wilde, R., Engstrom, P., and Fisher, E. R.: Further experimental observations on animals with arterialized livers, SURGERY 38: 181, 1955.
3. Fisher, B., Russ, C., and Updegraff, H.: Total arterialization of dog liver, SURGERY 35: 879, 1954.

4. Griffen, W. O., Bernstein, E. F., Nicoloff, D. M., Miller, E. O., Andersen, J. A., and Wangensteen, O. H.: The effect of liver arterialization upon ammonia clearance, Surg. Gynec. Obstet. **115:** 6, 1962.
5. Humphries, A. W., Young, J. R., De Wolfe, V. C., and Lefevre, F. A.: Complications of abdominal aortic surgery, Arch. Surg. **86:** 43, 1967.
6. McGredie, J. A., Doggart, J. R., and Welbourn, R. B.: Total arterialization of the liver, Brit. J. Surg. **45:** 83, 1957.
7. Maillard, J.-N., Benhamou, J. P., and Rueff, B.: Valeur pronostique de la mésure peropératoire du débit porte dans l'hypertension portale par cirrhose. Étude préliminaire de l'artérialisation du bout hépatique de la veine porte, 68è Congrès Français de Chirurgie, Paris, 1966, Presses Universitaires de France, Éditeurs, p. 593.
8. Matzander, U.: Verbesserung der Leberdurchblutung nach porto-cavalen Anastomosen, Ann. Univ. Sara. (Med.) **12:** 164, 1965.
9. Orloff, M.: Effects of side to side portacaval shunt on intractable ascites, sodium excretion and aldosterone metabolism in man, Amer. J. Surg. **112:** 287, 1966.
10. Schwartz, S. I., Morton, J. H., and McGovern, G. R.: Experimental arterialization of the liver, Surgery **49:** 611, 1961.
11. Zuidema, G. D., Gaisford, W. D., Abell, M. R., Brody, T. M., Neill, S. A., and Child, C. G.: Segmental portal arterialization of canine liver, Surgery **53:** 689, 1963.

Cystic degeneration of the popliteal artery

S. J. A. POWIS
D. M. MORRISSEY
E. L. JONES
EDGBASTON, BIRMINGHAM, ENGLAND
From the Queen Elizabeth Hospital

In a large series of patients suffering from intermittent claudication, Boyd and associates[3] described a group of young adult males in which primary thrombosis of the popliteal artery had occurred in the absence of arterial disease elsewhere. These patients may have been similar to the case described 5 years later by Ejrup and Hierton[4] to which they ascribed the diagnosis of cystic necrosis of the popliteal artery. This condition, which is a mucoid change in the adventitia of the artery, has since been described in 28 cases[9, 11] and in other arteries in 8 instances.[1, 2, 10]

The present report describes a further case with emphasis on the etiology and management, together with a review of the literature.

CASE REPORT

A 35-year-old male patient presented with a 5 week history of intermittent claudication in the left calf in April, 1966. At this time claudication occurred after walking 800 yards and was improving, all limb pulses were present, and no action was taken. After initial improvement, his condition deteriorated and he was admitted in October, 1966, with a claudication occurring after walking 350 yards, despite the presence of normal pulses in the left leg. Arteriography showed a block in the left popliteal artery and the absence of collaterals. At operation the vessel was distended and nonpulsatile. Incision of the adventitia released clear gel and allowed the pulse to return. Histological examination of the gel showed it to consist of mucin, containing a few swollen cells.

After operation he was asymptomatic for a year and then suffered occasional mild attacks of claudication for 12 months before presenting in October, 1968, with a claudicating distance of 400 yards. At this time there was also doubt about the distâl pulses. Repeat arteriography (Fig. 1) showed an 8 cm. block in the left popliteal artery. At operation (D. M. M. on September 26, 1968), 2 years after the original exploration, the vessel was distended (Fig. 2), and again gel was released on incision of the adventitia (Figs. 3 and 4). Histology of the cyst wall revealed thickened adventitia and outer media. The adventitia showed fibrous thickening, focal chronic inflammatory cell infiltration, and multiple cystlike clefts, which in places extended into the outer media (Fig. 5). These clefts were lined by swollen cells with a clear, fine granular cytoplasm and eccentrically placed nuclei (muciphages). The muscle coat of the remaining media was otherwise normal.

Results of histochemical staining, shown in Table I, indicated the mucin was either a neutral mucopolysaccharide or a mucoprotein and not an acid mucopolysaccharide, the usual connective tissue mucin.

Postoperative arteriogram (Fig. 6) showed the vessel to be patent, and clinically the patient remains symptom free.

DISCUSSION

Cystic necrosis of the popliteal artery affects males more than females in the ratio 8:1, at an average age of 36 years in the male.[9] The onset is usually sudden, but occasionally it is insidious or intermittent. The distal pulses may or may not be palpable, and in some cases the popliteal artery has been more readily palpable than on the normal side.[8] Ishikawa's sign[7] is usually present and is demonstrated by fully flexing the knee, an action which results in pallor, coldness, and pulselessness of the distal extremity.

Received for publication July 7, 1969.

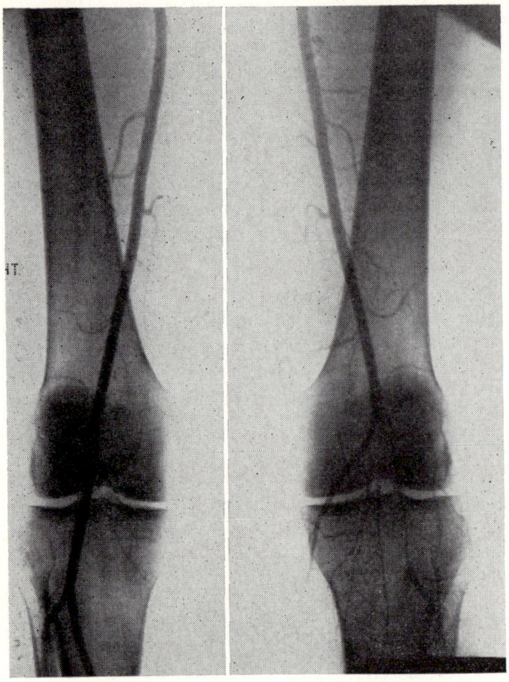

Fig. 1. Preoperative arteriogram showing block in left popliteal artery.

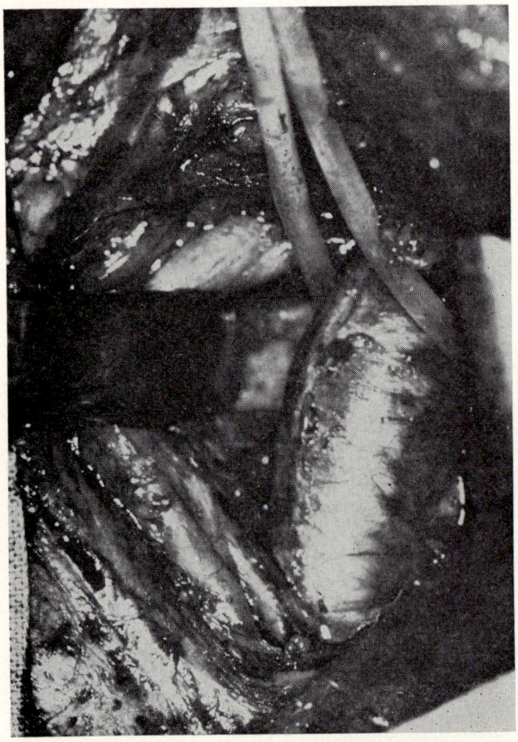

Fig. 2. Distended popliteal artery as seen at operation.

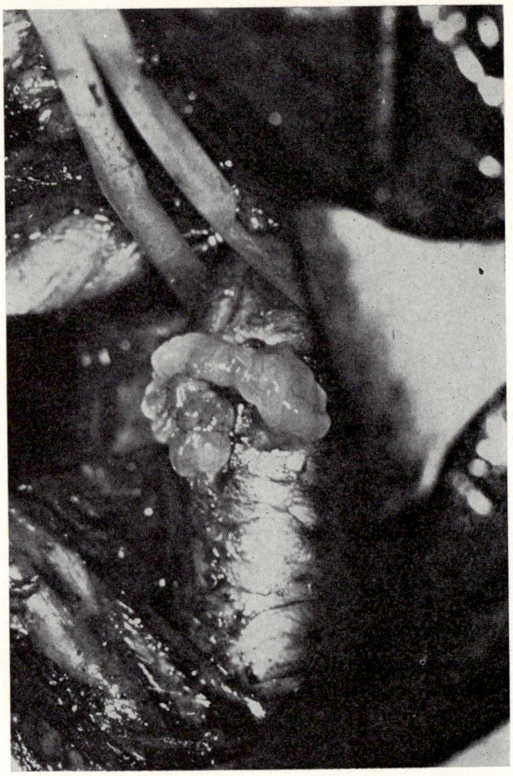

Fig. 3. Gel oozing from cystic space.

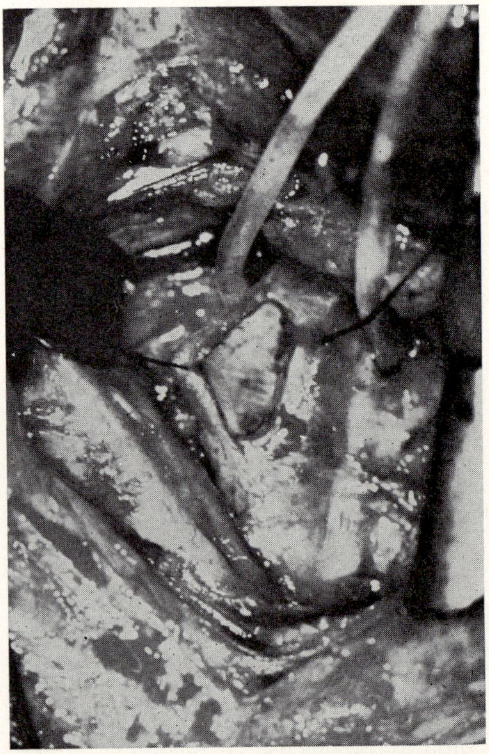

Fig. 4. Cavity left in vessel wall after removal of gel.

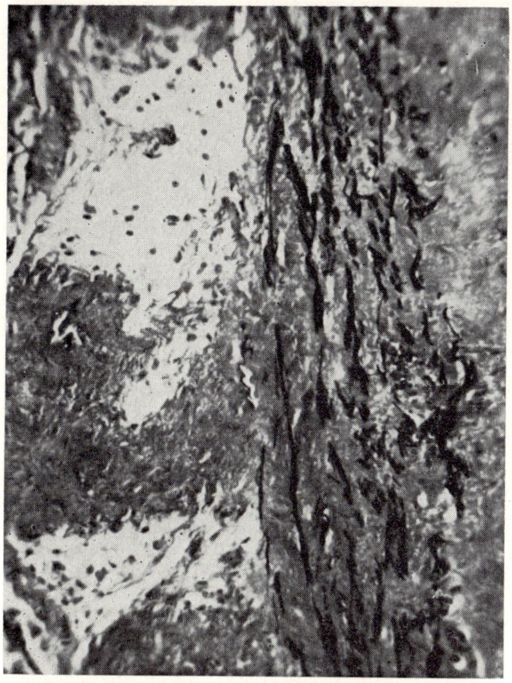

Fig. 5. Histological appearance of vessel wall demonstrating cystic space and dark staining elastic tissue.

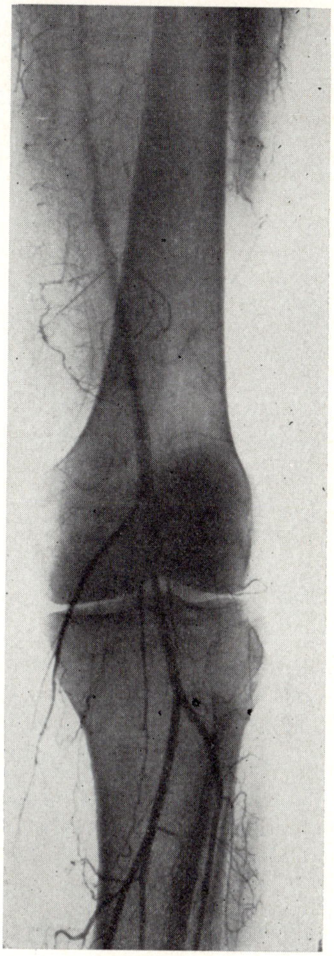

Fig. 6. Postoperative arteriogram demonstrating patency of popliteal artery.

Arteriography, including lateral views, shows a localized, smooth obstruction without post-stenotic dilatation, sometimes associated with displacement of the vessel. The obstruction is caused by either thrombosis superimposed on stenosis[9] or apposition of vessel walls.[6]

Cystic necrosis is unlikely to be of degenerative origin, as 2 cases have been reported in boys aged 11[5] and 13.[9]

Local trauma, such as may result from repeated movement, a possible event in the popliteal artery, does not account for an identical condition described in 8 cases,[1, 2, 10] affecting well-protected vessels, such as the iliac, radial, and ulna arteries; also the incidence is not increased in athletes and manual workers. As there is no evidence of inflammation or neoplasm, an alternative etiology must be sought. Mucin-secreting cells derived from the endothelial lining of the knee joint may be incorporated in the adventitia during development of the popliteal artery. These sequestrated cells may secrete

Table I. *Histochemical reactions of intracellular mucin from the lining of cyst wall*

Staining method	*Result*
Ehrlich's hematoxylin and eosin	±
Southgate's mucicarmine	±
Hale's dialyzed iron	–
Toluidine blue	–
Alcian blue	–
Hughesdon uranyl nitrate	–
Alcian blue—periodic acid-Schiff	–
Aldehyde fuchsin—alcian blue	–
Periodic acid-Schiff	±
Phenylhydrazine blockade with periodic acid-Schiff	–

± = weakly positive result.
– = negative result.

small amounts of mucin over the years and, eventually, give rise to cysts in the vessel wall. This theory would account for the presence of such cysts in many vessels, always in juxtaposition to a joint, and the 2 cases reported in 11- and 13-year-old boys supports this congenital inclusion theory.

Of 28 cases in the literature, 25 were followed up for periods varying between 6 months and 11 years. These 25 patients had 26 operations, following which 21 had unequivocably patent popliteal arteries. Three occluded, and of these, 2 had a prosthetic graft, and one had incomplete incision of the cyst, followed by a second operation performed for an asymptomatic narrowing.[9] Both who suffered narrowing of the affected artery had incision of the cyst.

Of the 21 who had unequivocably patent vessels, 15 had release of the gel, and 6 had excision of the narrowed segment and insertion of a graft. Of 8 grafted patients, 6 grafts were successful, and 2 occluded, while of 18 patients who had the gel released, 15 had successful results, 2 had narrowed arteries, and one had an occluded artery.

It would seem that if the gel is adequately released, the results are good and possibly preferable to excision and grafting. In the first instance, release of the gel should be advocated and if further occlusion occurs as the result of recurrence of a cyst, then this should also be released.

The present case is the first reported in which gel was released for a recurrence of symptoms with entirely satisfactory results.

SUMMARY

Cystic necrosis of the popliteal artery is a rare condition. The present case is only the twenty-ninth described during the last 15 years. The etiology is uncertain, but might well be due to congenital inclusion of mucin-secreting cells in the adventitia of the vessel affected. The most satisfactory surgical results are obtained by releasing the gel, without resection of part of the vessel.

REFERENCES

1. Atkins, H. J. B., and Key, J. A.: A case of myxomatous tumour arising in the adventitia of the left external iliac artery, Brit. J. Surg. **34:** 426, 1947.
2. Bäckstrom, C. G., Linnel, F., and Östberg, G.: Cystic myxomatous adventitial degeneration of the radial artery with development of ganglion in the connective tissue, Acta Chir. Scand. **129:** 447, 1965.
3. Boyd, A. M., Hall Ratcliffe, A., Jepson, R. P., and James, G. W. H.: Intermittent claudication, a clinical study, J. Bone Joint Surg. (Brit.) **31B:** 325, 1949.
4. Ejrup, B., and Hierton, T.: Intermittent claudication, Acta Chir. Scand. **108:** 217, 1954.
5. Harris, J. D., and Jepson, R. P.: Cystic degeneration of the popliteal artery, Aust. New Zeal. J. Surg. **34:** 265, 1965.
6. Hierton, T., Lindberg, K., and Rob, C.: Cystic degeneration of the popliteal artery, Brit. J. Surg. **44:** 348, 1957.
7. Ishikawa, K., Mishima, Y., and Kobayashi, S.: Cystic adventitial disease of the popliteal artery, Angiology **12:** 357, 1961.
8. Lambley, D. G.: Intermittent claudication due to cystic degeneration of popliteal artery, Brit. Med. J. **2:** 849, 1963.
9. Lewis, G. J. T., Douglas, D. M., Reid, W., and Kennedy Watt, J.: Cystic adventitial disease of the popliteal artery, Brit. Med. J. **3:** 411, 1967.
10. Parkes, A.: Intraneural ganglion of the lateral popliteal nerve, J. Bone Joint Surg. (Brit.) **43-B:** 784, 1961.
11. Savage, P. E. A.: Cystic disease of the popliteal artery, Brit. J. Surg. **56:** 77, 1969.

Renal artery thrombosis following blunt trauma: Report of four cases

OSCAR M. GRABLOWSKY, M.D.
RUDOLPH F. WEICHERT, III, M..D
JACOB B. GOFF, M.D.
JORGEN U. SCHLEGEL, M.D.
NEW ORLEANS, LA.
From the Department of Surgery, Tulane University School of Medicine

Renal artery thrombosis following blunt trauma is a rare condition which was first described by Von Recklinghausen[15] in 1861. Prior to this report, only ten cases of renal artery thrombosis secondary to blunt trauma have been reported. However, atrophic kidneys have been noted in a number of patients who have previously had blunt abdominal trauma, presumably caused by unrecognized renal artery injury. We describe here three cases of unilateral and one case of bilateral renal artery thrombosis. All the reported cases are summarized in Table I.

CASE REPORTS

Case 1 (A. E.). A 22-year-old seaman fell, striking his flank and head. He was examined at the United States Public Health Service Hospital in New Orleans for complaints of left chest and abdominal pain. Results of physical examination were normal, except for a small scalp laceration and abrasions over the left flank and buttocks. Vital signs were normal.

Hemoglobin was 13.6 Gm. per 100 ml. and urinalysis revealed albuminuria and microscopic hematuria. There was no function of the right kidney on an intravenous pyelogram. Cystoscopy was performed, and a normal collecting system was noted on a retrograde pyelogram. A retrograde aortogram through the femoral artery was interpreted as showing thrombosis of the right renal artery, demonstrated by decreased opacity of the artery beginning several centimeters distal to the aorta with a definite filling defect near the bifurcation of the distal renal artery (Fig. 1).

At operation, 24 hours after admission, a pulseless right renal artery was found. An attempt to restore vascular continuity failed because of extensive intraluminal thrombosis. A right nephrectomy was performed. The patient did well after operation and was discharged on the tenth postoperative day.

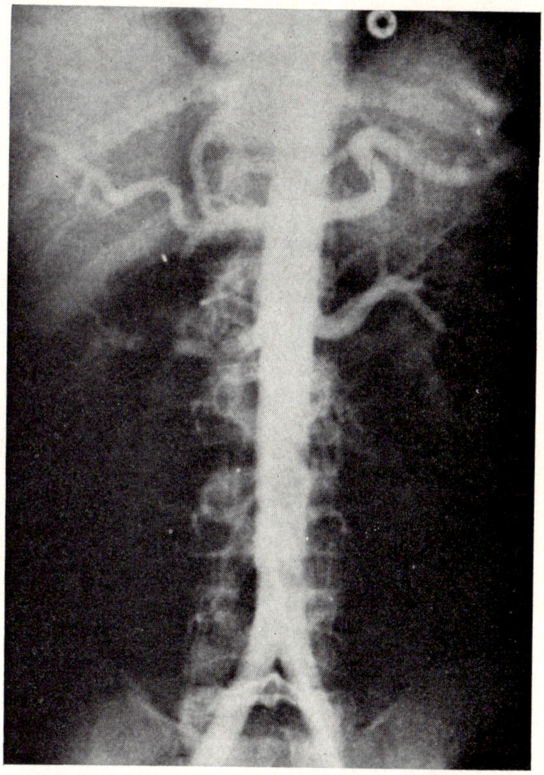

Fig. 1. Aortogram showing filling defect in the right renal artery several centimeters from the aorta, subsequently proved to be thrombosis.

Received for publication July 17, 1969.

Table I. *Clinical summary of 12 patients with renal artery thrombosis secondary to blunt trauma*

Reference	*Age and sex*	*Cause of injury*	*Associated injuries*	*Urinalysis*
Hirshberg and Soll[8] (1942)	48, male	Fall from truck	Abrasions of flank	Hematuria
Lichtenheld et al.[10] (1961)	10, male	Fall from bicycle	Abrasions of chest	Hematuria
Steiness and Thaysen[14] (1965)	18, male	Fall from motorcycle	None	Microscopic hematuria
Eliahou et al.[4] (1963)	33, male	Hit by bus	Abrasions of forehead and nose, contusions over lumbar area	Gross hematuria and albuminuria
Baichwal and Waugh[1] (1968)	26, male	Auto accident	Abrasions of face, back, and extremities; fractured clavicle	Microscopic hematuria
Collins and Jacobs[3] (1960)	—	Fall from tree	—	Hematuria
Owen and Pearlman[12] (1952)	36, female	Auto accident	Fractured ribs, pelvis, and clavicle; cerebral contusion	Hematuria
Von Recklinghausen[15] (1861)	13, male	Fall	Fractured leg and skull	—
Barney and Mintz[2] (1933)	Male	Fall from moving car	—	Hematuria
Grablowsky et al.	22, male	Fall	Scalp laceration and abrasions over flank and buttocks	Microscopic hematuria and albuminuria
Grablowsky et al.	37, male	Auto accident	Fractured mandible, abrasions of extremities and flanks	Microscopic hematuria
Grablowsky et al.	16, male	Motorcycle accident	Abrasions over body and mild lower abdominal tenderness	Microscopic hematuria
Grablowsky et al.	19, female	Car accident	Fractured mandible	Microscopic hematuria and albuminuria

*IVP = intravenous pyelogram.

Case 2 (J. C.). A 37-year-old male patient was involved in an automobile accident and was brought to Charity Hospital in New Orleans, Louisiana. Upon physical examination, a fractured mandible was found, as well as multiple abrasions of his extremities and flanks.

Urinalysis revealed 50 to 60 red blood cells per high-powered field. Hematocrit was 34 percent and blood urea nitrogen 23 mg. per 100 ml. There was no extravasation on cystogram and the intravenous pyelogram revealed a nonfunctioning left kidney.

Blood pressure on admission was 110/70 mm. Hg, but two days later rose to 230/110 mm. Hg. He became febrile with a temperature of 101 to 103° F. A translumbar aortogram showed complete occlusion of the left renal artery. At operation the only injury found was an intimal tear of the left renal artery with subintimal hematoma. A nephrectomy was performed. The patient did well following the operation and was discharged twelve days later, completely asymptomatic and normotensive.

Case 3 (A. G.). Three days prior to admission,

Diagnostic test	*Status of renal artery*	*Diagnosis verified by*	*Treatment*
IVP*: no visualization left kidney	Fragmentation of intima with thrombosis	Operation	Nephrectomy
IVP: no visualization left kidney; retrograde pyelogram: normal; aortogram: no visualization of left renal artery	No thrombosis renal artery	Operation	Nephrectomy
Retrograde pyelograms: normal; aortogram: both renal arteries almost completely occluded 2 cm. distal to aorta	Intimal tear on left with subintimal thrombosis; hematoma right renal artery	Operation	Left nephrectomy; segmental resection right renal artery and end-to-end anastomosis
Retrograde pyelograms: normal	Mural laceration right renal artery with thrombosis	Autopsy	—
IVP: no function left kidney; retrograde pyelograms: normal; aortogram: tapering of left renal artery 1 cm. from aorta	Intimal tear with thrombosis	Operation 38 days after injury	Nephrectomy
IVP: no function left kidney	—	Operation 4 days after injury	Nephrectomy
IVP: no function right kidney	Thrombosis	Operation 3 mo. after injury	Nephrectomy
—	—	Autopsy	—
—	Thrombosis	Autopsy	—
IVP: no function right kidney; retrograde pyelograms: normal; aortogram: occlusion right renal artery	Thrombosis	Operation 24 hr. after admission	Nephrectomy
IVP: no function left kidney; aortogram: complete occlusion left renal artery	Intimal tear with subintimal hematoma	Operation 48 hr. after admission	Nephrectomy
IVP: no function bilaterally; retrograde pyelograms: normal; aortogram: high-grade stenosis of both renal arteries 4 cm. from aorta	Bilateral intimal tears with distal thrombosis	Operation 12 hr. after admission	Bilateral aortorenal saphenous vein by-pass and renal transplantation
IVP: normal function left lower calyx and no function left upper calyx; aortogram: no visualization of arterial branch to left upper pole	Subintimal hematoma and thrombosis of segmental branch to left upper pole of kidney	Operation 18 hr. after injury	Exploration, no resection

a 16-year-old male patient was involved in a motorcycle accident. He was examined at a nearby hospital and released. After returning home, he voided only once during the following three days and became disoriented. He was then brought to Charity Hospital.

On physical examination, he was noted to be incoherent with a blood pressure of 160/110 mm. Hg. There were numerous abrasions over his body and mild lower abdominal tenderness.

On urinalysis there were 70 to 80 red blood cells per high-powered field. His hematocrit was 42 percent and blood urea nitrogen was 100 mg. per 100 ml. Paracentesis and carotid angiograms were normal. There was no function bilaterally on an intravenous pyelogram. Under general anesthesia, cystoscopy was performed and both ureters were catheterized. Approximately 2.5 ml. of bloody urine were obtained from the right ureter, and retrograde pyelograms were within normal limits. A translumbar aortogram showed high grade stenosis of both renal arteries 4 cm. from the aorta (Fig. 2).

Twelve hours after admission and three days

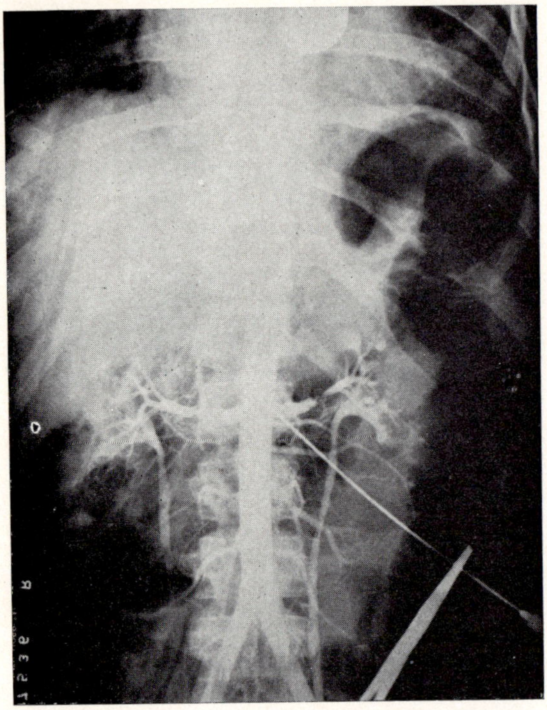

Fig. 2. Aortogram showing high-grade stenosis of both renal arteries. Subsequent operation showed these to be subintimal hematomas. Retained radiopaque medium from a previous retrograde pyelogram is noted in the pelvis of both kidneys.

after the initial accident, he was operated upon through a midline abdominal incision. Intimal tears with distal thrombosis were found in both renal arteries. Bilateral aortorenal artery saphenous vein bypasses were performed. Despite restoration of blood flow in the renal arteries, the kidneys remained mottled and cyanotic.

Following the operation, the patient remained anuric with a rising blood urea nitrogen. A Scribner shunt was inserted and hemodialysis was performed. On the twenty-first postoperative day, a transfemoral aortogram showed no function of the aortorenal saphenous vein bypasses.

The patient was then considered for renal transplantation. His father was found to be a compatible donor. Eighty-four days after the accident, the father's left kidney was implanted in the patient's right iliac fossa through a retroperitoneal approach.

Ten days after the transplant, he developed lower abdominal pain. A retrograde femoral arteriogram showed vascular integrity, but the excretory urogram showed extravasation at the ureteropelvic junction. On cystography, the bladder was compressed by urinary extravasation. An exploratory operation was performed and a portion of the ureter of the transplanted kidney was gangrenous. The transplanted ureter was removed and the patient's left ureter was anastomosed to the pelvis of the transplanted kidney. He later developed a cystocutaneous fistula and a ureteropelvic fistula which were successfully repaired. At present, ten months following injury, he is at home, but renal function shows evidence of steady deterioration in the functioning of the transplanted kidney.

Case 4 (L. J.). A 19-year-old female patient was admitted to Charity Hospital twelve hours after an automobile accident. On admission, she had bilateral mandibular fractures but no other evidence of injury. Her blood pressure was 132/78 mm. Hg and urinalysis revealed albuminuria and microscopic hematuria. Intravenous pyelogram showed a normal collecting system on the right and normal lower calyx on the left, but the left upper calyx did not function. There was no blood flow to the upper pole of the left kidney on aortogram. A paracentesis revealed hemoperitoneum. An exploratory operation was performed and a left retroperitoneal hematoma was found. The left renal artery bifurcated immediately upon leaving the aorta. There was a subintimal hematoma and thrombosis of the arterial branch to the left upper pole which began 4 cm. from the aorta. The upper half of the kidney was cyanotic and mottled, but the lower half was felt to be normal and therefore the kidney was not resected. Follow-up renal scan revealed minimal function of the left kidney. She remains normotensive three months after the original injury.

DISCUSSION

The extent of intra-abdominal injuries following blunt trauma is often difficult to determine. Abrasions were the only evidence of injury in six of thirteen cases of traumatic renal artery thrombosis. Admission urinalysis revealed albuminuria and hematuria in all the patients of this series and in all previously reported cases in which urinalysis was reported (Table I). If a patient has hematuria following trauma, an intravenous pyelogram should be obtained even though there are minimal signs of external injuries. If a kidney does not visualize on intravenous pyelograms, retrograde pyelograms should be done, and if they reveal a normal collecting system, renal arteriograms should be obtained. In each of our cases, the diagnosis was established by percutaneous retrograde femoral aortography using the Seldinger technique.

The mechanism of injury in renal artery

thrombosis following blunt trauma has been postulated by Collins and Jacobs.[3] They felt a sudden force may set the mobile kidney into motion and stretch its vascular pedicle. This ruptures the arterial intima, the least elastic component of the artery, and allows subintimal dissection and hematoma formation. An intimal disruption was identified in all of our cases and in four of the previously reported cases. The subintimal hematomas may cause partial or total occlusion of the artery. Prompt recognition is mandatory if repair is to be done before anoxic injury to the kidney has occurred. Partial occlusion must not be mistaken for spasm on arteriogram (Fig. 2) since delay in diagnosis decreases the chances of success following arterial reconstruction. Repair is feasible even with total occlusion of the renal artery, since the distal renal artery is usually patent.

In all cases, exploration should be performed through a transabdominal approach in an effort to restore vascular continuity and preserve renal function. Because of the sensitivity of the kidney to anoxia, immediate operation is imperative. When hematoma formation is extensive, a bypass graft from the aorta to distal renal artery may be possible. When the arterial injury is localized, thrombectomy and patch graft angioplasty may be sufficient. If the renal parenchyma is necrotic or if vascular reconstruction is impossible, a nephrectomy should be performed if the other kidney is normal. If renal artery thrombosis is bilateral, if the opposite kidney is missing or diseased, and if arterial reconstruction is impossible, implantation of an arterial-venous pedicle, such as the splenic artery and vein, into the renal parenchyma might be considered.[6, 7]

The prognosis in unilateral renal artery thrombosis is excellent following nephrectomy if the contralateral kidney is normal. If nephrectomy is not done initially, renal hypertension may necessitate nephrectomy at a later date. If both renal arteries are occluded, the situation is more serious and will require vascular reconstruction, splenic artery implantation, or, if these fail, chronic arterial dialysis and/or renal transplantation.

SUMMARY

Renal artery thrombosis following blunt trauma has been infrequently reported but may be more common than generally appreciated. Early recognition is mandatory for successful repair. All patients with hematuria following blunt trauma should have an intravenous pyelogram. If the kidney does not visualize on this study, then retrograde pyelograms and renal arteriograms should be performed. We have presented four patients with renal artery thrombosis following blunt trauma. Three patients had unilateral injuries. Two were treated by nephrectomy, while a third with ischemia to only the upper pole was treated without resection. The fourth patient had bilateral thrombosis initially treated by arterial reconstruction and subsequently by renal transplantation.

REFERENCES

1. Baichwal, L. S., and Waugh, D.: Traumatic renal artery thrombosis, J. Urol. **99:** 14, 1968.
2. Barney, J. D., and Mintz, E. R.: Infarcts of the kidney, J. A. M. A. **100:** 1, 1933.
3. Collins, H. A., and Jacobs, J. K.: Acute arterial injuries due to blunt trauma, J. Bone Joint Surg. **43-A:** 195, 1961.
4. Eliahou, H. E., Boichis, H., and Eden, E.: Traumatic renal infarction in a solitary kidney, J. Urol. **90:** 16, 1963.
5. Glenn, J. F., and Harvard, B. M.: The injured kidney, J. A. M. A. **173:** 1189, 1960.
6. Goldsmith, H. S., and Castillo, J.: A new method for kidney vascularization, Arch. Surg. **97:** 605, 1968.
7. Goldsmith, H. S., and Castillo, J.: Vascular implantation into kidney cortex to lower experimental renovascular hypertension, Ann. Surg. **169:** 127, 1969.
8. Hirshberg, H. A., and Soll, S. N.: Renal infarction of traumatic origin, J. A. M. A. **119:** 1088, 1942.
9. Knappenberger, S. T., Akers, R. E., and Galuszka, A. A.: Complete avulsion of the renal pedicle by nonpenetrating trauma, with survival, J. Urol. **89:** 316, 1963.
10. Lichtenheld, F. R., Franklin, S. S., and Serenati, Q. J.: Renal infarction due to trauma, J. Urol. **85:** 710, 1961.
11. Opit, L. J., McKenna, K. P., and Nairn, D.

E.: Closed renal injury, Brit. J. Surg. **48:** 240, 1960.
12. Owen, W. E., and Pearlman, C. K.: Hypertension due to thrombosis of the renal artery, J. Urol. **68:** 11, 1952.
13. Regan, F. C., and Crabtree, E. G.: Renal infarction: A clinical and possible surgical entity, J. Urol. **59:** 981, 1948.
14. Steiness, I., and Thaysen, J. H.: Bilateral traumatic renal artery thrombosis, Lancet **1:** 527, 1965.
15. Von Recklinghausen, F.: Hämorrhagische Niereninfarkte, Virchow. Arch. Path. Anat. **20:** 205, 1861.
16. Wilkey, J. L., Barson, L. J., Portney, F. R., and Turbow, B.: Acute renal artery thrombosis, J. Urol. **84:** 443, 1960.

Scoliosis and acute vascular compression of the duodenum

WILTON BUNCH, M.D.
JOHN DELANEY, M.D.*
MINNEAPOLIS, MINN.
From the Departments of Orthopedics and Surgery, University of Minnesota

Although Rokitansky[12] described superior mesenteric artery compression of the duodenum more than 100 years ago, skepticism regarding this syndrome still exists. The precise mechanism of obstruction is uncertain. Various descriptive terms have, therefore, been applied: arteriomesenteric duodenal compression, arteriomesocolic duodenal compression, superior mesenteric artery syndrome, duodenal ileus, Wilkie's syndrome, megoduodenum, and vascular compression of the duodenum. We prefer the last term. The common form of the condition is a chronic symptom complex characterized by recurrent abdominal distention, epigastric pain, and vomiting. Intervals of normal alimentation are interspersed with bouts of emesis that tend to progress in both frequency and severity. The subject of this report is the less common acute duodenal vascular compression, in particular that which is associated with scoliosis and its treatment.

The "cast syndrome" was first described by Willett[16] in 1878. His 17-year-old male patient began vomiting immediately after application of a plaster-of-paris cast intended to support a thoracolumbar "cyphosis." Vomiting persisted after removal of the cast, and the patient died five days later. At postmortem examination, the stomach was dilated. Buzzard[3] in 1880 reported fatal vomiting following application of a plaster body cast for treatment of Pott's disease. He postulated that the third portion of the duodenum had been compressed between the superior mesenteric artery and the distorted spine. The first report of the syndrome following casting for scoliosis is credited to Kelling,[10] whose 16-year-old female patient with a thoracolumbar curve was placed in a cast from neck to trochanters. She became acutely ill two days later but ceased vomiting after removal of the cast and survived. Operative or x-ray demonstration of the pathology was, therefore, not available. A body and neck cast applied to stabilize an injured spine led to persistent vomiting and death in a patient reported upon by Conley and Miller[5] in 1935. Sturtevant[15] in 1939 described three patients with duodenal compression, one of whom had scoliosis and had had intermittent vomiting since childhood with an increase in the frequency of vomiting following application of a cast. Beck[2] in 1946 reported four cases of acute duodenal obstruction. All patients were bedridden; two were supine in traction, and one was in a hyperextension jacket for treatment of a vertebral fracture. Dorph[7] reviewed the literature up to 1950 and added a case of his own, an 18-year-old girl who had been placed in a hip spica for treatment of a fractured femur. Nearly a month after application of the cast, she died as a result of persistent vomiting. Postmortem examination demon-

Requests for reprints to: John Delaney, M.D., University Hospitals, Minneapolis, Minn. 55455.

Submitted for publication July 17, 1969; resubmitted Aug. 25, 1969.

*Advanced Clinical Fellow American Cancer Society.

Table I

Case No.	*Age (yr.)*	*Sex*	*Cast*	*Position*	*X-ray findings*	*Treatment*	*Comments*
1	18	F	–	BR	Dilated duodenum	Prolonged NG suction	2 episodes relented with NG suction
2	24	F	+	A	Abrupt cutoff across duodenum at SMA level	Operation	2 previous episodes responded to NG suction
3	17	F	+	A	Outside hospital, no x-rays available	Partial removal of cast	Died—ruptured stomach
4	26	F	+	BR	Dilated stomach and duodenum, gastrografin passed through	Operation	First 2 episodes responded to NG suction
5	15	M	+	A	Dilated duodenum but contrast did empty	Cast removed	2 separate episodes relented with NG suction and cast removal
6	15	F	+	A	Sharp cutoff at mid-transverse duodenum	Operation	Late onset—4 wk. after casting
7	16	F	–	BR	Linear cutoff of duodenum at SMA crossing	Operation	Had upper GI bleeding during obstructive episode
8	15	F	+	A	Linear compression of duodenum at SMA level	Operation	Removal of cast necessitated bed rest; symptoms persisted
9	17	M	+	BR	Dilated stomach and duodenum	Remove cast, NG suction, position changes	Circle bed allowed position changes without strain on rod

SMA = superior mesenteric artery; NG = nasogastric; BR = bed rest; A = ambulatory; GI = gastrointestinal.

strated a dilated stomach and duodenum. A number of reports[8, 9, 13] since that time have been added to the literature on the "cast syndrome," but none has dealt specifically with the association of scoliosis and vascular compression of the duodenum.

The currently favored surgical treatment for the condition, duodenojejunal anastomosis, was first suggested by Stavely[14] in 1910.

Data on nine scoliotic patients developing duodenal obstruction during treatment are outlined in Table I.

ACUTE AND CHRONIC DUODENAL OBSTRUCTION

Barner and Sherman[1] summarized the subject of vascular compression of the duodenum in a review which should be studied by anyone interested in the problem. Of 281 collected cases, 32 were classified as acute, that is, the patients had symptoms for less than one month. Acute duodenal obstruction, in contrast to the chronic syndrome, was invariably marked by vomiting. Gastric dilatation was recorded in 72 percent of the acute cases but in only 18 percent of those with chronic recurrent symptoms. The vomiting, once having developed, tended to be persistent with acute duodenal compression, as opposed to the self-limited attacks of the chronic syndrome. Only those instances of acute duodenal obstruction with persistent symptoms would be recorded in the literature. A brief episode would be considered to be postoperative vomiting of unknown cause. The true frequency of acute duodenal compression has, therefore, probably been underestimated. All patients in the present series had the acute form of the syndrome.

SYMPTOMS AND SIGNS

In general, these patients complained of rather mild pain but a feeling of extreme distention. The pain was not crampy, nor was it well localized. The associated tenderness was confusing to physicians unfamiliar with this syndrome. In one instance, right lower quadrant tenderness led to inclusion of appendicitis in the differential diagnosis. One patient had rectal tenderness. Pseudo rebound tenderness, which was often noted, is due to compression and sudden release of a distended viscus rather than peritoneal irritation. All patients had abdominal distention, and all had bile-stained vomiting. One (Case No. 7) had upper gastrointestinal bleeding, which occurred after a second bout of acute duodenal obstruction and was accompanied by burning epigastric pain. Of the 281 patients reviewed by Barner and Sherman,[1] only four had gastrointestinal bleeding. Bowel sounds were normal to hypoactive in eight of our nine patients. This is to be contrasted with lower intestinal obstruction, which is invariably accompanied by abnormal bowel sounds. All patients testified to passing flatus throughout the episode, an indication that the obstruction is partial.

X-RAY FINDINGS

Abdominal distention and vomiting are common postoperative problems. Vascular compression of the duodenum is a relatively rare source of these symptoms. The essential radiologic finding is a dilated duodenum. Reverse peristalsis, the so-called "writhing duodenum," has been said to be pathognomonic of duodenal obstruction, but it is more striking in patients with chronic duodenal obstruction than in those with the acute syndrome. Furthermore, fluoroscopy is difficult in patients who have been recently operated upon for scoliosis or immobilized in plaster.

Contrast studies can provide useful information. To accomplish an adequate examination, however, the dilated stomach is first emptied by nasogastric suction. When this is done, the duodenum may also decompress and thus obscure the major finding. Contrast studies showed a linear obstruction at the level where superior mesenteric vessels cross the duodenum in four of the six patients so examined. An example is illus-

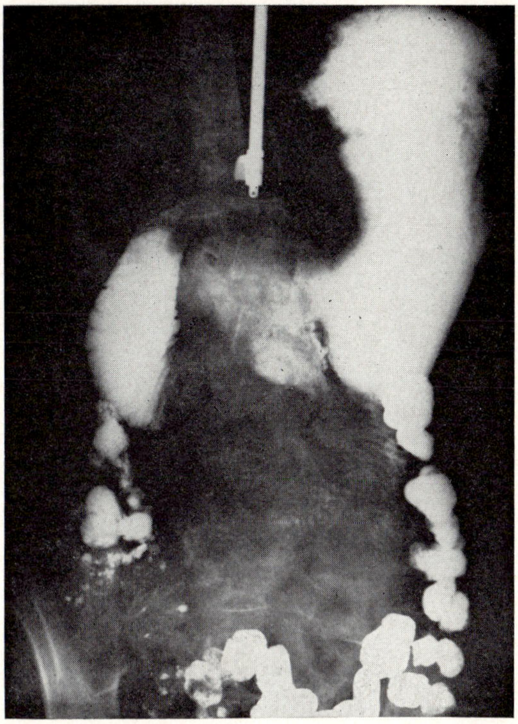

Fig. 1. Retained fluid in the stomach with linear compression of the duodenum.

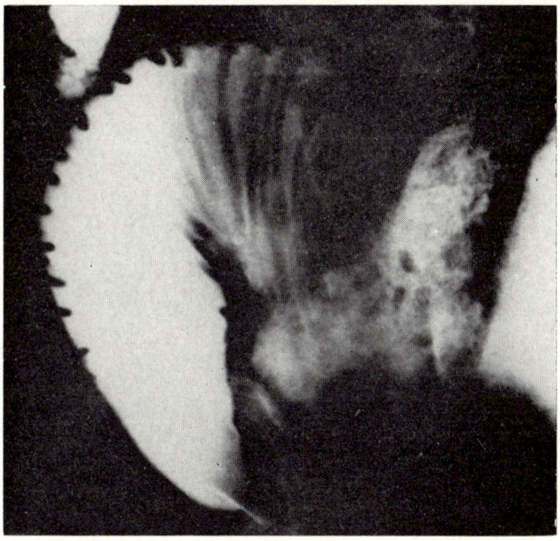

Fig. 2. The sharp cutoff of contrast in the duodenum coincides with the crossing of the superior mesenteric artery.

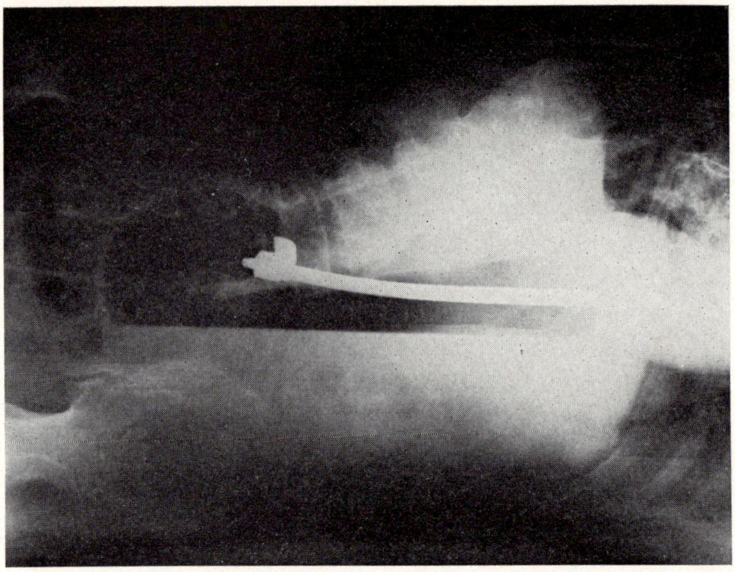

Fig. 3. Both duodenum and stomach are dilated as shown in the right lateral decubitus position.

trated in Figs. 1 and 2. One patient (Case No. 2) had a superior mesenteric arteriogram, which, superimposed upon the barium-filled duodenum, showed that the obstruction was at the point where the artery crossed the duodenum. The barium often passed through the area of compression, probably as the result of the position change temporarily relieving the obstruction. The fluoroscopist sometimes could demonstrate temporary relief of the obstruction by placing the subject in prone, knee-chest, or left lateral positions.

A rewarding radiologic study, not emphasized in the literature, is a lateral decubitus examination of the abdomen with the patient's right side up. This view reveals a dilated duodenal loop with a long air fluid level not well seen in other positions (Fig. 3). In this clinical setting, with the appropriate history and physical findings, radiologic demonstration of a dilated duodenum is virtually pathognomonic. The majority of patients in the present series also had gastric dilatation, although this finding is not essential to the diagnosis.

ETIOLOGIC CONSIDERATIONS

Many of the factors which have been implicated as possible causes are present in the patient being treated for scoliosis. These include weight loss, weak abdominal musculature, lumbar lordosis, prolonged bed rest, the supine position, and immobilization in plaster. Codman[4] in 1908 first pointed out the association of obstructive vascular compression of the duodenum with weight loss and injury. Other authors have since noted the etiologic role of prolonged bed rest, especially in the supine position.

Vascular compression of the duodenum has not been described in obese individuals. Müller[11] demonstrated that fat elevates the mesenteric vessels from the anterior surface of the duodenum. He was unable to compress the duodenum of obese cadavers until the fat was excised from around the base of the mesenteric vessels. The young victims of scoliosis are almost invariably thin.

Normally, the intestine is maintained in its position, not by the mesentery, but by the abdominal musculature. A lax abdominal wall permits the intestine to sag into the lower abdomen and even into the pelvis and thus to exert traction on the mesenteric vascular pedicle. The patient with paralytic scoliosis often has weak musculature and may actually have paralyzed abdominal muscles.

Duodenal compression has generally been assumed to be the primary event initiating this symptom complex, with the gastric dilatation being secondary. The reverse sequence has also been postulated. As early as 1907, Conner[6] recognized the relationship of duodenal dilatation and gastric dilatation. In his review, 55 percent of the patients with acute gastric dilatation undergoing autopsy were noted additionally to have duodenal distention, stopping at the superior mesenteric vessels. He showed in cadavers that distending the stomach can lead to duodenal compression. Presumably, the dilated stomach depresses the transverse mesocolon, putting the middle colic and superior mesenteric arteries on caudad stretch, with a resultant narrowing of the space between the superior mesenteric artery and the aorta.

Case No. 5 clearly illustrates the importance of the cast itself. Duodenal obstruction was twice relieved by simply removing the cast. The explanation for a body cast abetting vascular duodenal compression is obscure. The mechanism may be that restriction of abdominal distention forces the dilating stomach to expand caudally and put the mesenteric vessels on stretch. Seven of these nine patients were in body casts at the time of symptom onset.

Prolonged supine bed rest may be an important factor in initiating duodenal compression. Treatment in traction requires partial immobilization and makes assumption of the prone position particularly difficult. During the immediate postoperative period after spinal correction and insertion of the stabilizing metal rod (Harrington), the patient is at bed rest and allowed very little movement. Five of these nine patients, however, were ambulatory at the time symptoms started.

Lumbar lordosis, which often accompanies scoliosis, displaces the duodenum anteriorly and may serve to decrease the space between the mesenteric artery and the aorta. Either anatomic alteration tends to enhance vascular compression of the duodenum.

Spinal fusion and placement of Harrington rods are intended to alter the spinal configuration. As a result of correction of the curve, spinal lengthening occurs. The origin of the superior mesenteric artery thus is displaced cephalad at the expense of lateral mobility, possibly altering its relationship to the duodenum.

TREATMENT

If, in fact, gastric dilatation is the primary event, duodenal compression may be aborted by early institution of nasogastric suction. In four of our nine patients, symptoms and signs relented with gastric decompression.

The simple expedient of removing the cast may completely eliminate vascular compression of the duodenum. Unfortunately, after operation maintenance of spinal alignment demands that the patient be at bed rest when the cast is removed. In Case No. 9, the circle bed proved to be a valuable adjunct for providing position changes without putting stress on the spinal correction. Other measures employed are position changes, particularly assumption of the prone position following oral intake, ambulation, and restriction of diet to liquids. Frequently, for the postoperative scoliosis patient, ambulation and position changes are impossible.

Because some of the patients with scoliosis look forward to prolonged immobilization, repeated back operations, and body casts, we now tend toward early operative intervention. Five of the nine patients in this series underwent operation, side-to-side duodenojejunal anastomosis. All were completely relieved of symptoms.

Our current therapeutic regimen is to institute nasogastric suction and parenteral alimentation as soon as the diagnosis is established. Procrastination can only lead to further duodenal compression. If feasible, the cast should be removed and position changes accomplished on a circle bed.

Should the symptoms persist or recur when oral intake is resumed after a trial of conservative measures, we recommend doing a side-to-side duodenojejunostomy for definitive relief.

SUMMARY

Operative correction of scoliosis is occasionally associated with acute obstructive vascular compression of the duodenum. Factors contributing to this relationship are: immobilization in bed, the asthenic habitus, body casts, spinal distortion, and weak abdominal muscles. Distention, epigastric pain, and vomiting are the cardinal manifestations. The obstruction is only partial, and bowel sounds are usually normal. Radiologic demonstration of a dilated duodenum is pathognomonic. Initial treatment involves nasogastric suction, position changes and cast removal, if feasible. Should the obstruction persist or recur, it is bypassed by a duodenojejunal side-to-side anastomosis.

REFERENCES

1. Barner, H. B., and Sherman, D. C.: Vascular compression of the duodenum, Surg. Gynec. Obstet. **117:** 103, 1963.
2. Beck, W. C.: Acute gastroduodenal obstruction (dilatation), Arch. Surg. **52:** 538, 1946.
3. Buzzard, T.: Case of paraplegia from Pott's disease; Treatment by Sayre's jacket; intestinal obstruction; death from kink in duodenum, Trans. Clin. Soc. (London) **13:** 57, 1880.
4. Codman, E. A.: Chronic obstruction of the duodenum at the root of mesentery, Boston Med. Sci. J., **158:** 503, 1908.
5. Conley, A., and Miller, D. S.: Acute dilatation of stomach with perforation following body cast application, Industr. Med. **4:** 185, 1935.
6. Conner, L. A.: Report on acute dilatation of the stomach and its relation to mesenteric obstruction of the duodenum, Trans. Ass. Amer. Physicians **21:** 579, 1906.
7. Dorph, M. H.: The cast syndrome, New Eng. J. Med. **243:** 440, 1950.
8. Kaiser, G. C., McKain, J. M., and Shumacker, H. B.: The superior mesenteric artery syndrome, Surg. Gynec. Obstet. **110:** 133, 1960.
9. Kauffman, R. R., and Gerbode, F.: Arteriomesenteric duodenal ileus; report of 3 cases, Stanford Med. Bull. **9:** 262, 1951.
10. Kelling, G.: Uber den Mechanismus der acuten Magendilatation, Arch. Klin. Chir. **64:** 393, 1901.
11. Müller, R.: Uber akute postoperative Magendilatation, hervorgerufen durch arteriomesenteriale Duodenalkompression, Deutsch. Z. Chir. **56:** 486, 1900.
12. Rokitansky, C.: Lehrbuch der pathologischen Anatomie, ed. 1, Wein, 1842, W. Braumuller, vol. III.
13. Rosenburg, S. A., and Sampson, A.: The syndrome of mesenteric vascular compression of the duodenum, Arch. Surg. **73:** 296, 1956.
14. Stavely, A.: Chronic gastromesenteric ileus, Surg. Gynec. Obstet. **11:** 288, 1910.
15. Sturtevant, M.: Megoduodenum and duodenal obstruction, Radiology **33:** 185, 1939.
16. Willett, A.: Fatal vomiting following application of plaster-of-paris bandage in case of spinal curvature, St. Bartholomew Hosp. Rep. (London) **14:** 333, 1878.

Clinical and experimental use of thoracic impedance plethysmography in quantifying myocardial contractility

JOHN H. SIEGEL, M.D.*
MIKLOS FABIAN
CHARLES LANKAU, M.D.
MICHAEL LEVINE, M.D.
ANDREW COLE, M.D.
MICHEL NAHMAD, M.D.
BRONX, N. Y.
From the Department of Surgery, Albert Einstein College of Medicine, Yeshiva University

One of the more difficult problems facing the physician responsible for the care of the critically ill patient is how to evaluate myocardial function in a rapid and reliable manner which does not expose the patient to undue risk. It has become increasingly apparent that adequate care of such patients demands that the physician obtain an estimate of myocardial muscle function as distinguished from myocardial pump function,[1, 12] because in many critical illnesses significant increases in cardiac output can occur at a time when myocardial contractility appears to be deteriorating.[12] Indeed, there are a number of high-output shock states, such as that associated with septic shock[10, 17] and the hyperdynamic state seen in severe hepatic cirrhosis with portal hypertension,[18] in which a high-output cardiac failure is often the event leading to the patient's death.

Recently Kubicek and associates[7] have suggested that the use of a newly designed impedance cardiograph may enable the computation of cardiac output by thoracic impedance plethysmography without percutaneous instrumentation.

Supported in part by National Institute of Health Grants HE 10033 and HE 10415.

Submitted for publication July 2, 1969; resubmitted Aug. 26 and Nov. 14, 1969.

*Career Scientist, Health Research Council of the City of New York.

The present studies demonstrate that the clinical use of impedance plethysmography to measure cardiac output yields information about directional changes only. However, evaluation of the dynamic aspects of the thoracic impedance plethysmograph tracing appears to provide a guide to the myocardial contractile state in the intact animal and in man with the use of nondestructive, or minimally destructive, techniques.

METHODS

A dog preparation anesthetized with light pentobarbital anesthesia (25 mg. per kilogram) was used. An intracardiac micromanometer (Statham Model SF1) was positioned at the root of the ascending aorta, just above the aortic valve, and the second was placed into the left ventricular cavity via the apical dimple. This enabled the measurement of intraventricular dynamics simultaneously with the aortic pressure pulse, without interfering with aortic valve function. The heart was approached transabdominally through a diaphragmatic incision, so as not to violate the chest wall. After the intraventricular catheter tip manometer had been inserted, the chest was evacuated of air and maintained under a constant negative pressure of 14 cm. of water. In some animals, only the aortic catheter tip manometer was utilized, so as not to

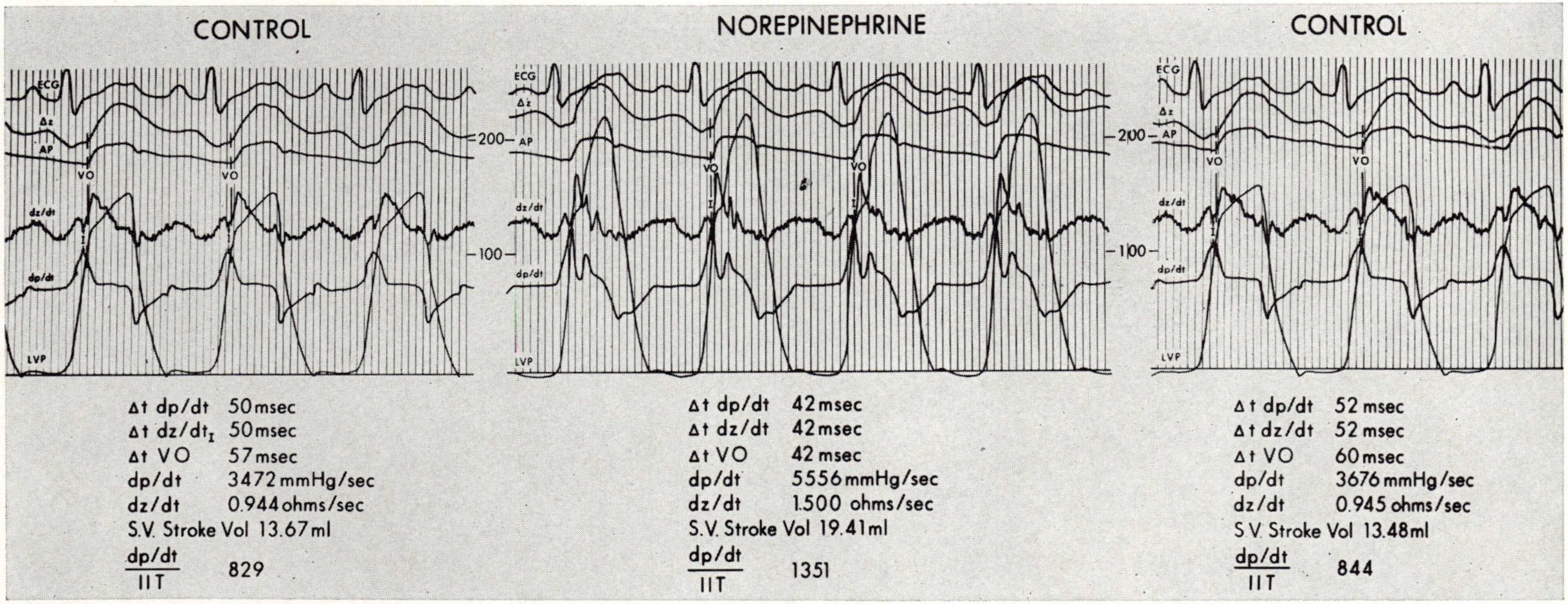

Fig. 1. Simultaneous tracing of the intraventricular pressure pulse (LVP) and its first derivative with regard to time (dp/dt), the central aortic pressure (AP), the thoracic impedance pulse (ΔZ) and its first derivative with regard to time (dz/dt), and the ECG. Pressure scale applies to LVP only. The DC component of the aortic pressure (AP) is held constant and is used in this record for timing purposes only. Paper speed 200 mm. per second.

alter intrathoracic dynamics in any way and to simulate the clinical situation. The animals were artificially respired with room air and all baro- and chemoreceptors were left intact. The thoracic impedance changes were measured by using the impedance cardiograph developed by Kubicek and associates.[7] In this instrument, two electrodes are placed circumferentially around the neck and two about the abdomen just below the xiphoid process. Alternating current is sent through the outer electrode of each pair and the change in voltage between the inner electrodes measured throughout the cardiac cycle. The change in impedance (ΔZ), indicated by the fluctuation in the voltage, corresponds to volume shifts between the two inner electrodes spanning the thorax. This technique measures pulmonary and cardiac volumes, but the slower respiratory cycle variations are electronically buffered, leaving only the rapid dynamic changes corresponding to events in the cardiac cycle. The electrocardiogram (ECG), the intraventricular pressure pulse, the aortic pressure pulse, and the impedance changes were recorded (Fig. 1). The change in impedance (ΔZ) and the first derivative of the impedance change (dz/dt) were compared with the first derivative of the intraventricular pressure pulse (dp/dt) and the electrocardiogram. Myocardial contractility and vascular tone were altered by the use of an inotropic vasoconstrictor (norepinephrine), an inotropic vasodilator (isoproterenol), and a noninotropic vasoconstrictor (methoxamine). In addition, two negative inotropic agents, pentobarbital and *E. coli* endotoxin, were also used to challenge the animals.

CLINICAL STUDIES

Six high-risk patients undergoing hemodynamic studies as part of a pre- or postoperative cardiovascular evaluation had a simultaneous determination of cardiac output by both thoracic impedance plethysmography[7, 8] and indicator dilution techniques with the use of cardiogreen dye. In order to evaluate the impedance cardiac outputs, they were compared to indicator dilution outputs computed by both the standard Stewart-Hamilton method,[5] which utilizes both the forward area under the dye curve plus an exponential replot of the downslope, and the gamma variate method of Thompson and associates,[24] which relies entirely on measurements made during the rising portion of the indicator dilution curve. In all instances, the bolus of dye was injected into the right atrium and the arterial samples were taken from the femoral artery.

Four of the six were studied under a variety of conditions which frequently resulted in alterations in cardiac output, and one of these, a hyperdynamic cirrhotic patient,[15] was re-evaluated on four different occasions during his postoperative recovery following portal venous decompression for portal hypertension.

In three additional patients, a long Teflon catheter was placed in the aortic arch via the femoral artery by the use of the Seldinger technique. Comparison of impedance and indicator dilution outputs was not done in this group, but determinations of impedance force-velocity relationships and the durational aspects of the impedance pulse were compared to more standard cardiovascular parameters, i.e., heart rate, central aortic blood pressure, and the Stewart-Hamilton cardiac output.

RESULTS

Experimental observations.

Myocardial isometric time-tension relations. Studies in ten animals revealed that there was a consistent relationship between the peak first derivative of the isovolumetric portion of the ventricular contraction (dp/dt maximum), and the inflection point in the impedance first derivative ($dz/dt_{(I)}$). Both of these points occurred before the time of valve opening in the control nonstimulated animal (Fig. 1). The time from the peak of the *r* wave of the ECG to the peak first derivative of the pressure pulse (Δt dp/dt) is shown below each panel and has been compared with the time to the inflection point of the first derivative of the impedance pulse ($\Delta t\ dz/dt_{(I)}$) and the time to valve opening

(Δt VO). The calculated value of the first derivative of the isometric pressure (dp/dt) and the first derivative of the impedance pulse (dz/dt) are shown, as well as the calculated stroke volume. Also, under each panel is the value of the computed isometric time-tension index $\frac{dp/dt}{IIT}$, which has been previously shown to also be an index of myocardial contractility independent of changes in fiber length.[13, 14] This index and the related Δt dp/dt are altered only by those interventions which also alter the duration of myocardial active state and change the maximum velocity of shortening.[13, 14, 21]

The administration of norepinephrine to this animal (Fig. 1) resulted in an increase in the peak pressure generated in the ventricle as well as an increase in dp/dt. There was a corresponding shortening of the time from activation to the peak dp/dt (Δt dp/dt), and this corresponded with a shortening in the Δt $dz/dt_{(I)}$. With the increase in contractility produced by norepinephrine, there was a tendency for the time to valve opening (Δt VO) to also shorten, and this tended to approach the time to maximum dp/dt, as is shown here. The isometric time-tension relation $\frac{dp/dt}{IIT}$ also increased. After the administration of norepinephrine had been stopped, all parameters of contractility and the Δt $dz/dt_{(I)}$ tended to return to the control state, which suggests that this is a reproducible alteration and that it follows directionally the changes in myocardial contractility in the intact heart.

Fig. 2 shows the interrelation between the time to maximum dp/dt (Δt dp/dt) and the time to the inflection point in the first derivative of the impedance pulse (Δt $dz/dt_{(I)}$ under a variety of conditions. These data represent 150 observations in seven animals and show a relationship between these two, such that increasing Δt dp/dt is associated with an increase in the Δt $dz/dt_{(I)}$. This change is a function of the state of contractility of the myocardium. When isoproterenol or norepinephrine were used, there was a decrease in both of these values associated with an increase in contractility. When agents which produce a decrease in myocardial contractility, such as *E. coli* endotoxin[16] or pentobarbital,[12] were used, there

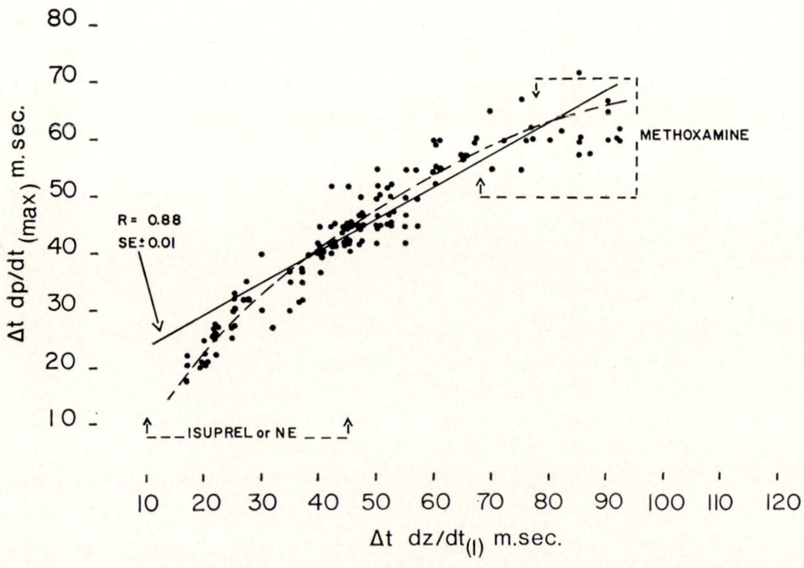

Fig. 2. Impedance isometric time-tension relationship. Temporal relation between maximum dp/dt (Δt dp/dt) and the inflection point in the first derivative of the thoracic impedance (Δt $dz/dt_{(I)}$).

was an increase in both values over the control range. The major departure from a linear relationship between these values occurred with the use of methoxamine, which in these innervated preparations resulted in a decrease in contractility, as the result of the reflex withdrawal of sympathetic activity to the myocardium associated with the increase in systemic pressures.[2, 15] There was also a marked disparity between the Δt dp/dt and the time of valve opening, as the aortic diastolic pressure was raised progressively. Under these circumstances, the period of electrical diastasis, represented by the Δt dz/dt inflection point, lengthened as valve opening and maximum dp/dt separated widely in time. The signal-to-noise ratio becomes significant during this period and it was somewhat difficult to ascertain the exact point of the inflection of Δt dz/dt. As a result of this and perhaps other factors which are less well defined, there was a tendency for the Δt $dz/dt_{(I)}$ to lengthen to values greater than the values of Δt dp/dt. However, there still appears to be a good general correlation, even when all the points, including those produced by methoxamine, are taken as a whole. The best linear approximation is shown here by the calculated value for the linear regression line (R = 0.88) with its standard error of estimate of the mean (± 0.01).

Table I shows the results of an experiment in which all of the pertinent relationships have been compared in response to positive and negative inotropic agents in an innervated preparation with intact baro- and chemoreceptor reflexes.

These data show that both the pre-ejection interval (Δt VO) and the time course of ejection (Δt dz/dt peak) can be influenced by changes in the myocardial contractile state and also by noninotropic factors which alter aortic outflow resistance. However, alterations in the Δt $dz/dt_{(I)}$, which occurs either before or at the time of valve opening (Δt VO), are only slightly influenced by outflow effects and correspond in the main rather closely to alterations in Δt dp/dt and therefore to the duration of the active state of the myocardial contractile process. This index, therefore, appears to provide an empiric correlate of the level of myocardial contractility and its directional changes without requiring intravascular instrumentation.

Myocardial force-velocity relations. With the use of thoracic impedance plethysmography, it is also possible to gain direct information concerning myocardial force-velocity relationships which delineate the velocity-dependent aspects of contraction,[19, 21] provided that, with the use of a catheter tip micromanometer, an accurate central aortic pressure pulse with a high frequency response can be obtained simultaneously with the impedance pulse. In this treatment, the impedance pulse (ΔZ) is evaluated as a

Table I

					Milliseconds				
Intervention	*HR**	*Stroke* vol.	*CO*	*dp/dt*	Δ*t* dp/dt	Δ*t* $dz/dt_{(I)}$	Δ*t* *VO*	Δ*t* $dz/dt_{(peak)}$	*BP*†
Control	151	16.90	2.55	3846	45	45	60	87	178/145
Norepinephrine	141	19.84	2.79	6250	27	25	32	55	220/148
Control	142	19.43	2.75	3571	45	47	62	82	180/149
Methoxamine	116	13.78	1.59	1968	62	82	107	147	223/178
Control	113	19.31	2.18	1960	62	77	95	137	177/153
Isuprel	146	20.70	3.02	5952	20	20	27	47	150/102
Control	144	15.47	2.22	3125	45	45	62	112	179/154
Endotoxin	164	11.90	1.95	2173	65	70	85	127	87/76

*HR = heart rate.

† BP = blood pressure.

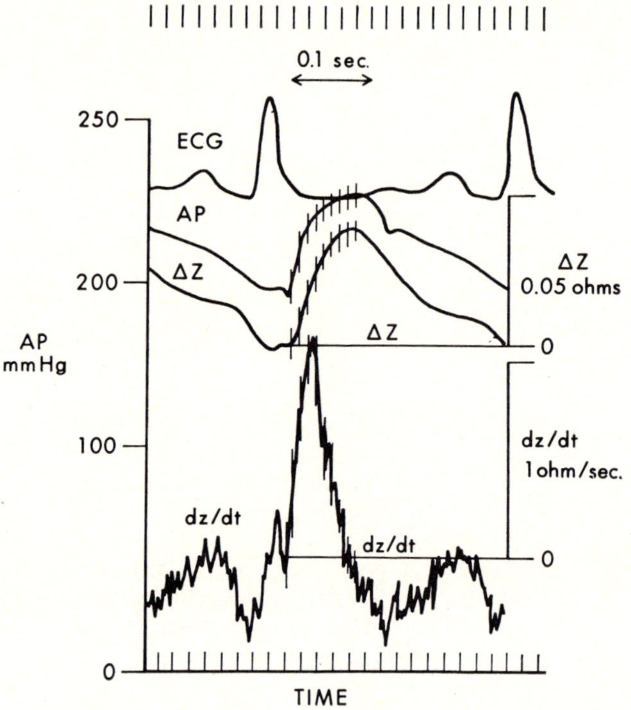

Fig. 3. Method of computing impedance force-velocity relation on basis of single beat. Afterload: aortic pressure (AP) times change in impedance pulse (ΔZ) in mm. Hg ohms; considered as function of the change in the velocity of the thoracic impedance pulse (dz/dt) in ohms per second and evaluated at 10 msec. intervals.

function of the aortic blood pressure at 10 msec. intervals during the systolic ejection period (Fig. 3). The impedance pulse during early systole is directly related to the ejected volume,[5-7] and the aortic pulse pressure to the resistance and capacitance factors opposing ejection. Together they reflect the afterload against which myocardial shortening (ejection) is occurring.[12] This afterload value in mm. Hg ohms is plotted against the instantaneous velocity of the impedance change (dz/dt) in ohms per second at each corresponding 10 msec. interval (Fig. 4), beginning from the point of valve opening. This portion of the dz/dt pulse is related to the velocity of aortic flow.[7,8] By extrapolating the exponential portion of the downslope of this impedance force-velocity curve back to zero load based on the log-log slope occurring at peak dz/dt, a function closely approximating a true myocardial force-velocity relationship is seen. This extrapolated maximum velocity (Vmax) changes in the same direction as cardiac contractility does.

Application to man.

Cardiac output. The observations of Kubicek and associates[7,8] and Harley and Greenfield[6] have suggested that a correlation exists between cardiac output determinations performed in man by impedance cardiography and by indicator dilution or pressure pulse methods. Their observations were made on normal subjects[7] or on patients with chronic cardiac disease[6] studied while the patients were in the erect position. In our hands, simultaneously performed flow studies of high risk general surgical patients, evaluated while the patients were in the supine position either pre- or postoperatively, revealed a poor quantitative correlation between cardiac outputs determined by impedance plethysmography and by standard indicator dilution techniques. However, there

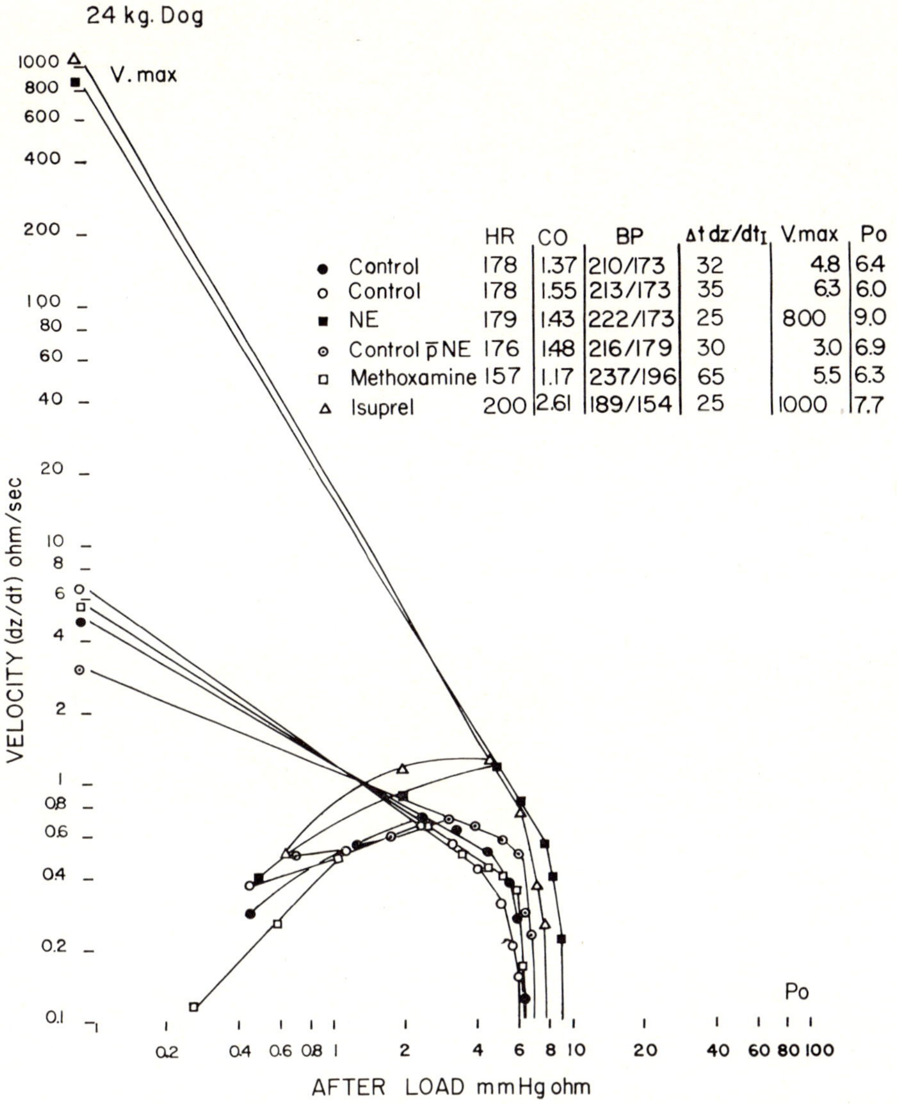

Fig. 4. Impedance force-velocity relationship. Change in impedance velocity as function of increasing impedance afterload in the presence of cardiac inotropic and noninotropic interventions.

was a qualitative trend which suggested that directional changes might be validly indicated by the impedance technique (Fig. 5, *A*). The quantitative aspects were improved if an initial impedance–CO/dye–CO ratio was used to correct subsequent impedance outputs (Fig. 5, *B*). Nevertheless, even this relationship tended to change with time and with some interventions which are known to alter myocardial function, perhaps as a function of alterations in pulmonary blood volume[11] or of differences in electrode placement on subsequent days. There was no consistent improvement in the CO_Z/CO dye ratio if the gamma variate[24] method of computation was used in preference to the Stewart-Hamilton[5] method for the indicator dilution curve.

Contractility. In contrast to the difficulty in quantifying the flow-related aspects of impedance plethysmography in man, the durational and velocity-related aspects of indi-

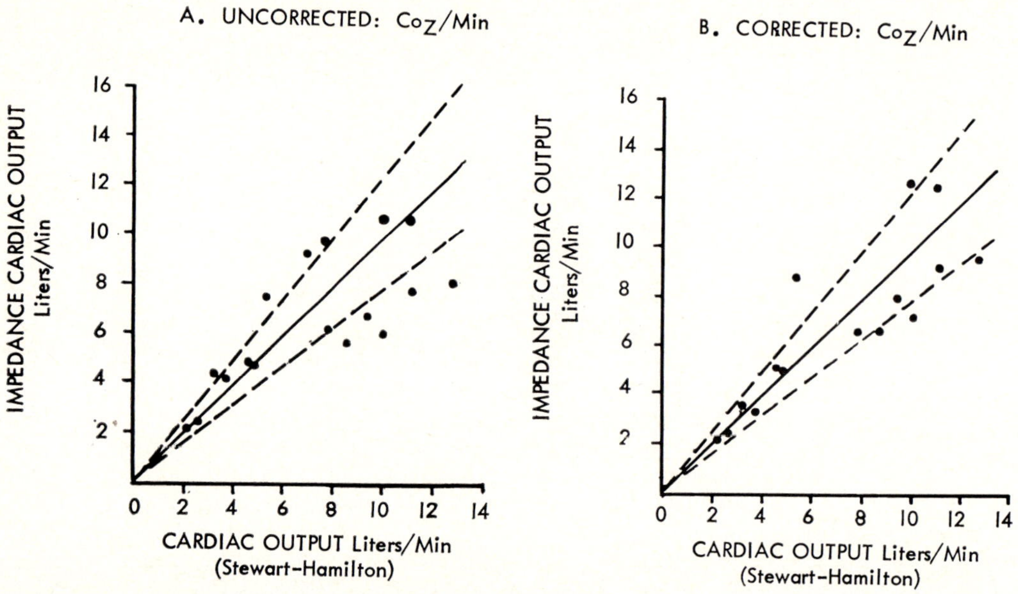

Fig. 5. *A,* Uncorrected cardiac output values in man obtained by the impedance and indicator dilution techniques (Stewart-Hamilton computation). *B,* Corrected impedance cardiac output values plotted against the original indicator dilution values obstained by the Stewart-Hamilton method.

vidual myocardial contractions were more satisfactorily delineated by this method. It was possible to evaluate relative changes in $\Delta t\ dz/dt_{(I)}$ in all but one patient, who showed ECG evidence of a right bundle branch block. In this patient, the conduction defect produced abnormalities in the impedance pulse such that no clear-cut inflection point could be determined. As is shown in Fig. 6, when a central aortic pressure is also obtained, it is possible to evaluate both the $\Delta t\ dz/dt_{(I)}$ interval and the extrapolated impedance Vmax, provided no major conduction abnormality or ventricular asynergy exists.

In Fig. 6 is shown the response of a 69-year-old woman studied prior to the operative resection of a recurrent sigmoid volvulus. The alteration in heart rate, cardiac output (via Stewart-Hamilton calculation of the cardiogreen indicator dilution curve), blood pressure, $\Delta t\ dz/dt_{(I)}$, and impedance Vmax and peak afterload (Po) are presented in the box. The method of extrapolation of the impedance Vmax is shown in the main part of Fig. 6. Very little change in the impedance force-velocity relation occurred during two control periods. A fifteen-minute period of inhalation of 100 percent oxygen produced a fall in heart rate and cardiac output and a lengthening of the durational aspects of contraction, $\Delta t\ dz/dt_{(I)}$. The impedance Vmax fell. After re-equilibration on room air, the cardiac output rose as did the Vmax, and the duration of $\Delta t\ dz/dt_{(I)}$ shortened even though no significant increase in heart rate occurred. The intravenous administration of 4 mg. of glucagon at this new control level produced a progressive increase in the impedance Vmax and a decrease in $\Delta t\ dz/dt_{(I)}$ over a five-minute period. These alterations in the contractile response were accompanied by a significant increase in the Stewart-Hamilton cardiac output five minutes after the administration of this inotropic agent. The impedance Vmax was increased to nearly five times the original control level after glucagon administration, which suggests that at least a part of the increase in cardiac output was due to a true increase in myocardial contractility.

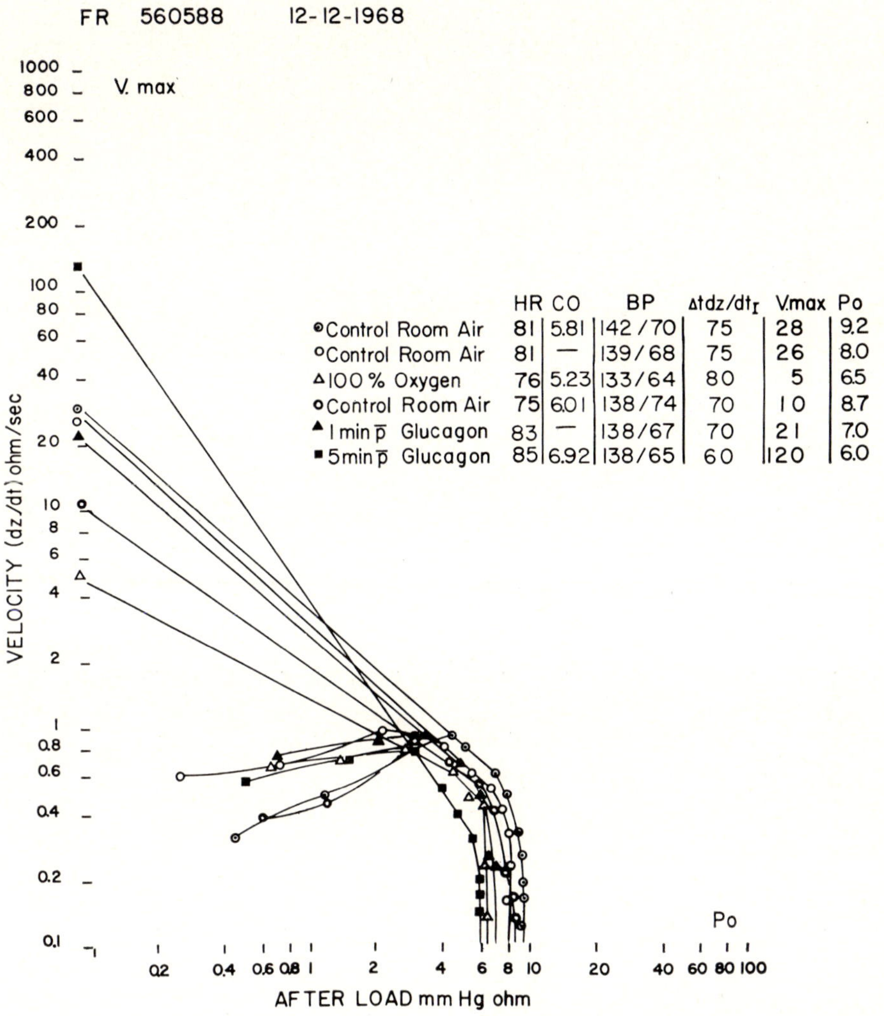

Fig. 6. Determination of impedance force-velocity relation in man. Comparison with Stewart-Hamilton cardiac output and with the durational aspects of the impedance pulse ($\Delta t\ dz/dt_{(I)}$).

DISCUSSION

The studies of Sonnenblick and associates[19-23] have indicated that the best description of myocardial contractility is contained in the myocardial force-velocity relationship which describes the alterations in the velocity of myocardial shortening as a function of the increasing afterload imposed on the myocardial fiber. Siegel and associates,[14] evaluated the interrelationships between the isometric and isotonic portions of contraction in papillary muscle fibers and in the intact heart. Their studies demonstrated that the durational aspects of the isometric contraction are a function of the force-velocity relationship in that alterations in the time from the onset of contraction to the peak isometric force and to the maximum first derivative of isometric tension development (Δt dp/dt) are directly related to the duration of myocardial contractile element activation and vary inversely with changes in the maximum velocity of isotonic shortening (Vmax). The interrelationship between myocardial contractile velocity, force, and active state which characterize changes in contractility are summarized in Table II.

The importance of attempting to measure myocardial contractility in intact man has

Table II

Aspects of contractility *Intervention*	*Velocity* *Vmax*	*Force* *Po*	*Active state* dp/dt	*Duration of active state*	
				$\Delta t\ dp/dt$	$\Delta t\ dz/dt_{(I)}$
A. Noninotropic agents	Constant	Increase proportional to ΔL	Increase proportional to ΔL	Constant	Constant
Increasing fiber length (ΔL)	0	+	+	0	0
B. Weak inotropic agents	Increase	No change or small increase	Increase	Decrease	Decrease
Increasing myocardial activation rate (ΔR)	+	0 or +	+	–	–
C. Strong inotropic agents	Large increase	Large increase	Large increase	Large decrease	Large decrease
Positive inotropic agents, norepinephrine, Isuprel, digitalis	++	++	++	– –	– –
D. Negative inotropic agents	Decrease	Decrease	Decrease	Increase	Increase
Barbiturates, endotoxin, anoxia	–	–	–	+	+

become obvious with the realization that stroke work and filling pressure relationships are "lumped" parameters of cardiovascular function. They do not solely reflect the contractile state of the heart, because myocardial work is not only a function of intrinsic myocardial contractility but is also a product of the ejected volume and the total peripheral resistance to flow (the afterload).[12, 14, 15, 19-23] Since, at any contractile state, the absolute velocity of cardiac muscle shortening decreases as a function of an increasing afterload,[22, 23] in order to delineate a change in contractility, elaborate techniques have been devised to determine a substantial portion of the velocity-load curve in the contracting heart, so as to extrapolate the maximum velocity of shortening.[1, 3, 4, 9] The determination of either the Vmax or the durational parameters of the myocardial active state is necessary to establish on which force-velocity relationship the heart is operating. This is especially true when there are significant alterations in the resistance load against which the myocardium pumps,[12, 23] as may occur in shock states[10, 14] in which there may be wide alterations in outflow resistance and fiber length. With this in mind, an attempt has been made to apply thoracic impedance plethysmography as a benign method of evaluating myocardial contractility which may be applicable to use in the critically ill patient. This noninvasive technique also offers the possibility of being able to determine whether a decrease in myocardial contractile function precedes a clinically apparent rejection crisis in patients with cardiac allografts.

SUMMARY

Studies have been directed toward evaluating the usefulness of cardiac output determinations by thoracic impedance plethysmography in the critically ill surgical patient, and an attempt has been made to determine whether dynamic aspects of the thoracic impedance pulse may also permit quantification of myocardial contractility. It has been shown that, while only qualitative changes in cardiac output can be delineated, the temporal aspects of the impedance pulse reflect alterations in the time course of isovolumetric pressure development. In this way an estimate of myocardial contractility related to the isometric time-tension index can be obtained and quantified in the intact animal by a totally noninvasive technique.

By simultaneously evaluating the thoracic impedance pulse and a central aortic blood pressure, an impedance force-velocity relation can also be obtained. Both of these techniques have been applied to the estimation of myocardial contractility in the critically ill surgical patient. Evaluation of the dynamic aspects of the thoracic impedance pulse appears to permit determination of the basic myocardial contractile state and enables quantification of the response to cardiac inotropic agents.

REFERENCES

1. Covell, J. W., Ross, J., Jr., Sonnenblick, E. H., and Braunwald, E.: Comparison of the force-velocity relation and the ventricular function curve as measures of the contractile state of the intact heart, Circ. Res. **19:** 364, 1966.
2. Downing, S. E., and Siegel, J. H.: Baroreceptor and chemoreceptor influences on sympathetic discharge to the heart, Amer. J. Physiol. **204:** 471, 1963.
3. Fry, D. L., Greggs, D. M., and Greenfield, J. C.: Myocardial mechanics: Tension-velocity-length relationships of heart muscle, Circ. Res. **4:** 73, 1964.
4. Gault, J. H., Ross, J., Jr., Sonnenblick, E. H., and Braunwald, E.: Characterization of myocardial contractility in patients with and without cardiac dysfunction by the instantaneous tension-velocity relation, (P), Circulation **33** (Suppl. 3): 108, 1966.
5. Hamilton, W. F., Moore, J. W., Kinsman, J. M., and Spurling, R. G.: Studies on the circulation. IV. Further analysis of injection methods and of changes in hemodynamics under physiologic and pathologic conditions, Amer. J. Physiol. **99:** 534, 1932.
6. Harley, A., and Greenfield, J. C. Jr.: Determination of cardiac output in man by means of impedance plethysmography, Aerospace Med. **39:** 248, 1968.
7. Kubicek, W. J., Karnegis, J. N., Patterson, R. P., Witsoe, D. A., and Mattson, R. H.: Development and evaluation of an impedance cardiac output system, Aerospace Med. **37:** 1208, 1966.
8. Kubicek, W. G., Witsoe, D. A., and Patterson, R. P.: Development and evaluation of an impedance cardiograph system to measure cardiac output and other parameters, Report to National Aeronautics and Space Administration, Contract No. NAS 9-4500, 1968.
9. Levine, H. J., and Britman, N. A.: Force-velocity relations in the intact dog heart, J. Clin. Invest. **43:** 1383, 1964.
10. MacLean, L. D., Mulligan, W. G., McLean, A. P. H., and Duff, J. H.: The patterns of septic shock in man—a detailed study of 56 patients, Ann. Surg. **116:** 543, 1966.
11. Pomerantz, M., Lauridson, J., Baumgartner, R., and Eiseman, B.: Early detection of pulmonary edema using transthoracic electrical impedance, Surgery **66:** 260, 1969.
12. Siegel, J. H.: The role of the myocardial contractile state in the response to anesthesia and surgery, Anesthesiology **30:** 519, 1969.
13. Siegel, J. H., and Sonnenblick, E. H.: Isometric time-tension relations as an index of myocardial contractility, Circ. Res. **12:** 597, 1963.
14. Siegel, J. H., Sonnenblick, E. H., Judge, R. D., and Wilson, W. S.: The quantification of myocardial contractility in dog and man, Cardiologia (Basel) **45:** 189, 1964.
15. Siegel, J. H., Sonnenblick, E. H., Judge, R. D., and Wilson, W. S.: Occult myocardial failure and vasopressors in shock, Cardiologia (Basel) **47:** 353, 1965.
16. Siegel, J. H., and Fabian, M.: Therapeutic advantages of an inotropic vasodilator in endotoxin shock, J. A. M. A. **200:** 696, 1967.
17. Siegel, J. H., Greenspan, M., and Del Guercio, L. R. M.: Abnormal vascular tone, defective oxygen transport and myocardial failure in human septic shock, Ann. Surg. **165:** 504, 1967.
18. Siegel, J. H., Greenspan, M., and Del Guercio, L. R. M.: The prognostic implications of altered physiology in operations for portal hypertension, Surg. Gynec. Obstet. **126:** 249, 1968.
19. Sonnenblick, E. H.: Implications of muscle mechanics in the heart, Fed. Proc. **21:** 975, 1962.
20. Sonnenblick, E. H.: Force-velocity relations in mammalian heart muscle, Amer. J. Physiol. **202:** 931, 1962.
21. Sonnenblick, E. H.: Determinants of active state in heart muscle: Force, velocity, instantaneous muscle length, time, Fed. Proc. **24:** 1396, 1965.
22. Sonnenblick, E. H.: Instantaneous force-velocity-length determinants in the contraction of heart muscle, Circ. Res. **16:** 441, 1965.
23. Sonnenblick, E. H., and Downing, S. E.: Afterload as a primary determinant of ventricular performance, Amer. J. Physiol. **204:** 604, 1963.
24. Thompson, H. K., Jr., Starmer, C. F., Whalen, R. E., and McIntosh, H. D.: Indicator transit time considered as a gamma variate, Circ. Res. **14:** 502, 1964.

Decompression of the colon with complete diversion of the fecal stream by an in situ colonic catheter: A pilot study

NORMAN H. SCHULMAN, Lieutenant Commander (MC) USNR*
HOWARD G. PRITHAM, Lieutenant (MC) USN
STANTON G. POLIN, Commander (MC) USNR
PORTSMOUTH, VA.
From the Department of Surgery, Naval Hospital

Current surgical practice of managing perforations of the distal half of an unprepared fecal-laden colon consists of exteriorizing the injured segment or repairing the site of injury and diverting the fecal stream with a proximal colostomy. Either method leaves the patient with a colostomy which is subsequently closed in a second formal procedure. This clinical situation is now quite common in the military hospital patient population.

A system is herein described which is intended to obviate the need for operative colostomy closure by the use of an in situ removable colonic catheter.

METHODS AND MATERIALS

The catheter was constructed from a flexible rubber corrugated tube 15 mm. internal diameter (Foregger breathing tube), cut to a length of approximately 12 cm. and shaped to a right angle by suturing together several corrugations on one side with a horizontal mattress suture of No. 3-0 nylon. The noncorrugated connector end of the catheter was fitted with a 12 mm. cuffed balloon (Rusch) (Fig. 1).

The opinions or assertions contained herein are those of the authors and are not to be construed as official or reflecting the views of the Navy Department or of the Naval Service at large.

Submitted for publication July 5, 1969; resubmitted July 31, 1969.

*Reprint address: 15-65 209th St., Bayside, N. Y. 11360.

Ten adult pedigree beagle hounds were used. All dogs were operated on in a similar fashion. They were anesthetized with intravenous pentobarbital, and with the exception of the first two dogs, received 50 mg. per kilogram of intravenous cephalosporin during the surgical operation. A loop of transverse or proximal descending colon was exposed and exteriorized through a midline abdominal incision. The fecal contents were milked proximally and distally from the region of the bowel loop into which the catheter would be placed. Noncrushing clamps (sterilized hairclips) were placed about this isolated loop to minimize the chance of fecal contamination from the unprepared bowel. A nonabsorbable pursestring suture was then placed in the antimesocolic edge of the isolated bowel segment and the lumen entered longitudinally through it with an electrocutting scalpel. After cultures were taken of the lumen, the catheter was inserted, and the pursestring suture secured snugly about it and the protruding balloon filler tube. The balloon was then slowly inflated with 7 to 10 c.c. of water and the filler tube sealed with multiple ligatures. A triple-thick band of elastic Silastic sheeting (Dow-Corning nonreinforced 0.01 single thickness) was cut to fit about the exterior of the colon between the inflated balloon and the pursestringed catheter and was fastened about

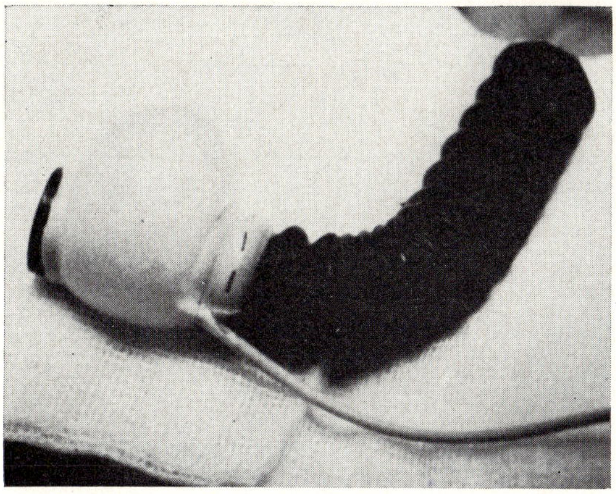

Fig. 1. The catheter and balloon.

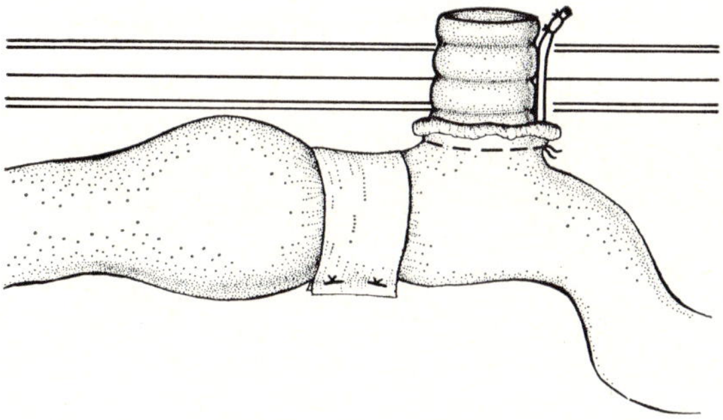

Fig. 2. Catheter and Silastic band in situ.

the bowel by nonabsorbable transmesocolon sutures (Fig. 2). The pressure exerted on the bowel by the Silastic was minimal. It was adjusted to remove slack from the sheeting and to insure a smaller diameter to the ensheathing Silastic than the proximal inflated balloon. The bowel and catheter were then replaced into the peritoneal cavity, the distal end of the catheter and balloon filler tube exteriorized via a stab wound, a Penrose drain placed at the bowel-catheter interface, and the midline incision closed. The excess length on the distal end of the catheter was trimmed so that no more than 1 cm. of the catheter protruded above the skin (Fig. 3). Postoperative care consisted of bowel softeners, daily catheter irrigations, and cephalosporin 50 mg. per kilogram for one week. Catheters were removed from 5 to 11 days and fistula closure observed. Radiographic, bacteriologic, gross, and histologic examinations, as well as reoperation, were used to supplement observations.

RESULTS AND DISCUSSIONS

The first two dogs were starved 48 hours preoperatively and given neomycin and Azulfidine; however, they both succumbed

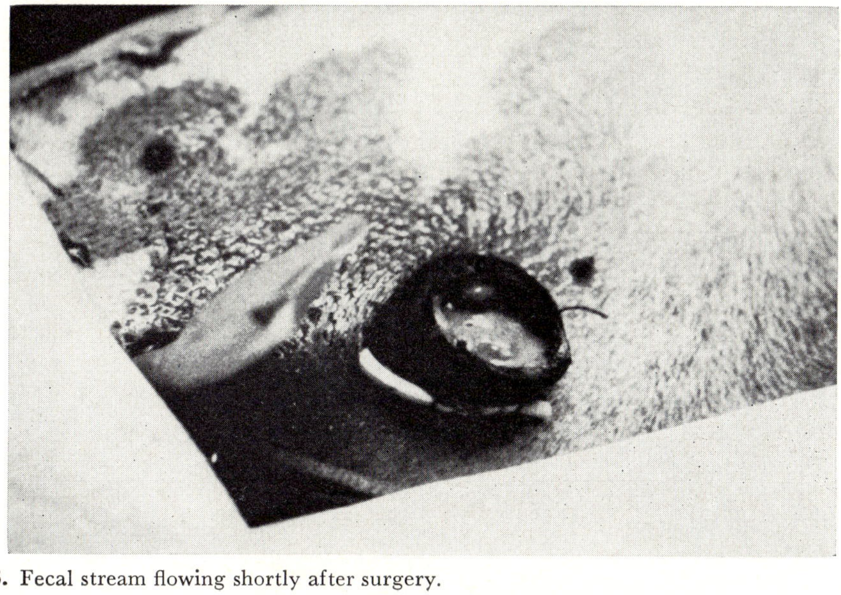

Fig. 3. Fecal stream flowing shortly after surgery.

Table I

Dog No.	*Catheter*	*Catheter retention (days)*	*Technical problem*	*Animal restraints*
1, 2	Died secondary to sepsis within the first postoperative week			
3	Nonballooned	7	Expelled; peristalsis	Canvas dog body jacket
4	Nonballooned	5	Expelled; peristalsis	Canvas dog body jacket
5	Ballooned, air filled	11	Pulled out by dog	Canvas dog body jacket
6	Ballooned, air filled	6	Pulled out by dog	Canvas dog body jacket plus repellent spray
7	Ballooned, air filled	10	Balloon air leak; expelled	Dog muzzle
8	Ballooned, water filled	9	Pulled out by dog	Dog muzzle, not replaced one evening
9	Ballooned, water filled	7	Balloon water leak; expelled	Flanged, padded, wooden collar
10	Ballooned, water filled	6	Separation of filter tube from balloon with resultant leak; expelled	Flanged, padded, wooden collar

to sepsis within the first postoperative week. The next three dogs received mechanical preparations of the bowel with enemas and laxatives, as well as the aforementioned preoperative medications. The remaining five dogs, to simulate actual potential clinical emergencies, received no preparation of the bowel whatsoever. In these latter two groups, sepsis was ultimately successfully managed by intra- and postoperative cephalosporin (50 mg. per kilogram per day for one week) as borne out by intraoperative cultures and sensitivities.

In the eight surviving animals, bowel wall viability, complete fecal diversion, and catheter retention were achieved with minimal balloon and Silastic cuff pressures. The only force on the system after the bowel accommodated the inflated balloon was that resulting from peristalsis, forcing the balloon against the distal external restraining Silastic cuff—as in a ball valve, thereby limiting distensibility and preventing distal fecal leakage. Peristalsis being the only dynamic pressure source and decompression being adequate (as described below), bowel wall viability was never in question.

Tract formation and peritoneal sealing about the catheter occurred as early as 48 hours after catheter placement, provided that a minimal margin (3 to 4 mm.) of exposed bowel wall (serosa) remained between Silastic cuff and bowel-catheter interface.

The diameter of the catheter was selected at 15 mm., since this most nearly approximated the resting lumen of the dog colon. This consideration, plus bowel softeners with daily catheter irrigations from the third postoperative day, provided adequate decompression, as judged by productive enemas and the absence of vomiting or abdominal distension.

Catheter retention and circumstances of removal were as follows: Dog No. 3, expelled in 7 days, nonballooned catheter; Dog. No. 4, expelled in 5 days, ballooned catheter (ballooned catheters were used in all subsequent dogs); Dog No. 5, pulled out by dog after 11 days; Dog No. 6, pulled out by dog after 6 days (muzzles and/or flanged, padded, wooden collars were used in subsequent dogs); Dog No. 7, expelled after 10 days as the result of slow air leak-

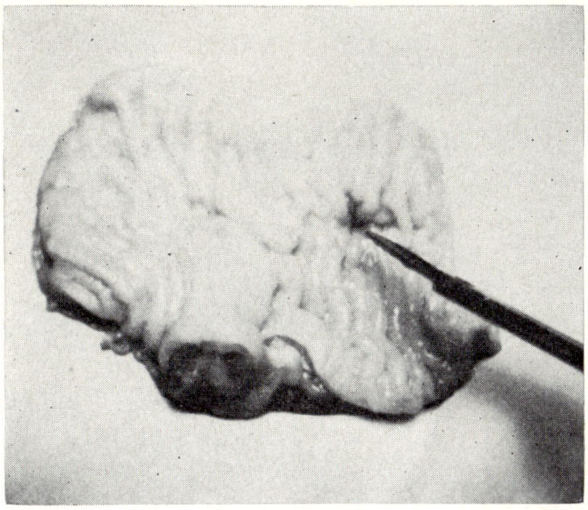

Fig. 4. Dimple marks site of fistula closure. To the left is seen the ridge caused by muscularis hypertrophy under the Silastic band, seven weeks after catheter placement.

age from the balloon (subsequent balloons filled with water and sealed with multiple ligatures); Dog No. 8, pulled out catheter after 9 days (left unattended without muzzle or collar one night); Dog. No. 9, expelled after 7 days as the result of development of leak in balloon; and Dog No. 10, expelled the catheter after 6 days as the result of separation of the filler tube from the balloon with resultant leak. The final limiting factor appeared to be the integrity of the rubber of the balloon and its filler tube (Table I).

In all the dogs, anal evacuation was noted within 24 hours of catheter removal, fistula closure was 80 to 90 percent at two weeks and 100 percent by the end of one month; no hernias demonstrated. Barium enemas and reoperation revealed no apparent bowel stricture as the result of fistula closure (Fig. 4).

The Silastic sheeting (Dow-Corning) selected is a nonreinforced medical grade silicone rubber specifically designed for implantation purposes. It has been shown to be nonantigenic, to cause minimal tissue reaction, and to be noncorrosive and noncarcinogenic.[1] In this study, with one exception, tissue reaction and stricture resulting from the now permanent Silastic cuff after catheter removal was considered to be minimal. There was no proximal bowel dilatation and no more than about five percent narrowing of the resting lumen, as observed by barium enemas and reoperation at periods of two and three months after catheter removal. Histological examination of the bowel wall under the Silastic sheet showed slight serosal thickening and muscularis hypertrophy, accounting for the observed minimal narrowing. In Dog No. 4, a nonballooned catheter was used and the Silastic cuff was tightened to the point of bowel blanching in order to maintain catheter retention. The catheter was expelled in five days and the fistula closed as noted above. However, the animal died in six weeks and postmortem examination revealed an 80 percent constriction of the bowel lumen at the site of the Silastic cuff with marked proximal bowel dilatation.

SUMMARY

It has been shown that it is possible to maintain a temporary semirigid catheter in unprepared bowel for at least 11 days, achieving complete fecal diversion as well as decompression with return to normal function upon simple catheter removal without encountering vascular compromise or unmanageable sepsis.

The reason for failure of retention after 11 days was not due to physiologic incompatibility, but rather to the physical characteristics of the rubber used in the balloon and its filler tube.

A workable colonic catheter system has been demonstrated, and it is suggested that this be used as a basis for the development of a long-term functional catheter suitable for clinical use.

REFERENCES

1. Brown, J. B., Fryer, M. P., and Ohlwiler, D. A.: Study and use of synthetic materials, such as silicones and Teflon, as subcutaneous prostheses, Plast. Reconstr. Surg. **26:** 264, 1960.

Diverticulosis of the appendix

ALFREDO R. ESPARZA, M.D.
CHARLES M. PAN, M.D.*
PROVIDENCE, R. I.
From the Department of Pathology, Rhode Island Hospital

Diverticula of the vermiform appendix are rarely encountered. They are of two types: (1) the congenital, or true, diverticula, which are exceedingly rare, and (2) the relatively more common, acquired, or false, type of diverticula. Their classification into these two types is based on the anatomical structure of the wall of the pouch. True diverticula contain all the tissue layers of the appendix, including a well-developed muscular coat. Less than 40 congenital diverticula have been reported,[4, 5] some being associated with other congenital malformations,[5] others with fibrocystic disease of the pancreas.[6] Acquired, or false, diverticula are thought by many to be secondary to inflammation, and the wall has, as a characteristic feature, the absence of the muscularis. Acquired diverticula have been reported at an incidence rate ranging from 0.08 to 2.8 percent.[2, 8] These figures are, however, of questionable validity, since it has been repeatedly noted that their frequency is proportional to the care and effort with which they are sought.[3, 8]

In this paper, we described a series of 18 cases found in the files of the Rhode Island Hospital.

REPORT OF CASES

Seventeen of the 18 cases herein reported were from patients whose appendices were surgically removed; one was found at autopsy. The significant clinical and pathological findings are summarized in Table I.

There were nine women and nine men; the ages varied from 22 to 79 years, most cases being found between the second and fourth decades, as noted in other series.[8, 10] Symptoms of acute appendicitis prompted the surgical intervention in 12 patients, while in five, appendectomy was incidental to other surgical procedure. In 11 of the 12 patients, a diagnosis of acute appendicitis was made, and in one (Patient No. 2), the appendectomy was performed two weeks after initial drainage for a perforated appendicitis with periappendiceal abscess. Patient No. 4, with a preoperative diagnosis of acute appendicitis, was discovered at operation to have a ruptured corpus luteum. The appendix showed no evidence of acute inflammation. Patient No. 16 is of interest because he presented with the clinical picture of acute appendicitis and yet at surgery the appendix appeared normal; but there was an inflamed mass, 4 cm. in diameter, anterior to the cecum and ascending colon, with the "appearance of diverticulitis" as described by the surgeon.

Pathological study of these 12 patients revealed that in eight instances, there was in effect an acute appendicitis with diverticulitis (Fig. 1). In two of these patients, the inflammatory reaction was exclusively found in the diverticula.

Evidence of inflammation was also seen in three other patients diagnosed as healed appendicitis (Patient Nos. 4, 5, and 11),

Received for publication July 7, 1969.

*Present address: Department of Pathology, St. Joseph's Hospital, Fort Wayne, Ind. 46802.

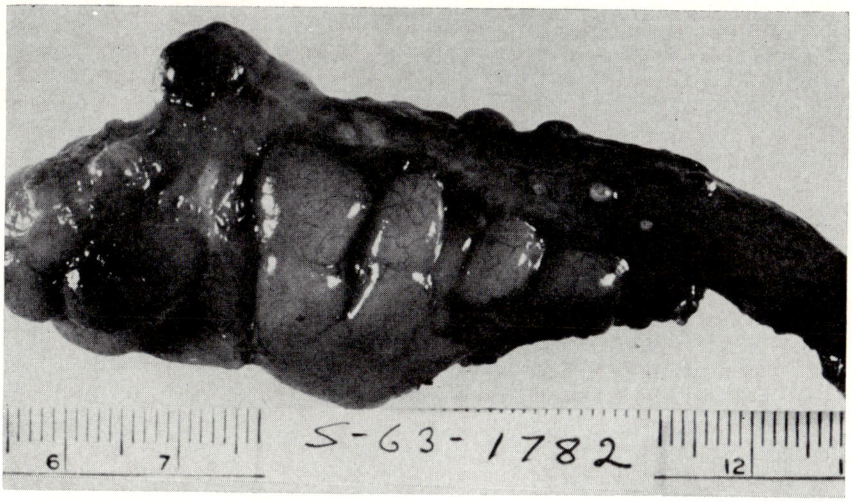

Fig. 1. Diverticulosis and acute diverticulitis of the appendix. Note the presence of diverticula on all surfaces of the wall and the hyperemia and fibrinous exudate.

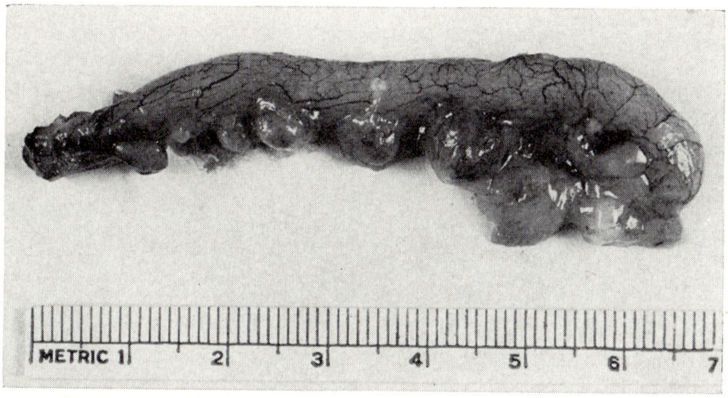

Fig. 2. Multiple appendiceal diverticula along the mesenteric border (the adipose tissue was partially removed for better exposure of the outpouchings). No evidence of inflammation was found, grossly or microscopically.

where there was scarring and atrophy of the appendiceal wall as well as a fibroblastic reparative reaction of the subserosal tissue and fibrous adhesions. This makes a total of 11 patients in whom evidence of inflammation was found. The other seven patients showed no evidence of acute or healed inflammatory reaction (Fig. 2).

In nine patients the diverticula were multiple, and in nine a single diverticulum was found. Most were found in the distal one third and tip, but some were also found in the proximal and middle thirds. In two instances, they were distributed throughout the entire length of the appendix. There was no significant predilection for the mesenteric border, because the lateral surfaces as well as the antimesenteric border were also sites of the diverticula.

From a histological point of view, most diverticula showed a thin wall with a rather flattened mucosal surface resting on a layer of fibroadipose tissue, continuation of the submucosa, and an external layer of fibrous tissue (Figs. 3 and 4).

In some instances a very thin layer of smooth muscle fibers was observed, particularly around the neck of the diverticular sac.

Table I

Patient No.	*Age, sex*	*Clinical diagnosis*	*Duration*	*Pathological description*	*Pathological diagnosis*
1	22, F	Acute appendicitis	3 days	Multiple diverticula, distal 1/3	Subsiding acute appendicitis with diverticulitis
2	48, F	Acute appendicitis	24 hr.	Single diverticulum, 0.5 cm. on distal 1/3; acutely inflamed	Acute diverticulitis of appendix
3	73, M	Acute appendicitis	3 days	Multiple diverticula, largest 1.5 cm. in diameter	Acute subsiding appendicitis and diverticulosis
4	33, F	Acute appendicitis	48 hr.	Single diverticulum 0.7 cm., tip and lateral; microscopically filled with mucus, no definite mucosal lining; not acutely inflamed	Ruptured corpus luteum; healed appendicitis with diverticulosis (mucocele ?)
5	?, F	Appendicitis ?	7 days	Single, bullous, at tip; fibrous adhesions	Healed appendicitis with diverticulosis
6	79, F	Chronic cholecystitis	N.A.	Single 0.6 cm. diverticulum at tip; no evidence of inflammation	Chronic cholecystitis and cholelithiasis; appendix with diverticulosis
7	45, F	Acute exacerbation of chronic appendicitis	24 hr.	Multiple small diverticula (largest 0.4 cm.), distal 1/3, lateral, and tip; stenosis of appendix in mid 1/3; healing and acute inflammation of appendix and diverticula	Recurrent acute appendicitis with diverticulitis
8	66, F	Adenocarcinoma of cecum	N.A.	Single, small diverticulum, distal 1/3	Adenocarcinoma of cecum with metastasis to regional lymph nodes; diverticulosis of appendix
9	32, M	Acute appendicitis	30 hr.	Multiple diverticula, tip and distal 1/3, largest 0.6 cm.; acutely inflamed	Acute diverticulitis of appendix
10	52, M	Inguinal hernia	N.A.	Multiple, largest, 0.5 cm., proximal and mid 1/3; mesenteric and lateral borders; no inflammation	Tissue consistent with hernial repair, containing adrenal rest, diverticulosis of appendix
11	67, F	Postdrainage of appendiceal abscess	2 wk.	Single, mid 1/3; healed inflammation with stenosis proximal to diverticulum; distorted appendix with kinking and adhesions	Healed appendicitis with diverticulosis
12	41, M	Carcinoma of transverse colon		Single, small diverticulum at tip; no evidence of inflammation	Cancer of colon with peritoneal carcinomatosis; diverticulosis of appendix
13	43, F	Acute appendicitis	12 hr.	Multiple, largest 1 cm., all length of appendix and all surfaces; acutely inflamed	Acute appendicitis with diverticulitis

Table I—*Cont'd*

Patient No.	*Age, sex*	*Clinical diagnosis*	*Duration*	*Pathological description*	*Pathological diagnosis*
14	40, M	Acute appendicitis	18 hr.	Single 0.8 cm. diverticulum, distal end, antimesenteric border; segmental area of stenosis just proximal to diverticulum; acutely inflamed diverticulum and appendix	Acute appendicitis with diverticulitis
15	56, M	Lymphoma of duodenum ?	N.A.	Multiple diverticula (0.3-1.5 cm.); all length mesenteric border; no evidence of inflammation	Biopsy of duodenum—no evidence of pathology; biopsy of liver—malignant lymphoma; diverticulosis of appendix
16	28, M	Acute appendicitis	24 hr.	Multiple 0.5 cm. diverticula; proximal 1/3, mesenteric border; no evidence of inflammation	Diverticulosis of appendix; at operation diverticulitis of ascending colon not resected
17	47, M	Acute appendicitis	48 hr.	Multiple, all length, mesenteric border; acute inflammation of appendix and diverticulum	Acute appendicitis with diverticulitis
18*	75, M	Myocardial infarct	N.A.	Single, 0.3 cm. diverticulum, distal 1/3, antimesenteric; obliterated lumen; healed inflammation	Diverticulosis of appendix

*Autopsy.

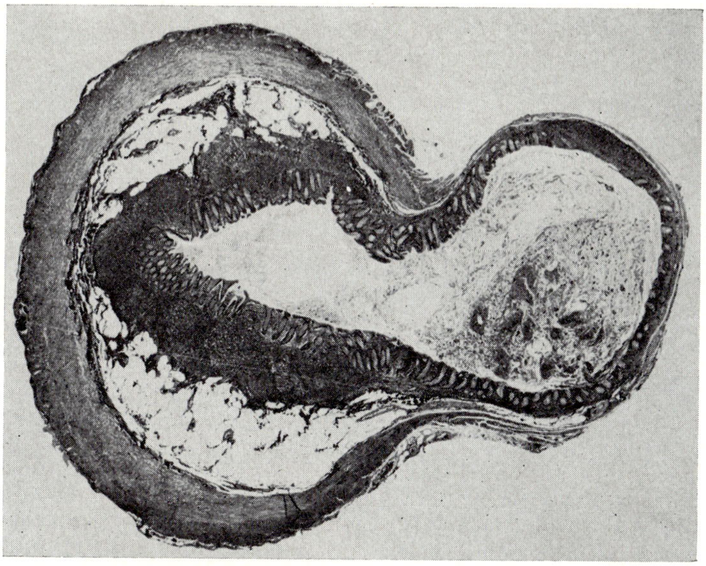

Fig. 3. Appendix with wide-mouthed diverticulum. Note the attenuated wall and lack of muscularis. (Gomori trichrome stain; ×16.)

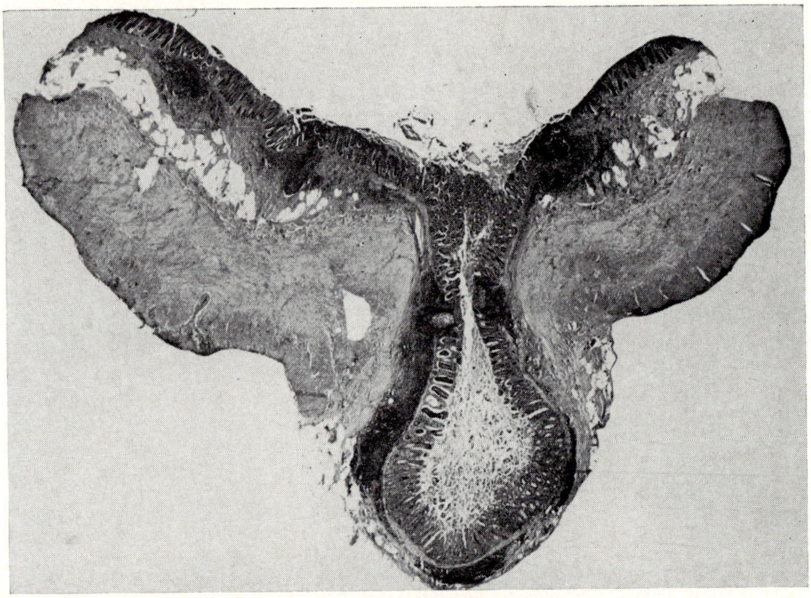

Fig. 4. Appendix with diverticulum. Here the diverticular sac has a narrow opening and long neck. The abrupt interruption of the muscle coat of the appendix wall at the site of the diverticulum is well demonstrated. (Hematoxylin and eosin; ×16.)

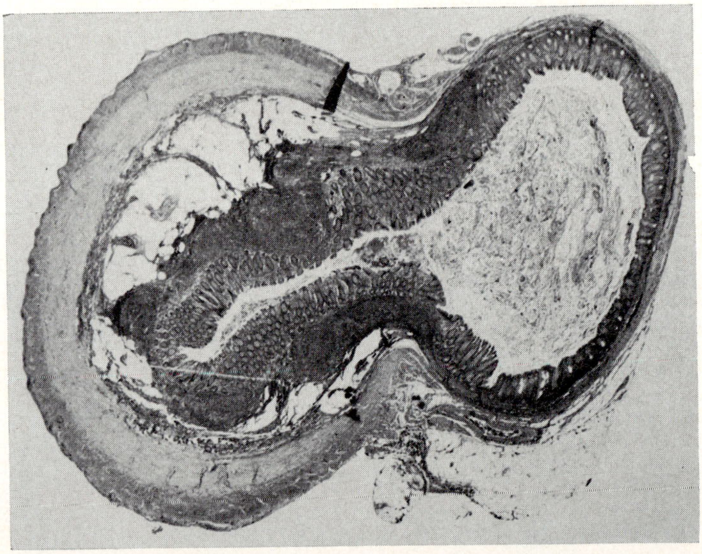

Fig. 5. Appendix with diverticulum on the mesenteric border. A good-sized arteriole is seen piercing the wall at one side of the diverticulum. No evidence of inflammation seen. (Hematoxylin and eosin; ×16.)

These fibers seemed to be a prolongation of the muscularis mucosa, for in all cases the muscular coat of the appendix was interrupted abruptly at the origin of the diverticula.

In those diverticula arising from the mesenteric border of the appendix, there was often found a good-sized vessel in relation to the neck of the diverticulum (Fig. 5).

Most diverticula contained fecaliths which occluded the ostium and distended their lumina (Fig. 6). In two instances the diver-

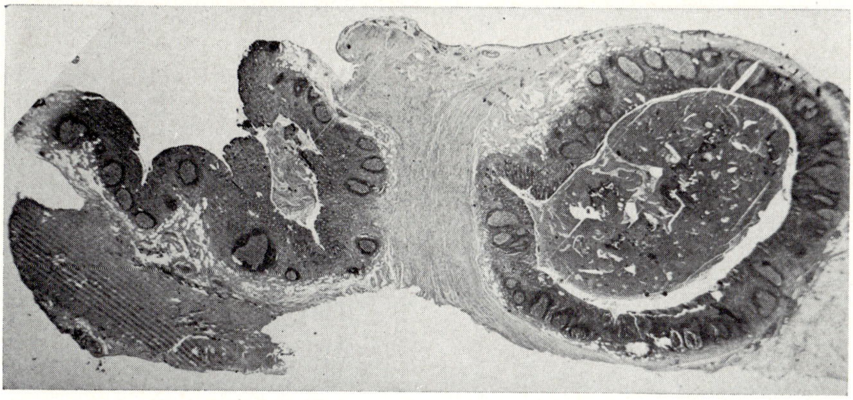

Fig. 6. Healed appendicitis and diverticulosis. The appendiceal wall is thickened and shows a dense condensation of collagen on the serosal surface. The diverticulum contains a fecalith. (Hematoxylin and eosin; ×16.)

ticular cavity appeared distended and filled with mucus. Their mucosal lining was greatly attenuated and had an appearance similar to a mucocele. In these two patients, there was definite evidence of a burned-out inflammatory reaction.

COMMENTS

Diverticula of the appendix are infrequently encountered, as it may be assessed by the various published reports of small series[3, 10] or individual cases.[1] Their frequent small size, their location along the mesenteric border where they may be buried in the adipose tissue, and the often associated acute inflammatory reaction with hemorrhage and fibrinous exudate, are all factors which contribute to making their detection difficult. In addition, some cases may be coded in the records only as "appendicitis" so that in retrospective analysis they may not become available. Technical improvements and increased alertness on the part of the radiologists have resulted in a feasible preoperative diagnosis of appendiceal diverticulosis,[9] and this undoubtedly will help the pathologist in the search for and discovery of diverticula.

Several theories have been postulated in order to explain the pathogenesis, and all are in agreement that areas of localized weakness in the appendix wall are an essential factor for the formation of diverticula. Some authors[3, 11] ascribe these areas of weakness to an inherent anatomical characteristic of the appendiceal wall, resulting from the passage of blood vessels. For others[1, 11] these areas of lesser resistance are the result of past episodes of focal necrosis which have subsided with reconstitution of the mucosal and submucosal layers, but not the muscularis. Re-epithelization of a previous perforation with abscess formation has also been suggested.[7]

The role of luminal obstruction, be it by an area of stenosis, fecalith, or even a foreign body, has been invoked as a factor causing distention of the lumen and therefore causing herniation of the mucosa and submucosa through the areas of lesser resistance.[2, 3, 10, 12] Experimental studies have been performed in an attempt to reproduce the naturally occurring disease and have lent support to some of the above views.[2, 11, 12]

From the evidence accumulated in the various published series,[2, 7, 8] one can conclude that inflammation does play a significant role in a great majority of cases, but perhaps other factors, which escape our detection, may be involved since no adequate explanation can be given for many of the acquired diverticula found at incidental appendectomies with no anatomical or clinical evidence of past appendicitis.

SUMMARY

Eighteen new cases of acquired appendiceal diverticula are reported.

The majority, eleven patients, showed evidence of acute or healed appendicitis, supporting the widely accepted theory that inflammation is an essential factor in the development. There were, however, seven cases where no trace of recent or past inflammatory reaction was found, which suggests that other as yet undetected mechanisms may be operative.

REFERENCES

1. Braunstein, L.: Diverticulosis of the vermiform appendix, J. Abdom. Surg. **41:** 136, 1962.
2. Collins, D. C.: Diverticula of the vermiform appendix, Ann. Surg. **104:** 1001, 1936.
3. Chenard, J., and Clement, J.: Diverticules acquis de l'appendice, Canad. Med. Ass. J. **88:** 1212, 1963.
4. Evertz-Suarez, E. A., and Noteboom, G.: Congenital diverticula of the appendix, Penn. Med. **64:** 1454, 1961.
5. Favara, B. D.: Multiple congenital diverticula of the vermiform appendix, Amer. J. Clin. Path. **49:** 60, 1968.
6. Kissane, J. M., and Smith, M. D.: Pathology of infancy and childhood, St. Louis, 1967, The C. V. Mosby Company, chap. 10.
7. Kline, B. S., Young, A. M., and Straus, R.: False diverticulum formation following acute perforative appendicitis, Arch. Path. **31:** 25, 1941.
8. Ladin, P.: Diverticulosis and diverticulitis of the vermiform appendix, Arch. Surg. **62:** 514, 1951.
9. Ochsner, S. F.: Diverticulosis of the appendix, Radiology **77:** 100, 1963.
10. Rabinovitch, J., Arlen, M., Barnett, T., Cuello, R., and Rabinovitch, P.: Diverticulosis and diverticulitis of the vermiform appendix, Ann. Surg. **155:** 434, 1962.
11. Stout, A. P.: A study of diverticulum forma- 1923.
12. Wilson, R. R.: Diverticula of the appendix, tion in the appendix, Arch. Surg. **6:** 793, Brit. J. Surg. **38:** 65, 1950.

Anterior mediastinitis as a complication of median sternotomy incisions: Diagnostic and surgical considerations

MANUEL JIMÉNEZ-MARTÍNEZ*
RUBÉN ARGÜERO-SÁNCHEZ
JUAN JOSÉ PÉREZ-ALVAREZ
PEDRO MINA-CASTAÑEDA
MEXICO CITY, MEXICO
From the Departments of Cardiovascular and Pediatric Surgery, Hospital de Pediatría, Centro Médico Nacional

Infections occurring in median sternotomy incisions represent a serious problem because they spread readily into the anterior mediastinum. Mediastinitis has been treated in the past by either of two methods: drainage of the infected space by means of a tube[10, 11] or by the open wound method with free drainage in addition to irrigation with antiseptic or antibiotic solutions.

The latter is inconvenient in that it takes a long time for the infection to be controlled and granulation tissue to form before secondary closure is indicated. In addition, proper ventilatory and coughing mechanisms are seriously impaired when inadequate mechanical support provided by the separated sternal bars is present for a long time.

In our experience, early surgical intervention, thorough cleansing of all necrotic and infected tissue, and closure of the wound followed by continous irrigation with antibiotic solutions make the control of the infection safer, improve the prognosis, and reduce the hospitalization time for the patient.

MATERIAL AND METHODS

A group of 19 patients with wound infections and anterior mediastinitis, from a total of 421 patients subjected to heart surgery by median sternotomy incision, were seen at the Hospital de Pediatría, Centro Médico Nacional of Mexico City, between May, 1963, and November, 1968. The age of the patients varied between one month and 15 years. Fourteen patients were male and 5 were female.

Before operation, 12 patients received oxacillin and 7 received procaine penicillin, beginning the day before operation and continuously in the postoperative period for at least five days or longer, when indicated. Also the following antibiotics were employed alone or in combination with the abovementioned drugs: novobiocin in 13 cases, kanamycin in 12 cases, ampicillin in 7 cases, penicillin G in 7 cases, cephalothin in 4 cases, lincomycin in 3 cases, Coly-Mycin in 3 cases, and leucomycin, bacitracin, erythromycin, and chloramphenicol in one case each.

The method for skin preparation was the same in all cases. The operative region was washed with hexachlorophene one day before and again on the day of operation, followed by application of benzalkonium chloride in alcohol 1:400.

The sternum was closed with stainless steel wire in all patients but the first four, in whom No. 2 silk was employed. The muscular layer over the sternum was closed with No. 3-0 silk, the subcutaneous tissue with No. 3-0 chromic catgut, and the skin with No. 4-0 silk. Electrocoagulation was used in all cases.

The diagnosis of mediastinitis was based

Submitted for publication July 16, 1969; resubmitted Aug. 18, 1969.

*Present address: Department of Cardiovascular Surgery, Hospital General I.M.S.S. Guadalajara, Jal., Mexico.

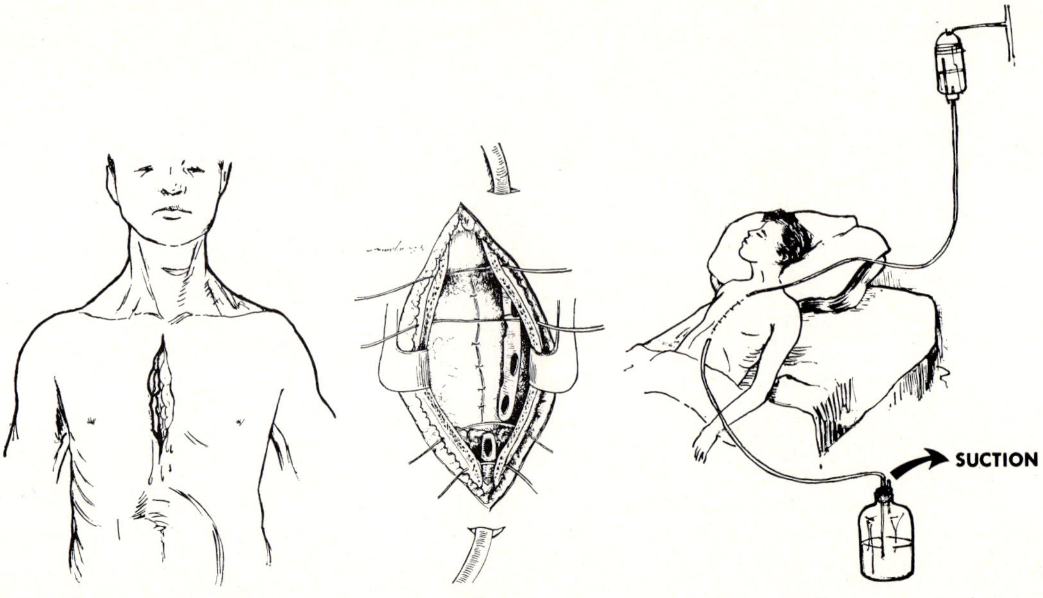

Fig. 1. *A,* Appearance of wound dehiscense. *B,* One tube is inserted above the upper end of the incision, 3 cm. into anterior mediastinum. A larger Nélaton's tube is placed in the mediastinum through a contralateral incision in the lower part. The wound is closed with wire sutures. *C,* Irrigation with antibiotic solutions is done through the upper tube, and the lower one is connected to suction through a water seal collecting bottle.

on drainage of purulent material from the wound and bubbling of the same material through the sternum, regardless of the presence of fever, elevated white blood cell count, and positive cultures, which were not always present, even in cases of obvious infection. When the diagnosis was established, it constituted a surgical indication for reoperation.

Washing of the wound was done with hexachlorophene and generous amounts of saline solution. The wound was opened wide, and debris and purulent material were removed by tailoring all necrotic-looking tissues. Washing of the cavity, or cavities if any pleural space was opened, was done with antibiotic solutions.

A No. 12 to 16 Nélaton's tube was inserted 3 to 5 cm. through a skin incision 1 cm. above the sternum into the anterior mediastinum. A larger Nélaton's tube was inserted from below into the anterior mediastinum through another incision below the xiphoid (Fig. 1). The sternum was approximated with No. 1 or 2 stainless steel wire and the skin with a No. 4-0 wire or 4-0 silk, leaving a Penrose drain in the subcutaneous space through a contralateral incision in the lower part. Tubes were secured to skin with No. 4-0 wire or silk. If any communication with a pleural space was found, another Nélaton's tube was used for pleural drainage. The upper tube was used to irrigate continuously the space with antibiotic solution; rifomycin, in doses of 1 to 1.5 Gm. diluted in saline solution, was used as a daily dose. In one case, kanamycin, 0.5 Gm. in 500 ml. of saline solution, was employed. The lower tube or tubes were connected to a water seal collecting bottle and suction.

The antibiotic irrigation through the upper tube was maintained for four to five days, or longer when osteomyelitis of the sternum was found, and then the tube was removed. The lower tube in the mediastinum was progressively withdrawn when the pleural space was not drained. In such a case, the withdrawal of the pleural and mediastinal tubes was done simultaneously around the seventh postoperative day. The skin sutures were removed 8 days after operation.

RESULTS

Of the 421 median sternotomies, 257 were operated upon under extracorporeal circulation. Thirteen of these (5 percent) developed wound infection and mediastinitis. One hundred and sixty-four patients underwent surgical procedures in which no extracorporeal circulation was used, and six patients (3.6 percent) developed the same complications (Table I). Sixteen patients had fever above 38° C. In 11 patients, the onset was from the third to the fifth day. Thirteen patients had purulent drainage—most of them between the seventh and fourteenth postoperative day; in only three patients, it appeared before the sixth day.

The white blood cell count was elevated in 11 patients, 72 percent of them (8 patients) with counts from 10,000 to 20,000 per cubic millimeter. White blood cell counts above 20,000 per cubic millimeter were recorded in three patients without spontaneous purulent drainage (Patients Nos. 1, 10, and 15). Only the last case showed radiological evidence of widening of the mediastinum in the posteroanterior projection. Cultures taken from the wound were positive in five patients: *Staphylococcus aureus* in 3 cultures, *Klebsiella* in 1, and *Pseudomona aeruginosa* in 1. Surgical drainage and closed irrigation with antibiotic solutions was performed in 16 cases with excellent results.

Fourteen patients are alive and two patients died of pulmonary complications; one died of staphylococcal pneumonia and the other of aspiration pneumonia (Patients Nos. 4 and 19, respectively). The living patients had a mean hospital stay of 16.5 days after reoperation, with a minimum of 11 days and a maximum of 30 days. Osteomyelitis was present in five patients. Three patients were not treated surgically (Patients Nos. 1, 2, and 10), and all three died: one with massive bleeding from the aorta, one with cardiac tamponade, and the last one with a mycotic aneurysm of the aorta which ruptured into the right bronchus.

DISCUSSION

The incidence of wound infections after clean thoracotomies[1, 9] varies between 0.3 to 22 percent, regardless of the use of prophylactic antibiotics in open-heart surgery cases.[7] When infection occurs in median sternotomies, it may extend to the deep spaces, since there is a lack of protective layers in comparison with other thoracotomies.

Any loss of continuity and water-tight closure over the sternum may draw the infected material through negative thoracic pressure into the anterior mediastium. Our incidence of mediastinitis in patients subjected to extracorporeal circulation was higher (5 percent) than that in cases operated without (3.6 percent). Protein denaturation and destruction of defensive mechanisms by the extracorporeal machine may play a role in the higher incidence of infection.

The first sign of infection was fever above 38° C. within the first week in most of our patients, followed by collection of purulent material and by dehiscence of the wound in the second postoperative week. When infection was not controlled by washing the infected region and massive antibiotic therapy, it was followed by mobility of the sternal bars and/or formation of a sinus into the anterior mediastinum. Bubbling through the sternum was indicative of communication of the infection to the anterior mediastinum. This was confirmed in all cases with the operative findings.

The white blood cell count varied between 10,000 to 20,000 in patients in whom the purulent material had free drainage. In those with encapsulated mediastinitis and no drainage, the white blood cell count varied from 20,000 to 25,000 cells per cubic millimeter (Patients Nos. 1, 10, and 15).

The diagnosis of anterior mediastinitis following median sternotomy is easy to establish when purulent material is obtained from the wound and when there is a communica-

Table I

Patient No.	Sex	Age (yr.)	Bypass	Clinical picture: Onset of fever above 38° C. (P.O. day)	Clinical picture: Drainage appeared (P.O. day)	Clinical picture: W.B.C. above 10,000
1	M	7	Yes	4	—	25,400
2	M	12	Yes	—	—	—
3	M	10	Yes	2	4	13,500
4	M	3	Yes	4	15	17,900
5	M	9	No	5	10	—
6	M	10	No	4	13	—
7	F	9	Yes	5	—	16,700
8	F	10	No	4	8	17,500
9	M	4	Yes	11	6	—
10	M	7	Yes	6	—	23,000
11	M	4	Yes	5	11	15,600
12	M	8	Yes	3	12	16,900
13	M	5	Yes	5	—	13,200
14	F	6	Yes	3	5	11,700
15	M	4	Yes	6	—	23,700
16	M	1/12	No	—	10	—
17	F	15	No	3	7	—
18	F	5	Yes	14	14	—
19	M	6/12	No	—	7	—

P.O. = postoperative.
W.B.C. = white blood cell count.

tion to the deep spaces, but it may impose a diagnostic problem when there is no outside evidence of wound infection. In these cases, persistent fever may be present and leukocytosis may be above 20,000. Roentgenograms of the chest may be misleading, although in some cases a widening of the mediastinum in the posteroanterior projection may be present. Retrosternal puncture may be of some help, but it may be negative in localized septic processes. If all sources of infection are ruled out, we feel that an exploratory thoracotomy is indicated.

The classical treatment of obvious mediastinitis with free drainage was to leave wide open the mediastinal space and perform mechanical washings of all necrotic and purulent material. This, we think, is satisfactory, but it is time-consuming and may favor respiratory infection as the result of improper ventilation, lack of forceful coughing, and extension of infection by continuity.

Infection in other closed areas has been treated by closed irrigation with success. In 1942, Brantigan and Owens[3] reported the use of tetradecyl sulfate in the treatment of infection of the pleural cavity. In 1960, Goldman and associates[6] reported the use of continuous or intermittent closed irrigation in 5 cases of osteomyelitis, and McElveny[8] in 1961 described the technique in another 12 cases in chronically infected, acutely infected, or potentially infected wounds. Campere[5] in 1962 reported the use of a combination of a detergent and antibiotic in sodium chloride solution for closed irrigation in chronic osteomyelitis and wound infections; and Bianchi[2] in 1963 used rifomycin as irrigation solution in the treatment of 15 cases of chronic osteomyelitis with good results. We thought that infection in the anterior mediastinum could be treated in the same way, and since 1964 we have used this method. Recently, Bryant and associates[4] reported a series of 5 cases treated by a method similar to the one described here. The only two patients who were treated surgically and died developed respiratory complications which were the cause of death.

Treatment		*Result*		
Surgical (P.O. day)	*Medical (daily irrigation)*	*Died (P.O. day)*	*Cured & discharged (P.O. day)*	*Remarks*
—	Yes	12	—	Autopsy—pancarditis
—	Yes	13	—	—
6	—	—	30	*St. aureus,* sternum osteomyelitis, P.O. pneumonia
14	—	25	—	Staphylococcal pneumonia
11	—	—	15	—
30	—	—	20	P.O. pneumonia
7	—	—	22	P.O. pneumonia
9	—	—	13	P.O. pneumonia
17	—	—	12	Sternum osteomyelitis
—	Yes	54	—	Autopsy—aortic mycotic aneurysm open to right bronchus
12	—	—	14	—
13	—	—	11	—
13	—	—	17	P.O. pneumonia, sternum osteomyelitis
8	—	—	14	—
49	—	—	20	—
13	—	—	14	—
17	—	—	12	—
60	—	—	11	Sternum osteomyelitis
8	—	8	—	Aspiration pneumonia, sternum osteomyelitis

Five cases complicated by respiratory infection after reoperation could be managed in a satisfactory manner. We think that the stability of the sternal bars contributed to the better result.

Hospitalization time is shorter with closed irrigation than with other methods. It was less than 15 days in two thirds of the patients and longer (15 to 30 days) only when complicated by osteomyelitis of the sternum, pneumonia, or both.

SUMMARY

Of 421 patients having undergone median sternotomies for heart surgery, a group of 19 patients with complications caused by anterior mediastinitis are studied. Thirteen of them had been operated upon under cardiopulmonary bypass. The clinical picture is analyzed and discussed. The method employed of closed irrigation with antibiotics is described.

Out of 16 patients treated by this method, 14 had excellent results; the other two patients died of respiratory complications after the mediastinal infection had been controlled. Three patients on whom conservative methods were employed died of complications secondary to mediastinitis.

The conclusion is drawn that early surgical intervention and closed irrigation with antibiotic solutions, once the diagnosis of anterior mediastinitis is established, is the best and shortest method of treatment.

REFERENCES

1. Altemeier, W. A.: C.I.O.M.S. Seminar on hospital infections, London, England, Sept. 24-28, 1962, SURGERY **54:** 419, 1963.
2. Bianchi, M. A.: Drenaggio continio e applicazione locale di rifamicina SV nell'osteomielite cronica, Chemoterapia **7:** 344, 1963.
3. Brantigan, O. C., and Owens, J. C.: Sodium tetradecyl sulfate used in the treatment of acute pyogenic empyema of the pleural cavity, Bull. Sch. Med. Univ. Maryland **26:** 247, 1942.
4. Bryant, L. R., Spencer, F. C., and Trinkle, J. K.: Treatment of median sternotomy infection by mediastinal irrigation with antibiotic solution, Ann. Surg. **169:** 914, 1969.
5. Campere, E. L.: Treatment of osteomyelitis and infected wound by closed irrigation with

a detergent-antibiotic solution, Acta Orthop. Scand. **32:** 324, 1962.

6. Goldman, M. A., Johnson, R. K., and Grossberg, N. B.: A new approach to chronic osteomyelitis, Orthopaedics **2:** 63, 1960.
7. Kittle, C. F., and Reed, W. A.: Antibiotics and extracorporeal circulation, J. Thorac. Cardiovasc. Surg. **41:** 34, 1961.
8. McElvenny, R. T.: The use of closed circulation and suction in treatment of chronically infected, acutely infected, and potentially infected wounds, Amer. J. Orthop. **3:** 86, 1961.
9. Nelson, J. C., and Nelson, R. B.: The incidence of hospital wound infection in thoracotomies, J. Thorac. Cardiovasc. Surg. **54:** 586, 1967.
10. Pacheco, R. C.: Neumología, Chap.—Diagnóstico y tratamiento quirúrgico, Mexico, 1968, Editores La Prensa Médica Mexicana, p. 311.
11. Webb, W. R., and Burford, T. H.: Current concepts of the management of acute mediastinitis, Amer. Surg. **28:** 309, 1962.

Influence of hemodialysis on a myocardial depressant factor in hemorrhagic shock

STEPHEN L. WANGENSTEEN, M.D.
J. DAVID DEHOLL, B.S.
STEPHEN F. KIECHEL, A.B.
JULIAN MARTIN, B.A.
ALLAN M. LEFER, PH.D.
CHARLOTTESVILLE, VA.
From the Departments of Surgery and Physiology, University of Virginia School of Medicine

The production of toxic factors in hemorrhagic shock has been postulated for many years.[6, 7] Recently Brand and Lefer[1] have described the presence of a myocardial depressant factor (MDF) in the plasma of cats in late hemorrhagic shock. MDF has been shown to decrease the developed tension of isolated cat papillary muscles[1, 9] as well as to depress reticuloendothelial function.[10] MDF has been shown to be a small polypeptide with a molecular weight in the range of 800 to 1,000[11, 12] and appears to be released in large part from the pancreas during severe ischemia and accumulates to toxic concentrations.[13]

The purposes of the present studies were to determine: (1) whether hemodialysis effectively removed MDF from plasma in the postoligemic stage of hemorrhagic shock; (2) if hemodialysis did remove MDF from the plasma, whether this had any significant effect on cardiac function; and (3) whether MDF is produced prior to reinfusion of shed blood.

This investigation was supported by the United States Army Medical Research and Development Command, Department of the Army, under Research Contract 17-67-C-7039, Grant HE-09924 from the National Heart Institute, National Institutes of Health, and a Grant-in-Aid from the American Heart Association. Dr. Lefer is an Established Investigator of the American Heart Association.

Received for publication Dec. 15, 1969.

MATERIALS AND METHODS

Mongrel dogs with a mean body weight of 26 kilograms were anesthetized with sodium pentobarbital (25 to 30 mg. per kilogram) administered intravenously. Hemorrhagic shock was produced by allowing the animals to bleed into an elevated reservoir through a polyethylene catheter inserted in the left femoral artery. The height of the reservoir was lowered in steps to allow the arterial blood pressure to decrease from control levels to 50 mm. Hg in approximately 30 minutes. Reservoir height was maintained at a level which permitted the arterial blood pressure to remain at 40 mm. Hg until the animals had spontaneously taken up 20 per cent of the maximum shed blood volume. When the dog spontaneously took up 20 per cent of its shed blood, all the remaining shed blood was reinfused slowly so as to avoid the production of cardiac failure.

The animals were divided into three groups (Table I).

Group 1 consisted of eight dogs subjected to the hemorrhagic shock protocol as described above. At the time of reinfusion, hemodialysis was begun and continued for a period of four hours with the use of a Dialung artificial kidney which had 33 dialyzing membranes (Couprophane-Bemberg Pt. 150) with a total exchange area of 0.5 $M.^2$

Table I. *Influence of hemodialysis on hemodynamics in hemorrhagic shock*

	Initial	*End-oligemic*	*End-dialysis*
Group I. Shock + dialysis (8 animals)			
MABP* (mm. Hg)	153 ± 6	50 ± 0.0	125 ± 7.0
CO (L./min.)	2.7 ± 0.3	0.6 ± 0.1	1.2 ± 0.1
CVP (mm. Hg)	1 ± 0.7	−2 ± 0.6	1 ± 0.8
TPR (PRU)	59 ± 6.5	80 ± 11	102 ± 12.0
Arterial pH	7.37 ± 0.02	7.21 ± 0.05	7.35 ± 0.02
Arterial L/P	13.7 ± 2.4	29.1 ± 2.0	18.5 ± 2.3
Group II. Shock + sham dialysis (8 animals)			
MABP (mm. Hg)	144 ± 7	50 ± 0.0	61 ± 15
CO (L./min.)	2.2 ± 0.1	0.6 ± 0.3	0.5 ± 0.2
CVP (mm. Hg)	1 ± 1.3	−1 ± 0.9	2 ± 0.7
TPR (PRU)	77 ± 16	115 ± 29	122 ± 26.0
Arterial pH	7.36 ± 0.03	7.17 ± 0.06	7.14 ± 0.10
Arterial L/P	10.4 ± 1.6	35.6 ± 13.2	25.4 ± 7.1
Group III. Sham shock + dialysis (5 animals)			
MABP (mm. Hg)	131 ± 10	—	124 ± 7.0
CO (L./min.)	2.2 ± 0.4	—	1.5 ± 0.3
CVP (mm. Hg)	3 ± 0.5	—	3 ± 0.5
TPR (PRU)	66 ± 9	—	94 ± 31
Arterial pH	7.34 ± 0.05	—	7.56 ± 0.03
Arterial L/P	17.2 ± 2.1	—	16.3 ± 2.1

*MABP, Mean arterial blood pressure; CO, cardiac output; CVP; central venous pressure; TPR, total peripheral resistance; PRU, peripheral resistance units; L/P, lactate/pyruvate ratio.

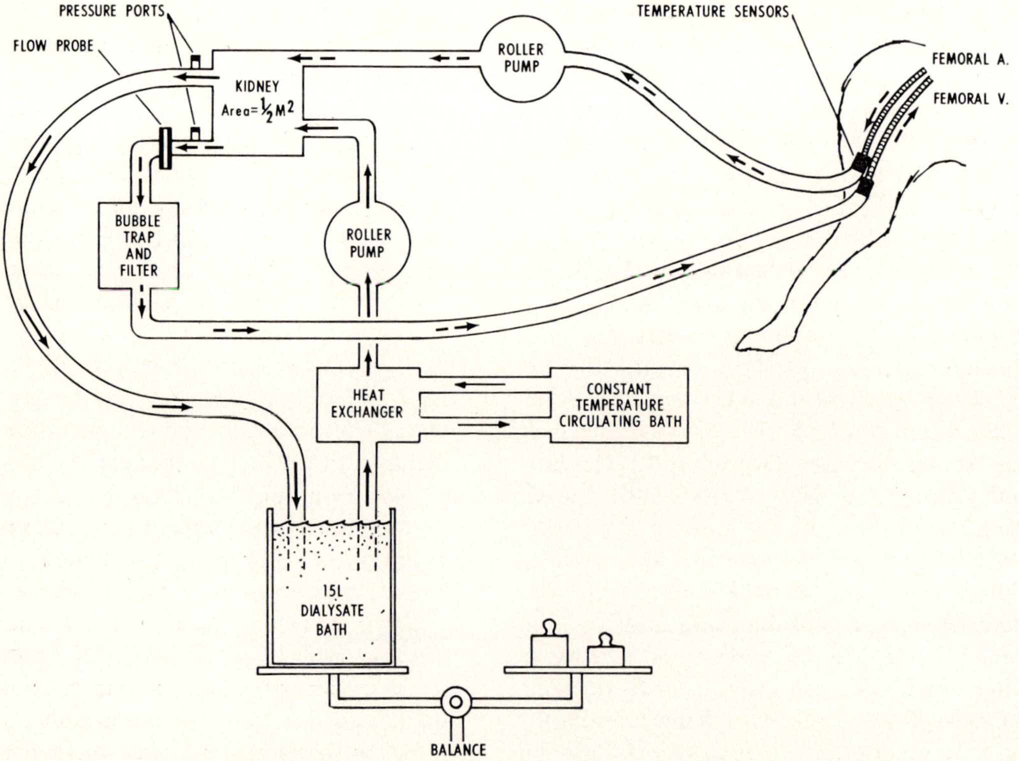

Fig. 1. Schematic diagram of the hemodialysis model.

Fig. 1 is a schematic diagram illustrating the experimental model. Blood was withdrawn by a variable speed roller pump from a femoral artery and returned via a femoral vein. Temperatures of outflowing and returning blood were continuously monitored and zero differential was maintained by heating incoming dialysate to the artificial kidney with a constant temperature bath and heat exchanger. The dialysate was recirculated through the artificial kidney from a 15 L. bath, which was changed after two hours of dialysis. A positive pressure of 70 to 100 mm. Hg (blood > dialysate) was maintained across the dialyzing membrane in order to achieve ultrafiltration of plasma. Blood flow rates from the femoral artery were maintained at 4 ml. per kilogram of body weight per minute (average flow rate 120 ml. per minute). Dialysate flow rates were adjusted to maintain the proper blood/dialysate pressure differential across the membrane, and averaged 90 ml. per minute. Both dialysate and blood were pumped through the kidney with variable speed roller pumps inside siliconized Tygon tubing. All tubing was sterile, and only new tubing was used in each experiment. The Dialung kidneys were sterilized by filling with 10 percent formaldehyde solution for 24 hours. Dialysate was freshly prepared from a Mallinckrodt hemodialysis concentrate and calcium was added. The composition of the dialysate was as follows: calcium 6 mEq. per liter, magnesium 1 mEq. per liter, potassium 2 mEq. per liter, sodium 130 mEq. per liter, chloride 101 mEq. per liter, acetate 35 mEq. per liter, and glucose 2,000 mg. per liter. The priming volume of the blood side of the kidney including all tubing was 200 ml., and the system was primed with lactate Ringer's solution. At the time of reinfusion, blood from the reservoir and the artificial kidney was pumped back into the animal. Central venous pressures were closely monitored during the 15 minutes of reinfusion. After reinfusion, animals received an additional 400 ml. of lactate Ringer's solution by slow intravenous drip to compensate for the 200 ml. of blood in the artificial kidney which was effectively lost to the animal during the dialysis period.

Group II consisted of eight animals in which hemorrhagic shock was carried out in a manner identical to Group I, except that at the time of reinfusion sham dialysis was performed. During sham dialysis, all procedures were the same as in Group I with the exception that connections to the dialysate bath were short circuited and only the priming volume (200 ml. of dialysate) circulated within the artificial kidney. Sham dialysis was conducted for a period of four hours.

Group III consisted of five animals that were subjected to a sham shock procedure and then dialyzed for a period of four hours. In these animals, the bleedout reservoir was not opened, so that no hemorrhage occurred. However, the hemodialysis was identical to that of Group I.

In all animals, cardiac output, arterial blood pressure, central venous pressure, blood P_{O_2} and P_{CO_2}, blood pH, plasma lactate and pyruvate concentrations were determined. An initial set of data was obtained before the period of dialysis. During the period of dialysis, the flow rates through the artificial kidney were monitored with Biotronex electromagnetic extracorporeal flow transducers and a pulsed-logic blood flow meter. The dialysate bath was positioned on a beam balance which was accurate to ±1 G. Fluid lost by the animals to the bath of ultrafiltration of plasma was monitored by measuring the weight change in the bath. Fluid loss by ultrafiltration averaged 60 ml. per hour and was replaced hourly by an intravenous infusion of the amount lost with sterile lactate Ringer's solution.

Cardiac output was measured by the dye-dilution technique using indocyanine green dye and a Gilford densitometer. Arterial blood pressure was obtained via a polyethelene catheter placed in the aortic arch. Central venous pressures were measured from a catheter placed in the right atrium via a jugular vein. Total peripheral vascular resistance (TPR) was calculated from arterial pressure, central venous pressure, and cardiac output values by the formula:

$$\frac{\text{MABP (mm. Hg)} - \text{CVP (mm. Hg)}}{\text{C.O. (liters/minute)}}$$

and was expressed in arbitrary units (PRU units). Pressures were recorded on a multichannel Honeywell recorder with the use of Statham P-23 transducers. Arterial blood gases and pH were determined on a Beckman Model 160 gas analyzer. Lactate and pyruvate plasma concentrations were determined by the enzymatic spectrophotometric method of Rosenberg and Rush[17] and were expressed as lactate/pyruvate ratios. Serum electrolyte determinations (sodium, potassium, calcium, bicarbonate, chloride) before and after dialysis were performed on Group III animals only.

Processing shock plasma and dialysate. Arterial blood samples were promptly centrifuged at 2,200 g and 4° C. for 20 minutes. The plasma was removed and placed inside dialysis tubing (Nojax tubing, viscose process, Union Carbide Corp. 30 mm. flat width) at 4° C. under a pressure of 200 mm. Hg for 20 to 36 hours. The plasma ultrafiltrates were clear solutions which have been shown to contain all the MDF activity of raw plasma, and have all the advantages of a protein-free solution.[2] Ultrafiltrates of plasma were stored at –10° C. until the time of the assay when they were thawed to room temperature and gently bubbled with 95 percent O_2 + 5 percent CO_2. The pH of these ultrafiltrates was 7.2 to 7.3. The ultrafiltrates were incubated at 37° C. just prior to assay.

Assays of MDF activity were performed on isolated cat papillary muscles according to previous described techniques.[8, 9] All assays were performed twice and compared with appropriate controls. MDF activity was expressed as percent decrease in developed tension of the isolated papillary muscles. One MDF unit is equal to a 1 percent decrease in developed tension.

In addition to the assay of the plasma ultrafiltrates, all ultrafiltrates were lyophilized to dryness, reconstituted to 20 percent of their original volume, applied to gel filtration columns, and eluted in Krebs-Henseleit solution as previously described.[12] The Bio-gel P-2 columns separate plasma ultrafiltrates into six peaks, one of which contains all the MDF activity. This has been termed peak D. In this manner, the purified peptide peak activity can be correlated with the activity of whole plasma ultrafiltrate. Similar assays were performed with samples of dialysate, which were lyophilized to dryness, reconstituted to 20 percent of original volume, lyophilized a second time, and reconstituted to 20 percent of the second volume. This concentrated sample was centrifuged at 2,000 g for 30 minutes and the supernatant fluid applied to the Bio-gel P-2 column.

All column elutions were performed at 4° C. and eluates were periodically checked for bacterial contamination. Fractions were collected in 3 ml. tubes and each tube was read in a Beckman Model DU spectrophotometer at 230 mμ in quartz cuvettes.

RESULTS

Group I. Shock and dialysis. Of the eight dogs in this group, seven dogs survived the hemodialysis period; one dog died during hemodialysis. The initial mean arterial blood pressure was 153 mm. Hg prior to hemorrhage. After reinfusion of all shed blood, the arterial blood pressure rose to 122 mm. Hg and then increased slightly to 125 mm. Hg at the end of the four-hour period of dialysis. Before hemorrhage, the average cardiac output was 2.7 L. per minute. During oligemia the cardiac output fell to 0.6 L. per minute but in the seven survivors rose to 1.2 L. per minute after four hours of hemodialysis.

The arterial blood pH was 7.21 late in the oligemic period, and it rose to 7.34 by the end of dialysis. The mean lactate/pyruvate ratio rose to 29.1 during oligemia from a control value of 13.7. After four hours of hemodialysis the lactate/pyruvate ratio had fallen to 18.5.

Central venous pressure remained essentially unchanged throughout the experiment and the calculated total peripheral resistance

(TPR) rose steadily from an average control value of 59 PRU to 102 PRU at the end of dialysis.

The mean survival time for the entire group was 24 ± 9.6 hours. The average period of oligemia before uptake of 20 percent of shed blood occurred was 5.5 ± 0.8 hours.

Group II. Shock and sham dialysis. The initial mean arterial blood pressure was 144 mm. Hg. The average blood pressure was 101 mm. Hg after reinfusion, but it steadily declined to an average value of 61 mm. Hg in those animals that survived the four-hour period of sham dialysis. The average cardiac output was 2.2 L. per minute before bleeding, and it fell to 0.6 L. per minute during oligmia. The mean cardiac output was 0.5 L. per minute in surviving dogs at the termination of sham dialysis.

In Group II dogs the arterial pH fell to 7.17 in late oligemia and remained at 7.14 after sham dialysis. The lactate/pyruvate ratio rose to 35.6 during oligemia and declined to 25.4 after reinfusion and at the end of sham dialysis.

The central venous pressure was –1 mm. Hg prior to bleeding; after sham dialysis the mean value was –2 mm. Hg. Calculated total peripheral vascular resistance rose from a control value of 77 PRU to 122 PRU after sham dialysis.

Four of these animals died during the period of sham dialysis and the average survival time after reinfusion of blood was 15 ± 9.6 hours.

The average period of oligemia at the point of 20 percent spontaneous uptake of shed blood was 8.5 ± 1.5 hours.

There were no significant differences in arterial blood Po_2 and Pco_2 values between Groups I and II.

Group III. Sham shock and dialysis. The mean arterial blood pressure was 131 mm. Hg prior to hemodialysis, and it declined only 7 mm. Hg after four hours of hemodialysis. The average initial cardiac output was 2.2 L. per minute and it declined to 1.5 L. per minute, a change which was not statistically significant.

The control arterial pH was 7.34; the pH increased to 7.56 during dialysis. The lactate/pyruvate ratio and the central venous pressure remained unchanged over the four-hour experimental period. Total peripheral resistance rose from a control value of 66 PRU to 94 PRU at the end of dialysis.

All Group III dogs survived for at least 72 hours.

Serum electrolyte determinations indicated no significant alterations in sodium, potassium, calcium, chloride, and bicarbonate concentrations during the course of hemodialysis.

Myocardial depressant activity (MDF) results. Fig. 2 depicts typical results of the Bio-gel column separation of ultrafiltrate samples from the plasma of a shocked dog and from the plasma of a control dog. The column separated the plasma ultrafiltrate into six peaks. Peak D contained all of the MDF activity, and it can be seen that peak D from the shocked dog has a considerably larger area than does peak D obtained from the control sample. Table II summarizes the results of myocardial depressant assays of plasma and dialysates. The MDF activity of a series of five control dogs (sham shock procedure for six hours) was 25.9 ± 5.2 MDF units. This represents a low level of MDF activity.

Group I. Shock and hemodialysis. The average myocardial depressant activity of plasma was 45.8 units during the oligemic period and was cleared to near control values of 29.6 units by the end of four hours of dialysis. In contrast, samples of dialysate had myocardial depressant activity which appeared soon after beginning dialysis to a mean level of 56.7 units and rose further to 75.3 units by the termination of dialysis.

Group II. Shock and sham dialysis. The mean plasma myocardial depressant activity was 46.3 units in late oligemia and became more elevated to 69.0 units at the end of the sham dialysis period. There were no dialysate samples in sham dialysis experiments.

Group III. Sham shock and dialysis. The average myocardial depressant activity of plasma after dialysis was 25.8 units and the

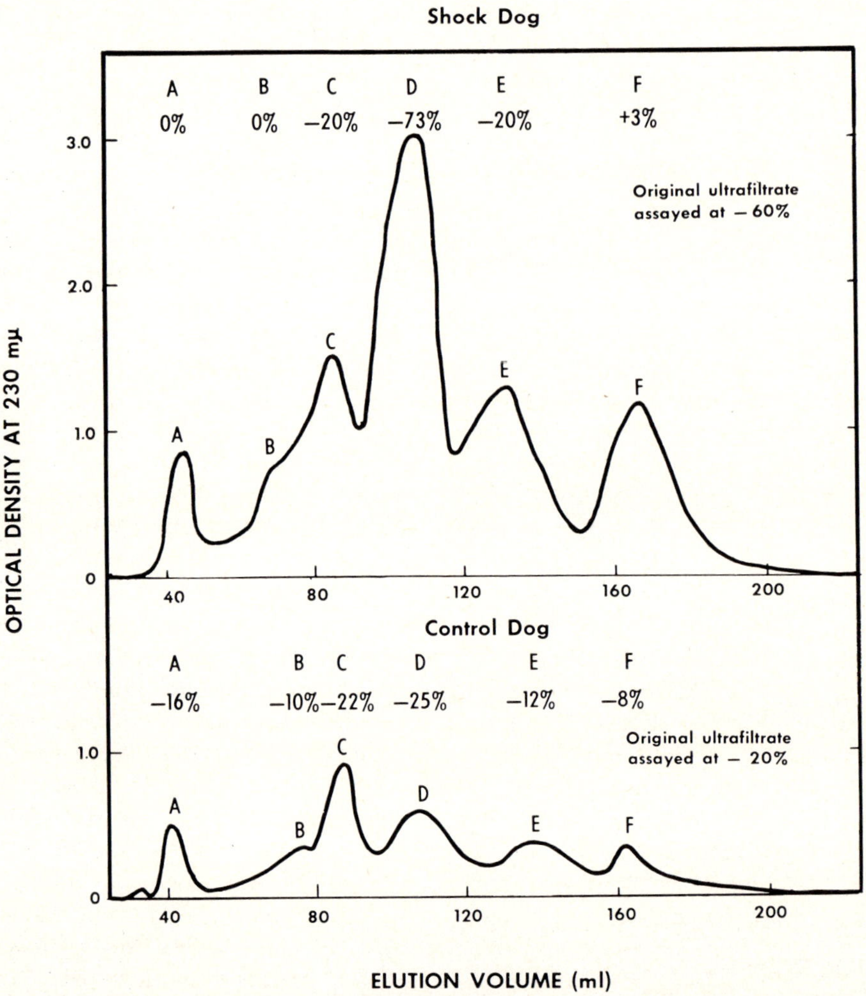

Fig. 2. Bio-gel P-2 column separation of plasma ultrafiltrates into six peaks. At the top of the figure are typical results from a shocked dog with a large peak D. At the bottom are shown results from a typical control dog sample.

Table II. *Myocardial depressant activities of column eluates (peak D) from plasmas and dialysates of dogs in hemorrhagic shock*

Group	No.	Plasma*		Dialysate*	
		Oligemic	Postoligemic	Early postoligemic	Late postoligemic
I. Shock + dialysis	8	45.8 ± 4.0	29.6 ± 3.4†	56.7 ± 5.3	75.3 ± 3.8*
II. Shock + sham dialysis	8	46.3 ± 3.2	69.0 ± 4.4‡	—	—
III. Sham shock + dialysis	5	25.8 ± 3.7§	—	13.3 ± 2.1§	—

*All values are means ± standard error of the means. MDF activities are given in percent depression of developed tension of isolated cat papillary muscles.
†$P < 0.02$ when compared to earlier control.
‡$P < 0.01$ when compared to earlier control.
§Normotensive.

mean activity of the dialysate after hemodialysis was 13.3 units. Krebs-Henseleit solution itself after passing through the Bio-gel column has a myocardial depressant activity of 12 units. Therefore, the depressant activity of plasma of 13.3 units after dialysis represents virtually no activity.

Statistical evaluation of the data. There were significant differences in the results between Group I and Group II in arterial blood pressure, cardiac output, and myocardial depressant activities. The mean arterial blood pressure at the end of dialysis in Group I animals was significantly higher than the blood pressure of sham-dialyzed animals in Group II ($P < 0.05$). More importantly, the cardiac output of dialyzed animals was significantly elevated over shocked sham-dialyzed animals ($P < 0.01$). Since central venous pressures were essentially unchanged, these alterations were probably the result of myocardial depression. In this respect it is notable that in Group I dogs, after dialysis, the MDF activity of the plasma was significantly decreased ($P < 0.01$) from oligemic levels, and concomitantly the MDF activity significantly increased in the dialysate ($P < 0.02$). In Group II shocked sham-dialyzed dogs, the MDF activity in the plasma increased significantly during sham dialysis ($P < 0.01$).

DISCUSSION

The results obtained in the present experiments demonstrate that myocardial depressant activity was removed from plasma of shocked dogs by hemodialysis and that MDF appeared in significant amounts in the dialysate. Removal of myocardial depressant activity was associated with a higher cardiac output after hemorrhagic shock. MDF was also shown to accumulate in the oligemic phase before reinfusion of shed blood. Previous studies demonstrated significant plasma activities of MDF only in the postoligemic period after reinfusion.[2, 9] In the present experiments, hemodialysis led to slightly longer survival time after shock, but not to the level of statistical significance. Perhaps one reason why a greater improvement in survival in the dialyzed dogs was not observed was that hemodialysis undoubtedly removed substances other than MDF, some of which may have been beneficial to the animal in shock.

The mechanisms responsible for circulatory collapse in the postoligemic phase of hemorrhagic shock remain unanswered. Although the initial mechanism which triggers circulatory collapse is still unknown, some of the intermediate steps are becoming clear. Most investigators agree that during postoligemic shock a progressive impairment of myocardial performance occurs so that in the late phases a severe impairment is present.[3, 8, 16, 18, 19] Many metabolic disturbances occur in shock so that cardiac depression may be a consequence of several events. In this connection, it is intriguing to speculate that MDF is the humoral link between the metabolic events of oligemia and the postoligemic cardiac depression.

The arterial pH increased toward normal in the postoligemic period by hemodialysis whereas the pH in sham-dialyzed dogs remained at low levels. However, arterial P_{O_2} and P_{CO_2} values were similar in dialyzed and sham-dialyzed dogs. We believe that the lower cardiac outputs in Group II animals cannot be accounted for on the basis of a more severe metabolic acidosis alone, since it is generally agreed that a reduced cardiac output results from myocardial hypoxia and not metabolic acidosis per se.[4, 15]

MDF has been postulated to play a role in the pathogenesis of hemorrhagic shock.[1, 2, 8, 9] Since MDF accumulates during the oligemic phase of hemorrhagic shock there would be adequate time for it to exert a negative inotropic effect which could initiate or exacerbate an already existing myocardial depression. It was previously shown that MDF is not produced in the extracorporeal blood which is in the reservoir[20] but is a product of the hypovolemic animal. MDF is produced to a large extent by the ischemic pancreas of the animal in shock.[13] Recently the presence of MDF in the ischemic splanchnic circulation has been confirmed by Williams and associates.[20] The precise trigger mechanism for the activation of MDF is not presently known.

MDF is now known to be produced in dogs as well as cats. In cats, the MDF molecule has been shown to be a peptide[12] in the molecular weight range of 800 to 1,000 as judged from the elution patterns of the gel filtration column[11] and selective membrane ultrafiltration.[12]

Hemodialysis with an artificial kidney has been tried previously in hemorrhagic shock. In 1952, Frank and his associates[5] reported that although the artificial kidney prolonged survival in dogs subjected to hemorrhagic shock, when compared to shocked controls, the dogs ultimately relapsed into shock and died. They concluded that their data offered no evidence of a readily diffusible depressant substance in the circulating blood of dogs in hemorrhagic shock. No cardiac output data were included in their study and they did not look for a specific depressant substance. Thus, the results of the present study are not in direct conflict with this earlier study, but extend the findings of Frank and associates.[5]

Moyo, Dossetor, and MacLean[14] performed hemodialysis experiments in dogs subjected to endotoxin and hemorrhagic shock. These investigators found decrease in mortality rates in dogs given endotoxin and hemodialysis when compared to controls. However, dialysis did not lead to a significant improvement in survival in hemorrhagic shock. The dialysis period was only one hour in their experiments, and cardiac output was not measured. They believed that their data suggested the presence of a dialyzable substance (toxin) in endotoxin shock, but that it was not endotoxin itself. They reasoned that the phospholipid-polysaccharide-protein complex could not be dialyzed because of its very large molecular weight, and therefore the improved survival was postulated to be due to removal of a small molecular weight toxic substance.

SUMMARY

The effect of hemodialysis on myocardial depressant activity (MDF) was studied in dogs subjected to hemorrhagic shock. Dogs in Group I were subjected to hemorrhagic shock and four hours of dialysis. Dogs in Group II were subjected to hemorrhagic shock and were sham dialyzed. Group III dogs were sham shocked and dialyzed for four hours.

Group I animals had a significantly greater arterial blood pressure and cardiac output at the end of the dialysis period when compared to the values at the same time in Group II animals. Group III animals showed no significant hemodynamic alterations during dialysis.

Myocardial depressant activity accumulated during the oligemic phase of hemorrhagic shock and was removed from the plasma of Group I dogs in significant amounts by hemodialysis. Furthermore, MDF reached high levels in the dialysates from Group I dogs. In shock without dialysis (Group II) MDF activity continued to accumulate in the plasma during the sham procedure. In Group III dogs dialysis decreased myocardial depressant activity from control levels to negligible activity.

The data suggest that removal of MDF activity by hemodialysis from the plasma of dogs subjected to hemorrhagic shock led to an impovement in cardiac performance.

REFERENCES

1. Brand, E. D., and Lefer, A. M.: Myocardial depressant factor in plasma from cats in irreversible postoligemic shock, Proc. Soc. Exp. Biol. Med. **122:** 200, 1966.
2. Brand, E. D., Cowgill, R., and Lefer, A. M.: Further characterization of a myocardial depressant factor present in hemorrhagic shock, J. Trauma **9:** 216, 1969.
3. Crowell, J. W., and Guyton, A. C.: Evidence favoring a cardiac mechanism in irreversible hemorrhagic shock, Amer. J. Physiol. **201:** 893, 1961.
4. Downing, S. E., Talner, N. S., and Gardner, T. H.: Cardiovascular responses to metabolic acidosis, Amer. J. Physiol. **208:** 237, 1965.
5. Frank, H. A., Frank, E. D., Jacob, S., Glotzer, P., Persky, L., Friedman, E. W., Schwartz, A., Rutenburg A. M., Milrod, S., and Fine, J.: Traumatic shock. XX. The course of hemorrhagic shock in dogs treated by peritoneal irrigation or by an artificial

kidney, Amer. J. Physiol. **168:** 140, 1952.
6. Fukuda, T.: Endogenous shock-inducing factor in canine hemorrhagic shock, Nature **205:** 392, 1965.
7. Gomez, O. A., and Hamilton, W. F.: Functional cardiac deterioration during development of hemorrhagic circulatory deficiency, Circ. Res. **14:** 327, 1964.
8. Lefer, A. M., Craddock, G. B., Cowgill, R., and Brand, E. D.: Performance of papillary muscles isolated from cats in postoligemic shock, Amer. J. Physiol. **211:** 687, 1966.
9. Lefer, A. M., Cowgill, R., Marshall, F. F., Hall, L. M., and Brand, E. D.: Characterization of a myocardial depressant factor present in hemorrhagic shock, Amer. J. Physiol. **243:** 492, 1967.
10. Lefer, A. M., and Blattberg, B.: Comparison of the effects of two factors present in the plasma of shocked animals, J. Reticuloendothel. Soc. **5:** 54, 1968.
11. Lefer, A. M., and Martin, J.: Relationship of plasma peptides to the depressant factor in hemorrhagic shock, Circ. Res. **26:** 59, 1970.
12. Lefer, A. M., and Martin, J.: Mechanism of the protective effect of corticosteroids in hemorrhagic shock, Amer. J. Physiol. **216:** 314, 1969.
13. Lefer, A. M., and Martin, J.: Studies on the origin of the myocardial depressant factor in hemorrhagic shock. In press.
14. Moyo, C. T. B., Dossetor, J. B., and MacLean, L. D.: Hemodialysis in the treatment of shock, J. Surg. Res. **4:** 380, 1964.
15. Opie, L. H., Kadas, T., and Gevers, W.: Effects of pH on the function and glucose metabolism of the heart, Lancet **2:** 551, 1963.
16. Regan, T. J., LaForce, F. M., Teres, D., Block, J., and Hellems, H. K.: Contribution of left ventricle and small bowel in irreversible hemorrhagic shock, Amer. J. Physiol. **208:** 938, 1965.
17. Rosenberg, J. C., and Rush, B. F.: An enzymatic spectrophotometric determination of pyruvic and lactate acid in blood, Clin. Chem. **12:** 299, 1966.
18. Rothe, C. F., and Selkurt, E. E.: Cardiac and peripheral failure in hemorrhagic shock in the dog, Amer. J. Physiol. **207:** 302, 1964.
19. Wiggers, C. J.: Myocardial depression in shock—A survey of cardiodynamic shock, Amer. Heart J. **33:** 622, 1947.
20. Williams, L. F., Jr., Goldberg, A. H., Polansky, B. J., and Byrne, J. J.: Myocardial effects of intestinal ischemia, J. Surg. Res. **9:** 319, 1969.

Successful 24 hour renal perfusion-preservation with monitoring by surface electrometry during the storage interval

J. L. ALEXANDER, M.D.
J. R. DMOCHOWSKI, M.D.
J. E. MURRAY, M.D.
N. P. COUCH, M.D.
WITH THE TECHNICAL ASSISTANCE OF
A. M. MACEY, B.S.
N. A. PRENTISS, B.S.
BOSTON, MASS.
From the Department of Surgery, Harvard Medical School and the Peter Bent Brigham Hospital

Organ preservation for unlimited intervals would help to relieve the prevalent shortage of transplantable organs, but until such a method is realized, shorter term storage should be perfected to utilize maximally the organs currently available.[11] During the era since human renal transplants began, such short-term methods have been evolved in various laboratories over the past eleven years[1, 4, 5, 6, 8, 9, 10, 14] and have been applied clinically in a limited way.[5]

As regional and national organ "banks" develop from metropolitan clearinghouses, a need will grow for completely reliable methods of whole-organ storage for at least 24 hours. To date, no such method exists, for there is no way to store a kidney for this period without partially compromising its immediate, posttransplantation function.[1, 4, 5, 15] One avenue to improved methodology is to apply better techniques for continuous surveillance of critical metabolic events in the renal tissue itself during the storage period. The degree of lactic acidosis, as an index to anaerobic glycolysis, is one such factor.

This work was supported by United States Public Health Service Grants FR-05489-05 and AI04-606, and grants from the United States Army, the Atomic Energy Commission, and the John A. Hartford Foundation.

Submitted for publication Sept. 10, 1969; resubmitted Oct. 30, 1969.

To this end, the present study details a method for organ perfusion, using a system somewhat similar in design to that of Belzer and associates,[4] that enables preservation of dog kidneys for 24 hours. Emphasis is placed on detailed study of metabolic events, particularly as reflected by continuous electrometry of hydrogen ion activity at the renal surface. A major objective of the study was to measure precisely and atraumatically the pH of the stored tissue as a new approach to closer monitoring of the perfusion method.

MATERIAL AND METHODS

Animals. The experimental animals were conditioned mongrel dogs which weighed 12 to 24 kilograms.

Apparatus. The preservation system was completely closed and free of air-perfusate interfaces. Its essential components were a Silastic* membrane oxygenator,[3] pulsatile pump,† refrigerator unit,‡ and heat exchanger (Fig. 1). The perfusion circuit tubing was medical grade Silastic* (inside diameter ¼ inch, outside diameter ⅜ inch).

Perfusate. Blood was obtained from nor-

*Dow Corning Corporation, Midland, Mich.
†Harvard Apparatus Company, Inc., Millis, Mass.
‡Cincinnati Sub-Zero Products, Inc., Cincinnati, Ohio.

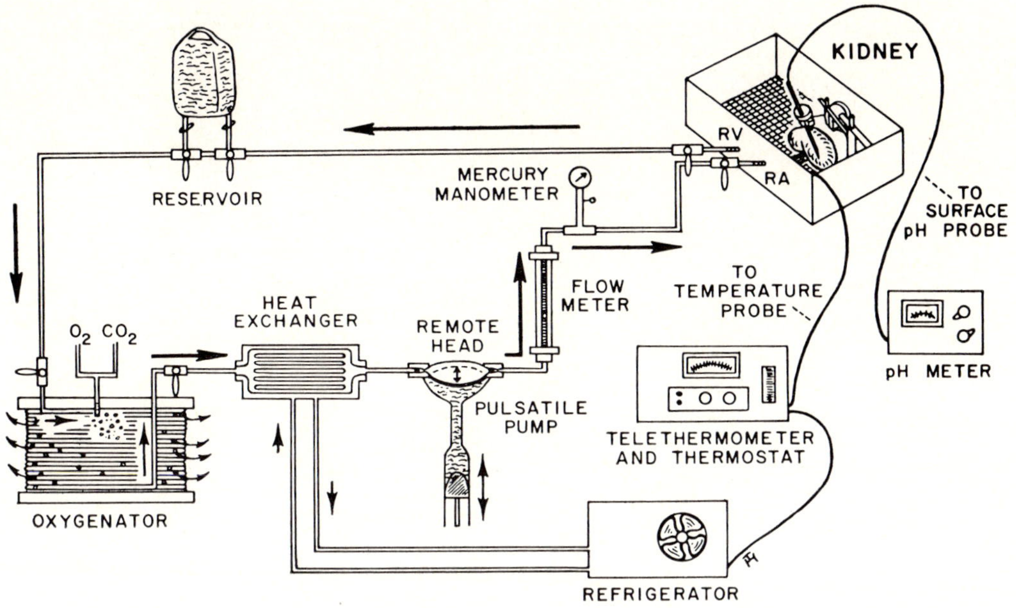

Fig. 1. Diagram of kidney perfusion-preservation apparatus designed and constructed with the technical assistance of (1) Cardiovascular Inst., Inc., Wakefield, Mass., and (2) The Wrangell Engineering Company, East Norwalk, Conn.

mal, normotensive[15] animals and collected in Fenwal* packs containing acid citrate dextrose (ACD) U.S.P. formula A solution, and the plasma was separated. The perfusate was prepared according to the method of Belzer and colleagues[6] with the following modifications: (1) omission of additional dextrose and phenol red and (2) addition of neomycin (0.5 mg. per liter). After filter† sterilization (minimum pore size 0.22 μ), the perfusate was collected in transfer packs* and the apparatus was primed. All air was evacuated from the system (Fig. 1) before a kidney was placed in the circut.

Technique. The animal was anesthetized with sodium pentobarbital; the kidney was removed for preservation, was flushed with 50 to 75 c.c. of cold (4° C.) Ringer's solution, Solucortef‡ (100 mg. per liter), and heparin (50 mg. per liter), and placed on the apparatus (Fig. 1). The renal vein was cannulated and connected to a reservoir whose level was kept about 5 cm. above the hilum. The plasma was recirculated, cooled to between 8° and 10° C. and allowed to equilibrate with a mixture of 1 to 5 percent carbon dioxide and 99 to 95 percent oxygen at one atmosphere. This required about twenty minutes. The priming volume was 600 ml. for the 4 and 8 hour experiments and 1,000 ml. for the 24 hour experiments. The kidney preperfusion ischemic time ranged from 8 to 12 minutes.

During perfusion the surface temperature of the organ was kept between 8° and 10° C. and the flow at approximately 1 ml. per gram per minute. No attempt was made to control the perfusion pressure, which never rose above 50 mm. Hg systolic and averaged 30/10 mm. Hg.

Surface pH[12] was monitored continuously by means of a tip-sensitive glass electrode (suspended from a constant pressure balance) and an electrometer.*

Perfusate pH, Po_2, Pco_2, potassium, sodium, glucose, osmolality, and lactate and

*Travenol Laboratories, Inc., Morton Grove, Ill.
†Millipore Filter Corporation, Bedford, Mass.
‡The Upjohn Company, Kalamazoo, Mich.

*Instrumentation Laboratory, Inc., Lexington, Mass.

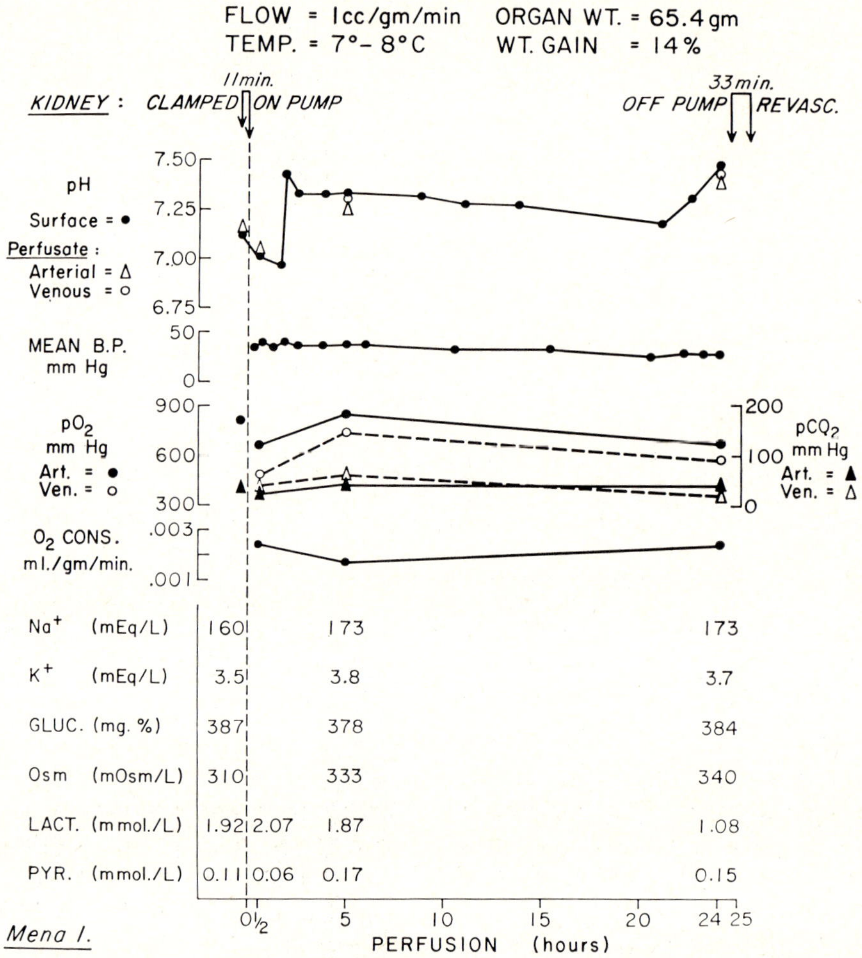

Fig. 2. Intraperfusion data of a 24 hour experiment. Note the close agreement between surface and perfusate pH and the constancy of mean perfusate pressure. The high sodium concentration and osmolality are discussed in the text.

pyruvate concentrations were measured before the organ was placed on the apparatus, and at 30 minutes, 4, 6 to 7, and 24 hours thereafter, depending on the duration of the perfusion.

Perfusion pressure was measured by an anaeroid manometer. The organs were weighed before and after perfusion, after being drained of blood or perfusate. Immediately after reimplantation of the kidney into the iliac fossa a contralateral nephrectomy was done.

Postoperatively, blood urea nitrogen was determined three times per week and urinary specific gravity and protein were measured at least twice weekly. All animals were killed at thirty days and complete autopsies were performed.

RESULTS

All of the perfused kidneys developed normal color and turgor upon revascularization and produced urine within a few minutes. These kidneys were life sustaining. There were 7, 3, and 3 experiments in the 4, 8, and 24 hour preservation groups, respectively. During perfusion there was a gradual but slight drop in pressure at the constant flows (Fig. 2).

The arterial oxygen tension ranged from 500 to 600 mm. Hg, with an average arterial-venous Po_2 difference of 100 mm.

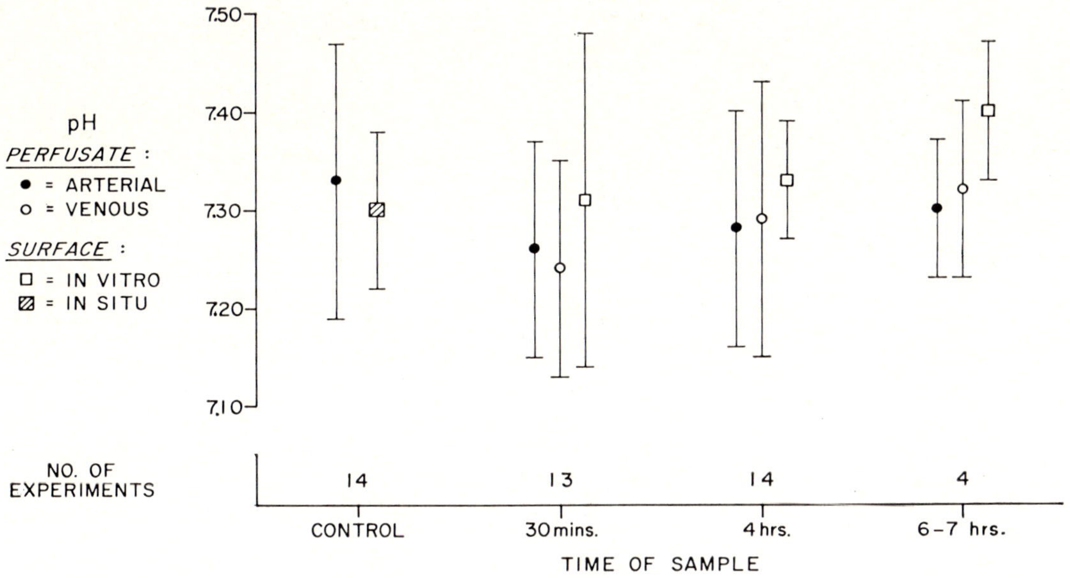

Fig. 3. Comparison of simultaneously determined surface, arterial, and venous perfusate pH; values are means and one standard deviation. The control arterial pH pertains to the perfusate immediately prior to insertion of the kidney. Note that the control surface pH pertains to the organ in situ (or in vivo).

Hg. The oxygen consumption ranged from 0.002 to 0.005 ml. per gram per minute and there was no difference in the mean values after 4, 8, and 24 hours of perfusion. The partial pressure of carbon dioxide in the perfusate varied from 40 to 60 mm. Hg. The perfusate pH was held in physiologic range by the addition of sodium bicarbonate or by varying the carbon dioxide content in the gas mixture bathing the oxygenator. During the later experiments it was rarely necessary to add bicarbonate because the pH could be controlled entirely by adjusting the carbon dioxide flow.

Under these conditions there was no significant difference between the surface and perfusate pH (Fig. 2) but the surface pH, for any given experiment, varied over a somewhat wider range than that of the perfusate (Fig. 3).

Perfusate lactate concentrations remained unchanged, whereas pyruvate concentrations were higher at 4, 6 to 7, or 24 hours than at 30 minutes (Fig. 4); thus the lactate-pyruvate ratios, which were almost all elevated at 30 minutes, returned toward control levels. Perfusate potassium concentration was relatively constant up to 24 hours. The increase in sodium and total osmolality during perfusion reflected the addition of sodium bicarbonate buffer (Table I and Fig. 3). There was a mean weight gain of 6, 9, and 13 percent after 4, 8, and 24 hours, respectively.

Postoperatively, the blood urea nitrogen became elevated in almost all animals (Table II); it reached its peak at about 5 days, and gradually returned to normal during the second and third postoperative weeks. Meanwhile, these autografts regained their ability to raise urine specific gravity while the proteinuria disappeared or returned to preoperative levels.

DISCUSSION

This series of experiments, wherein a microfiltered plasma was used, enabled preservation of dog kidneys for 24 hours, and thereby confirmed the results of Belzer and associates.[4] The reasonably simple and reliable system differed from that of Belzer on a number of counts: (1) the inclusion of the surface pH monitor, (2) the use of a small, efficient helical membrane

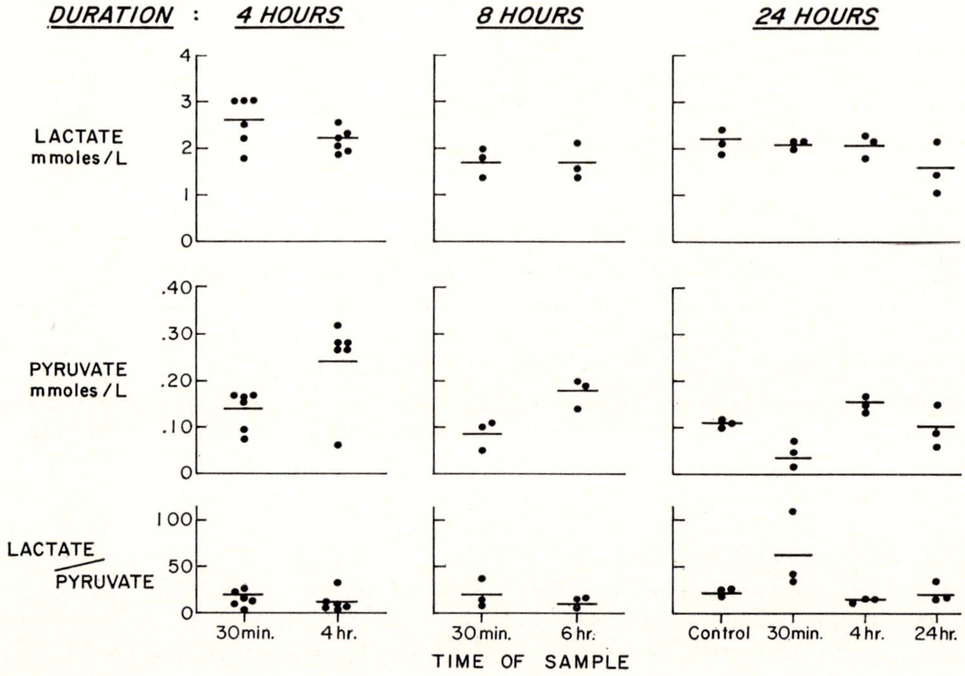

Fig. 4. Lactate and pyruvate concentrations in mMoles per liter and lactate/pyruvate ratios obtained at various intervals during 4, 8, and 24 hour preservation experiments. Note the constancy of lactate concentrations whereas pyruvate concentrations rise after 30 minutes.

Table I. *Canine kidney perfusion-preservation: sodium, potassium, osmolality (mean values)*

Duration (hr.)	*No. of experiments*	*Na+ (mEq./L.)*		*K+ (mEq./L.)*		*Osmolality (mOsm./L.)*	
		30 min.	*Final*	*30 min.*	*Final*	*30 min.*	*Final*
4	7	174	183	3.3	3.7	343	344
8	3	186	182	3.2	4.1	346	348
24	3	156	170	3.6	3.6	3.4	342

Table II. *Canine kidney perfusion-preservation: blood urea nitrogen (mean values)*

Duration (hr.)	*No. of experiments*	*Blood urea nitrogen (mg. percent)*			
		At 5 days		*At 30 days*	
		Mean	*Range*	*Mean*	*Range*
4	7	62	25 – 159	29	21 – 49
8	3	103	58 – 132	35, 36	(2 dogs)
24	3	156	123 – 183	27	23 – 42

oxygenator, and (3) the use of a completely closed design in order to avoid air-fluid interfaces.[16, 19] Beyond these features, the Belzer perfusate was modified by omitting the addition of glucose (the average 300 ml. unit of fresh dog ACD plasma contains about 1700 mg. of glucose) and by the addition of neomycin (because of the risk of proliferation of gram-negative organisms during the long perfusions).

The surface pH measurements were an accurate means for monitoring the renal pH, presumably an index of anaerobic glycolysis and lactic acidosis. The maintenance of renal pH within relatively normal ranges was correlated with eventual satisfactory renal function, although the data are insufficient to allow more precise correlations with quality of function. This finding accords well with previous studies of renal surface pH as related to duration of ischemia and temperature, two other determinants of tissue injury.[12] The finding was also supported by the fact that the oxygen consumption was in the normal range for temperatures of 8° to 10° C.[17, 20] The oxygen content of the perfusate ranged from 0.008 to 0.012 ml. of O_2 per milliliter of perfusate; therefore the amount of oxygen presented to the kidney per minute (at a flow of 50 ml. per minute) was approximately 0.4 to 0.6 ml., which is 16 to 24 times its hypothetical requirement. Of particular interest was the failure of the oxygen consumption to decline even after 24 hours (Fig. 2). The data for lactate and pyruvate concentrations and for lactate/pyruvate ratios also indicated that the metabolism was predominantly aerobic,[13] i.e., after an initial rise in the lactate/pyruvate ratios at 30 minutes, these values returned to baseline levels at 4 hours and remained there for the rest of the perfusion (Fig. 4).

The stable or gradually decreasing perfusion pressures at constant flows supports the findings of others, and may be explained by either slow vasodilatation or the opening of A-V shunts (perhaps in the juxtamedullary zone). The weight gain was only 13 percent at 24 hours, comparing favorably with 6 and 9 percent at 4 and 8 hours, respectively. Although this degree of weight gain is not excessive, it still indicates the need for improvement of the method.

The constancy of the perfusate potassium concentration after 24 hours is still another indication that cellular injury was minimal. The markedly elevated sodium levels in the earlier experiments simply reflected the addition of sodium bicarbonate buffer.

The final criterion for success of the storage was, of course, survival of the animals by the stored kidney alone until they were put to death at 30 days. The initial renal function was characterized by variable azotemia, proteinuria, and loss of concentrating power, but function became virtually normal within two to three weeks.

This system has also been successfully used to preserve dog livers for 8 to 10 hours.[2] Our present objective is to refine the method for 24 hour storage, rather than to attempt preservation for longer periods, because this interval is more than adequate to enable tissue typing and other preparations for the transplant. In experienced hands, it is possible to match a prospective donor against several potential recipients prior to the donor's death, since the majority of donors are patients with brain injury whose deaths are predictable several hours, or even a few days, ahead.[11]

SUMMARY

Dog kidneys were perfused at normal atmospheric pressure with modified undiluted plasma up to 24 hours at 8° to 10° C. The system was completely closed and the pulsatile flow was approximately 1 ml. per gram per minute. Organ surface pH was measured continuously and proved to be a simple, accurate means for monitoring the hydrogen ion activity of the organ.

There was a mean organ weight gain of 13 percent after 24 hours' preservation which, in view of normal oxygen consumption, relatively normal surface pH, stable lactate/pyruvate ratios, and perfusate potassium concentration, indicated that tissue injury was minimal. This interpretation is supported by the fact that all 13 animals with preserved autografts survived immediate contralateral nephrectomy and had good renal function at 30 days.

We are grateful for the invaluable advice and encouragement of Dr. Francis D. Moore. We are also indebted to the personnel of his laboratory, including Misses Ruth Raila, Virginia Vilnis, Lynn Hiskock, and Lourdes Budejen, under the supervision of Miss Margaret Ball.

REFERENCES

1. Ackerman, J. R., and Barnard, C. N.: Successful storage of kidneys, Brit. J. Surg. **53:** 525, 1966.
2. Alexander, J. L., et al.: Data to be published.
3. Bartlett, R., Ischerwood, J., Moss, R., Olszewski, W., Polat, H., and Drinker, P.: Toroidal flow membrane oxygenator: 4-day partial bypass in dogs, Surg. Forum **20:** 1969. In press.
4. Belzer, F. O., Ashby, B. S., and Dunphy, J. E.: 24-hour and 72-hour preservation of canine kidneys, Lancet **2:** 536, 1967.
5. Belzer, F. O., Ashby, B. S., Gulyassy, P. F., and Powell, M.: Successful seventeen hour preservation of human cadaver kidney, New Eng. J. Med. **278:** 608, 1968.
6. Belzer, F. O., Ashby, B. S., Huang, J. S., and Dunphy, J. E.: Etiology of rising perfusion pressure in isolated organ perfusion, Ann. Surg. **168:** 382, 1968.
7. Berkowitz, H. D., Miller, L. D., Itskovitz, H. D., and Bovee, K. C.: Renal function in the isolated perfused kidney, Surg. Gynec. Obstet. **127:** 1257, 1968.
8. Brettschneider, L., Daloze, P. M., Huguet, C., Porter, K. A., Groth, C. G., Kashiwagi, N., Hutchison, D. E., and Starzl, T. E.: The use of combined techniques for extended storage of orthotopic liver homografts, Surg. Gynec. Obstet. **126:** 263, 1968.
9. Cassie, G. F., Couch, N. P., Dammin, G. V., and Murray, J. E.: Normothermic perfusion and replantation of the excised dog kidney, Surg. Gynec. Obstet. **109:** 721, 1960.
10. Couch, N. N., Cassie, G. F., and Murray, J. E.: Survival of the excised dog kidney perfused in a pump oxygenator system, SURGERY **44:** 666, 1958.
11. Couch, N. P.: Supply and demand in kidney and liver transplantation: A statistical survey, Transplantation **4:** 587, 1966.
12. Couch, N. P., Maginn, R. R., Middleton, M. K., Appleton, D. R., and Dmochowski, J. R.: Effects of ischemic interval and temperature on the renal surface hydrogen ion concentration, Surg. Gynec. Obstet. **125:** 521, 1967.
13. Huckabee, W. E.: Relationship of pyruvate and lactate during anaerobic metabolism. I. Effects of infusion of pyruvate or glucose and of hyperventilation, J. Clin. Invest. **37:** 244, 1958.
14. Humphries, A., Jr., Russell, R., Stoddars, L. D., and Moretz, W. H.: Three day kidney preservation: Perfusion of kidneys with hypothermic diluted blood or plasma, SURGERY **63:** 646, 1968.
15. Kane, J. F., and Edwards, E. C.: Renal vascular shutdown during perfusion of the isolated kidney, Brit. J. Urol. **38:** 664, 1966.
16. Lee, W. H., Jr., Krumhaar, D., Fonkalsrud, E. W., Schjeide, O. A., and Maloney, J. V., Jr.: Denaturation of plasma proteins as a cause of death after intracardiac operations, SURGERY **50:** 29, 1961.
17. Levy, M. N.: Oxygen consumption and flow in the hypothermic perfused kidney, Amer. J. Physiol. **197:** 1111, 1959.
18. Lotke, P. A.: Lysosome stabilizing agents for hypothermic kidney preservation, Nature **212:** 512, 1966.
19. Owens, G., Adams, J. E., and Scott, H. W., Jr.: Embolic fat as a measure of various oxygenators, J. Appl. Physiol. **15:** 999, 1960.
20. Semb, G., Kreg, J., and Johansen, K.: Renal metabolism and blood flow during local hypothermia studied by means of renal perfusion *in situ,* Acta Chir. Scand. **253:** 196, 1960.

Collagen arterial graft of bovine origin: Seven-year observations in the dog

NORMAN ROSENBERG, M.D.
GEOFFREY H. LORD, D.V.M., PH.D.
JOHN HENDERSON, M.D.
JAMES W. BOTHWELL, PH.D.
EUGENE R. L. GAUGHRAN, PH.D.
NEW BRUNSWICK, N. J.
From the Vascular Surgical Service, Middlesex General Hospital, and the Johnson & Johnson Research Foundation

In 1956, we[7] first reported on the use of enzyme-treated bovine arterial heterografts as segmental aortic substitutes in the dog. Previous to that communication, it was generally accepted that untreated heterografts would provoke an intense reaction by the

Received for publication Sept. 19, 1969.

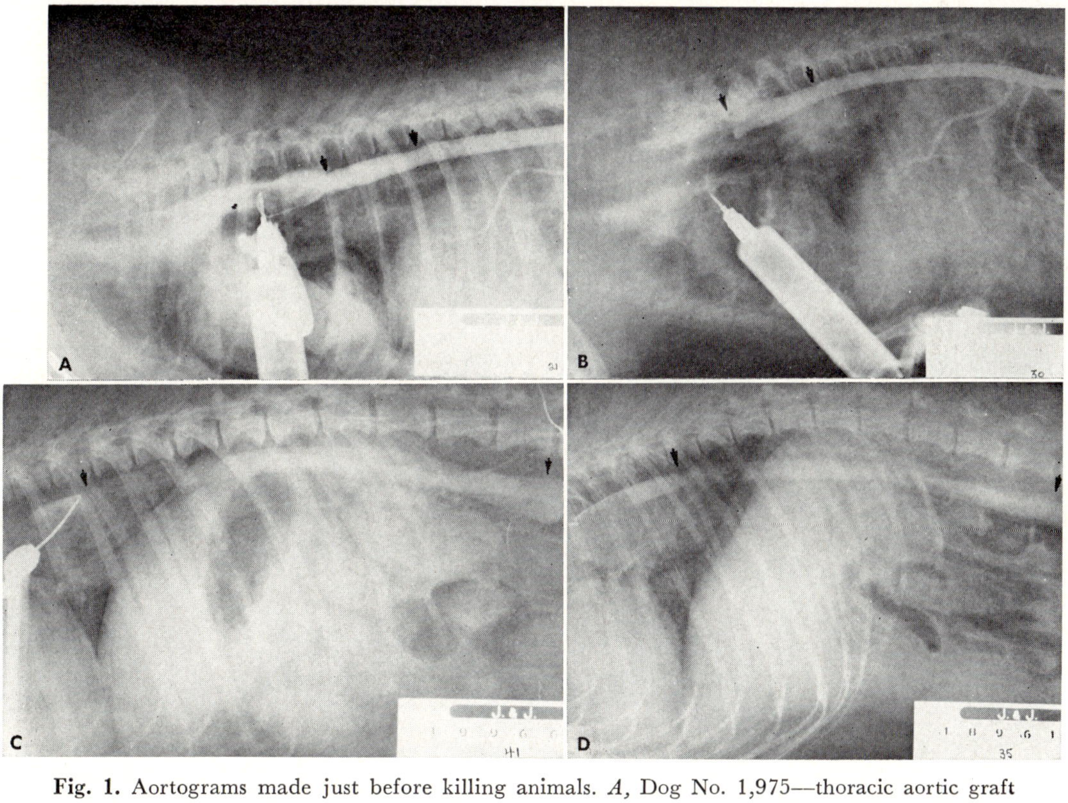

Fig. 1. Aortograms made just before killing animals. *A,* Dog No. 1,975—thoracic aortic graft at 7 years, 3 months. *B,* Dog No. 1,984—thoracic graft at 7 years, 3 months. *C,* Dog No. 1,996—thoracoabdominal graft at 7 years, 2 months. *D,* Dog No. 1,896—thoracoabdominal graft at 7 years, 5 months.

recipient, resulting in severe inflammatory and degenerative changes within the graft, which would lead to failure by thrombosis, rupture, or aneurysm formation.[1]

The modified heterografts prepared by us were converted by chemical processing into minimally reactive collagen tubes which are shown to have functioned as arterial conduits in dog and man for several years. More than 200 of these implants have since been inserted in man,[4] and long-term clinical results of up to five years' duration will be reported elsewhere.[10]

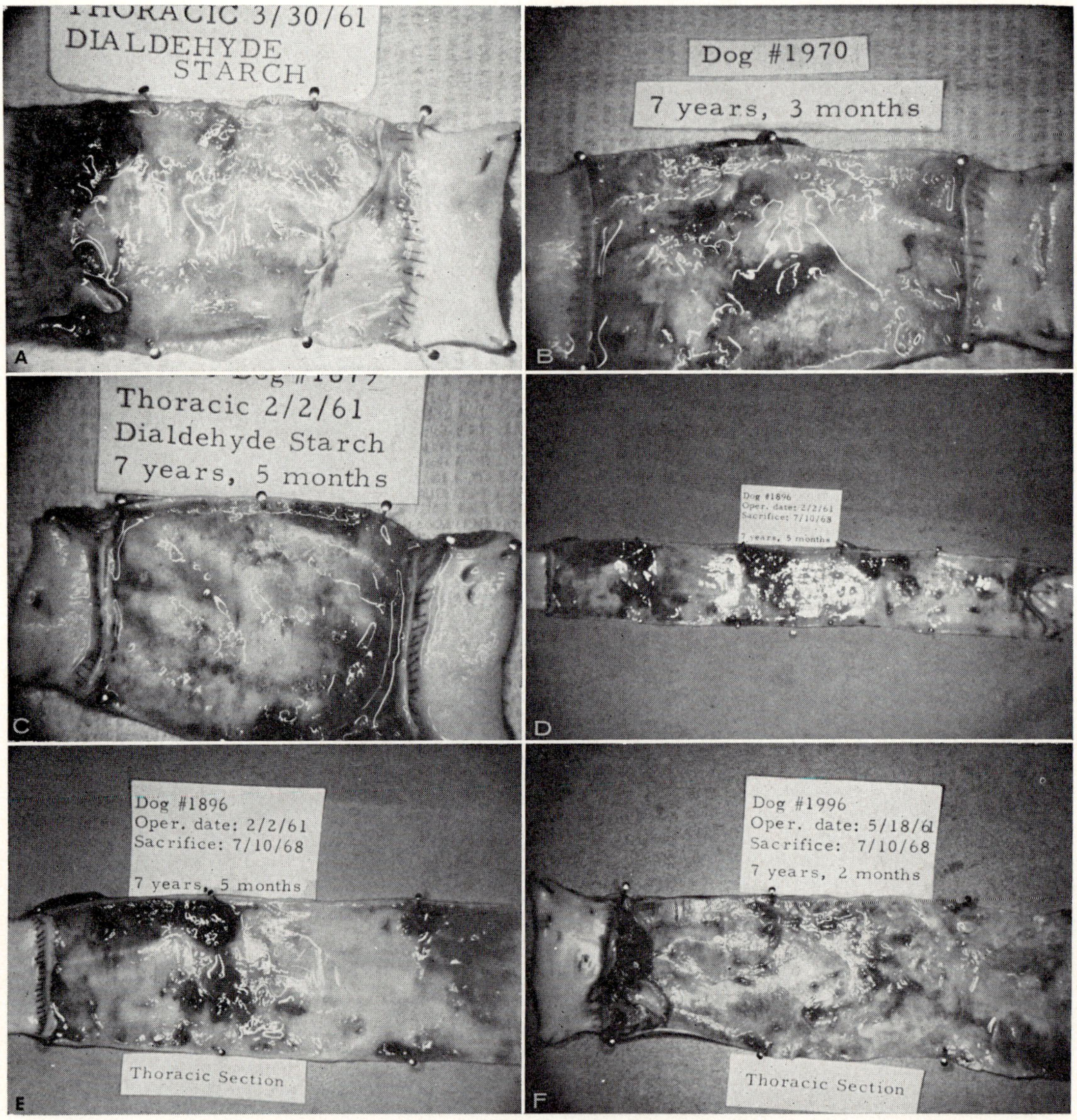

Fig. 2, *A-F.* Gross appearance of representative aortic grafts (intimal aspect). *A, B,* and *C* are thoracic implants (Dogs No. 1,975, 1,970, and 1,879, respectively). *D* and *E* represent an over-all view and close-up, respectively, of a thoracoabdominal implant at seven years, five months (Dog No. 1,896). *F* and *G* are views of thoracic and abdominal graft sections (Dog No. 1,996). Reproduced from Kodachrome transparencies. See Table I for gross descriptions of specimens.

TECHNIQUE

Bovine carotid arteries were enzymatically stripped of their reactive parenchymatous proteins and elastica by using the protease, ficin. This was followed, in a subsequently improved method, by tanning of the arteries with dialdehyde starch. A strong nonreactive tube resulted, composed mainly of collagen. Details are given in an earlier report.[8] When implanted in the rat or dog, the material evoked a mainly fibroblastic reaction in marked contrast to that seen with control material. Extensive testing revealed it to be essentially nonantigenic.[3]

The technique of bovine artery modification was refined to its present status by 1961, and a series of grafts were implanted into dogs as segmental aortic substitutes. Some animals received short thoracic segments (4.4 to 6.6 cm.) inserted end to end. Others were grafted in accordance with the technique of McCune and Blades,[5] which permits the use of long, 25 to 28 cm., thoracoabdominal implants. The suture material used was No. 5-0 Mersilene, employed in each anastomosis as an over-and-over continuous suture, interrupted twice. Animals were cooled to 29 to 30° C. for most of the procedures.

Serial aortograms performed by percutaneous puncture, or terminally by thoracotomy and direct puncture, were obtained in all animals, with the use of 75 percent Hypaque (sodium and meglumine diatrizoates).

The seven dogs reported herein represent the last in a series of animals commented on in previous communications[6, 8] and, until they were killed, constituted all our long-term survivors. All received their aortic implants from seven years, two months to seven years, five months ago.

RESULTS

Aortography. Terminal aortograms revealed no dilatation or aneurysm formation in any of the animals. The inner wall appeared, for the most part, to be smooth, with no x-ray evidence of filling defects. Slight suture-line constriction was occasionally noted (Fig. 1).

Gross findings. All but one of seven grafts were flexible at necropsy, there being some stiffness in the abdominal portion of one thoracoabdominal graft (Dog No. 1996) resulting from focal chondrification and osteoid metaplasia. Intimization was, for the most part, complete except for small areas of erosion and thin mural thrombus deposition. Suture-line pannus was limited in most animals but was occasionally noted as "prominent" at the proximal suture-line. There was no dilatation or aneurysm for-

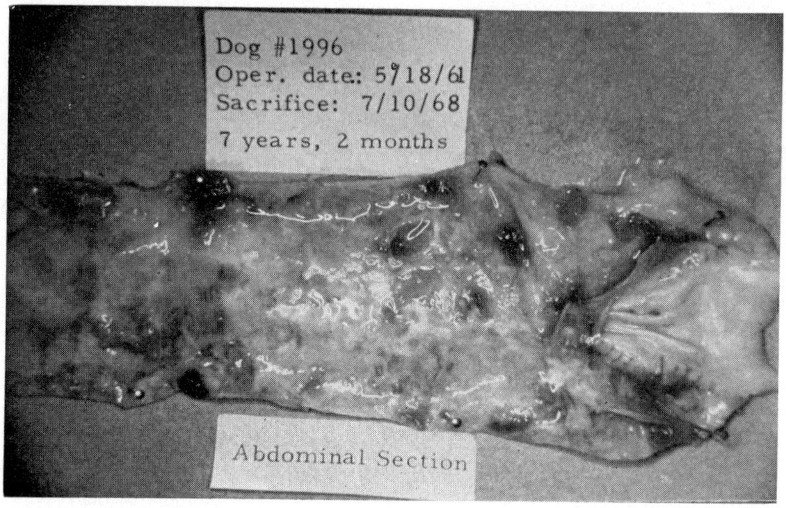

Fig. 2*G*. See legend under Fig. 2, *A-F*.

mation. Two animals showed foci of what could be considered gross atheroma formation (Fig. 2).

Microscopic findings. The grafts were externally invaded and encased in host fibrous tissue which had become compacted and acellular. There was no significant cellular reaction or infiltration. Graft fibers were prominent and identifiable in some animals but not to as significant a degree as in others. Microscopic calcification was seen in three dogs, being grossly evident in only one. In this latter animal (Dog No. 1996), the implant wall was architecturally disorganized by metaplastic foci of chondrification and osteoid formation.

Except for areas of erosion and thin (Fig. 3). A more detailed description of mural thrombi, intimization was evident microscopic findings is found in Table I.

A

B

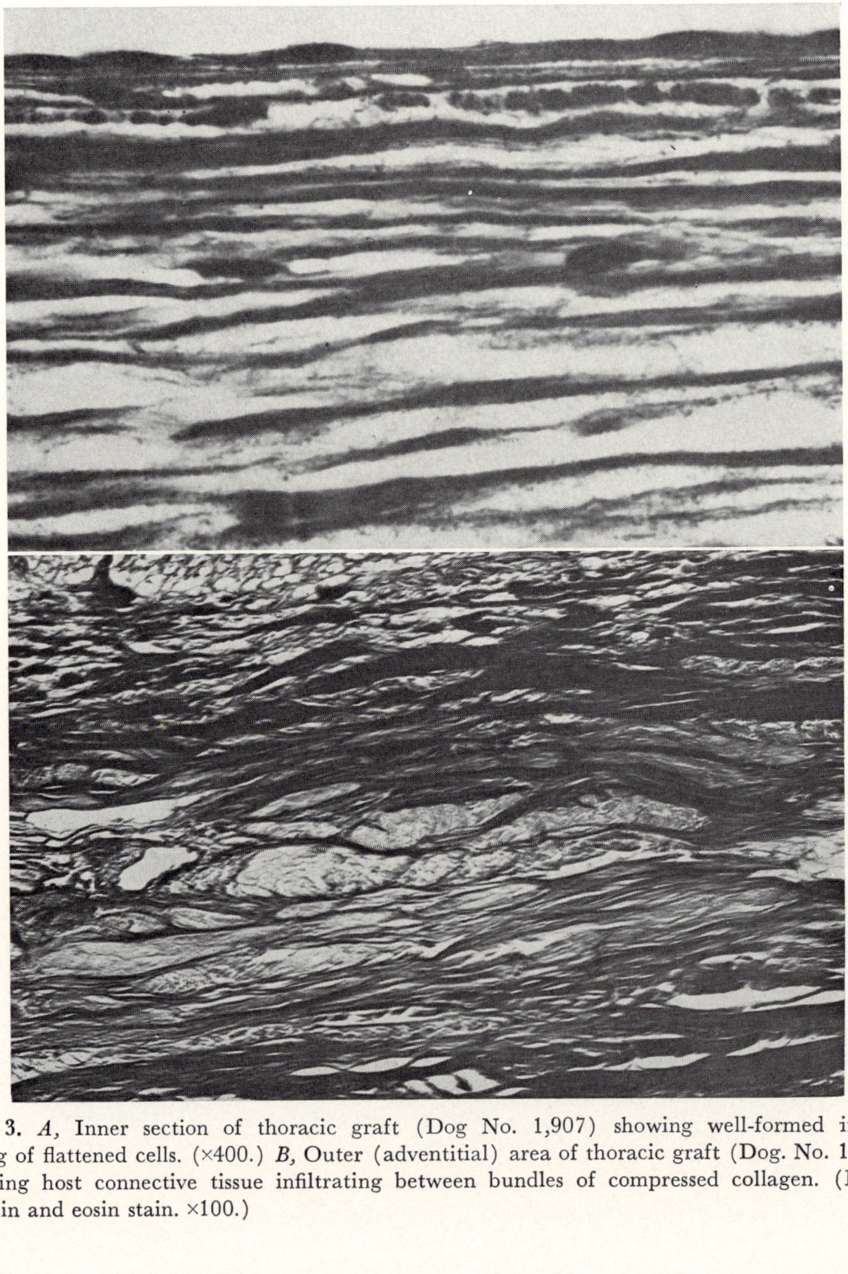

Fig. 3. *A,* Inner section of thoracic graft (Dog No. 1,907) showing well-formed intimal lining of flattened cells. (×400.) *B,* Outer (adventitial) area of thoracic graft (Dog. No. 1,879), showing host connective tissue infiltrating between bundles of compressed collagen. (Hematoxylin and eosin stain. ×100.)

Table I

Dog No.	*Type of graft*	*Length (cm.)*	*Time of death*	*Gross findings*	*Microscopic findings*
1879	Thoracic	5.3	7 yr., 5 mo.	Slightly larger than host, not dilated; firm but flexible, no calcification; narrow pannus at both suture lines; surface granular; small mural thrombus	50-75 percent of wall is dense compact host collagen; implant and host collagen are relatively acellular; no reaction, only encapsulation and integration; fibrous tissue did not extend into media; intimal surface smooth with superficial erosions; intima shows a few flattened nuclei; graft fibers identifiable
1896	Thoraco-abdominal	25.0	7 yr., 5 mo.	Outer surface smooth, graft soft and pliable; no dilatation; no calcification; small irregular patches of mural thrombus, mostly in thoracic section; major portion of intima smooth and glistening; small pannus at both anastomoses	Abdominal section: Similar to above; graft fibers more prominent, completely encased; intima smooth Thoracic section: No cellular reaction; fewer graft fibers present
1907	Thoracic	4.4	7 yr., 4 mo.	Firm but flexible, no calcification or dilatation; very little suture-line pannus; most of intima smooth, but some mural thrombus	Graft acellular; surface irregular (mural thrombus); graft identified in some areas, not in others
1970	Thoracic	6.6	7 yr., 3 mo.	Larger, but not dilated; firm but flexible, no calcification; narrow pannus at both suture lines; inner surface granular with irregular whitish areas suggesting atheroma	Difficult to recognize graft fibers; no cellular reaction; uneven intimal surface (erosion and mural thrombosis); focal calcification
1975	Thoracic	5.5	7 yr., 3 mo.	Proximal pannus 1 cm. wide and not firmly attached; inner surface partly granular, partly smooth and glistening	Difficult to recognize graft fibers, prominent suture line granulomas; center of graft thin-walled, acellular, with smooth surface
1984	Thoracic	5.5	7 yr., 3 mo.	Firm but flexible; 4.0 mm. proximal pannus; most of inner surface was granular and covered with mural thrombus	Original graft fibers (only few identified); foci of chondrification; fibrinous thrombi in foci; many areas in adventitia calcified with osteoid changes
1996	Thoraco-abdominal	28.0	7 yr., 2 mo.	Thoracic section soft and flexible; abdominal section more rigid and partly calcified; narrow pannus at thoracic end, more extensive at abdominal end; most of inner surface smooth with scattered foci of mural thrombus; irregular whitish unraised areas on intimal aspect of abdominal section	Abdominal section: Extensive irregular erosions; graft media recognized in only a few areas; graft adventitia not seen; chondrification and osteoid changes visible throughout giving disoriented structure; foci of epithelioid cells; rare focal atheroma Thoracic section: Same changes, but less common

DISCUSSION

The introduction of a new arterial prosthesis of biologic origin requires the assumption of awesome responsibility, which has not escaped the authors of this report. Work on enzymatically modified bovine arteries was begun some 15 years ago, and more than 300 implantations have been made in dogs over this period of time. It was not until seven years ago (April, 1962) that the first clinical implantation was undertaken.[9] The total number of grafts inserted in man by various investigators has now exceeded 300.[4] As these patients who have undergone operation more recently become "long-term" patients, the clinical efficacy of the modified bovine graft can receive more appropriate statistical scrutiny, and comparisons can be made between it and either autogenous saphenous vein or plastic prostheses. A few clinical reports have already appeared.[2, 9, 10]

Currently, one can conclude from seven-year observations in the dog that: (1) The implant has been shown to resist the stress imposed by a continually pulsating system without evidencing fatigue. (2) It does not induce an acute response in the early post-implantation period in contrast to the reaction seen with untreated heterografts. (3) The late reaction to the graft is one of fibrous invasion, substitution, and integration. (4) Antibodies to the graft have not been detected in the blood sera of animals after a period of six years.[3] (5) While the modified graft is biologically acceptable to the dog, and fibers of the original graft can still be identified in some dogs after seven years, other animals show few such remnants, without, however, undergoing dilatation. (6) Intimization is not a static event but is a dynamic and everchanging process. (7) "Atheromatous" lesions seem to be frequently, but entirely, the end products of resorbing subintimal thrombi. (8) Chondrotic, osteoid, and other bizarre metaplastic changes are seen in occasional long-term grafts.

CONCLUSIONS

1. Bovine carotid arteries can be modified by enzymatic removal of reactive parenchymatous proteins and subsequent tanning. The resulting collagen tube induces little to no inflammatory reaction and seems not to be antigenic.

2. When implanted as segmental arterial substitutes for over seven years in the dog, they are well incorporated in host tissue and function satisfactorily as arterial replacements.

REFERENCES

1. Creech, O., Jr., De Bakey, M. E., Self, M., and Halpert, B.: The fate of heterologous arterial grafts: An experimental study, SURGERY **36:** 431, 1954.
2. Dale, W. A., and Lewis, M. R.: Modified bovine heterografts for arterial replacement, Ann. Surg. **169:** 927, 1969.
3. DeFalco, R. S.: Immunologic studies of untreated and chemically modified bovine carotid arteries, J. Surg. Res. **10:** 95, 1970.
4. Henderson, J., Director, Medical Affairs, Johnson & Johnson. Personal communication.
5. McCune, W. S., and Blades, B.: The viability of long blood vessel grafts, Ann. Surg. **134:** 769, 1951.
6. Rosenberg, N.: Arterial heterografts and their modifications, *in* Wesolowski, S. A., and Dennis, C., editors: Fundamentals of vascular grafting, New York, 1963, McGraw-Hill Book Company, Inc., chap. 15.
7. Rosenberg, N., Gaughran, E. R. L., Henderson, J., Lord, G. H., and Douglas, J. F.: The use of segmental arterial implants prepared by enzymatic modification of heterologous blood vessels, Surg. Forum **6:** 242, 1956.
8. Rosenberg, N., Henderson, J., Lord, G. H., and Bothwell, J. W.: An arterial prosthesis of heterologous vascular origin, J. A. M. A. **187:** 741, 1964.
9. Rosenberg, N., Martinez, A., Sawyer, P. N., Wesolowski, S. A., Postlethwait, R. W., and Dillon, M. L.: Tanned collagen arterial prosthesis of bovine carotid origin in man, Ann. Surg. **164:** 247, 1966.
10. Additional references:

    Rosenberg, D. M., Glass, B., Rosenberg, N., Lewis, M., and Dale, W. A.: Experiences with modified bovine heterografts in arterial surgery, SURGERY. To be published.

    Keshishian, J. M., Smyth, N. P. D., Atkins, P. C., Camp, F., and Yahr, W. Z.: Clinical experience with the modified bovine arterial heterograft, Ann. Surg. To be published.

Prolonged left ventricular bypass by transvalvular aortic catheterization. I. Physiologic effects and rationale of surgical concept

R. E. SCHUHMANN*
L. A. GEDDES
H. E. HOFF
HOUSTON, TEXAS
From the Department of Physiology, Baylor College of Medicine

The heart-assist (left ventricular bypass) method of Geddes and associates[23] has provided total extracorporeal circulatory support in the living subject (dogs) without thoracotomy. More recently it has come to our attention that an identical investigation has been made independently by Zwart and associates[54, 55] in Amsterdam (Dr. Zwart is now at the University of Utah College of Medicine). The procedure has been applied in animals with a standard clinical roller pump (Sarns, Inc., Ann Arbor, Mich.) and two newly designed collapsing-bag pulsatile pumps.[11, 42] With these pumps, total left ventricular bypass has been provided for periods extending from one to 13 hours in anesthetized dogs in which ventricular fibrillation was induced. The principle of the method employs a combination of vacuum withdrawal of blood from the left ventricle via carotid artery–aortic valvular catheterization, and positive-pressure reinfusion into the femoral artery and cephalic end of the same catheterized carotid artery. Thus a total left ventricular bypass has been effected without thoracotomy.

To guarantee that total circulatory support was provided, ventricular fibrillation was induced and permitted to continue throughout the period of extracorporeal maintenance of the circulation. Proof of support under this condition means that any lesser degree of partial bypass could also be provided in the presence of a heartbeat.

The purpose of this paper is to present the description of this method of left ventricular bypass, to present additional information on the method, and to present some of the physiological observations and preliminary results that demonstrate the efficacy and rationale of this heart-assist procedure for circulatory maintenance.

METHOD AND PROCEDURE

The principle employed is shown in Fig. 1. The left ventricle was catheterized by passing a catheter down the carotid artery, through the ascending aorta, and then through the aortic valve into the ventricle, in a direction retrograde to the flow of blood. Vacuum withdrawal of blood from the left ventricle was accomplished via the carotid catheterization; reinfusion was accomplished via the carotid and femoral arteries. By means of this extracorporeal system, partial or total removal of the pumping (work) load of the left ventricle of the heart can be achieved by virture of the pumping rate selected.

This investigation employed dogs which ranged in weight from 15 to 26.5 kilograms. The animals were anesthetized with pento-

Supported in part by Grant 5-T1-HE 05125.10 from the United States Public Health Service, and in part by Public Health Service Fellowship 1-F3-HE 34825.01 and Fellowship 5-F3-HE 34825.02 from the National Heart Institute.

Submitted for publication Sept. 18, 1969; resubmitted Dec. 29, 1969.

*Address for reprints: Robert E. Schuhmann, Ph.D., Southwest Research Institute, Artificial Organs Research, 8500 Culebra Rd., San Antonio, Texas 78228.

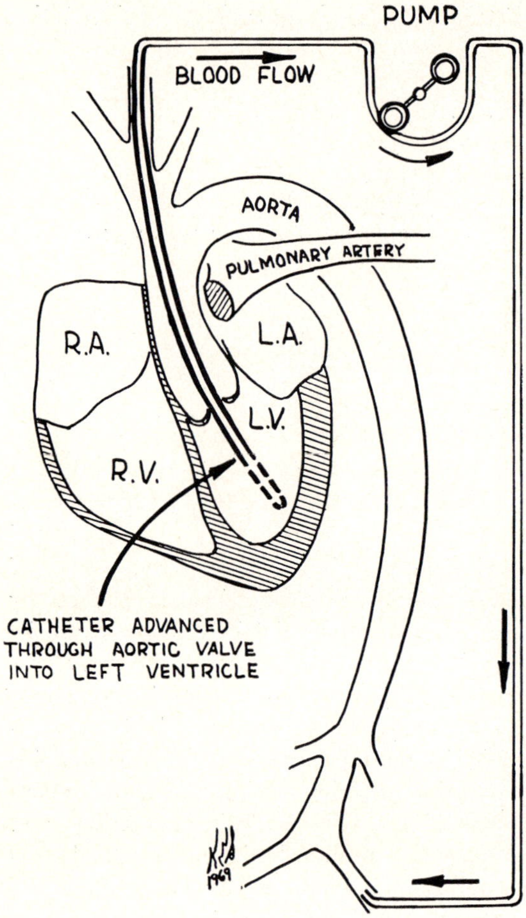

Fig. 1. Principle of left ventricular bypass by transvalvular aortic catheterization.

barbital sodium (30 mg. per kilogram) and maintained under sedation as necessary with morphine sulfate (2 mg. per kilogram) injected subcutaneously. Other than oxygen, maintenance doses of morphine, and sodium bicarbonate in some of the experiments, no other drug or pressor support was used. Clotting was inhibited by heparin, 2.5 mg. per kilogram plus 15 mg. in the priming fluid for the extracorporeal circuit. The extracorporeal system was primed with 380 ml. of 5 percent dextrose in saline at room temperature. Extracorporeal blood flow and cardiac output were determined by pump calibration and by the saline-dilution methods.[48, 49]

Either a tracheal cannula or cuffed endotracheal tube was employed for respiration with 100 percent oxygen or 95 percent oxygen–5 per cent carbon dioxide. The respiration (Bird Mark 7, Palm Springs, Calif.) was triggered by the animal's spontaneous respiratory movements. The inspiratory pressure limits on the respirator were generally maintained within the range of 3 to 10 cm. of water, as opposed to higher values. In this manner a minimum of intratracheal pressure was maintained, since excess respiratory pressure or insufflation of the lungs impaired the return of blood to the left ventricle.[1, 12, 13, 30] Because there was no active output from the right ventricle it was advantageous to make this adjustment with care. Therefore, the present objective during bypass with ventricular fibrillation was to maintain with the respirator an insufflation pressure into the lungs compatible with a maximum systemic blood pressure. Respiration was recorded by the impedance pneumograph.[19-22]

Plasma hemoglobin was measured by the cyanmethemoglobin method.[50] Blood pH and the acid-base status were determined by the Astrup method and the Siggaard-Andersen nomogram respectively.[2-6, 43-47]

The catheter used for withdrawal of blood from the left ventricle was a polytetrafluoroethylene (Teflon) tube, 0.180 inch in outside diameter, 0.115 inch in inside diameter, and 10 inches long. A metal catheter tip was found to be necessary in order to maintain patency of the catheter; the tip was multiholed, machined from bar stock, with the total area of the holes equal to seven times the cross-sectional area of the catheter lumen. Details of the catheter and tip are shown in Fig. 2.

The waxlike surface of the Teflon catheter provided lubrication for movement of the catheter within the carotid artery. Arterial constriction upon the catheter during insertion prevented easy advancement of the catheter in some cases of small-diameter arteries in the smaller animals. Topical anesthesia eliminated this difficulty. Procaine hydrochloride, 40 mg. of 2 percent solution, was applied to the tunica externa vasorum (adventitia) prior to making a quarter-inch

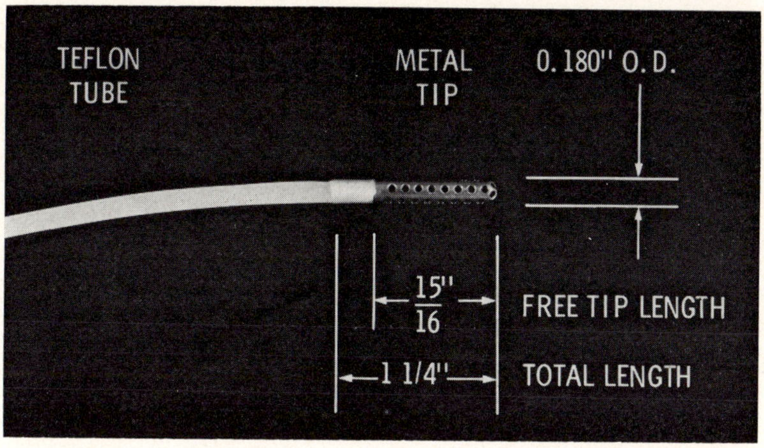

Fig. 2. Left ventricular catheter. Dimensions of the catheter are shown in the figure. The total area of the holes is seven times the cross-sectional area of the catheter lumen.

longitudinal arterial incision, thence immediately to the tunica interna vasorum between atraumatic arterial hemostats (or between ligature and proximal hemostat); the excess procaine was then drained off. With this procedure the catheter could be advanced or retrieved with relative ease of movement within the lumen of the artery. Care was taken at all times to avoid damage to the aortic valve cusps during entry into the ventricle.

The catheter was at all times connected to a blood-pressure transducer and pressure was recorded continuously to signal entrance of the catheter into the left ventricle. In no case was fluoroscopy used. The median time required for catheterization was 6½ minutes in 54 trials.*

The optimum pumping rate was found to occur at an inlet pressure no lower than –350 mm. Hg at the entrance to the extracorporeal pump; that is, vacuum of approximately half an atmosphere measured at the point in the catheter where it emerged from the carotid artery. In most of the experiments the extracorporeal pumping was performed with the roller pump because of its ease of adjustment. To establish the fact that any pumping system should be applicable to this new method of bypass, both nonpulsatile and pulsatile flow of blood were provided to the animal via the presence or absence, respectively, of a pulse-damping chamber (bubble trap). In some experiments either of two newly designed collapsing-bag pulsatile pumps were employed in order to demonstrate the same purpose.[11, 42]

*In a recent communication from Dr. W. J. Kolff, it was suggested that the aortic valve could be opened at the desired moment for entry by initiating pumping, thus lowering the local aortic pressure at the catheter tip within the root of the ascending aorta, and in turn causing the aortic valve to open. This technique has not yet been used in our laboratory.

At the time for termination of the period of extracorporeal maintenance of the circulation, defibrillation was carried out and the pumping rate was gradually decreased and then stopped. Most animals could be weaned from the pump within a two-minute period. Returning the pumping load to the heart too rapidly produced extrasystoles. In one instance a weaning time of 15 minutes was required in order for the heart to accept the load without the production of extrasystoles.

RESULTS

Fig. 3 is a typical plot of blood pressure, plasma hemoglobin, and arterial blood pH (animal No. 15) during 3¼ hours of extracorporeal maintenance of the circulation; throughout this period the ventricles were fibrillating. The curve shows the mean arterial blood pressure, and the vertical lines

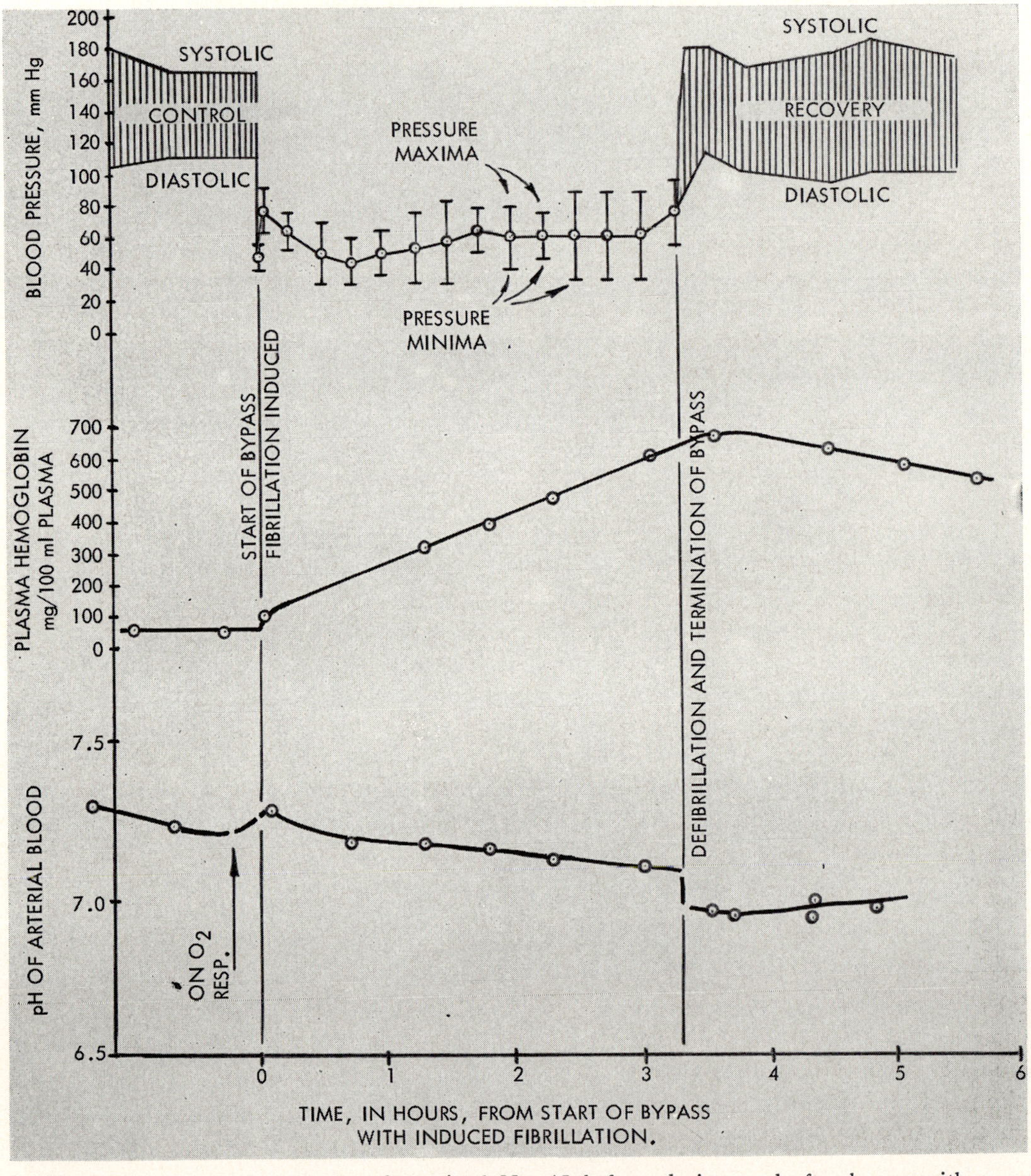

Fig. 3. Physiological parameters for animal No. 15 before, during, and after bypass with a pulsatile pump. The vertical bars on the blood pressure plot represent the maxima and minima of the rhythmic fluctuations in blood pressure, or Mayer waves. The mean blood pressure remained essentially stable during bypass with ventricular fibrillation in this animal, as opposed to the somewhat more typical pattern of a rise to a stable plateau. No pressor drugs or sodium bicarbonate were administered in this animal at any time. The lowest pH of the blood was observed after bypass, as was the highest plasma hemoglobin level. Normal recovery was observed.

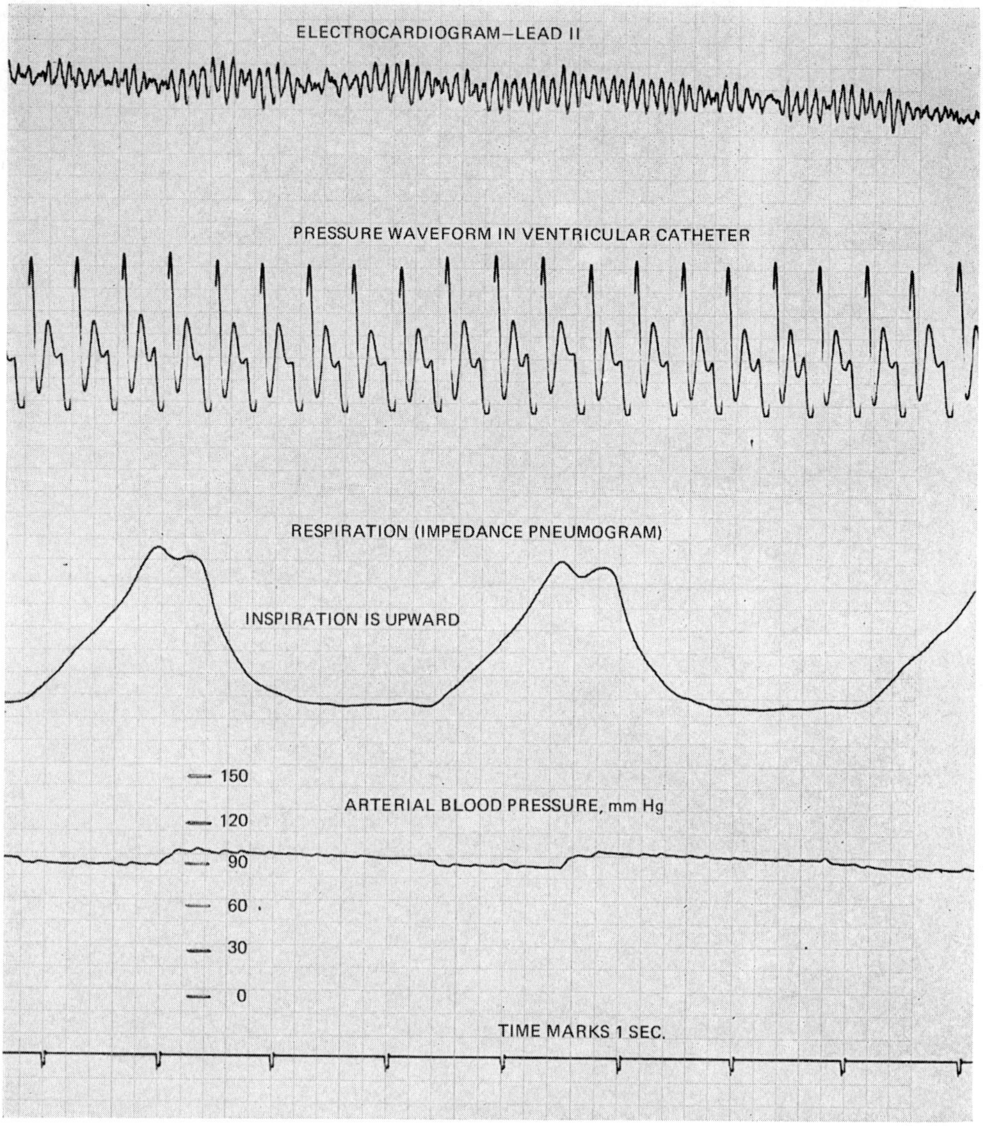

Fig. 4. Recording during second hour of bypass in dog No. 2 using the roller pump and nonpulsatile perfusion.

denote the maxima and minima of slow rhythmic variations in blood pressure (Mayer waves) which were often seen. Fig. 4 is a typical physiographic record (animal No. 2) taken during the second hour of pumping, using the roller pump in nonpulsatile configuration. Fig. 5 is a combined high-speed and low-speed physiographic record of the same animal (No. 2) exhibiting a normal recovery after defibrillation and termination of two hours of bypass.

Table I summarizes the typical respiratory and blood pressure data obtained. In nearly all animals there was a definite pattern of variation in the blood pressure with the passage of time. Immediately after the precipitation of ventricular fibrillation, the pump output was quickly increased, the blood pressure thus increased and showed respiratory variations. The mean pressures during pumping were usually less than the control mean values. In about half an hour,

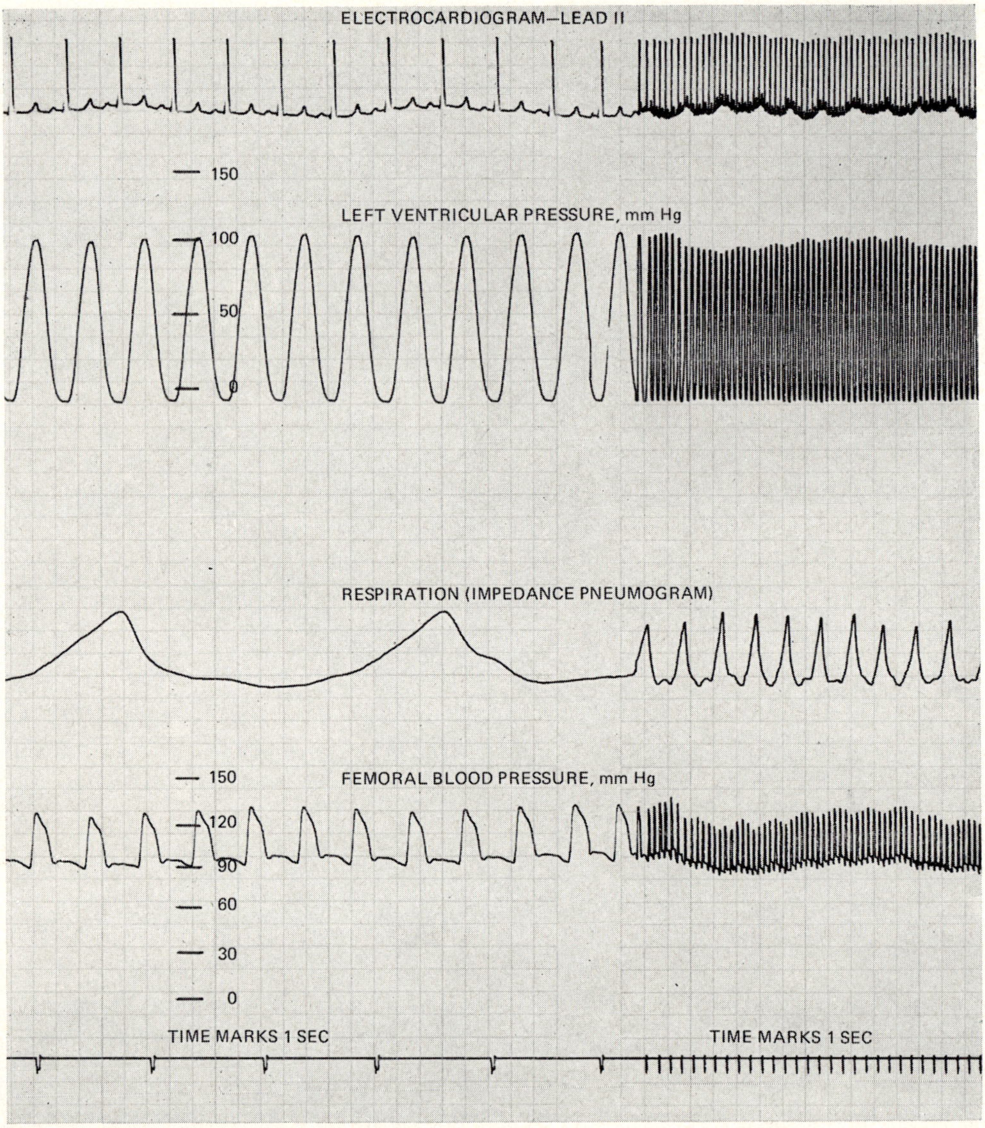

Fig. 5. Postbypass recovery in dog No. 2. Recording taken three minutes after pump off. Animal is breathing room air.

Mayer waves appeared. In about one hour or less, the blood pressure began to increase, and after approximately four hours it started to fall exponentially. Thereafter, the inlet gauge pressure fell from about –350 to about –400 mm. Hg, and the pump outlet pressure started to decrease. Frequently at these times pumping was terminated. In many instances, however, pumping was terminated for reasons unrelated to the condition of the animal.

It was noted that the knee-jerk reflex was the most consistently reliable indicator of the physiological status of the animal. The ability to breathe spontaneously was in every instance accompanied with an active knee-jerk reflex, as was the ability to defibrillate. Defibrillation, or effective cardiac contraction following the defibrillation procedure, was generally unsuccessful when the patellar reflex was absent.

Table II shows the hematocrit levels and

the amount of free hemoglobin in the plasma after different durations of pumping. Plasma hemoglobin increased during pumping, although not at a linear rate through the entire period. In some cases, hemoglobin continued to increase for 15 to 30 minutes after bypass. During the recovery period there was a progressive clearance of hemoglobin from plasma by physiological mechanisms.

The hematocrit usually decreased abruptly prior to pumping as a result of hemodilution by the equilibration procedure. During the period of extracorporeal pumping a relatively small further decrease in hematocrit was observed. With the pulsatile collapsible-bag pump the hematocrit increased in three experiments, decreased in four experiments, and remained constant in two experiments. Of the three experiments in which an increase in hematocrit was observed during pulsatile pumping, the values rose from 33, 32, and 33 up to final values of 47, 44, and 38 percent, respectively.

Use of the demand respirator to provide adequate oxygenation of the lungs was generally found to preclude respiratory acidosis and occasionally induced a mild respiratory alkalosis at various times during the period of bypass and recovery. The consistent finding during bypass was that of metabolic acidosis. In some of the experiments, however, the condition of metabolic acidosis was either corrected or precluded through the use of sodium bicarbonate administered intravenously. From these studies it was established that acid-base control within normal boundaries could be easily maintained, and the maintenance of a normal acid-base factor presented no adverse problem to use of the bypass procedure.

DISCUSSION

The studies reported in this paper demonstrate that the physiological requirements of the total circulation can be provided by this new method of closed-chest left ventricular bypass. It was found that a pressure gradient adequate to drive blood through the pulmonary circuit can be attained by the use of negative pressure applied to a catheter in the right carotid artery and continuing into the left ventricle. The pulmonary blood circuit pressure gradient in this study was equal to the difference between venous pressure and that actually existing in the left ventricle; calculations show that the largest portion of the pressure drop was through the catheter itself. Thus although the actual negative pressure in the left ventricle was unknown, it must have been numerically a small number. With the method described in this study the pump outflow was limited by the pulmonary blood flow, left ventricular inflow, and catheter resistance, i.e., due to length and diameter of the catheter. The flow provided by the extracorporeal pump was lower than normal cardiac output, and mean blood pressure was generally lower than normal but obviously above the critical level at which deterioration in vital function was manifest. Venous pressure in most experiments ranged from 10 to 15 mm. Hg during bypass with the fibrillating heart. It has been found by Bain and Mackey,[7] Galletti and Brecher,[18] and others[28, 32] that elevated venous pressures can be tolerated in dogs and man during (cardiopulmonary) bypass, and in fact is intentionally elevated by the investigator in some instances.

An interesting parameter in left ventricular bypass with ventricular fibrillation is the aspect of the nonfunctioning right ventricle. It was found in the present study that the fibrillating right ventricle did not affect the flow of blood through the pulmonary circulation to detract from the efficacy of the bypass. Regarding cardiovascular dynamics with the nonfunctioning right ventricle, the maintenance of total circulation through the pulmonary system in an intact subject (i.e., not on extracorporeal bypass) with compromised right ventricular function was first investigated by Starr and co-workers[50] in 1943 and later by others; only minimal rise in venous pressure was noted.[14, 50] More recently, Robicsek and colleagues,[33-37] Sanger and colleagues,[39-41] Glenn and colleagues,[25, 26] as well as others[8, 16, 28, 38, 51, 53] have de-

Table I. *Respiration and blood pressure*

Animal No.	Weight (Kg.)	Hours on pump	Control data: Blood pressure (mm. Hg)	Blood pressure mean (mm. Hg)	Heart rate per min.	Resp. rate per min.
1	20	1.1	190/100	130	140	12
		0.3				
2	21	2.0	165/120	135	150	12
		0.7				
3	19	1.1	80/ 60	65	114	14
4	22	4.5	120/ 80	95	140	16
		2.0				
5	26.5	13.2	120/ 65	83	170	13
6	22	3.9	240/140	170	170	30
7	22.5	10.0	215/160	178	198	62
8	21.5	8.7	180/100	125	210	26
9	25.5	3.8	200/120	145	200	56
10	21	6.5	200/130	153	190	24
11	20	1.5	180/120	140	192	10
12	21.5	2.5	180/ 90	120	125	21
13	18.5	1.0	150/100	115	140	29
14	20	1.1	190/120	140	210	18
15	17.5	3.2	180/120	140	182	8
16	25.5	2.0	170/120	135	150	9
17	21.5	1.1	220/135	160	186	20
18	21.5	1.1	220/120	153	204	54
19	20.5	2.2	150/ 90	110	142	13
20	25	4.0	180/ 95	123	174	21

*B, Beginning or early in run; M, middle or during run; E, end of run.

Table II. *Hemoglobin and hematocrit (bypass with ventricular fibrillation)*

Animal No.	Duration of pumping (hr. : min.)	Values at end of pumping period: Hematocrit (percent)	Hemoglobin (mg./100 ml. plasma)	Hemoglobin (mg./100 ml./hr.)
Roller pump; (damped) nonpulsatile perfusion				
5	13:12	46	300	280
6	3:52	48	100	25
7	10:00	36	300	30
8	8:40	41	500	60
9	3:45	46	500	135
10	6:27	44	650	100
11	1:33	42	400	260
Collapsible bag pump; pulsatile perfusion				
12	2:26	50	600	250
13	1:00	33	300	300
14	1:11	47	400	340
15	3:15	23	625	185
16	2:04	42	100	50
17	1:07	34	160	145
18	1:05	40	140	130
19	2:13	44	180	80
20	4:04	32	600	150

During fibrillation			Recovery data		
Blood pressure					
Max. (mm. Hg)	Min. (mm. Hg)	Resp. rate per min.	Blood pressure (mm. Hg)	Heart rate per min.	Resp. rate per min.
45 (M)*	30 (E)	15	165/ 75	140	35
45 (B)	30 (E)	28	140/ 75	110	30
106 (B)	70 (M)	13	135/ 90	125	19
63 (M)	52 (M)	13	120/ 70	144	24
15 (B)	10 (M)	29	180/110	132	23
82 (M)	70 (M)	16	120/ 80	130	15
80 (M)	65 (M)	20	120/ 80	120	13
85 (M)	42 (B)	30	135/ 70	130	50
28 (B)	25 (M)	18	120/ 40	192	16
110 (M)	35 (E)	50	130/ 70	150	70
80 (B)	32 (E)	36	170/ 80	190	26
65 (M)	32 (E)	37	160/100	166	43
100 (M)	60 (E)	27	170/120	205	61
50 (M)	10 (B)	24	150/ 70	150	20
90 (M)	40 (M)	16	150/ 90	105	11
100 (M)	40 (M)	43	150/ 95	116	55
105 (M)	30 (B)	29	200/120	192	25
100 (E)	30 (M)	17	170/ 90	108	18
95 (M)	55 (M)	36	155/110	168	29
70 (B)	25 (M)	17	80/ 25	102	27
90 (M)	15 (E)	24	120/ 70	168	32
65 (E)	15 (M)	24	190/ 90	99	17
80 (M)	27 (B)	24	140/ 80	159	25

scribed long-term circulatory exclusion of the right ventricle by atrial or caval anastomoses to the pulmonary artery permitting at most only coronary flow to pass through the right ventricle. The functioning left ventricle provided total circulatory support, with a nominal rise in venous pressure of 4 to 8 mm. Hg, and with some animals living a year or longer.[37] They believed that the blood circulation was facilitated by the respiratory movements of the thoracic cage and the pressure changes in the lung itself. These findings have corroborated the results of the present study, demonstrating the feasibility of total circulatory support by bypassing the left ventricle only and using the animal's own lungs for oxygenation.

Hypotensive episodes at the start of bypass were generally minimal. Observations revealed that when fluid (usually dextrose in saline) in the extracorporeal system was mixed with the animal's blood simultaneously with the beginning of bypass, the usual result was a precipitous drop in blood pressure. A loss of blood pressure with the start of bypass has been reported by other investigators also.[17, 24, 31] It was further observed in the present study, however, that either (a) the hemodilution, or (b) the start of bypass, when imposed singly, did not induce such a response. Therefore, slow equilibration to mix blood with the pump-priming solution homogeneously through the extracorporeal and intracorporeal systems prior to bypass was established as a practical procedure which could be completed in as little as two minutes without adverse effects, even with a mean priming volume of 380 ml., which is an appreciable percentage of the animal's blood volume.

In this study, no pressor drugs were employed before, during, or after pumping. Except for the cardiac effects of pentobarbital sodium, the heart rate, blood pressure, and cardiac output were therefore unadulterated in this series of experiments.[27]

No attempt was made to discover how long blood pressure could be maintained by this method of cardiac bypass. The time course of blood pressure evolved spontaneously in each experiment, and is characteristically shown in Fig. 3. A noteworthy observation regarding some of the animals was an apparent absence of untoward effects following prolonged circulatory maintenance at relatively low blood pressure, i.e., at shock-inducing levels. Mean blood pressure of dog No. 9 (killed at 3 days after bypass) remained at 60 mm. Hg in excess of 3 hours during bypass; dog No. 8 exhibited a mean pressure of 40 to 50 mm. Hg during the latter 3 hours of bypass; and dog No. 6 exhibited a mean pressure of 25 to 30 mm. Hg during nearly 4 hours of bypass which was followed by recovery.

The blood flow attainable in this series of experiments was usually one half of resting cardiac output or slightly less. Cardiac output after bypass generally trended toward normal resting levels, with some transient variations; notably, an initial overshoot which varied in time and amplitude to a minimal extent. The peak occurred several minutes after defibrillation and cessation of extracorporeal flow. This type of response has not been previously described by other investigators.

Postmortem examination of the hearts of the animals used in this study revealed a few subendocardial hemorrhagic areas. In many cases no hemorrhagic areas or bruises or other damage was visible on gross inspection. A common finding in the fibrillation-bypass experiments, however, were the pinpoint hemorrhagic areas over the surface of the left ventricle and frequently the right ventricle. Ecchymotic or petechial hemorrhagic areas have been observed by other investigators also in cardiac bypass procedure.[9, 10, 15, 29]

A most important consideration in applying this technique of left ventricular bypass is the use of a catheter as large in diameter as the carotid artery will permit, since total extracorporeal flow must move through the left ventricular catheter. Another important feature of the pumping system is the use of the special catheter tip (Fig. 2) which guarantees that flow will continue regardless of its location in the left ventricle. By use of multiple holes (which have a cross-sectional area equal to seven times that of the catheter cross-sectional area), patency is assured and the pressure gradient at the catheter tip is distributed over a large area. With this device, there was no evidence of the catheter being sucked against the ventricular walls, papillary muscles, or chordae tendinae. This did indeed happen in early catheter-design experiments in which a plastic catheter with only a few holes was employed.

SUMMARY AND CONCLUSIONS

The new method of Schuhmann and Geddes for left ventricular bypass without thoracotomy has been shown to be capable of providing total circulatory support in dogs in which ventricular fibrillation was precipitated. The animal's own lungs were used for oxygenation, and spontaneous respiration continued throughout the periods of extracorporeal pumping.

Prolonged physiological support of the circulation by means of left ventricular–arterial bypass has been demonstrated in this investigation to be a feasible procedure. Of practicable surgical importance is the convenience of application of the concept of catheterization.

Because the technique described in this paper has provided blood flow in the total absence of ventricular function, it should be ideally applicable to relieving the workload of a failing but beating left ventricle; and may be of some value in left ventricular bypass procedures in man because it employs a minimum of surgery and does not require thoracotomy.

REFERENCES

1. Andersen, M. N., and Kuchiba, K.: Depression of cardiac output with mechanical ventilation. Comparative studies of intermittent positive, positive-negative, and assisted ventilation, J. Thorac. Cardiovasc. Surg. **54:** 182, 1967.
2. Astrup, P.: On the recognition of disturbance in the acid-base metabolism, Danish Med. Bull. **2**(5)**:** 136, 1955.
3. Astrup, P.: Ultra-micro-methods for deter-

mining pH, pCO_2 and standard bicarbonate in capillary blood, CIBA Foundation Research Forum, London, Dec. 2-3, 1958.
4. Astrup, P., Siggaard-Andersen, O., Jorgensen, K., and Engel, K.: The acid-base metabolism. A new approach, Lancet **1:** 1035, 1960.
5. Astrup, P.: A new approach to acid-base metabolism, Clin. Chem. **7:** 1, 1961.
6. Bach, J. R.: The Astrup method. A micromethod for determination of pH and other acid-base values in blood, Manual AS 16, Radiometer A/S, Copenhagen, Denmark, 24 pp., 1963.
7. Bain, W. H., and Mackey, W. A.: Extracorporeal circulation, J. Roy. Coll. Surg. Edinb. **5:** 45, 1959.
8. Bakos, A. C. P.: The question of the function of the right ventricular myocardium: An experimental study, Circulation **1:** 724, 1950.
9. Bell, J. W., and Beretta, F. F.: Prolonged ventricular fibrillation. An experimental study in the closed chest animal utilizing a pump-oxygenator, J. Thorac. Cardiovasc. Surg. **38:** 17, 1959.
10. Bernstein, E. F., Castaneda, A. R., Blackshear, P. L., and Varco, R. L.: Prolonged mechanical circulatory support: Analysis of certain physical and physiologic considerations, SURGERY **57:** 103, 1965.
11. Bruner, J. D., Schuhmann, R. E., Geddes, L. A., Hoff, H. E., and Moore, A. G.: An active-valve, vacuum reservoir pump for use with left ventricular bypass without thoracotomy, 21st ACEMB, Nov. 1968, Paper 20.7.
12. Cannard, T. H.: Ventilation and ventilators, *in* Fredericks, L. E., and Morse, D. P., editors: Anesthesia for open heart surgery, Springfield, Ill., 1966, Charles C Thomas, Publisher, pp. 63-70.
13. Clowes, G. H. A., Jr., Cook, W. A., Vujovic, V., and Albrecht, M.: Patterns of circulatory response to the use of respirators, Circulation **31**(Suppl. 1): 157, 1965.
14. Donald, D. E., and Essex, H. E.: Pressure studies after inactivation of major portion of canine right ventricle, Amer. J. Physiol. **176:** 155, 1954.
15. Dubbelman, C. P.: Experiments with an artificial heart-lung apparatus, Acta Physiol. Pharmacol. Neerl. **2:** 465, 1951/2.
16. Edmunds, L. H., Jr., Austen, W. G., Shaw, R. S., and Kozminski, S.: Clinical and physiologic considerations of left heart bypass during cardiac arrest, J. Thorac. Cardiovasc. Surg. **41:** 365, 1961.
17. Gadboys, H. L., Slonin, R., and Litwak, R. S.: Homologous blood syndrome. I. Preliminary observations on its relationship to clinical cardiopulmonary bypass, Ann. Surg. **156:** 793, 1962.
18. Galletti, P. M., and Brecher, G. A.: Heart-lung bypass, New York and London, 1962, Grune & Stratton, Inc., 391 pp.
19. Geddes, L. A., Hickman, D. M., and Moore, A. G.: The impedance pneumograph, Aerospace Med. **33:** 28, 1962.
20. Geddes, L. A., Hoff, H. E., Hickman, D. M., Hinds, M., and Baker, L.: Recording respiration and the electrocardiogram with common electrodes, Aerospace Med. **33:** 791, 1962.
21. Geddes, L. A., and Hoff, H. E.: The measurement of physiologic events by electrical impedance. A review, Amer. J. Med. Electronics **3**(1): 16, 1964.
22. Geddes, L. A.: The transduction of physiological events, *in* Alt, F., editor: Advances in bioengineering and instrumentation, New York, 1966, Plenum Press, Chap. 2, pp. 71-181.
23. Geddes, L. A., Schuhmann, R. E., Hoff, H. E., Moore, A. G., and Peters, J. L.: Total maintenance of circulation in the closed-chest animal with ventricular fibrillation, Cardiovasc. Res. Cent. Bull. **6**(1): 33, 1967.
24. Gibbon, J. H., Jr.: Maintenance of cardiorespiratory functions by extracorporeal circulation. Circulation **19:** 646, 1959.
25. Glenn, W. W. L., and Patina, J. F.: Circulatory bypass of the right side of the heart. I. Preliminary observations on direct delivery of vena caval blood into pulmonary arterial circulation: azygos vein-pulmonary artery shunt, Yale J. Biol. Med. **27:** 147, 1954.
26. Glenn, W. W. L.: Circulatory bypass of the right side of the heart. IV. Shunt between superior vena cava and distal right pulmonary artery, New Eng. J. Med. **259:** 117, 1958.
27. Goodman, L. S., and Gilman, A.: The pharmacological basis of therapeutics, ed. 3, New York, 1965, The Macmillan Company, 1785 pp.
28. Kagan, A.: Dynamic responses of the right ventricle following extensive damage by cauterization, Circulation **5:** 816, 1952.
29. Lefemine, A. A., Bickel, R., Smith, G. T., Lunzer, S., and Harken D. E.: Circulatory arrest. II. Alkalosis in total circulatory arrest of two hours' duration, Angiology **17:** 353, 1966.
30. Maulsby, R. L., and Hoff, H. E.: Hypotensive mechanisms of pulmonary insufflation in dogs, Amer. J. Physiol. **202:** 505, 1962.
31. McGoon, D. C., Moffitt, E. A., Theye, R. A., and Kirklin, J. W.: Physiologic studies during high flow normothermic, whole body perfusion, J. Thorac. Cardiovasc. Surg. **39:** 275, 1960.
32. Osborn, J. J.: Perfusion techniques of car-

diopulmonary bypass, *in* Norman, J. C., editor: Cardiac surgery, New York, 1967, Appleton-Century-Crofts, Inc., pp. 91-98.

33. Robicsek, F., Magistro, R., Foti, E., Robicsek, L., and Sanger, P. E.: Vena cava–pulmonary artery anastomosis for vascularization of the lung, J. Thorac. Surg. **35:** 440, 1958.

34. Robicsek, F., Sanger, P. W., and Taylor, F. H.: Three year follow-up of a patient with transposition of the great vessels, atrial septal defect, and pulmonary stenosis treated by vena cava–pulmonary artery anastomosis, J. Thorac. Cardiovasc. Surg. **44:** 817, 1962.

35. Robicsek, F., Sanger, P. W., and Taylor, F. H.: The azygos "steal" syndrome in cava-pulmonary anastomosis, Ann. Surg. **158:** 1007, 1963.

36. Robicsek, F., Sanger, P. W., Taylor, F. H., Najib, A., and Tarana, M.: Complete bypass of the right heart, Amer. Heart J. **66:** 792, 1963.

37. Robicsek, F., Sanger, P. W., and Gallucci, V.: Long term complete circulatory exclusion of the right side of the heart, Amer. J. Cardiol. **18:** 867, 1966.

38. Rose, J. C., Cosimano, S. J., Hufnagel, C. A., and Massullo, E. A.: The effects of exclusion of the right ventricle from the circulation in dogs, J. Clin. Invest. **34:** 1625, 1955.

39. Sanger, P. W., Robicsek, F., and Taylor, F. H.: Vena cava–pulmonary artery anastomosis. III. Successful operation in case of complete transposition of great vessels with interatrial septal defect and pulmonary stenosis, J. Thorac. Cardiovasc. Surg. **38:** 166, 1959.

40. Sanger, P. W., Robicsek, F., Robicsek, L. K., and Galucci, V.: The clinical application of cava-pulmonary anastomosis, Dis. Chest **48:** 145, 1965.

41. Sanger, P. W., Robicsek, F., Taylor, F. H., and Galucci, V.: Observations on partial and complete circulatory exclusion of the right heart, J. Cardiovasc. Surg. **6:** 30, 1965.

42. Schuhmann, R. E., Bruner, J. D., Geddes, L. A., Hoff, H. E., Moore, A. G., and Peters, J. L.: Push-pull active valve pump for total left ventricular bypass in the closed-chest animal, Proc. 20th Ann. SWIEEECO Conf., 1968, pp. 9B1-9B8.

43. Siggard-Andersen, O.: A graphic representation of changes of the acid-base status, Scand. J. Clin. Lab. Invest. **12:** 311, 1960.

44. Siggard-Andersen, O., and Engel, K.: A new acid-base nomogram. An improved method for the calculation of the relevant blood acid-base data, Scand. J. Clin. Lab. Invest. **12:** 177, 1960.

45. Siggaard-Andersen, O.: Sampling and storing of blood for determination of acid-base status, Scand. J. Clin. Lab. Invest. **13:** 196, 1961.

46. Siggaard-Andersen, O.: Acute experimental acid-base disturbances in dogs. An investigation of the acid-base and electrolyte contents of blood and urine, Scand. J. Clin. Lab. Invest. **14** (Suppl. 66): 1, 1961.

47. Siggaard-Andersen, O.: Blood acid-base alignment nomogram. Scales for pH, pCO_2, base excess of whole blood of different hemoglobin concentrations, plasma bicarbonate, and plasma total-CO_2, Scand. J. Clin. Lab. Invest. **15:** 211, 1963.

48. Smith, McK., Geddes, L. A., and Hoff, H. E.: Cardiac output determined by the saline conductivity method using an extra-arterial conductivity cell, Cardiovasc. Res. Cen. Bull. 5(4): 123, 1967.

49. Smith, McK., Geddes, L. A., and Hoff, H. E.: Electrical calibration for the saline-dilution method for cardiac output, Cardiovasc. Res. Cen. Bull. **6**(4): 142, 1968.

50. Starr, I., Jeffers, W. A., and Meade, R. H., Jr.: The absence of conspicuous increments of venous pressure after severe damage to the right ventricle of the dog, with a discussion of the relation between clinical congestive failure and heart disease, Amer. Heart J. **26:** 291, 1943.

51. Uhl, H. S. M.: A previously undescribed congenital malformation of the heart: Almost total absence of the myocardium of the right ventricle, Bull. Johns Hopkins Hosp. **91:** 197, 1952.

52. Wintrobe, M. M.: Clinical hematology, ed. 6, Philadelphia, 1967, Lea & Febiger, Publishers, 1287 pp.

53. Zaus, E. A., and Kearns, W. M., Jr.: Massive infarction of the right ventricle and atrium. Report of a case, Circulation **6:** 593, 1952.

54. Zwart, H. H. J.: Doctoral dissertation. Complete left heart bypass without thoracotomy; An experimental study in dogs, Unpublished, Amsterdam, 1967.

55. Zwart, H. H. J., Kralios, A., Collan, R., and Kolff, W. J.: Transarterial closed-chest left ventricular (TaCLV) bypass and coronary flow, 8th ICMBE, July 1969, Paper 26-7.

Circulating lymphocyte depletion: Effect on renal allograft survival in calves

JAY C. FISH, M.D.
KENNETH R. T. TYSON, M.D.
GERALD A. BEATHARD, M.D.
HARRY E. SARLES, M.D.
AUGUST R. REMMERS, JR. M.D.
STEPHAN E. RITZMANN, M.D.
GALVESTON, TEXAS
From the Departments of Surgery, Pathology, and Medicine, The University of Texas Medical Branch and Shriners Burns Institute

Improved survival of skin allografts in rats following lymph drainage was demonstrated in 1964 by McGregor and Gowans.[7] Franksson[5] used the same technique to prepare a patient for renal allografting. Since these initial efforts were made, a number of investigators have studied the effects of lymphocyte depletion upon allograft survival. Some improvement in survival of allografts was demonstrated in several animal species after five to ten days of lymph depletion. In the clinical studies, it has been difficult to assess the effect of the lymph fistula because the patients were also given immunosuppressive agents.[6, 9]

A small series of patients with chronic thoracic duct fistulas have now been studied at this institution.[4] Pretransplant depletion of lymphocytes by the technique described in this paper eliminated the need for other immunosuppressive therapy during the first three to seven weeks after a cadaveric renal allograft. Azathioprine and prednisone were given at maintenance dosage at the time of discharge from the hospital or when acute rejection was suspected.

In this study, the single effect of depletion of lymphocytes upon the survival of unmatched renal allografts was evaluated in calves. The results indicate that little effect is achieved with pretransplant depletion for seven days, but a marked improvement in survival may follow 14 days of the pretransplant lymphocyte depletion.

METHODS

The techniques for housing, administration of anesthesia, and cannulation of the thoracic duct were previously reported.[2] Briefly, Hereford calves weighing from 100 to 200 kilograms were restrained in stanchions. Fluothane anesthesia was administered with the use of a cuffed endotracheal tube. The thoracic duct was isolated at the base of the left side of the neck and cannulated with a Silastic catheter. Two venous tributaries were similarly cannulated with Silastic catheters for intravenous infusions. Lymph was collected in sterile 12 L. glass flasks to which heparin was added. The lymphocytes were removed in a continuous flow centrifuge[3] and the cell-free lymph was reinfused each day.

Lymphocytes in fasting lymph were counted daily by means of a hemocytometer. Blood lymphocytes were counted three times weekly by the same technique. Serum and lymph proteins were measured weekly by a

Supported in part by National Institutes of Health grants AM-11143-03, AM-13114-03, and AI-09278-01 and the Moody Foundation.

Submitted for publication Aug. 8, 1969; resubmitted Nov. 20, 1969.

refractometer. The various protein fractions were separated and quantitated by microzonal electrophoresis.

Following transplantation, blood was analyzed three times a week for urea nitrogen, creatinine, sodium, potassium, and osmolarity. Twenty-four hour collections of urine from the transplanted kidney were analyzed for volume, sediment, osmolarity, sodium, potassium, and creatinine.

Lymph nodes were removed for histological study at the time the thoracic duct cannulas were inserted and at the time of transplantation. Complete autopsies were performed at the time when the animal died or was put to death.

The kidney transplant was biopsied within one hour after establishing vascular perfusion, and serially thereafter. All transplants were biopsied on the day the animal died or was killed. Biopsies were obtained percutaneously with a modified Menghini needle. In Group I, five animals received transplants after seven days of depletion of lymphocytes. Depletion was continued in some animals for as long as 18 days after transplantation (Table I). In Group II, the transplants were performed after 14 days of depletion. Post-transplant depletion was continued for as long as 7 days.

Unrelated donor and recipient calves were matched only by blood cross match compatibility. The donor kidney was perfused and cooled prior to implantation. The animals were operated upon in pairs with each animal serving as the other's donor. In all but three calves, the kidney was placed in the right side of the neck of the recipient. The renal artery was anastomosed end-to-end to the carotid artery and the renal vein placed end-to-side to the jugular vein. The ureter was cannulated with a Silastic catheter and connected to a sterile collection flask.

The recipient's own kidneys were removed in stages. Usually one kidney was used in paired operations as a donor kidney. After recovery from this operation, the second kidney was removed.

RESULTS

Two lymph fistulas in each group failed to drain following the transplantation procedure. In the remainder of the animals the fistulas functioned for 3 to 18 days. Those that drained less than 21 days became occluded and could not be restarted and those that drained 21 or more days were electively discontinued (Table I). There was no significant difference in the average lymph flow

Table I

	Lymph flow		*Lymphocyte counts (per mm.^{3})*				*Lymphocytes removed (×10^9)*		*Transplant function*	
			Lymph		*Blood*					
	Total days	*L./day (avg.)*	*Day 0*	*Day Tx*	*Day 0*	*Day Tx*	*Pre Tx*	*Total*	*(days)*	*Cause of failure*
Group I										
27	10	11.4	60,000	1,030	3,590	1,455	1,302	302	0	Obst. ureter
38	13	23.1	15,100	2,020	1,850	1,350	644	796	5	Pulmonary
40	25	12.5	58,000	3,480	3,800	970	864	1,390	14	Rejection
42	16	18.7	26,500	2,860	2,290	970	870	1,175	4	Rejection
44	6	7.3	34,000	1,140	2,060	1,020	482	482	6	Rejection
Group II										
29	21	11.8	36,900	1,950	4,090	1,290	1,060	1,167	2	Vas. occlusion
37	19	15.3	32,800	1,100	3,500	1,030	780	911	315	Alive
41	21	14.4	40,000	1,500	2,420	1,200	966	1,099	21	Obst. ureter
43	14	12.6	16,800	920	1,970	1,420	682	682	95	Obst. ureter
46	21	8.5	25,000	1,280	3,340	660	949	980	11	Obst. ureter
47	12	10.0	20,000	2,420	2,310	960	802	802	0	Obst. ureter
51	21	13.2	47,700	1,760	4,430	730	929	1,061	14	Obst. ureter
57	21	12.2	22,220	2,200	4,800	1,030	664	763	60	Alive

per day between Group I (14.6 L./day) and Group II (12.3 L./day).

The rate of decline of lymph lymphocytes was relatively constant for each animal although the initial lymphocyte count in lymph ranged between 16,800 and 60,000/mm.[3] The average initial lymphocyte count was 38,720 for Group I and 31,400/mm.[3] for Group II. These figures are within the normal range established from previous studies.[2] During the first 5 days of drainage a very rapid decline occurred in the lymphocyte count (Table I and Fig. 1). There was no significant difference in the lymph lymphocyte count between Group I and II at the time of transplantation or on the last day of lymph drainage.

Since the lymphocyte counts in lymph decline rapidly during the first five days and stabilized at a relatively low level, there was little difference between the two groups in the calculated number of cells removed prior to transplantation or in the total number of cells removed.

Blood lymphocyte counts generally declined coincident with lymphocyte depletion, but to a lesser degree and with less regularity than in the lymph (Fig. 1).

The lymph nodes, spleen and gut showed marked depletion of the thymic dependent areas in all animals that were sacrificed or biopsied in this study. These changes were documented in a previous report.[1]

In the Group I animals transplanted after 7 days of depletion of lymphocytes, one graft failed to function due to obstruction of the ureteral catheter (Table I). Another animal died on day 5 with extensive pneumonitis and massive pleural effusions. The transplanted kidney functioned well up to death and there was no histological evidence of rejection at the time of autopsy. The transplants in the remaining three animals ceased to function on days 4, 6 and 14 respectively. The cause of allograft failure was rejection.

In the Group II animals transplanted after 14 days of lymphocyte depletion, one graft was lost on the second day from thrombosis of the renal artery and vein. Five other animals lost their transplants due to obstruction of the ureteral catheter and recurrent

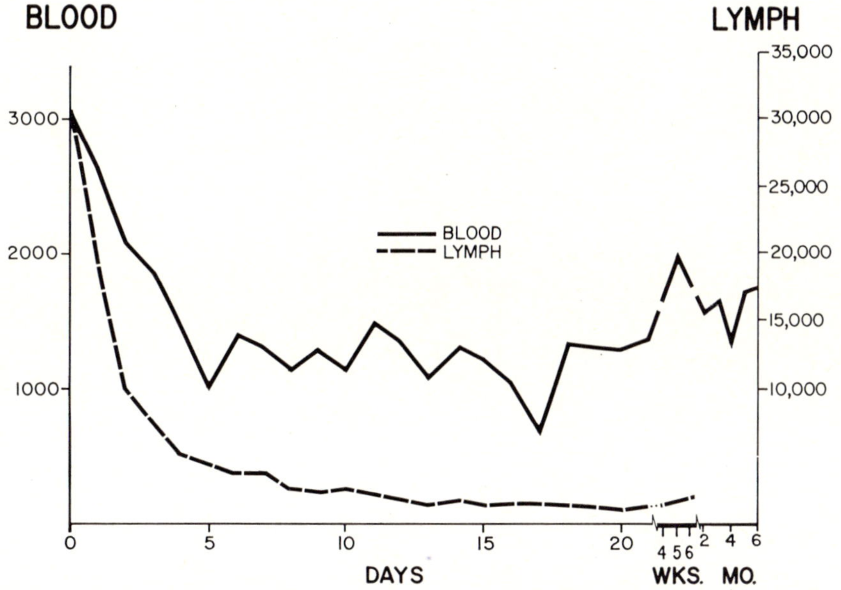

Fig. 1. This curve depicts the average daily blood and lymph lymphocyte counts for 13 calves undergoing lymphocyte depletion via a thoracic duct fistula. Lymph drainage was terminated after 21 days.

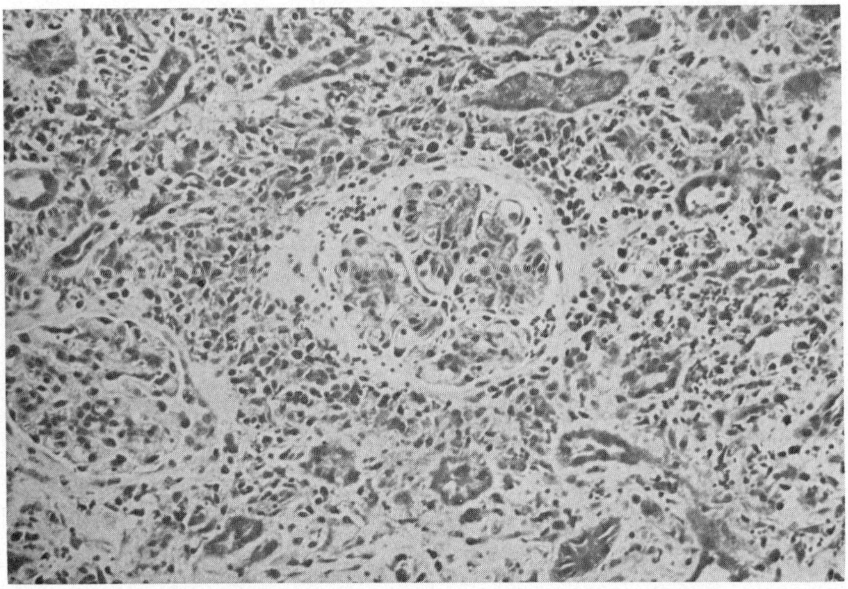

Fig. 2. Biopsy of renal transplant in Group I calf. Note the interstitial edema. A marked lymphocytic infiltrate is present in the interstitium and in the periglomerular region. (800×, hematoxylin and eosin.)

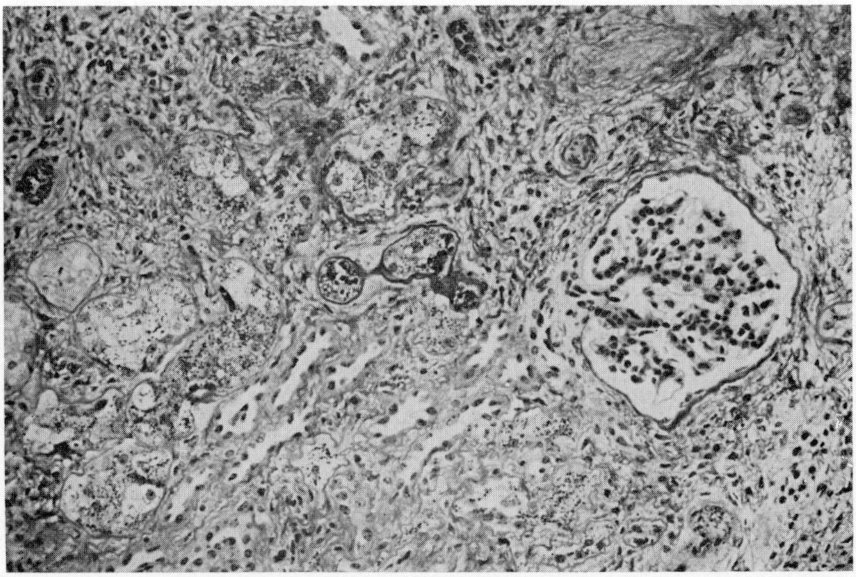

Fig. 3. The biopsy of renal transplant in calf 37 (Group II) on day 100 demonstrates interstitial fibrosis with tubular atrophy and a paucity of mononuclear cells. (800×, periodic acid methenamine with hematoxylin and eosin counter stain.)

pyelonephritis. Survival in these animals was 0, 11, 14, 21 and 95 days respectively.

Two animals were alive 60 and 315 days after transplantation. In the latter calf, the kidney has suffered four episodes of ureteral obstruction with pyelonephritis. On day 247, the ureteral catheter was removed and a dependent cutaneous ureterostomy was constructed.

Serial needle biopsies were taken from the grafts that survived for more than 7 days. The characteristic features of cellular rejection were observed in the last three animals of Group I (Fig. 2). The histological evaluation of serial biopsies of animals in Group II consisted primarily of lymphocytes attached to the endothelial lining of peritubular capillaries and an interstitial lymphocyte infiltrate. The transplants that survived for long periods of time developed interstitial fibrosis, intimal proliferation in small arteries, and a mild increase in glomerular cellularity (Fig. 3). All of these changes fluctuated from one biopsy to the next, except for the vascular and interstitial changes which were progressive. Interpretation of the histological changes were complicated by severe pyelonephritis which occurred in several of the kidneys that survived for more than a few days.

Serum proteins characteristically fell after the first day of drainage, reflecting the initial loss of lymph collected for centrifugation. The protein fractions stabilized after the initial drop. In calves 37 and 43, a remarkable increase in the gamma globulin fraction occurred after transplantation. The hypergammaglobulinemia persisted until a second and fatal episode of pyelonephritis in calf 43 and persisted at this time in calf 37.

DISCUSSION

The responses of blood and lymph lymphocytes to lymph lymphocyte depletion were similar in the animals reported in this study to an initial group of animals that were depleted, but not transplanted.[2] The prior studies document the depletion of circulating lymphocytes from lymph, blood, lymph nodes, spleen and gut. Studies of the thymus histology were not conclusive.

Because the lymphocyte counts in lymph are greater in the calf than in many other animals or man, marked depletion of lymphocytes can be produced rapidly in the calf.

The sterile collection, centrifugation and reinfusion of lymph permits the continuous collection of lymph over prolonged periods without interfering with serum protein or immunoglobulin levels.[6]

Despite the many technical difficulties in this study, it is apparent that profound depletion of lymph lymphocytes prior to transplantation favorably affects allograft survival. The average survival of renal allografts in unmodified calves is 4 days.[8] Little prolongation of allograft survival is achieved if it is introduced early in the course of lymphocyte depletion. Indicators of the optimal time for allotransplantation were not apparent in this study except for duration of the depletion prior to transplantation.

In the calves of Group I, allograft rejection occurred, but later than would be expected from survival date in unmodified calves. In Group II, long term survival was observed except in transplants lost from causes other than rejection. All of these allografts showed histological evidence of the rejection process, but of a low grade.

These findings suggest that lymphocyte depletion delays the rejection process and reduces the intensity of the reaction. This indicates that a quantitative rather than a qualitative change has occurred in the process of cellular rejection. There is no evidence to suggest that humorally mediated rejection mechanisms were altered. The rejection process as judged by the presence of a lymphocytic infiltrate, fluctuated as seen in serial biopsies in the allografts that survived for several months. This finding indicates that the histological evidence of cellular rejection may disappear without the influence of immunosuppressive agents.

If the problem of ureteral obstruction and pyelonephritis can be eliminated, the evaluation of allograft survival will be facilitated.

The culprit, of course, is the foreign body ureteral catheter. Early attempts with intra-abdominal placement of the renal allograft were complicated by the technical difficulties of obtaining exposure of the aorta, vena cava, and bladder in the calf. The last transplant in Group II was placed in the abdomen with the ureter anastomosed to the recipient's ureter. This animal has not had a urinary tract infection during the first eight weeks of observation. Further confirmation of these data is underway with renal allografts placed intra-abdominally.

At the present, one can only speculate about the immunological changes that occurred in these animals between the 7th and 14th days of depletion which permitted the long term survival of the allografts in the latter group. The only constant factor with a demonstrable effect was the duration of pre-transplant depletion of lymphocytes. The sequential changes in morphological and functional characteristics that occurred in the circulating lymphocytes are to be reported separately.

The experiences with the first five patients at the University of Texas Medical Branch prepared for renal allotransplantation by means of depletion of lymph lymphocytes were reported in 1969.[4] One patient receiving an ABO incompatible kidney suffered immediate hyperacute rejection. The other four patients were depleted for 39 to 108 days and tolerated their grafts without rejection crises or immunosuppressive drugs for 19 to 50 days following transplantation. After that, maintenance dosages of prednisone and azathioprine were begun and there have been no acute rejection crises.

Three subsequent patients were transplanted after 10 to 14 days of lymphocyte depletion. In two, the graft failed to function and the patients died within two weeks. The third patient survived but after five weeks he had a clear-cut acute rejection crises and eventually lost his transplant. Since that time, six patients have had at least 28 days of depletion prior to transplantation. One of the kidneys was lost with hyperacute rejection and the other five were well.

It is conclusive that depletion of lymphocytes via a thoracic duct fistula is an effective method for preparing patients for cadaveric organ transplants.

SUMMARY

Thirteen calves were prepared by either one week or two weeks of lymphocyte depletion via a continuously draining thoracic duct fistula. All lymph was reinfused after removal of the cells. Marked lymphocyte depletion was demonstrated within five days in the lymph, blood and lymphoid tissues. Renal allografts failed to survive beyond 14 days in the animals depleted for 7 days prior to transplant, regardless of the duration of depletion after transplantation.

Four of eight calves with 14 days of depletion survived for 21, 60, 95 and 315 days. Two of these animals died from urinary tract infections and two were alive at 60 and 315 days. The four other animals in this group lost their grafts from urinary tract infections and ureteral obstruction.

Analysis of data between the two groups of blood and lymph lymphocyte counts, number of cells removed, lymph flow rates, and lymphoid tissue morphology did not reveal any significant differences. The single determinate of prolonged graft survival was the duration of depletion of lymphocytes prior to allotransplantation.

Experiences with the depletion of lymph lymphocytes in 14 patients support these observations.

REFERENCES

1. Fish, J. C., Beathard, G., Sarles, H. E., Remmers, A. R., Jr., and Ritzmann, S. E.: Circulating lymphocyte depletion. Effect on lymphoid tissue, Surgery. In press.
2. Fish, J. C., Mattingly, A. T., Ross, M. V., Abston, S., Ritzmann, S. E., Sarles, H. E., and Remmers, A. R., Jr.: Circulating lymphocyte depletion in the calf. Effect on blood and lymph lymphocytes, Arch. Surg. **99:** 664, 1969.
3. Fish, J. C., Ross, M. V., Sarles, H. E., and Remmers, A. R., Jr.: Separation of lymphocytes from lymph by continuous flow centrifugation, Surgery **65:** 789, 1969.
4. Fish, J. C., Sarles, H. E., Remmers, A. R., Jr., Tyson, K. R. T., Canales, C. O., Beathard,

G. A., Fukushima, M., Ritzmann, S. E., and Levin, W. C.: Circulating lymphocyte depletion in preparation for renal allotransplantation, Surg. Gynec. Obstet. **128:** 777, 1969.

5. Franksson, C.: Letter to the Editor, Lancet **1:** 1331, 1964.
6. Franksson, C., editor: Kidney transplantation, Stockholm, 1968, Almqvist & Wiksell.
7. McGregor, D. D., and Gowans, J. C.: Survival of homografts of skin in rats depleted of lymphocytes by chronic drainage from the thoracic duct, Lancet **1:** 629, 1964.
8. Short, C. E., Cragle, R. G., Stone, W. H., Zukoski, C. F., and Swanson, E. W.: Techniques for successful renal transplants in cattle, Amer. J. Vet. Res. **28:** 1799, 1967.
9. Tilney, N. L., and Murray, J. E.: The thoracic duct fistula as an adjunct to immunosuppression in human renal transplantation, Transplantation **5:** 1204, 1967.

Reduction of postoperative thrombocytosis

PAUL ATKINS, M.S., F.R.C.S.*
ROBERT E. LEMPKE, M.D.
INDIANAPOLIS, IND.
From the Surgical Service, Veterans Administration Hospital and the Department of Surgery, Indiana University Medical Center

After an operation, the number of circulating blood platelets increases. Many investigators believe that this increase is a significant factor in causing postoperative thromboembolism.[2, 9, 10] The rise has variously been ascribed to tissue damage[10] and stress.[6] In a previous study, we[1] suggested that lowered arterial oxygen tensions seen after operation might also be etiologically related to this rise, because experimentally, a 24 hour period of hypoxia was found to produce a sustained elevation in the platelet count. This paper now describes an experimental attempt to modify this postoperative thrombocytosis by exposure to an oxygen-enriched atmosphere.

METHODS AND MATERIALS

Thirty-two rabbits were divided into two groups of sixteen. Four rabbits at a time were placed in an environmental chamber for 24 hours. After this, they were removed for 20 minutes, during which time a laparotomy was performed. They were then placed in the chamber for a further 24 hours. Alternate subgroups of four rabbits were exposed either to air delivered from a compressed air cylinder (control group) or to oxygen-enriched air (experimental group).

Thirteen other rabbits were studied; eight were exposed to oxygen-enriched air for 48 hours but a laparotomy was not performed, and five were used to study the relationship of arterial oxygen tension to environmental oxygen concentration.

The 32 rabbits of the main study were anesthetized with sodium pentobarbital (64.8 mg. per five pounds of body weight) given intraperitoneally and with ether by inhalation. A 10 cm. midline incision was made, hemostasis was obtained, and the small bowel was run through from the ileocecal junction to the duodenum. The linea alba and skin were each closed with a continuous No. 4-0 silk suture.

The environmental chamber used was as previously described[1] except that urine was absorbed on pelleted cellulose bedding (Pel-E-Cel*). Essentially, it consisted of a polythene-sealed cage into which gas was delivered through a short tube. A small polyethylene tube enabled samples of the chamber atmosphere to be taken and these were measured on a Beckman gas analyzer. Adequate food and water were provided.

Platelet counts were made according to the Sloan's[7] method. They were made immediately before the animals were placed in the chamber and on the third and seventh postoperative days. Counts were also made at corresponding times in the eight rabbits who did not undergo operation.

Blood samples were obtained in five rabbits to measure arterial oxygen tension. A long indwelling catheter filled with heparinized saline was placed in the femoral artery under local anesthesia so that samples could be obtained with the animal in the environ-

Submitted for publication May 1, 1969; resubmitted Jan. 5, 1970.

*Assisted by Wellcome Travel Award.

*Paxton Processing Company, Inc., Paxton, Ill.

mental chamber. These were promptly measured on a Beckman gas analyzer.

RESULTS

Platelet counts. One animal in the experimental group died during the course of the study and has been excluded from consideration. The results of the platelet counts of the remaining 15 rabbits in the experimental group and the 16 rabbits in the control group are shown in Fig. 1. Platelet counts of the control group were elevated after laparotomy was performed. The increase from the preoperative mean count of 516,000 to 771,500 and 743,400 platelets per cubic millimeter on the third and seventh days, respectively, is statistically highly significant by Student's t test ($p < 0.005$). The mean platelet count of the experimental group also rose on the third day, but the increase from 532,300 to 624,900 platelets per cubic millimeter was much smaller and statistically is not significant ($1 > p > 0.05$). On the seventh day the experimental group had a mean count of 528,500 platelets, which was lower than the initial count. The relative reduction in platelet count observed in the experimental group on the third and seventh days is statistically highly significant, ($p < 0.005$). The mean count of the eight rabbits not undergoing surgery but exposed to oxygen-enriched air was initially 500,750 platelets per cubic millimeter. It increased slightly on the third day to 512,250 ($p > 1$) but fell on the

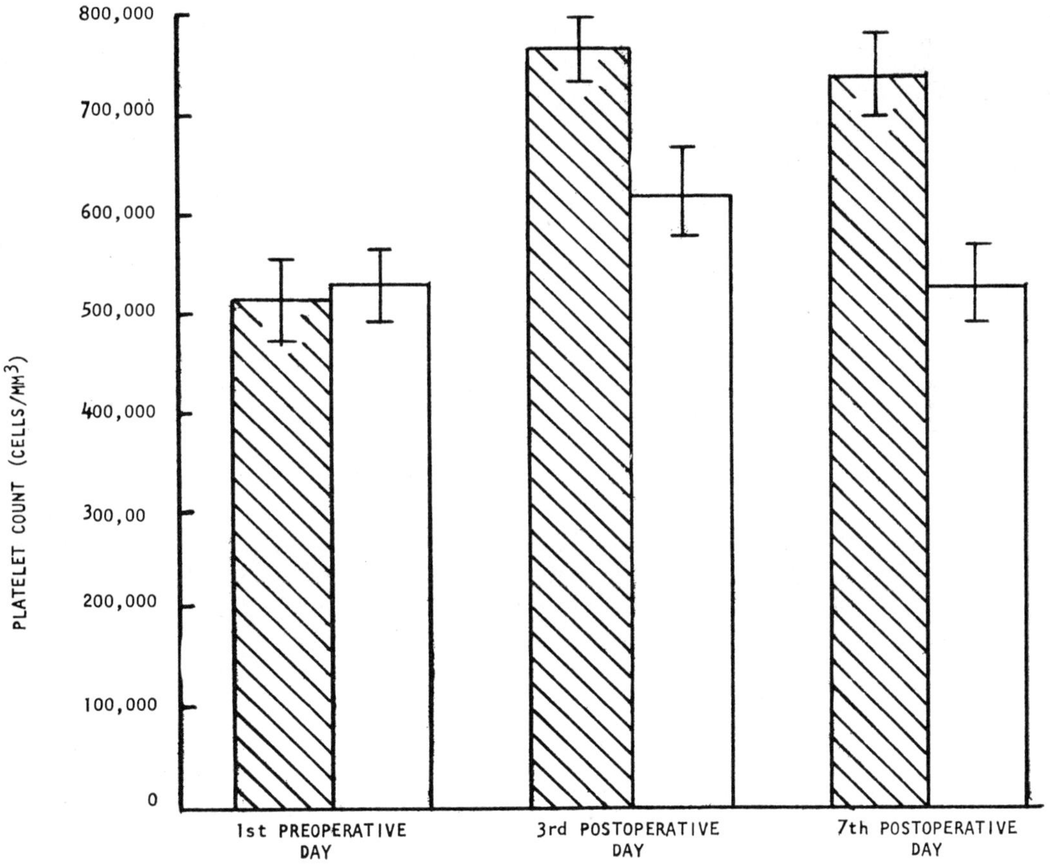

Fig. 1. Mean platelet count with standard error of the mean in rabbits exposed to air (cross-hatched columns) and oxygen-enriched air (open columns) for 24 hours before and after a standard exploratory laparotomy.

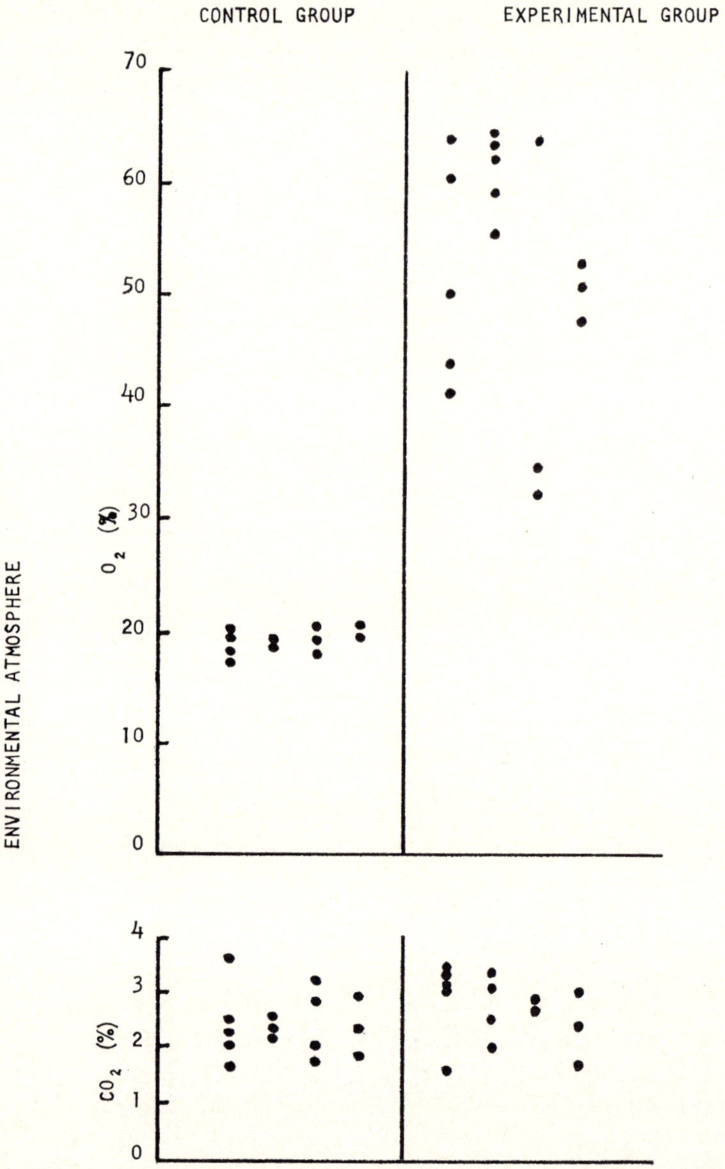

Fig. 2. Oxygen and carbon dioxide concentration of random samples of the atmosphere to which each lot of four rabbits was exposed for 24 hours before and after operation.

seventh day to 441,000 platelets ($1 > p > 0.05$).

Gas samples. Random gas analyses shown in Fig. 2 indicate that the oxygen concentration of the air inspired by the control group was approximately 18.5 percent (range 17.32 to 20.24 percent). In a previous study,[1] ten normal rabbits exposed to this range of oxygen concentration for 24 hours showed a small, statistically nonsignificant fall in the platelet count. The oxygen percentage of the air inspired by the experimental group was approximately 55 percent (range 31.45 to 64.1 percent). The carbon dioxide accumulated to a similar extent in both groups and it ranged from less than 1.40 to 3.69 percent.

Arterial oxygen tension. Arterial oxygen

tensions were measured in four rabbits not submitted to laparotomy but exposed to oxygen-enriched air. Two rabbits had arterial oxygen tensions of 170 and 180 mm. Hg when the atmospheric oxygen concentration was 54.8 percent. Two other rabbits had arterial oxygen tensions of 270 and 255 mm. Hg when the atmospheric oxygen concentration was 66.3 percent. In a rabbit studied during the first four hours after laparotomy arterial oxygen tensions of 170 to 180 mm. Hg were found when the atmosphere within the environmental chamber contained from 43 to 67 percent oxygen.

DISCUSSION

Thromboembolism is a major cause of postoperative morbidity and death.[5] Many factors probably combine to cause venous thrombosis, but the quantitative and qualitative changes which occur in platelets have received particular emphasis.[2, 6, 9] Indeed, detection of such changes has formed an important aspect of attempts to set up discriminatory tests for venous thrombosis.[3, 4] A simple way of modifying the postoperative behavior of platelets might have importance as a prophylactic measure.

Since moderate hypoxia of a degree and duration likely to be met in the postoperative period causes a considerable increase in platelets, it seemed possible that an increase of oxygen in the inspired air might also influence the platelet count. Although there are reports which suggest that oxygen might have a direct depressant effect on red cell production,[8] no information on its effect on platelets has been found in the literature. Our limited study of the effect in the normal rabbit of 55 percent oxygen for 48 hours shows that the platelets increase slightly by the third day but decrease even more by the seventh day. On neither day, however, is the difference from the initial count statistically significant.

The platelet counts made in the control group serve to confirm many previous studies which have shown a thrombocytosis after surgery. Here the counts were substantially the same on the third and seventh postoperative days. In man, an early fall preceding the increase in count has frequently been found. Counts in the early postoperative period are likely to vary, however, since they probably reflect a balance between increased production and increased loss from the circulation.

Increasing the oxygen content of inspired air, though it did not abolish the platelet increase seen on the third postoperative day, did substantially reduce it. It would appear to have had an even greater effect by the seventh postoperative day, when the mean count was fractionally lower than the initial count.

The manner in which oxygen influences platelet production in the postoperative period cannot be stated with certainty. It would seem most likely, however, that the avoidance of hypoxia after laparotomy is the main reason. The possibility that oxygen might exert a direct effect has not been excluded. Although an increased oxygen concentration of the inspired air would only raise the tissue-oxygen tension by a very small amount, the presence of megakaryocytes within the lung suggest the possibility that platelet production might be peculiarly sensitive to the level of oxygen in the inspired air.

The absence of an accurate method for detecting venous thrombosis has made it extremely difficult to evaluate the role of any of the supposed etiological factors in thrombolism. Proponents of the theory that platelets are important are as liable to this criticism as those who view other factors as being etiologically significant. Consequently, although this study has shown that increased O_2 in the inspired air decreases postoperative thrombocytosis, only a cautious hope is entertained that this fact will be found to be relevant to the prophylaxis of thromboembolism.

SUMMARY

A reduction in the postoperative rise of platelets by the use of increased oxygen in the inspired air is described. Fifteen rabbits breathing oxygen-enriched air for 48 hours had significantly lower platelet counts on the third and seventh days after a standardized exploratory laparotomy than did 16 rabbits breathing air.

REFERENCES

1. Atkins, P., and Lempke, R. E.: The effect of hypoxia on the platelet count. In preparation.
2. Dawbarn, R. U. F., Earlam, F., and Evans, W. H.: The relation of the blood platelets to thrombosis after operation and parturition, J. Path. Bact. **31:** 833, 1928.
3. Hume, M.: Platelet adhesiveness and other coagulation factors in thrombophlebitis, SURGERY **59:** 110, 1966.
4. Hume, M.: Blood coagulation in deep and superficial thrombophlebitis, Arch. Surg. **92:** 936, 1966.
5. MaLachlin, J., Richards, T., and Patterson, J. C.: An evaluation of clinical signs in the diagnosis of venous thrombosis, Arch. Surg. **85:** 738, 1962.
6. Pepper, H., and Lindsay, S.: Responses of platelets, eosinophils and leukocytes, Surg. Gynec. Obstet. **110:** 319, 1960.
7. Sloan, A. W.: The normal platelet count in man, J. Clin. Path. **4:** 37, 1951.
8. Tinsley, J. C., Jr., Moore, C. V., Dubach, R., Minnich, V., and Grinstein, M.: The role of oxygen in the regulation of erythropoiesis. Depression of the rate of delivery of new red cells to old blood by high concentration of inspired oxygen, J. Clin. Invest. **28:** 1544, 1949.
9. Wright, H. P.: Changes in the adhesiveness of blood platelets following parturition and surgical operations, J. Path. Bact. **54:** 461, 1942.
10. Wright, H. P.: Changes in number of circulating blood platelets following experimental traumata, J. Obstet. Gynaec. Brit. Comm. **52:** 253, 1945.

Body temperature monitoring via the tympanic membrane

WILLIAM THOMAS DICKEY
E. WARNER AHLGREN, M.D.
C. R. STEPHEN, M.D.
DALLAS, TEXAS
From the Department of Anesthesiology, Children's Medical Center, and University of Texas, Southwestern Medical School

The importance of body temperature monitoring has assumed greater significance recently, especially in the pediatric patient. It is well known that, under anesthesia in a modern air-conditioned operating room, the body temperature tends to fall—the smaller the patient, the greater and more rapid the fall.[7] This change occurs because the normal compensatory mechanisms for regulating body temperature are not active during anesthesia. The value of monitoring body temperature has received new impetus during the past few years with recognition of the syndrome of fulminant hyperthermia, in which for some unexplained reason an occasional patient in the younger age group develops a rapidly progressive, severe hyperthermia which, in most cases reported, has proved irreversible.[6]

Conventionally, body temperature is monitored by either a thermistor or a thermocouple placed in the rectum or the esophagus. The rectum reflects the peripheral temperature, as opposed to the esophagus, which tends to reflect core body temperature; the probe in the esophagus probably follows the temperature of the blood in the heart closely. However, there are certain esthetic objections to monitoring rectal temperature, and it is not always technically easy in the awake or anesthetized patient to insert a probe atraumatically into the esophagus. Therefore, through the years there have been attempts to evaluate the feasibility of monitoring body temperature from other areas, especially the axilla, nasopharynx, and forehead. It is the purpose of this presentation to discuss experiences which have been obtained in monitoring body temperature via the tympanic membrane. The feasibility of this method has been brought into focus by Benzinger and Taylor,[1] who have been interested, in temperature monitoring, as well as other topics, in association with projects of the National Aerospace Administration.

To indicate that the tympanic membrane is an acceptable place to monitor body temperature, one should look briefly at what part of the circulation is being monitored. The arteries of the tympanic membrane are derived from the deep auricular branch of the internal maxillary which ramifies beneath the cutaneous stratum and from both the stylomastoid branch of the posterior auricular and the tympanic branch of the internal maxillary, which are distributed on the mucus surface of the drum. Both the posterior auricular and internal maxillary are direct branches of the external carotid. It is generally believed that the tympanic membrane itself and the immediately surrounding structures have an abundant arteriolar and capillary supply.

As a result of considerable work under well-controlled conditions, Benzinger and Taylor[1] believe that, if a thermocouple is placed in juxtaposition to the tympanic

Submitted for publication Aug. 12, 1969; resubmitted Sept. 19, 1969.

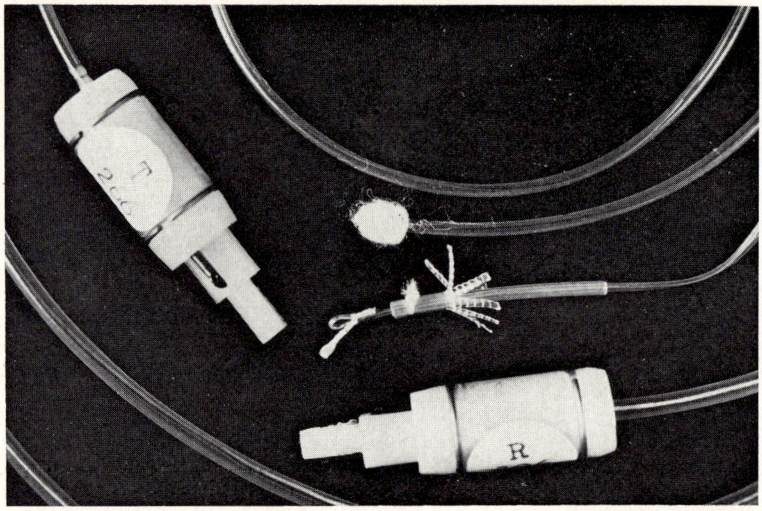

Fig. 1. Two types of tympanic membrane probe, both of which provided similar measurements of temperature.

membrane, it will accurately reflect the temperature of the blood coursing through the brain. Therefore, if one of the aims in monitoring body temperature is to monitor the temperature of blood in the temperature-regulating centers, then this source should be accurate. Animal work by Rawson and Hammel[5] showed that the tympanic membrane temperature closely paralleled the rapid fluctuations in hypothalamic temperature and that it was always below hypothalamic temperature by approximately 0.5° C. On short- and long-term utilization of the tympanic membrane probes, it has been shown that apposition of such a probe against the tympanic membrane is not injurious in man.[3] Simplicity of probe placement is a distinct advantage in this technique.

METHOD OF INVESTIGATION

In a group of 50 patients whose ages ranged from 48 hours to 90 years, body temperature measurements were made from a thermocouple placed against the tympanic membrance, and this source was compared with measurements from the esophagus and rectum. Periods of comparison ranged from two hours or more under anesthesia to 96 hours in patients receiving intensive care. It was shown that this technique of monitoring was stable for relatively long periods of time.

Two types of probes were utilized at the tympanic membrane; both were thermocouple in design (Fig. 1). One tip was of soft plastic looped back on itself. The other was plastic-tipped and covered with absorbent cotton in the manner of a "Q-tip." The rectal and esophagus probe was soft plastic without extra cover. Each thermocouple was connected to a monitoring recorder and the three temperatures being monitored were transcribed directly to a Leeds and Northrup Company* Speedomax continuous writer. In this way, one could compare from moment to moment the temperatures being recorded from the three sources. In all patients, no special preparations were made prior to inserting the tympanic probe. The technique was simply to advance the probe into the ear until resistance was met. Then it was held in place with adhesive tape.

Figs. 2 and 3 are representative of the results obtained in this study. The temperature monitored from the tympanic membrane followed closely that measured in the esophagus.

*Sumney Pike, North Wales, Pa. 19454.

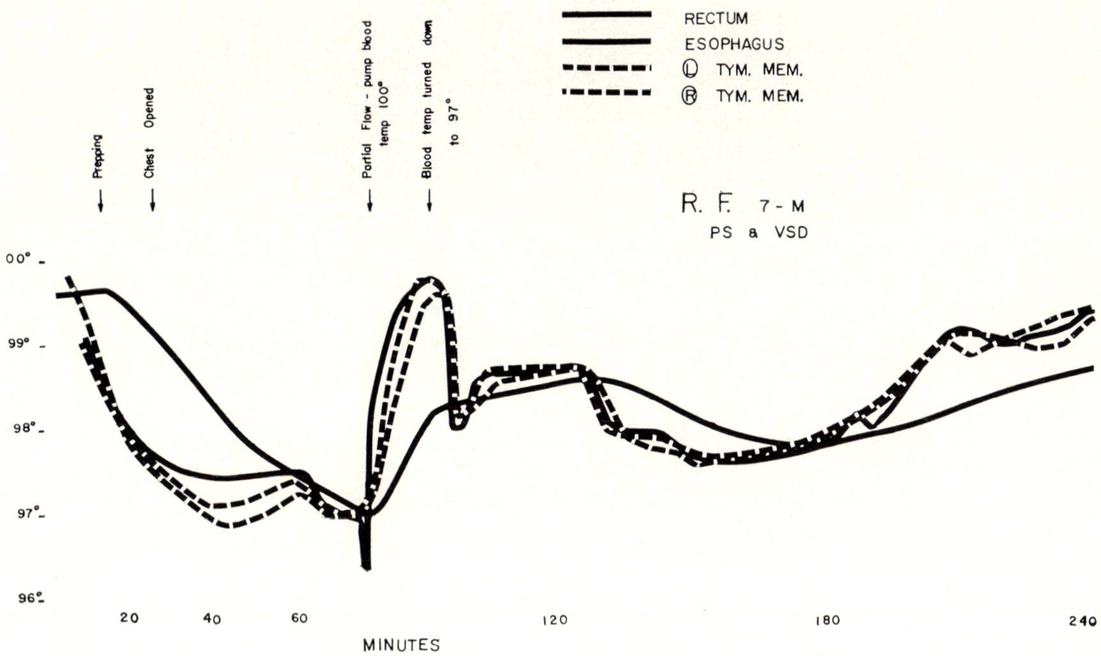

Fig. 2. Simultaneous monitoring of rectal, esophageal, and both tympanic membrane temperatures during repair of a pulmonary stenosis and ventricular septal defect under extracorporeal circulation in a 7-year-old boy. Note (1) the similarity of recordings from each tympanic membrane, (2) the lag in temperature changes recorded from the rectum, and (3) the close parallel between esophageal and tympanic membrane temperatures.

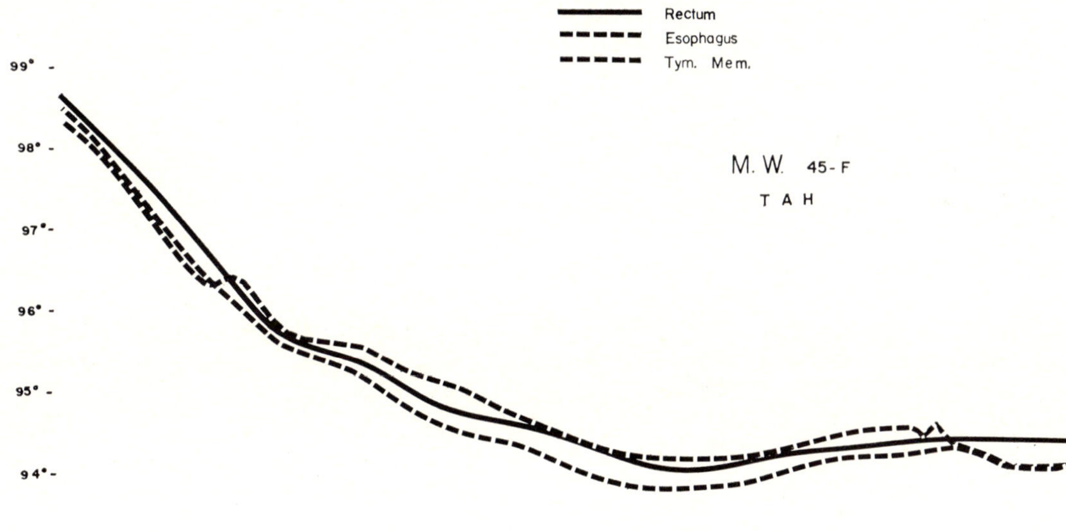

Fig. 3. Simultaneous monitoring of body temperature from rectum, esophagus and tympanic membrane in a 45-year-old woman during a total abdominal hysterectomy under nitrous oxide, oxygen, d-tubocurare, and hyperventilation anesthesia. Note the considerable reduction in body temperature indicated by all three sources.

DISCUSSION

It is our belief that the tympanic membrane is a suitable source clinically for monitoring body temperature during surgery and in patients receiving intensive care. The findings in this study indicate that the tympanic membrane temperature closely reflects that of the esophagus. In this respect, the observations parallel those of Pironen,[4] who compared esophageal and tympanic membrane temperatures in men during hyperthermia investigations. They also confirm the observations of Gibbons,[2] who established a positive correlation between tympanic membrane and oral temperatures in space-craft crews.

The investigative work of Benzinger and Taylor[3] has indicated that changes in tympanic membrane temperature reflect quickly and accurately those occurring in the hypothalamus and other parts of the brain. If one wishes to interpolate that the esophageal temperature accurately monitors the temperature of blood in the heart that is coursing directly to the brain, then it could be argued with merit that in these present investigations the temperature noted from the tympanic membrane also reflects closely the core body temperature and is close to the brain temperature.

This limited experience shows that body temperature can be monitored simply and easily from the tympanic membrane, and the records indicate that changes in body temperature are noted without lag when they develop. In the observations that have been made, the tympanic membrane temperature rarely has been more than 0.5° F. different from that recorded in the esophagus.

Early in the study, when a larger prototype aural probe was being used, two children who were receiving anticoagulant therapy during extracorporeal circulation developed oozing from the ear which persisted for 48 hours. There was no subsequent involvement. Since the employment of smaller probes, there have been no complications with this technique.

SUMMARY

The feasibility of monitoring body temperature by a thermocouple in proximity to the tympanic membrane has been evaluated in 50 patients and compared with simultaneous monitoring from the esophagus and the rectum. The recordings from the tympanic membrane in this study closely paralleled those obtained from the esophagus. The tympanic membrane is considered to be a realiable, practical, and clinically useful means of monitoring body temperature.

REFERENCES

1. Benzinger, T. H., and Taylor, G. W.: Cranial measurements of internal temperature in man. Temperature—its measurement and control in science and industry, New York, 1963, Reinhold Publishing Corporation, vol. 3, pp. 111-121.
2. Gibbons, L. V.: Body temperature monitoring in the external auditory meatus, Aerospace Med. **38:** 671, 1967.
3. Personal communication: Leeds and Northrup Company.
4. Pironen, P.: Effects of exposures to extremely hot environments on temperature of the tympanic membrane, the oesophagus and the rectum of men. Technical Documentary Report, Department of Physiology, Institute of Occupational Health, Helsinki, Finland, 1963.
5. Rawson, R. O., and Hammel, H. T.: Hypothalamic and tympanic membrane temperatures in rhesus monkey, Fed. Proc. **22:** 283, 1963.
6. Stephen, C. R.: Fulminant hyperthermia during anesthesia and surgery, J. A. M. A. **202:** 178, 1967.
7. Stephen, C. R., Dent, S. J., Hall, K. D., Knox, P. R., and North, W. C.: Body Temperature regulation during anesthesia in infants and children, J. A. M. A. **174:** 1579, 1960.

Coronary artery-right ventricular fistula with congestive heart failure: Surgical correction in the neonatal period

THOMAS M. DANIEL, M.D.
THOMAS P. GRAHAM, M.D.
DAVID C. SABISTON, Jr., M.D.
DURHAM, N. C.
From the Departments of Surgery and Pediatrics, Duke University Medical Center

Since the first coronary arteriovenous (A-V) fistula was described by Krause[17] in 1865, nearly 200 examples of this lesion have been reported in the literature. One of the serious complications which may ensue in the presence of this condition is congestive heart failure. Of 150 patients with isolated coronary A-V fistulas, 21 exhibited the clinical manifestations of congestive heart failure—an incidence of 14 percent.[2, 6, 10, 14, 19, 21, 22, 27, 30, 45, 48, 54, 57, 66, 67, 93, 97]

Recently, an infant with an unusually large left coronary–right ventricular fistula has been observed with the onset of congestive heart failure during the first month of life. The interesting features of this patient will be presented in this communication together with a review of those patients described in the literature in whom this lesion was associated with congestive heart failure.

CASE REPORT

E. T. S. (DUMC H1 6 994), a male infant who weighed seven pounds six ounces, was born on Sept. 16, 1967, the product of an uncomplicated pregnancy and delivery. A Grade II/VI continuous murmur was noted in the third and fourth left intercostal spaces at birth. One month later the infant was hospitalized because of persistent tachycardia, tachypnea, and an increase in the intensity of the murmur. The child weighed nine pounds, had a resting pulse rate of 160, and a variable respiratory rate of 40 to 80 per minute. There was a Grade IV/VI harsh, continuous murmur maximum in the third left intercostal space with apical radiation. Both femoral and brachial pulses were bounding. The liver edge was felt 1 cm. below the right costal margin. The electrocardiogram showed probable left atrial enlargement and biventricular hypertrophy (R_{V_2} = 32 mm., S_{V_2} = 34 mm., R_{V_6} = 34 mm.). A chest film demonstrated cardiomegaly, probable left atrial enlargement, and increased pulmonary vasculature (Fig. 1). The clinical impression was a large left-to-right shunt secondary to a patent ductus or an intracardiac A-V fistula with congestive heart failure and the infant was digitalized. Cardiac catheterization performed on Oct. 23, 1967, demonstrated a left-to-right shunt at the ventricular level with a 2.8/1 Qp/Qs ratio, minimal elevation of right-sided pressures, a normal pulmonary vascular resistance, and a wide aortic pulse pressure of 61 mm. Hg (Table I). Internal phonocardiography demonstrated a loud holosystolic murmur continuing into diastole in the right ventricle with no murmur in the pulmonary artery. An ascending aortogram showed a very large coronary A-V fistula from the left anterior descending coronary artery to the right ventricle (Fig. 2). No patent ductus arteriosus was present. Left heart volumes calculated from the levogram phase of a pulmonary artery biplane cineangiocardiogram are presented in Table II. The left ventricular end-diastolic volume and systolic index were both increased to over twice normal, the left ventricular wall mass and left atrial maximal volume were approximately 50 percent above normal, and the left ventricular ejection fraction was within the normal range.

At operation on Oct. 31, 1967, the heart was exposed through a left anterolateral thoracotomy. The anterior descending coronary artery measured 11 mm. in diameter and lay *within* the substance of the myocardium. It passed directly into the right ventricle at the apex and the opening could be palpated with the finger (Fig. 3). By the use of four transfixion ligatures it was possible to obliterate both the thrill and the palpable opening into the ventricular cavity. The postoperative recovery was uneventful and the child has since

Received for publication Nov. 17, 1969.

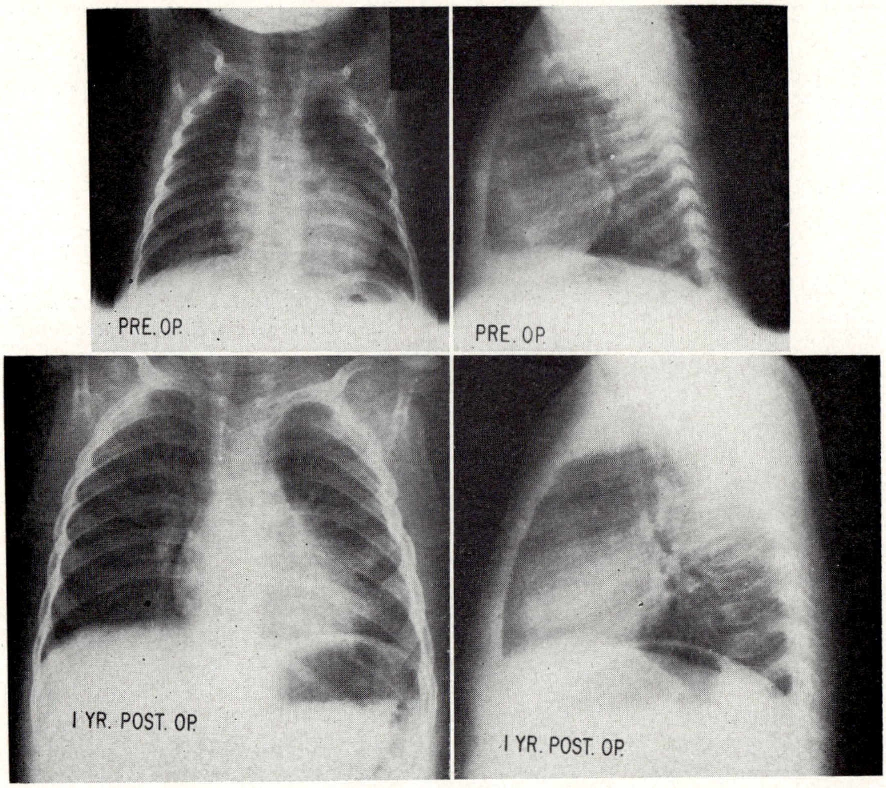

Fig. 1. Preoperative chest x-rays of infant with coronary artery fistula at five weeks of age. Interpretation was biventricular enlargement, left atrial enlargement, and increased pulmonary vasculature. X-rays one year after operation show relative decrease in cardiomegaly.

Table I. *Cardiac catheterization**

Site	*Percent O_2 saturation*	*Pressure (mm. Hg)*
Superior vena cava	76	
Right atrium	73	$\overline{2}$
Right ventricle	83	44/5
Pulmonary artery	87	40/18 $\overline{26}$
Aorta	95	108/47 $\overline{73}$
Left ventricle		105/10

*Left-to-right shunt, 64 percent. Qp/Qs, 2.8. Rp/Rs, 0.13.

remained well. The continuous murmur has been replaced by a well-localized Grade II/VI short systolic murmur in the third left intercostal space. The chest film shows a decrease in relative heart size (Fig. 1).

DISCUSSION

The finding of frank congestive heart failure in cases with a coronary artery fistula as

Table II. *Left heart volume data*

	Values in this patient	*Normal values*[40]
Left ventricular end-diastolic volume	92/c.c./M.^{2}	45 ± 9
Left ventricular ejection fraction	0.78	0.76 ± 0.07
Left ventricular systolic index	11.25 L./min./M.^{2}	4.51 ± 0.88
Left ventricular wall mass	114 Gm./M.^{2}	82 ± 10
Left atrial maximal volume	51 c.c./M.^{2}	34 ± 10

the sole cardiovascular anomaly has been described in 21 of 150 patients, representing an incidence of 14 percent (Table III). Nine additional cases with an isolated coronary artery fistula were excluded because the data reported were insufficient to assess the pres-

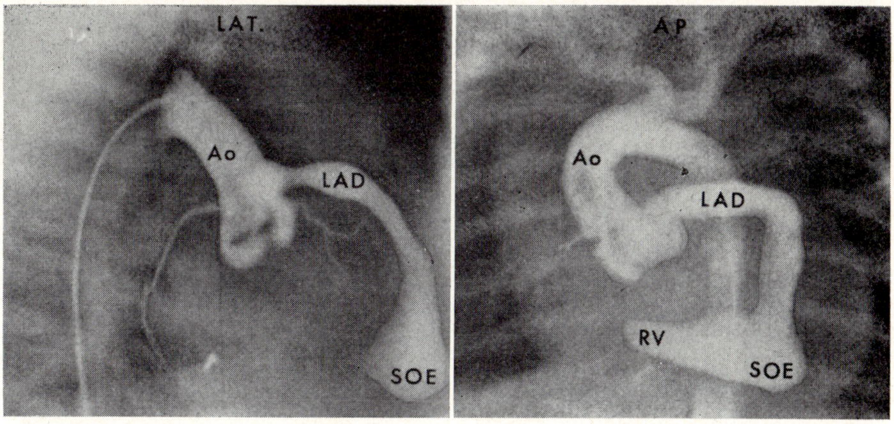

Fig. 2. Ascending aortogram of left coronary artery–right ventricular fistula showing lateral and anteroposterior views. *Ao,* Aorta; *LAD,* left anterior descending coronary artery; *SOE,* site of entry of fistula into the right ventricle; *RV,* incompletely opacified right ventricle.

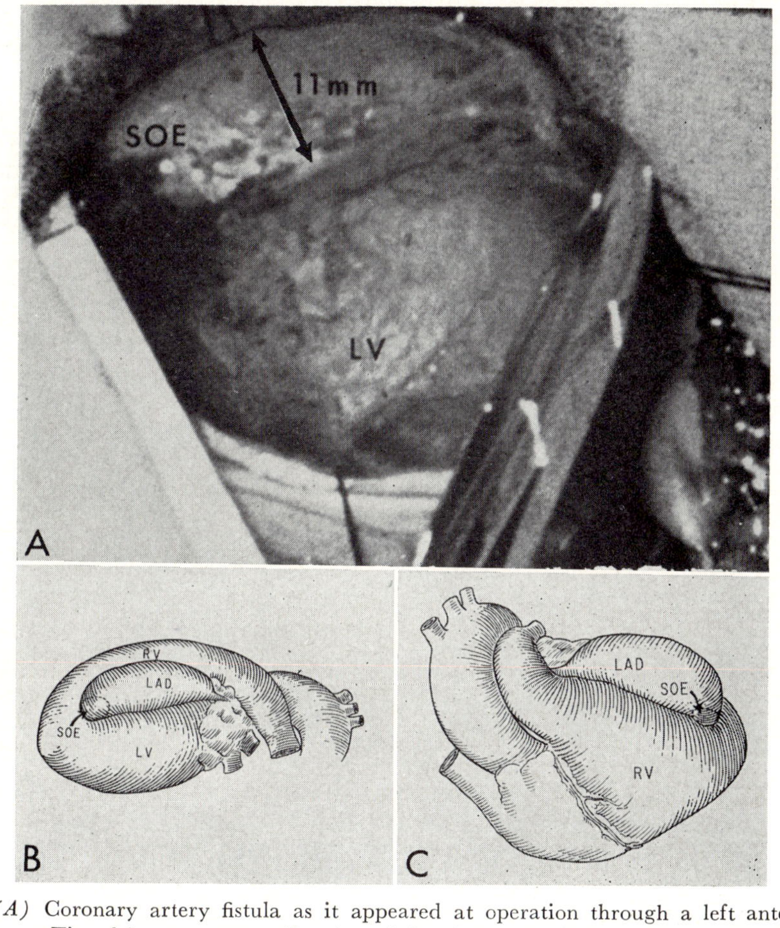

Fig. 3. *(A)* Coronary artery fistula as it appeared at operation through a left anterolateral thoracotomy. Tip of instrument overlies the origin of the anterior descending coronary artery which lay within the myocardium. Note the diameter of the artery, which is 11 mm. *SOE,* Site of entry of fistula into the apex of the right ventricle; *LV,* left ventricle; *LAD,* left anterior descending coronary artery; *RV,* right ventricle. *(B)* Sketch of heart as seen through left anterolateral thoracotomy. *(C)* Sketch of coronary artery fistula and right ventricle.

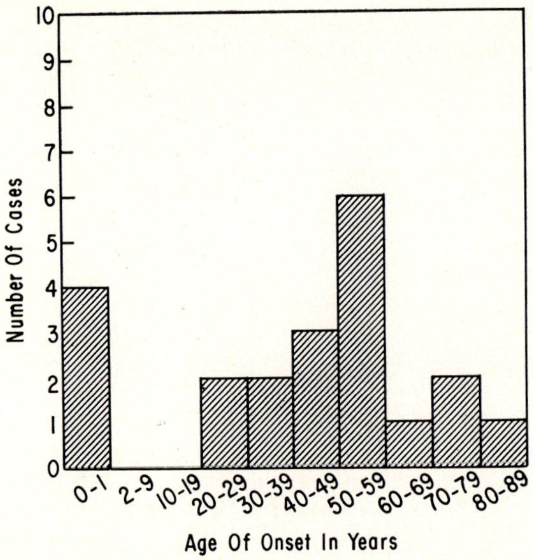

Fig. 4. Age of onset of congestive heart failure in patients with an isolated coronary artery fistula.

Table III. *Major presenting clinical pictures of coronary artery fistulas when present as sole cardiac anomaly*

	No. of cases	*Percent of total*
Asymptomatic murmur	67	45
Dyspnea on exertion, fatigue	34	22
Congestive heart failure	21	14
Angina or nonspecific chest pain	10	7
Bacterial endocarditis	9	6
Frequent upper respiratory infections	9	6
Total	150	

ence or absence of failure.[7, 17, 37, 45] It is interesting that approximately half of all cases of isolated A-V fistula were symptomatic. Of the 67 totally asymptomatic cases reported, 45 underwent surgical correction with no operative deaths.[4, 9, 14, 18, 20, 22, 26, 31, 32, 34-36, 41, 44, 46, 47, 49, 50, 53, 56, 58-60, 64, 67-76, 79, 83, 85, 89, 94]

Examination of the patients with congestive failure reveals a maximum distribution in the fifth and sixth decades (Fig. 4). Although there were four patients in the first year of life, there is a striking absence of this complication from the age of one to 20.

Three of the cases of heart failure in infants with coronary artery fistula were reported by Cooley and Ellis.[22] One of these was a 5-month-old boy who developed failure and pulmonary edema at one month. At operation, at 5 months of age, the fistula was not anticipated nor visualized and a pulmonary artery banding was performed. The infant died the day after the operation and the right coronary artery–right ventricular fistula was found at autopsy. Another infant died at the age of 2½ years after a course of intractable failure beginning at the age of 6 weeks. At autopsy a left coronary artery–right ventricular fistula with subendocardial fibroelastosis of the left ventricle and a patent foramen ovale were demonstrated. The third infant had onset of congestive failure at the age of 5 months. She responded to digitalization and at the age of 4 years successful ligation of a right coronary artery–right ventricular fistula was performed.

Our patient is the second one reported with congestive failure occurring in the first month of life and the first to undergo successful surgical treatment while still an infant. The demonstration of large increases in left atrial maximal volume and in left ventricular end-diastolic volume, systolic output, and wall mass at age five weeks attests to the large left-to-right shunt produced by the fistula and documents the remarkable myocardial response to the lesion during infancy.

Of the 21 patients described in the literature with congestive heart failure, eight underwent operative closure of the fistula and each survived. The rarity of failure in infants with this anomaly is apparent when it is noted that only four of 150 patients in this series developed failure in the first year of life. In contrast, the childhood morbidity and mortality rates of coronary artery fistula in the presence of additional cardiac anomalies are high. Of 22 infants reported, 16 died

Table IV. *Congestive heart failure (CHF) with coronary arteriovenous fistulas*

Case No.	*Age at onset of CHF*	*Sex*	*Origin of fistula**	*Termination of fistula†*	*Operation*	*Result*	*Reference*
1	60	F	RCA	Right coronary vein	None	Died age 62, CHF	57
2	76	F	LCA	PA	None	Died age 76, CHF	10
3	84	M	RCA	RA	None	Died age 85, CHF	21
4	57	F	LCA	RA	None	Palpitations age 48; atrial fibrillation age 57; died age 58, CHF	27
5	55	M	LCA	?	None	Hypertension and CHF; died age 55, subarachnoid hemorrhage	54
6	21	F	RCA	RA	Exploratory thoracotomy	Palpitations age 17; fistula not treated at operation; died age 25, CHF	93
7	56	F	LCA	RV	Ligation	Operation age 56 with disappearance of murmur; persistent CHF	66
8	48	F	RCA	RA	None	Died age 53, CHF	30
9	53	F	LCA	PA	Excision fistulous mass	Operation age 53; alive and well	6
10	30	F	RCA LCA	RA Great cardiac vein	None	Died age 43, CHF	19
11	75	F	RCA	Coronary sinus	None	Atrial fibrillation; died age 75, CHF	97
12	53	F	LCA	PA	Yes	Operation age 53; alive and well	67
13	43	M	LCA	RA	None	Died age 43, CHF	67
14	5 mo.	F	RCA	RV	Ligation	Digitalized age 5 mo.; surgery age 4; alive and well	22
15	6 wk.	F	LCA	RV	None	Died age 2½, CHF	22
16	5 mo.	M	RCA	RV	PA band	Died 1 day after operation; fistula discovered at autopsy	22
17	31	M	RCA	RV	None	Died age 31, CHF	48
18	40	F	RCA	RA	Ligation, division	Surgery age 40; alive and well	14
19	20	?	RCA	RV	Yes	Surgery age 20; alive and well	45
20	51	M	RCA	RV	Ligation, division	Surgery age 51; alive and well	2
21	4 wk.	M	LCA	RV	Ligation	Surgery age 6 wk; alive and well	Present case

*RCA, Right coronary artery; LCA, left coronary artery.
†PA, Pulmonary artery; RA, right atrium; RV, left ventricle.

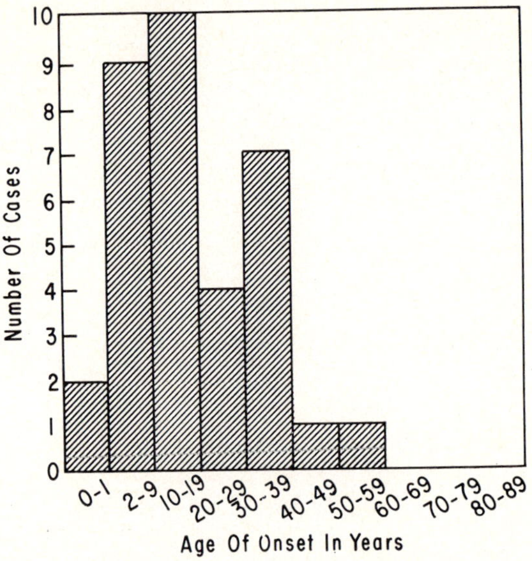

Fig. 5. Age of onset of dyspnea on exertion or fatigue in patients with an isolated coronary artery fistula.

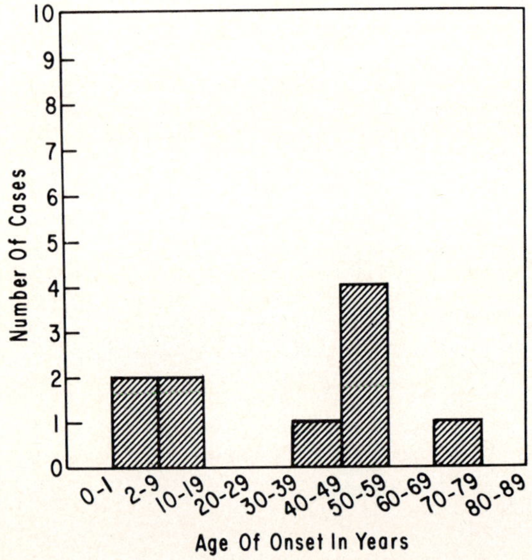

Fig. 6. Age of onset of angina or chest pain in patients with an isolated coronary artery fistula.

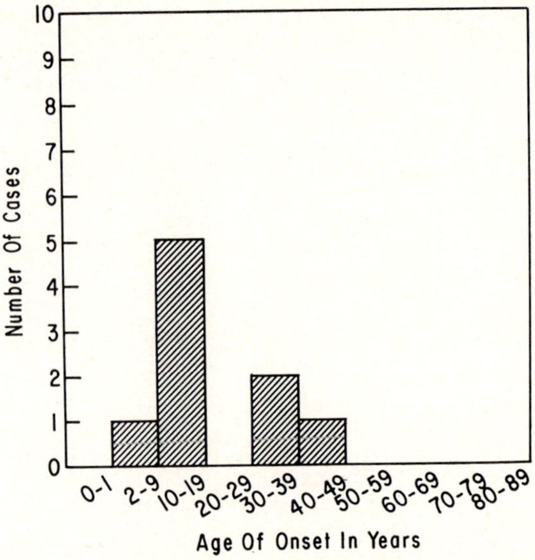

Fig. 7. Age of onset of bacterial endocarditis in patients with an isolated coronary artery fistula.

by the third year of life.[5, 8, 11, 14-16, 23, 25, 28, 42, 51, 55, 59, 62, 78, 80, 82, 95, 96]

A review was made of the anatomic features in those patients who developed congestive heart failure (Table IV). Whereas fistulous connections do occur with the left atrium and ventricle, all patients with failure had connections to the right side of the heart. In other words, no patient with a left-to-left shunt as the result of a coronary artery fistula has been reported to develop cardiac failure. Moreover, each of the four cases of failure in infants with this anomaly occurred with fistulas that entered the *right ventricle.*

An examination was made of all case reports of patients who presented with dyspnea or fatigue but without frank heart failure (Fig. 5).[1, 13, 19, 22, 28, 29, 33, 35, 36, 38, 39, 52, 59-61, 63, 64, 67, 68, 70, 75, 77, 81, 83, 86, 89, 92, 98] These symptoms characteristically occur beyond one year of age but within the first four decades of life. Whether these individuals were exhibiting the prodromes of congestive heart failure and would have progressed to failure is unclear, as 29 of the 34 with these symptoms underwent operation. There have been two postoperative deaths in this group. Only two infants were in this series.[36, 60] One, a 5-month-old girl described clinically as tachypneic and in a poor clinical state, underwent ligation of a left coronary artery–right ventricular fistula. She died suddenly 24 hours postoperatively of undetermined cause. The second infant developed moderate dyspnea at age 3½ months and underwent successful closure of a right coronary artery–right ventricular fistula at the age of two years.

In the ten patients in the present series who presented with angina or chest pain, the pain appeared either between the fifth and thirteenth year of life or not until the fifth decade (Fig. 6).[3, 24, 31, 43, 59, 65] There have been nine cases of bacterial endocarditis associated with coronary artery fistula with a maximal incidence in the second decade (Fig. 7).[12, 59, 60, 75, 76, 84, 88, 90, 91] No fatalities occurred in eight patients following surgical correction; one other died without operation in 1912. All nine of the patients presenting with the sole symptom of frequent upper respiratory infections underwent surgery.[19, 22, 67, 76, 87] There were no fatalities in this group.

SUMMARY

Congestive heart failure is one of the more serious complications of a coronary arteriovenous fistula. Successful surgical treatment of a left coronary artery–right ventricular fistula in a 6-week-old infant with congestive heart failure, a massive left-to-right shunt, and large increases in left heart volume and mass is presented. A review of the literature reveals the incidence of congestive heart failure in patients with congenital coronary artery fistula to be 14 percent. Of those developing heart failure, 80 percent were over the age of 20. It is interesting that patients who did develop failure before 20 were all less than one year of age. All patients with a coronary artery fistula and failure had shunts into their right ventricle. All eight patients with this anomaly and congestive heart failure who underwent surgical correction survived.

Coronary arteriovenous fistulas can now be diagnosed accurately and surgical treatment is curative. The high incidence of complications as well as the low operative morbidity indicates the need for early diagnosis followed by surgical closure.

REFERENCES

1. Abbott, O. R., Rivarola, C. H., and Logue, R. B.: Surgical correction of coronary arteriovenous fistula, J. Thorac. Cardiovasc. Surg. **42:** 660, 1961.
2. Abrams, L. D., Evans, D. W., and Howorth, F. H.: Coronary artery–right ventricular fistula treated surgically, Brit. Heart J. **29:** 132, 1967.
3. Agusti, R., Liebman, J., Ankeney, J., MacLeod, C. A., Linton, D. S., and Wiltsie, R.: Congenital right coronary artery to left atrium fistula, Amer. J. Cardiol. **19:** 428, 1967.
4. Aitken, G. J.: Coronary arterio-venous fistula, case report and discussion of the clinical picture, Scot. Med. J. **4:** 27, 1959.
5. Alexander, W. S., and Green, H. C.: Coronary blood vessel arising from cardiac ventricle, Arch. Path. **53:** 187, 1952.
6. Amplatz, K., and Aguirre, J.: Coronary arteriovenous fistula into main pulmonary artery, J. A. M. A. **172:** 1384, 1960.
7. Araya, I.: Two operated cases of coronary arteriovenous fistula, Jap. J. Thorac. Surg. **19:** 281, 1966.
8. Baker, W. P., Vogel, J. H. K., and Blount, S. G.: Coronary artery right ventricular communication associated with pulmonary atresia and ventricular septal defect, Circulation **35:** 923, 1967.
9. Barcia, A., Kincaid, O. W., Swan, H. J. C., Weidman, W. H., and Kirklin, J. W.: Coronary artery to right ventricle communication: report of two cases studied by selective angiography, Proc. Staff Meet. Mayo Clin. **37:** 623, 1962.
10. Baylis, J. H., and Campbell, M.: An unusual cause for a continuous murmur, Guy's Hosp. Rep. **101:** 174, 1952.
11. Bellet, S., and Gouley, B. A.: Congenital heart disease with multiple cardiac anomalies. Report of a case showing aortic atresia, fibrous scar in myocardium and embryonal sinusoidal remains, Amer. J. Med. Sci. **183:** 459, 1932.
12. Berman, D. A., Alexander, C. S., Adicoff, A., and Sako, Y.: Coronary arteriovenous fistula: report of an unusual case simulating atrial septal defect, Amer. J. Cardiol. **15:** 853, 1965.
13. Biorck, G., and Crafoord, C.: Arteriovenous aneurysm of the pulmonary artery simulating patent ductus arteriosus botalli, Thorax **2:** 65, 1947.
14. Bjork, V. O., and Bjork, L.: Coronary artery fistula, J. Thorac. Cardiovasc. Surg. **49:** 921, 1965.
15. Blakeway, H.: A hitherto undescribed malformation of the heart, J. Anat. **52:** 354, 1918.
16. Bosher, L. H., Jr., Vabli, S., McCue, C. M., and Belter, L. F.: Congenital arteriovenous fistula associated with large patent ductus arteriosus, Circulation **20:** 254, 1959.

17. Brooks, H. St.J.: Two cases of an abnormal coronary artery of the heart arising from the pulmonary artery, J. Anat. Physiol. **20:** 26, 1885.
18. Brown, R. C., and Burnett, J. D.: Anomalous channel between aorta and right ventricle: report of a case, Pediatrics **3:** 597, 1949.
19. Carmichael, D. B., and Davidson, D. G.: Congenital coronary arteriovenous fistula, Amer. J. Cardiol. **8:** 846, 1961.
20. Chalnot, P.: Grosdidier, J., Cherrier, F., and Mathieu, P.: Un cas de fistule coronaro-ventriculaire droite, Ann. Chir. Thorac. Cardiovasc. **3:** 281, 1964.
21. Colbeck, J. C., and Shaw, J. M.: Coronary aneurysm with arteriovenous fistula, Amer. Heart J. **48:** 270, 1954.
22. Cooley, D. A., and Ellis, P. R.: Surgical considerations of coronary arterial fistula, Amer. J. Cardiol. **10:** 467, 1962.
23. Craig, J. M.: Congenital endocardial sclerosis, Bull. Int. Amer. Med. Mus. **30:** 15, 1949, *as quoted in* Kauffman, S. L., and Andersen, D. H.: Amer. Heart J. **66:** 664, 1963.
24. Croom, R. D., Wilcox, B. R., and Abney, R. L.: Right coronary artery-coronary sinus arteriovenous fistula, Ann. Thorac. Surg. **4:** 182, 1967.
25. Currarino, G., Silverman, F. N., and Landing, B. H.: Abnormal congenital fistulous communications of the coronary arteries, Amer. J. Roentgenol. **82:** 392, 1959.
26. Davis, C., Fell, E. H., Gasul, B. M., and Dillon, R.: Congenital vascular lesions imitating the patent ductus, Arch. Surg. **72:** 838, 1956.
27. Davison, P. H., McCracken, B. H., and McIlveen, D. T. S.: Congenital coronary arteriovenous aneurysm, Brit. Heart J. **17:** 569, 1955.
28. Dedichen, H., Skalleberg, L., and Chappellen, C., Jr.: Congenital coronary artery fistula, Thorax **21:** 121, 1966.
29. Dubost, C., Chevrier, J. L., and Metianu, C.: Congenital communication between the right coronary artery and the right atrium, J. Cardiovasc. Surg. **2:** 60, 1961.
30. Edwards, J. E., Gladding, T. C., and Weir, A. B., Jr.: Congenital communication between the right coronary artery and the right atrium, J. Thorac. Surg. **35:** 662, 1958.
31. Effler, D. B., Sheldon, W. C., Turner, J. J., and Groves, L. K.: Coronary arteriovenous fistulas: diagnosis and surgical management, Surgery **61:** 41, 1967.
32. Effler, D. B., and Welti, H.: A propos d'une fistule arterioveineuse entre artère coronaire gauche et ventricule droit, Arch. Mal. Coeur **56:** 164, 1963.
33. Engle, M. A., Goldsmith, E. I., Holswade, G. R., Goldberg, H. P., and Glenn, F.: Congenital coronary arteriovenous fistula, diagnostic evaluation and surgical correction, New Eng. J. Med. **264:** 856, 1961.
34. Ernst, C. B., Klassen, K. P., and Ryan, J. M.: Vascular malformation overlying the pulmonary artery simulating a patent ductus arteriosus, Circulation **23:** 759, 1961.
35. Fell, E. H., Weinberg, M., Gordon, A. S., Gasul, B. M., and Johnson, F. R.: Surgery for congenital coronary artery arteriovenous fistulae, Arch. Surg. **77:** 331, 1958.
36. Gasul, B. M., Arcilla, R. A., Fell, E. H., Lynfield, J., Bicoff, J. P., and Luan, L. L.: Congenital coronary arteriovenous fistula, Pediatrics **25:** 531, 1960.
37. Gasul, B. M., Fell, E. H., Moreano, M., and Weinberg, M., Jr.: Congenital coronary arteriovenous aneurysm, Arch. Surg. **78:** 203, 1959.
38. Gensini, G. G., Palacio, A., and Buonanno, C.: Fistula from circumflex coronary artery to superior vena cava, Circulation **33:** 297, 1966.
39. Gerisch, R. A., Dodrill, F. D., Carmoney, W. J., and Krabbenhoft, K. L.: Anomalous coronary artery communicating with right atrium; case report, Harper Hosp. Bull. **21:** 215, 1963.
40. Graham, T. P., Jr., Jarmakani, M. M., Canent, R. V., Jr., Capp, M. P., and Spach, M. S.: Characterization of left heart volumes and mass in normal children and in infants with intrinsic myocardial disease, Circulation **38:** 826, 1968.
41. Grob, M., and Klob, E.: Congenital aneurysm of the coronary artery, Arch. Dis. Child. **34:** 8, 1959.
42. Guidici, C., and Becu, L.: Cardio-aortic fistula through anomalous coronary arteries, Brit. Heart J. **22:** 729, 1960.
43. Haberman, J. H., Howard, M. L., and Johnson, E. S.: Rupture of the coronary sinus with hemopericardium, a rare complication of coronary A-V fistula, Circulation **28:** 1143, 1963.
44. Haller, J. A., and Little, J. A.: Diagnosis and surgical correction of coronary artery-coronary sinus fistula, Circulation **27:** 939, 1963.
45. Hallman, G. L., Cooley, D. A., and Singer, D. B.: Congenital anomalies of the coronary arteries: anatomy, pathology and surgical treatment, Surgery **59:** 133, 1966.
46. Halpert, B.: Arteriovenous communication between the right coronary artery and the coronary sinus, Heart **15:** 129, 1930.
47. Harris, P. N.: Aneurysmal dilatation of the cardiac coronary arteries: review of the lit-

erature and report of a case, Amer. J. Path. **13:** 89, 1937.
48. Honey, M.: Coronary arterial fistula, Brit. Heart J. **26:** 719, 1964.
49. Hudspeth, A. S., and Linder, J. H.: Congenital coronary arteriovenous fistula, Arch. Surg. **96:** 832, 1968.
50. Humblet, L., Delvigne, J., Kulbertus, H., Collignon, P., and Joris, H.: Arteriovenous fistula involving both coronary arteries and main pulmonary trunk, Brit. Heart J. **31:** 136, 1969.
51. Kauffman, S. L., and Andersen, D. H.: Persistent venous valves, maldevelopment of the right heart, and coronary artery-ventricular communications, Amer. Heart J. **66:** 664, 1963.
52. Kitiyakara, K., Jumbala, B., and Sukrojana, K.: Congenital fistula between a coronary artery and the right atrium, Acta Chir. Scand. **129:** 663, 1965.
53. Kittle, C. F. (discussion), Arch. Surg. **78:** 204, 1959.
54. Knoblich, R., and Rawson A. J.: Arteriovenous fistula of the heart, Amer. Heart J. **52:** 474, 1956.
55. Kreutzer, R., Becu, L. M., Mosquera, J. E., and Caprile, J. A.: Una rara anomalia coronaria, Arch. Argent. Pediat. **24:** 40, 1953, *as quoted in* Kauffman, S. L., and Andersen, D. H.: Amer. Heart J. **66:** 664, 1963.
56. Lovitt, W. V., Jr., and Lutz, S., Jr.: Embryological aneurysm of the myocardial vessels, Arch. Path. **57:** 163, 1954.
57. Lowenheim, I.: Eine seltene Missbildung der Coronargefasse, Frankfurt Z. Path. **43:** 63, 1932.
58. McIntosh, H. D., Sleeper, J. C., Thompson, H. K., Sealy, W. C., and Young, W. G.: Preoperative evaluation of a continuous murmur in the chest, Arch. Surg. **52:** 74, 1961.
59. McNamara, J. J., and Gross, R. E.: Congenital coronary artery fistula, SURGERY **65:** 59, 1969.
60. Michaud, P., Froment, R., Viard, H., Gravier, J., and Verney, R. N.: Les fistulae coronaro-ventriculaires droites, Arch. Mal. Coeur **56:** 143, 1963.
61. Mozen, H. E.: Congenital cirsoid aneurysm of a coronary artery with associated arterio-atrial fistula treated by operation: a case report, Ann. Surg. **144:** 215, 1956.
62. Muir, C. S.: Coronary arterio-cameral fistula, Brit. Heart J. **22:** 374, 1960.
63. Munkner, T., Petersen, O., and Vesterdal, J.: Congenital aneurysm of the coronary artery with an arteriovenous fistula, Acta Radiol. **50:** 333, 1958.
64. Murray, R. H.: Single coronary artery with fistulous communication: report of two cases, Circulation **28:** 437, 1963.
65. Nagoya, M., and Takahashi, H.: Aneurysma serpentinum der linken koron arterie. Trans. Jap. Path. Soc. **22:** 583, 1932.
66. Neill, C., and Mounsey, P.: Auscultation in patent ductus arteriosus with a description of two fistulae simulating patent ductus, Brit. Heart J. **20:** 61, 1958.
67. Neufeld, H. N., Lester, R. G., Adams, P., Jr., Anderson, R. C., Lillehei, C. W., and Edwards, J. E.: Congenital communication of a coronary artery with a cardiac chamber or the pulmonary trunk, Circulation **24:** 171, 1961.
68. Newcombe, C. P., Whitaker, W., and Keates, P. G.: Coronary arterio-venous fistulae, Thorax **19:** 16, 1964.
69. Noonan, J. A., and Spencer, F. C.: Single coronary artery with coronary arteriovenous fistula communicating with the right ventricle, Amer. J. Cardiol. **15:** 848, 1965.
70. Nunn, D. B., Thrower, W. B., Boone, J. A., and Lipton, M.: Coronary arteriovenous fistula simulating patent ductus arteriosus, Amer. Surg. **28:** 476, 1962.
71. Papaioannou, A., Agdrogiannis, S., Nihoyanopoulos, J., and Lazzaridis, D.: Congenital coronary artery fistula, Amer. J. Cardiol. **10:** 588, 1962.
72. Paul, O., Sweet, R. H., and White, P. D.: Coronary arteriovenous fistula: case report, Amer. Heart J. **37:** 441, 1949.
73. Puyau, F. A., and Collins, H. A.: Congenital coronary arteriovenous fistula, Amer. J. Dis. Child. **106:** 65, 1963.
74. Reed, W. A., and Kittle, C. F.: Congenital coronary artery fistula, Arch. Surg. **93:** 772, 1966.
75. Sabiston, D. C., Jr., Ross, R. S., Criley, J. M., Gaertner, R. A., Neill, C. A., and Taussig, H. B.: Surgical management of congenital lesions of the coronary circulation, Ann. Surg. **157:** 908, 1963.
76. Sakakibara, S., Yokoyama, M., Takao, A., Nogi, M., and Gomi, H.: Coronary arteriovenous fistula, Amer. Heart J. **72:** 307, 1966.
77. Sanger, P. W., Taylor, F. H., and Robicsek, F.: The diagnosis and treatment of coronary arteriovenous fistula, SURGERY **45:** 344, 1959.
78. Schultz, J.: Coronary arteriovenous aneurysm: review of the literature, Amer. Heart J. **56:** 431, 1958.
79. Scott, D. H.: Aneurysm of the coronary arteries, Amer. Heart J. **36:** 403, 1948.
80. Shaffer, A. B., St. Ville, J., and Mackler, S. A.: Coronary arteriovenous fistula with patent ductus arteriosus, Amer. Heart. J. **65:** 758, 1963.
81. Sloman, G., MacPhee, A., and Fairley, K.:

An unusual arteriocameral fistula, Amer. J. Cardiol. **15:** 856, 1965.
82. Sondergaard, T.: Henry Ford Hospital international symposium in cardiovascular surgery, Philadelphia, 1955, W. B. Saunders Company, p. 490.
83. Soulie, P., Mathey, J., DiMatteo, J., Vernant, P., Piton, A., Bouchard, and Neveux, J. Y.: Communications congénitales entre artères coronaires et cavités cardiaques, Arch. Mal. Coeur **56:** 121, 1963.
84. Stansel, H. C., Jr., and Fenn, J. E.: Coronary arteriovenous fistula between the left coronary artery and persistent left superior vena cava complicated by bacterial endocarditis, Ann. Surg. **160:** 292, 1964.
85. Steinberg, I., Baldwin, J. S., and Dotter, C. T.: Coronary arteriovenous fistula, Circulation **17:** 372, 1958.
86. Stephenson, H. E.: Discussion of Effler, D. B., Sheldon, W. C., Turner, J. J., and Groves, L. K.: Coronary arteriovenous fistulas, SURGERY **61:** 41, 1967.
87. Swan, H., Wilson, J. N., Woodwark, M. B., and Blount, S. G.: Surgical obliteration of a coronary artery fistula to right ventricle, Arch. Surg. **79:** 820, 1959.
88. Symbas, P. N., Schlant, R. C., Hatcher, C. R., Jr., and Lindsay, J.: Congenital fistula of right coronary artery to right ventricle complicated by Actinobacillus actinomycetemcomitans endarteritis, J. Thorac. Cardiovasc. Surg. **53:** 38, 1967.
89. Taber, R. E., Gale, H. H., and Lam, C. R.: Coronary artery right heart fistulas, J. Thorac. Cardiovasc. Surg. **53:** 84, 1967.
90. Trevor, R. S.: Aneurysm of the descending branch of the right coronary artery situated in the wall of the right ventricle, Proc. Roy. Soc. Med. 5 (Sect. for Study of Dis. Child.): 20, 1912.
91. Tsagaris, T. J., and Hecht, H. H.: Coronary artery aneurysm and subacute bacterial endocarditis, Ann. Intern. Med. **57:** 116, 1962.
92. Upshaw, C. B.: Congenital coronary arteriovenous fistula—report of a case with an analysis of 73 reported cases, Amer. Heart J. **63:** 399, 1962.
93. Valdiva, E., Rowe, G. G., and Angevine, D. M.: Large congenital aneurysm of the right coronary artery, Arch. Path. **63:** 168, 1957.
94. Walther, R. J., Starkey, G. W. B., Zervopolus, E., and Gibbons, G. A.: Coronary arteriovenous fistula: clinical and physiologic report on two patients, with review of the literature, Amer. J. Med. **22:** 213, 1957.
95. Williams, R. R., Kent, G. B., Jr., and Edwards, J. E.: Anomalous cardiac blood vessel communicating with the right ventricle, Arch. Path. **52:** 480, 1951.
96. Wilson, J. G., and Grant, R. T.: A case of congenital malformation of the heart in an infant associated with partial heart block, Heart **12:** 295, 1926.
97. Yenel, F.: Coronary arteriovenous communication, New Eng. J. Med. **265:** 577, 1961.
98. Zuhdi, N., Kraft, D., Carey, J., and Greer, A.: Coronary arteriovenous-like communications, Arch. Surg. **80:** 178, 1960.

Studies of carbohydrate metabolism and serum electrolytes during surface-induced deep hypothermia with prolonged circulatory occlusion

EDWARD A. RITTENHOUSE, M.D.*
HITOSHI MOHRI, M.D., DR.MED.SCI.
K. ALVIN MERENDINO, M.D., PH.D.
SEATTLE, WASH.
From the Department of Surgery of the University of Washington School of Medicine and the First University Surgical Service of the University Hospital

A method of surface-induced deep hypothermia which allows safe cooling to 14° to 18° C. and total circulatory arrest up to 90 minutes has been developed at this institution. This technique consists of the use of deep ether anesthesia, respiratory alkalosis, and low molecular weight dextran[21, 22]; it has been successfully applied for open-heart surgery in 30 infants with severe congenital heart anomalies, such as transposition of the great vessels[10] and total anomalous pulmonary venous drainage.[9]

Various methods of surface-induced hypothermia were developed following the initial experimental work of Bigelow and associates[6] with subsequent clinical applications by Lewis and Taufic[19] and Swan and associates.[26] However, safe achievement of deep hypothermic levels was difficult because of the excessively high incidence of ventricular fibrillation during cooling with these methods; the permissible time for circulatory occlusion was thus limited to 10 or 15 minutes at moderate hypothermic levels. The clinical use of such methods was therefore gradually abandoned.

Numerous basic physiologic studies have been carried out and many controversial results obtained simply because experimental conditions, such as anesthetic agent, rate of ventilation, depth of anesthesia, and method of cooling, can significantly alter the variables being monitored.[8, 11, 27, 29, 31, 32]

The present studies were undertaken to evaluate carbohydrate metabolism, acid-base balance, and electrolyte changes during our hypothermic procedure because such information would contribute to the care of infants undergoing cardiac surgery with deep hypothermia.

MATERIAL AND METHODS

Twenty-four adult mongrel dogs weighing 10 to 15 kilograms were utilized after being fasted overnight.

Anesthesia and ventilation. The animals were anesthetized with Surital,* intubated, and maintained in the third plane of the third stage with ether. Ventilation was maintained with a constant-volume mechanical ventilator utilizing 100 percent oxygen and a closed system with a soda lime canister in the circuit. A normal tidal volume for normothermia was used during the entire procedure to produce the gradual development of respiratory alkalosis (pH 7.6 to 7.8 as body temperature reached approximately 18° C.).

Supported by Boeing Good Neighbor Fund, the Washington State Heart Association Grant No. 6970, and National Institutes of Health Grant No. HE03379-12.

Received for publication Nov. 8, 1969.

*Postdoctoral research fellow supported by United States Public Health Service Fellowship 1-F02-HE-39080-01.

*Sodium Thiamylal, Parke Davis & Co., Detroit, Mich.

Hypothermia. In three groups of animals, the hypothermic procedure with total circulatory occlusion for 40, 60, and 90 minutes was carried out. Hydrocortisone* (50 mg. per kilogram) was administered intravenously to the 90 minute occlusion group one hour prior to cooling in order to improve microcirculation. Rectal temperature was continuously monitored with a Yellow Springs thermistor. After cannulation of the femoral artery and vein for pressure monitoring, transfusion, and blood sampling, surface cooling was instituted by immersion in ice water.

Ten percent low molecular weight dextran† in dextrose (10 c.c. per kilogram) was administered as rectal temperature dropped from 35° to 25° C. Cooling was terminated at 22° C. and the temperature gradually drifted downward another 3 to 6° C. A right thoracotomy was performed under sterile conditions and circulatory arrest was achieved by cross-clamping both cavae, the ascending aorta, and the pulmonary artery. Aortic root injection of a known amount of Young's solution‡ resulted in mechanical arrest of the heart. In the 90 minute occlusion group the brain was additionally cooled by injection of 30 c.c. per kilogram of 4° C. saline into the left carotid artery after aortic occlusion.

Resuscitation was instituted by releasing inflow and outflow occlusion and gentle cardiac massage. Intravenous calcium chloride (300 mg.) neutralized the potassium injected in Young's solution and defibrillation was carried out with a 50 volt AC shock when necessary.

The animals were rewarmed in a tank of warm water (42° C.) with a plastic sheet interposed. Drug administration was avoided except in the 90 minute cardiac arrest group in which epinephrine and sodium bicarbonate were given for maximum assurance of survival. A normal hematocrit was maintained during rewarming by the intravenous infusion of isotonic saline in the carbohydrate study group and 5 percent dextrose and water in the electrolyte study group.

Chemical determinations. A series of blood samples was taken during the hypothermic procedure and postoperatively in all animals: (1) normothermic control, (2) 25° C. during cooling, (3) immediately prior to cardiac arrest, (4) end of circulatory occlusion period, (5) after three minutes of cardiac massage, (6) 25° C. during rewarming, (7) end of rewarming (35° C.), and (8) on the following day, approximately 16 hours after the procedure.

Carbohydrate metabolism was assessed by measuring blood glucose (glucose oxidase enzyme method[30]), pyruvate (Gloster and Harris'[12] method), and lactate (enzymatic fluorometric technique[20]) and calculation of the lactate/pyruvate ratio (L/P). Measurements of lactate content were carried out immediately following serum sampling.

Changes in serum electrolytes were determined by flame photometry (Baird Atomic Flame Photometer) for sodium and potassium and fluorometric methods for calcium[18] and magnesium.[25] Arterial blood pH was measured with a Radiometer pH meter and corrected for temperature according to the formula of Rosenthal.[24] Serum bicarbonate was determined by a method described by Van Slyke and colleagues.[28]

RESULTS

All animals recovered satisfactorily and were long-term survivors.

Glucose metabolism. Alterations in blood glucose, pyruvate, and lactate levels during hypothermia are illustrated in Fig. 1 (40 minute group), Fig. 2 (60 minute group), and Fig. 3 (90 minute group).

Serum glucose increased during cooling and reached a peak at 25° C. The elevated glucose levels dropped as body temperature reached around 18 to 19° C. Circulatory occlusion and cardiac massage did not significantly alter glucose levels. As the animals were rewarmed, mean serum glucose

*Solu-Cortef, Upjohn Co., Kalamazoo, Mich.

†Manufactured by Pharmacia Laboratories, Inc., Piscataway, N. J.

‡Young's solution contains 0.81 Gm. of potassium citrate, 2.46 Gm. of magnesium sulfate, 0.001 Gm. of neostigmine methyl sulfate, sufficient H_2O to make up to 100 c.c.; pH adjusted to 7.4 by $NaHCO_3$.

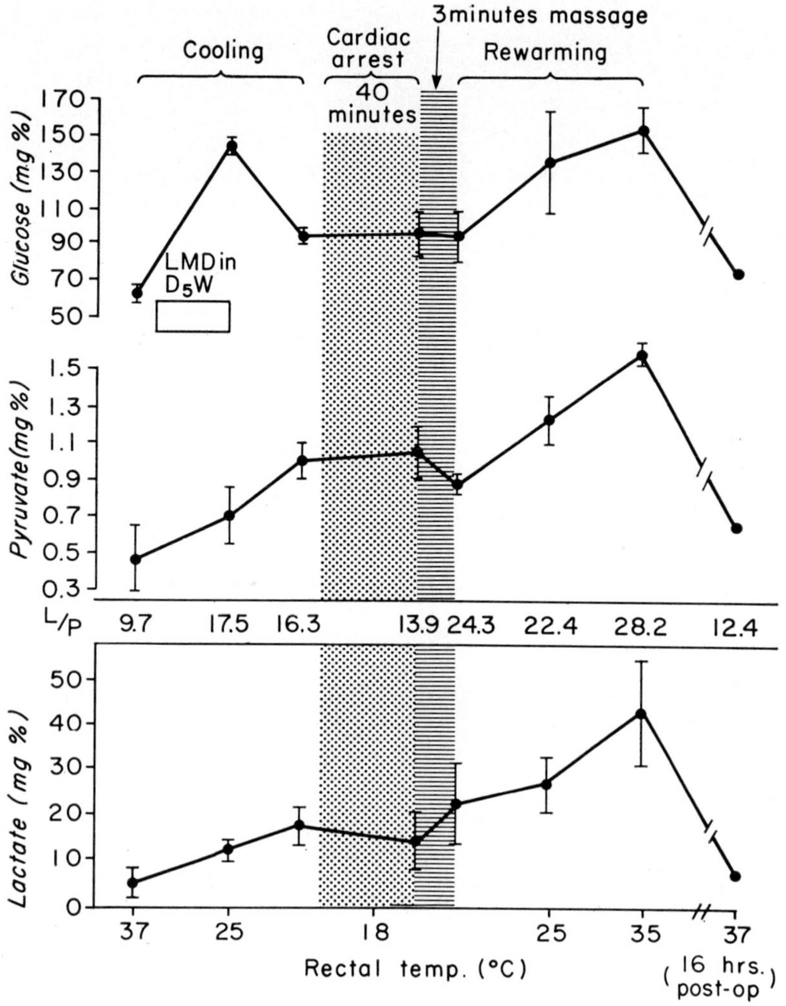

Fig. 1. Alterations in serum glucose, pyruvate, lactate, and lactate/pyruvate ratio (L/P) during the hypothermic procedure and after 40 minutes of cardiac arrest. Mean value and standard deviation (vertical bars) are plotted. Low molecular weight dextran in 5 percent dextrose and water (*LMD in D_5W*) was administered during cooling from 35° to 25° C.

tended to increase more in the 40 and 60 minute groups; in the 90 minute group, which had a higher glucose level at resuscitation, it decreased slightly, although it remained higher than control at the end of rewarming.

Mean pyruvate level prior to cooling was higher in the hydrocortisone group than the nonhydrocortisone group (average 0.74 vs. 0.50 mg. percent). Serum pyruvate during cooling tended to increase and reached about 100 percent above the control at the end of cooling but there was no consistency in these changes. With the re-establishment of circulation, pyruvate levels tended to decrease rather precipitously; they became fairly parallel to that of glucose as body temperature rose. In all groups pyruvate levels returned to normal by 16 hours postoperatively.

Changes in serum lactate levels varied. In the hydrocortisone group control lactate was higher than in the nonhydrocortisone group. With cooling, lactate alterations closely approximated the changes in pyruvate. In the nonhydrocortisone group it increased al-

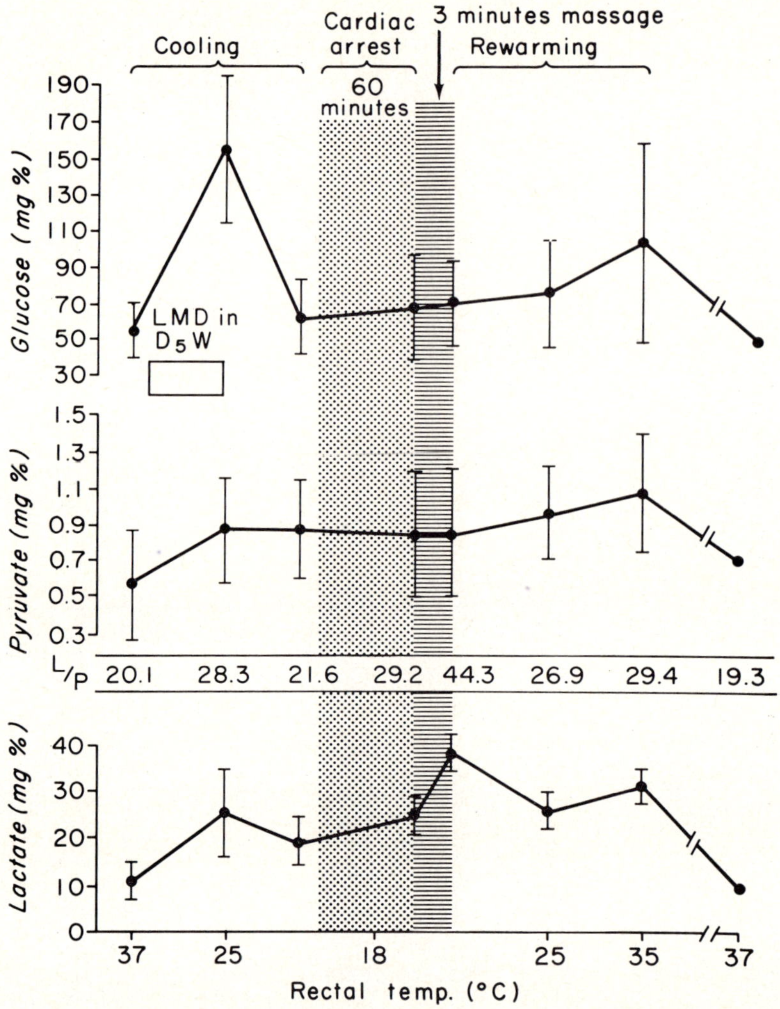

Fig. 2. Alterations in serum glucose, pyruvate, lactate, and lactate/pyruvate ratio (L/P) during the hypothermic procedure and after 60 minutes of cardiac arrest. Mean value and standard deviation (vertical bars) are plotted. Low molecular weight dextran in 5 percent dextrose and water (*LMD in* D_5W) was administered intravenously during cooling from 35° to 25° C.

most two times, reaching an average of 20 mg. percent, whereas in the hydrocortisone group the increase was almost three times and it reached 50 mg. percent at the end of cooling.

The increase in lactate levels following circulatory occlusion was directly related to the duration of cardiac arrest. During rewarming, it tended to increase, reaching 30 to 50 mg. percent at the end of rewarming in the 40 and 60 minute occlusion groups, and it reached as high as 70 mg. percent in the 90 minute occlusion group. The lactate levels in all groups also returned to normal by 16 hours postoperatively.

Control values of lactate/pyruvate (L/P) ranged from 10 to 20. During cooling the ratio tended to increase but remained close to the normal limit in the nonhydrocortisone group, whereas in the hydrocortisone group a precipitous rise was observed. After reestablishing circulation the ratio markedly rose in all groups. It decreased slightly at 25° C. of rewarming but rose again at the end of rewarming.

Electrolytes. Changes in serum electrolytes

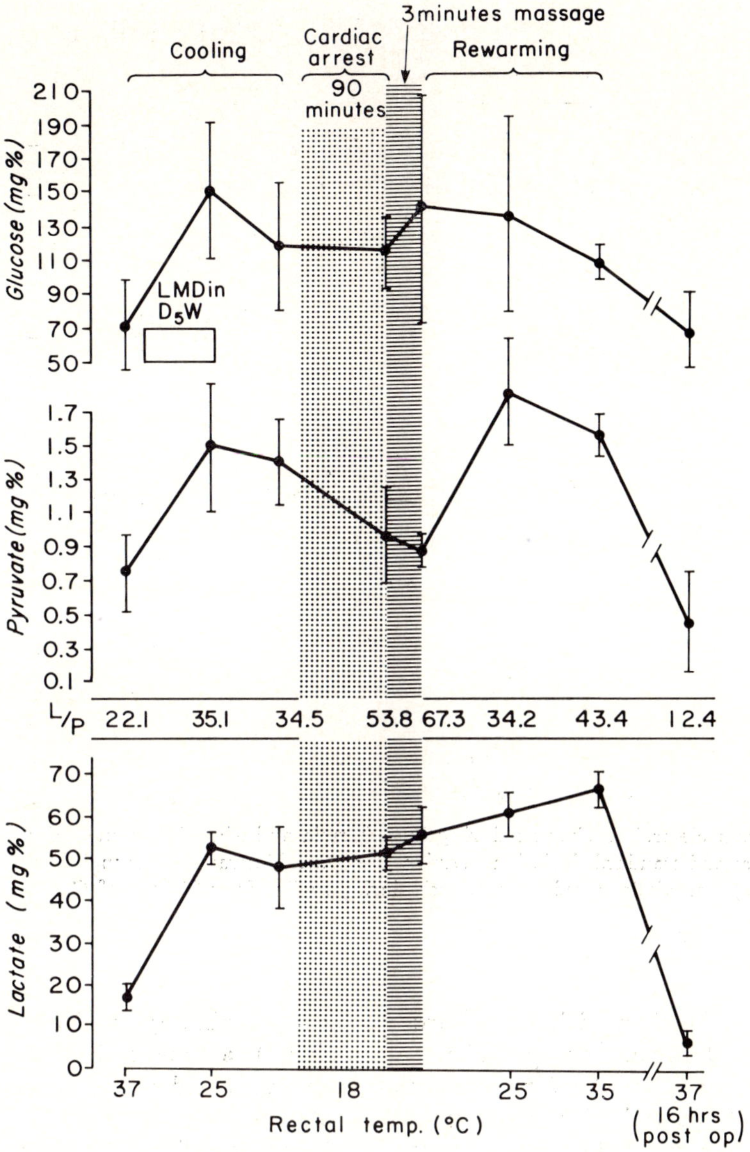

Fig. 3. Alterations in serum glucose, pyruvate, lactate, and lactate/pyruvate ratio (L/P) during the hypothermic procedure and after 90 minutes of cardiac arrest. Mean value and standard deviation (vertical bars) are plotted. Hydrocortisone (50 mg. per kilogram) was administered one hour prior to cooling and low molecular weight dextran in 5 percent dextrose and water (*LMD in* D_5W) was given intravenously as rectal temperature dropped from 35° to 25° C.

for the 60 and 90 minute cardiac arrest groups are illustrated in Figs. 4 and 5, respectively. Electrolyte changes in the 40 minute occlusion group were very similar to the 60 minute group. The alterations observed did not reflect the actual effect of hypothermia, except during cooling, because electrolyte-containing drugs were used for cardioplegia and resuscitation in this experimental setup.

Serum sodium decreased during cooling to 25° C., increased slightly prior to arrest, and changed little following circulatory occlusion. During rewarming, sodium tended

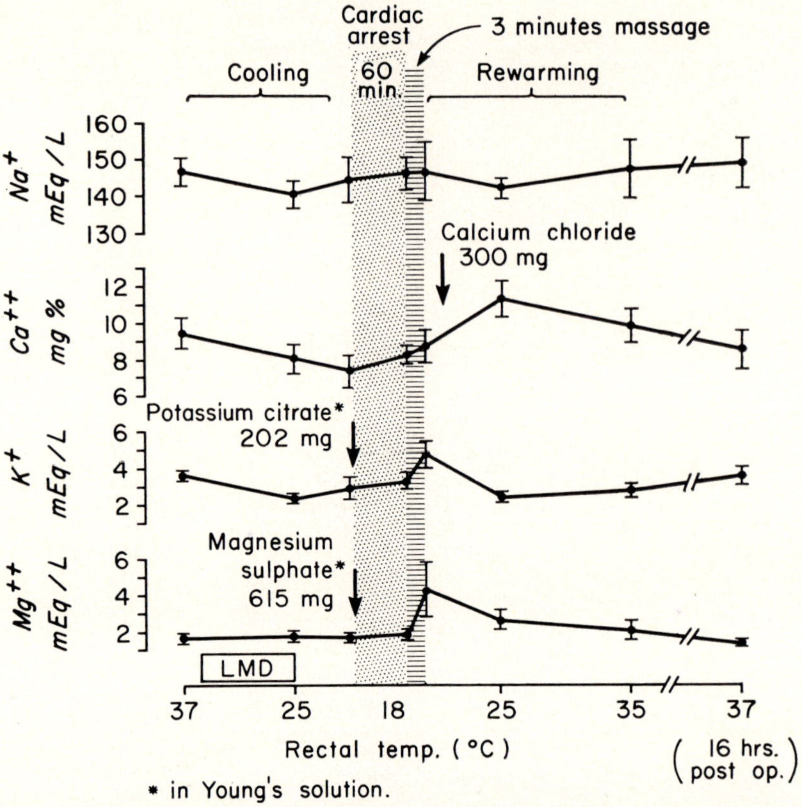

Fig. 4. Serum electrolyte changes during hypothermia and after 60 minutes of cardiac arrest. Mean values and standard deviation (vertical bars) are illustrated. Low molecular weight dextran (*LMD*) was administered intravenously during cooling from 35° to 25° C.

to decrease from the elevated levels toward normal in the 90 minute group while it slightly decreased at 25° C. of rewarming and increased at the end of rewarming in the 60 minute occlusion group. Sodium levels returned to nearly normal at 16 hours postoperatively.

Serum calcium levels declined steadily during cooling in both groups but the values for the hydrocortisone group were generally lower. At the end of cooling mean serum calcium was 4.0 mg. percent (hydrocortisone group) and 7.5 mg. percent (nonhydrocortisone group). Calcium increased markedly following the administration of calcium chloride, but decreased toward normal as rewarming continued.

Serum potassium progressively declined during cooling to a mean of 3.0 mEq. per liter (60 minute) and 2.2 mEq. per liter (90 minute) at the end of cooling. A sharp rise was noted at resuscitation due to circulation of the potassium contained in the Young's solution. Despite this marked elevation, potassium levels had dropped precipitously by rewarming to 25° C., and then gradually returned toward normal as rewarming progressed.

Serum magnesium remained within normal limits throughout the procedure except following the injection of Young's solution.

All electrolytes measured had returned to precooling levels by 16 hours postoperatively.

Acid-base balance. Continuous ventilation with normal tidal volume for normothermia produced the gradual development of respiratory alkalosis as rectal temperature de-

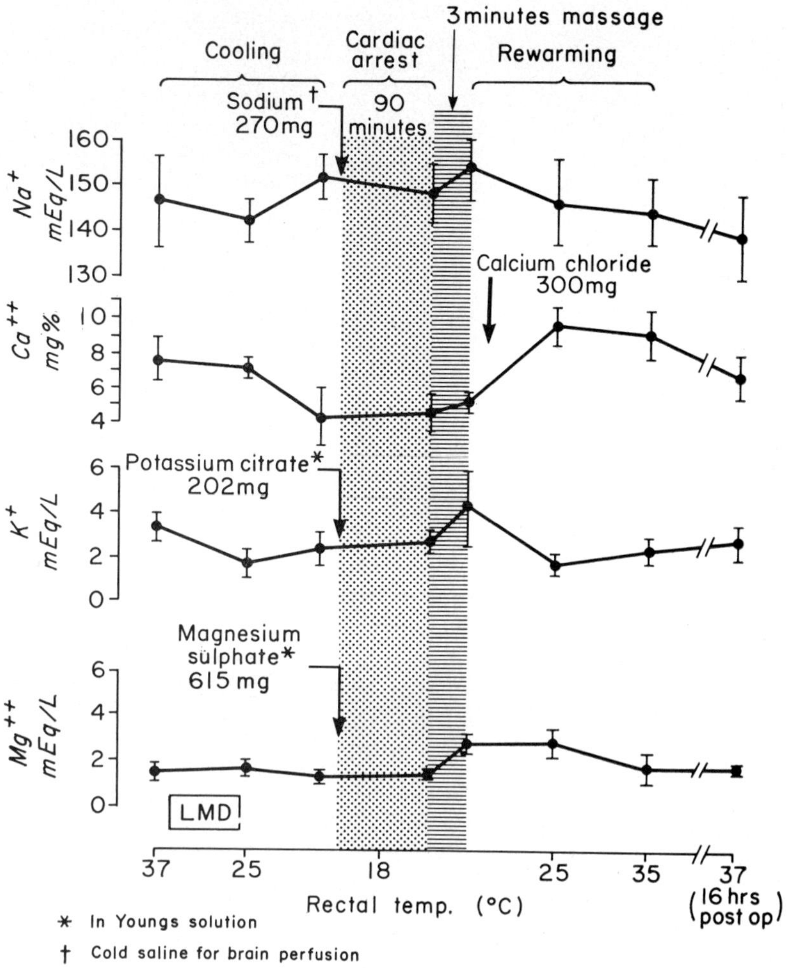

Fig. 5. Serum electrolyte changes during the hypothermic procedure and after 90 minutes of cardiac arrest. Mean value and standard deviation (vertical bars) are illustrated. Low molecular weight dextran (*LMD*) was administered during cooling from 35° to 25° C.

creased (Fig. 6). There was a drop in pH following circulatory occlusion but it remained above normal. In most instances, the pH was nearly normal after rewarming in the 40 and 60 minute circulatory occlusion groups. Occasional correction of pH by sodium bicarbonate injection was necessary in the 90 minute occlusion group.

DISCUSSION

Many physiologic alterations during hypothermia are the combined sequelae of hypothermia itself and other factors such as ventilation and anesthetic agents. The method utilized in the present study introduces several of these variables but they are considered necessary to assure maximum safety and obtain consistent survival.

Since all of the animals were fasted for almost 20 hours prior to operation the precooling blood sugar was less than 70 mg. percent in most cases. The sharp increase in glucose during cooling is most likely the result of dextrose infusion as well as the cold effect.[14] The reason for a drop in serum glucose as body temperature declined from 25° to 18° or 19° C. is not well understood. It may be related to ongoing glycolysis,

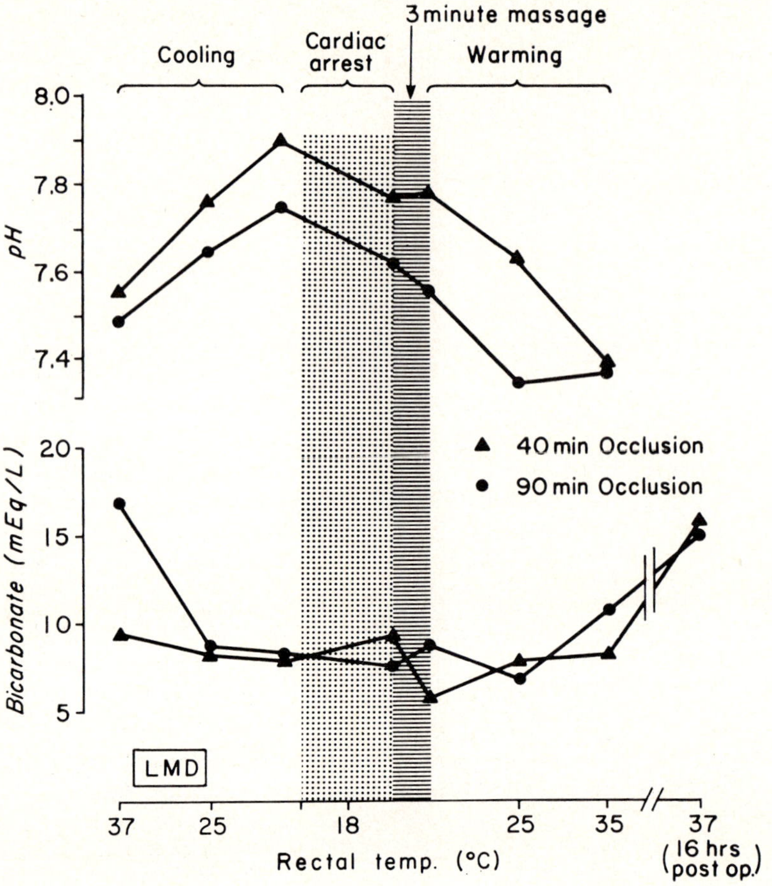

Fig. 6. Results of pH and bicarbonate determinations in animals subjected to the hypothermic procedure and cardiac arrest for 40 and 90 minutes. Low molecular weight dextran (*LMD*) was administered during cooling from 35° to 25° C.

although other investigators have reported diminished glucose utilization[14] and insulin release[3] during hypothermia. Excretion through the kidney is another possibility; however, our subsequent studies in experimental dogs indicate that there is no urine production during that period.

Hydrocortisone was administered to some animals prior to cooling in anticipation of a prolonged cardiac arrest of 90 minutes. Large doses of steroids are believed to improve cardiac contraction, increase peripheral perfusion, and stabilize lysosomal membranes during periods of hypoxia.[16, 17] Their effect on carbohydrate metabolism is well known and this property may be the reason for the higher blood levels of lactate and pyruvate in the group which received hydrocortisone.

Increased serum lactate during cooling is considered to result from depressed liver function.[1] Accelerated lactic acidosis can be expected if prolonged cardiac arrest is carried out even under hypothermia. The absolute value of serum lactate may not be representative of the degree of acidosis since the amount of lactate and pyruvate is a matter of chemical balance, and the ratio of these two parameters may be important. Huckabee[15] has stated that L/P is a biochemical parameter by which an approximate quantitation of cellular hypoxia can be obtained. With this ratio as a guideline, it could be determined that anaerobic metabolism was occurring after cardiac arrest and during rewarming. During cooling the L/P did not become remarkably elevated in the non-hydrocortisone group. In the hydrocortisone group there was an increase; however, in the presence of high doses of steroids it may not be possible to draw conclusions concerning the degree to which anaerobic metabolism is occurring.

The absence of late acidosis which has been proved experimentally and clinically[2] further supports the feasibility of this hypothermic method since persistent lactic acidosis has been reported with conventional hypothermia techniques.[5]

Serum electrolyte changes in this study were difficult to assess except during cooling because electrolytes were added with the injection of Young's solution and calcium chloride. Although there were wide fluctuations in electrolyte concentrations, it is important to note that all of these changes were reversible without any deleterious effect to the experimental subjects and with a return to near normal values at the end of rewarming.

There are many controversial observations concerning serum electrolyte changes under hypothermia due to the variation of methods utilized. Serum sodium is generally believed to remain unaltered by cooling to 25° C., and below that temperature an increase or decrease can occur.[11, 26] Furthermore, important shifts in total body sodium can take place but these may not be appreciated by measuring serum levels.[4] The effect of hypothermia on serum potassium is difficult to assess because anesthesia and artificial ventilation can produce significant changes.[7] Contrary to our findings, other investigators have reported a rise in serum magnesium[23] and no change in serum calcium[11] during cooling.

Myocardial damage has been ascribed to the injection of solutions containing potassium citrate to produce cardiac asystole.[13] However, we have not observed this phenomenon when Young's solution has been injected. If the cardiac injury is caused by potassium the development of hypokalemia during cooling with this method (due to hyperventilation) may be doing something to prevent such injury.

SUMMARY AND CONCLUSION

Alterations in carbohydrate and electrolyte metabolism during surface-induced hypothermia with total circulatory occlusion for 40, 60, and 90 minutes was studied in 24 dogs. The hypothermia method consisted of the use of deep ether anesthesia, respiratory alkalosis, and low molecular weight dextran.

Glucose increased during cooling to 25° C., presumably as the result of the administration of dextrose in dextran in addition to the cold effect itself. A drop occurred in serum glucose below 25° C., which suggested continuing metabolism of glucose. Lactate and pyruvate increased during cooling but the lactate/pyruvate ratio (L/P) remained within the normal range in the group which had not received hydrocortisone. Lactate reached a maximum of 70 mg. percent at the end of rewarming in the 90 minute arrest group; however, lactate and pyruvate returned to normal levels within 16 hours postoperatively and there was no late acidosis.

Sodium, potassium, and calcium decreased during cooling, whereas magnesium remained unchanged. Further alterations occurred following resuscitation but all parameters had returned to nearly normal levels at the end of warming without any deleterious effect on the animals. It has been suggested that hypokalemia secondary to respiratory alkalosis might prevent myocardial injury resulting from the potassium injected in Young's solution.

The use of hydrocortisone revealed some beneficial effect in experimental animals by decreasing the incidence of a gait disturbance which commonly developed in adult dogs after 50 or more minutes of total circulatory occlusion. The reason for this beneficial effect is not yet clear. It may simply be related to the relatively high blood pressure during cooling and especially at the early stage of resuscitation with the use of this drug or to the protective effect of hydrocortisone on the lysosomal membrane. Further studies with regard to this are now under way.

The present experimental study demonstrates that there are many and remarkable alterations in carbohydrate metabolism and electrolytes utilizing this particular method of hypothermia. However, all of these changes are well tolerated and are reversed in the early postoperative period. Our experience in the laboratory and with infants undergoing hypothermic cardiovascular surgery is that this method is safe and can provide adequate organ protection during circulatory occlusion.

The authors wish to express their appreciation to Mr. Murray P. Sands, the Department of Surgery chemistry personnel, Pharmacia Co., and Upjohn Co. for their assistance in performing this study.

REFERENCES

1. Ballinger, W. F., Vollenweider, H., Templeton, J. Y., and Pierucci, L., Jr.: Acidosis of hypothermia, Ann. Surg. **154:** 517, 1961.
2. Baum, D., Dillard, D. H., Mohri, H., and Crawford, E. W.: Metabolic aspects of deep surgical hypothermia in infancy, Pediatrics **42:** 94, 1968.
3. Baum, D., Dillard, D. H., and Porter, D.: Inhibition of insulin release in infants undergoing deep hypothermic cardiovascular surgery, New Eng. J. Med. **279:** 1309, 1968.
4. Beavers, W. R., and Rogers, J. T.: Hypothermia: alterations in cardiac and skeletal muscle electrolytes, Amer. J. Physiol. **196:** 706, 1959.
5. Belsey, R. H. R., Dowlatshahi, K., Keen, G., and Skinner, D. B.: Profound hypothermia in cardiac surgery, J. Thorac. Cardiovasc. Surg. **56:** 497, 1968.
6. Bigelow, W. G., Lindsay, W. K., and Greenwood, W. F.: Hypothermia: Its possible role in cardiac surgery; an investigation of factors governing survival in dogs at low body temperatures, Ann. Surg. **132:** 849, 1950.
7. Blair, E. A.: Surface immersion hypothermia, U. S. Army MNRL Report, 433519 and 433520, 1964.
8. D'Amato, H. E.: Thiocyanate space and the distribution of water in the musculature of the hypothermic dog, Amer. J. Physiol. **178:** 143, 1954.
9. Dillard, D. H., Mohri, H., Hessel, E. A., II, Anderson, H. N., Nelson, R. J., Crawford, E. W., Morgan, B. C., Winterscheid, L. C., and Merendino, K. A.: Correction of total anomalous pulmonary venous drainage in infants utilizing deep hypothermia with total circulatory arrest, Circulation **35, 36** (Suppl. 1): 105, 1967.
10. Dillard, D. H., Mohri, H., Merendino, K. A., Morgan, B. C., Baum, D., and Crawford, E. W.: Total surgical correction of transposition of the great arteries in children less than six months of age, Surg. Gynec. Obstet. **129:** 1258, 1969.
11. Fisher, B., Russ, C., Fedor, E., Wilde, R., Engstrom, P., Happel, J., and Prendergast, P.: Experimental evaluation of prolonged hypothermia, Arch. Surg. **71:** 431, 1955.
12. Gloster, J. A., and Harris, P.: Observations on an enzymic method for the estimation of pyruvate in blood, Clin. Chim. Acta **7:** 206, 1962.
13. Helmsworth, J. A., Kaplan, S., Leland, C. C., McAdams, A. J., Matthews, E. C., and Edwards, F. K.: Myocardial injury associated with asystole induced with potassium citrate, Ann. Surg. **149:** 200, 1959.
14. Henneman, G. H., Bunker, J. F., and Brewster, W. R.: Immediate metabolic response to hypothermia in man, J. Appl. Physiol. **12:** 164, 1968.
15. Huckabee, W. E.: Relationships of pyruvate and lactate during anaerobic metabolism. I. Effects of infusion of pyruvate or glucose and of hyperventilation, J. Clin. Invest. **37:** 244, 1958.
16. Ianz, R. D.: Inotropic actions of certain steroids upon cardiac tissue, *in* Martin, L., and Peirle, A., editors: Hormonal steroids, biochemistry, pharmacology and therapeutics, ed. 1, New York, 1964, Academic Press, Inc.
17. Janoff, A., Weissmann, G., Zweifach, B. W., and Thomas, L.: Pathogenesis of experimental shock. IV. Studies on lysosomes in normal and tolerant animals subjected to lethal trauma and endotoxemia, J. Exp. Med. **116:** 451, 1962.
18. Kepner, L., and Hercules, D. M.: Fluorometric determination of calcium in blood serum, Anal. Chem. **35:** 1238, 1963 (as modified by Turner, G. K., and associates).
19. Lewis, F. J., and Taufic, M.: Closure of atrial septal defects with the aid of hypothermia; experimental accomplishments and the report of one successful case, SURGERY **33:** 52, 1953.
20. Loomis, M. E.: An enzymatic fluorometric method for the determination of lactic acid in serum, J. Lab. Clin. Med. **57:** 966, 1961.
21. Mohri, H., Dillard, D. H., Crawford, E. W., Martin, W. E., and Merendino, K. A.: Method of surface-induced deep hypothermia

for open heart surgery in infants, J. Thorac. Cardiovasc. Surg. **58:** 262, 1969.

22. Mohri, H., Hessel, E. A., II, Nelson, R. J., Matano, I., Anderson, H. N., Dillard, D. H., and Merendino, K. A.: The use of Rheomacrodex and controlled hyperventilation in prolonged circulatory arrest under deep hypothermia induced by surface cooling. A method for open heart surgery in infants, Amer. J. Surg. **112:** 241, 1966.
23. Moulder, P. V., Eichelberger, L., Roma, M., Rams, J. J., Thurston, C., and Pinc, R.: Biochemistry of blood, heart, and skeletal muscle under induced controlled hypothermia, Arch. Surg. **78:** 37, 1959.
24. Rosenthal, T. B.: The effect of temperature on the pH of blood and plasma in vitro, J. Biol. Chem. **173:** 25, 1948.
25. Schacter, D.: The fluorometric estimation of magnesium in serum and urine, J. Lab. Clin. Med. **54:** 764, 1959, *as modified by Ralph E. Thiers in* Meites, S., editor: Standard methods of clinical chemistry, New York, 1965, Academic Press, Inc., vol. 5, p. 131.
26. Swan, H., Virtue, R. W., Blount, S. G., and Kircher, L. T., Jr.: Hypothermia in surgery, analysis of 100 clinical cases, Ann. Surg. **142:** 382, 1955.
27. Swan, H., Zeavin, I., Holmes, J. H., and Montgomery, V.: Cessation of circulation in general hypothermia. I. Physiologic changes and their control, Ann. Surg. **138:** 360, 1953.
28. Van Slyke, D. D., Stillman, E., and Cullen, G. E.: Carbon dioxide content (titrimetric) *in* Reiner, M., editor: Standard methods of clinical chemistry, New York, 1953, Academic Press, Inc., vol. 1, pp. 19-36.
29. Waddell, W. G., Fairley, H. B., and Bigelow, W. G.: Improved management of clinical hypothermia based upon related biochemical studies, Ann. Surg. **146:** 542, 1957.
30. Washko, M. E., and Rice, E. W.: Determination of glucose by improved enzymatic procedure, Clin. Chem. **7:** 542, 1961.
31. Willson, J. T., Miller, W. R., and Eliot, T. S.: Blood studies in the hypothermic dog, SURGERY **43:** 979, 1958.
32. Wynn, V.: Electrolyte disturbances associated with failure to metabolize glucose during hypothermia, Lancet **2:** 575, 1954.

Repair of aortic arch interruption in the neonate

KENNETH R. T. TYSON, M.D.
LEONARD C. HARRIS, M.D.
QUANG X. NGHIEM, M.D.
GALVESTON, TEXAS
From the Departments of Surgery and Pediatrics, University of Texas Medical Branch

Interruption of the aortic arch is an apparently uncommon but rapidly lethal form of congenital heart disease. Reports have been found of eight patients with aortic arch interruption successfully treated by operation.[1, 2, 5, 6, 10, 13, 14] The ages at operation ranged from 11½ months[5] to 16 years.[10] Though eighty percent of infants born with aortic arch interruption die within the first month of life,[12] no report of a successful operative procedure during the neonatal period for aortic arch interruption was found. A recent successful repair of Type A aortic arch interruption in a twelve-day-old neonate is the subject of this report.

CASE REPORT

S. W., a Negro female infant, was born Feb. 20, 1969, the product of an uncomplicated gestation and delivery, at the University of Texas Medical Branch Hospitals. Her birth weight was eight pounds nine ounces. A Grade 3/6 harsh systolic ejection murmur was heard best high at the left sternal border. Brachial and femoral pulses were normal. The liver was not enlarged. There was no cyanosis. The electrocardiogram was interpreted as normal for her age. Minimal cardiomegaly and prominent pulmonary vascular markings were seen on chest roentgenogram. Her condition during hospitalization in the newborn nursery was unremarkable, and she was discharged on the fourth day of life with a diagnosis of suspected patent ductus arteriosus, without evidence of congestive heart failure. Follow-up evaluation was planned on an outpatient basis.

She was seen again at seven days of age. Weight at that time was eight pounds six ounces. The mother reported that the baby had tired easily during feedings. The infant was in acute distress, with labored breathing and a respiratory rate of 120 per minute. The pulse rate was 180 beats per minute. The hands and face were puffy. She was not cyanotic. Brachial pulses were normal, and femoral pulses were absent. Flush pressure was 70 mm. Hg in the right arm and 30 mm. Hg in the right leg. Breath sounds were normal. A Grade 4/6 holosystolic murmur was maximal at the lower left sternal border. There was a long Grade 4/6 systolic ejection murmur extending through and obscuring the single second sound and heard best at the upper left sternal border. Presystolic and mid-diastolic flow murmurs were heard at the apex. The liver edge was palpable at the umbilical level. Chest x-ray demonstrated marked nonspecific cardiomegaly and prominent pulmonary vascular markings. The electrocardiogram showed a QRS axis of +120 degrees without evidence of ventricular hypertrophy or strain.

The baby was admitted with a provisional diagnosis of patent ductus arteriosus, coarctation of the aorta, and ventricular septal defect (VSD) with marked congestive heart failure. She was placed in the sitting position, given oxygen by mask, and treated with fluid restriction, intravenous ethacrynic acid and intravenous digoxin. Twenty-four hours later, the baby weighed seven pounds fifteen ounces. Breathing was less labored and the respiratory rate was 80 per minute. The liver edge was 1½ cm. below the right costal margin.

Cardiac catheterization was carried out when the patient was eight days of age. The results are summarized in Table I. Cineangiocardiography demonstrated a large VSD, filling of the descending aorta from the pulmonary artery, normal relationships of the great arteries to the ventricular chambers, and indistinct morphology of the aortic arch. Conclusions from the studies were as follows: (1) A large left-to-right shunt at the

Received for publication Nov. 19, 1969.

Table I. *Cardiac catheterization data*

Location	Pressure systolic/diastolic	Mean	O_2 Saturation (%)
Left atrium		15	94
Right brachial artery	129/67	90	80
Descending aorta	82/67	77	80
Pulmonary artery	120/45		82
Right ventricle	120/ - 6/12*		70 (Outflow) 73 (Midposition) 67 (Inflow)
Right atrium	a=14 v=17	13	55 (Low position) 59 (Midposition)
Inferior vena cava			63

*End-diastolic pressure.

ventricular level was present with equal pressures in the left and right ventricles, pulmonary artery, and right brachial artery; (2) a large right-to-left shunt was present from the pulmonary artery via a patent ductus arteriosus to the descending aorta with a 30 percent systolic gradient between the pulmonary artery and the descending aorta; (3) either a severe preductal coarctation of the aorta or an aortic arch interruption existed.

The treatment for congestive heart failure was continued, and at eleven days of age, the infant weighed seven pounds four ounces. The liver edge was at the right costal margin, and she appeared much more vigorous. A retrograde aortogram via the right brachial artery was attempted to delineate better the status of the aortic arch. There were prominent internal mammary and thyrocervical arterial collaterals. The descending aorta did not fill. It was not possible to distinguish between a severe preductal coarctation, atresia, or a Type A aortic arch interruption.

On March 4, 1969, at age twelve days, a left lateral thoracotomy was performed. The presence of a Type A aortic arch interruption was confirmed (Fig. 4). A moderately severe narrowing of a large patent ductus arteriosus was also found (Fig. 1). Even with extensive mobilization, the proximal and distal ends of the interrupted aortic arch could not be approximated. Fortunately, the diameter of the left subclavian artery was as great as that of the proximal and distal aortic arch. The left vertebral artery was ligated. A temporary band was placed about the main pulmonary artery, palpably diminishing the distal pulmonary artery pressure, to limit the left-to-right interventricular shunt prior to occlusion of the left subclavian artery and the ductus arteriosus. Clamps were placed across the proximal portion of the ductus, the descending aorta, and the proximal arch at the takeoff of the left subclavian artery. The left subclavian artery was ligated distally. It was transected, as was the distal segment of the ductus (Fig. 2). The transected end of the left subclavian artery and the end of the distal portion of the aortic arch were tailored obliquely to assure good anastomotic lumenal size and sutured together with the use of a continuous over-and-over suture for the posterior row and interrupted simple sutures for the anterior row, all of a No. 6-0 size. The clamps on the proximal and distal arch were released; the temporary pulmonary artery band was rapidly loosened and then sutured in place when a systolic pressure gradient of 50 percent between right ventricle and distal pulmonary artery was achieved. The ductus was excised and the pulmonary arterial end of the ductus was oversewn. The clamp was then removed, completing reconstruction of the interrupted aortic

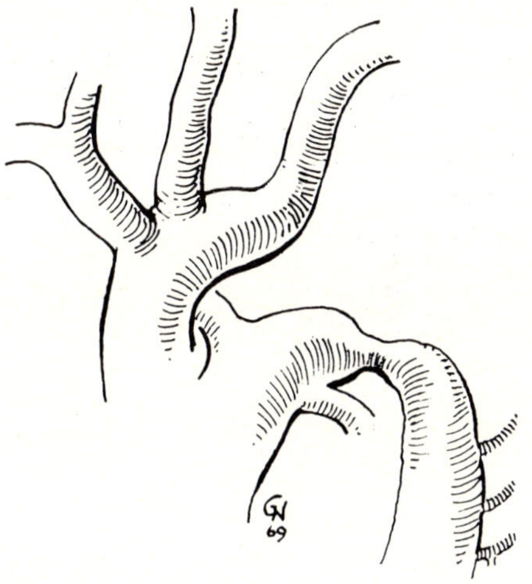

Fig. 1. Interruption of the aortic arch found in a twelve-day-old neonate. The aortic side of the large patent ductus was moderately stenotic.

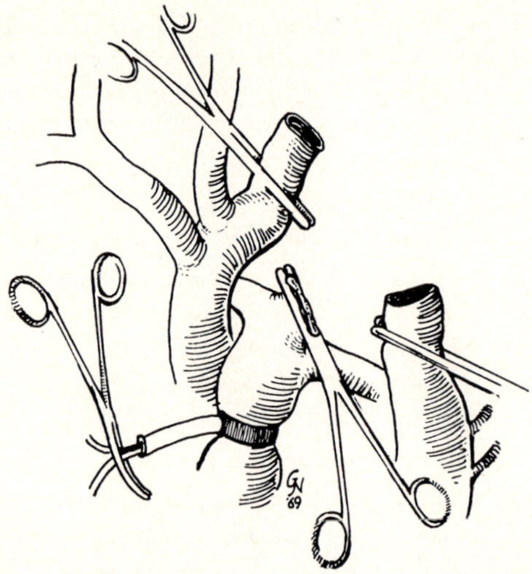

Fig. 2. A temporary band has been placed around the pulmonary artery to limit the left-to-right shunt through the large VSD as resistance to left ventricular ejection is increased by excision of the patent ductus and occlusion of the large left subclavian artery.

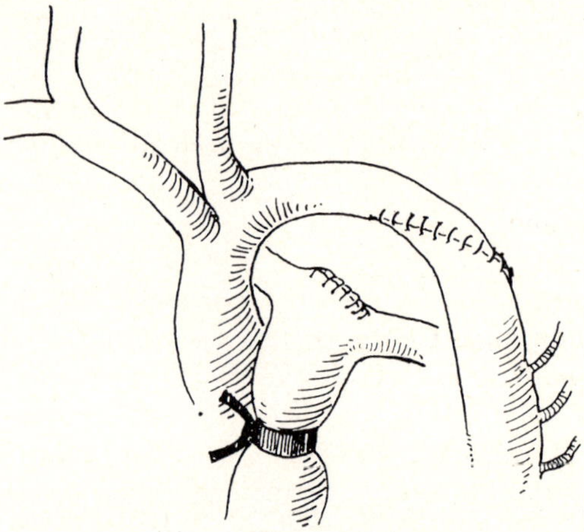

Fig. 3. Completed arch reconstruction by oblique anastomosis of left subclavian artery to descending aorta. The temporary pulmonary artery band was loosened upon release of the aortic clamps and then sutured in place when a 50 percent systolic pressure gradient was achieved.

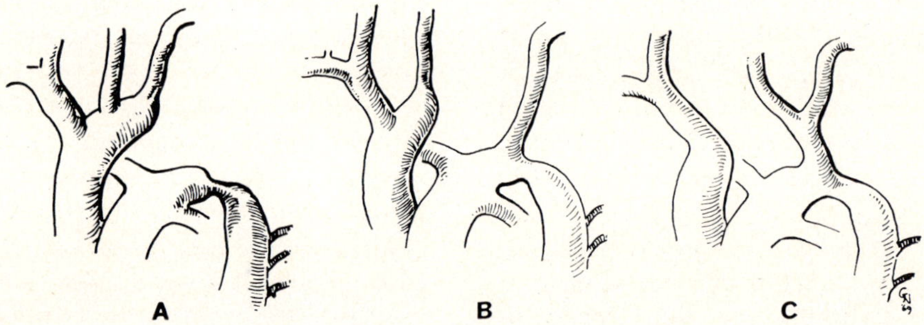

Fig. 4. Classification of interruptions of aortic arch, Types *A, B,* and *C,* according to Celoria and Patton.[4]

arch, division of the patent ductus arteriosus, and banding of the main pulmonary artery (Fig. 3). No pressure gradient could be detected between the ascending aorta and the descending aorta prior to wound closure. The baby's vital signs were stable throughout the procedure; operating time was one hour and fifteen minutes.

Twenty hours later, pulmonary compliance and diffusion capacity had improved sufficiently so that volume ventilator support and nasotracheal intubation were discontinued. Her postoperative course was uneventful. Arterial oxygen saturation was 98 percent. Flush pressures in the right arm and right leg were 75 mm. Hg and 80 mm. Hg, respectively. She was discharged on the tenth postoperative day on a maintenance dose of digoxin.

Eight months later, she weighed fifteen pounds eight ounces. She was acyanotic, very vigorous, and demonstrated no signs of congestive heart failure. Femoral pulsations were prominent. Brachial and femoral blood pressures by flush technique were normal.

DISCUSSION

Interruptions of the aortic arch have been classified by Celoria and Patton[4] into three types, based on the relationship of the interruption to the brachial and cephalic vessels.

The interruption occurs distal to the left subclavian artery in Type A, distal to the left common carotid artery in Type B, and distal to the innominate artery in Type C (Fig. 4). Moller and Edwards,[7] in a review of 95 classifiable cases of aortic arch interruption, found that 44 were Type A, 47 were Type B, and 4 were Type C.

Of major importance is the association of intracardiac anomalies, particularly VSD, with interruption of the aortic arch. The vast majority of neonates with interruption of the aortic arch die with uncontrollable left ventricular failure. The failure may be on the basis either of increased resistance to left ventricular ejection or of left ventricular volume overload from interventricular left-to-right shunting, or of both. Ventricular ejection resistance in a neonate with aortic arch interruption may be increased by associated ventriculoaortic obstruction[9] and partial or complete closure of the ductus arteriosus. Except when the VSD is quite small, increased left ventricular ejection resistance results in increased left-to-right shunting at the ventricular level and accentuation of left ventricular volume overload.

In neonates with interruption of the aortic arch and congestive heart failure, a rational operative approach can be derived by analysis of the hemodynamic situation. Prompt and precise cardiologic evaluation, including cardiac catheterization and angiocardiography, must be performed. The complex of severe preductal coarctation, patent ductus arteriosus, and VSD frequently cannot be distinguished in preoperative diagnosis or in hemodynamic effect from interruption of the aortic arch. Intensive medical management of the heart failure should be instituted. Because of the poor prognosis,[12] nonoperative therapy of congestive heart failure in neonates with interruption of the aortic arch should not be doggedly maintained after the period of improvement. Surgical management should then be employed, tailored to the specific hemodynamic situation at hand.

The following surgical plan is advocated. With equal or nearly equal left and right ventricular pressures, a large left-to-right interventricular shunt, and no aortic outflow obstruction, the main pulmonary artery should be temporarily banded first in order to reduce left atrial venous return and to relieve left ventricular failure. Arch reconstruction with division of the ductus should then be rapidly accomplished. Following release of the aortic clamps, the temporary band must be loosened and then reapplied to an extent that reduces pulmonary artery systolic pressure to 50 percent of right ventricular systolic pressure. If the right ventricular systolic pressure is two thirds or less than that of the left ventricle, indicating a relatively small VSD, it should be possible to divide the ductus and reconstruct the arch without preliminary pulmonary artery banding. If right ventricular systolic pressure remains at or near two thirds of the systemic level after arch reconstruction, pulmonary artery banding should be employed.

Since, in Moller and Edwards'[7] series, the right common carotid artery arose from the proximal arch segment regardless of associated great vessel and arch anomalies in each case reviewed, it seems the logical vessel in which to assess aortic pressure proximal to the aortic interruption. If a pressure gradient between the left ventricle and the right common carotid artery exists, some form of ventriculoaortic obstruction can be assumed to coexist. Left ventricular angiocardiography may, as well, help delineate the associated lesion. When there is evidence of ventriculoaortic obstruction, thoughts of arch reconstruction in the neonate should be abandoned. Instead, branch pulmonary artery banding, as suggested by Muller and Dammann[8] and successfully applied by Hairston and associates,[5] should be employed. Adequate, gradient-free communication between the pulmonary artery and the descending aorta must be assured at the time of branch pulmonary artery banding. Branch pulmonary artery banding should be applied, as well, to those cases of aortic arch interruption associated with a persistent truncus arteriosus. If left ventricular hypoplasia is demonstrated, a Rashkind[11] interatrial septostomy at the time of initial cardiac catheterization may be life saving.

The method of aortic arch reconstruction is of some importance. Prosthetic materials have been used successfully in older children to bridge the gap between proximal and distal segments of the arch[2, 10, 13] but probably have little application in neonates because of size and growth limitations. Certainly in Type A arch interruptions, if the left subclavian artery is of good size, as in the case here reported, it alone will suffice to reconstitute the arch when primary anastomosis is not feasible.[3] Tawes and associates[15] have recently reported successful use of this method in treating atresia of the aortic arch. The method of using both the left common carotid and left subclavian arteries, as described by Sirak and associates,[14] is applicable when the left subclavian alone is of insufficient size.

SUMMARY

A case of Type A aortic arch interruption is reported in a neonate. It was associated with a large VSD and incomplete closure of a patent ductus arteriosus, which caused congestive heart failure. It was successfully repaired by arch reconstruction and pulmonary artery banding when the child was twelve days old. Though 80 percent of infants born with aortic arch interruptions die within one month from birth, the patient reported is the first known to have been successfully repaired during neonatal life.

A discussion of the pertinent hemodynamic considerations in aortic arch interruptions is presented, and therapeutic approaches based on those considerations are suggested.

REFERENCES

1. Asano, K., Shiozaki, K., Eguchi, S., and Irisawa, T.: Congenital aortic arch interruption, Jap. Heart J. **8:** 196, 1967.
2. Blake, H. A., Manion, W. C., and Spencer, F. C.: Atresia or absence of the aortic isthmus, T. Thorac. Cardiovasc. Surg. **43:** 607, 1962.
3. Blalock, A., and Park, E. A.: The surgical treatment of experimental coarctation (atresia) of the aorta, Ann. Surg. **119:** 445, 1944.
4. Celoria, G. C., and Patton, R. B.: Congenital absence of the aortic arch, Amer. Heart J. **58:** 407, 1959.
5. Hairston, P., Webb, H., and Lee, W. H., Jr.: Aortic arch interruption: Treatment with pulmonary artery banding, J. Thorac. Cardiovasc. Surg. **54:** 50, 1967.
6. Merrill, D. L., Webster, C. A., and Samson, P. C.: Congenital absence of the aortic isthmus, J. Thorac. Surg. **33:** 311, 1957.
7. Moller, J. H., and Edwards, J. E.: Interruption of the aortic arch; anatomic patterns and associated cardiac malformations, Amer. J. Roentgen. **95:** 557, 1965.
8. Muller, W. H., Jr., and Dammann, J. F., Jr.: Results following the creation of pulmonary artery stenosis, Ann. Surg. **143:** 816, 1956.
9. Noonan, J. A., and Nadas, A. S.: The hypoplastic left heart syndrome, Pediat. Clin. N. Amer. **5:** 1029, 1958.
10. Pillsbury, R. C., Lower, R. R., and Shumway, N. E.: Atresia of the aortic arch, Circulation **30:** 749, 1964.
11. Rashkind, W. J., and Miller, W. W.: Creation of an atrial septal defect without thoracotomy, J. A. M. A. **196:** 991, 1966.
12. Rochette, M., Stanley, P., F.-Ethier, M., and Davignon, A.: Complete interruption of the aortic arch in infancy, Can. Med. Ass. J. **98:** 131, 1968.
13. Concepcion Ruiz Villalobos, M., De Balderrama, D. P., Lopez y Lopez, J., and Castellanos, M.: Complete interruption of the aorta, Amer. J. Cardiol. **8:** 664, 1961.
14. Sirak, H. D., Ressallat, M., Hosier, D. M., and de Lorimier, A. A.: A new operation for repairing aortic arch atresia in infancy, Circulation **37** (Suppl. 2): 43, 1968.
15. Tawes, R. L., Jr., Panagopoulos, P., Aberdeen, E., Waterson, D. J., and Bonham-Carter, R. E.: Aortic arch atresia and interruption of the aortic arch: Experience in 11 cases of operation. J. Thorac. Cardiovasc. Surg. **58:** 492, 1969.

Aortic arch atresia with transposition of the great vessels: Physiologic considerations and surgical management

J. B. NORTON, Jr., M.D.
DANIEL J. ULLYOT, M.D.
EDWARD T. STEWART, M.D.
A. M. RUDOLPH, M.D.
L. HENRY EDMUNDS, Jr., M.D.
SAN FRANCISCO, CALIF.
From the Departments of Pediatrics, Surgery, and Radiology, and the Cardiovascular Research Institute, University of California, San Francisco Medical Center

Atresia, or interruption of the aortic arch, rarely occurs as an isolated anomaly.[4, 10-12] Most commonly, a ventricular septal defect, patent ductus arteriosus, and abnormal arrangements of the brachiocephalic arteries occur together with the arch anomaly.[10] Rarely, more complex abnormalities, such as transposition of the great vessels are coexistent.[2, 4-6, 8, 9] The management of infants with arch atresia or coarctation has been a matter of controversy for many years. Medical therapy has been generally unsuccessful if additional cardiac anomalies have been present; however, operation may be successful in such neonates.[1, 12-15, 17] We present the case of an infant with transposition of the great vessels, ventricular septal defect, atresia of the aortic isthmus, and an associated patent ductus arteriosus in whom a successful surgical palliative operation was performed on the fourth day of life.

CASE REPORT

Clinical findings. This male infant was born after a 38 week gestation complicated only by cystitis in the third trimester. The birth weight was 3,480 grams and the length was 50.2 cm. The one- and five-minute Apgar scores were 8 and 9, respectively. At 18 hours of age, the physical examination was unremarkable, and the infant was considered normal until 72 hours of age. At that time, tachypnea of 120 per minute was noted and the heart rate was found to be 160 per minute. There was no cyanosis. The lungs were clear to auscultation and a Grade 1/6 early ejection systolic murmur was heard for the first time at the lower sternal border. At 74 hours of age, femoral pulses were difficult to palpate, although they had previously been normal. The liver had enlarged to 4 cm. below the right costal margin, and the murmur was louder. The electrocardiogram had a QRS axis of +115 degrees and normal right ventricular forces. The chest roentgenogram showed a heart generally enlarged, and with a narrow base. There was increased pulmonary vascularity. With the patient breathing room air, a temporal arterial sample showed a P_{O_2} of 51 mm. Hg, pH of 7.4, and a P_{CO_2} of 31 mm. Hg. When the patient breathed 100 percent oxygen, arterial P_{O_2} was 84 mm. Hg. By 82 hours of age, generalized cyanosis was apparent for the first time. Differential cyanosis was not observed. The clinical impression was transposition of the great vessels with a ventricular septal defect and possibly coarctation of the aorta. Because of rapidly increasing congestive heart failure and progressive cyanosis, cardiac catheterization was performed at 84 hours of age. Ethacrynic acid, 3.4 mg., was given intravenously preceding the study. Digitalis was given following it.

Cardiac catheterization. Local anesthesia was administered and catheterization was carried out from the right superficial femoral artery and vein. Representative pressure and oxygen saturation data are presented in Table I.

Fig. 1 shows the pressures recorded as the arterial catheter was withdrawn from the pulmonary artery across the patent ductus arteriosus

This study was supported in part by United States Public Health Service Grants HE-11231 and HE-06285.
Received for publication Feb. 4, 1970.

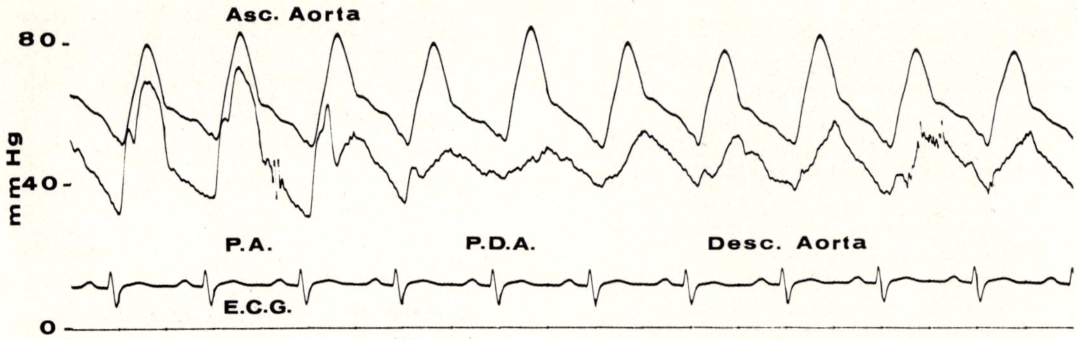

Fig. 1. Simultaneous pressure recordings from the ascending aorta and pulmonary artery *(PA)* as the catheter was withdrawn across the patent ductus arteriosus *(PDA)* into the descending aorta.

Table I

*Site**	*Pressure (mm. Hg)*	*Oxygen saturation (percent)*	*Comments*
Superior vena cava (SVC)	m = 10	69	
Right atrium (RA)	a = 12, v = 13, m = 8	72	Pressure obtained on withdrawal from LA
Right ventricle (RV)	70/18	82	
Aorta (ascending)	80/50, m = 65	85	Saturation simultaneous with PA of 88 percent
Pulmonary vein (PV)		91	
Left atrium (LA)	a = 12, v = 15, m = 8	89	
Left ventricle (LV)	70/18 to 80/16	89	Saturation simultaneous with PA of 87 percent
Pulmonary artery (PA)	70/40, m = 55	87, 88	On withdrawal from LV
Aorta (descending)	60/35, m = 50	86	On withdrawal from PA

*Samples obtained from SVC, RA, RV, LA were obtained in rapid succession. Considerable time elapsed between the RV sample and the ascending aorta and PA samples. The venous catheter was manipulated from the RA into the RV and anteriorly into the ascending aorta. This catheter was also passed into the LA and PV from the RA and across the mitral valve into the LV. The retrograde catheter could not be manipulated into the ascending aorta but passed easily across a patent ductus arteriosus into the pulmonary artery. The left ventricle was entered across the pulmonic valve.

into the descending aorta. The ascending aortic pressure was measured with the venous catheter which had been passed into the ascending aorta from the right ventricle.

Figs. 2, 3, and 4 show the pertinent angiographic data. The great vessels were transposed, the aorta originated anteriorly from the anatomic right ventricle, and the pulmonary artery arose posteriorly from the anatomic left ventricle. The pulmonary and aortic valves were normal. Contrast medium flowed from the left atrium to the right atrium across an atrial septal defect. Bidirectional shunting was demonstrated across a high ventricular septal defect. Brachiocephalic vessels arose normally from the aortic arch, but the aorta was not visible beyond the left subclavian artery. The descending aorta was on the left and communicated with the pulmonary artery by a patent ductus arteriosus.

The catheterization and angiographic data were consistent with the diagnosis of complete transposition of the great vessels with a large atrial communication (atrial septal defect or patent foramen ovale), ventricular septal defect, and either severe coarctation or atresia of the aortic isthmus. The descending aorta filled from a patent ductus arteriosus.

Operation. While oxygen was administered by

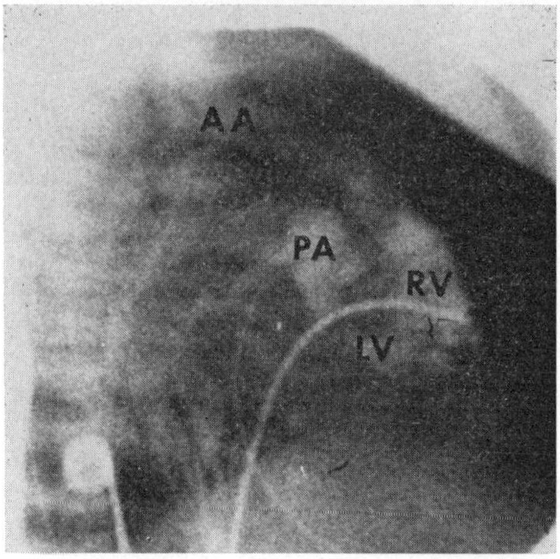

Fig. 2. Lateral right ventricular angiogram demonstrating the transposed aorta *(AA)* and filling of the left ventricle *(LV)* and pulmonary artery *(PA)* through the ventricular septal defect.

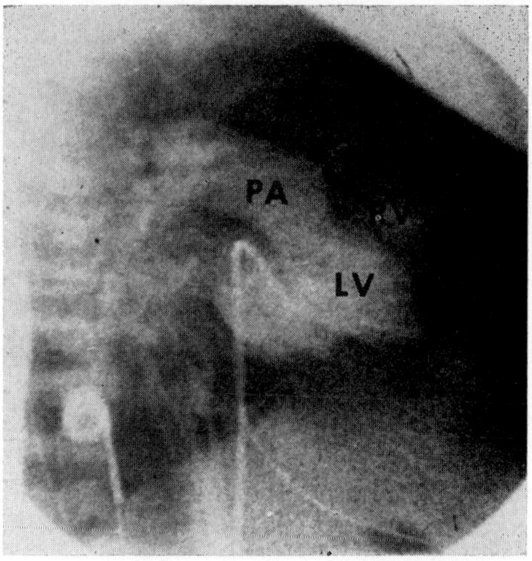

Fig. 3. Lateral left ventricular injection demonstrating the transposed pulmonary artery *(PA)* and faint opacification of the right ventricle *(RV)* by way of the ventricular septal defect.

mask, and the patient was given local anesthesia, silicone rubber catheters were inserted in the radial artery and antecubital vein. A base deficit of 13.5 mEq. per liter was corrected before induction with halothane. The radial arterial pressure, rectal temperature, and electrocardiogram were monitored throughout the procedure.

A left lateral thoracotomy was performed in the fourth intercostal space. The descending aorta was atretic for a distance of 2 cm. distal to the left subclavian artery (Fig. 5). A small fibrous cord connected the transverse arch with the descending aorta. The patent ductus arteriosus, 6 mm. in external diameter, was equal in diameter to the descending aorta. The left subclavian artery was 4 mm. in external diameter. An end-to-side anastomosis between the proximal stump of the divided left subclavian artery and the descending thoracic aorta was made with interrupted No. 6-0 dacron sutures. Blood flow through the ductus was not impeded during the construction of the anastomosis. The ductus was then occluded for five minutes without evidence of any difficulty and then divided. Finally, a 5 mm. Teflon band was placed around the posterior, transposed, main pulmonary artery. The pressure distal to the band was monitored by direct puncture of the main pulmonary artery with a No. 22 needle. As the band was tightened, the peak systolic pressure rose from 60 to 90 mm. Hg in the radial artery and fell from 60 to 40 mm. Hg in the distal pulmonary artery.

Postoperatively, the infant required ventilatory assistance for 18 hours. Digitalis was not given

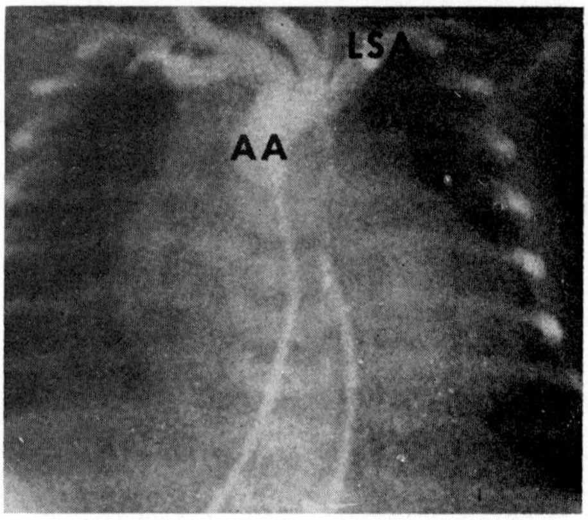

Fig. 4. Anteroposterior angiograms of the aortic injection demonstrating the ascending aorta *(AA)* and brachiocephalic vessels. The descending aorta did not opacify. *LSA,* Left subclavian artery.

after operation, although intravenous isoproterenol (0.1 μg per kilogram per minute) was given for four hours and then discontinued. Respiratory rate had returned to normal by the fifth postoperative day, and with the patient breathing room air the arterial Po_2 was 32 mm. Hg. He was discharged ten days after operation. One month later cyanosis was minimal, the femoral pulses were normal, and the flush blood pressure in the upper and lower extremities was 80 mm. Hg.

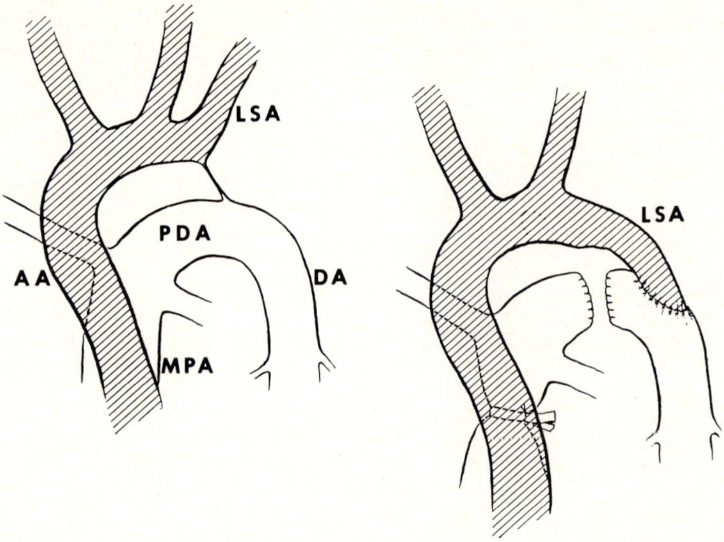

Fig. 5. Diagram of the anatomy before and after operation. *AA,* ascending aorta; *LSA,* left subclavian artery; *MPA,* main pulmonary artery; *PDA,* patent ductus arteriosus; *DA,* descending aorta.

DISCUSSION

From a physiologic and diagnostic view, several points in this case deserve consideration. Although the fetal circulation in this anomaly has not been studied, the ascending aorta, which arises from the right ventricle, must supply blood to the upper body and head. The pulmonary artery and patent ductus arteriosus supply blood to the descending thoracic aorta and placenta. Mixing at the atrial and ventricular septal defects allows part of the oxygenated placental venous return to reach the head and upper body from the right ventricle and ascending aorta.

After birth, blood flows through the lungs normally, but blood flow to the descending thoracic aorta must come through the patent ductus arteriosus. Pulmonary arterial blood is a mixture of venous blood from both the systemic and pulmonary circulations. Adequate mixing of the two circulations occurs through the atrial and ventricular septal defects. The similar oxygen saturations which are found in the ascending and descending thoracic aorta are evidence of this mixing.

In the immediate neonatal period, pulmonary blood flow is not excessive because neonates normally have a high pulmonary vascular resistance. However, as this resistance falls, pulmonary blood flow increases and raises the volume load on the left ventricle. When the ductus is large, the relationship between the systemic vascular resistance in the lower body and the pulmonary vascular resistance determines the amount of blood which enters the descending thoracic aorta. It is not unusual for infants with aortic atresia, mitral atresia with an intact septum, or hypoplastic left heart to have good femoral pulses and adequate perfusion of the lower body as long as the ductus arteriosus remains patent and the pulmonary vascular resistance is high.

As pulmonary vascular resistance decreases, more blood perfuses the lungs and less blood reaches the lower body. Partial constriction of the patent ductus arteriosus, which occurred in this case, further reduces blood flow to the descending thoracic aorta. These events cause relative ischemia of the lower body, overcirculation of the lungs, and failure of the left ventricle.

Changes in circulatory dynamics during operation are of interest. Banding alone in the presence of a patent ductus arteriosus and preductal atresia of the aorta is contraindicated because blood flow through the ductus is obligatory. Thus adequate flow to the descending aorta must be provided prior to the division of the ductus arteriosus. In this case, after the subclavian artery–descending aorta anastomosis was completed, pulmonary arterial and aortic pressures were equal. This allowed division of the ductus arteriosus without causing an abrupt change in either pulmonary blood flow or flow to the lower body. Once the ductus was divided, pulmonary blood flow could be reduced by banding. As the band was tightened, more blood was shunted across the ventricular septal defect to the right ventricle and the aorta; this increased systemic blood pressure. If flow through the ductus arteriosus had been impeded during the subclavian–aortic anastomosis, ischemia of the lower body might have developed. Recently, we observed postoperative anuria after a 20 minute repair of a severe coarctation of the aorta in an 18-day-old infant.

The subclavian arterial bypass procedure was utilized in this patient with aortic atresia because of the need to maintain flow to the descending aorta. This operation was devised by Blalock and Park[3] and first used clinically by Clagett.[7] Continuous monitoring of radial arterial pressure and measurement of distal pulmonary arterial pressure during the banding permitted the operation to achieve its objectives without episodes of bradycardia or hypotension.

Of the cases reported with atresia or interruption of the aortic arch in association with transposition of the great vessels, most died in the first months of life[2, 4-6, 8-10, 15] and those who lived beyond early childhood developed pulmonary vascular disease. Castellanos and associates[6] reported the case of a patient who had a patent ductus arteriosus and differential cyanosis at age six, but who had a closed ductus arteriosus when death occurred at age nine years. This child had developed considerable collateral circulation around the atretic aorta.

Operation has rarely been attempted in infants with the combination of aortic atresia and transposition of the great arteries. Tawes and associates[15] reported a case in which correction of the arch atresia and division of the patent ductus arteriosus was performed during early infancy. The patient died after a second operation at which the pulmonary artery was banded. Waldhausen and associates[16] reported successful repair of aortic atresia, division of a patent ductus arteriosus, and banding of the pulmonary artery in an 11-month-old child.

SUMMARY

The diagnosis of atresia of the aortic arch associated with transposition of the great arteries and ventricular septal defect was made in a newborn infant and confirmed by cardiac catheterization and angiography. A palliative operation (subclavian–aortic anastomosis, division of the patent ductus, and pulmonary artery banding) was successfully performed at four days of age. The circulatory physiology of this lesion during fetal life, at birth, during the neonatal period, and during operation is discussed.

REFERENCES

1. Adam, M., Johnson, A. F., Jr., Davis, M. V., and Mitchell, B. F.: Surgical management of coarctation of the aorta in infancy, Ann. Thorac. Surg. **2:** 188, 1966.
2. Blake, H. A., Manion, W. C., and Spencer, F. C.: Atresia or absence of the aortic isthmus, J. Thorac. Cardiovasc. Surg. **43:** 607, 1962.
3. Blalock, A., and Park, E. A.: The surgical treatment of experimental coarctation (atresia) of the aorta, Ann. Surg. **119:** 445, 1944.
4. Bowers, D. E., Schiebler, G. L., and Krovetz, L. J.: Interruption of the aortic arch with complete transposition of the great vessels, Amer. J. Cardiol. **16:** 442, 1965.
5. Buckley, M. J., Mason, D. T., Ross, J., Jr., and Braunwald, E.: Reversed differential cyanosis with equal desaturation of the upper limbs, Amer. J. Cardiol. **15:** 111, 1965.
6. Castellanos, A., Garcia, O., and Gonzalez, E.: Complete interruption of the aortic arch with transposition of the great vessels, Cardiologia **34:** 53, 1959.
7. Clagett, O. T.: Coarctation of the aorta:

Surgical aspects, Proc. Staff Meet. Mayo Clin. **22:** 137, 1947.

8. Hamburger, L. P., Jr.: Congenital cardiac malformation presenting complete interruption of the isthmus aortae with transposition of the great arteries, Bull. Johns Hopkins Hosp. **61:** 421, 1937.
9. Mehrizi, A., and Morrish, H. F.: Interruption of the aortic arch, Bull. Johns Hopkins Hosp. **111:** 127, 1962.
10. Moller, J. H., and Edwards, J. E.: Interruption of aortic arch: Anatomic patterns and associated cardiac malformations, Amer. J. Roentgen. **95:** 557, 1965.
11. Roberts, W. C., Morrow, A. G., and Braunwald, E.: Complete interruption of the aortic arch, Circulation **26:** 39, 1962.
12. Rochette, M., Stanley, P., Ethier, M. F., and Darignon, A.: Complete interruption of the aortic arch in infancy, Canad. Med. Ass. J. **98:** 131, 1968.
13. Sinha, S., Kardatzke, M. L., Cole, R. B., Muster, A. J., Wessel, H. U., and Paul, M. H.: Coarctation of the aorta in infancy, Circulation **40:** 385, 1969.
14. Tawes, R. L., Aberdeen, E., Waterston, D. J., and Bonham-Carter, R. E.: Coarctation of the aorta in infants and children: A review of 333 operative cases, including 179 infants, Circulation **39** (Suppl. 1): 173, 1969.
15. Tawes, R. L., Panagopoulos, P., Aberdeen, E., Waterston, D. J., and Bonham-Carter, R. E.: Aortic arch atresia and interruption of the aortic arch, J. Thorac. Cardiovasc. Surg. **58:** 492, 1969.
16. Waldhausen, J. A., Boruchow, I., Miller, W. W., and Rashkind, W. J.: Transposition of the great arteries with ventricular septal defect: Palliation by atrial septostomy and pulmonary artery banding, Circulation **39** (Suppl. 1): 215, 1969.
17. Waldhausen, J. A., Kind, H., Nahrwold, D. L., Lurie, P. R., and Shumaker, H. B., Jr.: Management of coarctation in infancy, J. A. M. A. **187:** 270, 1964.

The surgical treatment of peptic ulcer: A critical analysis of results from subtotal gastrectomy and from vagotomy plus partial gastrectomy*

ALTON OCHSNER, M.D.
PAUL R. ZEHNDER, M.D.
SHIRLEY W. TRAMMELL, B.A.
NEW ORLEANS, LA.
From the Department of Surgery, Ochsner Clinic and Ochsner Foundation Hospital

In a study of the surgical treatment of peptic ulcer, a historical look at the various procedures used helps to bring one's thinking into proper perspective.

SURGICAL PROCEDURES

Gastroenterostomy. Early in this century the ideal surgical treatment for peptic ulcer disease was gastroenterostomy and many patients were relieved and apparently cured by it. I recall when I was a surgical house officer in the early twenties, gastroenterostomy was so common that it was said that it was indicated if the patient belched. By the thirties, however, the bad results from gastroenterostomy became evident. Although in many patients there were no recurrences of duodenal ulcer, a new ulcer developed at the anastomotic stoma or in the jejunum and was even worse than the original ulcer. When I first came to Tulane University, in 1927, as Professor of Surgery, I was astounded to observe the large number of stomal and jejunal ulcers in patients who had been subjected to gastrojejunostomies 20 to 25 years previously. The most frequent gastric operation I did at that time was to take down the gastrojejunostomy and re-establish the normal gastrointestinal continuity. We thus learned that gastroenterostomy was a bad operation; but it had one great advantage—it could be taken down.

Gastric resection. Although I had been originally taught that gastroenterostomy was the ideal surgical treatment for peptic ulcer, when I served as an exchange surgical resident for three years in Zürich, Switzerland, under Prof. Clairmont and in Frankfurt-am-Main under Prof. Schmieden, I became convinced that wide gastric resection was the best procedure. The first gastric resection for ulcer was performed by Rydygier[49] on Nov. 21, 1881, on a 30-year-old woman with a stenosing ulcer; the operation resulted in complete relief of symptoms for 19 years. However, gastric resection for ulcer disease did not become popular until the first decade of the present century in Europe (von Eiselsberg,[14-16] Finsterer,[19-23] von Haberer,[27-31] Clairmont,[9-10] and Schmieden[53-54]). In the United States, Strauss[59-62] in Chicago, Berg,[3] and Lewisohn[44] in New York early did gastrectomy for ulcer. In 1915 Strauss[61] presented six successful cases of subtotal gastrectomy for peptic ulcer before the Chicago Surgical Society, at which time he was so severely criticized by his colleagues that he refrained from doing any more resections until 1917. Having observed the bad results following gastrojejunostomy in the United States and be-

Received for publication Dec 20, 1969.

*Abridged version of paper presented as the Grey Turner Lecture at the International Surgical Society, Buenos Aires, Argentina, September, 1969.

cause of the safety with which subtotal gastric resection could be done, producing sufficient reduction in the gastric acidity to prevent recurrent ulceration, I have routinely done subtotal resection for chronic peptic ulcer since 1925.

Vagus resection. Although vagus resection had been advocated in 1901 by Jaboulay[38] and performed by Exner[17, 18] and Bircher[5] for peptic ulcer, it was used only sporadically until Dragstedt and his associates popularized the method. Dragstedt's classical and fundamental investigations demonstrating the role of acid in the genesis of peptic ulcer and the part played by the vagi will rightfully go down in the annals of medical history as one of the finest experimental and clinical investigations. I wish I could look back on my life and think I had accomplished as much as has Lester Dragstedt by this work. In 1943 Dragstedt and Owens[13] reported the results in two cases of peptic ulcer treated by supradiaphragmatic vagus resection (the first one performed on Jan. 18 and the second on Jan. 22, 1943). Since then, there has been a tremendous increase in the number of patients with peptic ulcer treated with vagus resection, particularly in the United States and, to a lesser extent, in Latin America and England. This is undoubtedly due to two factors: (1) the prominence of Dr. Dragstedt and the importance of the experimental work that he and his associates have done in demonstrating the role of acid in the genesis of peptic ulcer and (2) because the operation is easier to perform than is gastrectomy and, in the hands of less competent surgeons, less hazardous. With very few exceptions, subtotal gastrectomy remains the method of choice in the treatment of peptic ulcer on the European continent, particularly in the Germanic countries. In France, about half the surgeons still do subtotal gastric resection.

Because I had observed the popularity of gastrojejunostomy come and go and because I appreciated, as most people do, that to evaluate any therapy for peptic ulcer requires a long period of observation (at least 25 years), I have refrained from doing vagus resection for peptic ulcer. It took approximately 25 years for the bad results following gastrojejunostomy to become evident. Also, the results from gastrectomy for intractable ulcer are so satisfactory that I felt that considerable time should elapse before final evaluation of this new procedure. I was also concerned that truncal vagus resection results in denervation of not only the stomach and duodenum (the viscera involved), but also the biliary tract and enteric tube to the midportion of the transverse colon. For this reason, I would have less objection to selective vagus resection if it can be accomplished. Another factor that disturbed me about vagus resection is that, since its original popular use in the mid-forties, there have been frequent modifications of the technique employed. First, it was only vagus resection, and then because of gastric stasis, it was combined with gastrojejunostomy. After a short period of time (approximately five years), probably because the results were not quite satisfactory, vagus resection was combined with pyloroplasty. More recently, the operation has been modified to combine vagus resection with partial gastrectomy. Even more recently, the operation of selective vagus resection has been employed. An operative procedure that requires modification every four to five years must have some inherent defect.

PEPTIC ULCER DISEASE

Genesis. Because of our experience with so many patients with gastrojejunal ulcers seen at Charity Hospital when I first came to New Orleans, it was decided that a better understanding of the genesis of peptic ulcer was necessary. An experimental program was begun by several members of the surgical staff (Ochsner, Gage, De Bakey, Graves, Hosoi[12, 24, 26, 48]). These studies demonstrated that the precipitating factor in the production of gastroduodenal disease was acid; also, that the tissue susceptibility to acid peptic digestion varies in different parts of the stomach and different parts of the enteric tube. The lesser curvature was found to be more vulnerable than the greater curvature, and when anastomoses were made between the stomach and the various portions of the enteric tube, the susceptibility of the mucosa to acid gastric chyme increased with the distance from the pylorus. It was found that the alkaline fluids in the duodenum (succus entericus, bile, and pancreatic juice) were protective. Because approximately ten percent of the normal population have hyperacidity but no ulcer, it was postulated that peptic ulcer in man resulted from two factors: (1) predisposition (susceptibility) which is inherent in the individual—he is born with it, lives with it, and will die with it; (2) acid, the precipitating factor.

Medical therapy. All methods of treating ulcer are designed to control gastric acidity, which is the controllable of the two etiologic factors. Generally, there is little difficulty in obtaining prompt healing of an ulcer if acid secretion is controlled. Unfortunately the ulcer, which is in fact a symptom and not a disease, usually recurs after healing and frequently with periodic regularity. This occurs because the patient, whose ulcer has healed, is allowed to revert to his usual mode of living which causes the return of uncontrolled acid secretion. If, however, the patient with the healed ulcer is instructed to avoid the factors which increase gastric acidity (gastric distension by overeating, alcohol, caffeine, tobacco, and emotional tension), he usually remains well and does not have an ulcer recurrence. We are convinced that the treatment of duodenal ulcer is primarily medical and that operative treatment is indicated only in patients with surgical complications, such as perforation, massive hemorrhage, and pyloric obstruction, and in those with intractable lesions.

Surgical therapy. It is difficult to determine what percentage of patients with peptic ulcer require surgical treatment. In our own institution 14 percent of patients with duodenal ulcer are operated upon, but this percentage is undoubtedly much higher than is generally necessary because our institution serves as a referral center to which only difficult and complicated cases are admitted. Probably not more than one in a thousand patients with duodenal ulcer disease requires surgical treatment. If one accepts our criteria concerning the treatment of peptic ulcer, that is, to operate only on those who have surgical complications or in whom conservative therapy has failed, the patients who are treated by surgical therapy are therefore those whose condition is most severe because it has resisted conservative therapy. Since surgical therapy is limited to those cases with intractable or complicated conditions, it is obligatory to employ the surgical procedure which will best control gastric acidity with minimal sequelae and fewest recurrences.

RESULTS OF GASTRIC RESECTION

Subtotal gastric resection has stood the test of time. It is an operation that has been done for over 50 years, and sufficient time has elapsed to evaluate it and to determine the possible sequelae which may develop after the resection of a large portion of the stomach.

Mortality rate. In the early twenties before antibiotics were available and before much was known about prevention of pulmonary infection, the mortality rate following gastric resection was relatively high (approximately five percent). However, Strauss and associates[62] in 1952 reported their results from a series of 1,796 patients with peptic ulcer treated over a period of 35 years who were divided into two groups: (1) those treated between 1917 and 1938 with a mortality rate of 3.5 percent and (2) those treated between 1930 and 1950 with a mortality rate of 1.4 percent!

Recurrence rate. The recurrence rate following subtotal gastrectomy for peptic ulcer disease is low. It varies from zero to two to three percent. Strauss and associates[62] in 1952 reported a recurrence rate of one percent. In 1964, Hoffman[37] reported on 800 patients who had been treated by gastrectomy for ulcer disease and who had been followed for 15 to 16 years and demonstrated a 1.1 percent recurrence rate; he also reported on 336 patients treated surgically since 1939 and followed for five to ten years with a one percent recurrence rate. Toole[64] in 1965 reported on 14,670 patients treated surgically who demonstrated a 1.34 percent recurrence rate. Stojanovic[58] in 1967 reported on 1,312 patients who had undergone resections with a one percent recurrence rate, and Späth and Kronberger[57] in the same year reported a 0.1 percent recurrence in 1,351 patients having undergone gastrectomy.

Dumping. Dumping syndrome is occasionally seen in patients with subtotal gastrectomy; however, it is usually of short duration. Zenker and Rueff[68] in 1967 in a series of 1,533 patients observed dumping in 6.48 percent, 2.5 percent of whom had temporary dumping and 3.9 percent had persistent dumping. Stojanovic[58] in 1967 in a series of 1,312 patients had 2.5 percent incidence of dumping. Krause[43] stated, "The incidence of pronounced postcibal symptoms is low at examination 10 years after operation (gastrectomy), 4 to 5 percent."

Diarrhea. Diarrhea is seldom a problem following gastric resection. Schlicke[52] in 1963 reported on 176 patients, 7.9 percent of whom had subsequent diarrhea, which was mild in all patients; Goligher and associates[25] in 117 patients observed subsequent diarrhea in 10.7 percent; Clark[11] reported its occurrence in 20.5 percent of 331 patients; only 1.5 percent were disabled by it. Burge and associates[7] reported on 200 patients with a 20 percent incidence of diarrhea, which was severe in none of them.

End results. The end results following gastrectomy have been good. In 1923, Burk[8] in a series of 83 cases of gastrectomy reported good results in 90.4 percent, fair in 6.1 percent, and poor in 3 percent. Strauss[61] in 1952 reported 1,200 cases with 95 percent good results. Lindenschmidt and Schwabe[45] in 1961 determined the ability of 6,771 patients to work after gastric resection: 75 to 97 percent were able to work; and of the twelve reports, in eight, over 90 percent were able to work following gastrectomy. Zarubin[67] determined the work capability of 650 patients who had undergone gastrectomy: 81.2 percent were able to work; 58 percent were able to do heavy work; 68 percent were able to do moderately heavy work; and 95 percent were able to do light work. Späth and Kronberger[57] in a series of 1,351 cases of gastrectomy found that 88.8 percent of the patients were able to work. Vara-Lopez and Vara-Thorbeck[65] in 1967 reported on 995 patients, of whom 93.8 percent had good results. Kissler and associates[39] reported good results in 98 percent and poor results in two percent in a series of 1,074 patients. Kourias[40] reported on 5,666 patients; of those treated before 1955, 89 percent had good results, five percent fair results, and six percent poor results. Of those treated between 1956 and 1966, 91 percent had good results, four percent fair results, and five percent poor results.

Generally the results in patients who have intractable symptoms for a long time are better than in patients in whom the operation has been done as an emergency measure, such as in cases of massive bleeding. This may be because the individual with an intractable ulcer has suffered so much that when he is operated upon, he is so motivated that any minor disturbance he might have is of little or no significance, and he obtains complete relief. In any case, relief is permanent. Krause,[43] in discussing postcibal symptoms after gastrectomy, stated, "If patients are operated upon with insignificant preoperative subjective symptoms, the incidence of postcibal symptoms is certainly higher. The patient can be said to be 'psychologically immature' for operation." Papo and associates[49] stated, "The longer the history, the more severe the complaints, the older the patients, the better are the results of surgery."

RESULTS OF VAGOTOMY

Mortality rate. It has been stated that the great advantage of vagotomy over gastric resection is that it results in a lower mortality rate. This is not necessarily true, although we are convinced that in the hands of surgeons with insufficient training and experience, it is lower than that following subtotal gastrectomy. Herrington[35] had a 2.8 percent mortality rate in 1,073 patients who underwent vagus resection. Bruce[6] in 184 patients subjected to vagectomy and gastroenterostomy had a 2.7 percent mortality rate, and of 99 patients treated surgically by vagotomy and Polya resection, 4.04 percent died.

Recurrence rate. The incidence of recurrence after vagus resection is definitely higher than that following subtotal gastric resection. Tanner[63] in 319 patients who were followed up to five years after operation had a 3.3 percent recurrence. In patients in whom vagus resection and drainage operation were done for duodenal ulcer, Zahn and associates[66] had a 10 percent recurrence rate, and when the procedure was done for gastric ulcer, 40 percent. Rhea and associates[50] in a collected series of 1,920 patients with peptic ulcer disease treated by vagus resection and gastric drainage and followed from one to 14 years, found a recurrence rate of 9.4 percent, ranging from 2.7 to 19.2 percent. Nobles[46] in 1966 reported on 102 patients treated by vagotomy and gastrojejunostomy with recurrence in 24 within ten years after an average interval of 8.5 years. The recurrence rate at the end of 15 years was 28 percent. Nobles further reported that in 110 postvagotomy patients with intact gallbladders, 18.2 percent developed gallstones after an average of 12 years or had to have a cholecystectomy because of acute noncalculous cholecystitis.

Dumping. Dumping occurs more frequently in patients subjected to vagus resection than in those treated with gastrectomy. Kraft and associates[42] found that, in 50 patients treated by truncal vagotomy, dumping occurred in 29 percent, and in the 50 treated with selective vagotomy, it occurred in 39 percent. Harkins and associates[33] observed dumping in 38 percent of 60 patients treated with truncal vagotomy and antrectomy, and in 46 percent of 52 treated with selective vagotomy and antrectomy. Dumping, however, is likely to be relatively mild, easily controlled with dietary measures, and is usually not of much consequence.

Diarrhea. The most severe sequel after vagus resection is diarrhea. In 1961 Clark,[11] in 161 patients followed for five to ten years after vagotomy and gastroenterostomy, observed diarrhea in 67, or 22 percent (12 percent mild, 7.4 percent moderate, and 2.6 percent severe). Of 77 patients subjected to vagotomy and partial gastrectomy, 13 percent had diarrhea (10.4 percent mild and 2.6 percent moderate). In 17 patients treated with vagotomy for jejunal ulcer, 41 percent had diarrhea (11.7 percent mild, 17.6 percent moderate, and 11.7 percent severe). Kraft and associates[41] in 47 cases treated by truncal vagotomy and drainage, observed diarrhea in 38 percent, and in 40 patients treated with selective vagotomy, observed diarrhea in 19 percent. Harkins and associates[33] and Smith and Farris[56] similarly noted a lower incidence of diarrhea after surgical treatment with selective vagotomy (29 and 12 percent, respectively) than after surgical treatment with truncal vagotomy (68 and 28 percent, respectively). Clark[11] stated, "It is significant that severe cases of diarrhea are associated with vagotomy and in these patients it represents a serious disability." Burge and associates,[7] discussing the incidence of diarrhea after vagotomy and gastrectomy as reported by Clark, stated, "We found as he had, that diarrhea was a much milder affair after gastrectomy than after vagotomy." Ballinger,[1] discussing the diarrhea in vagotomized patients, stated, "Certainly since the type of diarrhea was only rarely seen occurring after the usual gastric resection before the advent of vagotomy, it seems likely that vagotomy itself is involved." Hendry and Abdulla[34] in 1969 stated, "We agree with Burge and others (*Annals Royal College of Surgeons,* 1966) that there is no effective treatment for postvagotomy diarrhea. We have tried all methods of treatment with no real success." Nuboer[47] stated, "In a series of about 80 cases in which I, myself, used the procedure (vagotomy) there were a number of postvagotomy patients who although the ulcer symptoms had disappeared were worse off than before as a result of diarrhea and abdominal symptoms." Barrie and associates[2] in 1968 stated, "A Dragstedt procedure although effective and relatively safe is thus far from harmless when compared to the results of classic gastrectomy."

It has indeed distressed us that a procedure which at times requires the most unphysiologic of all operations we know, namely reversing a loop of jejunum in order to decrease the rapid transit of intestinal content, is so widely used. Obviously, it has inherent defects. Herrington and associates[36] reported on seven patients requiring the reversed jejunal loop because of intractable diarrhea. The patients had from ten to 25 copious, watery stools daily and had lost from 20 to 80 pounds.

It is interesting that Smith and Farris[56] in 1963 advocated selective vagus resection because the subsequent diarrhea was less than that following truncal vagotomy (12 and 28 percent, respectively). However, in 1969 they[55] stated, "Since the performance of selective vagotomy is infinitely more difficult than that of truncal vagotomy and since its benefits are open to serious question by several observers, consideration should be given to omit its routine employment in the surgical treatment of peptic ulcer disease."

EXPERIENCE AT OCHSNER CLINIC

Our experience is based upon a series of 4,489 cases of peptic ulcer of which 3,747 (83 percent) were duodenal ulcer and 742 (17 percent) gastric ulcer. Of the duodenal ulcer patients, 528 were operated upon (14 percent), and of the gastric ulcer patients, 253 were operated upon (34 percent). Although it is our belief that a duodenal ulcer should be treated conservatively and probably not more than one in a thousand cases should be operated upon, gastric ulcers are primarily surgical conditions because of the difficulty in distinguishing between a benign and malignant ulcer. Moreover, approximately ten to 15 percent of lesions which are believed to be benign prove to be malignant. The burden of proof is upon the physician who elects to treat a gastric ulcer conservatively to prove that it is not malignant. Our gastroenterologists insist that the patient with gastric ulcer, being treated conservatively, be hospitalized and on a strict dietary regimen. If, at the end of three weeks, the ulcer is not completely or almost completely healed, the patient is operated upon. If, however, at the end of three weeks, the ulcer is healed or almost healed, the patient is discharged, kept upon the dietary regimen, and re-examined in a month. If the ulcer is not completely healed at that time, operation is done. If it is healed, the patient is re-examined at monthly intervals for another two months and then at three-month intervals for a year. The simple healing of an ulcer does not mean that the lesion is not malignant because, in an individual in whom there is gastric acidity, it is possible for a superficial carcinoma to undergo peptic digestion, just as normal gastric mucosa can, and if such an individual is placed upon a dietary regimen which controls gastric acidity, the ulcer can heal. We have observed this in a number of instances.

Duration of ulcer. A total of 815 patients have been operated upon, 65 percent for duodenal ulcer, 31 percent for gastric ulcer, and four percent for gastrojejunal ulcer. The known duration of ulcer varied a good deal in the several types of ulcer (Table I). Over half of the gastric ulcer patients (56 percent) had symptoms for less than six months and only ten percent had symptoms over ten years. Contrariwise, 28 percent of

Table I. *Peptic ulcer—Ochsner Clinic: Known duration of ulcer*

	Duodenal (%)	*Gastric* (%)	*Gastrojejunal* (%)
Less than 6 mo.	28	56	3
6 mo.–2 yr.	17	15	12
2 yr.–10 yr.	29	19	41
Over 10 yr.	25	10	44

the patients with duodenal ulcer had symptoms less than six months, and 25 percent had symptoms for over ten years.

Operative indications. The indications for operation varied according to the type of ulcer; 52 percent of the patients with gastric ulcer were operated upon because of the possibility of malignant change, whereas 52 percent of the duodenal ulcer patients had intractable symptoms (Table II). The complicating factors at the time of operation were extremely important and greatly influenced the risk. Of the 528 patients operated on for duodenal ulcer, 28 percent had obstruction at the time of operation, 13 percent were bleeding massively, and eight percent had preperforation (Table III).

Types of operative procedures. Our experiences consist primarily of the classic 75 percent gastric resection because until relatively recently practically all of the peptic ulcer cases were so treated. In recent years, however, some of the younger members of the staff have done vagus resection, usually with a 50 percent gastric resection. Sixty patients (6.5 percent) had Billroth I procedure, 675 (74 percent) had Billroth II procedure (most of which were of the Hoffmeister-posterior), 152 patients underwent vagotomy (16 percent) of whom 140 had as associated partial gastrectomy (Table IV). Of those patients in whom a resection was done, either with or without vagotomy, the group was divided into those with radical resection (75 percent or more of the stomach removed) and those with conservative resection (approximately 50 percent). Of the entire group, 62 percent had radical resection and 38 percent had conservative resection (Table V). Gastric ulcers do not require as wide a resection to secure good results as do duodenal ulcers.

Mortality rate. One of the supposedly great advantages of vagus resection is that

Table II. *Peptic ulcer—Ochsner Clinic: Indications for operation*

	Duodenal (%)	Gastric (%)	Gastrojejunal (%)
Hemorrhage	27	21	32
Perforation	6	4	2
Obstruction	26	13	11
Intractable symptoms	52	31	76
Fear of possible malignancy	5	52	0

Table III. *Peptic ulcer—Ochsner Clinic: Complicating factors at time of operation*

	Duodenal (528 cases)		Gastric (253 cases)		Gastrojejunal (34 cases)	
	No.	%	No.	%	No.	%
Obstruction	148	28	34	13	8	23
Hemorrhage	70	13	38	14	6	18
Perforation	40	8	17	7	1	3

Table IV. *Peptic ulcer—Ochsner Clinic: Type of operation*

	No. of patients	%
Billroth I	60	6.5
Billroth II		
Polya—anterior	1	
Polya—posterior	18	
Hoffmeister—anterior	30	
Hoffmeister—posterior	626	
Total	675	74
Total gastrectomy	3	
Segmental resection	3	
Gastroenterostomy	3	
Closure of perforation	16	
Vagotomy		
Alone	2	
With drainage	9	
With subtotal gastrectomy	141	
Total	152	16

Table V. *Peptic ulcer—Ochsner Clinic: Subtotal gastrectomy*

	Radical		Conservative	
	No. of patients	%	No. of patients	%
Duodenal	309	64	170	36
Gastric	129	56	100	44
Gastrojejunal	23	72	9	28
Total	461	62	279	38

it is a safer procedure and carries a lower mortality rate. As mentioned previously, we believe this is probably true when performed by relatively inexperienced surgeons. However, in our series of cases, this is not borne out. The mortality rate following gastric resection alone was 1.4 percent; whereas that following gastric resection associated with vagotomy was four percent (Table VI). The greatest risk is in patients in whom operation is necessary because of massive hemorrhage. The mortality rate in this group was 5.8 percent. Recently vagus resection has been advocated as the treatment of choice for massive hemorrhage. This seems illogical to us and our opinion is substantiated by our results. The patients with massive hemorrhage treated by subtotal gastrectomy alone had a three percent mortality rate; whereas, of the patients treated with vagotomy and gastrectomy, it was 13.6 percent. Obviously vagotomy in our experience has been a poor operation for massive bleeding in peptic ulcer (Table VII).

Table VI. *Peptic ulcer—Ochsner Clinic: Mortality following gastric resection*

Procedure	*Mortality rate (%)*
Without vagotomy	1.4
With vagotomy	4

Table VII. *Peptic ulcer—Ochsner Clinic: Massive hemorrhage at time of operation (13 percent)*

Type of operation		*Deaths (%)*	
Gastrectomy alone	(57%)	3	5.8
Gastrectomy and vagotomy	(43%)	13.6	

Length of follow-up. In evaluating the results from any method of therapy in the treatment of peptic ulcer, the length of follow-up is extremely important. In our series, follow-up was less than one year in 20 percent, one to five years in 41 percent, and more than five years in 39 percent. Evaluation of results in our cases showed that the incidences of dumping, diarrhea, gastric retention, vomiting, and recurrence were higher in patients subjected to vagotomy and gastric resection than it was in individuals having gastric resection without an associated vagotomy (Table VIII).

Recurrence. The incidence of recurrent ulceration varied as to the type of ulcer treated: gastric, zero percent; duodenal, two percent; gastrojejunal, three percent. The recurrence was three times more frequent following conservative than radical gastrectomy, three and one percent, respectively.

Dumping. Dumping is an uncomfortable postoperative sequel. In our patients, it occurred in 31 percent of those having a radical resection and in 26 percent of those having a conservative resection; however, in most patients it was mild (23 and 16 percent, respectively). Dumping was, however, much more common in patients treated with vagotomy associated with resection than with gastric resection alone (Table IX), 35 and 14 percent, respectively. Even more important was the fact that only 3.8 percent of the patients subjected to gastric resection without vagotomy had persistent dumping, whereas 26 percent of those treated with vagotomy had persistent dumping.

Diarrhea. Diarrhea is one of the most troublesome of manifestations following vagus resection (Table X). Forty-four percent of patients had diarrhea; 22 percent of the patients had persistent diarrhea as

Table VIII. *Peptic ulcer—Ochsner Clinic: Long-term sequelae*

	Dumping (%)	*Diarrhea (%)*	*Gastric retention (%)*	*Vomiting (%)*	*Recurrent ulcer (%)*
Gastric resection without vagotomy	14	6.5	1.4	4	2.1
Vagotomy	35	44	3	15	5.4

contrasted with an incidence of 6.5 percent in patients with gastric resection without vagotomy, 4.8 percent of whom had persistent diarrhea.

Weight loss. Weight loss has been considered undesirable in individuals who have been subjected to gastric resection. It is always of interest to us that, although obesity is considered undesirable generally, individuals who have had a gastric operation are thought not to be well unless they get fat again. We have had a large number of patients who have had radical subtotal gastrectomies and failed to gain weight after the operation but who have remained perfectly well, in that they were able to eat and drink everything without any symptoms. In our study, weight loss was observed in both groups of patients (Table XI). Of those with a weight loss of more than 15 pounds, 25 percent had not undergone vagotomy and 30 percent had undergone vagotomy. In those that lost less than 15 pounds, these respective percentages were 58 and 33 percent. The weight loss was greater in patients subjected to radical gastric resection than in those having less radical gastrectomies, 20 and 17 pounds, respectively.

Variation in results. The satisfactory results vary somewhat in the different types of ulcer treated, being best in gastric ulcer (Table XII) and also according to the extent of the gastric resection. Of those who had radical resection, 93 percent had satisfactory results and of those treated by conservative resection, 90 percent (Table XIII). The results generally were better in men than in women (Table XIV).

Patients' evaluation. There is no operation which I have done through the years which has given me so much satisfaction because it has relieved so many patients so completely as has the 75 percent resection of the stomach for intractable ulcer of the duodenum. Almost invariably the only criticism patients have when they return is, "Why did we not do the operation sooner?" We have classified our cases into these

Table IX. *Peptic ulcer—Ochsner Clinic: Long-term sequel*

Dumping	*Gastric resection without vagotomy (%)*	*Vagotomy (%)*
Mild	11	14
Moderate	2	15
Severe	0.5	3
Total	14	35
Persistent	3.8	26

Table X. *Peptic ulcer—Ochsner Clinic: Long-term sequel*

Diarrhea	*Gastric resection without vagotomy (%)*	*Vagotomy (%)*
Mild	3.4	14
Moderate	3.4	27
Severe	0.4	2
Total	6.5	44
Persistent	4.8	22

Table XI. *Peptic ulcer—Ochsner Clinic: Weight*

	Gastric resection without vagotomy (%)	*Vagotomy (%)*
Loss		
Less than 15 lb.	58	33
More than 15 lb.	25	30
No change	16	15
Gain	11	13

Table XII. *Peptic ulcer—Ochsner Clinic: Results following subtotal gastrectomy*

	Satisfactory (%)	*Unsatisfactory (%)*
Duodenal	89	11
Gastric	92	8
Gastrojejunal	90	10

Table XIII. *Peptic ulcer—Ochsner Clinic: Results following subtotal gastrectomy*

	Satisfactory (%)	*Unsatisfactory (%)*
Radical (93%)	Good 87 Fair 13	7
Conservative (90%)	Good 81 Fair 19	10

Table XIV. *Peptic ulcer—Ochsner Clinic: Final result according to sex*

Sex	*Type of resection*	*Satisfactory (%)*	*Unsatisfactory (%)*
Male	Radical	97	3
	Conservative	91	9
Female	Radical	94	6
	Conservative	90	10

Table XV. *Peptic ulcer—Ochsner Clinic: Long-term results*

	Gastric resection without vagotomy (%)	*Vagotomy (%)*
Excellent	80	21
Good	13	48
Fair	4.3	19
Poor	2.5	12

categories: "excellent," those who are completely relieved, have no symptoms at all, and are able to eat and do anything they want; "good," those who are much improved but require some dietary restriction to carry on their usual work; "fair," those who are improved but still have definite limitation as to what they can eat; and "poor" those who are as bad or worse than they were before the operation. Of those treated by gastric resection without vagotomy (Table XV), 80 percent were "excellent"; whereas, of those treated with vagotomy with gastric resection, 21 percent were "excellent."

CONCLUSION

Although these results demonstrate the superiority of the long-term effects following a subtotal gastrectomy for treatment of peptic ulcer disease over those following a vagus resection, one presumes that surgeons will still continue to do vagus resection because of the supposedly decreased risk from the operation, which is undoubtedly true when performed by inadequately trained surgeons. Whether this is a justification for using a procedure which is likely to be associated with prolonged, uncomfortable, and disabling sequelae is open to question. As mentioned previously, we believe that an operation which denervates the biliary tract and the enteric tube down to the midportion of the transverse colon is undesirable.

This study is particularly valid because all the patients were treated by well-trained, competent surgeons and in both series, with the exception of a very few patients treated by vagus resection and drainage, gastric resection was performed. In those treated with truncal vagotomy, approximately 50 percent of the stomach was resected; whereas in the remainder a wider portion—usually 75 percent was removed—the principal difference between the two groups being the gastroenteric-biliary denervation.

If vagus resection continues to be used, hopefully those who use it in the future will limit the denervation to the selective procedure so that possibly fewer side effects will be obtained. The statistics at the present show that gastric resection is preferable to vagus resection. The results are better than those following vagus resection and the sequelae fewer. We hope that the longer period of observation will not demonstrate that the undesirable sequelae persist and become more frequent because, unfortunately, in contradistinction to gastroenterostomy, which proved to be a bad operation but could be corrected, one cannot put back vagus nerves.

Because of the intensive study on the treatment of peptic ulcer in the United States and in other countries and because of our own experience, we are more convinced than ever that subtotal gastrectomy is the ideal method for treating intractable ulcer disease. Furthermore, we predict that in another ten to fifteen years, when the final bad results from vagus resection will have been evaluated, the operation will be in the same category as gastroenterostomy is at present.

REFERENCES

1. Ballinger, W. F.: Post-vagotomy changes in the small intestine, Amer. J. Surg. **114:** 382, 1967.
2. Barrie, J., Miguet, J., Latreille, R., Bocchio,

J. J., and Ronzy, J.: Ulcère du duodénum non compliqué, Gastrectomie ou opération de Dragstedt? Lyon Chir. **64:** 341, 1968.
3. Berg, A. A.: Radical surgical cure of gastric and duodenal ulcer, Surg. Clin. N. Amer. **5:** 49, 1925.
4. Bergmann, v.: *In* Schmieden, V.: Über die kausale Behandlung des Magengeschwür, Arch. Klin. Chir. **118:** 1, 1921.
5. Bircher, E.: Die Resektion von Aesten der N. vagus zur Behandlung gastrischer Affektionen, Schweiz. Med. Wschr. **50:** 519, 1920.
6. Bruce, Sir John: The surgical treatment of peptic ulceration, 22nd Congrès de la Société Internationale de Chirurgie, 1967, pp. 201-211.
7. Burge, H., Hutchison, J. S. F., Longland, C. J., Miln, D. C., McLennan, L., Rudick, J., and Tombin, A. M.: Selective nerve section in the prevention of post-vagotomy diarrhea, Lancet **1:** 577, 1964.
8. Burk, W.: Zur operativen Behandlung des Magen—und Zwölffinger darmgeschwürs, Zbl. Chir. **50:** 1569, 1923.
9. Clairmont, P.: Die Technik der Duodenalresektion wegen Ulkus, Wien. Klin. Wschr. **29:** 733, 1916.
10. Clairmont, P.: Ergebnisse der operatinen Behandlung der Ulcuskrankheit, Schweiz. Med. Wschr. **54:** 209, 1924.
11. Clark, C. G.: Vagotomy for peptic ulcer, Brit. Med. J. **1:** 1250, 1961.
12. De Bakey, M. E.: Peptic ulceration: Relative protective value of alkaline duodenal juices, Arch. Surg. **34:** 230, 1937.
13. Dragstedt, L. R., and Owens, F. M.: Supradiaphragmatic section of the vagus nerves in treatment of duodenal ulcer, Proc. Soc. Exp. Biol. Med. **53:** 152, 1943.
14. Eiselsberg, A. v.: The choice of the method of operation in the treatment of gastric and duodenal ulcer: With a review of my experiences in the past 10 years, Surg. Gynec. Obstet. **19:** 555, 1914.
15. Eiselsberg, A. v.: Die chirurgische Behandlung des Ulcus ventriculi et duodeni, Wien. Klin. Wschr. **34:** 108, 1921.
16. Eiselsberg, A. v.: Die chirurgische Behandlung des Magenulcus, Acta Chir. Scand. **59:** 71, 1925.
17. Exner, A.: Ein neues Operationsverfahren bei tabischen "crises gastriques," Deutsch. Z. Chir. **111:** 576, 1911.
18. Exner, A., and Schwarzmann, E.: Tabische Krisen, Ulcus ventriculi und vagus, Wien. Klin. Wschr. **25:** 1405, 1912.
19. Finsterer, H.: Ausgedehnte Magenresektion bei Ulcus duodeni statt der einfachen Duodenalresektion bzw Pylorus-ausschaltung, Zbl. Chir. **45:** 434, 1918.
20. Finsterer, H.: Fernresultate der operativen Behandlung des Ulcus duodeni, Wien. Klin. Wschr. **34:** 11, 1921.
21. Finsterer, H.: Über die Bedeutung des Pylorusringes für das Ulcusrezidiv und das Ulcus pepticum jejuni, Arch. Klin. Chir. **120:** 111, 1922.
22. Finsterer, H.: Ist die ausgedehnte Resektion des Magens beim Ulcus duodeni erlaubt oder nicht? Zbl. Chir. **50:** 1566, 1923.
23. Finsterer, H.: Duodenal ulcer and its surgical treatment, New Orleans Med. Surg. J. **76:** 459, 1924.
24. Gage, M., Ochsner, A., and Hosoi, K.: Relationship of gastric acidity to peptic ulceration, Arch. Surg. **32:** 1019, 1936.
25. Goligher, J. C., Pulvertaft, C. N., and Watkinson, G.: Controlled trial of vagotomy and gastroenterostomy, vagotomy and antrectomy, and subtotal gastrectomy in elective treatment of duodenal ulcer: Interim report, Brit. Med. J. **1:** 455, 1964.
26. Graves, A. M.: Combined and separate effects of bile, pancreatic secretion, and trauma in experimental peptic ulcer, Arch. Surg. **30:** 833, 1935.
27. Haberer, H. v.: Meine Erfahrungen mit 183 Magenresektionen, Arch. Klin. Chir. **106:** 533, 1915.
28. Haberer, H. v.: Ulcus duodeni und postoperatives peptisches Jejunalgeschwür, Arch. Klin. Chir. **109:** 413, 1918.
29. Haberer, H. v.: Anwendungsbreite und Vorteil der Magenresektion nach Billroth I, Arch. Klin. Chir. **114:** 127, 1920.
30. Haberer, H. v.: Operative Behandlung des Ulcus duodeni, Med. Klin. **16:** 275, 1920.
31. Haberer, H. v.: Ulcus ventriculi, ulcus duodeni, ulcus pepticum jejuni mit besonderer Berüschschtigüng der chirurgischen Therapie, Deutsch. Z. Chir. **172:** 1, 1922.
32. Harkins, H. N., Stavney, L. S., Griffith, C. A., Savage, L. E., and Nyhus, L. M.: Selective gastric vagotomy, Scientific Exhibit, 112th Annual Meeting of the American Medical Association, Atlantic City, 1963.
33. Harkins, H. M., Stavney, L. S., Griffith, C. A., Savage, L. E., and Nyhus, L. M.: Selective gastric vagotomy, Postgrad. Med. **35:** 289, 1964.
34. Hendry, W. G., and Abdulla, K. H.: Diarrhea after vagotomy. A comparative study of truncal and bilateral selective vagotomy, Brit. J. Surg. **56:** 1, 1969.
35. Herrington, J. L., Jr.: Antrectomy-vagotomy for duodenal ulcer: A fifteen year appraisal, New York J. Med. **63:** 2489, 1963.
36. Herrington, J. L., Jr., Edwards, W. H., Carter, J. H., and Sawouyers, J. L.: Treatment of severe postvagotomy diarrhea by reversed jejunal segment, Ann. Surg. **168:** 522, 1968.

37. Hoffman, V.: Die Krankheiten nach Magenresektion wegen Geschwürs (Billroth II) in meinen Nachuntersuchungen, Langenbecks Arch. Klin. Chir. **308:** 371, 1964.
38. Jaboulay, M.: La chirurgie du sympathique abdominal et sacré, Zbl. Chir. **28:** 227, 1901.
39. Kissler, F., Kissler, V., and Kyrle, P.: Operatives Vorgehen, Fruh und Spatergebnisse bei 1042 (1953-1967) Fällen von Gastroduodenalulcus, 22nd Congrès de la Société Internationale de Chirurgie, 1967, pp. 282-287.
40. Kourias, B. G.: Le problème actuel: gastrectomie ou vagotomie. Résultats de la gastrectomie, 22nd Congrès de la Société Internationale de Chirurgie, 1967, pp. 221-229.
41. Kraft, R. O., Fry, W. J., and Ransom, H. K.: Selective gastric vagotomy, Arch. Surg. **85:** 687, 1962.
42. Kraft, R. O., Fry, W. J., Wilhelm, K. G., and Ransom, H. K.: Selective gastric vagotomy, Arch. Surg. **95:** 625, 1967.
43. Krause, U.: Long term results of medical and surgical treatment of peptic ulcer, Acta Chir. Scand. Suppl. 310, 1963.
44. Lewisohn, R.: Resection of the stomach for chronic gastric and duodenal ulcer, Ann. Surg. **78:** 507, 1923.
45. Lindenschmidt, T. O., and Schwabe, G.: Das Ulcuscarcinom des Magens, Klinishcher Erfahrungsbericht über 156 Patienten, Langenbecks Arch. Klin. Chir. **319:** 306, 1967.
46. Nobles, E. R., Jr.: Vagotomy and gastroenterostomy. 15-year follow-up of 175 patients, Amer. Surg. **32:** 177, 1966.
47. Nuboer, J. F.: Gastrectomy or vagotomy in the treatment of duodenal ulcer, 22nd Congrès de la Société Internationale de Chirurgie, 1967, pp. 233-235.
48. Ochsner, A., Gage, M., and Hosoi, K.: Treatment of peptic ulcer based on physiological principles, Surg. Gynec. Obstet. **62:** 257, 1936.
49. Papo, I., Bervar, M., Jankuloski, A., Atanasijević, T., Spasojević, P., and Smiljanie: Classical gastric resection, a favorite operation for gastroduodenal ulcer, 22nd Congrès de la Société Internationale de Chirurgie, 1967, pp. 347-352.
50. Rhea, W. G., Jr., Killen, D. A., and Scott, H. W., Jr.: Long term results of partial gastric resection without vagotomy in duodenal ulcer disease, Surg. Gynec. Obstet. **120:** 970, 1965.
51. Rydygier, L.: Die erste Magenresektion beim Magengeschwür, Klin. Wschr. (Berlin) **19:** 39, 1882.
52. Schlicke, C. P.: Complications of vagotomy, Amer. J. Surg. **106:** 206, 1963.
53. Schmieden, V.: Über die Exzision der Magenstrasse, Zbl. Chir. **48:** 1534, 1921.
54. Schmieden, V.: Über die kausale Behandlung des Magengeschwürs, Arch. f. Klin. Chir. **118:** 1, 1921.
55. Smith, G. K., and Farris, J. M.: Reappraisal of the long-term effects of selective vagotomy, Amer. J. Surg. **117:** 222, 1969.
56. Smith, G. K., and Farris, J. M.: Some observations upon selective gastric vagotomy, Arch. Surg. **86:** 716, 1963.
57. Späth, F., and Kronberger, L.: Chirurgie des Magen-Duodenal-ulcus, 22nd Congrès de la Société Internationale de Chirurgie, 1967, pp. 316-320.
58. Stojanovic, V. K. Expérience clinique dans le traitement chirurgical de l'ulcère gastroduodénal, 22nd Congrès de la Société Internationale de Chirurgie, 1967, pp. 236-252.
59. Strauss, A. A.: Longitudinal resection of the lesser curvature with resection of pyloric sphincter: An experimental and clinical study, J. A. M. A. **82:** 1765, 1924.
60. Strauss, A. A.: Reminiscence of half a century of gastric surgery, Rev. Surg. **23:** 305, 1966.
61. Strauss, A. A., Block, L., Friedman, J. C., Meyer, J., and Parker, M. L.: Subtotal gastrectomy for duodenal ulcer. Ten years' experience and clinical end-results, J. A. M. A. **95:** 1883, 1930.
62. Strauss, A. A., Strauss, S. F., Schwartz, A. H., Kram, D. D., and Masur, W. W.: Results of subtotal gastrectomy for gastric and duodenal ulcer since 1917, J. A. M. A. **149:** 1095, 1952.
63. Tanner, N. C.: Management of peptic ulcer, Ann. Roy. Coll. Surg. Eng. **37:** 150, 1965.
64. Toole, H.: Über die Haüfigkeit des Ulcus pepticum nach Magenresektion in Griechenland, Langenbecks Arch. Klin. Chir. **313:** 372, 1965.
65. Vara-Lopez, R., and Vara-Thorbeck, R.: Tratamiento de la úlcera gástrica y sus resultados, 22nd Congrès de la Sociètè Internationale de Chirurgie, 1967, pp. 437-441.
66. Zahn, R. L., Stemmer, E. A., Hom, L. W., and Cowndley, J. E.: Delayed recurrence of gastric ulcer following vagotomy and drainage procedures, Amer. Surg. **34:** 757, 1968.
67. Zarubin, S. A.: Work capacity in a long term follow-up following gastric resection for ulcer, Vestn. Khir. Grekov. **80:** 28, 1958.
68. Zenker, R., and Rueff, F.: Ergebnisse der chirurgischen Behandlung des Magen-Duodenalgeschwürs, 22nd Congrès de la Sociètè Internationale de Chirurgie, 1967, pp. 258-261.

Technique of gastric mobilization for esophageal replacement

E. P. SIMKIN, M.CHIR., F.R.C.S.
P. M. STELL, M.B., F.R.C.S.*
LIVERPOOL, ENGLAND
From the United Liverpool Hospitals and the University of Liverpool

Mobilization of the entire stomach, with its blood supply intact, in order to restore continuity of the resected esophagus has been described on several occasions. This paper describes a technique of mobilizing the stomach to replace the pharynx and esophagus after resection of a carcinoma of the cervical esophagus. This technique makes mobilization of the stomach particularly easy.

The basic principle of the operation is to obtain a visceral tube, long enough to reach the pharynx without any tension, not damaged or twisted during advancement to the neck, and still supplied by blood from its normal connections through intact vascular arcades, which functions normally, allowing for peristalsis.

TECHNIQUE

The abdomen is opened through a long midline epigastric incision, prolonged well over the xiphisternum, so that when deepened the incision can be extended well into the left costoxiphisternal angle. This procedure gives the best possible abdominal exposure of the diaphragm.

After a full examination of the abdominal contents to exclude secondary deposits and to ascertain the integrity of the stomach's vascular arcades, mobilization is begun. Mobilization starts from above and proceeds downward, rather than beginning below or in the middle of the stomach. This gives easy control of the upper portion of the stomach and gastrosplenic omentum. The surgeon carries out the more difficult part of the operation first, working toward the easier part.

As a first step, the left triangular ligament of the liver is divided, and the left lobe of the liver, thus mobilized, is retracted downward and to the right (Fig. 1). The stomach is then gently pulled downward and the abdominal esophagus is displayed. The peritoneum overlying this area is divided transversely with long dissecting scissors and the esophagus is mobilized slightly. A soft tube is passed around the esophagus and held with a hemostat, giving complete control of the lower esophagus and upper stomach (Fig. 2). This displays three folds of peritoneum: the gastrohepatic fold on the right containing the ascending branch of the left gastric artery; the gastrosplenic fold on the left containing an inconstant branch from the uppermost vasa brevis; and finally the upper portion of the main gastrosplenic omentum, seen as a crescentic margin stretching between the gastric fundus and the spleen.

The first two of these folds are easily clamped, divided, and ligated. The vessels on the stomach side are transfixed, as elsewhere on both curvatures, to prevent them being pulled off when the stomach is drawn upward into the neck.

This procedure enables the lesser omentum

Received for publication July 5, 1969.

*Reprint requests: Department of Oto-rhino-laryngology, Ear, Nose and Throat Infirmary, Myrtle Street, Liverpool 7, England.

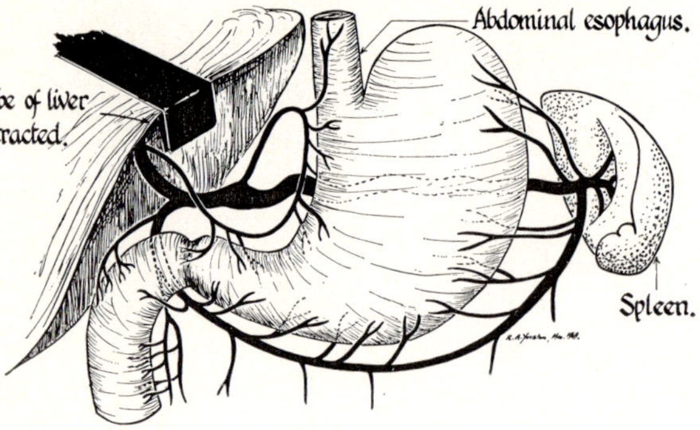

Fig. 1.

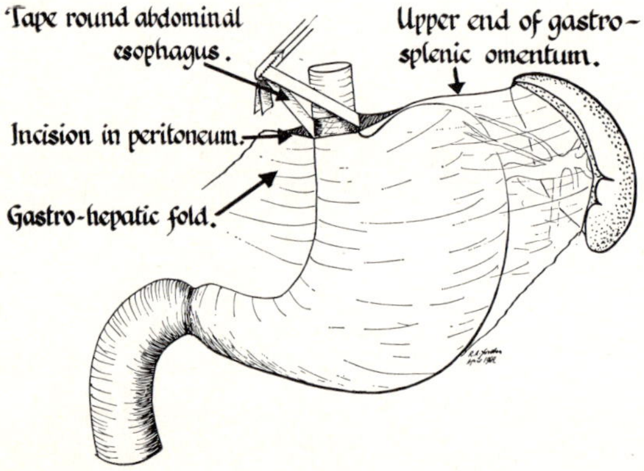

Fig. 2.

to be easily mobilized, clears the upper aspect of the left gastric pedicle, and allows easy access to the free upper border of the main gastrosplenic omentum. The latter allows the short gastric vessels to be seen and divided easily, minimizing the chance of injury to the spleen.

The vessels in the gastrosplenic omentum are then progressively displayed and divided from above downward until the gastroepiploic arcade appears. The greater omentum is then divided carefully (keeping outside the vascular arcade) as far down as the first part of the duodenum, where the middle colic artery and the right gastroepiploic vein must be preserved.

This procedure leaves the greater curvature of the stomach free; the only vascular connection still needing division is the left gastric artery. The stomach is lifted upward and to the right, dividing inconstant avascular adhesions between the posterior surface of the stomach and the pancreas. The gastropancreatic fold containing the left gastric artery above the upper border of the pancreas is then easily seen from below, and, by slipping a finger around it on either side, the surgeon easily mobilizes it into the space developed when the abdominal esophagus was mobilized.

After ensuring that no accessory or aberrant hepatic artery is arising from the left gastric artery, the surgeon divides it between ligatures close to its origin.

The avascular tissue of the lesser omentum above the vascular arcade is then easily divided; a pyloroplasty is performed, and Kocher's maneuver is carried out to mobilize the duodenal loop and head of the pancreas. This not only gives a greater length of stomach to draw up into the neck and chest, but, should rotation of the stomach occur, prevents kinking of the duodenum.

The hand is now passed through the hiatus, and the esophagus is mobilized by blind finger dissection up to the aortic arch.

While the abdominal operation is in progress, the larynx and pharynx are mobilized in the neck. The esophagus above the aortic arch is then mobilized by finger dissection from above.

With traction on the esophagus from above, the stomach, guided from below, is now drawn up through the posterior mediastinum. The pharynx, larynx, and esophagus are removed, the esophageal opening into the stomach is closed, and the fundus of the stomach is anastomosed to the pharynx.

This technique is relatively simple and allows one-stage reconstruction of the pharynx and esophagus with immediate restoration of swallowing.

The authors wish to acknowledge their gratitude to Dr. R. A. Yorston, E.N.T. Department, Dundee Royal Infirmary, for drawing the illustrations.

An electromagnetic probe for the quantitation of intracardiac flows

BRYN T. WILLIAMS, M.D.*
ROBERT K. WORMAN, M.D.*
RAE R. JACOBS, M.D.*
WORTHINGTON G. SCHENK, JR., M.D.
BUFFALO, N. Y.
From the Department of Surgery, State University of New York at Buffalo, and the Surgical Research Laboratory, E. J. Meyer Memorial Hospital

With the introduction of the use of the cardiac catheter by Forssmann[1] in 1929, the cardiac function in normal and disease states could be scientifically assessed. Since that time, the development of the technique has become a valuable routine clinical and experimental procedure in the study of intracardiac pressures.

The similar development of indicator dilution techniques can measure cardiac output and even intracardiac shunt flows.

The accuracy of dye dilution techniques has recently been questioned by Jacobs and associates,[2] and in addition, they provide no means of estimating cyclical flows or flow wave form either across a normal intracardiac structure, such as a valve, or across an abnormal one, such as a septal defect.

Currently, the most accurate technique of measuring flow is by means of an electromagnetic flowmeter. Recently, Nolan and associates[3, 4] described the flow characteristics across an in vivo ball-valve prosthesis fitted with an electromagnetic flow probe. The device described here is at present being used experimentally to measure flow characteristics across normal and abnormal valves and through septal defects.

Supported in part by Grants-in-Aid from the Institute of General Medical Sciences (GM-15768) and the National Heart Institute (HE-03181) of the United States Public Health Service.

Received for publication Aug. 29, 1969.

*Buswell Fellow in Surgical Research, State University of New York at Buffalo.

METHOD AND INSTRUMENTS

Technical description. The electronic components are of standard square wave elec-

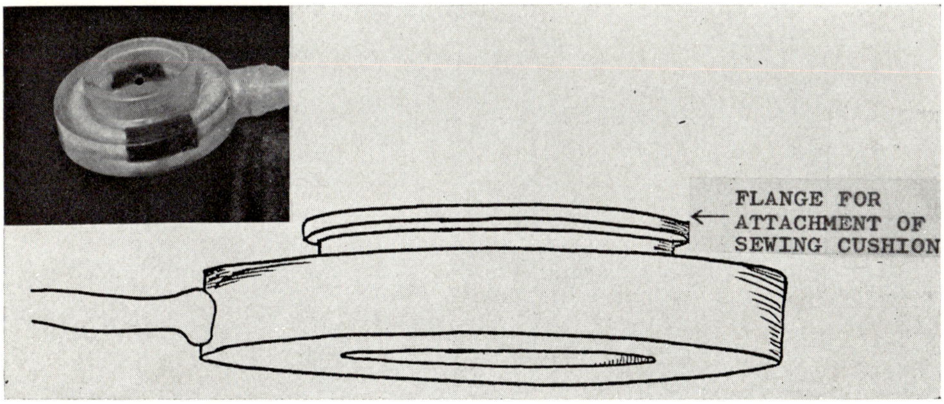

Fig. 1. Intracardiac flow probe.

tromagnetic design consisting of a twin-coiled electromagnet with a soft iron core.

The induced electromotive force is collected by two electrodes placed at right angles to the magnetic field. The molded epoxy housing is circular, with a raised flange around one side of the orifice (Fig. 1). To this may be attached a woven Teflon cuff, secured in place by a circumferential ligature.

Insertion of flow probe. In the laboratory, the probes described above are being used

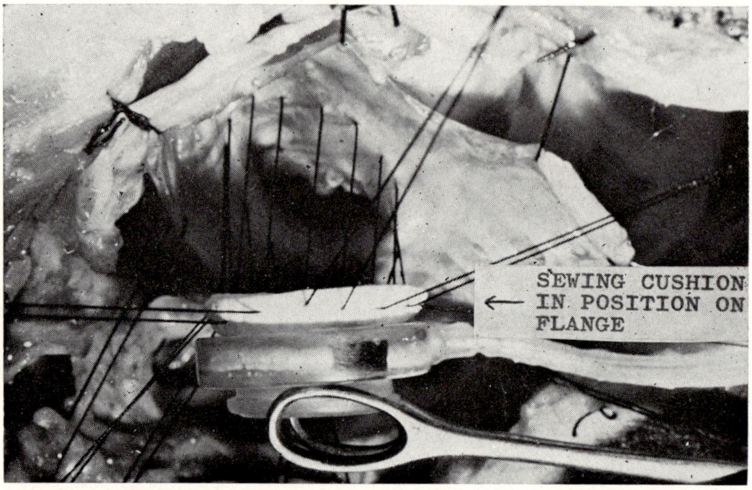

Fig. 2. Intracardiac probe; techniques of insertion on atrial side of mitral valve.

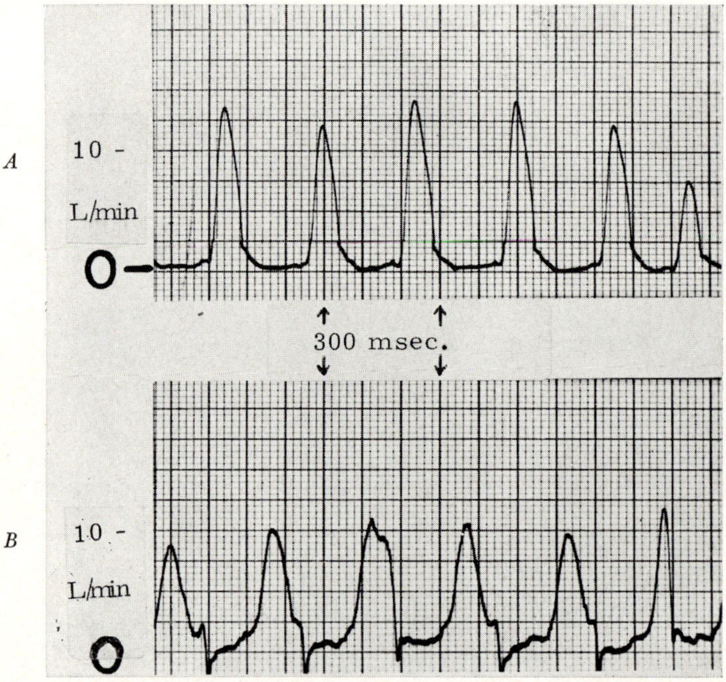

Fig. 3. Simultaneous recordings of aortic root flow (*A*) and normal mitral valvular blood flow (*B*).

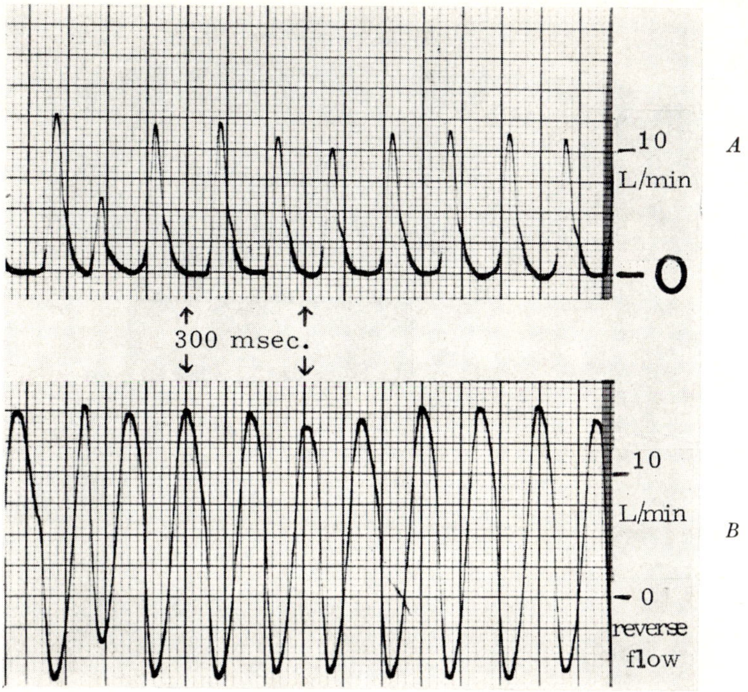

Fig. 4. Simultaneous recordings of blood flow through an aortic root (*A*) and incompetent mitral valve (*B*).

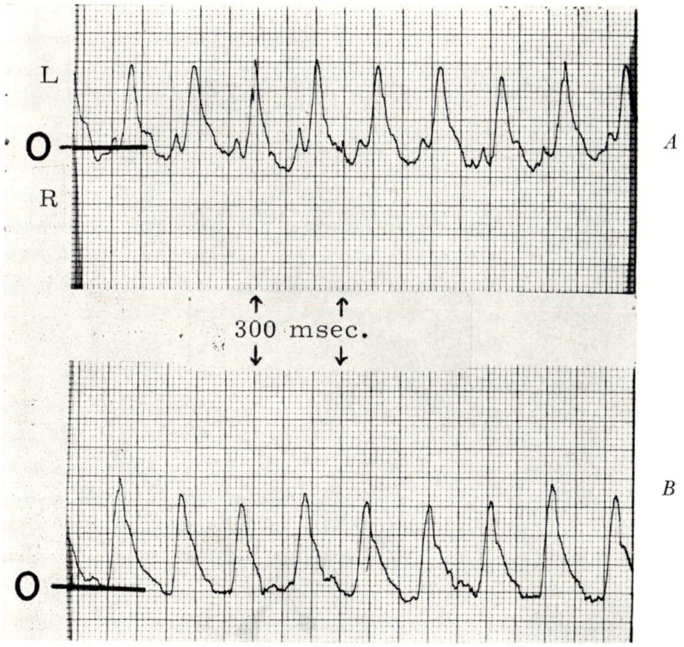

Fig. 5. Simultaneous recordings of right-to-left flow across an atrial septal defect (*A*) and aortic blood flow (*B*).

to study directly intracardiac blood flows in experimental animals by positioning the probe within the heart during cardiopulmonary bypass.

Through a transatrial approach, the probes are sutured into position with the use of interrupted sutures placed through the Teflon cushion (Fig. 2).

The cable is led out through the end of the atrial incision which is extended into the auricular appendage. After the incision has been closed, an encircling ligature is placed around the tip of the appendage at the point where the cable emerges leakproof. Zero flow is obtained by temporary occlusion of the probe by indentation of the atrial wall from the outside.

RESULTS

After the probe has been sutured to the atrial side of the mitral annulus, flow patterns across the normal valve and across a valve made incompetent by rupture of the chordae tendineae can be obtained.

In Fig. 3, simultaneous recordings of normal mitral valve flow and normal aortic root flow are shown. Here it can be seen that maximum flow across the mitral orifice occurs exactly midway between peak aortic flows in contrast to peak atrial pressure which occurs just before ventricular systole.

Fig. 4 demonstrates simultaneous flow through the aortic root and through an incompetent mitral valve. Maximum reverse flow can be seen to occur at the onset of ventricular ejection.

Fig. 5 shows simultaneous recordings of aortic flow and flow across an atrial septal defect.

The aortic flow traces, with the absence of valve-closing transients, are characteristically those seen in low cardiac output states resulting from the early postbypass time of the studies.

SUMMARY

An electromagnetic flow probe is designed to be applicable to the experimental study of intracardiac blood flows. Early results of some of these continuing studies are presented.

REFERENCES

1. Forssmann, W.: Die Sondierung des Rechten Herzens, Klin. Wschr. **8:** 2085, 1929.
2. Jacobs, R. R., Schmitz, U., Heyden, W. C., Roding, B., and Schenk, W. G., Jr.: A comparison of the accuracies of the electromagnetic flowmeter and the cardio-green dye dilution blood flow measurement techniques in a model, Surg. Forum **19:** 113, 1968.
3. Nolan, S. P., Stewart, S., Fogarty, T. J., and Morrow, A. G.: Instantaneous blood flow through ball valve prostheses in the tricuspid position: Effects of heart rate and atrial contraction, Arch. Surg. **97:** 969, 1968.
4. Nolan, S. P., Stewart, S., Fogarty, T. J., Dixon, S. K., and Morrow, A. G.: In vivo studies of instantaneous blood flow across mitral ball valve prostheses: Effects of cardiac output and heart rate on transvalvular energy loss, Ann. Surg. **169:** 551, 1969.

Editorial

Conducted by EDWIN H. ELLISON, M.D.

This editorial is one of a series designed to discuss items of significance and current importance which define the context rather than the content of surgical practice and surgical education. These thoughts about the social, surgical, and scientific scene of the 1970's are expected to stimulate discussion, rebuttal, or concurring editorial comments from surgical colleagues, and it is hoped that presentation of these ideas will create the dialogue and criticism which may provide solutions to some of the problems that currently beset surgical education.

THE EDITORS

Considerations regarding the coming of National Health Insurance

C. BARBER MUELLER, M.D.
HAMILTON, ONTARIO, CANADA
From the Department of Surgery, McMaster University

In recent weeks, there have been several significant articles which predict the early advent of National Health Insurance. In October, Walter Reuther challenged sixty-five health organizations to view the health care system which is "faced with catastrophic collapse," and to advise the United Auto Workers to create a position paper on National Health Insurance to be used for drafting legislation for a national health insurance plan. These suggestions called for the inclusion of the entire United States population, an end to the "dual system" of charity medicine, an emphasis on preventive medicine, a "louder and clearer" voice for the consumer, a broader base of health workers with new criteria for their credentials, an emphasis on outpatient care, and reimbursement to institutions on the basis of "legitimate" rather than total cost. At the same time that President Nixon charged a committee to establish a program for Health Cost Control, a task force to study "Medicaid and Related Problems" was established by Blue Cross, and the American Hospital Association formed a committee to review the possibilities inherent in a national health insurance program. At the recent meeting of the Association of American Medical Colleges, the assembly reacted favorably to the principle of universal health insurance and proposed a committee to work out a position statement. All of these presage an inevitable move toward a federal plan of health care in the near future; with it, will come alterations in the traditional patient-doctor relationship which has characterized medical practice on the North American continent since its inception.

The basic arrangement between patient and doctor has been created on an employer-employee framework in which the patient, the employer, petitions for care from the

Received for publication Jan. 12, 1970.

doctor, the employee, who as the giver of health responds upon appropriate request. His role in society has been determined by those who request or are able to buy his service, not by those who neither seek his personal help nor are unable to afford it. He goes when called, particularly if there is prestige involved in the transaction, and he has the privilege of giving his service to those whom he enjoys and with whom he is comfortable. There are written and unwritten laws and medical ethical practices which perpetuate this role for the physician. The patient is the employer, the doctor is the employee in a very particular and confidential relationship. The public who can afford it, like it; the doctor enjoys it, and any contingency about social gain, education, clinical research, social betterment, or responsibility to the remainder of society is at a minimum in this relationship. By the initiation of the actions described above, United States society of the 1970's suggests that the current arrangement is not a sufficiently adequate framework upon which to provide total health care for a nation which prides itself on equality and nondiscrimination.

Western civilization has been given the promise of better life and more health by the scientific, technologic, and humanitarian advances of the past twenty-five to fifty years. The elimination of major diseases, successful treatment of many others, and the management of many human ills have not been lost upon all observers. Everyone wishes to enjoy some of this largesse, expects it, demands it, and society at large intends that all shall share it. Man's unprecedented scientific and technologic developments have, for the first time in his history, freed him from the continual search for food and shelter. For the first time, his capabilities have reached the point at which, with twenty to thirty percent of the population at work, there are sufficient resources to feed, clothe, and house practically everyone. Political evolution has decreed that all of the people shall share society's wealth to some degree, and political systems that fail to provide this are no longer acceptable and will not survive unless imposed by armed might. With the development of this scientific and technologic affluence has come the need to redesign the social framework for the delivery of health care and redefine its objectives. Current social thought generates infectious ideas about human values in a humane social setting and creates concepts of social justice for those who *live in* a society, rather than for those who *rule* the society.

In their affluence, all of the western nations have assumed the conjoint responsibility to be socially sensitive and to create states which are able to minister to the needs of all citizens. By so doing, the state attempts to see that no member goes without food, then clothing, then shelter, then education, then health care, then personal dignity, and finally a guaranteed annual wage. Food, clothing, and shelter are availabue on an international and commercial market. The items can be fair-traded, bought and sold, and are commodities in a commodity-oriented society. Education, previously a religious-private prerogative, is now becoming solely a state affair. Some church schools remain, some universities are "private" in a small sense, but most teachers receive a state paycheck—either city, county, state, or federal—and in large measure have become state employees to deliver education on behalf of the society that lives on and by the educated product. The forces which mold state ownership of education, state determination of educational content, the state's demands for the educational product, and state social concepts arise in many ways. Bussing of students, ghetto reclamation, conflicts on campus over the military-industrial complex, education's role as a social force in urban reorganization, its role in redefinition of the job force, and recreation of our national ideal are a portion of these current stresses.

Medical care as a social benefit is now on the horizon and in fact has already begun to arrive. For a significant portion of our people, the state has become the third party payer—the insurance carrier—and it is actively concerned that all who are covered shall receive adequate and high quality care. It not only expects that care shall never be refused if requested, but anticipates that health professionals will actively promote health and aggressively supply adequate disease management. Under this system, the doctor can no longer wait until someone petitions for his service. The petition is demeaning. Institutional organization will become important and society expects that its doctors will actively "rescue the perishing and care for the dying." The physician must be alert to the needs of society as society perceives those needs, not as he, the physician, may perceive them.

The employer-employee relationship is changing from patient-physician to state-physician, as it has largely become a state-educator relationship. The complexities of current medical practice require smooth, swift, effective consultations, hospital-based health centers, complex team organizations which create an associate relationship between the physician and other health professionals, a view of new social and technologic horizons, and the creation of new definitions and new dimensions of health. As we enter the 1970's, it is apparent that the physician is losing out as "captain of the team" by his inability to conceive more than a one-man team. He appears to be standing idly by as an observer despite his technologic advances and scientific skills, or he becomes a reactionary fighting to stay in society's yesterday for which his ethical practices and his limited concepts of the organization required for the delivery of health care have fitted him.

Current social needs and current societal moral bases require a new and updated set of medical practice patterns. The fee for service method of remuneration, solo general practice, departmental autonomy, and medical autocracy are now becoming outdated. There is developing a new relationship for the medical practitioner with a dual responsibility. As he must always remain sensitive to individual patient needs and bring new skills and new technocracy to the patients he treats, so must he simultaneously create a relationship to the third party payer—the state—and be sensitive to its direction, its goals, and its obligations to the many people it serves. This is a new, difficult, and demanding role which, by comparison, makes the "state-educator" role look simple.

In October, 1969, Ontario entered into the strange waters created by compulsory health insurance. During the early portions of the decade of the 70's, universal health insurance is certain to be a major item in the party platforms of the 1972 or 1976 campaigns, if it has not already been adopted by the Nixon administration. The advent of universal health insurance brings great alterations in the funding of medical care, and for the first time, it obligates a review of cost-benefit and cost-effectiveness in what constitutes health, health care, and health care delivery systems. Prior to the advent of universal health insurance with its restricted budget for health expenditures, the nature and direction of health care have been largely determined by the health professional as he views the health needs of society. These views have frequently failed to coincide with the views of the public or nonhealth professional who has had little or no say in health direction, except as he participates through voluntary health agencies.

Regional programs of heart disease, cancer, and stroke have not been particularly imaginative, and it is apparent that they have been moderately well refused by the medical schools, but their lesson is clear. Society shall help define our medical ends; there will be a ceiling on money spent on health, and the allocation of our resources and efforts will be made by joint consultation between society and medicine as corporate bodies. The terms of reference in which the physician treats his patient will no longer be referable only to patient benefit as conceived by the physician. Social considerations of equality, humanity, benevolence, social benefit, nondiscrimination, evaluation of cost-effectiveness, and the creation of social worth will enter into society's program for the delivery of health care. It will mandate systems that provide the same quality of care to those living in ghetto poverty as to those living in suburban affluence.

In order to participate as a partner in the creation of this new scheme of health activity we, as physicians, must provide acceptable dimensions for medicine and health. We may not be content with the mere treatment of disease without regard for the presence of societal needs and social goals. It is hoped that medicine will be wise enough and participate willingly in order to preserve a profession, not create a trade. For despite the physician's ultimate dual relationship to the state as well as to the patient, it is health, compassion, understanding, scientific skill, and humaneness which must be received by the humanity, the other partner; all of this must be given in the fullness of an understanding of our heritage as well as the new social contract which the physician will shortly make with his society.

REFERENCE

1. Kramer, J.: Medical care: As costs soar, support grows for major reform, Science **166:** 1126, 1969.

Index to volume 67

AUTHOR INDEX*

A

AABY, GENE V. (*See* Berman, Lemieux, and Aaby), 507
ABERDEEN, EOIN. (*See* Stark et al.), 536
ADAR, RAPHAEL. (*See* Mozes et al.), 452
ADIARTE, EDGARDO. (*See* Rosenberg et al.), 437
AGRAWAL, GIRHAR P. (*See* Boley et al.), 350
AHLGREN, E. WARNER. (*See* Dickey, Ahlgren, and Stephen), 981
ALEXANDER, J. L., DMOCHOWSKI, J. R., MURRAY, J. E., AND COUCH, N. P. Successful 24 hour renal perfusion-preservation with monitoring by surface electrometry during the storage interval, 944
ALEXANDER, RAYMOND H. (*See* Folse and Alexander), 114
ALPERT, JOSEPH. (*See* Parsonnet, Alpert, and Brief), 26
ALTEMEIER, WILLIAM A., BARNES, BENJAMIN A., PULASKI, EDWIN J., SANDUSKY, WILLIAM R., BURKE, JOHN F., AND CLOWES, GEORGE H. A., JR. Infections: Prophylaxis and management—a symposium, 369
AMATO, J. J. (*See* Shoemaker et al.), 754
ANDERSON, CARL F., O'KANE, HUGH O., SHORTER, ROY G., JOHNSON, WILLIAM J., AND HALLENBECK, GEORGE A. Use of diuretic agents during oliguria after renal transplantation, 249
APPERT, HUBERT E. (*See* Daniele et al.), 484
ARAVENA, LUIS A., KAPLAN, LEO, GOLDING, ARTHUR, GORDON, ARTHUR, AND MAXWELL, MORTON H. Improved surgical technique for arteriovenous shunt implantation: Experiences with an all-Silastic shunt, 593
ARGÜERO-SANCHEZ, RUBÉN. (*See* Jiménez-Martínez et al.), 929
ARMSTRONG, RAYMOND G., LINDBERG, EVAN F., STANFORD, WILLIAM, TAKAMOTO, ROBERT M., WOLFE, RICHARD D., AND DIETZ, JAMES W. Traumatic pseudodiverticulum of the esophagus in the newborn infant, 844
ARMSTRONG, RICHARD P. (*See* Brant, Armstrong, and Vetto), 650
ARNER, ORED, AND FERNSTRÖM, INGMAR. The value of pneumoperitoneum in the diagnosis of hernia in the inguinal region, 741
ATKINS, PAUL, AND LEMPKE, ROBERT E. Reduction of postoperative thrombophlebitis, 976
ATKINS, ROBERT, TRIMBLE, CLEVE, AND EISEMAN, BEN. A technique for prolonged splenic perfusion, 306
AUSTEN, W. G. (*See* Mundth et al.), 168
AUSTIN, DALE J. (*See* Thompson et al.), 212

*January, pp. 1-248; February, pp. 249-402; March, pp. 403-560; April, pp. 561-726; May, pp. 727-882; June, pp. 883-1058.

B

BACKWINKEL, KLAUS D. (*See* Rosenberg et al.), 437
BALFOUR, JOHN F. (*See* Strode and Balfour), 527
BARKER, WILEY F. (*See* Pilcher, Barker, and Cannon), 5
BARNES, BENJAMIN A. (*See* Altemeier et al.), 369
BARNETT, WILLIAM O. (*See* McMullan and Barnett), 432
BAUE, ARTHUR E. (*See* Donawick and Baue), 667
BEATHARD, GERALD. (*See* Fish et al.), 658, 969
BENEVENTANO, THOMAS C. (*See* Schein and Beneventano), 255
BENHAMOU, JEAN-PIERRE. (*See* Maillard, Benhamou, and Rueff), 883
BERGER, KNUTE. (*See* Sauvage et al.), 151
BERMAN, IRWIN R., LEMIEUX, MICHAEL D., AND AABY, GENE V. Responses of skeletal muscle pH to injury: A new technique for determination of tissue viability, 507
BERNSTEIN, MICHAEL. (*See* Schimert et al.), 129
BEVEN, EDWARD G. (*See* Esselstyn et al.), 34
BHAGAVAN, BELUR S., RAO, D. R. GOVINDA, AND WEINBERG, TOBIAS. Carcinoma of thyroglossal duct cyst: Case reports and review of the literature, 281
BIALOSTOZKY, LEÓN, LEGASPI, RAÚL, RISH F., LORENZO, AND MORALES M., FEDERICO. Contralateral arterial grafts, 442
BLAIR, EMIL, HUNZIKER, ROBERT, AND FLANAGAN, MARTIN E. Catheter embolism, 457
BLANCHARD, HERVE. (*See* Ono et al.), 322
BLUM, LESTER. (*See* Nabatoff, Blum, and Touroff), 272
BOEREMA, I., KLOPPER, P. J., AND HOLSCHER, A. A. Transabdominal ligation-resection of the esophagus in cases of bleeding esophageal varices, 409
BOGOKOWSKY, HARRY. (*See* Mozes et al.), 452
BOLEY, SCOTT J., KAMIL, NEIL, LEVOWITZ, BERNARD S., TREIBER, WILLIAM F., JR., AGRAWAL, GIRHAR P., AND VEITH, FRANK J. Potassium vasoactivity—a biphasic effect, 350
BONHAM-CARTER, RICHARD E. (*See* Stark et al.), 536
BOOKSTEIN, JOSEPH J. (*See* Frey, Reuter, and Bookstein), 548
BOTHWELL, JAMES W. (*See* Rosenberg et al.), 951
BOYDEN, EDWARD A. (*See* Hessel et al.), 624
BRANT, BOLEK, ARMSTRONG, RICHARD P., AND VETTO, R. MARK. Vasodepressor factor in declamp shock production, 650
BREMNER, CEDRIC G., SCHLEGEL, JERRY F., AND ELLIS, F. HENRY, JR. Studies of the "gastroesophageal sphincter mechanism": The role of the phrenoesophageal membrane, 735
BRIEF, DONALD K. (*See* Parsonnet, Alpert, and Brief), 26

Britton, Richard C., Voorhees, Arthur B., Jr., and Price, John B., Jr. Selective portal decompression, 104
Bruckner, Walter L., Snow, Harold D., and Fonkalsrud, Eric W. Gastric secretion in the canine fetus following maternal stimulation: Experimental studies on placental transfer of insulin, histamine, and gastrin, 360
Buchwald, Henry. (*See* Gebhard and Buchwald), 474
—. (*See* Schwartz, Moore, and Buchwald), 346
Buckley, M. J. (*See* Mundth et al.), 168
Bujdoso, Leslie J. (*See* Rosenberg et al.), 437
Bunch, Wilton, and Delaney, John. Scoliosis and acute vascular compression of the duodenum, 901
Bunnell, Ivan L. (*See* Schimert et al.), 129
Burke, John F. Isolation techniques and their effectiveness, 373
—. (*See* Altemeier et al.), 369

C

Callow, Allan D., Resnick, Robert H., Chalmers, Thomas C., Ishihara, Albert M., Garceau, Arthur J., and O'Hara, Edward T. Conclusions from a controlled trial of the prophylactic portacaval shunt, 97
Cannon, Jack A. (*See* Pilcher, Barker, and Cannon), 5
Carey, J. S. (*See* Shoemaker et al.), 754
Castaneda, Aldo. (*See* Rees et al.), 141
—. (*See* Zamora et al.), 706
Cerruti, Marcial. (*See* Garzon et al.), 633
Chalmers, Thomas C. (*See* Callow et al.), 97
Chapman, Kenneth. (*See* Litwin, Chapman, and Stoliar), 342
Chávez-Peón, Federico, Gonzalez, Eduardo, and Malt, Ronald A. Vena cava catheter for asanguineous liver resection, 694
Civetta, Joseph M., Williams, M. J., and Richie, Robert E. Diagnostic peritoneal irrigation—a simple and reliable technique, 874
Claman, Henry N. (*See* Ono et al.), 322
Clark, William R., Jr., and Leather, Robert P. Hemostasis during liver resections, 556
Clatworthy, H. William, Jr. (*See* Grosfeld and Clatworthy), 519
—. (*See* Kilman et al.), 197
Clowes, George H. A., Jr. Survival or death from sepsis, 374
—. (*See* Altemeier et al.), 369
Cohn, Lawrence H., Moore, Wesley S., and Hall, Albert D. Extra-abdominal management of late aortofemoral graft thrombosis, 775
Cole, Andrew. (*See* Siegel et al.), 907
Collins, Dale. (*See* Salerno, Collins, and Redmond), 863
Corley, R. D. (*See* Shoemaker et al.), 754
Couch, N. P. (*See* Alexander et al.), 944
Coupland, G. A. E., and Reeve, T. S. Recurrent pulmonary emboli following inferior vena caval plication, 639
Cowen, D. (*See* Eiseman et al.), 725
Craenen, Josepha. (*See* Kilman et al.), 197
Crawford, E. Stanley, Fenstermacher, James M., Richardson, William, and Sandiford, Frank. Reappraisal of adjuncts to avoid ischemia in the treatment of thoracic aortic aneurysms, 182
Cross, Robert A. (*See* Nelsen et al.), 826

D

Dale, W. Andrew. Ligation, stripping, and excision of varicose veins, 389
—, and Lewis, R. Malcolm. Management of ischemia of the hand and fingers, 62
Daniel, Thomas M., Graham, Thomas P., and Sabiston, David C., Jr. Coronary artery–right ventricular fistula with congestive heart failure: Surgical correction in the neonatal period, 985
Daniele, Ronald, Singh, Hira, Appert, Hubert E., Pairent, Frederick W., and Howard, John M. Lymphatic absorption of intraperitoneal endotoxin in the dog, 484
Das Gupta, Tapas K. Scapulectomy: Indications and technique, 601
Dean, David C. (*See* Schimert et al.), 129
Deckers, Peter J., Fraley, Elwin E., Paulson, David F., and Harbert, John C. Vascular obstruction of the superior renal infundibulum in children, 856
Dedomenico, Mark. (*See* Sauvage et al.), 151
deHoll, J. David. (*See* Wangensteen et al.), 935
Delaney, John. (*See* Bunch and Delaney), 901
Derrick, John R. The retrievable error, 881
DeWeese, Bob M. (*See* Mays, Ransdell, and DeWeese), 780
DeWeese, M. S. (*See* Ridenhour et al.), 614
deWolfe, Victor G. (*See* Esselstyn et al.), 34
Diaz-Ordaz, Manuel Matos. (*See* Pérez Alvarez et al.), 355
Dickey, William Thomas, Ahlgren, E. Warner, and Stephen, C. R. Body temperature monitoring via the tympanic membrane, 981
Dietz, James W. (*See* Armstrong et al.), 844
Dietzman, Ronald H. (*See* Motsay et al.), 577
DiGiglia, John W. D., Leonard, George L., and Ochsner, John L. Local irrigation with an antibiotic solution in the prevention of infection in vascular prostheses, 836
Dinsmore, R. E. (*See* Mundth et al.), 168
Dmochowski, J. R. (*See* Alexander et al.), 944
Donawick, William J., and Baue, Arthur E. The immunologic response to intravascular skin allografts, 667
Doty, Donald B., Kugler, Heinz W., and Moseley, Roger V. Control of the hepatic parenchyma by direct compression: A new instrument, 720
—. (*See* Moseley and Doty), 455, 765
Dowell, V. R., Jr. (*See* Yale and Dowell), 478
Drapanas, Theodore. "Letters to the Editors," 401
Dressler, Donald P., and Skornik, William A. Silver sulfadiazine and Sulfamylon Cream in the burned rat model: A comparative evaluation, 644
Dye, William S. (*See* Javid et al.), 80

E

Eckert, Gerald. (*See* Salinas Izaguirre, Haggerty, and Eckert), 607
Edmunds, L. Henry, Jr. (*See* Norton et al.), 1011
Egdahl, Richard H. A fork in the road: The geographic full-time system, 878

Ehrenfeld, W. K., Hamilton, F. N., Larson, C. P., Jr., Hickey, R. F., and Severinghaus, J. W. Effect of CO_2 and systemic hypertension on downstream cerebral arterial pressure during carotid endarterectomy, 87
Eiseman, B., Pomerantz, M., Merkel, F., and Cowen, D. Experiments in delivery of surgical care, 725
—. (*See* Atkins, Trimble, and Eiseman), 306
—. (*See* Novak et al.), 678
Eisenberg, M. Michael. (*See* Isaza et al.), 462
Eliahou, Heskel E. (*See* Mozes et al.), 452
Ellis, F. Henry, Jr. (*See* Bremner, Schlegel, and Ellis), 735
Ellison, Edwin H. "Letters to the Editors," 401
Enright, Lee P. (*See* Hannah, Enright, and Reis), 831
Ersek, Robert A. (*See* Motsay et al.), 577
Esparza, Alfredo R., and Pan, Charles M. Diverticulosis of the appendix, 922
Esselstyn, Caldwell B., Jr., Humphries, Alfred W., Young, Jess R., Beven, Edward G., and deWolfe, Victor G. Aneurysmectomy in the aged? 34
Ewing, J. Burke. (*See* Tanga and Ewing), 418

F

Fabian, Miklos. (*See* Siegel et al.), 907
Fadali, A. Moniem. (*See* Nelsen et al.), 826
Falsetti, Herman L. (*See* Schimert et al.), 129
Fenstermacher, James M. (*See* Crawford et al.), 182
Fernström, Ingmar. (*See* Arner and Fernström), 741
Fink, George. (*See* Thieme and Fink), 403
Fish, Jay C., Beathard, Gerald, Sarles, Harry E., Remmers, August R., Jr., and Ritzmann, Stephan E. Circulating lymphocyte depletion: Effect on lymphoid tissue, 658
—, Tyson, Kenneth R. T., Beathard, Gerald A., Sarles, Harry E., Remmers, August R., and Ritzmann, Stephan E. Circulating lymphocyte depletion: Effect on renal allograft survival in calves, 969
Fishman, Noel H., Hutchinson, John C., and Roe, Benson B. Prevention of prosthetic cardiac valve detachment, 867
Flanagan, Martin E. (*See* Blair, Hunziker, and Flanagan), 457
Folse, Roland, and Alexander, Raymond H. Directional flow detection for localizing venous valvular incompetency, 114
Fonkalsrud, Eric W. (*See* Bruckner, Snow, and Fonkalsrud), 360
—. (*See* Momma et al.), 799
Fraley, Elwin E. (*See* Deckers et al.), 856
Frey, Charles F., Reuter, Stewart R., and Bookstein, Joseph J. Localization of gastrointestinal hemorrhage by selective angiography, 548
Fulton, Robert L., and Peter, Edward T. The progressive nature of pulmonary contusion, 499

G

Gage, Andrew A. (*See* Schimert et al.), 129
Garceau, Arthur J. (*See* Callow et al.), 97
Garzon, Antonio A., Cerruti, Marcial, Gourin, Anatole, and Karlson, Karl E. Pulmonary resection for massive hemoptysis, 633
Gaughran, Eugene R. L. (*See* Rosenberg et al.), 951
Gaylis, H. The duplicated saphenous vein in femoropopliteal bypass grafting, 277
Gebhard, Roger L., and Buchwald, Henry. Cholesterol absorption following reversal of the upper and lower halves of the small intestine, 474
Geddes, L. A. (*See* Schuhmann, Geddes, and Hoff), 957
Goff, Jacob B. (*See* Grablowsky et al.), 895
Golding, Arthur. (*See* Aravena et al.), 593
Gonzales, Eduardo. (*See* Chávez-Peón, Gonzales, and Malt), 694
Goodhead, Bernard. (*See* Wright and Goodhead), 807
Gordon, Arthur. (*See* Aravena et al.), 593
Gott, Vincent L. (*See* Nelsen et al.), 826
Gourin, Anatole. (*See* Garzon et al.), 633
Grablowsky, Oscar M., Weichert, Rudolph F., III, Goff, Jacob B., and Schlegel, Jorgen U. Renal artery thrombosis following blunt trauma: Report of four cases, 895
Graham, Gerald R. (*See* Stark et al.), 536
Graham, Thomas P. (*See* Daniel, Graham, and Sabiston), 985
Greene, David G. (*See* Schimert et al.), 129
Griffith, Charles A. (*See* Legros and Griffith), 654
Grosfeld, Jay L., and Clatworthy, H. William, Jr. Intrauterine midgut strangulation in a gastroschisis defect, 519
Gutiérrez-Bosque, Ramón. (*See* Pérez Alvarez et al.), 355

H

Haggerty, James T. (*See* Salinas Izaguirre, Haggerty, and Eckert), 607
Hall, Albert D. (*See* Cohn, Moore, and Hall), 775
Hallenbeck, George A. (*See* Anderson et al.), 249
Hamilton, F. N. (*See* Ehrenfeld et al.), 87
Hanlon, C. Rollins. Presidential address: Standards in vascular surgery, 1
Hannah, Hamner, III, Enright, Lee P., and Reis, Robert L. The effect of epicardiectomy on the function and diastolic compliance of the normal canine left ventricle, 831
Harbert, John C. (*See* Deckers et al.), 856
Harris, Leonard C. (*See* Tyson, Harris, and Nghiem), 1006
Harthorne, J. W. (*See* Mundth et al.), 168
Hellström, Ingegerd E. (*See* Pierce et al.), 328
Henderson, John. (*See* Rosenberg et al.), 951
Hengesh, John W. (*See* Javid et al.), 80
Henzel, J. H. (*See* Ridenhour et al.), 614
Hessel, Eugene A., II, Boyden, Edward A., Stamm, Stanley J., and Sauvage, Lester R. High systemic origin of the sole artery to the basal segments of the left lung: Findings, surgical treatment, and embryologic interpretation, 624
Hickey, R. F. (*See* Ehrenfeld et al.), 87
Hill, J. Donald, and Johnson, Elmer E. An intensive care bed for the initial diagnosis and treatment of severely ill patients, 414
Hill, L. (*See* Novak et al.), 678
Hirooka, Masao. (*See* Ishigami et al.), 620

HOFF, H. E. (*See* Schuhmann, Geddes, and Hoff), 957
HOLSCHER, A. A. (*See* Boerema, Klopper, and Holscher), 409
HOLSWADE, GEORGE R. (*See* Rees et al.), 141
HOSIER, DON M. (*See* Kilman et al.), 197
HOWARD, JOHN M. (*See* Daniele et al.), 484
HUMPHRIES, ALFRED W. (*See* Esselstyn et al.), 34
HUNTER, JAMES A. (*See* Javid et al.), 80
HUNZIKER, ROBERT. (*See* Blair, Hunziker, and Flanagan), 457
HURWICH, BARUCH. (*See* Mozes et al.), 452
HUTCHINSON, JOHN C. (*See* Fishman, Hutchinson, and Roe), 867

I

ISAZA, JAIME, SUGAWARA, KYOJI, TIONGCO, RICHARD, AND EISENBERG, M. MICHAEL. Studies on the effect of 2-phenyl-2-(2-pyridyl)-thioacetamide (antigastrin) on canine gastric acid secretion, 462
ISHIGAMI, KOICHI, YOSHIDA, YOSHIYUKI, HIROOKA, MASAO, AND MOHRI, KIKUO. A new operation for varicocele: Use of microvascular anastomosis, 620
ISHIHARA, ALBERT M. (*See* Callow et al.), 97
IZUKAWA, T. (*See* Simpson et al.), 697

J

JACOBS, RAE R. (*See* Williams et al.), 1031
JACOBS, ROBERTA. (*See* Kashiwagi et al.), 789
JACOBSON, JULIUS H., II. (*See* Yasargil, Krayenbuhl, and Jacobson), 221
JAVID, HUSHANG, OSTERMILLER, WILLIAM E., JR., HENGESH, JOHN W., DYE, WILLIAM S., HUNTER, JAMES A., NAJAFI, HASSAN, AND JULIAN, ORMAND C. Natural history of carotid bifurcation atheroma, 80
JIMÉNEZ-MARTÍNEZ, MANUEL, ARGÜERO-SÁNCHEZ, RUBÉN, PÉREZ-ALVAREZ, JUAN JOSÉ, AND MINA-CASTAÑEDA, PEDRO. Anterior mediastinitis as a complication of median sternotomy incisions: Diagnostic and surgical considerations, 929
JOHNSON, ELMER E. (*See* Hill and Johnson), 414
JOHNSON, GEORGE, JR. (*See* McDaniel and Johnson), 394
JOHNSON, WILLIAM J. (*See* Anderson et al.), 249
JOHNSTON, PAUL W. (*See* Michaelian, Mahour, and Johnston), 703
JONES, E. L. (*See* Powis, Morrissey, and Jones), 891
JULIAN, ORMAND C. (*See* Javid et al.), 80

K

KAHN, DONALD R., REYNOLDS, ERNEST W., JR., WALTON, JOSEPH A., JR., KIRSH, MARVIN M., VATHAYANON, SATHAPORN, AND SLOAN, HERBERT. Human heart transplantation for cardiomyopathy, 122
KAMIL, NEIL. (*See* Boley et al.), 350
KAPLAN, LEO. (*See* Aravena et al.), 593
KAPUR, BRIJ. (*See* Kashiwagi et al.), 789
—. (*See* Pacache, Kapur, and Starzl), 319
KARLSON, KARL E. (*See* Garzon et al.), 633
KASHIWAGI, NOBORU, SCHERER, DAVID, TOWNSEND, COURTNEY M., JACOBS, ROBERTA, ONO, KEIJI, KAPUR, BRIJ, AND STARZL, THOMAS E. Antibody localization in horse, rabbit, and goat antilymphocyte sera, 789
—. (*See* Ono et al.), 322
KERR, S. EARL. (*See* Ridenhour et al.), 614
KIECHEL, STEPHEN F. (*See* Wangensteen et al.), 338, 935
KILMAN, JAMES W., SIRAK, HOWARD D., CLATWORTHY, H. WILLIAM, JR., CRAENEN, JOSEPHA, AND HOSIER, DON M. The case for the early closure of a patent ductus arteriosus, 197
KIRSH, MARVIN M. (*See* Kahn et al.), 122
KLOPPER, P. J. (*See* Boerema, Klopper, and Holscher), 409
KOCK, NILS G. (*See* Tibblin, Kock, and Schenk), 816
KOEHNLEIN, H. E., AND LEMPERLE, G. Experimental studies on the effect of dimethyl sulfoxide on pedicle flaps, 672
KORENEV, NICOLAY N. (*See* Petrov and Korenev), 574
KRAMER, SCOTT G., AND LIPSON, CHARLES S. Intensive care unit flow sheet, 590
KRAYENBUHL, HUGO A. (*See* Yasargil, Krayenbuhl, and Jacobson), 221
KUGLER, HEINZ W. (*See* Doty, Kugler, and Moseley), 720
KWONG, K. H. (*See* Ong and Kwong), 293

L

LAJOS, THOMAS Z. (*See* Schimert et al.), 129
LANKAU, CHARLES. (*See* Siegel et al.), 907
LARSON, C. P., JR. (*See* Ehrenfeld et al.), 87
LAWRENCE, WALTER, JR. (*See* Sokol et al.), 748
LEATHER, ROBERT P. (*See* Clark and Leather), 556
LEFER, ALLAN M. (*See* Wangensteen et al.), 935
LEGASPI, RAÚL. (*See* Bialostozky et al.), 442
LEGROS, GUY, AND GRIFFITH, CHARLES A. The permanence of adequate incomplete vagotomy: A preliminary study in dogs, 654
LEININGER, BERNARD, PEACOCK, HOWARD, AND NEVILLE, WILLIAM E. Esophageal mucosal regeneration following experimental prosthetic replacement of the esophagus, 468
LEMIEUX, MICHAEL D. (*See* Berman, Lemieux, and Aaby), 507
LEMPERLE, GOTTFRIED, MICHAELIS, WOLF, AND WIECZOREK, ULF. Autoradiographic studies on the incorporation of foreign DNA and RNA into kidney allografts, 332
—. (*See* Koehnlein and Lemperle), 672
LEMPKE, ROBERT E. (*See* Atkins and Lempke), 976
LEONARD, GEORGE L. (*See* DiGiglia, Leonard, and Ochsner), 836
LEVINE, MICHAEL. (*See* Siegel et al.), 907
LEVINSON, SHAUL. (*See* Vidne, Levinson, and Levy), 279
LEVOWITZ, BERNARD S. (*See* Boley et al.), 350
LEVY, MORRIS J. (*See* Virne, Levinson, and Levy), 279
LEWIS, R. MALCOLM. (*See* Dale and Lewis), 62
LILLEHEI, C. WALTON. (*See* Rees et al.), 141
LILLEHEI, RICHARD C. (*See* Motsay et al.), 577
LINDBERG, EVAN F. (*See* Armstrong et al.), 844
LINDE, LEONARD M. (*See* Momma et al.), 799
LINTON, ROBERT R., AND WILDE, W. LAWRENCE. Modifications in the technique for femoropopliteal saphenous vein bypass autografts, 234
LIPSON, CHARLES S. (*See* Kramer and Lipson), 590

LITWIN, MARTIN S., CHAPMAN, KENNETH, AND STOLIAR, J. BRUCE. Blood viscosity in the normal man, 342
LORD, GEOFFREY H. (*See* Rosenberg et al.), 951
LOTKE, PAUL A., AND SCHWARTZ, SORELL L. Studies on the functional and biochemical changes during kidney preservation, 488
LUCAS, RUSSELL V., JR. (*See* Zamora et al.), 706
LUDEWIG, ROBERT M. (*See* Wangensteen et al.), 338
LUNDBORG, RICHARD O. (*See* Tarhan et al.), 584

M

McDANIEL, W. JASON, AND JOHNSON, GEORGE, JR. A method of salvaging the bifurcated saphenous vein for use in femoral-to-popliteal bypass grafts, 394
McMULLAN, MARTIN H., AND BARNETT, WILLIAM O. The clinical use of intraperitoneal cephalothin, 432
McSHERRY, CHARLES K. (*See* Parsons, Miscall, and McSherry), 841
MACSWEEN, RODERICK N. M. (*See* Ono et al.), 322
MADDEN, JAMES J., JR. (*See* Wangensteen et al.), 338
MAHOUR, G. H. (*See* Michaelian, Mahour, and Johnston), 703
MAILLARD, JEAN-NOËL, BENHAMOU, JEAN-PIERRE, AND RUEFF, BERNARD. Arterialization of the liver with portacaval shunt in the treatment of portal hypertension due to intrahepatic block, 883
MALT, RONALD A. (*See* Chávez-Peón, Gonzales, and Malt), 694
MANNICK, JOHN A. The current status of immunosuppressive therapy, 711
MARTIN, JULIAN. (*See* Wangensteen et al.), 935
MAXWELL, MORTON H. (*See* Aravena et al.), 593
MAYS, E. TRUMAN, RANSDELL, HERBERT T., AND DEWEESE, BOB M. Metabolic changes in surgical delirium tremens, 780
MAZZARIELLO, R. Removal of residual biliary tract calculi without reoperation, 566
MENDES, N. F. (*See* Seigler, Mendes, and Metzgar), 261
MERENDINO, K. ALVIN. (*See* Pierce et al.), 328
—. (*See* Rittenhouse, Mohri, and Merendino), 995
MERKEL, F. (*See* Eiseman et al.), 725
METZGAR, R. S. (*See* Seigler, Mendes, and Metzgar), 261
MEYEROWITZ, BASIL R. The crisis in surgical training, 399
MICHAELIAN, MELVYN J., MAHOUR, G. H., AND JOHNSTON, PAUL W. Torsion of the testis in the newborn infant, 703
MICHAELIS, WOLF. (*See* Lemperle, Michaelis, and Wieczorek), 332
MINA-CASTAÑEDA, PEDRO. (*See* Jiménez-Martínez et al.), 929
MISCALL, BRIAN G. (*See* Parsons, Miscall, and McSherry), 841
—. (*See* Rees et al.), 141
MOES, C. A. F. (*See* Simpson et al.), 697
MOFFITT, EMERSON A. (*See* Tarhan et al.), 584
MOHR, P. A. (*See* Shoemaker et al.), 754
MOHRI, HITOSHI. (*See* Pierce et al.), 328
—. (*See* Rittenhouse, Mohri, and Merendino), 995
MOHRI, KIKUO. (*See* Ishigami et al.), 620
MOLLER, JAMES H. (*See* Zamora et al.), 706
MOMMA, KAZUO, LINDE, LEONARD M., FONKALSRUD, ERIC W., STEVENS, GARY H., RANGEL, DECIO M., AND YAKEISHI, YOZO. Hemodynamics and blood gas exchange in allografted canine lungs. I. Immediate effects, 799
MONSON, D. O. (*See* Shoemaker et al.), 754
MOORE, RICHARD B. (*See* Schwartz, Moore, and Buchwald), 346
MOORE, THOMAS C., SALZBERG, ARNOLD M., AND TALMAN, E. ARMISTEAD. Jejunoileocolic intubation and plication for intestinal obstruction caused by massive adhesions in infancy, 364
—. (*See* Patton and Moore), 513
MOORE, WESLEY S. (*See* Cohn, Moore, and Hall), 775
MORALES M., FEDERICO. (*See* Bialostozky et al.), 442
MORGAN, A. (*See* Nicholas, Morgan, and Zachary), 847
MORGAN, W. W. (*See* White and Morgan) 522
MORRISSEY, D. M. (*See* Powis, Morrissey, and Jones), 891
MORTON, DONALD L. Cancer immunology and the surgeon, 396
MOSELEY, ROGER V., AND DOTY, DONALD B. Hypoxemia during the first twelve hours after battle injury, 765
— and —. Long-term arterial catheterization for repeated blood sampling, 455
—. (*See* Doty, Kugler, and Moseley), 720
MOSS, GERALD. A simple and accurate manometer for monitoring central venous pressure, 773
MOTSAY, GEORGE J., DIETZMAN, RONALD H., ERSEK, ROBERT A., AND LILLEHEI, RICHARD C. Hemodynamic alterations and results of treatment in patients with gram-negative septic shock, 577
MOZES, MARK, HURWICH, BARUCH J., ADAR, RAPHAEL, ELIAHOU, HESKEL E., AND BOGOKOWSKY, HARRY. Arteriovenous vein graft for chronic hemodialysis: A preliminary report, 452
MUELLER, C. BARBER. Considerations regarding the coming of National Health Insurance, 1035
MUNDTH, E. D., HARTHORNE, J. W., BUCKLEY, M. J., DINSMORE, R. E., AND AUSTEN, W. G. Direct coronary arterial revascularization for segmental occlusive disease, 168
MURRAY, J. E. (*See* Alexander et al.), 944
MUSTARD, W. T. (*See* Simpson et al.), 697

N

NABATOFF, ROBERT A., BLUM, LESTER, AND TOUROFF, ARTHUR S. Long-term sequelae of common femoral vein ligation in the treatment of thromboembolic disease, 272
NAHMAD, MICHEL. (*See* Siegel at al.), 907
NAJAFI, HASSAN. (*See* Javid et al.), 80
NAKAYAMA, KOMEI. (See Oi, Takemoto, and Nakayama), 561
NELSEN, LITA, CROSS, ROBERT A., VOGEL, MARY ANN, GOTT, VINCENT L., AND FADALI, A. MONIEM. Synthetic thromboresistant surfaces from sulfonated polyelectrolyte complexes, 826
NELSON, RUSSELL M. (*See* Vaughn, Warner, and Nelson), 204

NEMANICH, GEORGE J., AND NICOLOFF, DEMETRE M. Perforated duodenal ulcer: Long-term follow-up, 727
NEVILLE, WILLIAM E. (*See* Leininger, Peacock, and Neville), 468
NGHIEM, QUANG X. (*See* Tyson, Harris, and Nghiem), 1006
NICHOLAS, J. L., MORGAN, A., AND ZACHARY, R. B. Idiopathic edema of scrotum in young boys, 847
NICOLOFF, DEMETRE M. (*See* Nemanich and Nicoloff), 727
NORTON, J. B., JR., ULLYOT, DANIEL J., STEWART, EDWARD T., RUDOLPH, A. M., AND EDMUNDS, L. HENRY, JR. Aortic arch atresia with transposition of the great vessels: Physiologic considerations and surgical management, 1011
NOVAK, V., HILL, L., ROTHWELL-JACKSON, R., VELASQUEZ, A., WRIGHT, R., AND EISEMAN, B. Auxiliary homotransplantation of the porcine liver into the retroperitoneal space, 678

O

OCHSNER, ALTON, ZEHNDER, PAUL R., AND TRAMMEL, SHIRLEY W. The surgical treatment of peptic ulcer: A critical analysis of results from subtotal gastrectomy and from vagotomy plus partial gastrectomy, 1017
OCHSNER, JOHN L. (*See* DiGiglia, Leonard and Ochsner), 836
O'HARA, EDWARD T. (*See* Callow et al.), 97
OI, ITARU, TAKEMOTO, TADAYOSHI, AND NAKAYAMA, KOMEI. "Fiberduodenoscopy"—early diagnosis of cancer of the papilla of Vater, 561
O'KANE, HUGH O. (*See* Anderson et al.), 249
O'NEILL, JAMES A., JR. The influence of thermal burns on gastric acid secretion, 267
ONG, G. B., AND KWONG, K. H. Management of malignant esophagobronchial fistula, 293
ONO, KEIJI, BLANCHARD, HERVE, KASHIWAGI, NOBORU, MACSWEEN, RODERICK N. M., CLAMAN, HENRY M., AND STARZL, THOMAS E. Effects of phytohemagglutinin in humoral antibody response, delayed hypersensitivity, and homograft rejection, 322
—. (See Kashiwagi et al.), 789
OSTERMILLER, WILLIAM E., JR. (See Javid et al.), 80

P

PAIRENT, FREDERICK W. *See* Daniele et al.), 484
PAN, CHARLES M. (*See* Esparza and Pan), 922
PARSONNET, VICTOR, ALPERT, JOSEPH, AND BRIEF, DONALD K. Femorofemoral and axillofemoral grafts—compromise or preference, 26
PARSONS, JOHN M., MISCALL, BRIAN G., AND MCSHERRY, CHARLES K. Appendicitis in the newborn infant, 841
PATMAN, R. DON (*See* Thompson et al.), 212
PATTON, JAMES J., AND MOORE, THOMAS C. Massive megacolon and megaileum in childhood due to tuberculous stenosis of the ascending colon, 513
PAULSON, DAVID F. (*See* Deckers et al.), 856
PEACOCK, HOWARD. (*See* Leininger, Peacock, and Neville), 468
PENNEYS, RAYMOND, AND WILKINSON, J. HENRY. Elevation of serum creatine kinase following amputation of the leg, 302
PÉREZ ALVAREZ, JUAN J., VARGAS-ROSENDO, RUBÉN, GUTIÉRREZ-BOSQUE, RAMÓN, DIAZ-ORDAZ, MANUEL MATOS, AND SANTOS-ATHERTON, DAVID. A new type subcutaneous arteriovenous fistula for chronic hemodialysis in children, 355
PÉREZ-ALVAREZ, JUAN JOSÉ. (*See* Jiménez-Martínez et al.), 929
PETER, EDWARD T. (*See* Fulton and Peter), 499
PETROV, BORIS A., AND KORENEV, NICOLAY N. Local gastric hypothermia in gastroduodenal hemorrhage, 574
PICACHE, REGINALDO S., KAPUR, BRIJ M. L., AND STARZL, THOMAS E. The effect of liver disease on the need for venous decompression during the anhepatic phase of canine orthotopic liver transplantation, 319
PIERCE, GEORGE E., HELLSTRÖM, INGEGERD E., MOHRI, HITOSHI, REICHENBACH, DENNIS D., AND MERENDINO, K. ALVIN. Demonstration of humoral immunity against aortic leaflet heterografts, 328
PILCHER, DAVID B., BARKER, WILEY F., AND CANNON, JACK A. An aortoiliac endarterectomy case series followed 10 years or more, 5
POLIN, STANTON G., WALKLETT, WILLIAM D., AND SAYLER, OSBEY L. Arteriography as an adjunct to the diagnosis of splenic injury, 313
—. (*See* Schulman, Pritham, and Polin), 918
POMERANTZ, M. (*See* Eiseman et al.), 725
POWIS, S. J. A., MORRISSEY, D. M., AND JONES, E. L. Cystic degeneration of the popliteal artery, 891
PRICE, JOHN B., JR. (*See* Britton, Voorhees, and Price), 104
PRINTEN, K. J. (*See* Shoemaker et al.), 754
PRITHAM, HOWARD G. (*See* Schulman, Pritham, and Polin), 918
PULASKI, EDWIN J. Newer antibiotics and hospital-acquired infections, 370
—. (*See* Altemeier et al.), 369

R

RAO, ALLOJU M. (*See* Sauvage et al.), 151
RAO, D. R. GOVINDA. (*See* Bhagavan, Rao, and Weinberg), 281
RAFFENSPERGER, JOHN G. Letter to the Editors, 401
RANGEL, DECIO M. (*See* Momma et al.), 799
RANSDELL, HERBERT T. (*See* Mays, Ransdell, and DeWeese), 780
RAUT, P. S. (*See* Thompson et al.), 212
REDMOND, DANIEL C. (*See* Salerno, Collins, and Redmond), 863
REES, J. RICHARD, MISCALL, BRIAN G., HOLSWADE, GEORGE R., CASTANEDA, ALDO, AND LILLEHEI, C. WALTON. Late results of valve replacement, 141
REEVE, T. S. (*See* Coupland and Reeve), 639
REICHENBACH, DENNIS D. (*See* Pierce et al.), 328
REIS, ROBERT L. (*See* Hannah, Enright, and Reis), 831
REMIGIO, PATERNO, AND ZAINO, EDWARD. Polyarteritis nodosa of the gallbladder, 427
REMMERS, AUGUST R. (*See* Fish et al.), 658, 969
RESNICK, ROBERT H. (*See* Callow et al.), 97

Reuter, Stewart R. (*See* Frey, Reuter, and Bookstein), 548
Reynolds, Ernest W., Jr. (*See* Kahn et al.), 122
Richardson, William. (*See* Crawford et al.), 182
Richie, Robert E. (*See* Civetta, Williams, and Richie), 874
Ridenhour, C. E., Henzel, J. H., DeWeese, M. S., and Kerr, S. Earl. Thymoma arising from undescended cervical thymus, 614
Rish F., Lorenzo. (*See* Bialostozky et al.), 442
Rittenhouse, Edward A., Mohri, Hitoshi, and Merendino, K. Alvin. Studies of carbohydrate metabolism and serum electrolytes during surface-induced deep hypothermia with prolonged circulatory occlusion, 995
Ritzmann, Stephan E. (*See* Fish et al.), 658, 969
Robb, Douglas. A Pacific-wide view of surgery, 558
Robel, Stephen B. (*See* Sauvage et al.), 151
Roe, Benson B. (*See* Fishman, Hutchinson, and Roe), 867
Rosenberg, Norman, Adiarte, Edgardo, Bujdoso, Leslie J., and Blackwinkel, Klaus D. Mortality factors in major limb amputations for vascular disease: A study of 176 procedures, 437
—, Lord, Geoffrey H., Henderson, John, Bothwell, James W., and Gaughran, Eugene R. L. Collagen arterial graft of bovine origin: 7 year observations in the dog, 951
Ross, Michael A. (*See* Sauvage et al.), 151
Rothwell-Jackson, R. (See Novak et al.), 678
Rudolph, A. M. (*See* Norton et al.), 1011
Rueff, Bernard. (See Maillard, Benhamou, and Rueff), 883

S

Sabiston, David C., Jr. (*See* Daniel, Graham, and Sabiston), 985
Sako, Yoshio, and Varco, Richard L. Arteriovenous fistula: Results of management of congenital and acquired forms, blood flow measurements, and observations on proximal arterial degeneration, 40
Salerno, Felix, Collins, Dale, and Redmond, Daniel C. External iliac artery occlusion in a newborn infant, 863
Salinas Izaguirre, Saul F., Haggerty, James T., and Eckert, Gerald. Spontaneous rupture of the esophagus, 607
Salzberg, Arnold M. (*See* Moore, Salzberg, and Talman), 364
Sandiford, Frank. (*See* Crawford et al.), 182
Sandusky, William R. Spread of infection in hospitals, 372
—. (*See* Altemeier et al.), 369
Santoni, Ernesto. (*See* Tice and Santoni), 493
Santos-Atherton, David. (*See* Pérez Alvarez et al.), 355
Sarles, Harry E. (*See* Fish et al.), 658, 969
Sarti, Lorenzo. Total prosthetic transplantation of the inferior vena cava, with venous drainage restoration of the one remaining kidney on the graft, successfully performed on a child with Wilms' tumor, 851
Sauvage, Lester R., Viggers, Robert F., Berger, Knute, Wood, Stephen J., Rao, Alloju M., Dedomenico, Mark, Ross, Michael A., and Robel, Stephen B. Aortic ball valve design based upon healing and hydraulic considerations, 151
—. (*See* Hessel et al.), 624
Sayler, Osbey L. (*See* Polin, Walklett, and Sayler), 313
Schein, Clarence J., and Beneventano, Thomas C. Biliary manometry: Its role in clinical surgery, 255
Schenk, Worthington G., Jr. (*See* Tibblin, Kock, and Schenk), 816
—. (*See* Williams et al.), 1031
Scherer, David. (*See* Kashiwagi et al.), 789
Schimert, George, Lajos, Thomas Z., Bunnell, Ivan L., Greene, David G., Falsetti, Herman L., Gage, Andrew A., Dean, David C., and Bernstein, Michael. Operation for cardiac complications following myocardial infarction, 129
Schlegel, Jerry F. (*See* Bremner, Schlegel, and Ellis), 735
Schlegel, Jorgen U. (*See* Grablowsky et al.), 895
Schuhmann, R. E., Geddes, L. A., and Hoff, H. E. Prolonged left ventricular bypass by transvalvular aortic catheterization. I. Physiologic effects and rationale of surgical concept, 957
Schulman, Norman H., Pritham, Howard G., and Polin, Stanton G. Decompression of the colon with complete diversion of the fecal stream by an in situ colonic catheter: A pilot study, 918
Schwartz, Marshall Z., Moore, Richard B., and Buchwald, Henry. Cholesterol excretion following chronic ileal bypass, 346
Schwartz, Sorrell L. (*See* Lotke and Schwartz), 488
Seigler, H. F., Mendes, N. F., and Metzgar, R. S. Accelerated rejection of skin grafts in recipients sensitized with extracted human histocompatibility antigens, 261
Severinghaus, J. W. (*See* Ehrenfeld et al.), 87
Shoemaker, N. J. (*See* Shoemaker et al.), 754
Shoemaker, W. C., Carey, J. S., Yao, S. T., Mohr, P. A., Amato, J. J., Printen, K. J., Corley, R. D., Monson, D. O., Youssef, S., and Shoemaker, N. J. Hemodynamic alterations in acute cardiac tamponade after penetrating injuries of the heart, 754
Shorter, Roy G. (*See* Anderson et al.), 249
Siegel, John H., Fabian, Miklos, Lankau, Charles, Levine, Michael, Cole, Andrew, and Nahmad, Michel. Clinical and experimental use of thoracic impedance plethysmography in quantifying myocardial contractility, 907
Sigler, Luis. (*See* Thompson et al.), 212
Simkin, E. P., and Stell, P. M. Technique of gastric mobilization for esophageal replacement, 1029
Simpson, James S., Mustard, W. T., Moes, C. A. F., and Izukawa, T. Emergency separation of thoracopagus (twins conjoined at thorax) in the newborn period: Importance of careful preoperative evaluation, 697
Singh, Hira. (*See* Daniele et al.), 484
Sirak, Howard D. (*See* Kilman et al.), 197
Skornik, William A. (*See* Dressler and Skornik), 644
Sloan, Herbert. (*See* Kahn et al.), 122
Snow, Harold D. (*See* Bruckner, Snow, and Fonkalsrud), 360
Sokol, Ezri S., Walker, Barry, Terz, Jose J., and Lawrence, Walter, Jr. Role of mammography with palpable breast lesions, 748

SOMERVILLE, JANE. (*See* Stark et al.), 536
STAMM, STANLEY J. (*See* Hessel et al.), 624
STANFORD, WILLIAM. (*See* Armstrong et al.), 844
STARK, JAROSLAV, TYNAN, MICHAEL, ABERDEEN, EOIN, WATERSTON, DAVID J., BONHAM-CARTER, RICHARD E., GRAHAM, GERALD R., AND SOMERVILLE, JANE. Repair of intracardiac defects after previous constriction (banding) of the pulmonary artery, 536
STARZL, THOMAS E. (*See* Kashiwagi et al.), 789
—. (*See* Ono et al.), 322
—. (*See* Picache, Kapur, and Starzl), 319
STELL, P. M. (*See* Simkin and Stell), 1029
STEPHEN, C. R. (*See* Dickey, Ahlgren, and Stephen), 981
STEVENS, GARY H. (*See* Momma et al.), 799
STEWART, EDWARD T. (*See* Norton et al.), 1011
STOLIAR, J. BRUCE. (*See* Litwin, Chapman, and Stoliar), 342
STONEY, RONALD J., AND WYLIE, EDWIN J. Arterial autografts, 18
STRODE, J. E., AND BALFOUR, JOHN F. Surgery for duodenal and gastric ulcer in infancy and childhood, 527
SUGAWARA, KYOJI. (*See* Isaza et al.), 462

T

TAKAMOTO, ROBERT M. (*See* Armstrong et al.), 844
TAKEMOTO, TADAYOSHI. (*See* Oi, Takemoto, and Nakayama), 561
TALMAN, E. ARMISTEAD. (*See* Moore, Salzberg, and Talman), 364
TANGA, MANIKCHAND RUKMANAPPA, AND EWING, J. BURKE. Primary malignant tumors of the gallbladder: Report of 43 cases, 418
TARHAN, SAIT, MOFFITT, EMERSON A., LUNDBORG, RICHARD O., AND WALLACE, ROBERT B. Use of heparinized priming blood after whole-body perfusion, 584
TERZ, JOSE J. (*See* Sokol et al.), 748
THIEDE, HENRY A. Amniocentesis: A new approach to some old problems in obstetrics, 383
THIEME, E. THURSTON, AND FINK, GEORGE. A study of the danger of antibiotic preparation of the bowel for surgery, 403
THOMPSON, JESSE E., SIGLER, LUIS, RAUT, P. S., AUSTIN, DALE J., AND PATMAN, R. DON. Arterial embolectomy: A 20 year experience with 163 cases, 212
TIBBLIN, STEN, KOCK, NILS G., AND SCHENK, WORTHINGTON G., JR. Dissociation of the hyperglycemic and vascular effects of glucagon, 816
TICE, DAVID A., AND SANTONI, ERNESTO. Use of saphenous vein homografts for arterial reconstruction: A preliminary report, 493
TILSON, M. DAVID, AND WRIGHT, HASTINGS K. Adaptation of functioning and bypassed segments of ileum during compensatory hypertrophy of the gut, 687
TIONGCO, RICHARD. (*See* Isaza et al.), 462
TOUROFF, ARTHUR S. W. (*See* Nabatoff, Blum, and Touroff), 272
TOWNSEND, COURTNEY M. (*See* Kashiwagi et al.), 789
TRAMMELL, SHIRLEY W. (*See* Ochsner, Zehnder, and Trammell), 1017
TREIBER, WILLIAM F., JR. (*See* Boley et al.), 350
TRIMBLE, CLEVE. (*See* Atkins, Trimble, and Eiseman), 306
TYNAN, MICHAEL. (*See* Stark et al.), 536
TYSON, KENNETH R. T., HARRIS, LEONARD C., AND NGHIEM, QUANG X. Repair of aortic arch interruption in the neonate, 1006
—. (*See* Fish et al.), 969

U

ULLYOT, DANIEL J. (*See* Norton et al.), 1011

V

VARCO, RICHARD L. (*See* Sako and Varco), 40
VARGAS-ROSENDO, RUBÉN. (*See* Pérez Alvarez et al.), 355
VATHAYANON, SATHAPORN. (*See* Kahn et al.), 122
VAUGHN, CECIL C., WARNER, HOMER R., AND NELSON, RUSSELL M. Cardiovascular effects of glucagon following cardiac surgery, 204
VEITH, FRANK J. (*See* Boley et al.), 350
VELASQUEZ, A. (*See* Novak et al.), 678
VETTO, R. MARK. (*See* Brant, Armstrong, and Vetto), 650
VIDNE, BERNARD, LEVINSON, SHAUL, AND LEVY, MORRIS J. Venous pressure monitor, 279
VIGGERS, ROBERT F. (*See* Sauvage et al.), 151
VOGEL, MARY ANN. (*See* Nelsen et al.), 826
VOORHEES, ARTHUR B., JR. (*See* Britton, Voorhees, and Price), 104

W

WALKER, BARRY. (*See* Sokol et al.), 748
WALKLETT, WILLIAM D. (*See* Polin, Walklett, and Sayler), 313
WALLACE, ROBERT B. (*See* Tarhan et al.), 584
WALTON, JOSEPH A., JR. (*See* Kahn et al.), 122
WANGENSTEEN, STEPHEN L., DEHOLL, J. DAVID, KIECHEL, STEPHEN F., MARTIN, JULIAN, AND LEFER, ALLAN M. Influence of hemodialysis on a myocardial depressant factor in hemorrhagic shock, 935
—, KIECHEL, STEPHEN F., LUDEWIG, ROBERT M., AND MADDEN, JAMES J., JR. The role of vasoconstriction in the suppression of hemorrhage from arteries. I. The completely severed artery, 338
WARNER, HOMER R. (*See* Vaughn, Warner, and Nelson), 204
WATERSTON, DAVID J. (*See* Stark et al.), 536
WEICHERT, RUDOLPH F., III. (*See* Grablowsky et al.), 895
WEINBERG, TOBIAS. (*See* Bhagavan, Rao, and Weinberg), 281
WHITE, JOHN J., AND MORGAN, W. W. Improved operative technique for gastric duplication, 522
WIECZOREK, ULF. (*See* Lemperle, Michaelis, and Wieczorek), 332
WILDE, W. LAWRENCE. (*See* Linton and Wilde), 234
WILKINSON, J. HENRY. (*See* Penneys and Wilkinson), 302
WILLIAMS, BYRN T., WORMAN, ROBERT K., JACOBS, RAE R., AND SCHENK, WORTHINGTON G., JR. An electromagnetic probe for the quantitation of intracardiac flows, 1031
WILLIAMS, M. J. (*See* Civetta, Williams, and Richie), 874

WOLFE, RICHARD D. (*See* Armstrong et al.), 844
WOOD, STEPHEN J. (*See* Sauvage et al.), 151
WORMAN, ROBERT K. (*See* Williams et al.), 1031
WRIGHT, HASTINGS K. (*See* Tilson and Wright), 687
WRIGHT, PHILIP W., AND GOODHEAD, BERNARD. The value of dextrans in the treatment of experimental pancreatitis, 807
WRIGHT, R. (*See* Novak et al.), 678
WYLIE, EDWIN J. (*See* Stoney and Wylie), 18

Y

YAKEISHI, YOZO. (*See* Momma et al.), 799
YALE, C. E., AND DOWELL, V. R., JR. Intestinal strangulation in rats monocontaminated with *Sphaerophorus necrophorus,* 478
YAO, S. T. (*See* Shoemaker et al.), 754
YASARGIL, M. GAZI, KRAYENBUHL, HUGO A., AND JACOBSON, JULIUS H., II. Microneurosurgical arterial reconstruction, 221
YOSHIDA, YOSHIYUKI. (*See* Ishigami et al.), 620
YOUNG, JESS R. (*See* Esselstyn et al.), 34
YOUSSEF, S. (*See* Shoemaker et al.), 754

Z

ZACHARY, R. B. (*See* Nicholas, Morgan, and Zachary), 847
ZAINO, EDWARD. (*See* Remigio and Zaino), 427
ZAMORA, ROLANDO, MOLLER, JAMES H., LUCAS, RUSSELL V., JR., AND CASTANEDA, ALDO R. Complete transposition of the great vessels: Surgical results of emergency Blalock-Hanlon operation in infants, 706
ZEHNDER, PAUL R. (*See* Ochsner, Zehnder, and Trammell), 1017

SUBJECT INDEX*

A

Acid, gastric, secretion, canine, effect of antigastrin on (Isaza et al.), 462
  influence of thermal burns (O'Neill), 267
Adhesions, massive, in infancy, jejunoileocolic intubation and plication for intestinal obstruction caused by (Moore, Salzberg, and Talman), 364
Aged patient, aneurysmectomy in (Esselstyn et al.), 34
Allografted canine lungs, hemodynamics and blood gas exchange in (Momma et al.), 799
Allografts, kidney, incorporation of foreign DNA and RNA into, autoradiographic studies (Lemperle, Michaelis, and Wieczorek), 332
  skin, intravascular, immunologic response to (Donawick and Baue), 667
Amniocentesis, new approach to some old problems in obstetrics (Thiede), 383
Amputation of leg, elevation of serum creatine kinase following (Penneys and Wilkinson), 302
  limb, major, for vascular disease, mortality factors in, study of 176 procedures (Rosenberg et al.), 437
Anastomosis, microvascular, use in new operation for varicocele (Ishigami et al.), 620
Aneurysmectomy in aged (Esselstyn et al.), 34
Aneurysms, thoracic aortic, reappraisal of adjuncts to avoid in treatment of (Crawford et al.), 182
Angiography, selective, localization of gastrointestinal hemorrhage by (Frey, Reuter, and Bookstein), 548
Antibiotic(s), newer, and hospital-acquired infections (Pulaski), 370
  preparation of the bowel for surgery, study of danger of (Thieme and Fink), 403
  solution, local irrigation with, in prevention of infection in vascular prostheses (DiGiglia, Leonard, and Ochsner), 836
Antibody localization in horse, rabbit, and goat antilymphocyte sera (Kashiwagi et al.), 789
  response, humoral, effects of phytohemagglutinin (Ono et al.), 322
Antigastrin, effect on canine gastric acid secretion (Isaza et al.), 462
Antigens, histocompatibility, extracted human, accelerated rejection of skin grafts in recipients sensitized with (Siegler, Mendes, and Metzgar), 261
Antilymphocyte sera, horse, rabbit, and goat, antibody localization in (Kashiwagi et al.), 789
Aortic arch atresia with transposition of great vessels, physiologic considerations and surgical management (Norton et al.), 1011
Aortic—Cont'd
  ball valve design based upon healing and hydraulic considerations (Sauvage et al.), 151
  catheterization, transvalvular, prolonged left ventricular bypass by, physiologic effects and rationale of surgical concept (Schuhmann, Geddes, and Hoff), 957
  leaflet heterografts, humoral immunity against, demonstration (Pierce et al.), 328
Aortofemoral graft thrombosis, late, extra-abdominal management of (Cohn, Moore, and Hall), 775
Aortoiliac endarterectomy case series followed 10 years or more (Pilcher, Barker, and Cannon), 5
Appendicitis in newborn infant (Parsons, Miscall, and McSherry), 841
Appendix, diverticulosis (Esparza and Pan), 922
Arterial autografts (Stoney and Wylie), 5
  catheterization, long-term, for repeated blood sampling (Moseley and Doty), 455
  degeneration, proximal, in arteriovenous fistula (Sako and Varco), 40
  embolectomy, 20 year experience with 163 cases (Thompson et al.), 212
  graft, collagen, of bovine origin, 7 year observations in dog (Rosenberg et al.), 951
    contralateral (Bialostozky et al.), 442
  pressure, downstream cerebral, during carotid endarterectomy, effect of CO_2 and systemic hypertension (Ehrenfeld et al.), 87
  reconstruction, microneurosurgical (Yasargil, Krayenbuhl, and Jacobson), 221
    use of saphenous vein homografts for, preliminary report (Tice and Santoni), 493
Arterialization of liver with portacaval shunt in treatment of portal hypertension due to intrahepatic block (Maillard, Benhamou, and Rueff), 883
Arteriography as adjunct to diagnosis of splenic injury (Polin, Walklett, and Sayler), 313
Arteriovenous fistula: results of management of congenital and acquired forms, blood flow measurements, and observations on proximal arterial degeneration (Sako and Varco), 40
    subcutaneous, new type for chronic hemodialysis in children (Pérez Alvarez et al.), 355
  shunt implantation, improved surgical technique for, experiences with all-Silastic shunt (Aravena et al.), 593
  vein graft for chronic hemodialysis, preliminary report (Mozes et al.), 452
Artery, completely severed, suppression of hemorrhage from, role of vasoconstriction (Wangensteen et al.), 338
  coronary, direct revascularization, for segmental occlusive disease (Mundth et al.), 168

*January, pp. 1-248; February, pp. 249-402; March, pp. 403-560; April, pp. 561-726; May, pp. 727-882; June, pp. 883-1058.

Artery, coronary—Cont'd
–right ventricular fistula with congestive heart failure, surgical correction in neonatal period (Daniel, Graham, and Sabiston), 985
external iliac, occlusion in newborn infant (Salerno, Collins, and Redmond), 863
popliteal, cystic degeneration of (Powis, Morrissey, and Jones), 891
pulmonary, previous constriction (banding) of, repair of intracardiac defects after (Stark et al.), 536
renal, thrombosis following blunt trauma, report of 4 cases (Grablowsky et al.), 895
sole, to basal segments of left lung, high systemic origin of, findings, surgical treatment, and embryologic interpretation (Hessel et al.), 624
Atheroma, carotid bifurcation, natural history (Javid et al.), 80
Autografts, arterial (Stoney and Wylie), 5
femoropopliteal saphenous vein bypass, modifications in technique (Linton and Wilde), 234
Autoradiographic studies on incorporation of foreign DNA and RNA into kidney allografts (Lemperle, Michaelis, and Wieczorek), 332
Axillofemoral and femorofemoral grafts, compromise or preference (Parsonnet, Alpert, and Brief), 26

B

Ball valve design, aortic, based upon healing and hydraulic considerations (Sauvage et al.), 151
Battle injury, hypoxemia during first twelve hours after (Moseley and Doty), 765
Biliary manometry, role in clinical surgery (Schein and Beneventano), 255
tract calculi, residual, removal without reoperation (Mazzariello), 566
Blalock-Hanlon operation, emergency, in infants, in complete transposition of great vessels, surgical results (Zamora et al.), 706
Blood flow measurements in arteriovenous fistula (Sako and Varco), 40
gas exchange and hemodynamics in allografted canine lungs (Momma et al.), 799
heparinized priming, use after whole-body perfusion (Tarhan et al.), 584
sampling, repeated, long-term arterial catheterization for (Moseley and Doty), 455
viscosity in normal man (Litwin, Chapman, and Stoliar), 342
Bowel, antibiotic preparation for surgery, study of danger of (Thieme and Fink), 403
Breast lesions, palpable, role of mammography with (Sokol et al.), 748
Burned rat model, silver sulfadiazine and Sulfamylon Cream in, comparative evaluation (Dressler and Skornik), 644
Burns, thermal, influence on gastric acid secretion (O'Neill), 267

C

Calculi of biliary tract, residual, removal without reoperation (Mazzariello), 566
Cancer immunology and the surgeon (Morton), 396
Cancer—Cont'd
of papilla of Vater, early diagnosis, fiberduodenoscopy in (Oi, Takemoto, and Nakayama), 561
Carbohydrate metabolism and serum electrolytes during surface-induced deep hypothermia with prolonged circulatory occlusion (Rittenhouse, Mohri, and Merendino), 995
Carcinoma of thyroglossal duct cyst, case reports and review of literature (Bhagavan, Rao, and Weinberg), 281
Cardiac complications following myocardial infarction, operation for (Schimert et al.), 129
defects, repair of, after previous constriction (banding) of pulmonary artery (Stark et al.), 536
evaluation, importance of careful preoperative, in emergency separation of thoracopagus (Simpson et al.), 697
surgery, cardiovascular effects of glucagon following (Vaughn, Warner, and Nelson), 204
tamponade, acute hemodynamic alterations in, after penetrating injuries of heart (Shoemaker et al.), 748
valve, prosthetic, prevention of detachment (Fishman, Hutchinson, and Roe), 867
Cardiomyopathy, human heart transplantation for (Kahn et al.), 122
Cardiovascular effects of glucagon following cardiac surgery (Vaughn, Warner, and Nelson), 204
Care, intensive, bed for initial diagnosis and treatment of severely ill patients (Hill and Johnson), 414
Carotid bifurcation atheroma, natural history (Javid et al.), 80
endarterectomy, downstream cerebral arterial pressure during, effect of CO_2 and systemic hypertension (Ehrenfeld et al.), 87
Catheter embolism (Blair, Hunziker, and Flanagan), 457
Catheterization, arterial, long-term, for repeated blood sampling (Moseley and Doty), 455
Cephalothin, intraperitoneal, clinical use (McMullan and Barnett), 432
Cerebral arterial pressure, downstream, during carotid endarterectomy, effect of CO_2 and systemic hypertension (Ehrenfeld et al.), 87
Cervical thymus, undescended, thymoma arising from (Ridenhour et al.), 614
Cholesterol absorption following reversal of upper and lower halves of small intestine (Gebhard and Buchwald), 474
excretion following chronic ileal bypass (Schwartz, Moore, and Buchwald), 346
Circulatory occlusion, prolonged, with surface-induced deep hypothermia, carbohydrate metabolism and serum electrolytes during (Rittenhouse, Mohri, and Merendino), 995
Closure, early, of patent ductus arteriosus, case for (Kilman et al.), 197
CO_2 and systemic hypertension, effect on downstream cerebral arterial pressure during carotid endarterectomy (Ehrenfeld et al.), 87

Collagen arterial graft of bovine origin, 7 year observations in dog (Rosenberg et al.), 951
Colon, ascending, tuberculous stenosis of, massive megacolon and megaileum in childhood due to (Patton and Moore), 513
decompression with complete diversion of fecal stream by in situ colonic catheter, pilot study (Schulman, Pritham, and Polin), 918
Contusion, pulmonary, progressive nature of (Fulton and Peter), 499
Coronary arterial revascularization, direct, for segmental occlusive disease (Mundth et al.), 168
artery–right ventricular fistula with congestive heart failure, surgical correction in neonatal period (Daniel, Graham, and Sabiston), 985
Creatine kinase, serum, elevation following amputation of leg (Penneys and Wilkinson), 302
Cyst of thyroglossal duct, carcinoma of, case reports and review of literature (Bhagavan, Rao, and Weinberg), 281
Cystic degeneration of popliteal artery (Powis, Morrissey, and Jones), 891

D

Declamp shock production, vasodepressor factor in (Brant, Armstrong, and Vetto), 650
Decompression, portal, selective (Britton, Voorhees, and Price), 104
Delirium tremens, surgical, metabolic changes in (Mays, Ransdell, and DeWeese), 780
Dextrans, value in treatment of experimental pancreatitis (Wright and Goodhead), 807
Dimethyl sulfoxide, effect on pedicle flaps, experimental studies (Koehnlein and Lemperle), 672
Directional flow detection for localizing venous valvular incompetency (Folse and Alexander), 114
Diuretic agents, use of, during oliguria after renal transplantation (Anderson et al.), 249
Diverticulosis of appendix (Esparza and Pan), 922
DNA and RNA, foreign, incorporation into kidney allografts, autoradiographic studies (Lemperle, Michaelis, and Wieczorek), 332
Duodenal and gastric ulcer in infancy and childhood, surgery for (Strode and Balfour), 527
ulcer, perforated, long-term follow-up (Nemanich and Nicoloff), 727

E

Edema of scrotum, idiopathic, in young boys (Nicholas, Morgan, and Zachary), 847
Electrolytes, serum, and carbohydrate metabolism during surface-induced deep hypothermia with prolonged circulatory occlusion (Rittenhouse, Mohri, and Merendino), 995
Electromagnetic probe for quantitation of intracardiac flows (Williams et al.), 1031
Electrometry, surface, monitoring by, during storage interval, in successful 24 hour renal perfusion-preservation (Alexander et al.), 944
Embolectomy, arterial, 20 year experience with 163 cases (Thompson et al.), 212
Emboli, pulmonary, recurrent, following inferior vena caval plication (Coupland and Reeve), 639
Embolism, catheter (Blair, Hunziker, and Flanagan), 457
Endarterectomy, aortoiliac, case series followed 10 years or more (Pilcher, Barker, and Cannon), 5
carotid, downstream cerebral arterial pressure during, effect of CO_2 and systemic hypertension (Ehrenfeld et al.), 87
Endotoxin, intraperitoneal, in dog, lymphatic absorption of (Daniele et al.), 484
Epicardiectomy, effect on function and diastolic compliance of normal canine left ventricle (Hannah, Enright, and Reis), 831
Error, retrievable (editorial) (Derrick), 881
Esophageal mucosal regeneration following experimental prosthetic replacement of esophagus (Leininger, Peacock, and Neville), 468
replacement, gastric mobilization for, technique (Simkin and Stell), 1029
varices, bleeding, transabdominal ligation-resection of esophagus in cases of (Boerema, Klopper, and Holscher), 409
Esophagobronchial fistula, malignant, management (Ong and Kwong), 293
Esophagus, experimental prosthetic replacement, esophageal mucosal regeneration following (Leininger, Peacock, and Neville), 468
spontaneous rupture (Salinas Izaguirre, Haggerty, and Eckert), 607
transabdominal ligation-resection of, in cases of bleeding esophageal varices (Boerema, Klopper and Holscher), 409
traumatic pseudodiverticulum of, in newborn infant (Armstrong et al.), 844

F

Fecal stream, complete diversion by in situ colonic catheter, with decompression of colon, pilot study (Schulman, Pritham, and Polin), 918
Femoral-to-popliteal bypass grafts, method of salvaging bifurcated saphenous vein for use in (McDaniel and Johnson), 394
Femoral vein, common, ligation in treatment of thromboembolic disease, long-term sequelae (Nabatoff, Blum, and Touroff), 272
Femorofemoral and axillofemoral grafts, compromise or preference (Parsonnet, Alpert, and Brief), 26
Femoropopliteal bypass grafting, duplicated saphenous vein in (Gaylis), 277
saphenous vein bypass autografts, modifications in technique (Linton and Wilde), 234
Fiberduodenoscopy in early diagnosis of cancer of papilla of Vater (Oi, Takemoto, and Nakayama), 561
Fingers and hand, ischemia of, management (Dale and Lewis), 62

Fistula, arteriovenous: results of management of congenital and acquired forms, blood flow measurements, and observations on proximal arterial degeneration (Sako and Varco), 40
arteriovenous, new type subcutaneous, for chronic hemodialysis in children (Pérez Alvarez et al.), 355
coronary artery–right ventricle, with congestive heart failure, surgical correction in neonatal period (Daniel, Graham, and Sabiston), 985
malignant esophagobronchial, management (Ong and Kwong), 293
Flow, directional, detection, for localizing venous valvular incompetency (Folse and Alexander), 114
Fork in the road: geographic full-time system (editorial) (Egdahl), 878

G

Gallbladder, polyarteritis nodosa of (Remigio and Zaino), 427
primary malignant tumors of, report of 43 cases (Tanga and Ewing), 418
Gastrectomy, subtotal, and vagotomy plus partial gastrectomy, critical analysis of results from, in surgical treatment of peptic ulcer (Ochsner, Zehnder, and Trammell), 1017
Gastrin, placental transfer in canine fetus (Bruckner, Snow, and Fonkalsrud), 360
Gastric acid secretion, canine, effect of antigastrin on (Isaza et al.), 462
influence of thermal burns (O'Neill), 267
and duodenal ulcer in infancy and childhood, surgery for (Strode and Balfour), 527
duplication, improved operative technique for (White and Morgan), 522
hypothermia, local, in gastroduodenal hemorrhage (Petrov and Korenev), 574
mobilization for esophageal replacement, technique (Simkin and Stell), 1029
secretion in canine fetus following maternal stimulation (Bruckner, Snow, and Fonkalsrud), 360
Gastroduodenal hemorrhage, local gastric hypothermia in (Petrov and Korenev), 574
Gastroesophageal sphincter mechanism, studies of, role of phrenoesophageal membrane (Bremner, Schlegel, and Ellis), 735
Gastrointestinal hemorrhage, localization of, by selective angiography (Frey, Reuter, and Bookstein), 548
Gastroschisis defect, intrauterine midgut strangulation in (Grosfeld and Clatworthy), 519
Geographic full-time system (editorial) (Egdahl), 878
Glucagon, cardiovascular effects of, following cardiac surgery (Vaughn, Warner, and Nelson), 204
dissociation of hyperglycemic and vascular effects of (Tibblin, Kock, and Schenk), 816
Graft(s), aortofemoral, thrombosis, late, extra-abdominal management of (Cohn, Moore, and Hall), 775
arterial, collagen, of bovine origin, 7 year observations in dog (Rosenberg et al.), 951
contralateral (Bialostozky et al.), 442

Grafts—Cont'd
femorofemoral or axillofemoral, compromise or preference (Parsonnet, Alpert, and Brief), 26
femoropopliteal bypass, duplicated saphenous vein in (Gaylis), 277
skin, accelerated rejection of, in recipients sensitized with extracted human histocompatibility antigens (Seigler, Mendes, and Metzgar), 261
vein, arteriovenous, for chronic hemodialysis, preliminary report (Mozes et al.), 452

H

Hand and fingers, ischemia of, management (Dale and Lewis), 62
Healing and hydraulic considerations, aortic ball valve design based upon (Sauvage et al.), 151
Heart, acute penetrating injuries of, hemodynamic alterations in acute cardiac tamponade after (Shoemaker et al.), 748
human, transplantation for cardiomyopathy (Kahn et al.), 122
Hemodialysis, chronic, arteriovenous vein graft for, preliminary report (Mozes et al.), 452
in children, new type subcutaneous arteriovenous fistula for (Pérez Alvarez et al.), 355
influence on myocardial depressant factor in hemorrhagic shock (Wangensteen et al.), 935
Hemodynamic alterations in acute cardiac tamponade after penetrating injuries of heart (Shoemaker et al.), 748
and results of treatment in patients with gram-negative septic shock (Motsay et al.), 577
Hemodynamics and blood gas exchange in allografted canine lungs (Momma et al.), 799
Hemoptysis, massive, pulmonary resection for (Garzon et al.), 633
Hemorrhage from completely severed artery, role of vasoconstriction (Wangensteen et al.), 338
gastroduodenal, local gastric hypothermia in (Petrov and Korenev), 574
gastrointestinal, localization of, by selective angiography (Frey, Reuter, and Bookstein), 548
Hemorrhagic shock, influence of hemodialysis on myocardial depressant factor in (Wangensteen et al.), 935
Hemostasis during liver resections (Clark and Leather), 556
Heparinized priming blood, use after whole-body perfusion (Tarhan et al.), 584
Hepatic parenchyma, control by direct compression, new instrument (Doty, Kugler, and Moseley), 720
Hernia in inguinal region, diagnosis of, value of pneumoperitoneum in (Arner and Fernström), 741
Heterografts, aortic leaflet, humoral immunity against, demonstration (Pierce et al.), 328
Histamine, placental transfer in canine fetus (Bruckner, Snow, and Fonkalsrud), 360

Histocompatibility antigens, extracted human, accelerated rejection of skin grafts in recipients sensitized with (Seigler, Mendes, and Metzgar), 261
Homograft rejection, effects of phytohemagglutinin (Ono et al.), 322
saphenous vein, use of, for arterial reconstruction, preliminary report (Tice and Santoni), 493
Homotransplantation, auxiliary, of porcine liver into retroperitoneal space (Novak et al.), 678
Hospitals, spread of infections in (Sandusky), 372
Humoral antibody response, effects of phytohemagglutinin (Ono et al.), 322
immunity against aortic leaflet heterografts, demonstration (Pierce et al.), 328
Hydraulic and healing considerations, aortic ball valve design based upon (Sauvage et al.), 151
Hyperglycemic and vascular effects of glucagon, dissociation of (Tibblin, Kock, and Schenk), 816
Hypersensitivity, delayed, effects of phytohemagglutinin (Ono et al.), 322
Hypertension, portal, due to intrahepatic block, arterialization of liver with portacaval shunt in treatment of (Maillard, Benhamou, and Rueff), 883
systemic, and CO_2, effect on downstream cerebral arterial pressure during carotid endarterectomy (Ehrenfeld et al.), 87
Hypertrophy, compensatory, of gut, adaptation of functioning and bypassed segments of ileum during (Tilson and Wright), 687
Hypothermia, deep, surface-induced, carbohydrate metabolism and serum electrolytes during, with prolonged circulatory occlusion (Rittenhouse, Mohri, and Merendino), 995
gastric, local, in gastroduodenal hemorrhage (Petrov and Korenev), 574
Hypoxemia during first twelve hours after battle injury (Moseley and Doty), 765

I

Iliac artery, external, occlusion in newborn infant (Salerno, Collins, and Redmond), 863
Ileal bypass, chronic, cholesterol excretion following (Schwartz, Moore, and Buchwald), 346
Ileum, functioning and bypassed segments, adaptation of, during compensatory hypertrophy of gut (Tilson and Wright), 687
Immunity, humoral, against aortic leaflet heterografts, demonstration (Pierce et al.), 328
Immunologic response to intravascular skin allografts (Donawick and Baue), 667
Immunology, cancer, and the surgeon (Morton), 396
Immunosuppressive therapy, current status (Mannick), 711
Infarction, myocardial, cardiac complications following, operation for (Schimert et al.), 129
Infection(s), hospital-acquired, and newer antibiotics (Pulaski), 370
prophylaxis and management (Altemeier et al.), 369
spread of, in hospitals (Sandusky), 372
Inguinal region, hernia in, diagnosis of, value of pneumoperitoneum in (Arner and Fernström), 741
Insulin, placental transfer in canine fetus (Bruckner, Snow, and Fonkalsrud), 360
Insurance, National Health, considerations regarding coming of (Mueller), 1035
Intensive care bed for initial diagnosis and treatment of severely ill patients (Hill and Johnson), 414
unit flow sheet (Kramer and Lipson), 590
Intestinal obstruction caused by massive adhesions in infancy, jejunoileocolic intubation and plication for (Moore, Salzberg, and Talman), 364
strangulation in rats monocontaminated with *Sphaerophorus necrophorus* (Yale and Dowell), 478
Intestine, small, reversal of upper and lower halves, cholesterol absorption following (Gebhard and Buchwald), 474
Intracardiac flows, quantitation of, electromagnetic probe for (Williams et al.), 1031
Intubation, jejunoileocolic, and plication for intestinal obstruction caused by massive adhesions in infancy (Moore, Salzberg, and Talman), 364
Ischemia of hand and fingers, management (Dale and Lewis), 62
reappraisal of adjuncts to avoid, in treatment of thoracic aortic aneurysms (Crawford et al.), 182
Isolation techniques and their effectiveness (Burke), 373

J

Jejunoileocolic intubation and plication for intestinal obstruction caused by massive adhesions in infancy (Moore, Salzberg, and Talman), 364

K

Kidney allografts, incorporation of foreign DNA and RNA into, autoradiographic studies (Lemperle, Michaelis, and Wieczorek), 332
preservation, functional and biochemical changes during (Lotke and Schwartz), 488
Kinase, serum creatine, elevation following amputation of leg (Penneys and Wilkinson), 302

L

Leg, amputation, elevation of serum creatine kinase following (Penneys and Wilkinson), 302
Letters to the Editors, 401
Limb amputations, major, for vascular disease, mortality factors in, study of 176 procedures (Rosenberg et al.), 437
Liver, arterialization of, with portacaval shunt in treatment of portal hypertension due to intrahepatic block (Maillard, Benhamou, and Rueff), 883
disease, effect on need for venous decompression during anhepatic phase of canine orthotopic liver transplantation (Picache, Kapur, and Starzl), 319

Liver—Cont'd
porcine, auxiliary homotransplantation of, into retroperitoneal space (Novak et al.), 678
resection, asanguineous, vena cava catheter for (Chávez-Peón, Gonzalez, and Malt), 694
hemostasis during (Clark and Leather), 556
transplantation, canine orthotopic, need for venous decompression during anhepatic phase, effect of liver disease on (Picache, Kapur, and Starzl), 319
Lung(s), canine, allografted, hemodynamics and blood gas exchange in (Momma et al.), 799
left, basal segments, high systemic origin of sole artery to, findings, surgical treatment, and embryologic interpretation (Hessel et al.), 624
Lymphatic absorption of intraperitoneal endotoxin in dog (Daniele et al.), 484
Lymphocyte, circulating, depletion, effect on lymphoid tissue (Fish et al.), 658
on renal allograft survival in calves (Fish et al.), 969
Lymphoid tissue, effect on, of circulating lymphocyte depletion (Fish et al.), 658

M

Malignant esophagobronchial fistula, management (Ong and Kwong), 293
tumors, primary, of gallbladder, report of 43 cases (Tanga and Ewing), 418
Mammography, role of, with palpable breast lesions (Sokol et al.), 748
Manometer for monitoring central venous pressure, simple and accurate (Moss), 773
Manometry, biliary, role in clinical surgery (Schein and Beneventano), 255
Mediastinitis, anterior, as complication of median sternotomy incisions, diagnostic and surgical considerations (Jiménez-Martínez et al.), 929
Megacolon and megaileum, massive, in childhood, due to tuberculous stenosis of ascending colon (Patton and Moore), 513
Megaileum and megacolon, massive, in childhood, due to tuberculous stenosis of ascending colon (Patton and Moore), 513
Metabolic changes in surgical delirium tremens (Mays, Ransdell, and DeWeese), 780
Microneurosurgical arterial reconstruction (Yasargil, Krayenbuhl, and Jacobson), 221
Midgut strangulation, intrauterine, in gastroschisis defect (Grosfeld and Clatworthy), 519
Mortality factors in major limb amputations for vascular disease, study of 176 procedures (Rosenberg et al.), 437
Mucosal, esophageal, regeneration following experimental prosthetic replacement of esophagus (Leininger, Peacock, and Neville), 468
Muscle, skeletal, pH, responses to injury, new technique for determination of tissue viability (Berman, Lemieux, and Aaby), 507
Myocardial contractility, clinical and experimental use of thoracic impedance plethysmography in quantifying (Siegel et al.), 907

Myocardial—Cont'd
depressant factor in hemorrhagic shock, influence of hemodialysis on (Wangensteen et al.), 935
infarction, cardiac complications following, operation for (Schimert et al.), 129

N

Newborn infant, appendicitis in (Parsons, Miscall, and McSherry), 841
external artery occlusion in (Salerno, Collins, and Redmond), 863
traumatic pseudodiverticulum of esophagus in (Armstrong et al.), 844

O

Obstetrics, new approach to some old problems: amniocentesis (Thiede), 383
Obstruction, intestinal, caused by massive adhesions in infancy, jejunoileocolic intubation and plication for (Moore, Salzberg, and Talman), 364
Oliguria after renal transplantation, use of diuretic agents during (Anderson et al.), 249

P

Pacific-wide view of surgery (Robb), 558
Pancreatitis, experimental, value of dextrans in treatment of (Wright and Goodhead), 807
Papilla of Vater, cancer of, early diagnosis of, fiberduodenoscopy in (Oi, Takemoto, and Nakayama), 561
Parenchyma, hepatic, control by direct compression, new instrument (Doty, Kugler, and Moseley), 720
Patent ductus arteriosus, case for early closure (Kilman et al.), 197
Pedicle flaps, effect of dimethyl sulfoxide on, experimental studies (Koehnlein and Lemperle), 672
Peptic ulcer, surgical treatment (Ochsner, Zehnder, and Trammell), 1017
Perfusion, splenic, prolonged, technique (Atkins, Trimble, and Eiseman), 306
Peritoneal irrigation, diagnostic, simple and reliable technique (Civetta, Williams, and Richie), 874
2-Phenyl-2-(2-pyridyl)-thioacetamide (antigastrin), effect on canine gastric acid secretion (Isaza et al.), 462
Phrenoesophageal membrane, role of, in gastroesophageal sphincter mechanism (Bremner, Schlegel, and Ellis), 735
Phytohemagglutinin, effects on humoral antibody response, delayed hypersensitivity, and homograft rejection (Ono et al.), 322
Placental transfer of insulin, histamine, and gastrin in canine fetus (Bruckner, Snow, and Fonkalsrud), 360
Plethysmography, thoracic impedance, clinical and experimental use, in quantifying myocardial contractility (Siegel et al.), 907
Plication and jejunoileocolic intubation for intestinal obstruction caused by massive adhesions in infancy (Moore, Salzberg, and Talman), 364

Pneumoperitoneum, value of, in diagnosis of hernia in inguinal region (Arner and Fernström), 741
Polyarteritis nodosa of gallbladder (Remigio and Zaino), 427
Polyelectrolyte complexes, sulfonated, synthetic thromboresistant surfaces from (Nelsen et al.), 826
Popliteal artery, cystic degeneration of (Powis, Morrissey, and Jones), 891
Portacaval shunt and arterialization of liver in treatment of portal hypertension due to intrahepatic block (Maillard, Benhamou, and Rueff), 883
  prophylactic, conclusions from controlled trial (Callow et al.), 97
Portal decompression, selective (Britton, Voorhees, and Price), 104
  hypertension due to intrahepatic block, arterialization of liver with portacaval shunt in treatment of (Maillard, Benhamou, and Rueff), 883
Potassium vasoactivity, biphasic effect (Boley et al.), 350
Presidential address (Society for Vascular Surgery): Standards in vascular surgery (Hanlon), 1
Prostheses, vascular, infection in, local irrigation with antibiotic solution in prevention of (DiGiglia, Leonard, and Ochsner), 836
Prosthetic cardiac valve detachment, prevention (Fishman, Hutchinson, and Roe), 867
  transplantation of inferior vena cava, total, with venous drainage restoration of the one remaining kidney on the graft, successfully performed on child with Wilms' tumor (Sarti), 851
Pseudodiverticulum of esophagus, traumatic, in newborn infant (Armstrong et al.), 844
Pulmonary artery, previous constriction (banding) of, repair of intracardiac defects after (Stark et al.), 536
  contusion, progressive nature of (Fulton and Peter), 499
  emboli, recurrent, following inferior vena caval plication (Coupland and Reeve), 639
  resection for massive hemoptysis (Garzon et al.), 633

R

Renal allograft survival in calves, effect of circulating lymphocyte depletion (Fish et al.), 969
  artery thrombosis following blunt trauma, report of 4 cases (Grablowsky et al.), 895
  infundibulum, superior, vascular obstruction of, in children (Deckers et al.), 856
  perfusion-preservation, 24 hour, successful, with monitoring by surface electrometry during storage interval (Alexander et al.), 944
  transplantation, oliguria after, use of diuretic agents during (Anderson et al.), 249
Retroperitoneal space, auxiliary transplantation of porcine liver into (Novak et al.), 678
Revascularization, direct coronary arterial, for segmental occlusive disease (Mundth et al.), 168
RNA and DNA, foreign, incorporation into kidney allografts, autoradiographic studies (Lemperle, Michaelis, and Wieczorek), 332

S

Saphenous vein, bifurcated, method of salvaging, for use in femoral-to-popliteal bypass grafts (McDaniel and Johnson), 394
  bypass autografts, femoropopliteal, modifications in technique (Linton and Wilde), 234
  duplicated, in femoropopliteal bypass grafting (Gaylis), 277
  homografts, use of, for arterial reconstruction, preliminary report (Tice and Santoni), 493
Scapulectomy, indications and technique (Das Gupta), 601
Scoliosis and acute vascular compression of duodenum (Bunch and Delaney), 901
Scrotum, idiopathic edema of, in young boys (Nicholas, Morgan, and Zachary), 847
Segmental occlusive disease, direct coronary arterial revascularization for (Mundth et al.), 168
Sepsis, survival or death from (Clowes), 374
Septic shock, gram-negative, hemodynamic alterations and results of treatment in patients with (Motsay et al.), 577
Severely ill patients, initial diagnosis and treatment of, intensive care bed for (Hill and Johnson), 414
Shock production, declamp, vasodepressor factor in (Brant, Armstrong, and Vetto), 650
  septic, gram-negative, hemodynamic alterations and results of treatment in patients with (Motsay et al.), 577
Shunt, arteriovenous, implantation, improved surgical technique for, experiences with all-Silastic shunt (Aravena et al.), 593
  portacaval, and arterialization of liver in treatment of portal hypertension due to intrahepatic block (Maillard, Benhamou, and Rueff), 883
    prophylactic, conclusions from controlled trial (Callow et al.), 97
Silastic shunt, experiences with, in arteriovenous shunt implantation (Aravena et al.), 593
Silver sulfadiazine and Sulfamylon Cream in burned rat model, comparative evaluation (Dressler and Skornik), 644
Skeletal muscle pH, responses to injury, new technique for determination of tissue viability (Berman, Lemieux, and Aaby), 507
Skin allografts, intravascular, immunologic response to (Donawick and Baue), 667
  grafts, accelerated rejection of, in recipients sensitized with extracted human histocompatibility antigens (Seigler, Mendes, and Metzgar), 261
Sphaerophorus necrophorus, intestinal strangulation in rats monocontaminated with (Yale and Dowell), 478
Sphincter mechanism, gastroesophageal, studies of, role of phrenoesophageal membrane (Bremner, Schlegel, and Ellis), 735

Splenic injury, diagnosis, arteriography as adjunct (Polin, Walklett, and Sayler), 313
perfusion, prolonged, technique (Atkins, Trimble, and Eiseman), 306
Sternotomy, median, incisions, anterior mediastinitis as complication of, diagnostic and surgical considerations (Jiménez-Martínez et al.), 929
Strangulation, intestinal, in rats monocontaminated with *Sphaerophorus necrophorus* (Yale and Dowell), 478
intrauterine midgut, in gastroschisis defect (Grosfeld and Clatworthy), 519
Sulfadiazine, silver, and Sulfamylon Cream in burned rat model, comparative evaluation (Dressler and Skornik), 644
Sulfamylon Cream and silver sulfadiazine in burned rat model, comparative evaluation (Dressler and Skornik), 644
Sulfoxide, dimethyl, effect on pedicle flaps, experimental studies (Koehnlein and Lemperle), 672
Surgeon, cancer immunology and (Morton), 396
Surgery, Pacific-wide view of (Robb), 558
Surgical care, delivery, experiments in (Eiseman et al.), 725
training, crisis in (Meyerowitz), 399

T

Tamponade, cardiac, acute, hemodynamic alterations in, after penetrating injuries of heart (Shoemaker et al.), 748
Temperature, body, monitoring, via tympanic membrane (Dickey, Ahlgren, and Stephen), 981
Testis, torsion of, in newborn infant (Michaelian, Mahour, and Johnston), 703
Thermal burns, influence on gastric acid secretion (O'Neill), 267
Thoracic aortic aneurysms, reappraisal of adjuncts to avoid ischemia in treatment (Crawford et al.), 182
impedance plethysmography, clinical and experimental use, in quantifying myocardial contractility (Siegel et al.), 907
Thoracopagus, emergency separation in newborn period, importance of careful preoperative cardiac evaluation (Simpson et al.), 697
Thrombocytosis, postoperative, reduction of (Atkins and Lempke), 976
Thromboembolic disease, common femoral vein ligation in treatment, long-term sequelae (Nabatoff, Blum, and Touroff), 272
Thromboresistant surfaces, synthetic, from sulfonated polyelectrolyte complexes (Nelsen et al.), 826
Thrombosis, late aortofemoral graft, extra-abdominal management of (Cohn, Moore, and Hall), 775
of renal artery following blunt trauma, report of 4 cases (Grablowsky et al.), 895
Thymoma arising from undescended cervical thymus (Ridenhour et al.), 614
Thymus, cervical, undescended, thymoma arising from (Ridenhour et al.), 614
Thyroglossal duct cyst, carcinoma of, case reports and review of literature (Bhagavan, Rao, and Weinberg), 281
Tissue viability, new technique for determination (Berman, Lemieux, and Aaby), 507
Training, surgical, crisis in (Meyerowitz), 399
Transplantation, liver, canine orthotopic, need for venous decompression during anhepatic phase, effect of liver disease on (Picache, Kapur, and Starzl), 319
Tumor(s), malignant, primary, of gallbladder, report of 43 cases (Tanga and Ewing), 418
Wilms', total prosthetic transplantation of inferior vena cava in child with (Sarti), 851
Tuberculous stenosis of ascending colon, massive megacolon and megaileum in childhood due to (Patton and Moore), 513
Tympanic membrane, body temperature monitoring via (Dickey, Ahlgren, and Stephen), 981

U

Ulcer, duodenal and gastric, in infancy and childhood, surgery for (Strode and Balfour), 527
perforated, long-term follow-up (Nemanich and Nicoloff), 727
peptic, surgical treatment (Ochsner, Zehnder, and Trammell), 1017

V

Vagotomy, incomplete, adequate, permanence of, preliminary study in dogs (Legros and Griffith), 654
plus partial gastrectomy and subtotal gastrectomy, critical analysis of results from, in surgical treatment of peptic ulcer (Ochsner, Zehnder, and Trammell), 1017
Valve replacement, late results (Rees et al.), 141
Valvular incompetency, venous, directional flow detection for localizing (Folse and Alexander), 114
Varices, esophageal, bleeding, transabdominal ligation-resection of esophagus in cases of (Boerema, Klopper, and Holscher), 409
Varicocele, new operation for, use of microvascular anastomosis (Ishigami et al.), 620
Varicose veins, ligation, stripping, and excision (Dale), 389
Vascular compression, acute, of duodenum and scoliosis (Bunch and Delaney), 901
disease, major limb amputations for, mortality factors in, study of 176 procedures (Rosenberg et al.), 437
and hyperglycemic effects of glucagon, dissociation of (Tibblin, Kock, and Schenk), 816
obstruction of superior renal infundibulum in children (Deckers et al.), 856
protheses, infection in, local irrigation with antibiotic solution in prevention of (DiGiglia, Leonard, and Ochsner), 836
surgery, standards in (Hanlon), 1
Vasoconstriction, role in suppression of hemorrhage from completely severed artery (Wangensteen et al.), 338
Vasodepressor factor in declamp shock production (Brant, Armstrong, and Vetto), 650
Vater, papilla of, cancer of, early diagnosis of, fiberduodenoscopy in (Oi, Takemoto, and Nakayama), 561

Vein(s), femoral, common, ligation in treatment of thromboembolic disease, long-term sequelae (Nabatoff, Blum, and Touroff), 272
graft, arteriovenous, for chronic hemodialysis, preliminary report (Mozes et al.), 452
saphenous, bifurcated, method of salvaging, for use in femoral-to-popliteal bypass grafts (McDaniel and Johnson), 394
bypass autografts, femoropopliteal, modifications in technique (Linton and Wilde), 234
duplicated, in femoropopliteal bypass grafting (Gaylis), 277
homografts, use of, for arterial reconstruction, preliminary report (Tice and Santoni), 493
varicose, ligation, stripping, and excision (Dale), 389
Vena cava catheter for asanguineous liver resection (Chávez-Peón, Gonzalez, and Malt), 694
inferior, total prosthetic transplantation of, in child with Wilms' tumor (Sarti), 851
caval plication, inferior, recurrent pulmonary emboli following (Coupland and Reeve), 639
Venous decompression, need for, during anhepatic phase of canine orthotopic liver transplantation, effect of liver disease on (Picache, Kapur, and Starzl), 319
Venous—Cont'd
pressure, central, manometer for monitoring, simple and accurate (Moss), 773
monitor (Vidne, Levinson, and Levy), 279
valvular incompetency, directional flow detection for localizing (Folse and Alexander), 114
Ventricle, canine, left, normal, effect of epicardiectomy on function and diastolic compliance (Hannah, Enright, and Reis), 831
right–coronary artery, fistula with congestive heart failure, surgical correction in neonatal period (Daniel, Graham, and Sabiston), 985
Ventricular bypass, left, prolonged, by transvalvular aortic catheterization, physiologic effects and rationale of surgical concept (Schuhmann, Geddes, and Hoff), 957
Vessels, great, complete transposition of, surgical results of emergency Blalock-Hanlon operation in infants (Zamora et al.), 706
transposition of, with aortic arch atresia, physiologic considerations and surgical management (Norton et al.), 1011
Viscosity, blood, in normal man (Litwin, Chapman, and Stoliar), 342

W

Wilms' tumor, total prosthetic transplantation of inferior vena cava in child with (Sarti), 851